THERAPEUTIC EXERCISE

Moving Toward Function

THERAPEUTIC EXERCISE

Moving Toward Function

Carrie M. Hall, MHS, PT
Physical Therapist
Owner, Movement Systems Physical Therapy
Clinical Faculty
University of Washington
Seattle, Washington

Lori Thein Brody, MS, PT, SCS, ATC
Senior Clinical Specialist
University of Wisconsin Clinics Research Park
Madison, Wisconsin

with contributors

LIPPINCOTT WILLIAMS & WILKINS
A **Wolters Kluwer** Company
Philadelphia • Baltimore • New York • London
Buenos Aires • Hong Kong • Sydney • Tokyo

Acquisitions Editor: Margaret Biblis
Developmental Editor: Danielle DiPalma
Editorial Assistant: Amy Amico
Senior Project Editor: Sandra Cherrey Scheinin
Senior Production Manager: Helen Ewan
Senior Production Coordinator: Nannette Winski
Assistant Art Director: Kathy Kelley Luedtke

9 8 7 6 5 4 3 2

Library of Congress Cataloging-in-Publication Data

Hall, Carrie M.
Therapeutic exercise : moving toward function / Carrie M. Hall, Lori Thein Brody.
p. cm.
Includes bibliographical references and index.
ISBN 0-397-55260-2 (alk. paper)
1. Exercise therapy. I. Brody, Lori Thein. II. Title.
RM725.H33 1998 98-28903
615.8′2—dc21 CIP

Care has been taken to confirm the accuracy of the information presented and to describe generally accepted practices. However, the authors, editors, and publisher are not responsible for errors or omissions or for any consequences from application of the information in this book and make no warranty, express or implied, with respect to the contents of the publication.

The authors, editors and publisher have exerted every effort to ensure that drug selection and dosage set forth in this text are in accordance with current recommendations and practice at the time of publication. However, in view of ongoing research, changes in government regulations, and the constant flow of information relating to drug therapy and drug reactions, the reader is urged to check the package insert for each drug for any change in indications and dosage and for added warnings and precautions. This is particularly important when the recommended agent is a new or infrequently employed drug.

Some drugs and medical devices presented in this publication have Food and Drug Administration (FDA) clearance for limited use in restricted research settings. It is the responsibility of the health care provider to ascertain the FDA status of each drug or device planned for use in their clinical practice.

I would like to dedicate this book
to my husband, Glenn,
without whose inspiring wisdom and endless support,
this book would not have been possible to complete;
my daughter, Caroline,
whose natural inquisitiveness inspires me daily
and wonderful humor makes me laugh during the most trying of times;
and my mom and dad, Carol and Bob,
whose support and encouragement throughout my life
allowed me to achieve such an accomplishment.

—Carrie Hall

To my mom and dad, Bonnie and Jack, and my sister and brother, Jill and Scott,
for providing the foundation of integrity, hard work, persistence, and humor.
And to my husband, Marc, for his sage advice, endless energy, and enduring love.

—Lori Thein Brody

Contributors

Judith Aston, MFA
Director, Aston-Patterning
Aston-Patterning Center
Incline Village, Nevada

Donna F. Bajelis, PT
Certified Hellerwork Practitioner and Teacher
Physical Therapy and Bodywork
Hellerwork Institute of Washington
Seattle, Washington

Stuart Bell, MS
Certified Alexander Teacher
Certified Feldenkrais Practitioner
Certified Hellerwork Structural Integration Practitioner
Tulsa, Oklahoma

Kimberly D. Bennett, PhD, PT
Clinical Assistant Professor
University of Washington
Physical Therapist
Olympic Physical Therapy
Seattle, Washington

Dorothy J. Berg, MPT
Staff Physical Therapist
Virginia Mason Medical Center
Seattle, Washington

Jack Blackburn, LMP, MTS, RC
Trager Practitioner
Seattle, Washington

Lisa M. Dussault, OTR
Occupational Therapist
TMD Clinic
University of Wisconsin Hospitals and Clinics
Madison, Wisconsin

Daniel J. Foppes, CHP, LMT
Assistant Instructor, Hellerwork Training
Hellerwork International
Seattle, Washington

Jeff Haller, PhD
Trainer, Feldenkrais Method
Seattle, Washington

Chuck Hanson, PT, OCS
Board Certified Clinical Specialist in Orthopedic Physical Therapy
Owner, Therapeutic Associates, Inc.
North Lake Physical Therapy
Therapeutic Associates, Inc.
Seattle, Washington

Darlene Hertling, PT
Lecturer, Division of Physical Therapy
Department of Rehabilitation Medicine
University of Washington School of Medicine
Seattle, Washington

Carol N. Kennedy, BScPT, MCPA, FCAMT
Partner, Treloar Physiotherapy Clinic
Lecturer, School of Rehabilitation Medicine
University of British Columbia
Vancouver, British Columbia

Susan Lefever-Button, MA, PT, ATC
President
San Juan Physical Therapy, Inc.
Friday Harbor, Washington

Marilyn Moffat, PT, PhD, FAPTA
Professor, Physical Therapy
New York University
New York, New York

David Musnick, MD
Physician
Sports Medicine Clinic
The Northwest Center for Environmental Medicine
Bastyr University and University of Washington Medical Schools
Seattle, Washington

Sandra Rusnak-Smith, PT, MA, OCS
Partner
Queens Physical Therapy Associates
Forest Hills, New York

Elizabeth R. Shelly, PT
Specialist in Pelvic Floor Dysfunction
Woman's Hospital
Baton Rouge, Louisiana

M. J. Strauhal, PT
Physical Therapist
Clinical Specialist in OB-GYN and Women's Health
Providence St. Vincent Medical Center Rehabilitation Services
Portland, Oregon

Stan Smith, PT
Director
Newsome and Smith Physical Therapy
Shorewood, Illinois

Linda Tremain, PT, ATC-R
Personal Best Performance
Fitness Foundations
Oak Brook, Illinois

Reviewers

Cara Adams, PT, MS
Associate Professor
Department of Rehabilitation Sciences
Division of Physical Therapy
The University of Alabama at Birmingham
School of Health Related Sciences
Birmingham, Alabama

Patricia M. Adams, MPT
Assistant Professor of Clinical Physical Therapy
Master of Physical Therapy Program
UMDNJ
Stratford, New Jersey

Lisa M. Dussault, OTR
Occupational Therapist
TMD Clinic
University of Wisconsin Hospitals and Clinics
Madison, Wisconsin

Joan E. Edelstein, MA, PT, FISPO
Director of Programming in Physical Therapy
Associate Professor of Clinical Physical Therapy
Columbia University
College of Physicians and Surgeons
New York, New York

Susan E. George, MS, PT
Assistant Professor
Department of Physical Therapy
University of Pittsburgh
Pittsburgh, Pennsylvania

Diana Hunter, PhD, PT
Associate Professor
Department of Physical Therapy
Southwest Texas State University
San Marcos, Texas

Aimee Klein, MS, PT, OCS
Clinical Assistant Professor in Physical Therapy
MGH Institute of Health Professions
Senior Resource Rehabilitation Services
Beth Israel Descontes Medical Center
Boston, Massachusetts

Laura Knapp, MS, PT, OCS
Clinical Assistant Professor
Division of Physical Therapy
University of Utah
Salt Lake City, Utah

Robin L. Marcus, MS, PT, OCS
Clinical Assistant Professor
Division of Physical Therapy
College of Health
University of Utah
Salt Lake City, Utah

David J. Pezzullo, MS, PT, SCS, ATC
Clinical Assistant Professor
Department of Physical Therapy
University of Pittsburgh
Pittsburgh, Pennsylvania

Paul Rockar, MS, PT, OCS
Vice President, Human Resources
CORE Network, LLC
McKeesport, Pennsylvania

Richard Ruoti, PhD, PT, CSCS
Certified WATSU Practitioner
Cofounder of Aquatic Physical Therapy section of APTA
Doylestown, Pennsylvania

Amy Schramm, PT
Senior Physical Therapist
JFK Medical Center
Edison, New Jersey

Mary Sesto, MEIS, PT
Physical Therapist
Department of Occupational Medicine
University of Wisconsin
Assistant Researcher
Department of Industrial Engineering
University of Wisconsin
Madison, Wisconsin

Linda J. Tsoumas, MS, PT
Chairperson and Associate Professor of Physical Therapy
Department of Physical Therapy
Springfield College
Springfield, Massachusetts

Cynthia Watson, MS, PT, OCS
Instructor, Department of Physical Therapy
University of Texas
Southwestern Medical Center
Dallas, Texas

Nancy J. Whitby, OTR, CHT
Lead Therapist
Hospital and Clinics
University of Wisconsin
Madison, Wisconsin

Foreword

Therapeutic exercise is a key component of the physical therapy management of patients with a wide variety of impairment syndromes. The largest growth in delivery of physical therapy services has been in the treatment of patients who have musculoskeletal pain problems. Over the years, the methods of treating these patients have also grown. In recent years, there has been marked improvement in the understanding of the mechanisms underlying exercise as an intervention for pain problems. But often associated with an increase in the variety of available treatments is greater difficulty in devising a suitable strategy for selecting the appropriate treatment. Carrie Hall and Lori Thein Brody have tackled this very difficult issue by organizing the concepts of therapeutic exercise around the disablement model. Clearly, the key issue in physical therapy is relating the impairments that are addressed by therapeutic exercise to function and disability. The improvement of their patients' functional abilities to the highest possible level, has always been the ultimate goal of physical therapists. What has varied is whether or not that goal should be achieved by placing major emphasis on treating impairments or on functional activities with less direct effort to improve specific impairments. This book provides information designed to help therapists relate impairments to functional limitations.

In addition to the relationship between impairments and functional limitations, the relationship of disease to impairments is another issue that needs to be addressed. Physical therapists, once guided by the physician's diagnosis of disease, are recognizing that impairments must be further classified to provide a much more specific guide to the design of the therapist's treatment program. The editors have attempted to address these issues by providing a scheme for organizing the major impairments as well as addressing the impairments in specific detail. This book provides a structure that goes beyond the mere collection of a variety of techniques and exercises. The editors have integrated the current concepts of physical therapy management of patients who have musculoskeletal pain problems with the terminology that is being promoted by the American Physical Therapy Association. In the complex world of today's health care, the need to communicate in a way that facilitates the understanding of conditions, interventions, goals, and outcomes by health care providers and by patients is particularly important. The expectations for care today are that it is efficient and cost-effective, and that it enables the client to be an informed participant in his or her program. Providing a structure and guidelines for developing therapeutic intervention programs and promoting the use of terminology that is clear and consistent throughout the health care system is an important step in achieving the goal of cost-effective care. *Therapeutic Exercise: Moving Toward Function* is a step in that direction. I commend the editors for their effective efforts to address this challenging but most necessary task.

Shirley A. Sahrmann, PhD, PT, FAPTA
Professor Physical Therapy/Cell Biology
Associate Professor of Neurology
Director, Program in Movement Science
Washington University School of Medicine
St. Louis, Missouri

Preface

Choosing the title of this book was not easy, but once it was decided, the choice seemed obvious. *Therapeutic Exercise: Moving Toward Function* is the title that encapsulates the premise of this book. The emergence of managed care in the United States has altered the delivery of health care. Although value has always been important, its role in today's health care management is even more critical. Value can be defined as patient satisfaction (ie, functionally meaningful patient outcomes), divided by the financial and social costs of providing care (Kasman GS, Cram JR, Wolk SL. *Clinical Applications in Surface Electromyography*. Rockville, MD: Aspen; 1998). Physical therapists are challenged daily to provide value to their patients in delivering care to improve function and quality of life. Among the many interventions available to the physical therapist, therapeutic exercise is the cornerstone in providing patients with the means to improve their functional capabilities and, ultimately, their quality of life. Although other interventions can improve these elements, it is the assumption of this book that only through careful therapeutic exercise prescription can an individual make the permanent changes necessary to maintain, optimize, or prevent future loss of function. It is the premise of this book to use therapeutic exercise for patients with musculoskeletal dysfunction for the sole purpose of achieving functionally meaningful patient outcomes.

It was our decision to write this book as a textbook and not a manual of activities and techniques. The latter deals with providing activities and techniques without the theoretic framework to make decisions about what would or could be the best possible course of treatment and the possible alternatives. *Therapeutic Exercise: Moving Toward Function* attempts to provide a conceptual framework for learning how to make clinical decisions regarding the prescription of therapeutic exercise—from deciding which exercise(s) to teach, to how to teach them, to the dosage required for the best possible outcome. The common thread throughout the text is to treat, with the use of therapeutic exercise and related interventions, the impairments that correlate to functional limitations and disability and to work toward the most optimal function possible.

Because this book primarily was written as a textbook, decisions were made to provide the reader and instructor with a variety of educational features:

- Extensively illustrated. Therapeutic exercise is a visual intervention. This book uses photographs and line drawings to illustrate examples of therapeutic exercises.
- Selected Interventions. Featured at the end of pertinent chapters, these are activities or techniques written for the student as the audience and are included to provide examples of application of the therapeutic exercise intervention model presented in Chapter 2. Faculty can use the Selected Interventions as models for the student to develop exercise prescriptions.
- Self-Management boxes. These are activities or techniques written for the patient as the audience. These are included as examples to show the student how to write an exercise for a patient so that all the important features of an exercise prescription are clearly understood.
- Patient-Related Instruction boxes. These are similar to Self-Management boxes. The primary difference is that these are not exercises, but rather educational features to assist in the carryover of exercise into functional activities.
- Key Points. This feature summarizes key concepts the author wants to convey in the chapter. A thorough understanding of the Key Points should be realized following the reading of each chapter.
- Critical Thinking Questions. These were provided to stimulate the reader's thinking after studying the chapter. Case Studies are used to incite hypothetical situations to which concepts can be applied.
- Lab Activities. These provide examples of applied use of the concepts to practice teaching and execution of selected activities and techniques.
- Case Studies. The final unit of the book provides the reader with a description of 11 cases. These cases are used in Critical Thinking Questions and Lab Activities to provide the student with real-life situations in which to apply concepts learned in the relevant chapter.

The book is organized into seven units. The purpose of each unit is as follows:

- Unit 1 provides the foundations of therapeutic exercise, beginning with a presentation of the disablement model to provide conceptual clarity for the remainder of the book, and ending with concepts of patient management. In the second chapter, a proposed therapeutic exercise intervention model is presented. This model attempts to separate the clinical reasoning process into the individual, but cumulative steps to take in order to prescribe an effective therapeutic exercise. Chapter 3 describes two crucial elements of patient management: motor learning and self-management.
- Unit 2 provides the reader with a functional approach to therapeutic exercise for physiologic impairments. Although we attempted to include a somewhat extensive review of the scientific literature on muscle performance, balance, endurance, mobility, posture, movement, and pain, our purpose was not to publish a review of the material. Instead, we have selected pertinent literature to illustrate the concepts needed for a basic knowledge of physiologic impairments as it relates to therapeutic exercise prescription.

- Unit 3 presents special physiologic considerations to heed when prescribing therapeutic exercise. They include soft tissue injury, postoperative issues, arthritis, fibromyalgia syndrome and chronic fatigue, and obstetrics. Although this list is not comprehensive, we chose these special considerations because of the frequency with which the clinician encounters them.
- Unit 4 provides the reader with selected methods of intervention. Although there are numerous schools of thought regarding the prescription of exercise, we chose these methods to provide the reader with examples of a variety of contrasting methods—each has its own merits. The authors have attempted to illustrate how each method can be incorporated into a cohesive program of therapeutic exercise prescription.
- Units 5 and 6 provide the reader with a regional approach to therapeutic exercise prescription. Each chapter is organized into a brief review of anatomy and kinesiology, examination and evaluation guidelines, therapeutic exercise for common physiologic impairments affecting the region, and therapeutic exercise for common medical diagnoses affecting the region. The anatomy, kinesiology, and examination and evaluation sections set the foundation for prescription of therapeutic exercise for physiologic impairments. Therapeutic exercise for physiologic impairments provides the reader with examples of exercises to improve physiologic capability and ultimately function. Therapeutic exercise for common medical diagnoses provides the reader with examples of comprehensive interventions, including therapeutic exercise for common medical conditions affecting the region.
- Unit 7 consists of 11 Case Studies, which are used in Critical Thinking Questions and Lab Activities at the end of selected chapters. Faculty can use these Case Studies for a variety of learning experiences.
- Appendices 1 and 2 give the student a quick reference for red flags of serious pathology or visceral referred symptoms and clinical actions to take in the event of serious signs and symptoms in the exercising patient.

We worked diligently to provide a comprehensive textbook designed to prepare the foundation of knowledge and skills necessary to prescribe therapeutic exercise. We urge our readers to write to us in response to how well we accomplished our goal. We hope that subsequent editions can address your comments as well as the ever-changing needs of those involved in therapeutic exercise prescription.

Carrie M. Hall, MHS, PT
Lori Thein Brody, MS, PT, SCS, ATC

Acknowledgments

First and foremost, we wish to express our everlasting gratitude to family, friends, and colleagues who offered their emotional support and generosity of time to allow us to complete this project.

We would also like to express our appreciation to Danielle DiPalma and Sarah Kyle, whose intense developmental editing efforts persisted through their pregnancies and the births of their first children, and to Amy Amico who seamlessly stepped in during Danielle's maternity leave. A book of this magnitude with its large number of figures, displays, tables, references, and special features cannot be produced without cohesive editorial and production efforts. For this we thank the entire editorial and production staff and the art department at Lippincott Williams & Wilkins who assisted us in the timely production of this book. A special thanks is extended to Andrew Allen who had enough confidence in my knowledge and skills to ask me to head this project, and to Margaret Biblis who persisted in this support.

We would like to extend our appreciation to our colleagues at the University of Wisconsin Clinics Research Park for the donation of the facility, and to the models who donated their time for the photography in this text.

Over the course of a person's career, many individuals assist in the development of that person's knowledge and expertise. The people from whom we have learned the most and who should not go unrecognized, are the patients and students who have challenged our thoughts and actions. A topic of this magnitude requires intense critical thinking to transform concepts into written word. We are indebted to the patients and students who have assisted us in developing the conceptual framework with which to address this complex topic, and in providing us with the incentive to convey this information to others in a comprehensive text.

We are honored and grateful for the contributions of the following individuals whose knowledge brought greater breadth and depth to the writing in the chapters involving their expertise: Chuck Ratzlaff, BSc (PT), MCPA, COMP, and Diane Lee, BSR, MCPA, COMP, for their contributions to the lumbo-pelvic region section; Diane Lee, again, for her contribution to the section on the thoracic region; Glenn Kasman, MS, PT, for his contribution to the surface electromyography section of Chapter 2; Jim Zachazewski, MS, PT, SCS, ATC, for his contribution to Chapter 6, Mobility Impairment; Lisa Dussault, OTR; and Ann Kammein, PT, CHT; Cindy Glaenzer, PT, CHT; Christine Burridge, PT, CHT; Mary Sesto, MS, PT; Nancy Whitby, OT; and Jill Thein, MPT, ATC for their contributions to the elbow, wrist, and hand section.

Carrie Hall
Lori Thein Brody

Each coauthor would like to extend her personal acknowledgments:

Over the course of my career, I have had the good fortune to work with some of the most highly respected individuals in the field of physical therapy. Their greatest gift to me was not the delivery of facts and ideas, but rather how to use sound information to perform critical thinking. I would especially like to thank Shirley Sahrmann, PhD, PT, FAPTA and the late Steve Rose, PhD, PT for their role as my mentors, from the beginning of my career to the present, and for their continued inspiration to always ask "why" and never accept the status quo. And finally, this project would not have been possible to complete without my coauthor and editor, Lori Thein Brody. I extend my most sincere indebtedness for her commitment to see the fruition of this monumental project.

Carrie Hall

My life has been blessed with exceptional colleagues who have believed in and advocated for me through each phase of my career: Peg Houglam, MS, PT, ATC; Bill Flentje, PT, ATC; Susan Harris, PhD, PT, FAPTA; and Colleen McHorney, PhD. My deepest gratitude to them and to the many others who have helped me along this path. Brad Sherman, MS, ATC, has been my hero with his patience, tolerance, and flexibility at work; I am truly grateful. Finally, a heartfelt thanks goes to my sister, Jill Thein, MPT, ATC, for taking care of everything else while I worked on this book.

Lori Thein Brody

Brief Contents

Contents

CHAPTER 6

Mobility Impairment 87

LORI THEIN BRODY

CHAPTER 7

Balance Impairment 112

LORI THEIN BRODY

CHAPTER 8

Posture and Movement Impairment 128

CARRIE HALL

CHAPTER 9

Pain 145

LORI THEIN BRODY

UNIT 1

Foundations of Therapeutic Exercise

CHAPTER 1

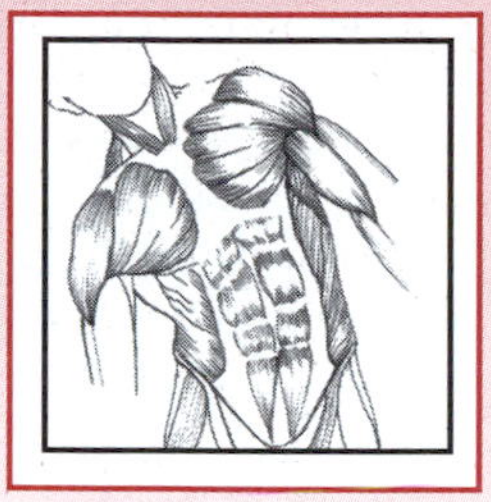

Introduction to Therapeutic Exercise and the Modified Disablement Model

Carrie Hall

DEFINITION OF PHYSICAL THERAPY

The Model Definition of Physical Therapy for State Practice Acts[1] was adopted by the American Physical Therapy Association (APTA) Board of Directors in March 1993 and revised in March 1995. *Physical therapy, which is the care and services provided by or under the direction and supervision of a physical therapist, includes*

1. *Examining patients with impairments, functional limitations, and disability or other health-related conditions to determine a diagnosis, prognosis, and intervention.* Examinations within the scope of physical therapy practice include, but are not limited to, tests and measures of the musculoskeletal system (eg, range of motion, manual muscle test, joint mobility, posture), neurologic system (eg, reflexes, cranial nerve integrity, neuromotor development, sensory integrity), cardiopulmonary system (eg, aerobic capacity or endurance, ventilation, circulation, respiration), and integumentary system (eg, integumentary integrity).
2. *Alleviating impairments and functional limitations by designing, implementing, and modifying therapeutic interventions.* Interventions include, but are not limited to, therapeutic exercise; manual therapy; prescription, fabrication, and application of assistive, adaptive, supportive, and protective devices and equipment; airway clearance techniques; physical agents and mechanical and electrotherapeutic modalities; and patient education.
3. *Preventing injury, impairments, functional limitations, and disability, including the promotion and maintenance of fitness, health, and quality of life in all age populations.*
4. *Engaging in consultation, education, and research.*

It is evident from this definition that physical therapists examine, evaluate, diagnose, and intervene at the level of impairment, functional limitation, and disability in the disablement process. The most critical message promoted by this definition is that physical therapists are primarily concerned with using knowledge and clinical skills to reduce or eliminate functional limitation and disability and enable individuals seeking their services to achieve the most optimal quality of life possible.

In the past, the focus on measuring and altering impairments superseded the more important goals of improving function and reducing disability. This text focuses on improving function and reducing disability through the use of therapeutic exercise. The emphasis is not on using therapeutic exercise to alter lists of impairments, but rather to use intervention to improve function and reduce disability that is meaningful to the individual seeking physical therapy services. A case is made for altering the line of thinking. Instead of considering "which exercise can be prescribed to improve an impairment," the therapist should consider "what impairments are related to reduced function and disability for *this patient* and which exercises can *enhance function* by addressing the appropriate impairments."

To understand the relationships among disease, pathology, impairment, functional limitation, and disability, and to avoid confusion caused by misunderstood terminology, a detailed description of the disablement process is necessary and is provided later in this chapter. The model proposed is based on two conceptual models and modifications thereof. The model presented is an attempt to compile modifications pertinent to the practice of physical therapy. It is not intended to serve as the definitive model for the disablement process, because it is too premature to reach consensus about any one conceptual approach. The reader is encouraged to use this model to think about the complex process of disablement and how the disablement process relates to decisions regarding therapeutic exercise intervention.

THERAPEUTIC EXERCISE INTERVENTION

Therapeutic exercise intervention is a health service provided by physical therapists to patients and clients. Patients are persons with diagnosed impairments or functional limitations. Clients are persons who are not necessarily diagnosed with impairments or functional limitations but who are seeking physical therapy services for prevention or enhanced performance, such as education provided to a group of persons involved in strenuous occupational activity, early education and exercise prescription geared toward prevention for persons diagnosed with a musculoskeletal disease such as rheumatoid arthritis, or exercise recommended for a group of high level athletes to prevent injury or enhance performance.[1]

Therapeutic exercise is considered a core element in most physical therapy plans of care, augmented by other interventions, to achieve improved function and reduced disability. It includes a broad scope of activities that

- *Improve* physical function, health status, and general sense of well-being of persons diagnosed with impairments, functional limitations, or disability (ie, patients)
- *Prevent* complications and decrease the use of health care resources during hospitalization or after surgery
- *Improve or maintain* physical function or health status of well individuals (ie, clients)
- *Prevent* or minimize future impairments, functional loss, or disability for any individual (ie, patient or client)

The methods of intervention that therapeutic exercise encompasses include, but are not limited to, activities or techniques to improve mobility, force or torque production, neuromuscular control, cardiovascular and muscular endurance, balance, coordination, breathing patterns, posture awareness, and movement patterns. Although therapeutic exercise can benefit numerous systems of the body, this text focuses primarily on treatment of the musculoskeletal system. Concepts of therapeutic exercise intervention specifically for the cardiopulmonary and neurologic systems are not covered in this text, except as they relate to impairments of the musculoskeletal system.

Decisions regarding therapeutic exercise intervention should be based on individual goals that provide patients or clients with the ability to achieve optimal functioning in the home, school, workplace, or community. To implement goal-oriented treatment, the physical therapist must

- Provide comprehensive and personalized patient management
- Rely on keen clinical decision-making skills
- Implement a variety of therapeutic interventions that are complementary (eg, heat application before joint mobilization and passive stretch, followed by active exercise to use new mobility in a functional manner)
- Promote patient independence whenever possible through the use of home treatment (eg, home spine traction, home heat or cold therapy), independent exercise programs (eg, in the home, community-sponsored group classes, school- or community-sponsored athletics), and patient-related instruction

Care must be taken to provide intervention sufficient to meet functional goals without providing extraneous interventions and to promote patient independence to contribute to the battle of health care cost containment. In some cases, patient independence is not possible, but therapeutic exercise intervention is necessary to improve or maintain health status or prevent complications. In these situations, training and educating family, friends, significant others, or caregivers to deliver appropriate therapeutic exercise intervention in the home can greatly reduce health care costs by limiting in-house physical therapy intervention.

THE DISABLEMENT PROCESS

Physical therapists intervene at the level of impairment, functional limitation, and disability of the disablement process. A practitioner's understanding of the process of disablement and the factors that affect its development is fundamental to achieving the goal of restoring or improving function and reducing disability in the individual seeking physical therapy services. This will become evident as the disablement process is defined and described. The specific relation to therapeutic exercise intervention is discussed throughout the explanation of the disablement process.

Purpose of Defining the Disablement Process

The purpose of defining the disablement process in a text on therapeutic exercise is to provide the reader with an understanding of the complex relationships of pathology and disease, impairments, functional limitation, and disability and an understanding of the complexity of the disablement process. The accepted definitions of impairments, functional limitations, and disability according to the APTA[1] are as follows:

- Impairments are losses or abnormalities of physiologic, psychological, or anatomic structure or function.
- Functional limitations are restrictions of the ability to perform a physical action, activity, or task in an efficient, typically expected, or competent manner.
- Disability is the inability to engage in age- and gender-specific roles in a particular social context and physical environment.

Therapeutic exercise intervention must not focus on pathology, disease, or impairments; it should instead focus on the functional loss and disability of the patient seeking physical therapy services. Although a specific therapeutic exercise intervention may be selected to treat an impairment, it must be selected in view of improving a functional outcome. One example is the scenario of a patient with low back pain. Examination reveals that this patient has impairments associated with excessive mobility of the lumbar spine in the direction of flexion and low back pain after prolonged flexion postures and movement patterns associated with repetitive flexion. A passive or active stretch technique may be chosen to apply to the hamstrings.

Stretching the hamstrings is an intervention at the impairment level of the disablement process. Improving the length of the hamstrings can increase hip range of motion and consequently improve mobility to bend forward at the hips before stressing the low back in a flexion movement pattern. Choosing to treat this impairment directly influences function by improving the mobility of a forward bend movement (ie, a functional movement pattern) and reducing pain during an activity of daily living (ADL) (eg, bending forward to wash one's face, make the bed, set the table, or reach into the refrigerator). Although weak abdominal muscles constitute a common impairment of patients with low back pain, treating weak abdominals with a partial curl-up exercise, for example, may not be appropriate for that patient. The flexion force on the low back may exacerbate symptoms, and the partial curl-up may not relate to a meaningful functional movement pattern for the patient. Understanding the disablement process for each patient enables the therapist to make sound decisions about therapeutic exercise intervention.

Evolution of the Disablement Model

The previous example is an oversimplification of the use of the disablement process in making decisions about therapeutic exercise. The relationships of the components along the continuum of disability are quite complex. The disablement process can be better understood by examining the evolution of the disablement model.

The most frequently presented models of the disablement process are the World Health Organization's (WHO) International Classification of Impairments, Disabilities, and Handicaps (ICIDH)[2] and a model developed by sociologist Saad Nagi[3] in the 1960s (Fig. 1-1). In both disablement models, the central theme is the description of a process from disease or active pathology toward functional limitations and the factors limiting a person's ability to interact as a normally functioning person in society.

INTERNATIONAL CLASSIFICATION OF IMPAIRMENTS, DISABILITIES, AND HANDICAPS (ICIDH)

"DISEASE" → IMPAIRMENT → DISABILITY → HANDICAP

NAGI SCHEME

ACTIVE PATHOLOGY → IMPAIRMENT → FUNCTIONAL LIMITATION → DISABILITY

FIGURE 1-1 Two conceptual models for the disablement process.

ACTIVE PATHOLOGY OR DISEASE

There is general agreement between the Nagi and ICIDH models in the definition of the first two concepts of disablement (see Fig. 1-1). For Nagi, active pathology involves the interruption of normal cellular processes and the efforts of the affected systems to regain homeostasis. Active pathology can result from infection, trauma, metabolic imbalance, degenerative disease process, or another cause.[4] ICIDH uses the term *disease* to refer to the biomechanical, physiologic, and anatomic abnormalities of the human organism.[5] Examples of active pathology and disease common to both models are the altered cellular processes found in osteoarthritis, cardiomyopathy, or ankylosing spondylitis.

IMPAIRMENT

Both models refer to the next stage in the continuum as impairment. Impairment refers to a loss or abnormality at the tissue, organ, or body system level. The effects of disease or pathology are found in impairments of the body systems in which the pathologic state is manifested. The clinical example of a person diagnosed with rheumatoid arthritis may help to clarify the difference between pathology and impairments. Rheumatoid arthritis represents the pathology or disease diagnosis. The primary physiologic impairments (defined later in this chapter) associated with rheumatoid arthritis are found chiefly in the alteration of normal structure and function of bones, joints, and soft tissues of the musculoskeletal system. The physiologic impairments resulting from this disease process relevant to the musculoskeletal system may include loss of mobility or reduced force or torque capability. Physiologic impairments of the neuromuscular system (eg, poor balance) or cardiopulmonary system (eg, decreased endurance) can also be detected, usually as sequelae of the musculoskeletal system impairments (ie, secondary conditions, which are explained later in this chapter).

FUNCTIONAL LIMITATION, DISABILITY, AND HANDICAP

The Nagi and ICIDH models diverge at the next two levels of the disablement model (see Fig. 1-1).

Nagi Model

The next level in the disablement model is functional limitation. For Nagi, this term represents a restriction in performance of basic tasks. It appears he is referring to *components* of more complex tasks of basic activities of daily living (BADL) (eg, personal hygiene, feeding, dressing) and instrumental activities of daily living (IADL) (eg, preparing meals, housework, grocery shopping). Examples of functional limitations for Nagi might include gait abnormalities, reduced tolerance to sitting or standing, difficulty climbing the stairs, or inability to reach overhead.

Disability is the final element in Nagi's model. Nagi describes disability as any restriction or inability to perform socially defined roles and tasks expected of an individual within a sociocultural and physical environment. Activities and social roles associated with the term disability include

- BADLs and IADLs
- Social roles, including those associated with an occupation or the ability to perform duties as a parent or student
- Social activities, including attending church and other group activities, and socializing with friends and relatives
- Leisure activities, including sports and physical recreation, reading, and travel[4]

Nagi reserves the term disability for social rather than individual functioning. In considering Nagi's definition of disability, not all impairments or functional limitations result in disability. For example, two persons diagnosed with the same disease with similar levels of impairment and functional limitation may have two different levels of disability. One person may remain very active in all aspects of life (ie, personal care and social roles), have support from family members in the home, and seek adaptive methods of continuing with his occupational tasks, whereas the other individual may choose to limit social contact, depend on others for personal care and household responsibilities, and have a job where it is not possible to use adaptive methods to participate in work tasks.

Nagi describes the distinction between functional limitation and disability as the difference between attributes and relational concepts. Attributes are defined by Nagi as phenomena that pertain to characteristics or properties of the individual. A functional limitation is primarily a reflection of the characteristics of the individual person. It is therefore unnecessary to go beyond the individual to measure a functional limitation. Disability, however, has a relational characteristic in that it describes the individual's limitation in relation to society and the environment. As the previous example demonstrated, persons with similar attribution profiles (eg, pathology, impairments, functional limitations) can present with different disability profiles. Factors such as age, general health status, personal goals, motivation, social support, and physical environment influence the level of disability the person experiences.

International Classification of Impairments, Disabilities, and Handicaps Model

The ICIDH model (see Fig. 1-1) does not discriminate between functional limitation and disability. According to ICIDH, the term disability describes any restriction or lack of ability to perform a task or an activity in the manner considered normal for a person, such as a disturbance in gait, BADLs, or IADLs. Handicap is the term used to describe the final element of the ICIDH model. It is a disadvantage resulting from an impairment or disability that limits or prevents fulfillment of an individual's normal role. The WHO stipulates that a handicap is not a classification of *individuals* but is a classification of *circumstances* that place such individuals at a disadvantage relative to peers when judged by the norms of society. The handicap represents the social and environmental consequences for the individual stemming from the presence of impairments and disabilities.[2]

A criticism of the ICIDH model is that it does not differentiate between limitations in *performing* societal roles and the *cause* of these limitations. The cause of societal limitations is clear in Nagi's model in that it is broken down into functional limitations (ie, attributes relating to the individual) and disability (ie, relational characteristics to society). In understanding the disablement process, it is important to identify the extent to which disability results from the social and physical environment or from factors within the individual. It is believed that the Nagi model does this more succinctly than the ICIDH model.

Modified Disablement Model

The previous two disablement models demonstrate that much of the discrepancy between the Nagi and ICIDH models is semantic and that neither model completely fulfills the description of the complexity of the disablement process. Several modifications of the two basic models of Nagi and ICIDH have been proposed,[4,6] and each has important contributions. The model described and used in this text combines elements from each basic model and their modifications to provide a model for physical therapy practitioners (Fig. 1-2).

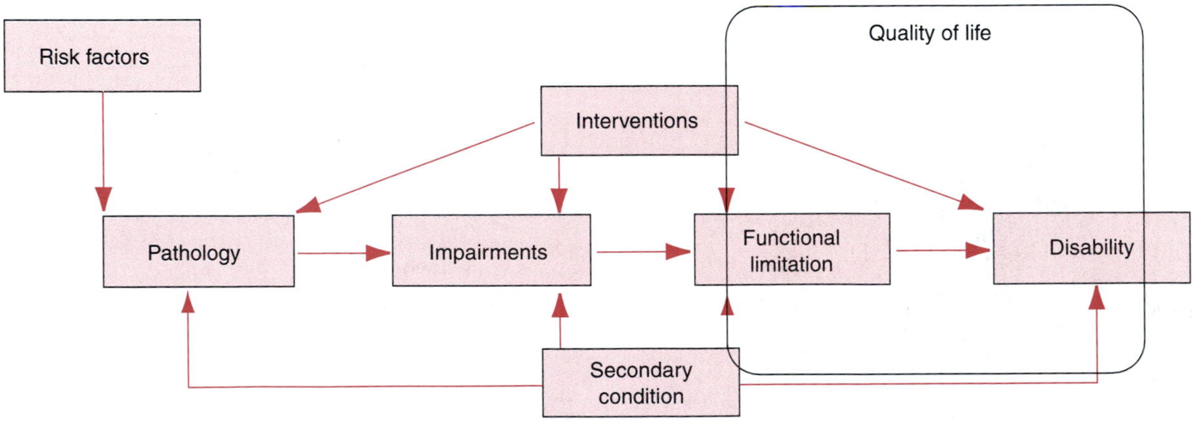

FIGURE 1-2 Modification of the disablement process.

PATHOLOGY

The main pathway of the modified disablement model follows Nagi's model closely, with some minor alterations in definitions of terminology. The first element of the modified model remains the same as in the Nagi model, with a minor addition to the definition. Pathology refers to biomechanical, anatomic, and physiologic abnormalities that are labeled as disease, injury, or congenital or developmental conditions.

IMPAIRMENTS

Similar to the Nagi and ICIDH models, impairments are defined as losses or abnormalities of physiologic, psychological, or anatomic structure or function (Fig. 1-3). Active pathology results in impairment, but not all impairments originate from pathology (eg, congenital anatomic deformity or loss). Throughout this text, physiologic, anatomic, and psychological impairments are differentiated (Display 1-1).

Physiologic Impairment

Physiologic impairment can be defined as an alteration in any physiologic function such as reduced force or torque production, reduced endurance, reduced mobility (ie, hypomobility), excessive mobility (ie, hypermobility), reduced balance and coordination, altered posture and movement patterns, pain, or altered muscle tone. It is this impairment that physical therapy interventions can most significantly modify. Unit 2 of this text provides a more thorough discussion of each of these physiologic impairments and examples of therapeutic exercise interventions to remedy these impairments.

Anatomic Impairment

Anatomic impairment is an abnormality or loss of structure, such as hip anteversion, structural subtalar varus, structural genu varum, or congenital or traumatic loss of a limb. Anatomic impairments cannot be remedied with physical therapy intervention, but modifications can be made to function in light of anatomic impairments. The physical therapist should be aware of the presence of anatomic impairments to be able to provide an appropriate prognosis and determine the best plan of care.

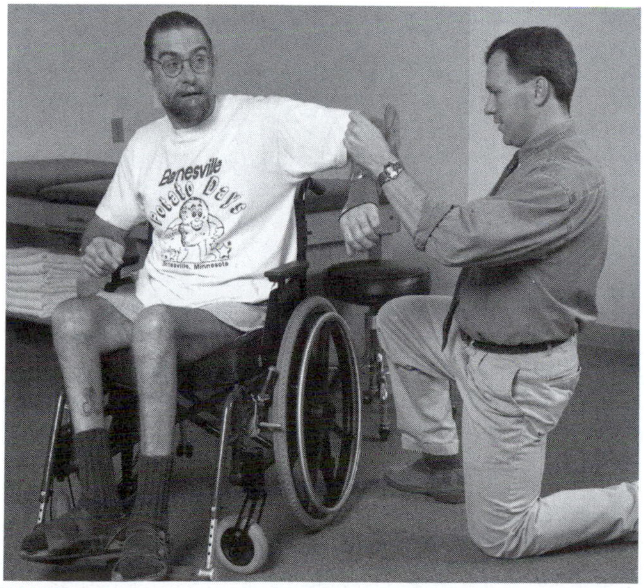

FIGURE 1-3 The patient shows a loss of medial rotation at the glenohumeral joint, which is a mobility impairment.

DISPLAY 1-1

Impairments

Physiologic impairment: an alteration in any physiologic function
Anatomic impairment: an abnormality or loss of structure
Psychological impairment: any abnormality related to the psychological system

Psychological Impairment

Psychological impairment is any abnormality related to the psychological system. Although most persons with any degree of disability are affected to some extent psychologically, it is beyond the scope of physical therapy practice to treat psychological impairments directly. It is the responsibility of the physical therapist to recognize when a psychological impairment is reducing the effectiveness of a physical therapy intervention and therefore requires referral to an appropriate health care practitioner. Because physical therapy intervention can greatly impact psychological impairments, it is important that the physical therapist understand basic psychological paradigms. However, it is not within the scope of this text to provide the details warranted for a thorough understanding of the topic. Proper screening for psychological impairments is the responsibility of the physical therapist, as is working with other members of the health care team to provide a consistent philosophic approach to the person's psychological impairment and disability.

Primary and Secondary Impairments

Primary impairments result from active pathology or disease (eg, pain, quadriceps atrophy and weakness, joint hypomobility secondary to osteoarthritis of the tibiofemoral joint). A secondary impairment results from primary impairments and pathology (eg, impairments associated with low back pain resulting from faulty repetitive movement patterns because of an inability to bend the knees due to osteoarthritis of the tibiofemoral joint). Primary impairments can create secondary impairments (ie, impairments associated with low back pain), and primary impairments (eg, weak quadriceps and stiff knees) can cause secondary pathology (eg, degenerative disk disease). The disablement process is not a unidirectional process, but one that is much more complex, interrelated, and cyclical.

The term applied to this concept and used in the modified disablement model is secondary conditions (see Fig. 1-2).[4] Secondary conditions occur as a result of a primary disabling condition. A secondary condition may be a type of pathology or impairment, as exemplified earlier, and it can designate additional functional limitations and disability. By definition, secondary conditions only occur in the presence of a primary condition. Other commonly encountered secondary conditions include pressure sores, contractures, urinary tract infection, cardiovascular deconditioning, and depression. Each of these secondary conditions can lead to additional functional limitations and disability.

FUNCTIONAL LIMITATIONS, DISABILITY, AND QUALITY OF LIFE

The final two elements of the main pathway, functional limitation and disability, remain unchanged from the definitions provided in the description of Nagi's model (Fig. 1-4). Beyond the main pathway of pathology toward disablement, a final outcome—quality of life—has been added.[4] Quality of life has been defined as generally corresponding to total well-being, encompassing several physical and psychological determinants:

- Performance of social roles
- Physical status
- Emotional status
- Social interactions
- Intellectual functioning
- Economic status
- Self-perceived or subjective health status[7]

Assessments of quality of life attempt to capture how limitations in function affect emotional, social, and physical roles as well as perceptions of health status.[8–10] A person may argue that issues related to quality of life are not distinct from disability, but it is considered broader than disability, encompassing more than well-being related to health such as education and employment. The model (see Fig. 1-2) displays quality of life overlapping components of the main pathway.

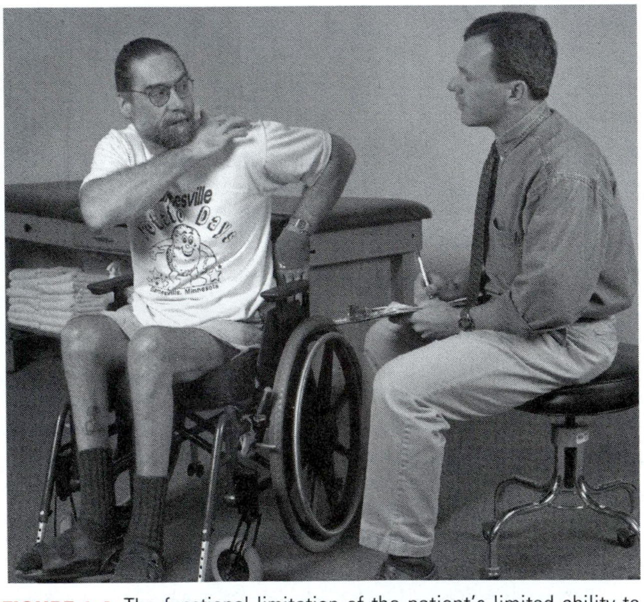

FIGURE 1-4 The functional limitation of the patient's limited ability to reach behind his back is related to his mobility impairment, which is loss of medial rotation at the glenohumeral joint. (The patient's disability may be the inability to perform wheelchair transfers safely.)

RISK FACTORS AND INTERVENTIONS

The main pathway from pathology to disability, including quality of life, can be modified by a host of factors such as age, gender, education, income, comorbidities, health habits, motivation, social support, and physical environment. Proper medical care and timely rehabilitation also can eliminate or reduce the impact of pathology on impairments, impairments on functional limitation, and functional limitation on disability. Conversely, improper medical care or rehabilitation along with other aforementioned factors can magnify the impact of each component in relation to the next or accelerate the disablement process. Education, age, gender, disease severity, duration of illness and treatment, and comorbidity modify the disablement process in persons diagnosed with rheumatoid arthritis,[11–13] and anxiety, depression, and coping style have been related to functional limitations in individuals with hip or knee osteoarthritis.[14] The model exhibits these components as risk factors and interventions (see Fig. 1-2).

Risk factors are predisposing in that they exist before the onset of the disablement process. There are several types of risk factors:

- Demographic, social, lifestyle, behavioral, psychological, and environmental factors
- Comorbidities
- Physiologic impairments (eg, short hamstrings, weak abdominal muscles, lengthened lower trapezius)
- Anatomic impairments (eg, congenital scoliosis, shallow glenoid fossa, hip anteversion)
- Functional performance factors (eg, less than optimal work station ergonomics resulting in poor posture at the work station, faulty gait kinetics or kinematics, inappropriate lifting mechanics)

The physical therapist must be aware of these factors for each individual, because they can greatly alter the individual's disablement profile. With respect to therapeutic exercise intervention, many of these factors can directly influence the choice of activities or techniques, dosage, and expected functional outcome. An example is the scenario of two individuals involved in a motor vehicle accident and diagnosed with an acceleration injury to the cervical spine with resultant sprain and/or strain to the cervical soft tissues. One individual is a sedentary, 54-year-old male smoker with diabetes who has a significant forward head and thoracic kyphosis and must return to a data entry job (which he dislikes) at a poorly designed work station. The other individual is an active and otherwise healthy, 32-year-old man who enjoys his job as a salesman and is engaged in activities such as sitting, standing, and walking throughout the day. The disablement profiles of these two individuals are quite different, and the prognoses, therapeutic exercise interventions, and functional outcomes differ accordingly.

In addition to the risk factors present before disability, interventions (see Fig. 1-2) can alter the disablement process at each juncture. Interventions may include factors outside of the individual (ie, extra-individual factors) such as medications, surgery, rehabilitation, supportive equipment, and environmental modifications or self-induced changes (ie, intra-individual factors) such as changes in health habits, coping mechanisms, and activity modifications. The expected outcome is that interventions modify the disablement process in a positive manner. However, interventions occasionally serve as exacerbators to the disablement process. Exacerbators may occur in the following ways:

- Interventions may go awry.
- Persons may develop negative behaviors or attitudes.
- Society may place environmental or attitudinal barriers in the path of the individual.

Therapeutic exercise as an intervention intends to eliminate or reduce the severity of impairment, functional limitation, and disability, and it intends to reduce the progression of pathology and prevent secondary conditions and recurrences from developing. Prevention must be a critical component of therapeutic exercise intervention at each juncture of the disablement process. Constant reevaluation combined with careful clinical decision making can detect when a therapeutic exercise intervention has caused or contributed to an exacerbation. Immediate modification of the exercise is necessary to prevent harm (see Chapter 2, Exercise Modification).

SUMMARY

The modified disablement model (see Fig. 1-2) exhibits the complexity of the relationships among pathology, impairments, functional limitations, disability, quality of life, risk factors, and interventions. A practitioner's understanding of this model is critical to developing a therapeutic exercise program that is effective, efficient, and meaningful for the individual seeking physical therapy services. The amount of data that can be collected during an initial examination or evaluation of an individual can be immense and often overwhelming. This model (see Fig. 1-2) allows the physical therapist to organize data pertaining to the patient's impairments, functional limitations, and disability. It also allows the physical therapist to categorize pertinent aspects of the patient's history, the effect of prior treatment, and the presence of risk factors. Most important, the clinical presentation can be classified in a way that identifies the impairments impeding the performance of certain functional tasks and activities, thereby focusing the treatment on only those impairments directly related to functional limitation and disability. It also enables the practitioner to clarify risk factors and interventions that may serve as impediments to improved functional performance, reduced disability, and improved quality of life. With this analysis, the practitioner can develop goals that are relevant to the individual's daily life, understand potential impediments to their achievement, develop a likely prognosis, and plan an appropriate intervention.

! Key Points

- Physical therapists examine patients with impairments, functional limitations, and disabilities or other health-related conditions to determine a diagnosis, prognosis, and intervention.
- Physical therapists are involved in alleviating and preventing impairments, functional limitations, and disability by designing, implementing, and modifying therapeutic interventions.
- Therapeutic exercise intervention engages the individual to become an active participant in the treatment plan.
- Therapeutic exercise should be a core intervention in most physical therapy treatment plans.
- As the health care industry continues to change, the practitioner must recognize that the third-party reimburser for medical care is seeking health care services that are efficient and cost-effective. Prudent use of therapeutic exercise can reduce health care costs by promoting patient independence and self-responsibility.
- A thorough understanding of the disablement process can assist the practitioner in developing an effective, efficient, and cost-contained therapeutic exercise intervention, meaningful to the person seeking physical therapy services.

? Critical Thinking

Develop a case defining each feature of the modified disablement model. Provide a brief history of the current condition. Include a brief description of each of the following features:

- Risk factors
- Previous interventions
  - Intra-individual
  - Extra-individual
- Interventions that have served as exacerbators
- Pathology
- Impairments
  - Anatomic
  - Psychological
  - Physiologic
- Functional limitations
- Disability

REFERENCES

1. American Physical Therapy Association. A guide to physical therapist practice, I: A description of patient management. *Phys Ther.* 1995;75:709–764.
2. *International Classification of Impairments, Disabilities, and Handicaps.* Geneva, Switzerland: World Health Organization; 1980.
3. Nagi SZ. *Disability and Rehabilitation.* Columbus, Ohio: Ohio State University Press; 1969.
4. Pope A, Tarlov A, eds. *Disability in America: Toward a National Agenda for Prevention.* Washington, DC: National Academy Press; 1991.
5. Verbrugge L, Jette A. The disablement process. *Soc Sci Med.* 1994;38:1–14.
6. *National Advisory Board on Medical Rehabilitation Research, Draft V: Report Plan for Medical Rehabilitation Research.* Bethesda, MD: National Institutes of Health; 1992.
7. Jette AM. Physical disablement concepts for physical therapy research and practice. *Phys Ther.* 1994;74:380–386.

8. DeHaan R, Aaronson N, Limburt M, et al. Measuring quality of life in stroke. *Stroke*. 1993;24:320–327.
9. Jette AM. Using health-related quality of life measures in physical therapy outcomes research. *Phys Ther.* 1993;73: 528–537.
10. Hollbrook M, Skillbeck CE. An activities index for use with stroke patients. *Age Ageing.* 1983;12:166–170.
11. Mitchell DM, Spitz PW, Young DY, et al. Survival, prognosis and cause of death in rheumatoid arthritis. *Arthritis Rheum.* 1986;29:706–714.
12. Sherrer YS, Bloch DA, Mitchell, et al. Disability in rheumatoid arthritis: Comparison of prognostic factors across three populations. *J Rheumatol.* 1987;14:705–709.
13. Mitchell JM, Burhouser RV, Pincus T. The importance of age, education, and comorbidity in the substantial earnings and losses of individuals with symmetric polyarthritis. *Arthritis Rheum.* 1988;31:348–357.
14. Summers MN, Haley WE, Reville JD, et al. Radiographic assessment and psychologic variables as predictors of pain and functional impairment in osteoarthritis of the knee or hip. *Arthritis Rheum.* 1988;31:348–357.

CHAPTER 2

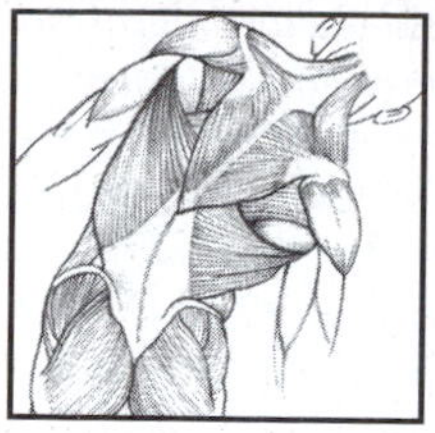

Patient Management

Carrie Hall

An understanding of the disablement process presented in Chapter 1 enables the clinician to provide optimal patient management by understanding the relationships among pathology, impairments, functional limitations, disabilities, quality of life, risk factors, and the effects of intra-individual and extra-individual interventions. Knowledge of the disablement process enables the clinician to

- Develop comprehensive but efficient examinations and evaluations of impairments and functional limitations relating to the patient's unique disability profile.
- Reach an appropriate diagnosis based on logical classification of impairments and functional limitations.
- Develop a prognosis based on the evaluation and the patient's goals.
- Create and implement effective and efficient interventions.
- Reach a desirable functional outcome for the patient as quickly as possible.

Each patient presents with unique physiologic, biomechanical, musculoskeletal, cognitive or affective, and environmental characteristics. Consideration of all these variables is necessary to develop an effective plan of care, but it can be overwhelming even for the experienced clinician. This chapter presents two additional models to assist in organizing the data and making the clinical decisions that are necessary to develop an effective and efficient therapeutic exercise intervention: the patient management model proposed by the American Physical Therapy Association (APTA)[1] and a therapeutic exercise intervention model.

PATIENT MANAGEMENT MODEL

The physical therapist's approach to patient management is described as the patient management model in Figure 2-1. The physical therapist integrates five elements of care in a manner designed to maximize the patient's outcome, which may be conceptualized as patient-related (eg, satisfaction with care) or associated with service delivery (eg, efficacy and efficiency).

Examination

The first two elements of patient management are examination and evaluation. Examination is defined as the process of obtaining a history, performing a relevant systems review, and selecting and administering specific tests and measures to obtain data.[1] Examination is a required element before any intervention. The history is expected to provide the physical therapist with pertinent information about the patient:

- Demographic profile and social history
- Occupation
- Living and working environments
- General health history
- Past and current history of the physical condition
- Past and current functional status
- Extra-individual and intra-individual interventions

This data can be obtained from the patient, family, significant others, caregivers, and other interested persons through interview or self-report forms, by consulting with other members of the health care team, and by reviewing the medical record. Display 2-1 summarizes the data generated from the history.

The systems review is a screening process that provides information about the bodily systems involved in the patient's current disability profile. Data generated from the systems review may affect tests performed during subsequent examinations and choices regarding interventions. Several major systems should be screened for involvement: cardiovascular, pulmonary, musculoskeletal, neuromuscular (including the autonomic nervous system), psychological, and integumentary. Display 2-2 summarizes the data generated from a systems review.

Depending on the data gathered from the history and systems review, the therapist may use one or more examinations, in whole or in part. The examination may be as brief or as lengthy as necessary to generate a diagnosis. For example, after taking the history and concluding a systems review, the physical therapist may determine that further examination is not appropriate and that the patient should

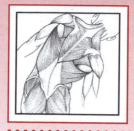

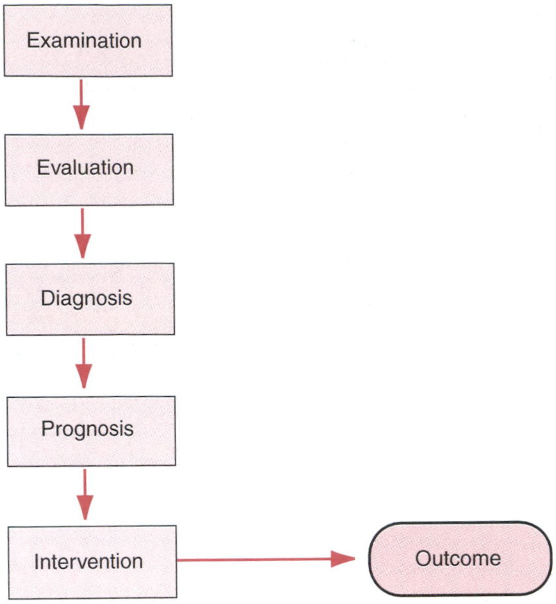

FIGURE 2-1 Patient management model.

be referred to another health care practitioner. Conversely, the physical therapist may determine that a detailed examination of several bodily systems is required to develop a thorough diagnosis. The specific tests and measures included in each examination generate data about the patient's impairments and functional limitations. Implementation of the examination is based on a prioritized order of tests and measures that depend on medical safety, patient comfort, and medical treatment priorities; the patient's physiologic, emotional, functional, social, and vocational needs; and financial resources. Although a complete list can be found elsewhere,[1] the relevant examinations performed by a physical therapist are given here:

- Aerobic capacity
- Gait and balance
- Joint integrity and mobility
- Motor function
- Muscle performance
- Posture
- Range of motion (ROM) and muscle length
- Ventilation, respiration, and circulation

DISPLAY 2-1

Data Generated From Client History[1]

General Demographics
- Age
- Sex
- Race
- Primary language

Social History
- Cultural beliefs and behaviors
- Family and caregiver resources
- Social interactions, social activities and support systems

Occupation
- Current or prior work (eg, job, school, play) or community activities

Growth and Development
- Hand and foot dominance
- Developmental history

Living Environment
- Living environment and community characteristics
- Projected discharge destination(s)

History of Present Condition
- Concerns that led the individual to seek the services of a physical therapist
- Concerns or needs of the individual requiring the services of a physical therapist
- Onset and pattern of symptoms
- Mechanism(s) of injury or disease, including date of onset and course of events
- Patient's, family's, or caregiver's perceptions of the patient's emotional response to the present clinical situation
- Current therapeutic interventions
- Patient's, family's, or caregiver's expectations and goals for the therapeutic intervention

Functional Status and Level of Activity
- Prior functional status, and self care and home management (ie, activities of daily living and instrumental activities of daily living)
- Behavioral health risks
- Sleep patterns and positions

Medications
- Medications for present condition
- Medications for other conditions

Other Tests and Measures
- Review of available records
- Laboratory and diagnostic tests

Past History of Present Condition
- Prior therapeutic interventions
- Prior medications

Past Medical or Surgical History
- Endocrine/metabolic
- Gastrointestinal
- Genitourinary
- Pregnancy, delivery, and postpartum
- Prior hospitalizations, surgeries, and preexisting medical and other health related conditions

Family History
- Familiar health risks

Social Habits (past and present)
- Level of physical fitness (self-care, home management, community, work [eg, job, school, play] and leisure activities)

DISPLAY 2-2
Systems Review Data That May Affect Subsequent Examinations and Interventions

Communication, affect, cognition, language, and learning style

Physiologic and anatomic system status
- Cardiopulmonary
- Musculoskeletal
- Neurological
- Integumentary

Other information may be required to complete the examination process:

- Clinical findings of other health care professionals
- Results of diagnostic imaging, clinical laboratory, and electrophysiologic studies
- Information from the patient's place of work regarding ergonomic, posture, and movement requirements

The examination is an ongoing process throughout the patient's treatment to determine the patient's response to intervention. Based on re-examination findings, the intervention may be terminated or modified by new clinical symptoms or failure to respond in the expected manner to the intervention. Exercise modification is discussed later in this chapter.

Evaluation

Evaluation is the dynamic process in which the physical therapist makes judgments based on data gathered during the examination. To make appropriate clinical decisions regarding the evaluation, the physical therapist must

- Determine the priority of problems to be assessed based on the medical history (and any other pertinent data collected through medical records or interactions with other health care providers) and systems review.
- Implement the examination.
- Interpret the data.

Interpretation of the data constitutes the evaluation. Interpretation of the examination findings is one of the most critical stages in clinical decision making. In interpreting the data to understand the sources or causes of the patient's impairments, functional limitations, and disabilities, all aspects of the examination must be considered and analyzed to determine the following:

- Progression and stage of the signs and symptoms
- Stability of the condition
- Presence of preexisting conditions (ie, comorbidities)
- Relationships among involved systems and sites

To remain consistent with the language of the disablement process and to link the patient management model with the disablement model, examples of examinations and evaluations are described for each element of the disablement model.

PATHOLOGY

Laboratory tests, radiologic studies, and neurologic examinations are used to assess the presence and extent of the pathologic process. Because some biochemical and physiologic abnormalities may be beyond the scope of medical testing, detection often relies on the evaluation of impairments. One of the frustrations for physical therapists following the disablement model is that underlying pathology accounting for the impairments, functional limitations, and resulting disabilities often cannot be identified. Radiologic, neurologic, or laboratory study results commonly are negative despite the presence of clinical signs and symptoms. However, the lack of an identifiable pathology should not lead the physical therapist to believe that an organic reason for the individual's impairments, functional limitation, or disability is not present. Even with a diagnosis of pathology, the physical therapist should concentrate on examination and evaluation of impairments, functional limitations, and disabilities, because the diagnosis may not provide much guidance.

IMPAIRMENTS

Medical procedures to evaluate impairments include clinical examinations, laboratory tests, imaging procedures, and the patient's medical history and symptom reports. Physical therapy procedures to examine and evaluate impairments should be based on bodily systems most treated by physical therapists: musculoskeletal, neuromuscular, cardiovascular, pulmonary, and integumentary systems (Fig. 2-2*A*). Many bodily systems are not within the scope of thorough and definitive examination by a physical therapist (eg, metabolic, renal, circulatory). However, if pertinent to the physical therapy intervention, this information should be gathered from the patient, other medical and health care professionals, or medical records. Specific tests (eg, pulse, blood pressure) indicating a system impairment that are within the scope of therapists should be performed (Fig. 2-2*B*).

Examinations may reveal a list of impairments, functional limitations, or disabilities that may or may not be amenable to physical therapy treatment. It is tempting to evaluate and treat lists of impairments, but this type of practice may not be the most effective or efficient use of health care dollars. It is therefore prudent to make simultaneous decisions about whether testing or measuring an impairment is pertinent to determining the cause of the functional limitation and disability. To facilitate this decision-making process, ask the following questions:

- Is the impairment related directly to a functional limitation? For example, reduced shoulder girdle mobility (ie, impairment) can be directly related to an inability to reach upward (ie, functional limitation).
- Is the impairment a secondary condition of the primary pathology or impairment? For example, a patient has complaints of shoulder pain and loss of mobility (ie, impairments) resulting in reduced function of the upper extremity (ie, functional limitation) for the activities of daily living (ADLs). However, the source of the shoulder pain is cervical disk disease (ie, primary pathology). Loss of mobility of the shoulder is a secondary impairment, and reduced use of the upper extremity during

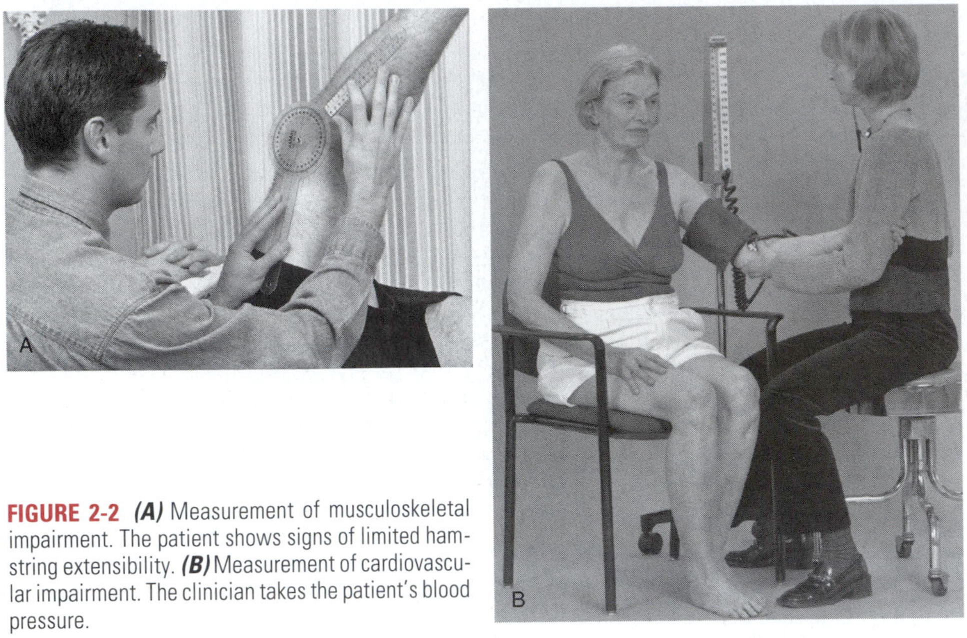

FIGURE 2-2 ***(A)*** Measurement of musculoskeletal impairment. The patient shows signs of limited hamstring extensibility. ***(B)*** Measurement of cardiovascular impairment. The clinician takes the patient's blood pressure.

ADLs is a secondary functional limitation, both of which developed because of pain in the shoulder originating from the primary condition of cervical degenerative disk disease.

- Can the impairment be related to future functional limitation? Studies have shown that a relationship can exist between current impairment findings and future functional limitations.[3,4] For example, loss of shoulder ROM in the absence of functional limitation may lead to functional limitation in the future from exaggeration of the impairment or the existing impairment leading to other impairments.
- Is the impairment unrelated to the functional limitation and disability and therefore should not be assessed or treated? For example, a patient complains of shoulder pain (ie, impairment) and reduced use of the shoulder girdle during ADLs. Hypomobility of the shoulder girdle may be an obvious impairment, but it may not be related to the functional limitation or disability. The patient's pain may occur in the midrange and is a result of impaired scapulohumeral rhythm, not hypomobility.

In summary, it is not useful to evaluate endless lists of impairments inconsequential to the person's current status in the disablement scheme. Prerequisites to an effective, efficient evaluation that leads the physical therapist toward a comprehensive, safe, effective, and efficient treatment include careful determination of tests before the evaluation process based on subjective history, self-report forms, review of charts, discussions with other members of the health care team and family members or significant others, and on clinical decision making throughout the evaluation process.

FUNCTIONAL LIMITATIONS

Rarely does the patient seen in the physical therapy department, clinic, or office describe specific complaints of weakness, loss of muscle length, or loss of joint mobility (ie, impairments). For example, the patient is probably more concerned about his ability to climb a flight of stairs (ie, functional outcome) than the adequate knee ROM and quadriceps force or torque production needed to climb the stairs (ie, impairments). Improved knee ROM and quadriceps force production may not result in the ability to climb a flight of stairs. The inability to climb stairs may be related to other impairments, such as physical impairments (eg, weak gluteal musculature, lack of ankle mobility) or psychological impairments (eg, fear).

One question must be addressed in daily practice and in physical therapy research: Which and to what degree are impairments linked to functional limitations? Few studies have attempted to establish the relationships among pathology, impairments, and functional limitations, but this question is clinically important to physical therapists. For example, the information gained from a descriptive study of individuals with arthritis indicates correlations among pathology (ie, arthritis), impairments (ie, knee ROM), and functional limitations (ie, performance of basic ADLs).[5] It was found that subjects with less than 70 degrees of knee flexion ROM had difficulty walking to the toilet, transferring to the toilet, getting in and out of a bathtub, and walking up and down stairs. This knowledge enables the physical therapist to feel confident that restoring at least 70 degrees of knee flexion can improve the patient's ability to perform selected basic ADLs.

Improving the impairments related to the functional outcome is necessary, but the measure of success is in the ability to achieve the functional outcome of climbing the stairs. To determine success in achieving functional outcome, valid, reliable, and sensitive tests must be used to measure functional performance. With standardized tests, no single assessment instrument can measure the full range of potential impairments, functional limitations, and disabilities. Adequate evaluation usually must rely on a battery of appropriate instruments. It is beyond the scope of this text to discuss the various standardized tests, but please refer to the appropriate references.[6–14]

Tests and measures of physical functional limitations have various formats:

- Self-reports or proxy reports (eg, spouse, parent, personal physician) of the level of difficulty performing tasks (eg, no difficulty, some difficulty, much difficulty, inability)[15,16]
- Observation of performance of functional tasks and rating the level of difficulty (eg, fully able, partially able, unable) or measuring distances, number of repetitions, or quality of motion based on kinesiologic standards[17,18]
- Equipment-based evaluation of performance (eg, use of a hand dynamometer to examine grip strength, computer-assisted assessment of balance, use of specialized grids to measure performance of closed chain activities)[8,13,14,16–23]

DISABILITY

Improvement in functional outcome may not be the only or most important measure of the positive effects of physical therapy intervention. Disability, as defined in the disablement model introduced in Chapter 1 (see Fig. 1-2), entails the social context of functional loss. Social function encompasses three domains: social interaction, social activity, and social role.[24] Each of these domains requires a certain degree of physical ability. For example, functional limitation in going up and down stairs may limit

1. A person's social interaction because of the inability to go outside the home to visit friends.
2. A person's social activity because of the inability to go to church with stairs to the front door.
3. A person's social role because of the inability to go to work and perform tasks that require going up and down stairs.

Understanding the relationships among physical impairments, functional limitations, and disabilities is relevant to the evaluation and treatment of a person seeking physical therapy services. Limitations in cognitive and affective abilities also affect the level of the person's physical function. Successful performance of complex instrumental ADLs such as personal hygiene, housekeeping, and dressing require integration of physical, cognitive, and affective abilities. As a result, measurement of disability requires tests that consider the complexity of variables that effect the person's ability to interact in society.

The standard and most economic procedure for measuring disability is self-reports or proxy reports, which include simple ordinal or interval scoring of the degree of difficulty in performing roles within the person's milieu. Questions regarding functional limitations, disability, and quality of life are included in many self-reports used by physical therapists.[13,18–21,25–29] Similar to tests and measures of functional limitation, no one self-report can encompass all aspects of disability from a physical therapist's perspective, and it is important to be aware of numerous reports pertinent to specific areas of practice. The appropriate self-report can offer comprehensive, concise information pertaining to functional limitations, disability, and quality of life, which can guide the physical therapist's evaluation and intervention.

Results of a disability measure often reveal aspects of the disability that are beyond physical impairments and functional limitations. Refer the patient to the appropriate health care professional if aspects of his disability are beyond your knowledge, expertise, or experience. Decide whether further physical therapy intervention is appropriate or physical therapy should be deferred until other aspects of disability are adequately dealt with. For example, a patient with low back pain may have a high level of anxiety or depression associated with the loss of function and the disability. Physical therapy may not be effective until the patient is treated for the anxiety or depression, or physical therapy concurrent with counseling may be determined to be most effective.

The time it takes to complete and interpret the self-report forms has been described as a methodologic and practical barrier to using self-reports. However, self-reports assist in determining whether functional limitations and disability exist beyond the scope of physical therapy practice and result in a referral to health care providers educated to evaluate and treat components outside the physical therapist's domain. This information may save financial resources and time spent attempting to treat physical impairments or functional limitations that cannot be resolved without more comprehensive intervention involving other health care practitioners, family members, or significant others. The time and cost savings to the patient and the health care system justifies the time spent completing and interpreting the form. It is beyond the scope of this text to discuss all of the standardized tests of disability. Please refer to the appropriate references.[14,15,22,25,30]

Diagnosis

Diagnosis is the next element in the patient management model. **Diagnosis** is the *process* and *end result* of information obtained in the examination and evaluation. The diagnostic process includes analyzing the information obtained in the examination and evaluation and organizing it into clusters, syndromes, or categories (Display 2-3) to help determine the most appropriate intervention strategy for each patient. The diagnostic process includes the following components[1]:

- Obtaining a relevant history (ie, examination)
- Performing a systems review (ie, examination)

DISPLAY 2-3

Definitions of Terms

Cluster: A set of observations or data that frequently occur as a group for a single patient.
Syndrome: An aggregate of signs and symptoms that characterize a given disease or condition.
Diagnosis: A label encompassing a cluster of signs and symptoms commonly associated with a disorder, syndrome, or category of impairment, functional limitation, or disability.

Adapted from American Physical Therapy Association. A guide to physical therapist practice, I: a description of patient management. Phys Ther. *1995;75:749–756.*

- Selecting and administering specific tests and measures (ie, examination)
- Interpreting all data (ie, evaluation)
- Organizing all data into a cluster, syndrome, or category (ie, diagnosis)

The end result of the diagnostic process is establishing a diagnosis. To reach an appropriate diagnosis, additional information may need to be obtained from other health care professionals. In the event that the diagnostic process does not yield an identifiable cluster, syndrome, or category, intervention may be guided by the alleviation of impairments and functional limitations. Caution should be taken in randomly treating impairments not associated with functional outcome. The purpose of a diagnosis made by a physical therapist is not to identify all of the patient's impairments, but to focus on which impairments are related to the patient's functional limitations and therefore should be addressed by the physical therapist. To ensure optimal patient care, the physical therapist may need to share the diagnosis determined from the physical therapy examination and evaluation process with other professionals on the health care team. If the diagnostic process reveals that the condition is outside of the therapist's knowledge, experience, or expertise, the patient should be referred to the appropriate practitioner.

Diagnosis in the physical therapy patient management model is synonymous with the term *clinical classification* and is not to be confused with the term *medical diagnosis*. Medical diagnosis is the identification of a patient's pathology or disease by its signs, symptoms, and data collected from tests ordered by the physician. Diagnosis established by a physical therapist is related to the primary dysfunction toward which the physical therapist directs treatment.[31–33] The medical diagnosis, in most cases, does not provide the physical therapist with enough information to proceed with intervention. For example, compare a medical diagnosis such as "cerebrovascular accident related to thrombolytic origin" to a diagnosis given by a physical therapist such as "nonfragmented volitional movement with severe tone dysfunction."[31] The physician diagnoses and treats the cause of cerebrovascular accident (ie, thrombosis), whereas the physical therapist diagnoses and treats the resulting impairments (ie, tone), functional limitations (ie, inability to walk), and disability (ie, inability to work). The physical therapist's diagnosis is reached only after performing a thorough examination and evaluation combined, if necessary, with the results of tests and measures ordered and performed by professionals from other disciplines and with the medical diagnosis itself.

DIAGNOSIS CLASSIFICATION

Diagnosis is one of the main decisional acts in the clinical decision-making process. Appropriate decisions regarding diagnostic classification are imperative, because the diagnosis directs the intervention. The ability to diagnose clusters, syndromes, or categories can foster the development of efficient treatment interventions and facilitate reliable outcomes research to present to the public, medical community, and third-party payers. For example, a common medical diagnosis of patients referred to outpatient physical therapy practices is low back pain, which is nothing more than a location of pain. If an outcomes study was performed that included all patients with the diagnosis of low back pain in a given practice, the results would not shed light on the best approach for treating low back pain because of the diverse causes, stages and severity of the condition, and comorbidities involved. Subclassification of patients based on diagnostic classification paradigms is necessary to provide more efficient patient management strategies and more meaningful outcome data.

The classification scheme developed by physical therapists does not mean that it is the exclusive domain of physical therapists. Avoid using the term *physical therapy diagnosis*; the phrase *diagnosis by a physical therapist* is preferred. The term physical therapy diagnosis reflects *ownership* of the condition and implies that it is unique to a physical therapist's knowledge and training. As physical therapists disseminate information about the diagnostic classifications they use, a variety of other practitioners would be expected to recognize the same signs and symptoms in their patients and to use these diagnoses when referring patients to physical therapists for confirmation of the presence of these conditions and for treatment.[31] In an integrated health care system, this kind of communication is essential.[34]

APTA's inclusion of diagnosis as an element of the patient management model is a testament to the importance of this aspect of patient care.[1,35] The field of physical therapy is strongly promoting the use of diagnosis to augment research regarding improved interventions and outcomes.[34] Several practitioners have developed or are developing diagnostic categories to provide effective and efficient interventions.[31–33,36–43]

For example, a diagnostic classification can be based on clusters of impairments in muscle balance and quality of movement (ie, movement impairment syndromes) that result in movement dysfunction and musculoskeletal pain.[41] Combinations of existing or preexisting impairments in muscle length-tension properties, timing and patterns of recruitment, structural alignment, and quality of movement can contribute to the development of movement dysfunction. It is theorized that movement dysfunction, if used repeatedly, can create microtrauma and eventually cause pathology.[41] Use of this theory of diagnostic classification fosters understanding of risk factors (eg, impairments in muscle length-tension properties, patterns of muscle recruitment, quality of movement), which can result in pathology and subsequent functional limitation and disability. If physical therapists could reliably group patients according to movement impairment syndromes, early diagnosis of movement impairment syndromes could *prevent* development of pathology and subsequent functional limitation and disability.

Another diagnostic classification method is based on treatment-oriented categories.[38] The first level of classification involves determining whether a patient can be managed predominantly and independently by a physical therapist or requires consultation with other services (eg, psychology) or referral to another health care practitioner (eg, medical physician because of serious pathology). After determining that the patient can be managed by a physical therapist, the next level of classification is to stage his condition with regard to severity. After making classification according to severity of the condition, a third level classification is used to classify patients into distinct categories that are treatment-based.

These two methods of diagnosis are certainly not inclusive of all diagnostic classifications in development, nor are they mutually exclusive. A case can be made for both types of classification. Physical therapy is in the early stages of developing impairment-based, functional limitation–based, and treatment-based diagnostic classifications. After classifications are developed, much work regarding validity, reliability, and sensitivity of diagnostic classifications needs to be done. Formulation and development of a useful classification design require the use of

- Measurement theory and advanced statistical techniques (ie, factor and cluster analyses) to validate clinical observations and systematize the complexities of clinical findings.
- Advanced technology that enables simultaneous collection, storage, and repeated acquisition of data that characterize multiple elements of movement.[42]

This text does not present clinical diagnoses made by a physical therapist, because this information has not yet been developed. Many leaders in the physical therapy community hope in the future to correlate effective and efficient treatment with the clinical diagnosis made by physical therapists to establish more efficient and cost-effective outcomes.[31,36,38,43] Only then can physical therapists promote the efficacy of the profession in today's cost-conscious health care environment.

Prognosis

Prognosis in the patient management model is defined as the determination of short-term improvements expected at various intervals during the course of intervention and of maximal improvement that may be attained and the time required to reach each level. For example, an expected short-term outcome for an otherwise healthy 65-year-old person after a hip fracture treated with open reduction and internal fixation may be the ability to walk 300 feet with partial weight bearing, using a walker, in 3 days; an expected long-term outcome may be the ability to walk independently without a gait deviation in 12 to 16 weeks. The prognosis should be based on the following factors:

- The patient's health status, risk factors, and response to previous interventions
- The patient's safety, needs, and goals
- The natural history and the expected clinical course of the pathology, impairment, or diagnosis
- The results of the examination, evaluation, and diagnostic processes

To ensure the prognosis is based on the patient's safety, needs, and goals, the physical therapist should confer with the patient and establish *patient goals*. During this discussion, the patient must be informed of the diagnosis or prioritized impairment list if a diagnosis cannot be developed. The patient should also be provided with an explanation of the relationship between the diagnosis or impairments and the functional limitations and disability. This information can assist the patient in developing realistic goals and understanding the purpose of the selected interventions. Agreement between the patient and therapist on the long- and short-term goals is imperative for successful treatment outcomes. When the physical therapist determines that physical therapy intervention is unlikely to be beneficial, the reasons should be discussed with the patient and other individuals concerned and documented in the medical record.

To ensure the prognosis is based on the natural history and the expected clinical courses of the pathology, impairment, or diagnosis, the physical therapist must rely on textbooks, lectures from instructors, literature reviews, research articles, and clinical experience. There are few reports regarding the natural history and the clinical course of specific diagnoses to which treatment should be directed, in part because of the limited development and use of diagnostic classification schemes by physical therapists.

The prognosis and goals can be modified as treatment progresses, based on the patient's response to intervention. Regardless of the diagnosis or prognosis, the physical therapist must develop a patient management program that promotes patient independence to the highest level that is possible.

Intervention

Intervention is defined as the purposeful and skilled interaction of the physical therapist with the patient using various methods and techniques to produce changes in the patient's condition consistent with the evaluation, diagnosis, and prognosis. Ongoing decisions regarding intervention are contingent on the timely monitoring of the patient's response and the progress made toward achieving outcomes.[1] The three major types of intervention are listed in Display 2-4. This text focuses on one aspect of direct intervention (ie, therapeutic exercise) and patient-related instruction as it relates to therapeutic exercise.

The key to a successful intervention and patient outcome is *to do the right things well*.[44] To determine the right things, the physical therapist must have a thorough understanding of the patient's disablement process and sound clinical decision-making skills.

DISPLAY 2-4

Types of Physical Therapy Interventions

- Direct intervention (eg, therapeutic exercise, manual therapy techniques, debridement, wound care)
- Patient-related instruction (eg, education provided to the patient and other caregivers involved regarding the patient's condition, treatment plan, information and training in maintenance and prevention activities)
- Coordination, communication, and documentation (eg, patient care conferences, record reviews, discharge planning)

CLINICAL DECISION MAKING FOR INTERVENTION

The physical therapist is educated and trained to effectively and efficiently treat physiologic and certain anatomic impairments related to functional limitations and to arrive at desirable functional outcomes for the patient. The choice of how to design and direct the treatment plan is based on the prognosis and functional goals. Recall that the ultimate functional goal of physical therapy is the achievement of optimal movement and functioning. Physical therapists generally develop treatment interventions with the intention of restoring function and reducing disability. However, strictly impairment-based interventions often do not achieve functional goals because the focus is not on the *right* impairment.

Treating the "Right" Impairments

An important clinical decision in the patient management process is to determine the impairment(s) that most closely relates to a functional limitation or disability. If the impairment is related to a functional limitation or disability, treat it directly. If the impairment is not directly or indirectly related to a functional limitation or disability, defer treatment of that specific impairment until it clearly correlates with a functional limitation or disability.

Physical therapists are often tempted to include impairments that do not correlate in their intervention plan because they assume that the reduction of any or all impairments leads directly to improvement in function.[45] In reality, the treatment of impairments can only lead to improvement in function if the impairments contribute to a functional limitation.

There are two instances, however, in which physical therapists must treat impairments that do not contribute to an identified functional limitation or disability. First, an impairment may not be related to a functional limitation, but it may be so severe that it impedes achievement of a functional goal. In this instance, the physical therapist must put aside the functional goal and alleviate the impairment. After the impairment is sufficiently resolved, treatment aimed at the functional goal may resume. This situation may occur where severe pain or profound weakness is present in an unrelated region from the one for which the patient is seeking treatment. Second, an impairment may not correlate with a functional limitation or disability, but if left untreated, it may lead to functional loss. In this instance, the physical therapist may treat the impairment as a preventive measure. For example, a patient has been prescribed a prone hip extension exercise to improve gluteal strength for treatment of hip pain. However, while he is extending his hip, his lumbar spine is moving into excessive extension. If the faulty movement pattern is left untreated, low back pain may develop. Exercises need to be prescribed to improve the stability of the low back to prevent the possibility of future episodes of low back pain.

If an impairment seems to be linked to a functional limitation or disability, the therapist must question whether the impairment is amenable to physical therapy intervention. To help determine the answer, the physical therapist should ask several questions:

- Will the patient benefit from the intervention (ie, can treatment improve functioning or prevent functional loss)?
- Are there any possible negative effects of the treatment (contraindications)?
- What is the cost–benefit ratio?

If the treatment cannot be justified, the physical therapist should consider other options such as the following:

- Discussing the decision to decline intervention with the patient to ensure patient agreement and understanding of the decision.
- Referring the patient to an appropriate practitioner or resource.
- Assisting in modifying the environment in which the individual lives, goes to school, or works to ensure maximal performance despite the impairment, functional limitation, or disability
- Teaching the individual to appropriately compensate for the impairment, functional limitation, or disability.

If the impairment is amenable to treatment, decide whether to treat the impairment, functional limitation, or both. For example a 72-year-old man after total knee replacement may present with weakness of the quadriceps and reduced mobility of the knee. The therapist may choose to treat the impairments with specific exercise instruction to increase quadriceps force or torque and knee mobility or to teach the patient the functional task of sit to stand that can resolve the impairments and restore function to the patient's satisfaction. The added benefit of choosing to focus on function rather than on specific exercise is that patient compliance may improve, because incorporating functional exercise into daily life is easier than finding time for specific exercise. However, the impairments may be too profound to allow adequate performance during a functional activity. For example, if the quadriceps strength in the previous example is less than fair, specific quadriceps strengthening may be necessary to achieve enough force or torque production to participate in a functional activity without compromising the quality of movement. Caution must be applied in prescribing functional activities prematurely to improve impairments.

Selecting and Justifying Treatment Interventions

When a decision has been made to treat a specific impairment or functional limitation, the next step is to select an appropriate treatment approach or combination of complementary approaches (eg, moist heat before joint mobilization, which is followed by stretching and ends with a functional task that employs the new mobility). The clinician must select and justify the chosen intervention.

Physical therapists may select an intervention from among the following possibilities[1]:

- Therapeutic exercise (including aerobic conditioning)
- Functional training in self-care and home management (including basic ADLs and instrumental ADLs)
- Functional training in community or work reintegration (including instrumental ADLs, work hardening, and work conditioning)
- Manual therapy techniques (including mobilization and manipulation)
- Prescription, fabrication, and application of assistive, adaptive, supportive, and protective devices and equipment

- Airway clearance techniques
- Wound management
- Physical agents and mechanical modalities
- Electrotherapeutic modalities

Numerous patient factors must be taken into consideration to determine which of the described interventions are correct. This information is obtained from the history and systems review (see Displays 2-1 and 2-2).

An awareness of the physical environment for living, working, or participating in recreational activities to which the patient wishes to return is important in developing functional activities and achieving functional outcomes. For example, a successful outcome may not be reflected in increased strength in the physical therapy office by a handheld dynamometer, but may be observed in the use of that strength in a functional manner in the patient's environment, such as walking up a flight of stairs with 20 pounds of groceries.

The process of selecting and justifying treatment intervention must include knowledge of research literature and the ability to interpret the literature as reliable and valid. The most credible source of *justification* is based on relevant research literature. Use caution when making decisions based on theory of pathophysiologic mechanisms and expert opinion not substantiated by credible clinical evidence. Knowledge of the literature combined with an accumulation of clinical experience facilitates the most sound choice.

PATIENT-RELATED INSTRUCTION

Patient-related instruction is the process of imparting information and developing skills to promote independence and to allow care to continue after discharge. It must be an integral part of any physical therapy intervention (Fig. 2-3).

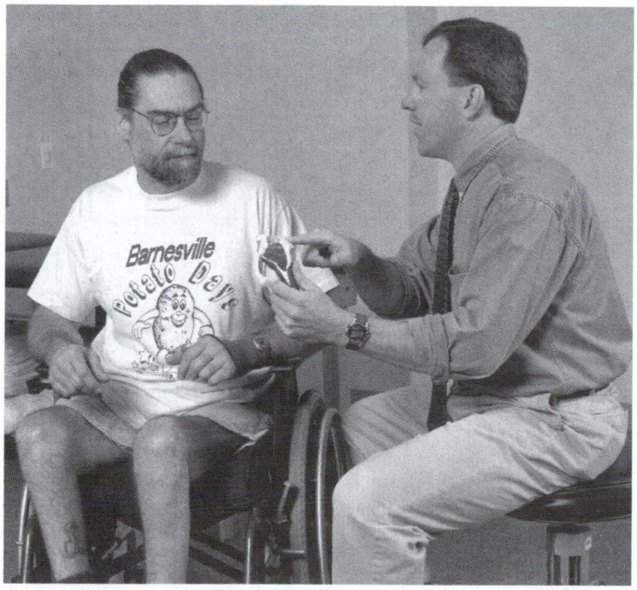

FIGURE 2-3 Patient-related instruction is an integral part of physical therapy intervention. By helping the patient understand his impairment and functional limitations, the clinician promotes patient compliance with the therapeutic intervention program.

When patient education is not possible (eg, the patient is an infant, comatose, or has a head injury), educating family members, significant others, friends, or other caregivers is essential. Patient-related instruction offered to a support person, even when educating the patient is possible, can promote compliance by teaching the support person to intervene in an appropriate manner and encouraging the display of appropriate attitudes toward the patient's functional limitations and disabilities.

Patient-related instruction is critical to enhance compliance in following through with interventions and preventing future disability. Imparting your knowledge of the patient's disablement process enables the patient to gain confidence in your skills, which further enhances compliance. Patient-related instruction may include the following:

- Education pertaining to the pathologic process and impairments contributing to functional limitation and disability; the prognosis; and the purposes and potential complications of the intervention
- Instruction and assistance in making appropriate decisions about management of the condition during the ADLs (eg, work station ergonomic modifications, altered movement patterns and body mechanics, altered sleep postures)
- Instruction and assistance in implementing interventions under the direction of the physical therapist (eg, training a support person in techniques of therapeutic exercise in the event that cognitive, physical, or resource status of the patient requires assistance to perform a home management program)

Patient-related instruction confers several benefits:

- Increased patient, significant other, family, and caregiver knowledge about the patient's condition, prognosis, and management
- Acquisition of behaviors that foster healthy habits, wellness, and prevention
- Improved levels of performance in employment, recreational, and sports activities
- Improved physical function, health status, and sense of well-being
- Improved safety for the patient, significant others, family, and caregivers
- Reduced disability, secondary conditions, and recurrence
- Enhanced decision making about the use of health care resources by the patient, significant others, family, or caregivers
- Decreased service use and improved cost containment

Patient-related instruction represents the first and most important step toward directing responsibility for treatment outcome from the physical therapist to the patient. A thorough understanding of the individual's disablement process and the factors that may impede improved functional outcome are necessary to provide comprehensive and personalized patient-related instruction. The successful practitioner is one who is skillful in the delivery of an active treatment approach based on treatment specific to the individual's disablement profile and on education that places the patient (or caregiver) in the position of taking responsibility for the outcome.

Outcome

Outcome is the result of physical therapy management expressed in five areas[1]:

1. Prevention or management of symptom manifestation
2. Consequence of disease (eg, impairment, functional limitation [basic ADLs]), disability (eg, instrumental ADLs, social roles)
3. Cost-benefit analysis
4. Health-related quality of life
5. Patient satisfaction

An outcome is considered successful when the following conditions are met:

- Physical function is improved or maintained whenever possible.
- Functional decline is minimized or slowed when the status quo cannot be maintained.
- The patient is satisfied.

At each step of the patient management process, the physical therapist considers the possible patient outcomes. This ongoing measurement of patient outcomes is based on the examination and evaluation of impairments, functional status, and level of disability. To evaluate the effectiveness of the intervention, the physical therapist must select criteria to be tested (eg, impairments or functional limitations) and interpret the results of the examination. Outcomes can be measured through outcome analysis. This is a systematic examination of patient outcomes in relation to selected patient variables (eg, age, sex, diagnosis, interventions, patient satisfaction). It can be part of a quality assurance program, used for economic analysis of a practice, or used to demonstrate efficacy of intervention.

Although positive outcomes are not synonymous with improved impairment measures, measurement of impairments and functional status should be performed to determine the efficacy of the intervention plan. By measuring both variables, the therapist can determine whether changes in the impairment are associated with changes in functional status.[45] If functional status has not changed, consider modifying the intervention plan. Modification of intervention is based on the status relative to the expected outcome and the rate of progress. Modification of an intervention is also based on the following considerations:

- Medical safety
- Patient comfort
- Patient's level of independence with the intervention (especially related to therapeutic exercise intervention)
- Effect of the intervention on the impairments and functional outcome
- New or altered symptoms due to intervention by other health care providers
- Patient finances, environment, and schedule constraints

The intervention may be modified by one of the following actions:

- Increasing or decreasing the dosage of the intervention, especially in the case of therapeutic exercise intervention (see the section on exercise modification in this chapter)
- Treating different impairments
- Changing the focus to functional limitations
- Consulting or referring to a more experienced physical therapist
- Referring the patient to a more appropriate health care provider
- Improving physical therapy techniques, verbal cues, and teaching skills

Prudent clinical reasoning assists the clinician in determining the need for modification and the best adjustments to implement. In determining and implementing revised goals and interventions, the clinician uses the additional data gathered from the re-evaluation. This re-evaluation and modification process continues until the decision to stop treatment is reached.

In an era of cost containment, there is an urgent need to document the effectiveness of physical therapy procedures. The field lacks studies regarding successful and cost-effective outcomes. Physical therapists have a responsibility to demonstrate to patients and third-party payers that physical therapy is efficient, cost effective, and provides patient satisfaction. In daily practice, physical therapists should adhere to the same principles of measurement used in research. Changes should be carefully documented in an effort to demonstrate that physical therapy intervention is related to successful outcomes in an efficient and cost-effective manner. Display 2-5 summarizes patient management concepts.

CLINICAL DECISION MAKING

At each juncture in the patient management model, clinical decisions are made. Appropriate decisions are crucial for a successful outcome. However, the clinical reasoning process involved in patient management presents the greatest challenge to the physical therapist, who often encounters difficulties with the following aspects of clinical decision making:

- Organization of evaluation findings into a diagnosis
- Development of a prognosis based on the patient's functional limitations and disabilities
- Development of realistic patient-based goals

DISPLAY 2-5

Patient Management Concepts

- Develop an examination or evaluation schema pertinent to the patient.
- Diagnose the patient's impairments, functional limitations, and disabilities.
- Develop a prognosis based on the patient's individual disablement process.
- Develop a plan of care designed to improve function (ie, the right things).
- Apply appropriate judgment and motor skills to provide the appropriate intervention.
- Continually use clinical reasoning to modify the intervention as needed for a positive outcome.

- Development and implementation of an intervention that is effective and efficient

Display 2-6 summarizes clinical decision-making tips in relation to patient management to help the physical therapist address some of these challenges. The effectiveness of clinical decision making is based on obtaining pertinent data. The physical therapist must possess

- Knowledge about what is pertinent
- The skill to obtain the data
- The ability to store, record, evaluate, relate, and interpret the data.

These actions require knowledge of the disablement process; clinical experience in treating impairments and functional limitations; and disciplined, systematic thought processes. Common to those who strive to excel in clinical decision making are the following characteristics:

- Wide range of knowledge
- Ongoing acquisition of knowledge
- Need for order or a plan of action
- Questioning unproven conventional solutions
- Self-discipline and persistence in work

Information regarding clinical decision making and the process involved warrant their own text. However, this text strives to include theoretical information and pertinent issues related to clinical decision making. This information empowers the physical therapist with some of the necessary tools to make appropriate clinical decisions regarding the design and application of treatment plans.

DISPLAY 2-6

Clinical Decision-Making Tips for Patient Management

Examination: Prioritize the problems to be assessed and the tests and measures to be implemented.

Evaluation: Consider and analyze all examination findings for relationships, including the progression and stages of the symptoms, diagnostic findings by other health care professionals, comorbidities, medical history, and treatment or medications received.

Diagnosis: Segregate findings into clusters of symptoms and signs by common causes, mechanisms, and effects. Refer to diagnosis classifications being developed by leading physical therapists.

Prognosis: Develop long-term and short-term goals based on patient safety, needs, and goals and on information regarding the natural history and expected clinical courses of the pathology, impairment, or diagnosis.

Intervention: Determine whether impairments correlate with a functional limitation or disability and are amenable to physical therapy treatment. Select and justify a method of intervention. The most credible source of justification is based on relevant research literature.

Outcome: Measure the success of the intervention plan according to functional gain and make appropriate modifications when necessary.

THERAPEUTIC EXERCISE INTERVENTION

Of the three components of physical therapy intervention (see Display 2-4), this text presents information regarding the direct intervention of therapeutic exercise and patient-related instruction associated with therapeutic exercise intervention.

After a thorough examination or evaluation has been performed; a diagnosis and prognosis have been developed; and the clinician understands the relationships among the pathology (if a disorder has been diagnosed), impairments, functional limitations, and disability, a plan of intervention is determined through the clinical decision-making process. In this text, the focus is on one intervention-therapeutic exercise. Therapeutic exercise may be the basis of the intervention or may be one component of the intervention, but it should be included to some extent in all patient care plans. Therapeutic exercise includes activities and techniques to improve physical function and health status resulting from impairments by identifying specific performance goals that allow a patient to achieve a higher functional level in the home, school, workplace, or community. It also incorporates activities to allow well clients to improve or maintain their health or performance status for work, recreation, or sports and prevent or minimize future potential functional loss or health problems.

To develop an efficient, effective therapeutic exercise intervention, consider these variables:

- Which elements of the movement system need to be addressed to restore function?
- Which activities or techniques are chosen to achieve a functional outcome, including the sequence within a given exercise session and the sequence of gradation in the total plan of care?
- What is the purpose of each specific activity or technique chosen?
- What are the posture, mode, and movement for each activity or technique?
- What are the dosage parameters for each activity or technique?

The following section presents a therapeutic exercise intervention model to assist in organizing all the details necessary to prescribe an effective, efficient exercise prescription.

Intervention Model

A three-dimensional model has been used to determine the appropriate exercise and the elements necessary to make a clinical decision about the appropriate therapeutic exercise intervention (Fig. 2-4). Three axes are used to visualize three components of exercise prescription and their relationships:

1. Elements of the movement system as they relate to the purpose of each activity or technique
2. The specific activity or technique chosen
3. The specific dosage

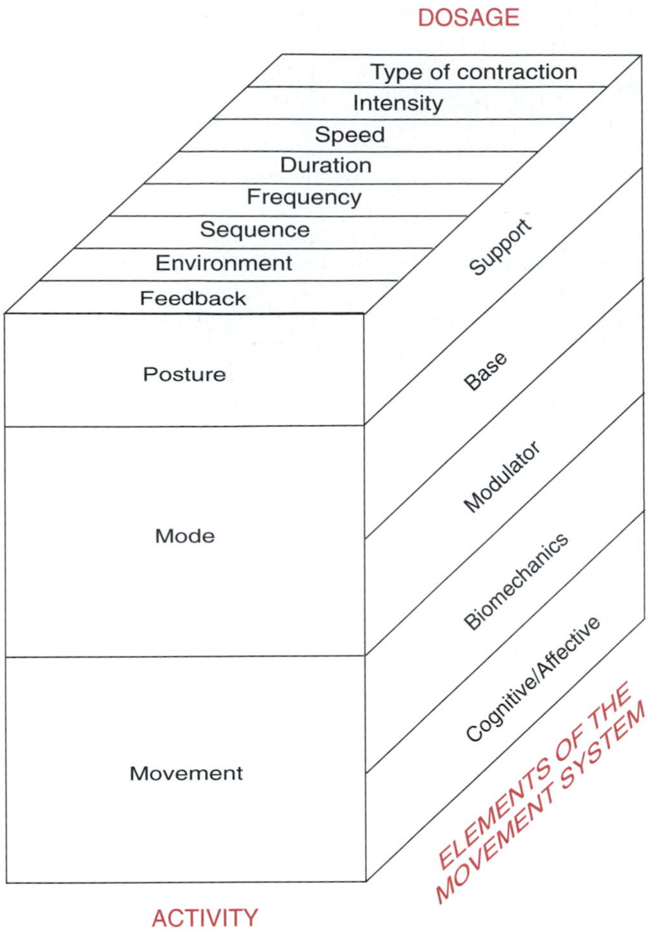

FIGURE 2-4 Therapeutic exercise intervention model.

ELEMENTS OF THE MOVEMENT SYSTEM

To prescribe the appropriate exercise, factors regarding the patient's disability profile must be considered. One critical factor is the patient's functional status. Often, the patient's functional status is related to movement. Whether the patient is a burn victim requiring passive ROM to prevent contractures, a patient requiring gradual active exercise and elevation on a tilt table to prevent orthostatic hypotension after prolonged bed rest, a high-performance athlete performing sport-specific drills to return to sport as a final stage of rehabilitation of a ligament tear, or an elderly patient performing posture exercises to prevent further collapse of the thoracic spine into kyphosis, each exercise prescription has a common goal: to restore functional movement as best as possible and prevent or minimize functional loss in the future.

Ideal movement can be thought of as the result of a complex interaction of several elements of the movement system. The proposed elements of the movement system are defined as follows[41]:

- *Support element:* the functional status of the cardiopulmonary system. This element provides energy for movement, such as
  - Breathing patterns
  - Physiologic status of the heart and lungs
- *Base element:* the functional status of the integumentary, musculoskeletal, and nervous systems. This element provides the basis for movement, such as
  - Extensibility properties of skin, muscle, fascia, and periarticular tissues
  - Mobility of neuromeningeal tissue and integrity of soft tissue and bones (eg, skin, muscle, ligaments, cartilage, subchondral bone, nerve)
  - Force or torque capability and endurance of muscle
  - Muscle length-tension properties
- *Modulator element:* the physiologic status of the neuromuscular system. This element is particularly related to motor control, such as
  - Patterns and synchronization of muscle recruitment
  - Feedforward and feedback systems
- *Biomechanical element:* the functional status of static and dynamic kinetics and kinematics, such as
  - Static forces involved in alignment
  - Dynamic forces involved in arthrokinetics, osteokinetics, and kinematics
- *Cognitive or affective element:* the functional status of the psychological system as it is related to movement, such as
  - The cognitive ability to learn
  - Compliance
  - Motivation
  - Emotional status

  (*Note:* The cognitive element is not an original element of the movement system as defined by Shirley Sahrmann)[41]

The elements of the movement system are along the horizontal axis of the therapeutic exercise intervention model (see Fig. 2-4). The diagnostic process can determine the impairments that are related to the patient's functional limitations and disability. To begin planning the therapeutic exercise intervention, the impairments should be related to an element of the movement system. This process guides the clinician toward the most appropriate activities or techniques and the dosage to treat the impairments related to the functional limitations and disability.

After evaluating a patient, it may be apparent that one, a few, or all elements of the movement system are involved. Most often, the interaction of the elements is critical, but one or two elements usually are pivotal to effect change. Determine *which* elements are involved in order to choose the appropriate activity or technique, to determine the proper dosage, and to determine in *what order* these elements should be prescribed to be most efficient at restoring normal movement. For example:

A 42-year-old woman is referred to you for treatment of an impingement syndrome of the shoulder. The functional limitation is an inability to raise the arm to groom her hair without pain. A pivotal impairment is determined to be a thoracic kyphosis that results in the scapula resting in an excessive anterior tilt (Fig. 2-5). The scapula, resting in anterior tilt, fails to posteriorly tilt during upper extremity flexion (Fig. 2-6). As a result, the glenohumeral joint mechanically impinges under the acromion process, and tissues in the subacromial space (eg, bursa, biceps tendon, rotator cuff tendons) undergo microtrauma resulting in pain (ie, impairment), inflammation (ie, pathology), and the inability to raise the arm without pain (ie, functional limitation). If left untreated, loss of mobility of the upper extremity may ensue, further affecting function and potentially leading to disability (eg, inability to pick up chil-

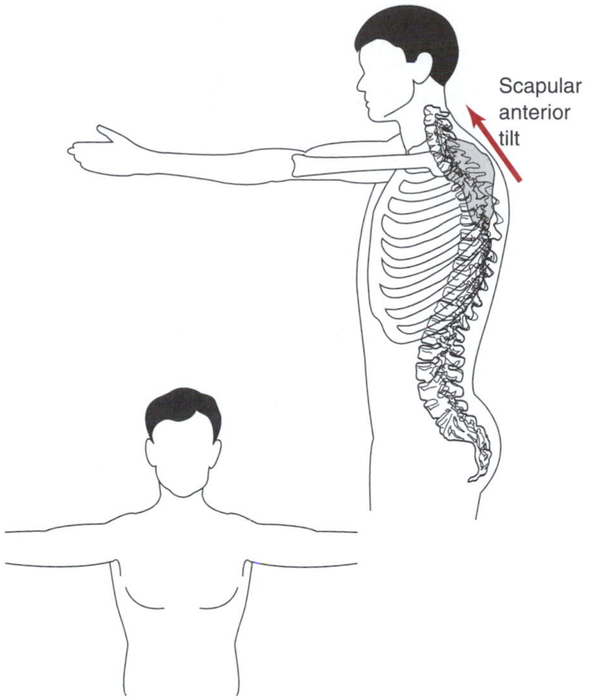

FIGURE 2-5 Thoracic kyphosis with excessive scapular anterior tilt.

dren, inability to perform work-related duties, inability to participate in desired recreational sports).

Impairments can be listed and categorized by the elements of the movement system, as exhibited in Display 2-7.

As can be seen from this example, a different impairment is correlated with each element of the movement system. A specific exercise can be prescribed to address each impairment associated with an element of the movement system (eg, stretching the pectoralis minor to address the base element). Most often, the interaction of elements is critical; therefore, one exercise may address numerous elements of the movement system. For example, wall slides (Fig. 2-7) can improve several features:

- Extensibility of the pectoralis minor (ie, base element)
- Force or torque capability (ie, base element) and recruitment of lower trapezius (ie, modulator element)
- Thoracic extension mobility to reduce the thoracic kyphosis (ie, biomechanical element)

When instructing a patient in the performance of this exercise, provide verbal, visual, or tactile feedback to focus on any one element of the movement system, or provide instruction to the patient regarding the interaction of elements. The order in which each exercise is prescribed is based on prioritizing which elements are pivotal to restoring function and which elements must be improved for other elements to follow. For example, it may be decided that the patient needs to take measures to improve her emotional status (ie, affective state) to address the physical manifestation of depression (ie, slumped posture), combined with exercise to improve postural habits (ie, biomechanical element) before any other intervention. Diaphragmatic breathing (ie, pulmonary system) may be pivotal to reduce the activity of the pectoralis minor and improve thoracic spine alignment and mobility to allow improved muscle balance to occur. Concurrent stretching for the pectoralis minor and strengthening (in the shortened range) for the lower trapezius (ie, base element) can also improve muscle length-tension properties of both muscles (see Chapter 4). Using the correct recruitment strategy (ie, modulator element) during specific exercise and during functional movement is necessary to achieve a functional outcome.

Display 2-8 summarizes the factors to consider before determining the relevant and prioritized list of the elements of the movement system.

DISPLAY 2-7

Elements of the Movement System Related to Impairments

- Biomechanical element impairment: Thoracic kyphosis contributing to the anterior tilted scapula
- Base element impairment: Short pectoralis minor and short head of biceps pulling coracoid process anteriorly, lengthened and weak lower trapezius not providing sufficient counterforce
- Modulator element impairment: Reduced recruitment of lower trapezius and inappropriate pectoralis minor recruitment during scapular upward rotation
- Support element impairment: Inappropriate breathing pattern using accessory muscles of respiration versus diaphragmatic breathing, leading to overuse and shortening of pectoralis minor
- Cognitive and affective element impairment: Patient is clinically depressed, and the physical manifestation is a slumped posture contributing to the thoracic kyphosis.

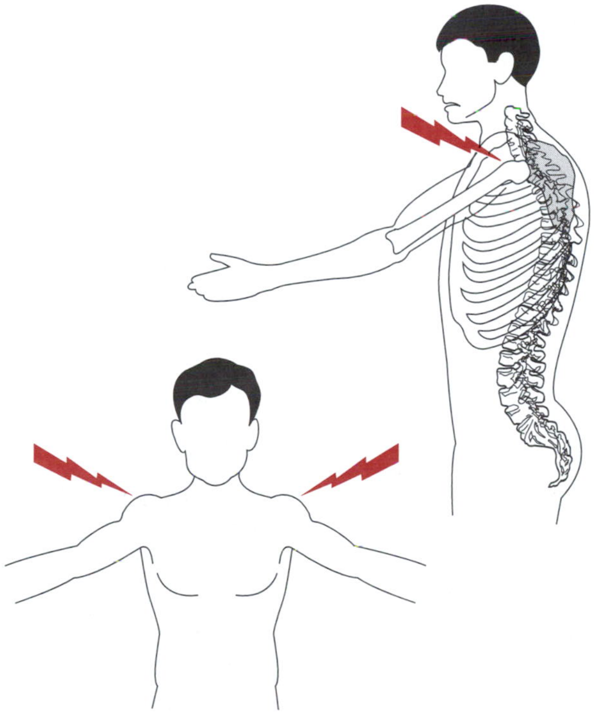

FIGURE 2-6 Lack of scapular posterior tilt leads to glenohumeral impingement.

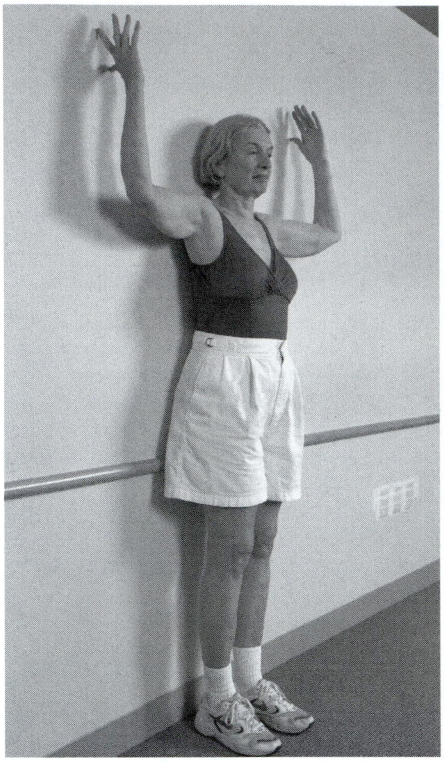

FIGURE 2-7 This exercise illustrates a patient performing a wall slide. The patient moves from the position shown here to the end position of the shoulders in full elevation.

ACTIVITY OR TECHNIQUE

Along the vertical axis is the activity or technique chosen to achieve the functional goal. Therapeutic exercise activities and techniques include the following:

- Stretching (passive and active)
- ROM exercises (eg, active assisted ROM, active ROM)
- Strengthening (eg, active assistive, active, and resistive exercise using manual resistance, pulleys, weights, hydraulics, elastics, robotics, and mechanical or electromechanical devices)
- Neuromuscular re-education
- Developmental activities
- Breathing exercises
- Aerobic or muscular endurance activities using cycles, treadmills, steppers, pools, manual resistance, pulleys, weights, hydraulics, elastics, robotics, and mechanical or electromechanical devices
- Aquatic exercise
- Gait training
- Balance and coordination training
- Posture awareness training
- Body mechanics and ergonomics training
- Movement training

To be successful in choosing the proper activity or technique, first determine the element of the movement system being addressed. For example, posture awareness training is associated with the biomechanical element, neuromuscular re-education is associated with the modulator element, breathing exercises and aerobic endurance activities are associated with the cardiovascular and pulmonary element, and stretching and strengthening are associated with the base element.

After identifying the elements of the movement system, the physiologic status of the impairments or functional limitations chosen to be treated must be considered. This information assists in determining the activity or technique, posture, movement, and mode parameters. For example, if the force or torque capability (ie, base element; see Chapter 4) is pivotal to a successful functional outcome, the chosen activity or technique depends on the force torque capability of the affected muscles. If the force or torque capability is less than fair in muscle strength as determined by Kendall et al.,[46] a gravity-lessened position active ROM activity or an against-gravity active assisted technique may be chosen. Another example may be related to reduced muscle recruitment from prolonged immobilization (ie, modulator element) or *muscle amnesia*. If the ability to recruit is poor, a gravity-lessened active ROM activity may be chosen with tactile feedback or against-gravity active ROM with neuromuscular electrical stimulation as an adjunctive intervention (discussed later in this chapter), both of which are chosen to augment muscle re-education.

Stage of Movement Control

Another factor to consider in choosing an activity is the stage of movement control (Display 2-9) focused on in the intervention. Mobility is defined as the presence of a functional range through which to move and the ability to initiate and sustain active movement through the range.[47] A person with musculoskeletal dysfunction may exhibit impairments in either or both parameters of mobility. For example, after total knee arthroplasty, a person may experience passive mobility restrictions caused by pain, swelling,

DISPLAY 2-8

Considerations in Clinical Decision Making Relevant to the Elements of the Movement System

- Identify the functional limitations and related impairments to be treated.
- Relate functional limitations and impairments to be treated with the appropriate elements of the movement system.
- Prioritize elements of the movement system.

DISPLAY 2-9

Stages of Movement Control

Mobility: A functional range through which to move and the ability to sustain active movement through the range
Stability: The ability to provide a stable foundation from which to move
Controlled mobility: The ability to move within joints and between limbs following the optimal path of instant center of rotation (PICR)
Skill: The ability to maintain consistency in performing functional tasks with economy of effort

and soft tissue stiffness or shortness and have decreased ability to initiate knee motion as a result of reduced muscle force or torque production or reduced recruitment capability. The cause of the mobility restriction must be determined on a case-by-case basis to determine the most appropriate exercise intervention (see Chapter 6).

Stability in the construct of stages of movement control is defined as the ability to provide a stable foundation from which to move.[47] A precursor to achieving the stability necessary for movement, or dynamic stability, is optimal posture. The individual must be able to maintain optimal posture without a load before optimal posture can be maintained during movement of a limb. Mobility and stability are not mutually exclusive. Achieving mobility before addressing stability is unnecessary; the two stages of movement control should occur concurrently. For example, as mobility after total knee arthroplasty is achieved passively, active motion must be prescribed. For optimal active motion, the knee requires a stable proximal base from which to move (ie, pelvis and trunk) and distal base for weight bearing (ie, foot and ankle). Stability must be achieved at these regions for optimal active motion to take place.

Controlled mobility is defined as the ability to move within joints and between limbs, following the optimal path of instant center of rotation (see Chapter 8). This requires proper recruitment of synergists that perform movement (ie, stability within a segment during movement) and proper length and recruitment, if necessary, of muscles providing a stable foundation for movement. The previous example would progress from exercises improving knee mobility and intrinsic stability, as well as pelvic-trunk and foot-ankle stability, to functional movement patterns. To walk, the knee must flex and extend at proper stages in the gait cycle. The trunk, pelvis, ankle, and foot must move into proper position at each stage of the gait cycle and provide proximal and distal stability for optimal knee function. The activity may involve the swing phase of gait, which requires a stable pelvis from which to swing the lower limb (Fig. 2-8*A*), or the stance phase of gait (Fig. 2-8*B*), which requires a stable foot for optimal knee loading.

The final progression in the stages of movement control is skill. Skill implies consistency in performing functional tasks with economy of effort.[48] Skill in the upper extremities

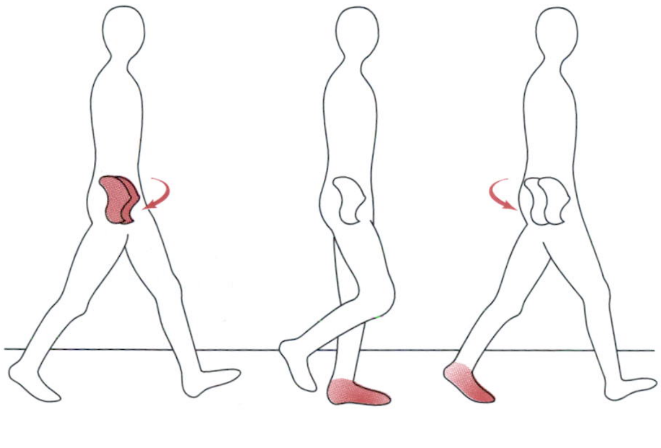

FIGURE 2-8 ***(A)*** Swing phase of gait requires a stable pelvis. ***(B)*** Stance phase of gait requires a stable foot.

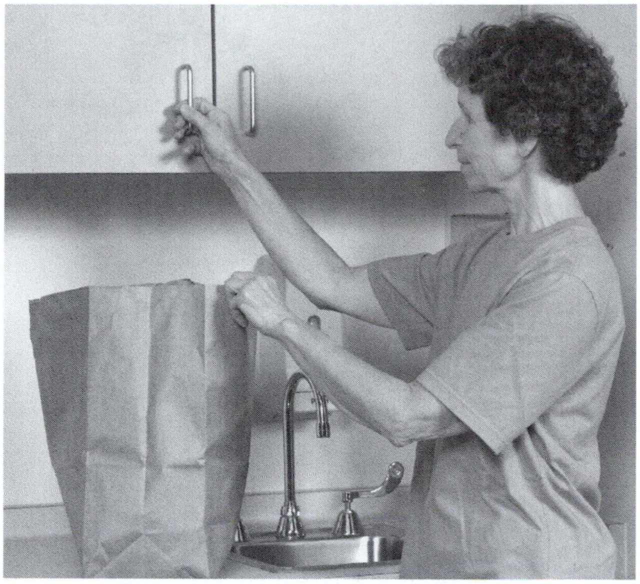

FIGURE 2-9 Grasping a cabinet door requires freedom of movement in space in a coordinated manner within and between the joints of the upper extremity, trunk, and pelvis.

most often requires freedom of movement in space in a coordinated manner within and between the hand, wrist, forearm, elbow, shoulder girdle, trunk, and pelvis (eg, grasping a cabinet door) (Fig. 2-9). Occasionally, closed chain (weight-bearing) movements are required in the upper extremity (eg, gymnast performing a handstand on the balance beam) (Fig. 2-10). Skill in the lower extremities requires coordination of open chain (nonweight-bearing) movements (eg, swing leg in kicking a soccer ball) (Fig. 2-11) and closed chain movements (eg, stance leg in kicking a soccer ball) within and between the foot, ankle, tibia, femur, pelvis, and trunk for movement on varied surfaces. For total body movement to be optimal, coordinated movement must

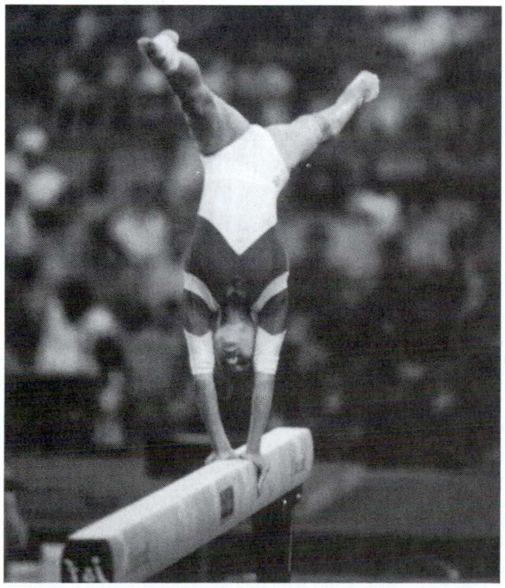

FIGURE 2-10 A gymnast performing on the uneven parallel bars represents an upper extremity closed chain movement.

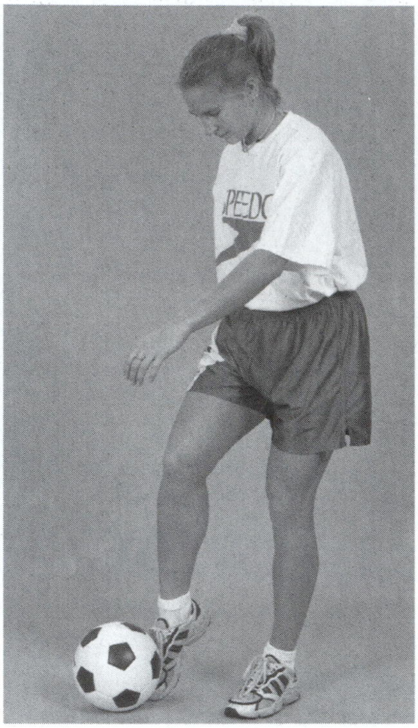

FIGURE 2-11 Skill in lower extremities requires coordination of open and closed chain movement. The swing leg performs an open chain movement, as the stance leg performs a closed chain movement.

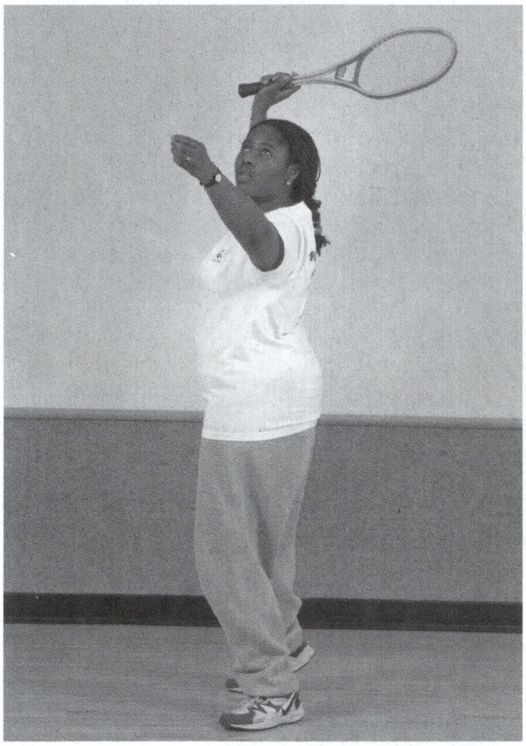

FIGURE 2-12 A tennis serve represents a total body movement, which is coordinated within and between each segment involved in the movement.

occur within and between each segment involved in the movement (eg, the tennis serve) (Fig. 2-12).

Commonly, patients are asked to perform skill-level activities without first developing proper foundations for functional movement control. Conversely, patients may be prescribed exercises developing the other stages of movement control without finalizing the intervention with skill-level activities during functional movements. Skill is a necessary stage of movement control despite the prognosis of the patient (eg, walk 10 feet with a walker versus run a marathon), which must be worked toward by achieving optimal function at each prior stage of movement control.

In summary, an activity can be as simple as performing a dynamic knee extension movement in supine (ie, mobility) or as difficult as an integrated movement pattern such as walking (ie, skill). An understanding of the level of involvement of the base, modulator, and cognitive or affective elements of the movement system help to determine the complexity of the task and the stage of movement control in which to intervene. Display 2-10 summarizes the factors to consider before determining the activity or technique.

Mode, Posture, and Movement

After choosing the activity or technique, further breakdown of the activity is necessary for precise prescription. The mode, which is the method of performing the activity or technique, must be chosen. For example, if aerobic exercise is chosen, the mode can be cycling, swimming, walking, or a similar activity. If strengthening is chosen, the mode can be weights, manual resistance, or active assisted exercise. If balance and coordination training is chosen, the mode can be a balance board, balance beam, or computerized balance device. The initial and ending *postures* (eg, standing, sitting, supine, prone, wide base of support, narrow base of support) need to be determined. Included in this information is proper hand placement and angle of application of the force if the activity is performed manually. When elastics, pulleys, mechanical, or electromechanical devices are used, proper equipment placement and angle of application of force must be determined, and these items are included in the beginning and ending posture information. The *movement* needs to be specifically defined (eg, partial squat through a 30-degree arc, unilateral arm raise through full-range, proprioceptive neuromuscular facilitation diagonal of the upper extremity to chest height).

The quality of performance of the exercise is critical to the outcome (ie, neuromuscular element of the movement system). In relation to base or modulator elements an obvious but often neglected example is that a muscle that is not recruited cannot be strengthened. Even if the correct activity is chosen and the mode, posture, and movement are

DISPLAY 2-10

Considerations Involved in Clinical Decision Making Related to Choice of Activity or Technique

- Determine the element of the movement system related to the impairment or functional limitation to be treated.
- Consider the physiologic status of the movement system.
- Determine the stage of movement control.

carefully selected, proper execution of the exercise is necessary to ensure a successful outcome. For example, hip abduction while sidelying can be performed with at least five different recruitment patterns (Fig. 2-13 and Display 2-11). Attention to precision of movement and recruitment patterns is vital and always must be promoted to the best of the individual's capability. Modify the exercise to achieve the best performance possible.

DOSAGE

The third axis is related to dosage parameters (see Fig. 2-4). When determining dosage, anatomic sites, and the physiologic status of the affected elements of the movement system, the patient's learning capability must be considered. The anatomic site comprises the specific tissues involved (eg, ligament, muscle, capsule, fascia). The physiologic status of the affected elements of the movement system includes the severity of the tissue damage (eg, partial versus complete tear), the irritability of the condition (eg, easily provoked and difficult to resolve versus difficult to provoke and easy to resolve), the nature of the condition (eg, chemical versus mechanical mediated pain), and the stage of the condition (eg, acute, subacute, chronic). For patients recovering from an injury, the dosage parameters are modified according to the tissues involved and the principles of tissue healing. In the early stages of healing, tissues tolerate low-intensity passive or active activities, but in the later stages, tissues tolerate more aggressive resistive activities (see Chapter 10).

The patient's ability to learn, or *learning capability*, influences the schedule and the amount of reinforcement, feedback, or sensory input needed to perform the activity successfully. If a patient has difficulty learning a motor task, the dosage may be altered according to the principles of learning (see Chapter 3). For example, various forms of feedback (eg, verbal, visual, tactile) combined with numerous, low-intensity repetitions may be required initially for optimal performance of an activity. As skill is acquired, feedback and repetitions may be reduced, and a more complex activity eventually may be prescribed.

After the anatomic and physiologic elements and the learning capabilities are understood, specific dosage parameters can be determined. Display 2-12 summarizes the factors to consider before determining dosage parameters. Parameters related to dosage include

- Type of contraction (ie, eccentric, concentric, isometric, dynamic, or isokinetic)
- Intensity (ie, amount of assistance or resistance required)
- Speed of the activity or technique
- Duration tolerated (ie, number of repetitions or number of sets, particularly related to endurance and stretching activities)
- Frequency of exercise (ie, number of exercise sessions in a given period)
- Sequencing of the exercise prescription (ie, stretch before strengthen, warm-up before stimulus, or simple before difficult)
- Environment in which the exercise is performed (ie, quiet, controlled environment of a private room in a physical therapy clinic versus a loud, chaotic, uncontrolled, outside environment)
- Amount of feedback necessary for optimal performance of the activity

In summary, numerous variables in this model must be considered in prescribing an exercise, and variables often overlap (eg, learning capabilities under dosage is similar to stages of movement control under activity, which is similar to modulator and cognitive or affective elements for the movement system). The task of organizing this data can be

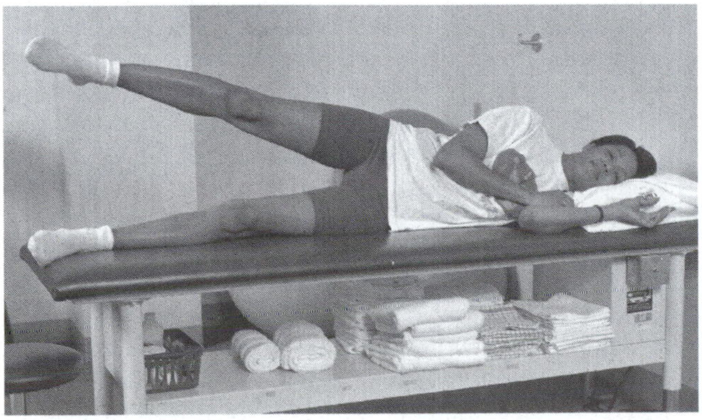

FIGURE 2-13 Hip abduction in the sidelying position. Optimal execution is with the pelvis in the frontal plane and the hip abducted with all of the hip abductors in synergy.

DISPLAY 2-11

Variations in Performing Sidelying Hip Abduction

1. Sidelying with pelvis in frontal plane and abducting the hip with all of hip abductors in synergy (See Fig. 2-13)
2. Sidelying with pelvis rotated backward and hip rotated laterally, causing the movement to move toward the sagittal plane and resulting in recruitment of hip flexors
3. Sidelying with pelvis in frontal plane with hip rotated medially and flexed, resulting in recruitment of tensor fascia lata
4. Sidelying with pelvis in frontal plane, but movement is at the pelvis (hip hike), resulting in recruitment of lateral trunk muscles
5. Sidelying with pelvis in frontal plane, but movement is abduction of opposite hip, resulting in recruitment of opposite hip abductors

DISPLAY 2-12

Considerations Involved in Clinical Decision Making Related to Choice of Dosage Parameters

- Determine the anatomic sites involved in the current condition.
- Determine the physiologic status of the tissue(s) involved.
- Consider the patient's learning capability.

overwhelming. The three-dimensional model may help to visualize the relationships among the components of exercise prescription. I hope this model assists in organizing the data necessary to develop an effective, efficient therapeutic exercise intervention.

Functional Outcomes

The key to a successful intervention by a physical therapist is the functional outcome. The therapist must determine early how the effect of a therapeutic exercise will be measured. Changes in impairments and functional limitations should be measured. By measuring both variables, the therapist can determine whether changes in the impairment are associated with changes in functional status.

When the desired patient outcome is not met in a reasonable time frame, modification is based on evaluating how the following possibilities affect the lack of progress achieved with the therapeutic exercise intervention:

- The physical therapist may choose the wrong activity, dosage of exercise, or both.
- The physical therapist may not be able to effectively implement or teach the exercise.
- The patient may not be able to learn the exercise well enough or misunderstand or forget the instructions or dosage.
- The patient may not follow through with the prescription.[44]

Understanding certain methods and principles can help to minimize the incidence of each of the confounding factors:

- Basic theory and research literature related to the activity and dosage of the exercise and to the condition being treated
- Motor learning and exercise instruction (see Chapter 3)
- Exercise modification
- Exercise adherence (see Chapter 3)

If you've paid careful attention to basic methods and principles, but the patient is not responding to the intervention, you must realize that all has been done within the scope of your therapeutic knowledge, expertise, and experience and that the patient should be discharged if you feel maximum improvement has been attained. If not, the patient should be referred to another practitioner for further treatment.

Exercise Modification

To be most effective and efficient with exercise prescription, constant re-examination and evaluation of changes in impairments and function are required. The exercises must be continually modified to increase or decrease the difficulty to ensure continual progress is being made with minimal setbacks. Numerous parameters can be modified to render an exercise more or less difficult. Four general parameters can be varied in an exercise prescription: biomechanical, physiologic, neuromuscular, and cognitive or affective. Display 2-13 outlines parameters that can be varied and provides examples for various types of exercise.

Numerous variables can be manipulated to increase or decrease the difficulty of an exercise. The clinical decision-making process used to determine the best strategy for modification of exercise parameters related to dosage and activity should consider the affected elements of the movement system combined with biomechanical, physiologic, neuromuscular, and cognitive or affective variables, as discussed in this section.

ADJUNCTIVE INTERVENTIONS

Although this is a textbook devoted to theory and practice of therapeutic exercise, other physical therapy interventions can be complementary to therapeutic exercise to achieve functional outcomes. This section focuses on interventions considered adjunctive to therapeutic exercise in that they are not considered essential to achieving a functional outcome. The adjunctive interventions include physical agents and mechanical modalities, electrotherapeutic modalities, and orthotics.

When choosing to use an adjunctive intervention, a decision must be made regarding the benefit of its use in conjunction with therapeutic exercise. The clinician should be reasonably sure that combining the adjunctive intervention with the therapeutic exercise will produce more rapid or optimal functional recovery. Make it clear to the patient that the adjunctive intervention is being used to augment the exercise and that the exercise and modified posture and movement habits will ultimately change the impairments and functional limitations for long-term improvement. There are conditions for which physical agents, mechanical and electrotherapeutic modalities, and orthotics are imperative to achieve improved physical function and health status, in which case these interventions are not considered adjunctive (eg, significant soft tissue inflammation, severe pain disorders, skin conditions, nerve injury, impaired motor function, structural abnormalities). The following section provides examples of selected physical agents and mechanical and electrotherapeutic modalities used as adjuncts to therapeutic exercise. The use of foot orthotics is presented in Chapter 22.

Physical Agents

Physical agents use ice, heat, sound, or light energy to increase connective tissue extensibility, modulate pain, reduce or eliminate soft tissue inflammation and swelling caused by musculoskeletal injury or circulatory dysfunction, increase the healing rate of open wounds and soft tissue, remodel scar tissue, or treat skin conditions. Examples of physical agents include ultrasound, moist heat, paraffin baths, cryotherapy (Fig. 2-15), and hydrotherapy.

Heat combined with stretch is an example of using physical agents as an adjunct to therapeutic exercise. Because collagenous tissue is a major factor in joint contracture, a method for elongating or stretching this tissue is important in changing a hypomobility impairment. Elevating the temperature of collagenous tissue has been shown to increase its extensibility; when combined with stretching procedures, it can produce permanent elongation. The combined

DISPLAY 2-13
Exercise Modification Parameters

Biomechanical

Stability

- Size of base of support
  Example: It is more difficult to balance with feet close together or in tandem than feet wide apart, and in sidelying rather than supine.
- Height of center of mass
  Example: Sit-ups may be done first with hands at the sides, progressed to forearms folded across the chest, progressed to hands clasped behind the neck. This upward shift of arm weight moves the center of mass toward the head by stages, progressively increasing the difficulty of the exercise.
- Support surface
  Example: The stability of the support surface can be progressed from a static or stable surface to a mobile base, such as a balance, board, or a trampoline.

External Load

- Magnitude
  Example: Increased magnitude of resistance alters the weight of the segment and thereby increases the difficulty of movement; however, it may also increase feedback from muscle and joint receptors and enhance the response.
- Gravitational forces
  Example: The force of gravity on a segment is maximal when the part is horizontal and diminishes as it moves toward the vertical. Knee flexion in prone is more difficult at the beginning of the movement and becomes easier as the motion progresses. Hip abduction is gravity reduced in prone or standing and against gravity in sidelying.
- Speed (see Chapter 4, page 48)
  Example: A medium rate is usually easier than very rapid or very slow.
- Length of lever arm
  Example: In prone exercises for scapular adductors (middle and lower trapezius), raising the arms with the elbows flexed gives less resistance than if the arms are nearly or completely straight.
- Point and angle of application of manual or mechanical resistance
  Example: A muscle pulling at or near a right angle to the long axis of the segment exerts its force more effectively than when its angle of pull is very small.

Number of Segments Involved

- Fewer segments may not always be easier than more segments, especially as in fine motor control.

Length of Muscle

- A muscle is better able to exert active tension when it is in a lengthened state than after it has undergone considerable shortening. When it is desirable to limit the participation of a given muscle in a movement, it is placed in a shortened position, or "put on slack." The active tension exerted by a muscle spanning more than one joint at a given joint depends on the position of the second joint over which it passes, because this determines the length of the muscle. For instance, the hamstrings are more effective as knee flexors when the hip is flexed and less effective when the hip is extended. Similarly, if the goal is to isolate the gluteus maximus during hip extension, the participation of the hamstrings is reduced if hip extension is done with the knee flexed compared with the knee extended.

Passive Tension of Two-Joint Muscles

- The hip can be flexed to only 70 to 90 degrees with the knee extended but considerably more if the hip and knee are flexed. Similarly, the ankle can dorsiflex far more when the knee is flexed than when the knee is extended. These considerations are particularly important in planning effective stretching activities and in analyzing stabilization of body segments in all types of exercise. Altering joint positions or the use of external supports such as pillows can reduce or increase the tension of two-joint muscles based on the goal of the exercise.

Open Versus Closed Kinetic Chain

- The kinetic chain is related mostly to specificity of exercise. If the desired activity is in the closed kinetic chain, this position should be used for training whenever possible. However, the closed kinetic chain often cannot isolate muscle function as well as a specific open kinetic chain exercise.

Stabilization (External or Within)

- If stability is required for a movement, use of external straps or prepositioning a limb may assist stabilization if the patient is unable to stabilize with proper patterns internally. For example, in supine, the trunk can stabilize with greater ease if the hip and knee are flexed and held in place by the hands while the other limb slides down and back during an abdominal strengthening exercise (Fig. 2-14) This is an example of prepositioning to offer external stability.

Physiologic

Duration

- Number of repetitions or sets performed

Frequency

- Number of exercise sessions in a given time period

Speed

- Slow is not necessarily easier (see earlier)

Intensity of Contraction or External Load

Type of Muscle Contraction

- Eccentric, isometric, concentric

Sequence of Exercise

- May require beginning with less complex tasks or less strenuous activity in early stages of learning or healing and progressing to less need for "warm-up" activities as skill is achieved and tissues are in more advanced stages of healing

Rest Between Repetitions and Sets

- As strength or endurance improves, less rest is necessary between repetitions and sets. Be cautious of overtraining, especially in presence of neuromuscular disease or injury.

Neuromuscular

Sensory input

- Visual, proprioceptive, and tactile inputs can be manipulated. If the eyes are closed, visual input is eliminated, leaving the vestibular, proprioceptive, and tactile receptors to detect any disurbance. The tactile and proprioceptive input can be varied by standing on soft foam.

(continued)

DISPLAY 2-13 (Continued)

Exercise Modification Parameters

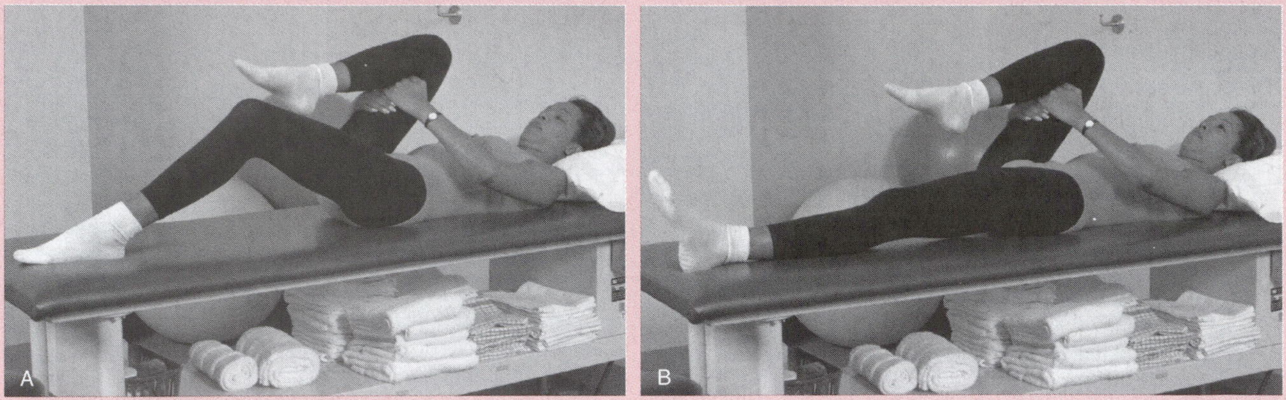

FIGURE 2-14 Lower abdominal leg slide. The hip and knee are flexed and held closer to the chest as the other limb slides down and back. ***(A)*** Starting position. ***(B)*** Ending position.

Sensory Facilitation or Inhibition

- Techniques such as cutaneous and pressure input, approximation, and traction can alter muscle responses. Prolonged pressure on the long tendons such as the quadriceps, biceps, hamstrings, or finger flexors seems to inhibit responses.[49] The placement of manual contacts is critical to facilitate the desired response. Contacts are placed in the direction toward which the segment is to move. Approximation or compression into or through a joint stimulates the joint receptors and may facilitate extensor muscles and stability around a joint.[50] Traction separates the joint surface and is incorporated if increasing range of motion around a joint is desired.

Number of Segments Involved

- In weight-bearing postures, joint involvement usually refers to the weight-bearing segments; for example, prone on elbows does not require participation of the forearm and hand or the lower body compared with quadruped. The placement of manual contacts or other external forces also influences the number of segments involved. For example, contacts placed on the scapula and pelvis in sidelying involve the entire trunk, whereas contacts positioned on the lumbar spine and pelvis result in more isolated activity of the lower trunk.

Stage of Movement Control

- Mobility, stability, controlled mobility, skill (see page 22 for examples of stages of movement control)

Cognitive or Affective

Frequency and Duration of the Activity

- Increased frequency and duration of the activity increases the practice schedule to enhance learning.

Initial Information Provided

- Care should be taken to provide enough information to perform the activity with the correct strategy, but not to give too much information, which may overwhelm the learner.

Accuracy Provided

- As skill is acquired, increased accuracy of cues is provided to "fine tune" a movement.

Variability of Environmental Conditions

- Initially reduced number of external distractions is provided with increasing external distractions toward a functional environment as skill is acquired.

Complexity of Activity

- Number of steps involved; as in breaking down components of gait into single tasks and then uniting them into the integrated complex motor task of gait with numerous steps

Anxiety Level

- Initially, greater focus on the activity is combined with the least emotional distractions to enhance early learning.

application of heat and stretching was found to be more effective in producing permanent increase in length than heat or stretching alone.[51] When motion is limited by collagenous tissue crossing the joint, the combined application of heat and stretch may be a useful intervention if the following considerations are observed:

- Stretch should be combined with the highest tolerable therapeutic temperature that can be achieved in the area to be treated.
- The application of stretch should be of long duration.
- Moderated forces should be used to take advantage of the viscous nature of the tissue.
- The tissue temperature should be elevated before applying stretch to reduce tissue damage.
- The tissue elongation achieved should be maintained while the tissue is allowed to cool. This takes approximately 8 to 10 minutes.[52]

Infrared radiation, electromagnetic radiation, and ultrasound are three sources of energy used for therapeutic heating. The choice of energy source depends on the treatment objective, because each of the three sources produces a different heating pattern in tissue. Please refer to the appropriate reference for further information regarding the choice of physical agent.[53]

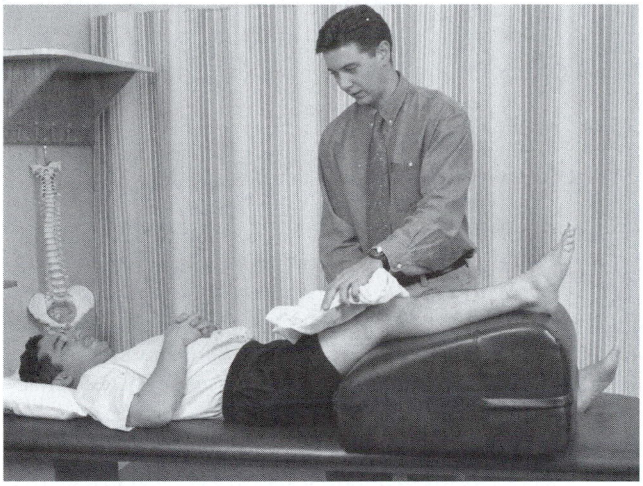

FIGURE 2-15 The clinician ices the patient's knee as an adjunct to therapeutic exercise.

Mechanical Modalities

Mechanical modalities include a broad group of procedures (eg, traction, continuous passive motion, tilt table, vasopneumatic compression devices, compression, taping) to modulate pain, stabilize an area that requires temporary support, increase ROM, or apply distraction, approximation, or compression. Candidates for mechanical modalities include patients with pain disorders, disk disorders, nerve compression or entrapment, sprains or strains, hypomobility or hypermobility, and hemodynamic impairments.

Although many mechanical modalities can assist therapeutic exercise in achieving functional outcome, taping is discussed in more detail because of its potential direct effect on enhancing the outcome of therapeutic exercise. The clinical indications for taping have expanded beyond the traditional taping to immobilize and protect a sprained or strained tissue. There are several indications for taping:

- Improvement of contact areas for weight-bearing cartilage
- Improvement of initial alignment, thereby assisting in restoration of normal movement patterns
- Alteration of length-tension properties of muscle tissue; progressive stretching of shortened tissue and shortening of lengthened tissue
- Unloading of inflamed or injured tissue

Specific techniques for taping are included in the relevant regional chapters. The techniques illustrated include patellofemoral joint taping, plantar fascia taping, scapulothoracic, and hip joint taping.

Electrotherapeutic Modalities

Electrotherapeutic modalities include a broad group of physical agents that use electricity to modulate pain, reduce or eliminate soft tissue inflammation, decrease muscle spasm, and assist in muscle re-education. Electrotherapeutic modalities include alternating direct and pulsed current, neuromuscular electrical stimulation (NMES), transcutaneous electrical nerve stimulation, and surface electromyography (SEMG). Although many electrotherapeutic modalities deal with the treatment of pain, inflammation, and soft tissue healing, this discussion focuses on the use of NMES and SEMG for treatment of muscle re-education.

NEUROMUSCULAR ELECTRICAL STIMULATION

NMES is a versatile modality that can be integrated into treatment plans for a variety of patient problems. NMES can be a safe and effective adjunct to treatment of disuse atrophy, ROM deficits, and muscle re-education.

Although studies have not shown NMES to be effective in preventing disuse atrophy, there is some evidence that it can retard the effects of immobilization and disuse.[54–56] Treatment protocols reported to decrease the effects of disuse atrophy vary considerably. The patient's diagnosis and preinjury condition influence the initial parameter settings and rate of progression. Table 2-1 illustrates suggested parameters for initiating a NMES program for patients with various degrees of atrophy.[57]

A patient with long-standing neurologic insult may experience severe atrophy. Moderate atrophy is observed in postsurgical patients such as after total knee replacement or after ligament reconstructive surgery. A lesser degree of atrophy is observed in the patient who experiences an acute injury and for whom NMES is initiated within the first week after injury.

Whenever possible, involve the patient in active exercise combined with NMES. For example, a patient with moderate disuse atrophy of the vastus medialis oblique (VMO) with patellofemoral pain may use NMES in conjunction with a closed chain isometric exercise for the VMO (see Fig. 21-26). The decision to discontinue a NMES program for disuse atrophy should be based on the patient's recovery of function. When the patient is able to voluntarily exercise effectively against resistance, NMES may be discontinued.

Patients who are weak or experience pain and joint swelling have difficulty moving a joint through its available ROM. In the absence of a fracture involving the joint itself, early motion is desirable to accelerate rehabilitation and prevent loss of motion. NMES may be used for patients with orthopedic or neurologic dysfunction to promote full return of joint mobility.[58–60]

Table 2-1. SUGGESTED TREATMENT PARAMETERS FOR PATIENTS WITH DISUSE ATROPHY

	SEVERE ATROPHY	MODERATE ATROPHY	MINIMAL ATROPHY
Frequency (pps)	3–10	10–30	30–50
On time (s)	5	5–10	10–15
Off time (s)	25–50	20–30	10–30
Session length (min)	5–10	15	15
Sessions per day	3–4	3–4	1–2

pps, pulses per second; s, seconds

Most patients who have difficulty regaining or maintaining ROM have been immobilized or have significant weakness and disuse atrophy, and similar guidelines with regard to disuse atrophy may be followed for frequency and duty cycle selection. NMES is ideally suited as an adjunct to active ROM exercises because of its cyclic, repetitive nature. NMES is not intended to replace passive stretching, active, or active assistive ROM exercises, or functional retraining of new ROM gained.

NMES can be used for muscle re-education and facilitation to reestablish voluntary control of body positions and movements after injury or disease has affected the motor control mechanism or when less than optimal movement patterns have been learned because of repetition of faulty movement patterns during ADLs, sport, recreation, or work. Improvement in motor control has been documented after NMES was used at a current intensity sufficient to evoke a muscle contraction (ie, motor threshold).[61,62] When using NMES for muscle reeducation and facilitation, the patient should attempt to perform a desired movement or contraction along with the stimulation. That way, NMES is used to augment the voluntary movement, not replace it. Use of NMES for muscle re-education and facilitation is limited only by the therapist's creativity.

SURFACE ELECTROMYOGRAPHY

SEMG is increasingly recognized by physical therapists as a tool to augment evaluation and treatment of a variety of musculoskeletal and neuromuscular conditions. Applications have been proposed for numerous conditions in which inappropriate patterns of muscle activity are thought to be contributory. SEMG can be used as a form of biofeedback to augment relaxation-based training, tension recognition training, postural training, body mechanics instruction, therapeutic exercise, and functional activity or work station modification. It can serve as an online biofeedback technique to ensure the desired response is elicited at the desired time. For example, it can augment a stretching technique by placing the electrodes on the muscle to be stretched and maintaining low or no activity during the stretch. It can be used during a specific exercise to ensure isolated recruitment of a muscle. For example, one electrode can be placed over the tensor fascia lata and one over the gluteus medius during prone hip abduction. If the desired muscle for recruitment is the gluteus medius, activity in the gluteus medius is expected with relative quiescence in the tensor fascia lata. SEMG also can be used to ensure the desired synergy and timing of muscles acting in a force couple during a functional movement pattern. For example, one electrode is placed over the upper trapezius, one over the lower trapezius, and one over the serratus anterior during upper extremity flexion. The proper recruitment pattern and timing of the muscles can be correlated with the path of motion at the scapula. If the scapula appears to be elevating, more activity is required under the lower trapezius and serratus anterior; likewise, if the scapula is not elevating enough, more activity is needed under the upper trapezius and serratus anterior.

Appropriate use of SEMG requires a thorough knowledge of instrumentation, set-up, and interpretation of data. Please refer to recommended reading on the topic.[63,64]

SURFACE ELECTROMYOGRAPHY–TRIGGERED NEUROMUSCULAR ELECTRICAL STIMULATION

Combining SEMG with NMES can more powerfully facilitate muscle than either modality alone.[65] In SEMG-triggered NMES, NMES is delivered to a target muscle once a prescribed EMG threshold is exceeded. The benefit of combining the two modalities is that the patient must activate the muscle to a predetermined threshold, thereby serving as an *active participant* in the process, which may not happen during traditional NMES. This modality is particularly useful for muscles in which volitional control is difficult (eg, gluteus medius, VMO, serratus anterior, lower trapezius). For example, during a step activity, the VMO is set up for EMG-triggered NMES. After the VMO has reached a predetermined level of activity as sensed by SEMG, the NMES is triggered to contract the muscle beyond its volitional capability. This approach can assist in treating disuse atrophy, muscle re-education, and synchronization of muscle activity.

Key Points

- The success of appropriate, safe, effective, and efficient therapeutic exercise prescription relies on the clinical decision making process from initial, subjective intake to re-evaluation of the intervention.
- The clinician's knowledge, expertise, experience, and ongoing acquisition of knowledge and experience are the determinants for successful patient management.
- An understanding of each component of the patient management model assists the clinician in maximizing patient satisfaction and in delivering the most effective and efficient services possible.
- Critical clinical decisions are those involved in determining which impairments from the list generated from the examination are most closely related to functional limitation and disability and therefore warrant intervention.
- Patient-related instruction must be an integral part of any physical therapy intervention.
- The three-dimensional therapeutic exercise intervention model is designed to help organize the data necessary to make clinical decisions regarding therapeutic exercise intervention.
- Exercises must be continually monitored to determine the need for modification to increase or decrease difficulty to ensure continual progress is being made with minimal setbacks. To be most effective with exercise modification, the clinician must possess thorough understanding of the parameters that can be modified.
- Therapeutic exercise can be complemented with adjunctive interventions if the additional intervention can lead to a higher level of functional outcome in a shorter period.

Critical Thinking Questions

1. Read Case Study #2 in Unit 7.
   a. List the physiologic, anatomic, and psychological impairments.
   b. List the functional limitations.
   c. Correlate the impairments to the functional limitations.
   d. Choose the impairments and functional limitations you feel warrant treatment.
   e. Correlate the impairments and functional limitations you have chosen to treat with the elements of the movement system.
   f. Prioritize the elements of the movement system.
2. Still using Case Study #2, you have decided to prescribe exercises to improve knee mobility, because you know she requires 70 degrees of knee flexion to perform simple ADLs. You would like to use a sit to stand movement to work on knee mobility. Recall that she requires moderate assistance with sit to stand transfers.
   a. Describe the posture, mode, and movement of the activity.
   b. Describe all pertinent parameters of dosage.
3. The patient has progressed to 70 degrees of flexion and no longer requires assistance with sit to stand transfers. How would you modify the mobility exercises to make them more difficult? Use the principles of exercise modification listed in Display 2-12.
4. The patient is having difficulty with recruitment of her quadriceps.
   a. What adjunctive intervention would you use?
   b. Describe the posture, mode, and movement of the activity.
   c. Describe all pertinent parameters of dosage.

REFERENCES

1. A guide to physical therapist practice. *Phys. Ther*. 1997;77: 1163–1165
2. Jette AM, Branch LG. Impairment and disability in the aged. *J Chronic Dis*. 1985:38:59–65.
3. Jette AM, Branch LG, Berlin J. Musculoskeletal impairments and physical disablement among the aged. *J Gerontol*. 1990: 45:M203–M208.
4. Bradley EM, Wagstaff S, Wood PHN. Measures of functional ability (disability) in arthritis in relation to impairment of range of joint movement. *Am Rheum Dis*. 1984:43:563–569.
5. Wade DT. *Measurement in Neurological Rehabilitation*. Oxford, England: Oxford University Press; 1992.
6. Mason JH, Anderson JJ, Meenan RF, et al. The Rapid Assessment of Disease Activity in Rheumatology (RADAR) Questionnaire: validity and sensitivity to change of a patient self-report measure of joint count and clinical status. *Arthritis Rheum*. 1992:35:156–162.
7. Meenan RF, Mason JH, Anderson JJ, et al. AIMS2: the content and properties of a revised and expanded Arthritis Impact Measurement Scales health status questionnaire. *Arthritis Rheum*. 1992:35:1–10.
8. Jette AM, Davies AR, Cleary PD, et al. The functional status questionnaire: reliability and validity when used in primary care. *J Gen Intern Med*. 1986:1:143–149.
9. Haley SM. Motor assessment tools for infant and young children: a focus on disability assessment. In: Forrsberg H, ed. *Treatment of Children with Movement Disorders: Theory and Practice*. Basel, Switzerland: S Karger; 1992:278–283.
10. Frey WD. Functional outcome: assessment and evaluation. In: Delisa JA, ed. *Rehabilitation Medicine: Principle and Practice*. Philadelphia: JB Lippincott; 1988:158–172.
11. Haley SM, Coster WJ, Ludlow LH. Pediatric functional outcome measures. In: Jaffe KM, ed. *Pediatric Rehabilitation*. Philadelphia: WB Saunders; 1991:689–723.
12. Law M. Evaluating activities of daily living: directions for the future. *Am J Occup Ther*. 1993:47:233–237.
13. Heinemann AW, Linacre JM, Wright BD, et al. Relationships between impairment and physical disability as measured by the Functional Independence Measure. *Arch Phys Med Rehabil*. 1993:74:566–573.
14. Mahoney FL, Barthel DW. Functional evaluation: the Barthel index. *Md State Med J*. 1965:14:61–65.
15. Hamilton BB, Laughlin JA, Granger CV, Kayton RM. Interrater agreement of the seven level Functional Independence Measure (FIM). *Arch Phys Med Rehabil*. 1991:72:790.
16. Berg K, Wood Dauphinee S, Williams JI, Maki B. Measuring balance in the elderly: validation of an instrument. *Can J Public Health*. 1992:2:S7–S11.
17. Butland RJA, Pang J, Gross ER, et al. Two, six, and twelve minute walking test in Respiratory disease. *BMJ*. 1982:284: 1604–1608.
18. Keith RA, Granger CV. The functional independence measure: a new tool for rehabilitation. In: Eisenberg MG, Greysiak RC, eds. *Advances in Clinical Rehabilitation*. New York: Springer Publishing; 1987:6–18.
19. Granger CV, Cotter AC, Hamilton RB, Fiedler RC. Functional assessment scales: a study of persons after stroke. *Arch Phys Med Rehabil*. 1993:74:133–138.
20. Gresham GE, Labi ML. Functional assessment instruments currently available for documenting outcomes in rehabilitation medicine. In: Granger CV, Gresham GE, eds. *Functional Assessment in Rehabilitation Medicine*. Baltimore: Williams & Wilkins; 1984:65–85.
21. Shields RK, Enioe LJ, Evans R, et al. Analysis of the reliability of clinical functional tests in total hip replacement patients. *Phys Ther*. 1992:72:S113.
22. Stewart A, Ware JE, eds. *Measuring Functioning and Well-Being: The Medical Outcomes Study Approach*. Durham, NC: Duke University Press; 1992.
23. Guccione AA, Cullen KE, O'Sullivan SB. Functional assessment. In: Sullivan SB, Schmitz TJ, eds. *Physical Rehabilitation: Assessment and Treatment*. 2nd ed. Philadelphia: FA Davis; 1988:219–236.
24. Guccione AA. Arthritis and the process of disablement. *Phys Ther*. 1994:74:408–414.
25. Bergner M, Babbitt RA, Carter WB, Gilson BS. The sickness impact profile: development and final revision of a health status measure. *Med Care*. 1981:19:787–805.
26. Roland M, Morris RA. A study of the natural history of back pain, part I: the development of a reliable and sensitive measure of disability in low back pain. *Spine*. 1983:8:141–144.
27. Fairbanks JCT, Couper J, Davies JB, et al. The Oswestry low back pain disability questionnaire. *Physiotherapy*. 1980:66: 271–273.
28. Waddell G, Main CJ, Morriss EW, et al. Chronic low back pain, psychological distress, and illness behavior. *Spine*. 1984: 9:209–213.
29. Lawliss GF, Cuencas R, Selby D, et al. The development of the Dallas pain questionnaire: an assessment of the impact of spinal pain on behavior. *Spine*. 1989:14:512–515.

30. Schuling J, de Hann R, Limburg M, Groenier KH. The Frenchay activities index: assessment of functional status in stroke patients. *Stroke*. 1993:24:1173–1177.
31. Sahrmann SA. Diagnosis by the physical therapist—prerequisite for treatment: a special communication. *Phys Ther*. 1988:68:1703–1706.
32. Rose SJ. Physical therapy diagnosis: role and function. *Phys Ther*. 1989:69:535–537.
33. Delitto A, Synder-Mackler L. The diagnostic process: examples in orthopedic physical therapy. *Phys Ther*. 1995:75:203–210.
34. Fosnaught M. A critical look at diagnosis. *Phys Ther*. 1996: 4:48–53.
35. Balla JL. *The Diagnostic Process: A Model for Clinical Teachers*. Cambridge, England: Cambridge University Press; 1985.
36. Guccione AA. Physical therapy diagnosis and the relationship between impairments and function. *Phys Ther*. 1191:71: 499–503.
37. Dekker J, Van Baar ME, Curfs EC, Kerssens JJ. Diagnosis and treatment in physical therapy: an investigation of their relationship. *Phys Ther*. 1993:73:568–577.
38. Delitto A, Ehrard RE, Bowling RW. A treatment-based classification approach to low back syndrome: identifying and staging patients for conservative treatment. *Phys Ther*. 1995: 75:470–485.
39. Delitto A, Cibulka MT, Ehrard RE, et al. Evidence for use of an extension-mobilization category in acute low back pain syndrome: a prescriptive validation pilot study. *Phys Ther*. 1993:73:216–228.
40. Delitto A, Shulman AD, Rose SJ, et al. Reliability of a clinical examination to classify patients with low back syndrome. *Physical Therapy Practice*. 1992:1:1–9.
41. Sahrmann SA. *Diagnosis and Exercise Management of Musculoskeletal Pain Syndromes.* St Louis: Mosby; in press.
42. Rose SJ. Description and classification: the cornerstone of pathokinesiological research. *Phys Ther*. 1986:66:379–381.
43. Jette AM. Diagnosis and classification by physical therapists: a special communication. *Phys Ther*. 1989:69:967–969.
44. Kane R. Looking for physical therapy outcomes. *Phys Ther*. 1995:74:425–429.
45. Rothstein JM. Outcome assessment of therapeutic exercise. In: Bajmajian JV, Wolf SL, eds. *Therapeutic Exercise*. 5th ed. Baltimore: Williams & Wilkins; 1990:93–107.
46. Kendall FP, McCreary EK, Provance PG. *Muscles Testing and Function.* 4th ed. Baltimore: Williams & Wilkins; 1993.
47. Sullivan PE, Markos PD. *Clinical Decision Making in Therapeutic exercise.* Norwalk, CT: Appleton & Lange; 1995.
48. Gentile AM. Skill acquisition: action, movement, and neuromotor processes. In: Carr JH, Shepherd RB, eds. *Foundations of Physical Therapy Rehabilitation. 1988.*
49. Stockmeyer SA. An interpretation of the approach of Rood to the treatment of neuromuscular dysfunction. *Am J Phys Med*. 1967:46:900–956.
50. Johansson H, Sjolander P, Sojka P. A sensory role for the cruciate ligaments. *Clin Orthop*. 1990:228:161–178.
51. Lehmann JF, Masock AJ, Warren CG, Koblanski JN. Effect of therapeutic temperature on tendon extensibility. *Arch Phys Med Rehabil*. 1970:51:481–487.
52. Warren CG, Lehmann JF, Koblanski JN: Elongation of rat tail tendon: effect of load and temperature. *Arch Phys Med Rehabil*. 1971:52:465–474, 484.
53. Hecox B, Tsega A, Weisberg J. *Physical Agents: A Comprehensive Text for Physical Therapists*. Norwalk, CT: Appleton and Lange; 1994.
54. Wiggerstad-Lossing I. Effects of electrical muscle stimulation combined with voluntary contractions after knee ligament surgery. *Med Sci Sport Exerc*. 1988:20:93.
55. Morrissey MC. The effects of electrical stimulation on the quadriceps during postoperative knee immobilization. *Am J Sports Med*. 1985:13:40.
56. Bohannon RW. Effect of electrical stimulation to the vastus medialis in a patient with chronically dislocating patellae. *Phys Ther*. 1983:63:1445.
57. DeVahl J. Neuromuscular electrical stimulation (NMES) in rehabilitation. In: Gersh MR, ed. *Electrotherapy in Rehabilitation*. Philadelphia: FA Davis; 1992:218–268.
58. Cannon NM, Strickland JW. Therapy following flexor tendon surgery. *Hand Clin*. 1985:1:147.
59. Haug J, Wood LT. Efficacy of neuromuscular stimulation of the quadriceps femoris during continuous passive motion following total knee arthroplasty. *Arch Phys Med*. 1988:69:423.
60. Baker LL. Electrical stimulation of wrist and fingers for hemiplegic patients. *Phys Ther*. 1979:59:1495.
61. Carnstam B, Larsson LE, Prevec TS. Improvement of gait following functional electrical stimulation. *Scand J Rehabil Med*. 1977:9:7.
62. Gracanin F. Functional electrical stimulation in control of motor output and movements. In: Cobb WA, Van Duijn H. eds. *Contemporary Clinical Neurophysiology (EEG Suppl)*. Amsterdam: Elsevier; 1978:355.
63. Cram JR, Kasman GS. *Introduction to Surface Electromyography*. Bethesda: Aspen; 1998.
64. Kasman GS, Cram JR, Wolf SL. *Clinical Applications in Surface Electromyography: Chronic Musculoskeletal Pain.* Bethesda: Aspen; 1998.
65. Fields RW. Electromyographically triggered electric muscle stimulation for chronic hemiplegia. *Arch Phys Med*. 1987:68: 407–414.

CHAPTER 3

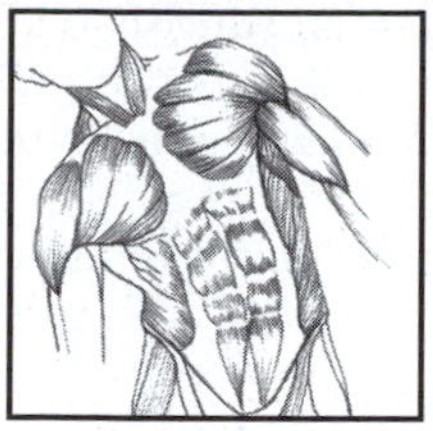

Principles of Self-Management and Exercise Instruction

Lori Thein Brody

Clinicians often minimize the importance of teaching in the clinic. Serving as a clinical mentor for a physical therapy intern or teaching parents how to assist their child in stretching exercises are obvious examples of teaching in the clinic. Clinicians spend much time teaching patients during the evaluation and treatment sessions. A study of the perceptions of physical therapists regarding their involvement in patient education showed that therapists educate 80% to 100% of their patients.[1] These therapists primarily recognized teaching range of motion (ROM) techniques, home exercise programs, and treatment rationales. Clinicians recognize but may underestimate the importance of educating their patients on various aspects of their physical conditions and symptoms, including the relationship between symptoms and the patient's daily routine and information on the expected response to the exercise program. Patients' satisfaction with treatment and willingness to adhere are often based on the fulfillment of their expectations. The more time spent educating the patient on prognosis and expectations from the rehabilitation program, the more likely the patient is to adhere to and be satisfied with the treatment program. Gahimer and Domholdt[2] found that therapists educated their patients primarily in the areas of information about illness, home exercises, and advice and information. Moreover, the patients reported attitudinal or behavioral changes ranging from 83.8% to 86.5% as a result of this education. Health education and stress counseling were addressed less frequently during the treatment session.

TEACHING IN THE CLINIC

Teaching in the clinic is a constant and ongoing process. As changes in health care occur, many clinicians are finding that their role has changed from full-time, hands-on providers of rehabilitation services to part-time educators, administrators, and clinicians.[2] Clinical teaching, particularly in the area of the home exercise program, is especially important, because in-house supervised physical therapy is often inadequate to achieve the patient's goals. For example, performing stretching exercises three times per week for 30 minutes under the clinician's supervision probably will be insufficient to produce a change. The development of a thorough, complementary home exercise program is essential. Exercise prescription for the home, workplace, or school can prove to be an interesting challenge for the clinician and patient. However, helping the patient establish a daily exercise program as routine can be a positive lifelong influence.

Safety

Depending on the specific circumstances, provision of rehabilitation services may be limited to a few visits. In this situation, the patient may be carrying out the rehabilitation program at home or at a local health club with intermittent rechecks for status and progression of the program. To ensure safety during exercise and improvement in the patient's symptoms, the exercise program must be executed properly. Frequently, the patient appears to understand proper performance of the exercises, but she subsequently forgets the instructions, resulting in improper technique. This problem can result in a lack of improvement and potentially in exacerbation, or worsening, of the symptoms. The patient should understand which signs and symptoms predict an exacerbation so she can modify the exercise program appropriately. This education can prevent an exacerbation and potential reinjury.

Self-Management

In addition to increasing the safety of the exercise program, educating the patient about the effects of the exercise program on specific symptoms can empower her to self-manage the situation. The more clearly patients understand the relationships among various activities (including the exercise program) and their symptoms, the better able they will be to regulate their activity levels. This makes the patient a partner in the rehabilitation program. The patient still looks to the clinician for guidance and education regarding the physical problem, but the clinician gives the patient some responsibility in the decision-making process.

This approach gently guides the patient in the self-management process.

ADHERENCE AND MOTIVATION

Adherence, or degree of patient compliance to the rehabilitation program, can be enhanced by educating the patient regarding the relationships among the injury or pathology, the exercise program, and the expected outcome. The clinician clearly sees the purpose of the exercise and the link to the patient's specific problem, but the patient often does not perceive this relationship. She should understand this relationship to ensure active participation in the treatment program. The best-designed rehabilitation program achieves little if the patient is not compelled to participate. A study by Sluijs et al.[3] demonstrated complete adherence rate of only 35%, with 76% of the patients "partly" compliant with their rehabilitation program. The factors related to nonadherence were barriers that patients perceived, lack of positive feedback, and the degree of helplessness.

Motivation is a key factor in exercise adherence. Every person experiences various influences on motivation. What motivates one person is unlikely to motivate another. The clinician should attempt to determine which factors motivate the patient to adhere with the exercise program and use these as the "carrot" or reward. These factors vary tremendously and may include return to activities the patient enjoys (eg, gardening, sports, leisure, recreational activities), return to work, return home (eg, from hospital or intermediary care facility), ability to shop or carry out instrumental activities of daily living, or the ability to care for a child. After the motivators are identified, the exercise program should be tailored to those activities. Inability to participate in these activities is often one of the primary reasons the patient sought medical attention initially.

When designing the rehabilitation program with motivation and adherence in mind, use caution when using "exercise files." If the exercise program seems nonspecific or unrelated to the patient's functional needs, adherence could become a problem. In the early rehabilitation phases, some exercises may not seem particularly "functional" to the patient, but they are important aspects of the treatment program. In this case, explaining the importance of the exercise educates the patient about the condition, assuring the patient of the clinician's understanding of the problem and the potential solution, and treats the patient as an educated participant in the rehabilitation process. Further explanation of how the exercises will be progressed to more functional activities or how a specific exercise is related to the motivating activity validates the importance of that activity and verifies that this is important to the patient.

As the exercise program progresses, it should reflect more and more closely the activity to which the patient will be returning. The same physical therapy goals can be achieved while increasing motivation and function by using functional activities as the exercise program. For example, for the individual recovering from shoulder surgery who is unable to unload the dishwasher, transferring dishes of increasing weight from the counter to shelf for progressively longer periods is more motivating and interesting than lifting a 1-pound weight (Fig. 3-1). This type of activity has the added benefit of requiring distal muscle function that more closely replicates the actual important activity than lifting a weight or using resistive tubing. Weights and tubing are useful adjuncts to the rehabilitation program and, when possible, should be used in a way that duplicates the functional activity. Rather than performing a series of cardinal plane shoulder exercises, mimicking activities such as a tennis swing, raking, sawing, or throwing a ball can increase strength and reinforce important motor programs.

An exercise program requiring the fewest lifestyle changes possible, increases the patient's adherence to it. Rather than trying to add more activities to the patient's day (often asking that exercise be performed several times per day), choosing exercises that can be incorporated into her day has many added benefits. If an exercise program requires a 15- or 30-minute time block carved out of a person's busy day once or twice daily, adherence is difficult despite the patient's desire to participate. If the exercises can be blended into activities that the patient already does during the day, adherence becomes much easier. A study by Fields et al.[4] examined the relationships among self-motivation or apathy, perceived exertion, social support, scheduling concerns, clinical environment, and pain tolerance to adherence to sport injury rehabilitation in college-age recreational athletes. Of the variables under consideration, significant differences were seen between adherers and nonadherers in self-motivation, scheduling concerns, and pain tolerance, and of these factors, scheduling concerns contributed most to the overall group difference. Sluijs et al.[3] found that the strongest factor in nonadherence was the barriers patients perceived. The most frequent

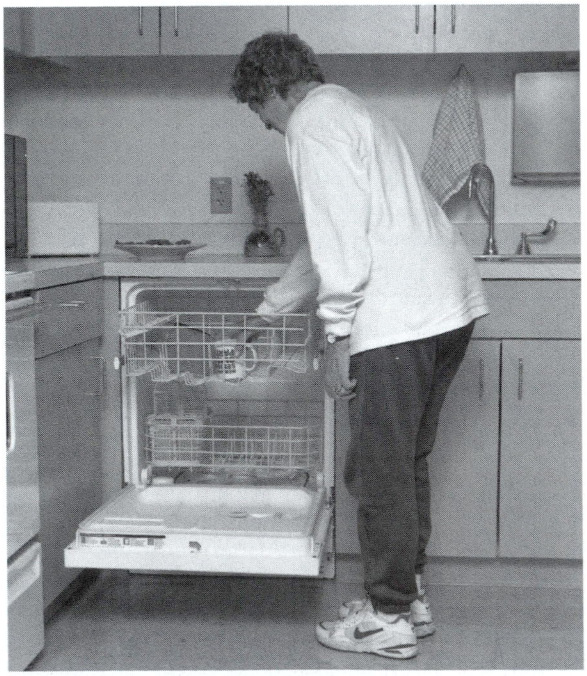

FIGURE 3-1 Choose home exercises reflective of the patient's usual activities.

complaint was that the exercise program required too much time and that the exercises did not fit into the patient's daily routine. An example of an exercise program for a patient with adhesive capsulitis can be found in Display 3-1.

Fitting exercise into the patient's daily routine establishes a conditioned response that may carry over after therapy is concluded. For example, if a patient needs to increase the length of the gastrocnemius-soleus complex by stretching several times each day, instructing that person to stretch for 20 to 30 seconds each time she ascends the stairs is less burdensome than doing this as part of an exercise routine at the day's end. For the individual needing to increase shoulder flexion ROM, leaning ahead with her arm forward and flexed on the desk or kitchen counter before making a phone call is a productive use of time. This may become a conditioned response, and whenever the phone rings, the individual associates that activity with stretching her shoulder, or whenever the patient climbs the stairs, she thinks of calf stretching. This technique works particularly well with postural re-education exercises (Fig. 3-2).

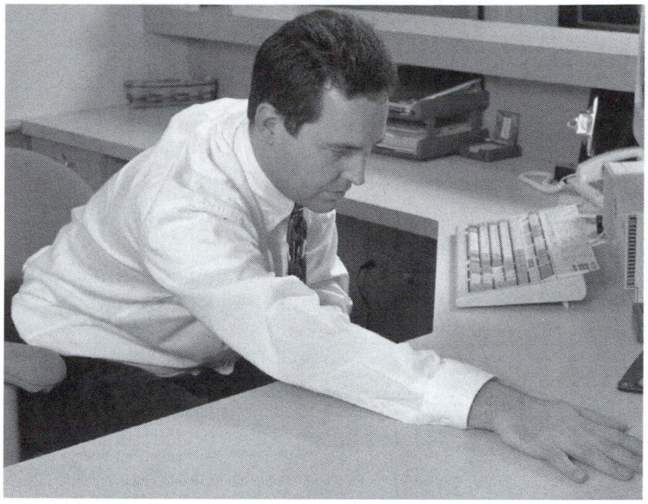

FIGURE 3-2 The clinician should prescribe exercises that can be performed during other home or work activities.

DISPLAY 3-1

Home Exercise Program for Office Worker with Adhesive Capsulitis

Impairments

1. Decreased range of motion in all directions in a capsular pattern
2. Decreased strength tested by manual muscle tests in all major shoulder muscle groups
3. Resting pain at 4 on 0–10 (0 = least; 10 = most pain); activity pain at 8 and 0–10.

Functional Limitations

1. Unable to use arm for activities of daily living
2. Unable to lift weight with arm held away from the body
3. Unable to get arm over head for work and daily activities

Disability

1. Unable to fulfill all roles at work because of limitations.
2. Unable to participate in leisure activities

Home Exercises

1. Stretching for shoulder elevation while in warm shower
2. Active use of arm for personal hygiene, including showering, combing hair, dressing, eating, pendulum exercises during dressing
3. Scapular retraction exercise with abduction in front of mirror during grooming 3 times per day, looking in the mirror each time
4. Shoulder flexion or abduction stretch on desk when talking on the phone
5. Passive shoulder external rotation stretch at file cabinet every time
6. Isometric exercise while reading morning mail
7. Walk with large arm swings during lunch hour
8. Supine overhead stretches on couch during the evening news
9. Use arm as much as possible for cooking, dishwashing, housework, and yardwork
10. Resistive tubing exercises sometime during the day; patient's choice.

CLINICIAN-PATIENT COMMUNICATION

Individual differences significantly affect the patient-clinician relationship. Fundamental personality differences, values, and teaching and learning styles influence communication and may ultimately affect adherence and outcome. Possessing important skills to assess the patient's willingness and style of communication and learning can enhance the rehabilitation program. These skills include the ability to actively listen and reflect the patient's reports and to provide appropriate feedback.[5,6] Sluijs et al.[3] found lack of positive feedback to be one of the primary factors related to lack of adherence with a rehabilitation exercise program.

Teaching in the clinic implies a willingness to participate by the patient and the clinician. The patient's readiness to learn depends on many factors, including the relationship with the health care provider. The clinician must be able to assess the patient's readiness and willingness to learn. The relationship is based on how the patient is coping with the particular situation. Schwenk and Whitman[6] described a control scale in which the control level of the patient and clinician inversely related. As the clinician uses less controlling or assertive behaviors, the patient's control of the situation increases. The converse is also true; the clinician who is very active and assertive is likely to push the patient into a more passive role. If the patient is unwilling to be in such a role, conflict will ensue, or the clinician will become more passive, relinquishing some control to the patient.

The clinician's attention to the patient's needs can guide the appropriate communication style. In the initial visits, a more passive listener role gives the patient an opportunity to explain her needs. This gives the clinician an opportunity to hear the patient's concerns, expectations, and goals. Fundamental skills necessary for active listening include close observation of the patient's words, intonation and body language. Eye contact, along with affirmation and reflection of the patient report, can clarify what the clinician heard and validate the patient report (Fig. 3-3). This gives the clinician an opportunity to discuss the recovery prognosis given

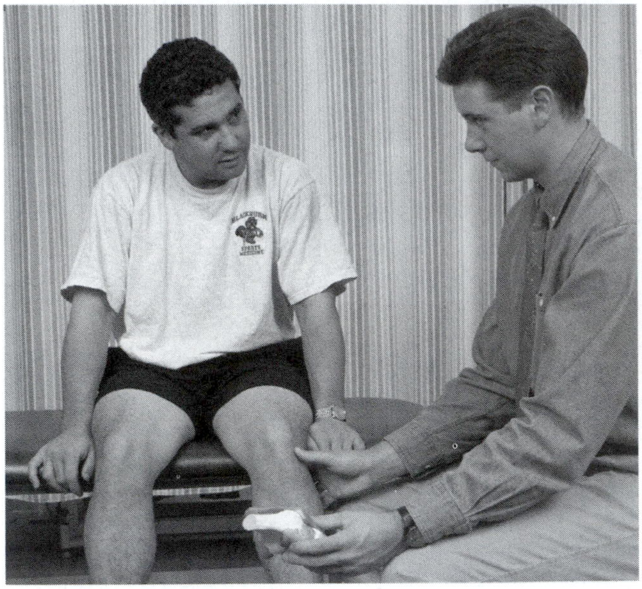

FIGURE 3-3 Good eye contact is essential to effective communication.

adherence to the treatment program, which, along with discussion of the clinician's expectations of the patient, can enhance communication and the rehabilitation process. Several studies have shown the "Pygmalion effect" in a variety of settings in which the instructors' expectations were matched by students' achievements.[7–10]

Although communicating the expectations of all involved participants is important, it is equally important to provide realistic expectations in the form of short-term and long-term goals. Setting reasonable and achievable goals can provide one form of positive feedback for the patient. Occasionally, the patient's motivation can be improved by education about reasonable goals. The ability to perform the same level of exercise or activity at a lower level of pain is a reasonable short-term goal. The patient may only see that she is performing at the same level and perceives this as a lack of progress. Clarification on how progress is defined and reasonable expectations regarding progress can improve patient adherence and satisfaction.

ISSUES IN HOME EXERCISE PROGRAM PRESCRIPTION

The home exercise program is an increasing component of the overall treatment program for most patients. In some cases, the patient performs the exercises independently, whereas in other cases, a family member or other health care provider assists in the exercise program. In either situation, clarity in goals and exercise procedures is essential to ensure an optimal outcome.

Understanding Instructions

One of the fundamental steps in ensuring a positive outcome after initiation of a rehabilitation program is the patient's ability to understand the therapist's instructions. Many variables affect this aspect of patient care, including language or cultural barriers, reading or comprehension levels, hearing impairment, and clarity of instructions. The best-designed rehabilitation program may fail because it has not been carried out well. Do everything possible to ensure that your instructions are clear and easy to understand.

CULTURAL BARRIERS

Identify any cultural barriers to understanding early in the rehabilitation course. Language differences may hinder the use of even the simplest terminology. Although an individual may appear to understand many words in English, communicating thoughts about medically related issues is likely to be difficult. Use of an interpreter, whether a professional or a family member, can minimize communication difficulties in this area.

Other cultural barriers to adherence may exist and should be identified to the best of your ability. Religious observances or customs or other cultural customs may prevent individuals from exercising on certain days or from wearing clothing that allows a body part to be visualized or palpated during exercise. Although these specific instances are difficult to know ahead of time, be alert to signs during the treatment session that the patient is unwilling or hesitant to participate.

CLARITY OF INSTRUCTION

Simple aspects of the exercise program such as clear descriptions and legible writing are also important for adherence. Although written exercise programs may provide a personalized touch to the program, it may prove detrimental if the patient is unable to read your writing. Busy schedules and too little time contribute to hastily written patient instructions. The specific exercise descriptions may make perfect sense to the clinician but confuse the patient. Baseline knowledge assumed by the therapist may be too much for the patient and may result in incorrect exercise performance. Although the patient may be extremely bright and appears to grasp many aspects of medical care, clarity about which direction is "forward" or "up" is still necessary. Directions should be lengthy enough to be comprehensive without overburdening the patient with details. Full sentences are unnecessary, but key phrases or bulleted points can improve the clarity.

Pictures of the exercises should be included and can ideally demonstrate the exercise in the start and finish positions. Communicating a three-dimensional movement on a single sheet of paper at a stationary point in time is difficult. Showing starting and ending positions or showing pictures from different angles helps clarify the three-dimensional nature of the movement. Arrows showing the direction of movement with marks clearly indicating the start and end positions can be helpful. Often exercise pictures show positions midway through the exercise and the patient is unclear as to the full excursion of the movement. Throughout this book, Self-Management boxes present examples of exercise instructions.

Many clinics provide file boxes of exercises with pictures, descriptions, and exercise prescriptions included. These are helpful for the clinician, particularly in providing pictures of the exercise, but the clinician should use caution with these for a number of reasons. First, the therapist frequently needs to modify the exercise in some way to adapt it to the specific patient needs. These modifications should be made on the patient's exercise record, not just verbalized. Do not assume that because an exercise is demonstrated in this file it is the best or only way to perform that exercise. Second, the exercise prescription should be individualized based on the patient's needs and ability to self-manage the problem, not necessarily prescribed as a certain number of sets and repetitions per day. This type of prescription may conflict with the goal of teaching the patient self-management skills. Exercises that appear to be "canned" or the standard sheet of exercises that is given to every patient with a certain diagnosis minimizes the individuality of the exercise program. Lack of individualization minimizes the skills of the therapist and may affect adherence if the patient feels her needs are not being met.

Communication with the patient regarding the exercise program should be written and verbal. Simply handing a patient the exercise program without having the patient perform each of the exercises increases the likelihood of nonadherence and incorrect performance. A study by Friedrich et al.[11] found that patients who received a brochure of exercises rather than supervised instruction had a lower rating of correctness of exercise performance. A strong correlation between the quality of exercise performance and a decrease in pain was found.[11] Although patients may say they can remember their exercises, it is best to document the exercises with a written description that is reinforced with verbal cuing as the exercises are performed.

The exercises should be organized and follow a logical sequence. A sequence of exercises requiring frequent position changes is time-consuming and burdensome for the patient. Exercises of a similar nature should be clustered together for ease of understanding and ease of performance. For example, all exercises performed in a supine position should be clustered together to minimize position changes, and shoulder rotation exercises should be grouped because of their similar nature. Be sure to organize the exercises to simplify their performance and minimize the impact on the patient's lifestyle.

Proper Exercise Execution

Although the patient may appear to follow the exercise instructions, the exercise may still be performed incorrectly. The patient may understand the instructions, but the instructions may be incomplete, the patient may read things into the instructions, or the patient may simply be unaware that she is not doing what the instructions call for. For example, the patient may be performing a trunk curl but still doing a full sit-up or performing a straight leg raise without the necessary quadriceps set first.

Ensuring proper performance can be maximized by having the patient perform each of the exercises under the clinician's direction and guidance, with verbal and tactile cuing for proper performance. Encouraging the patient to take her own notes during these sessions enhances participation, responsibility, and understanding of the exercise program. Although written and verbal instructions help ensure proper performance, more instruction is occasionally necessary. Other options include having a family member observe the clinician instructing the patient, so that this individual may guide the patient's home exercise performance. Videotaping the exercise session allows the patient to see herself performing the exercise, along with hearing the clinician's verbal cues and observing tactile cues for proper performance. The patient can replay this tape at home if a question regarding the exercise program exists.

When the patient returns for follow-up, ask her to demonstrate the home exercise program. If the patient has been performing the exercises on a daily basis, the exercises should nearly be committed to memory. The ability of the patient to quickly recall the exercises with or without the assistance of the handout may provide a clue about adherence. Moreover, this shows precisely how the patient has been executing the exercise. Frequently the exercise has been changed somewhat from the clinician's original intended performance, and this may affect the patient's progress since the last visit. Occasionally, the incorrect exercise performance can have negative consequences, such as increasing the patient's symptoms or hindering progress (Fig. 3-4).

Equipment and Environment

Along with determining what motivates the patient, determination of the motivation derived from use of exercise equipment is valuable as well. Although performing exercises using body weight, objects at the home or office, or work tools may be more functional, the patient may feel like this is not really exercise if it does not involve weights or resistive bands. Patient education is necessary to ensure the patient of the importance of these activities. However, preconceived ideas about exercise are frequently difficult to overcome, and adherence may be improved by use of some equipment. The financial cost of purchasing some equipment for home use may increase or decrease adherence. If money must be spent to carry out the exercise program, the patient may decline participation. However, some patients feel obligated to use equipment that they have purchased. The clinician should assess the patient's position on this issue before issuing or recommending purchase of equipment.

When designing an exercise program with some specific equipment, the clinician must ensure that the patient has a place to use the equipment (Fig. 3-5). Depending on the region of the country, homes may or may not have stairs. Other accommodations may be necessary if exercises require the use of a step. When prescribing exercises to be performed in a supine or prone position, a surface of the appropriate height and firmness must be available. Exercises often are easy to perform on the plinth in the clinic, but the quality or the ability to perform the exercise is negated at home because of the patient's environment. The patient must be able to comfortably transition positions to and from that surface. If the only available firm surface to carry out the exercise program is the floor, the patient must be able to easily get up and down from the floor. If not, the exercise

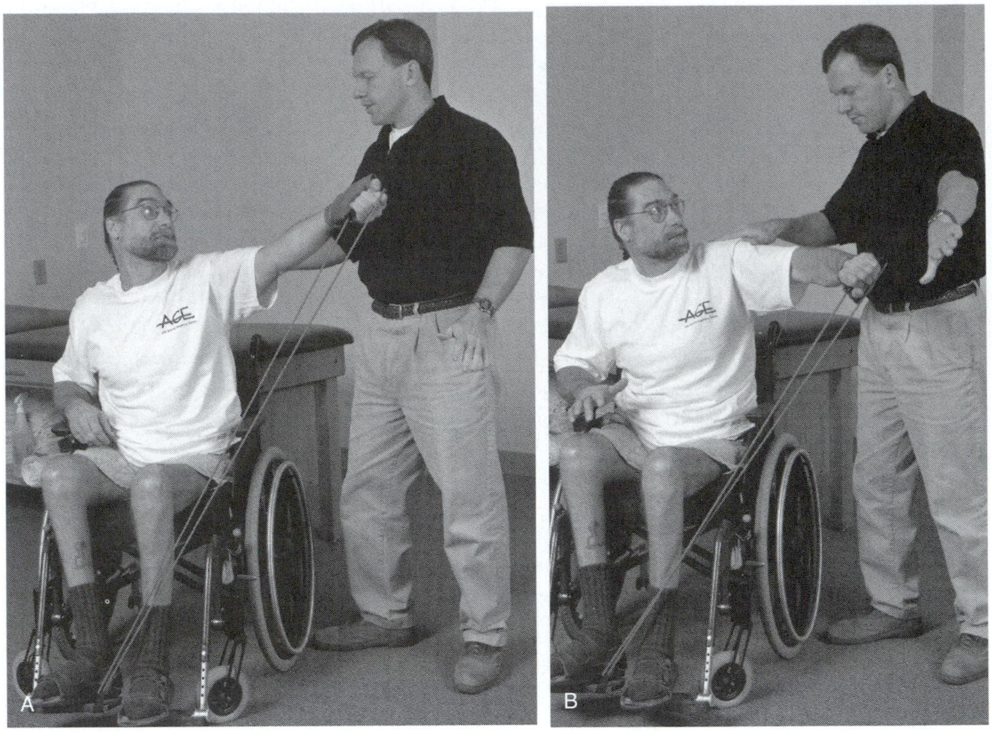

FIGURE 3-4 The exercise program must be reviewed at follow-up visits to ensure correct performance. ***(A)*** Incorrect position—substituting scapular movement for gleno-humeral movement and incorrect degree of rotation. ***(B)*** Correct position—clinician corrects exercise performance.

program should be modified to increase the ease of participation in the program.

A final aspect of the environment that the clinician has little control over but should consider is the presence of a supportive family. A supportive family can maximize the patient's opportunity to participate in medical care by being physically and emotionally supportive. Family members who take over duties normally carried out by the patient and advocate participation in the exercise program can enhance the patient's opportunity for improvement. A nonsupportive family who criticizes the patient for being injured or unable to carry out expected roles can create barriers to improvement. Always be alert to signs of this situation and make referrals as necessary to ensure optimal participation in the rehabilitation program.

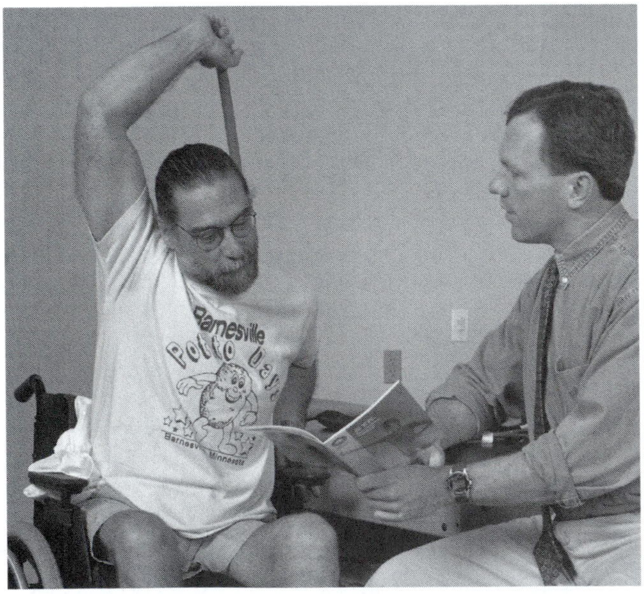

FIGURE 3-5 The clinician should choose equipment that can be easily used by the patient at home.

HOME EXERCISE PRESCRIPTION

Prescribing exercises for a home program is challenging. These exercises are performed without supervision, and patient education is critical to a successful home exercise program. Frequently, limited patient visit time further challenges the clinician to teach the patient all the necessary components of the self-management program. Providing a short, safe home exercise program is better than being too broad and overwhelming the patient with information on the first visit.

Considerations in Exercise Prescription

Exercise prescription can be difficult for several reasons. Determining the number of exercises and the quantity of repetitions, sets, bouts, and intensity is challenging. Too little exercise may not produce the desired result, but too much exercise may overwork the patient, resulting in a decline in progress. Many factors influence choices regarding the exercise prescription:

- Stage of healing
- Tissue irritability and symptom stability
- Patient's time and willingness to participate
- Time between physical therapy visits

STAGE OF HEALING

The acuity or chronicity of the injury affects the exercise prescription, including the regularity of supervised physical therapy and the time between visits. In the early stages, the patient will likely be given a few things to do at home between closely scheduled supervised visits because of the rapidity with which the patient's symptoms, impairments, and function are changing. The exercise program changes more frequently as goals are met and new goals established. In the early stage, the symptoms may be new to the patient, making determination of the appropriate exercise level difficult. Close follow-up of response to treatment is necessary to ensure forward progress. Conversely, in the intermediate to later stages, changes in the patient's symptoms and function occur more slowly, and the exercise program may be more extensive. The patient is often instructed in self-progression of activities.

TISSUE IRRITABILITY AND SYMPTOM STABILITY

Tissue irritability has a significant effect on the rehabilitation program choices. This factor is somewhat subjective and is determined through a complete subjective examination. Questions regarding the patient's symptoms provide the clinician with the best information on this issue (Display 3-2).

Before deciding on the choice or intensity of the exercises, the clinician must know what kinds of activities or positions worsen the patient's symptoms. These activities or positions may or may not need to be avoided. If the patient can tolerate the activity or position for some time, is able to detect the prodromal signs that the symptoms are going to worsen, and understands that stopping the activity or changing position can alleviate the symptoms, these activities or positions may be used therapeutically. For example, if a patient with carpal tunnel syndrome enjoys knitting and this is one of the patient's functional goals, knitting may be used as part of the rehabilitation program. The patient must be able to recognize the onset of symptoms and be able to alleviate them by taking a rest period or discontinuing the knitting. Similarly, if a patient with back pain enjoys and is able to tolerate some walking, this activity can be a component of the exercise program. The patient must be able to detect the onset of symptoms and be able to relieve them by discontinuation, stretching, icing, or some other self-management intervention. Conversely, if the patient reports an unmanageable, inevitable worsening of symptoms once irritated, the exercise program should expressly avoid any position or activity that may exacerbate symptoms.

The stability of the patient's symptoms is a component of tissue irritability that must be considered. Individuals may have significant unpredictable fluctuations in their symptoms over the course of the day or week. If symptom changes cannot be associated with the time of day, position, or any specific activity, the exercise prescription can be difficult. If the patient is unable to determine what kinds of things make her better or worse, assessing the effects of the exercise program becomes yet another variable in the symptomatology. Deciding whether a specific exercise prescription is beneficial or deleterious is challenging if the patient's symptoms fluctuate randomly. When possible, it is best to proceed with fewer exercise interventions until a stable baseline of symptoms is achieved. This baseline then serves as a gauge of the effect of the exercise program.

Other activities engaged in by the patient affect the exercise prescription. Understanding the behavior of a patient's symptoms over a 24-hour period and how her normal daily routine affects the symptoms helps the clinician gauge appropriate exercise levels. Frequently, the patient is unaware of the impact of certain routine activities on her problem, or she must perform some activities that worsen her symptoms. The individual with patellofemoral pain should be counseled about the importance of good shoes, particularly if standing for a large portion of the day. Despite the fact that standing behind a cash register for 8 hours may exacerbate the patient's symptoms, this work may be necessary to provide financial support for the family. The individual with back pain may need to lift a child out of a crib several times each day, despite the fact that this activity is painful. The clinician must educate the patient about the impact of these activities on her symptoms and provide suggestions to minimize their negative effects. Moreover, the clinician must educate the patient regarding modification of the exercise program based on the symptoms related to participation in these activities. On days when the patient's symptoms may be increased due to excessive standing, working, or lifting, she may need to decrease the rehabilitation exercise level. Failure to recognize the impact of daily activities on symptoms may cause the clinician to erroneously assume that a change in the patient's symptoms was caused by the exercise program alone.

> **DISPLAY 3-2**
> ### Questions Assessing Tissue Irritability
>
> 1. What activities or positions increase your symptoms?
> 2. How much time can you spend in that activity or position before your symptoms begin?
> 3. When you start feeling these symptoms, will they continue to progress despite discontinuing the activity or changing positions? Will changing the activity or position alleviate the symptoms?
> 4. After you begin experiencing your symptoms, how long do they last? How long until you return to "baseline"?
> 5. Is there anything you can do to relieve your symptoms?

TIME BETWEEN PHYSICAL THERAPY VISITS

The time between follow-up visits affects the exercise prescription. For the patient attending supervised physical therapy one or more times per week, the clinician may be more willing to give the patient more challenging exercises for her home program, knowing that the patient will be monitored more closely in the clinic. For those who live some distance away or who have longer time intervals between supervised visits for other reasons, the clinician should provide exercises less likely to overwork the patients. This program is supplemented with instructions on how to progress exercises if they become too easy (eg, increase time, repetitions, intensity), or an intermediate phone follow-up can take place.

PATIENT'S TIME AND WILLINGNESS

The amount of time the patient has available to exercise is an important factor affecting exercise prescription. If the patient claims to have little time available for the home exercise program, education by the clinician about the importance of this program is necessary. Make an effort to select exercises considered to be the most important for the exercise program. More is not always better, and giving thoughtful consideration to the core exercises is beneficial for the clinician and the patient. Choosing exercises that have the greatest impact for the least time commitment can minimize the time requirement and maximize the benefits. The patient will probably appreciate your concern and attention to her needs. This approach must be coupled with education regarding the importance of the home exercise program to achieve the determined goals in as expedient and efficient a time frame as possible. The patient's responsibility in achieving those goals must be emphasized.

Determining Exercise Levels

Determining the appropriate level of exercise can be difficult, particularly when the patient has had little or no experience with the specific problem previously or little previous experience with exercise. Although many individuals exercise regularly, many others have little experience with exercise. Knowing how to respond to different sensations felt during the rehabilitation exercises can prove frustrating to the patient. Many patients ask whether to continue exercising if the exercise produces pain. Despite the fact that pain is a subjective symptom, this sensation should be acknowledged by the clinician. Pain should be considered in the context of change from the patient's baseline symptom level and how the symptoms behave over the subsequent 24-hour period.

Curwin and Stanish[12] provide guidelines originally designed to help determine readiness to return to a sport. However, these same guidelines are nicely adapted to evaluation of the patient's exercise program (Table 3-1). The column in Table 3-1 entitled "Description of Pain" refers to the level of pain during rehabilitation exercise performance, and the category "Level of Sports Performance" could be retitled "Level of Exercise Program Performance." Activity levels that keep the patient within her optimal loading zone are generally levels 1 through 3. Occasionally, some patients may be able to tolerate exercise at level 4 without any residual effects. In these cases, progress may need to be reassessed on a weekly basis rather than on an exercise session to exercise session or a daily basis. Patients with adhesive capsulitis often experience pain at level 4, but this level of pain does not interfere with their overall function or progress. These guidelines provide the patient and the clinician common criteria with which the exercise program prescription is evaluated.

Despite the clinician's best efforts, some patients experience an exacerbation of their symptoms, which may or may not be related to the exercise program. Although the first response of the clinician and the patient may be some level of distress, an exacerbation is not always a negative experience. Valuable lessons can be learned from an exacerbation. At some point, whether days, weeks, months, or years later, most patients experience some type of symptoms related to the current problem. The patient with patellofemoral pain may experience a milder level of pain after a hiking vacation, or the individual with low back pain may notice some back discomfort after a long plane flight. Some patients experience a complete exacerbation of their symptoms at some future point. Patients must learn how to manage the exacerbation.

Frequently, several weeks have passed by the time the patient seeks medical attention and gets an appointment with the physician and a subsequent appointment with the therapist. The optimal time for intervention has passed, and the patient may be struggling with secondary problems due to compensation, or movement changes made because of pain or other impairments. One of the best services the clinician can offer the patient is instruction on how to manage a return of symptoms. Instruction may include the use of modalities such as ice, appropriate activity modifications or rest, changes in the maintenance exercise program, or education regarding when to seek medical attention.

In addition to possibly preventing reentry to the medical system through immediate, appropriate symptom management, self-management has the added benefit of enhancing

Table 3-1. CURWIN AND STANISH CLASSIFICATION FOR DETERMINING THE APPROPRIATE LEVEL OF DISCOMFORT ASSOCIATED WITH HOME EXERCISE PRESCRIPTION

LEVEL	DESCRIPTION OF PAIN	LEVEL OF SPORTS PERFORMANCE OR ACTIVITY
1	No pain	Normal
2	Pain only with extreme exertion	Normal
3	Pain with extreme exertion and 1–2 hours afterward	Normal or slightly decreased
4	Pain during and after any vigorous activities	Somewhat decreased
5	Pain during activity and forcing termination	Markedly decreased
6	Pain during daily activities	Unable to perform

From Curwin S, Stanish WD: Tendinitis: Its Etiology and Treatment. Lexington, MA: DC Heath and Co., 1984:64.

patients' confidence in their ability to resolve the symptoms. The exacerbation experience coupled with instruction in appropriate management under the clinician's guidance can greatly decrease the patient's anxiety. Patients are often fearful about participating in activities that may provoke their symptoms, afraid that they will be "back where they started" in the early stages of their injury. Learning that an exacerbation does not necessarily send them back to the initial phase and that they can successfully manage the problem empowers patients to make appropriate activity choices. Eventually, patients may choose to participate in activities they enjoy at the expense of getting a little sore, knowing that they can manage the symptoms successfully independently.

Formulating the Program

When possible, formulate the exercise program after the patient's baseline level of symptoms has stabilized and the previously mentioned factors (eg, tissue irritability) have been determined. Ensuring the patient's understanding of what the "baseline" feels like allows better communication between the clinician and patient regarding the behavior of their symptoms and the effects of the exercise program. Symptoms that are unstable or fluctuating without determinable cause make assessing the effects of intervention difficult. Asking the patient to articulate her "normal" level of symptoms can assist the patient in determining the stability of her symptoms. If patients have difficulty determining the stability of their symptoms, slow progression is necessary. When the patient is able to perform the same exercise program for three consecutive sessions without an increase in symptoms, progression is appropriate.

If intervention needs to be implemented before the establishment of a stable baseline, give the patient as few exercises as possible. This minimizes the impact of the exercise program, thereby lowering the possibility of exacerbating the symptoms. If the patient's symptoms do worsen, you'll have an easier time determining the cause, and changes can be made more appropriately. As symptoms resolve and the baseline stabilizes, activities can be increased systematically and gradually. This is done by increasing the time and repetitions or by adding new exercises slowly.

How the exercise program is progressed depends on each person's stage of injury, specific goals, and stability of symptoms. For the individual who is in the intermediate to late healing stages and has demonstrated stable symptoms, several exercises can be progressed simultaneously. For those with unstable symptoms and frequent exacerbations, only one change in the rehabilitation program should be made at a time. In this way, any positive or negative response to the change can be more easily identified and remedied.

Patients must be taught how to modify their exercise program based on their activity level on any given day. Put exercises in the context of their daily routine. On days when the patient is more active, (eg, working overtime, child care, shopping, yard work), the home exercise program should be modified to prevent overload. On days when the patient is more sedentary (eg, bad weather, day off from work), the exercise program may be increased. In this way, the patient begins to understand the impact of her overall activity level on her symptoms. This assists the patient in the self-management of her symptoms in the future.

Choosing exercises that can be incorporated into activities already performed during the day should be a fundamental of the exercise program. This can improve motivation and adherence. This type of exercise prescription results in short bouts of exercise performed several times throughout the day. In this case, the patient is unlikely to overwork in any single session, resulting in a lower chance of an exacerbation of symptoms. Moreover, the likelihood of exacerbation is decreased despite a greater volume of exercise than can be performed in any single session. For example, the individual with Achilles tendinitis may tolerate only two repetitions of 30 seconds of calf stretching at a time. If that individual performs those two repetitions six times spread out over the course of her day, the stretch has been performed 12 times. In contrast, if the patient tried to carry out the home exercise program in the evening after work and dinner, chances are only two repetitions would be performed that day.

Finally, teach the patient that some exercise is better than none, and if time limitations exist, a couple of key exercises should be performed. Occasionally, other life events prevent completion of the full home exercise program despite the patient's willingness to adhere. Educate the patient on the various exercises, highlighting those that are most important to complete if time does not permit completion of the entire program. Emphasize the importance of finishing all of the exercises when time permits, while suggesting that some exercise is better than none.

Key Points

- Changes in health care delivery systems require more patient education and self-management.
- Patient safety is the primary issue when designing a home exercise prescription.
- The best-designed treatment program is of little value if the patient does not adhere to the clinician's recommendations.
- The clinician must determine the patient motivators to enhance likelihood of adherence.
- Exercises requiring the fewest lifestyle changes and imposing changes that mimic the patient's usual activities can increase adherence.
- Patient-clinician communication is enhanced by determining the patient's willingness to learn and listening actively to the patient's needs.
- Written and verbal instructions should be included in a home exercise program. Written exercises should include beginning and ending positions and any precautions.
- On subsequent visits, the patient should demonstrate the home exercise program to ensure correct performance of all exercises.
- Home exercise choices are affected by the acuity of the injury, tissue irritability, stability of symptoms, time available for exercise, and factors affecting the length of follow-up.
- A symptom exacerbation can be a learning experience for the patient if educated properly about the experience.

LAB ACTIVITIES

1. Refer to Case Study 6 in Unit 7. Design a home program for this patient. Include written instructions and diagrams for all exercises. Teach your patient this home program while relaying the following emotions:
   a. Empathy
   b. Disinterest
   c. Hurry
   d. Insecurity
2. Using the exercises developed for the first question, modify each exercise to be performed throughout the day, incorporating the exercises into the patient's daily routine.
3. Using the exercises developed for the first question, prioritize the exercises for the patient, and explain your rationale for the prioritization to the patient. Use language the patient can understand.
4. Your patient desires to return to several sporting activities. Choose two of the exercises you have given the patient, and modify them to mimic a sporting activity to which the patient would like to return.
5. Teach someone else in the class who does not know how to tie a necktie how to do this without looking at each other and without using the words *yes* or *no*.

- Patients must be taught how to modify their home exercise program based on other activities and symptoms.
- Understanding the "normal" behavior of their symptoms allows patients to more easily recognize an exacerbation and be able to guide activity choice and intensity.
- Any cultural, language, education, visual, or hearing barriers should be identified early and appropriate accommodations made.
- Prioritize exercises so that the patient may perform at least some of her exercises on busy days.

Critical Thinking Questions

1. How would your home exercise instruction differ for patients who were
   a. Visual learners
   b. Auditory learners
   c. Kinesthetic learners
2. Consider the patient in Lab Activities question 1. How would you provide this patient with a home exercise program if she were blind?
3. A patient returns to see you and reports that the home exercise was not done because of a lack of time. How do you respond? What is your strategy and rationale?
4. A patient returns to see you and reports that the home exercise program was not done because the exercises hurt. How do you respond? What is your strategy and rationale?

REFERENCES

1. Chase L, Elkins JA, Readinger J, Shepard KF. Perceptions of physical therapists toward patient education. *Phys Ther*. 1993;73:787–796.
2. Gahimer JE, Domholdt E. Amount of patient education in physical therapy practice and perceived effects. *Phys Ther*. 1996;76:1089–1096.
3. Sluijs EM, Kok GJ, van der Zee J. Correlates of exercise compliance in physical therapy. *Phys Ther*. 1993;73:771–787.
4. Fields J, Murphey M, Horodyski MB, Stopka C. Factors associated with adherence to sport injury rehabilitation in college-age recreational athletes. *J Sport Rehab*. 1995;9:172–180.
5. Gieck J. Psychological considerations for rehabilitation. In: Prentice W, ed. *Rehabilitation Techniques in Sports Medicine*. 2nd ed. St. Louis: Mosby–Year Book; 1994:238–252.
6. Schwenk TL, Whitman N. *The Physician as Teacher*. Baltimore: Williams & Wilkins; 1987.
7. Brophy J. Research on the self-fulfilling prophecy and teacher expectations. *J Ed Psychol*. 1983;75:631–661.
8. Fisher A. Adherence to sports injury rehabilitation programmes. *Sports Med*. 1990;9:151–158.
9. Horn T. Expectancy effects in the interscholastic athletic setting: metholodogical concerns. *J Sport Psychol*. 1984;6:60–76.
10. Wilder KC. Clinician's expectations and their impact on an athlete's compliance in rehabilitation. *J Sport Rehab*. 1994; 3:168–175.
11. Friedrich M, Cermak T, Maderbacher P. The effect of brochure use versus therapist teaching on patients performing therapeutic exercise and on changes in impairment status. *Phys Ther*. 1996;76:1082–1088.
12. Curwin S, Stanish WD. *Tendinitis: Its Etiology and Treatment*. Lexington, MA: DC Heath; 1984.

UNIT 2

Functional Approach to Therapeutic Exercise for Physiologic Impairments

CHAPTER 4

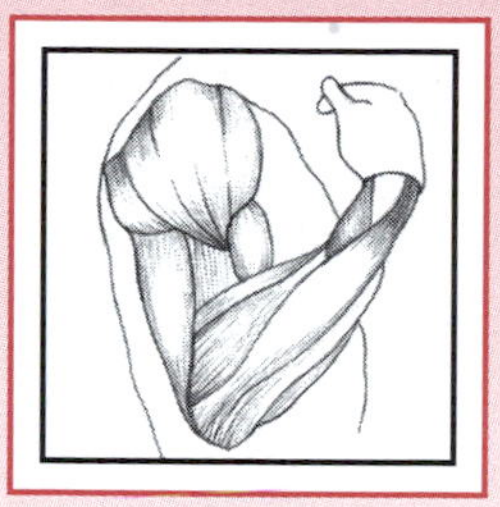

Impairment in Muscle Performance

Carrie Hall and Lori Thein Brody

Impaired muscle performance results from many conditions. Direct damage to the muscle, biomechanical factors, cardiovascular limitations, neuromuscular incoordination, or pathology can limit force production. Muscle performance impairment can be further classified by impairments in force, torque, power, or work production. These impairments must be directly or indirectly related to a functional limitation or prevention of a functional limitation to justify therapeutic exercise intervention. For example, an individual lacking the muscle performance to carry a bag of groceries into the house needs intervention to achieve this instrumental activity of daily living. A worker lacking the muscle performance to maintain efficient posture throughout the work day requires intervention to prevent work disability.

Although not all scientific and clinical information on force, torque, work, and power production can be covered in this text, this chapter provides the foundation for this important element of therapeutic exercise application. Fundamental terms and concepts are defined, the essential morphology and physiology of skeletal muscle relative to muscle performance are reviewed, and clinical applications are presented.

DEFINITIONS

Strength

Impaired muscle performance is commonly treated by clinicians and is usually described as a strength deficit. However, strength is a relative term and suffers from the lack of a clear definition. *Strength* is usually defined as the maximum force that a muscle can develop during a single contraction. However, strength is the result of complex interactions of neurologic, muscular, biomechanical, and cognitive systems. Strength can be assessed in terms of force, torque, work, and power. If appropriate decisions are to be made regarding these impairments, operational definitions are necessary.

Force

Force is an agent that produces or tends to produce a change in the state of rest or motion of an object.[1] For example, a ball sitting stationary on a playing field remains in that position unless it is acted on by a force. Force, described in metric units of newtons or British units of pounds, is displayed algebraically in the following equation:

force = mass × acceleration

Kinetics is the study of forces applied to the body. Some of the factors influencing muscular force production include the neural input, mechanical arrangement of the muscle, cross-sectional area, fiber-type composition, age, and gender.[1]

Torque

All human motion involves rotation of body segments about their joint axes. These actions are produced by the interaction of forces from external loads and muscle activity. The ability of a force to produce rotation is *torque.* Torque represents the rotational effect of a force with respect to an axis:

torque = force × moment arm

The *moment arm* is the perpendicular distance from the line of action of the force to the axis of rotation. The metric unit of torque is the newton-meter; the foot-pound is used in the older British system of units.

Clinically, the word *strength* is often used synonymously with torque. Large amounts of torque are produced by the musculoskeletal system during everyday functional activities such as walking, lifting, and getting out of bed. It is incorrect to conclude that a person is "strong" only because his muscles generate large forces. It would be just as erroneous to conclude that a person is strong only because he has large moment arms.

Torque can be altered in biomechanics through three strategies:

- Changing the force magnitude
- Changing the moment arm length
- Changing the angle between the direction of force and momentum

In the human musculoskeletal system, changing the force magnitude (ie, tension-producing capability of muscle) can be altered by training. The moment arm can be decreased by positioning a load closer to the body, and the angle between the force and moment arm may be changed by altering joint alignment through postural education. This chapter is devoted to variables affecting the tension-producing capability of muscle.

Work and Power

Work is the magnitude of a force acting on an object multiplied by the distance through which the force acts. The unit used to describe work is the joule, which is equivalent to 1 newton-meter (the foot-pound unit is used in the British system). Work is algebraically expressed in this equation:

work = force × distance

Power is the rate of performing work. The unit of power in the metric system is the watt, which is equal to 1 joule/second (foot-pound/second in the British system). Power can be determined for a single body movement, a series of movements, or for a large number of repetitive movements, as in the case of aerobic exercise. Power is algebraically expressed in this equation:

power = work/time

For the simple movement of lifting or lowering a weight, the muscle must overcome the weight of the limb and the weight, acting some distance from the axis of rotation through a range of motion (ROM) during a certain time. This example summarizes the practical aspects of force, torque, work, and power in resistance training.

Muscle Actions

Poorly defined muscle actions can be a source of confusion and inaccuracy. Resistive exercise uses various types of muscle contraction to improve impaired muscle performance. Muscle actions can be divided into two general categories: static and dynamic. A static muscle action, traditionally referred to as *isometric,* is a contraction in which force is developed without any motion about an axis, so no work is performed.

All other muscle actions involve movement and are called dynamic or isotonic. An *isotonic contraction* is a uniform force throughout a dynamic muscle action. No dynamic muscle action uses constant force because of changes in mechanical advantage and muscle length. Isotonic is therefore an inappropriate term to describe human exercise performance, and the term *dynamic* is preferred.

Dynamic muscle action is further described as concentric or eccentric action. The term *concentric* describes a shortening muscle contraction, and the term *eccentric* describes a lengthening muscle contraction. Eccentric contractions differ from concentric and isometric contractions in several important ways. Per contractile unit, more tension can be generated eccentrically than concentrically and at a lower metabolic cost (ie, less use of ATP-derived energy).[2] Eccentric contractions are an important component of a functional movement pattern (eg, required to decelerate limbs during movement), are the most energy-efficient form, and can develop the greatest tension of the various types of muscle actions.

The term *isokinetic* refers to a concentric or eccentric muscle contraction in which a constant velocity is maintained throughout the muscle action. A person can exert a continuous force by using an isokinetic device, which provides a resistive surface that restricts movement to a set, constant velocity. Some acceleration and deceleration occurs as the individual accelerates the limb from a resting position to the preset velocity and decelerates the limb to change directions. By constraining the speed of the isokinetic device, the limb moves at a constant velocity. Because the device cannot be accelerated beyond the preset speed, any unbalanced force exerted against it is resisted by an equal and opposite force. This muscular force may be measured, displayed, recorded, or used as concurrent visual feedback. Although the isokinetic device may be moving at a constant velocity, it does not guarantee that the user's muscle activation is at a constant velocity. Despite this inaccuracy, the terms isokinetic and isotonic to describe muscle action are likely to be employed for pragmatic reasons.

During functional movement patterns, combinations of static and dynamic contractions occur. Trunk muscles contract isometrically to stabilize the spine and pelvis during movements of the extremities such as reaching or walking. Lower extremity muscles are subjected to impact forces requiring combinations of concentric and eccentric contractions, sometimes within the same muscle acting at two different joints. Muscles commonly perform eccentric contractions against gravity, as in slowly lowering the arm from an overhead position.

Muscles often act eccentrically and then contract concentrically. The combination of eccentric and concentric actions forms a natural type of muscle action called a *stretch-shortening cycle* (SSC).[3,4] The SSC results in a final action (ie, concentric phase) that is more powerful than a concentric action alone. This phenomenon is called *elastic potentiation*.[4] The SSC is discussed in more detail later in this chapter.

MORPHOLOGY AND PHYSIOLOGY OF MUSCLE PERFORMANCE

Improving muscle performance often translates into improvements in functioning by the patient. A thorough understanding of muscle morphology and physiology is required to prescribe an appropriate exercise program that proceeds to the ultimate goal of a functional outcome for each patient.

Gross Structure of Skeletal Muscle

Each of more than 430 voluntary muscles in the body consists of various layers of connective tissue. Figure 4-1 illustrates a cross section of a muscle consisting of thousands of muscle cells called muscle fibers. These multinucleated muscle fibers lie parallel to one another and are separated by the innermost layer of connective tissue, called the endomysium. As many as 150 fibers are arranged into bundles called fasciculi and are surrounded by the perimysium, the next layer of connective tissue. The entire muscle is encased by the outermost layer of connective tissue, called the epimysium. This connective tissue sheath tapers at the ends as it blends into and joins the intramuscular tissue sheaths forming the tendons. The tendons connect to the outermost covering of the bone, the periosteum. The force of muscle contraction is transmitted directly from the muscle's connective tissue to the point of attachment on the bone.

Beneath the endomysium and surrounding each muscle fiber is a thin, elastic membrane, called the sarcolemma, enclosing the fiber's cellular contents. The aqueous protoplasm or sarcoplasm contains the contractile proteins, enzymes, fat and glycogen particles, the nuclei, and various specialized cellular organelles. Embedded in the sarcoplasm is an extensive network of interconnecting tubular channels known as the sarcoplasmic reticulum. This highly specialized system provides the cell with structural integrity and also serves important functions in muscular contractions.

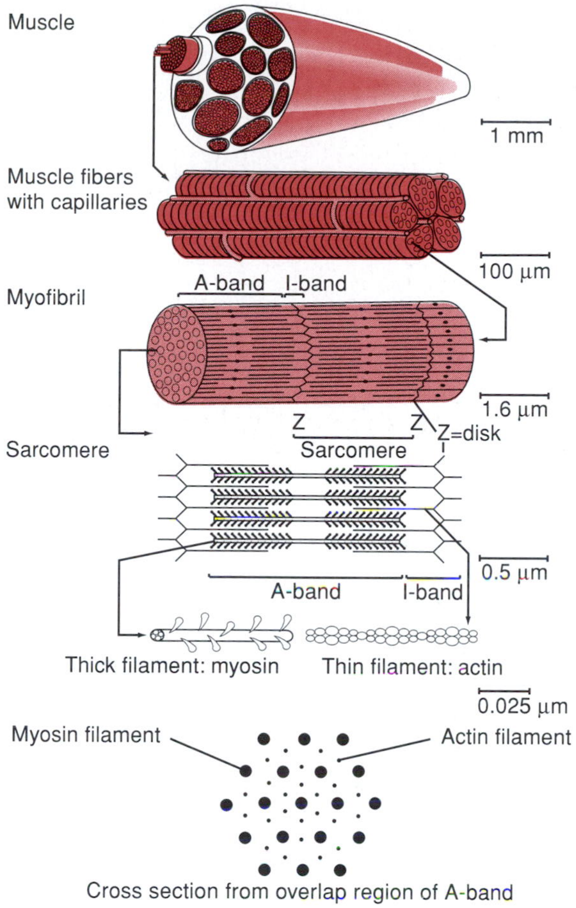

FIGURE 4-1 Structure of skeletal muscle.

Ultrastructure of Skeletal Muscle

The ultrastructure of skeletal muscle consists of different levels of subcellular organization (see Fig. 4-1). Each muscle fiber consists of small fibers called myofibrils. Myofibrils are composed of even smaller threads called myofilaments. The myofilaments are composed primarily of two proteins, actin and myosin. Six other proteins have been identified that have a structural or physiologic purpose. The contractile unit of the entire myofibril is known as the sarcomere.

THE SARCOMERE

Figure 4-1 illustrates the structural pattern of myofilaments within a sarcomere. The lighter area is referred to as the I band, and the darker zone is known as the A band. The Z line bisects the I band and adheres to the sarcolemma to give the entire structure stability. The repeating unit between two Z lines represents the sarcomere. The actin and myosin filaments within the sarcomere are primarily involved in the mechanical process of muscular contraction and therefore in force development. Each myosin crossbridge is an independent force generator.

ACTIN-MYOSIN ORIENTATION

Figure 4-2 illustrates the actin–myosin orientation within a sarcomere at resting and contracted lengths. Figure 4-3 illustrates the spatial orientation of the various proteins

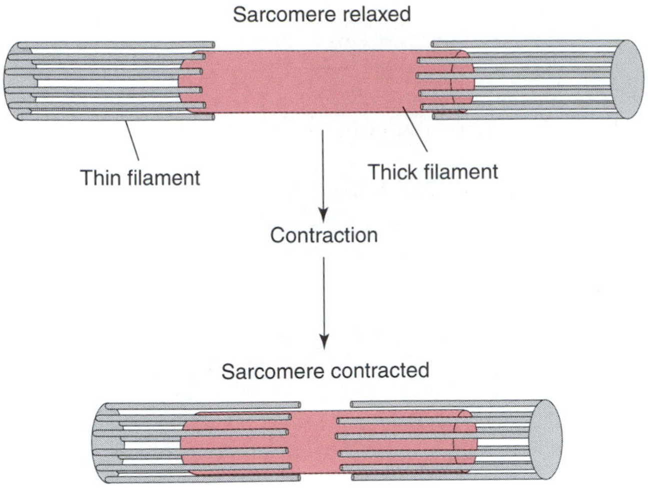

FIGURE 4-2 Actin–myosin relationships in relaxed and contracted position.

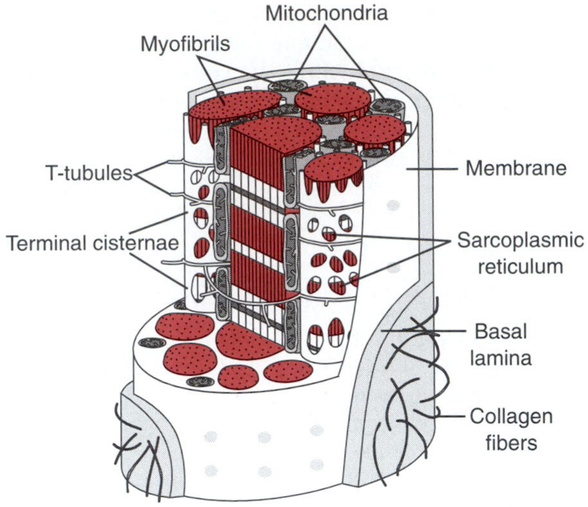

FIGURE 4-4 Relationships of the sarcoplasmic reticulum, T-tubule system, and myofibrils.

that constitute the contractile filaments. Cross-bridges spiral about the myosin filament at the region where the filaments of actin and myosin overlap. Tropomyosin and troponin are two important proteins that appear to regulate the make-and-break contacts between the myofilaments during contraction.

INTRACELLULAR TUBULE SYSTEM

The sarcoplasmic reticulum and transverse tubule (T-tubule) system within the muscle fiber can be seen in Figure 4-4. The sarcoplasmic reticulum lies parallel to the myofibrils, whereas the T-tubule system runs perpendicular to the myofibril. The lateral end of the sarcoplasmic reticulum terminates in a saclike vesicle that stores calcium. The T-tubule system appears to function as a microtransportation network for spreading the action potential (ie, wave of depolarization) from the fiber's outer membrane inward to the deep regions of the cell.

Chemical and Mechanical Events During Contraction and Relaxation

The sliding filament theory, which explains the events that occur during muscle contraction, proposes that a muscle shortens or lengthens because the thick and thin myofilaments slide past each other without the filaments themselves changing length.

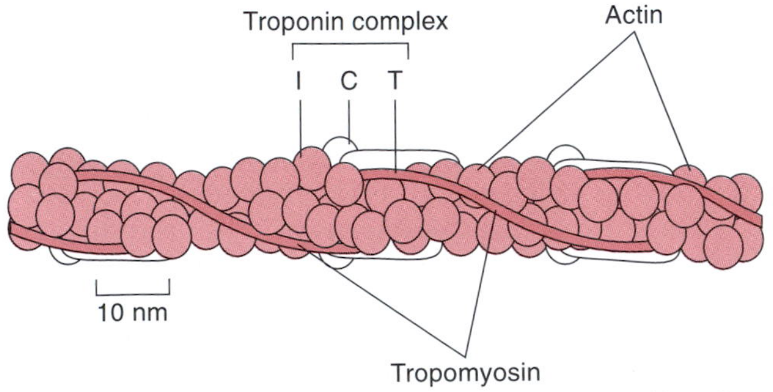

FIGURE 4-3 Diagram of a thin filament shows the relationships of troponin, tropomyosin, and actin.

Excitation-contraction is the physiologic mechanism whereby an electric discharge at the muscle initiates the chemical events that lead to contraction. When a muscle fiber is stimulated to contract, there is an immediate increase in the intracellular calcium concentration. Arrival of the action potential at the T-tubules causes calcium to be released from the lateral sacs of the sarcoplasmic reticulum. The inhibitory action of troponin (ie, preventing actin-myosin interaction) occurs when calcium ions bind rapidly with troponin in the actin filaments. The globular head of the myosin cross-bridge provides the mechanical means for the actin and myosin filaments to slide past each other. During contraction, each cross-bridge undergoes many repeated but independent cycles of movement.

At any one time, only about one half of the bridges are in contact with the actin filaments, forming the protein complex actomyosin. Myosin ATPase is an enzyme that splits ATP so that its energy can be used for muscle contraction. When the active sites on the actin and myosin are joined, myosin ATPase is activated and splits the ATP molecule. When ATP is combined with the actomyosin complex, actin and myosin detach. ATP also provides energy for cross-bridge movement. The transfer of energy causes movement of myosin cross-bridges, and the muscle generates tension. The cross-bridges uncouple from actin when ATP binds to the myosin bridge. Coupling and uncoupling continues as long as the calcium concentration remains at a sufficient level to inhibit the troponin-tropomyosin system. When the nerve stimulus is removed, calcium moves back into the lateral sacs of the sarcoplasmic reticulum, restoring the inhibitory action of the troponin-tropomyosin, and actin and myosin remain separated as long as ATP is present (Display 4-1).

Muscle Fiber Type

Skeletal muscle is not a simple homogenous group of fibers with similar metabolic and functional properties. Distinct fiber types have been identified and classified by their contractile and metabolic characteristics.

DISPLAY 4-1

Sequence of Events in Muscular Contraction

The following is a list of the main events in muscular contraction and relaxation. The sequence begins with the initiation of an action potential by the motor nerve. This impulse is propagated over the entire surface of the muscle fiber as the cell membrane becomes depolarized.

1. Depolarization of the T-tubules causes release of calcium from the lateral sacs of the sarcoplasmic reticulum.
2. Calcium binds to the troponin-tropomyosin complex in the actin filaments, releasing the inhibition that prevented actin from combining with myosin.
3. Actin combines with myosin-activated myosin ATPase, which splits ATP. The energy that is created produces movement of the cross-bridge, and tension is created.
4. ATP binds to the myosin bridge. This action breaks the actin-myosin bond and allows the cross-bridge to dissociate from actin, causing the thick and thin filaments to slide past each other, and the muscle shortens.
5. Cross-bridge activation continues as long as the concentration of calcium remains high enough to inhibit the action of the troponin-tropomyosin system.
6. When stimulation ceases, calcium moves back into the lateral sacs of the sarcoplasmic reticulum.
7. Removal of calcium restores the inhibitory action of troponin-tropomyosin. In the presence of ATP, actin and myosin remain in the dissociated, relaxed state.

Slow-twitch fibers, or type I fibers, are characterized by slow speed of contraction, low activity of myosin ATPase, and glycolytic capacity that is less well developed than that of their fast-twitch counterparts. Slow-twitch fibers are well suited for prolonged aerobic exercise.

Fast-twitch fibers are divided into fast oxidative-glycolytic, or type IIA, and fast-glycolytic, or type IIB, fibers. Generally, fast-twitch fibers have a high activity level of myosin ATPase associated with their ability to generate energy rapidly for quick, forceful contractions. Fast oxidative-glycolytic fibers are a hybrid between slow-twitch and fast-glycolytic fibers. These fibers combine the ability to produce quick, forceful contractions and sustain them for longer than fast-glycolytic fibers (though not as long as slow-twitch fibers). Compared with fast oxidative-glycolytic fibers, the fast-glycolytic fibers possess a greater anaerobic potential. A third fast-twitch fiber, type IIC, has been identified. The type IIC fiber is normally a rare and undifferentiated fiber that may be involved in reinnervation or motor unit transformation.[5]

Motor Unit

The motor unit consists of the motor neuron, its axon, and the muscle fibers supplied by the motor neuron. The number of muscle fibers belonging to a single motor unit can vary from 5 to 10 to more than 100. As a general rule, small muscles responsible for precision tasks (eg, intrinsic hand muscles) are composed of motor units supplying few muscle fibers, whereas trunk and proximal limb muscles contain motor units supplying a large number of muscle fibers.

Human motor units with the following characteristics tend to be classified as tonic motor units: long contraction times, low-twitch tension, high resistance to fatigue, small-amplitude action potentials, and slow conduction velocities. Conversely, phasic motor units tend to be recruited at high levels of voluntary contraction, display short contraction times and high-twitch tensions, are not fatigue resistant, and show large-amplitude action potentials and fast conduction velocities.

Force Gradation

Motor units are activated to increase force production or deactivated to decrease force production. Force gradation can be likened to a rheostat, through which more motor units are brought on line as the need for force increases or taken off line as the need for force decreases. Force increases can occur by increasing the rate of discharge (ie, rate coding) or by graded recruitment of higher threshold motor units (ie, size principle).[6] Rate coding implies high-frequency discharge when high forces are needed, and low-frequency pulses are delivered when low forces are necessary.[7] The size principle states that, during activation of motor neurons, those with the smallest axons have the lowest thresholds and are recruited first, followed by larger cells with higher thresholds.

In most voluntary everyday contractions, slow (type I) motor units are the first to be recruited. With increasing power output, more fast (type II) units are activated. Trained persons can activate all the motor units in a large limb muscle during a static, maximal, voluntary contraction, whereas this is not possible for untrained persons. The fastest (type IIB) motor units are preferentially activated in fast corrective movements and reflexes. Explosive maximal contractions are thought to activate fast and slow motor units simultaneously.

There is some evidence that violations of the size principle occur. Two departures occur through neural adaptations related to the specificity of velocity and movement pattern in strength training. High-threshold, fast-twitch motor units are preferentially activated during brief, rapid concentric actions in which the intent is to relax quickly.[8] It has also been demonstrated that fast-twitch motor units are preferentially recruited in eccentric actions performed at moderate to high velocities.[9]

Factors Affecting Muscle Performance

The clinician requires knowledge about muscle performance to make clinical decisions regarding the use of resistive exercise to achieve a desired functional outcome. The functional outcome must be related to the need to improve force, torque, work, or power production.

FIBER TYPE

Sedentary men and women and young children possess 45% to 55% slow-twitch fibers.[10] Persons who achieve high levels of sport proficiency have the fiber predominance and distributions characteristic of their sport. For example, those who train for endurance sports have a higher distribution of slow-twitch fibers in the significant muscles, and sprint athletes have a predominance of fast-twitch fibers. Other studies show that men and women who perform in middle-distance events have an approximately equal percentage of the two types of muscle fibers.[11] Any resistive rehabilitation program should be based on the probable distribution of fiber type of the individual.

Clear-cut distinctions between fiber type composition and athletic performance are true only for *elite* athletes. However, a person's fiber composition is not the sole determinant of performance. This is not surprising, because performance capacity is the end result of the blending of many physiologic, biochemical, and neurologic components, not simply the result of a single factor such as muscle fiber type.[12]

FIBER DIAMETER

Although the different fiber types show clear differences in contraction speed, the force developed in a maximal static action is independent of the fiber type but is related to the fiber's cross-sectional diameter. Because type I (slow) fibers tend to have smaller diameters than type II (fast) fibers, a high percentage of type I fibers is believed to be associated with a smaller muscle diameter and therefore lower force development capabilities.[13]

MUSCLE SIZE

When adult muscles are trained at intensities that exceed 60% to 70% of their maximum force generating capacity, adaptations occur that increase the total muscle cross-sectional area and force production capability. The increase in muscle size may result from increases in fiber size (ie, hypertrophy), fiber number (ie, hyperplasia), interstitial connective tissue, or some combination of these factors.[14,15]

Although the major mechanism for increased muscle size in adults is hypertrophy, ongoing controversy surrounds evidence of hyperplasia. Mammalian skeletal muscle does possess a population of reserve or satellite cells that, when activated, can replace damaged fibers with new fibers.[16,17] A mechanism exists for the generation of new fibers in the adult animal. Scientific models of exercise and stretch overload have shown significant increases in fiber number.[14] The mechanisms for fiber hyperplasia probably are the result of satellite cell proliferation and longitudinal fiber splitting.[14]

Despite few investigations of the effect of strength training on interstitial connective tissue, it appears that, because it occupies a relatively small proportion of the total muscle volume, its potential to contribute substantial changes in muscle size is limited.[18]

FORCE–VELOCITY RELATIONSHIP

Muscle can adjust its active force to precisely match the applied load. This property, which differentiates it from a simple elastic body, is based on the fact that active force continuously adjusts to the speed at which the contractile system moves. When the load is small, the active force can be made correspondingly small by increasing the speed of shortening appropriately. When the load is high, the muscle increases its active force to the same level by slowing the speed of shortening sufficiently[19] (Fig. 4-5).

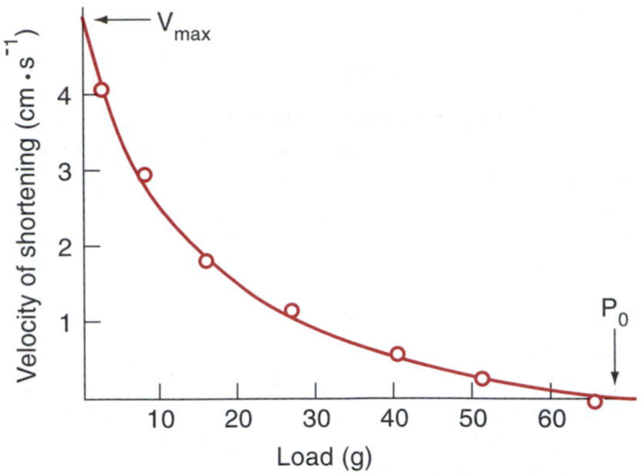

FIGURE 4-5 Relationship between the force and velocity of a shortening muscle contraction.

Slowing the speed of contraction allows a patient to develop more tension during concentric contractions. However, during eccentric contractions, increased speed of lengthening produces more tension. This appears to provide a safety mechanism for limbs excessively loaded. Increasing the speed of a concentric contraction (ie, increasing the speed of an isokinetic device) significantly lowers the amount of concentric torque developed. In contrast, increasing the speed of an eccentric contraction until a plateau is reached increases the amount of torque developed.

LENGTH–TENSION RELATIONSHIP

A muscle's capacity to produce force depends on the length at which the muscle is held with maximum force delivered near the muscle's normal resting length (Fig. 4-6). The number of sarcomeres in series determines the distance through which the muscle can shorten and the length at which it produces maximum force. Sarcomere number is not fixed, and in adult muscle, this number can increase or decrease[20] (Fig. 4-7). Regulation of sarcomere number is an adaptation to changes in the functional length of a muscle.

Length-associated changes can be induced by postural malalignment or immobilization.[21,22] In muscles chronically maintained in a shortened range because of faulty posture or immobilization, sarcomeres are lost, and the remaining sarcomeres adapt to a length that restores homeostasis; the new length enables maximum tension development at the

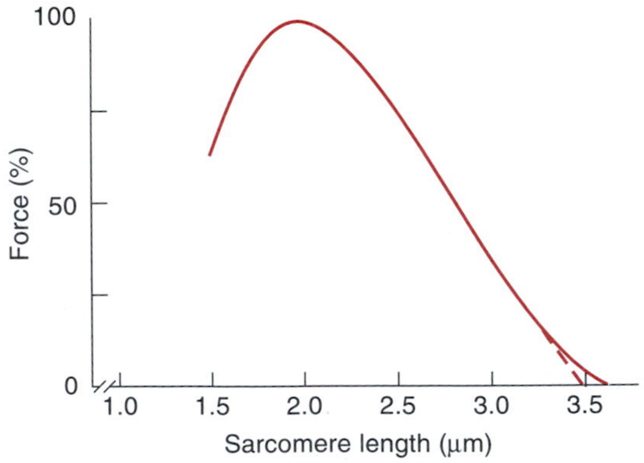

FIGURE 4-6 Relationship between muscle length and force development.

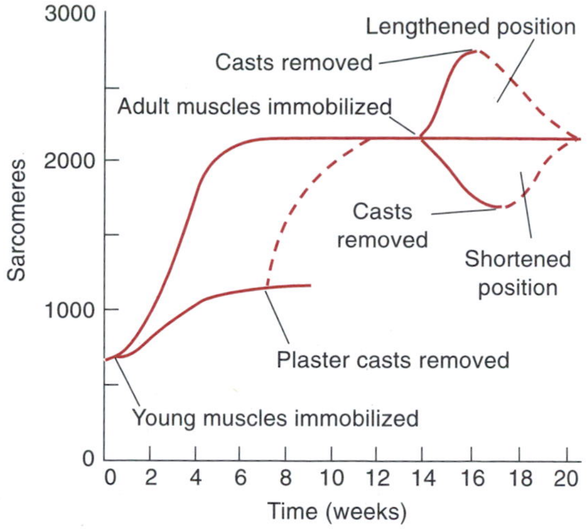

FIGURE 4-7 Changes in the number of sarcomeres in various conditions.

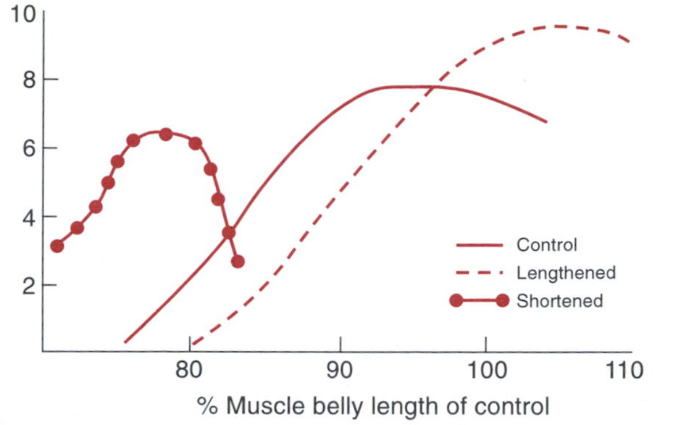

FIGURE 4-8 Changes in the length-tension relationship caused by length changes associated with immobilization.

new immobilized, shortened position.[23] In muscles immobilized or posturally held in a lengthened position, sarcomeres are added, and maximum tension is developed at the new increased length. When a cast is removed or posture restored, the sarcomere number returns to normal. The stimulus for sarcomere length changes may be the amount of tension along the myofibril or the myotendon junction, with high tension leading to an addition of sarcomeres and low tension to a subtraction of sarcomeres.[24]

The clinical implication of the length–tension relationship is that the evaluation of muscle "strength" must be reconsidered. Muscles that are shortened (eg, hip flexors) may test as strong as normal-length muscles, because the manual muscle test position is a shortened position.[25] Conversely, the lengthened muscle (eg, gluteus medius on the high iliac crest side) tests weak, because the manual muscle test occurs at a relatively shortened range, which is an insufficient position. According to animal studies,[26] the short muscles should develop the least peak tension, followed by the normal-length muscle and the lengthened muscle, which develops the greatest peak tension. This finding reflects the greater number of sarcomeres in series (Fig. 4-8). The lengthened muscle may be interpreted as weak although it is capable of producing substantial tension at the appropriate point in the range. This phenomena is called *positional strength*. A muscle should be tested at multiple points in the range to determine whether the muscle is positionally weak or weak throughout the range. The relationship between strength and length is called the length-tension property of muscle.

The emphasis of therapeutic exercise intervention should be on restoring normal length and tension development capability at the appropriate point in the range, rather than just strengthening the muscle. The positionally weak muscle should be strengthened isometrically in the shortened range, and the weak muscle should be strengthened dynamically throughout the range.

MUSCLE ARCHITECTURE

Fiber arrangements in different muscles vary according to whether the muscle is designed for high force generation or for a high rate of shortening (Fig. 4-9). Gans and Bock have provided an excellent review of the theoretical effects of muscle architecture and function (see Additional Reading).

To increase the effective cross-sectional area of muscles such as those in the lower leg, the muscle fibers are arranged in a chevron pattern. These are referred to as pennate or multipennate muscles. The penniform fiber allows more sarcomeres to be arranged in parallel at the expense of sarcomeres arranged in series, enhancing the muscle's force-producing capability. Given equal fiber lengths, the range of excursion through which a pennate muscle operates at an efficient sarcomere length is greater than that of a nonpennate muscle. A muscle that has pennate fibers can use the length-tension relationship more effectively than one in which the muscle fibers are arranged in parallel to the line of muscle action.[27]

Understanding muscle architecture is important in designing a rehabilitation program. Highly pennate muscles with short fibers and high cross-sectional areas are best suited for force production, and muscles with long fibers and smaller cross-sectional areas (ie, parallel fibers) are best suited for excursion; these fibers have a greater absolute working range than highly pennate muscles.[7] Parallel muscles are trained through a greater ROM than pennate muscles.

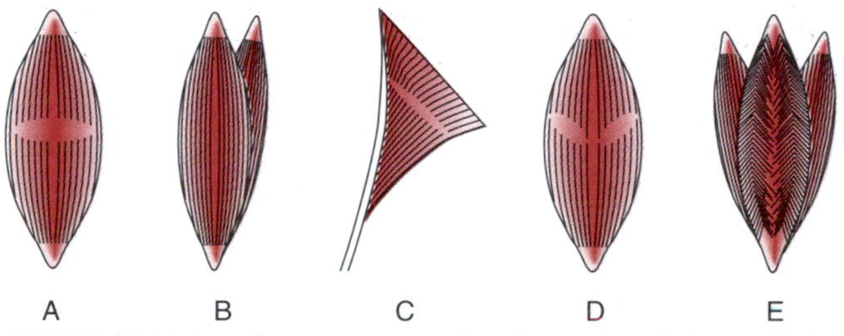

FIGURE 4-9 Various fiber arrangements found throughout the human body. ***(A** and **B)*** muscles adapted for a high overall rate of shortening have parallel fibers and are arranged in a fusiform manner. The fibers in muscles adapted for high force generation are arranged in a chevron-like fashion, which provides a larger effective fiber cross-sectional area, shown by the area encircled by the dotted lines. These are referred to as ***(C)*** pennate, ***(D)*** bipennate, or ***(E)*** multipennate muscles.

TRAINING SPECIFICITY

Training specificity suggests that "you get what you train for." This specificity is particularly significant in terms of training velocity.[28,29] The greatest training effects are evident when the same exercise type is used for testing and training, although this principle varies by muscle contraction types. A study of concentric and eccentric quadriceps training found specificity was related to eccentric training but not concentric training.[30] Concentric training showed increases only in concentric and isometric strength.[31] Studies have shown bilateral transfer; training one limb resulted in strength gains in the contralateral limb.[32] Further studies of bilateral versus unilateral training have shown improved bilateral scores when training bilaterally and improved unilateral scores when training unilaterally. These findings were consistent for upper extremity and lower extremity training.[33]

ROM specificity also exists; strength improvements are greatest at the joint angles exercised.[28] A study of eccentric training showed isometric strength gains that were joint angle specific, and a similar study of concentric training showed improvements throughout the range.[32]

The effects of posture on the specificity of training was assessed using squat and bench press lifts as the training tool. A variety of tests followed an 8-week training session that included skills such as vertical jump, 40-meter sprint, isokinetic tests, and a 6-second bout on a power bicycle. The authors found results to support the concept of posture specificity, because the exercise postures similar to the training postures enabled the greatest improvements.[34]

NEUROLOGIC ADAPTATION

Muscle performance is determined by the type and size of the involved muscles and by the ability of the nervous system to appropriately activate muscles. Activities requiring high force development require coordinated input from the neurologic system. The muscles responsible for producing the large force in the intended direction, called agonists, must be fully activated. Muscles that assist in coordinating the movement, called synergists, must be appropriately activated to ensure precision of rotating parts. Muscles producing force in the opposite direction of the agonists, called antagonists, must be appropriately activated or relaxed. For example, during a squat or step-up, the joint alignment and muscular recruitment patterns at the trunk, pelvis, hips, knees, ankles, and feet can alter which muscles are trained. The nervous system control for resistive exercises such as the squat is complex. When an unfamiliar exercise is introduced into the resistive exercise program, the early increase in strength partially results from adaptive changes in the nervous system control. The clinician must ensure appropriate nervous system control over the movement pattern for the desired outcome. Inappropriate instruction or failure to monitor the exercise can render it ineffective or detrimental to the expected outcome.

DeLorme and Watkins[35] hypothesize that the initial increase in strength after progressive resistance exercise occurs at a rate greater than can be accounted for by muscle morphologic changes. The initial rapid increases in strength probably result from motor learning. When a new exercise is introduced, neural adaptation predominates in the first several weeks of training as the individual masters the coordination necessary to perform the exercise efficiently. Subsequently, hypertrophic factors gradually dominate over neural factors in the gain in muscle performance.[36] Although neurologic adaptations were once thought to dominate in the first few weeks of training, Staron and colleagues[37] found that morphologic changes begin to occur in the second week of training.

Other adaptations, such as the ability to fire motor units at very high rates to develop power, may require a longer period of training to attain and be lost more rapidly during detraining.[38] In the long term, further improvement in performance critically depends on the way the muscles are activated by the nervous system during training.[39]

MUSCLE FATIGUE

Muscle fatigue may be defined as a reversible decrease in contractile strength that occurs after long-lasting or repeated muscular activity.[40] Human fatigue is a complex phenomenon that includes failure at more than one site along the chain of events that leads to muscle fiber stimulation. Fatigue involves a central component, which puts an upper limit to the number of command signals that are sent to the muscles, and a peripheral component. Peripheral changes in cross-bridge function associated with fatigue include a slight decrease in number of interacting cross-bridges, reduced force output of the individual cross-bridge, and reduced speed of cycling of the bridges during muscle shortening.

It is beyond the scope of this text to review the complex mechanisms related to muscle fatigue. More specific information regarding muscle endurance prescription can be found in Chapter 5. When the patient is performing resistive training, the clinician must be alert for signs of fatigue. Fatigue can lead to substitution or injury. The dosage for resistive exercise is often limited to form fatigue, the point at which the individual must discontinue the exercise or sacrifice exercise form.

Quality of motion usually is the most important factor in prescribing any exercise. With resistive exercise, the patient cannot expect gains in force or torque production unless the muscle is recruited during the movement pattern. Because synergists can readily dominate a movement pattern, allowing the motion to occur but compromising the quality of motion, care must be taken to ensure precision of motion during all exercise prescription. After the form is compromised (ie, form fatigue), the exercise should stop. Continuing to exercise with poor form compromises the outcome and may be detrimental.

An example of the importance of form is the traditional sit-up and the effect of holding the feet down while the trunk raises forward. Kendall[25] provides a detailed analysis of muscle function during the sit-up. For the curled-trunk sit-up to be used as a technique or test of abdominal strength, the ability to flex the trunk must be differentiated from the ability to flex the hips. The trunk flexion phase must precede the hip flexion phase in the trunk raising movement (Fig. 4-10). When the feet are free, the pelvis tilts posteriorly as the head and shoulders are raised to initiate trunk flexion. With the feet held down, the hip flexors are given distal fixation, and the trunk raising may become a hip flexion activity with minimal trunk flexion (Fig. 4-11). The trunk flexion phase is bypassed, and the motion is pri-

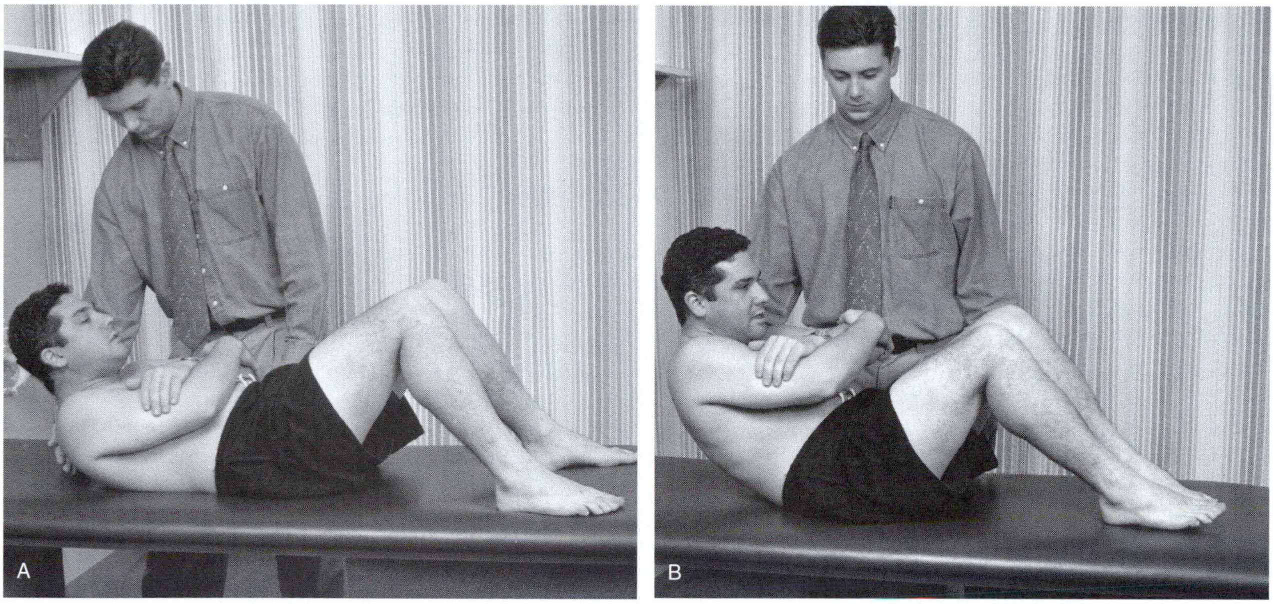

FIGURE 4-10 Two phases of a sit-up. ***(A)*** Trunk curl phase. ***(B)*** Hip flexion phase.

marily hip flexion. Recruitment of the abdominals is minimized, and recruitment of the hip flexors is maximized. When performing abdominal curls (especially with the feet held), the individual may exhibit proper technique for a few repetitions but then slip into faulty technique, or form fatigue, when the abdominal muscles fatigue. With the feet free, abdominal muscle fatigue results in an inability to complete the trunk curl. The feet raise in an attempt to use the hip flexors, but without distal fixation, they are rendered insufficient and unable to lift the trunk upward. To ensure testing or training of the abdominal muscles' ability to flex the trunk before the hip flexion phase is initiated, the feet must not be held down during the trunk flexion phase.

As in the previous example, the proper exercise may be prescribed but performed incorrectly, therefore not achieving the desired result of increased abdominal strength. It is not good enough to perform the exercise; it must be performed correctly and with the appropriate recruitment pattern. A person cannot strengthen a muscle that is not being recruited.

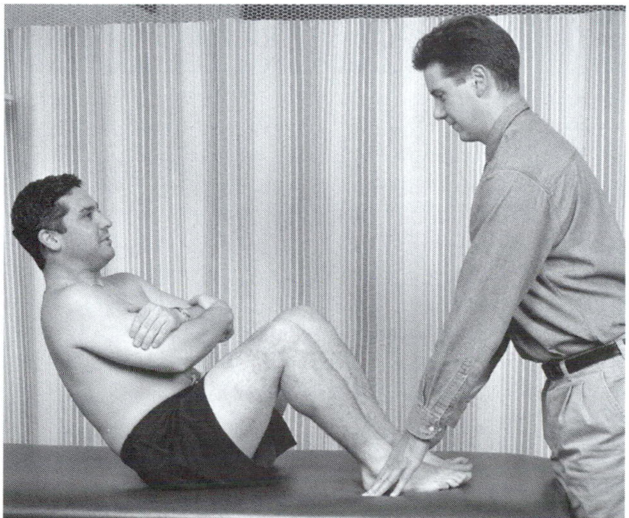

FIGURE 4-11 Improperly performed sit-up, with only a hip flexion phase.

AGE

Prepuberty

Only about 20% of a newborn child's body mass is muscle tissue. The infant is weak, and muscular strengthening in the first months takes place by spontaneous movements. These movements should not be limited by tight clothes or constant bundling of the newborn. However, the infant and toddler should not be burdened with systematic resistive training; normal developmental progression provides an appropriate stimulus for the development of an optimal amount of muscular strength.

In the prepubertal phase, muscle mass increases parallel to body mass. Moderate strength training is recommended, but higher burdens should be avoided because of the sensitivity of joint structures, especially at the epiphyses of bones. Resistive training at this age should focus on technique and the neurologic aspects of training. Maximum lifts are contraindicated, and submaximal resistive training focused on form is indicated (8 to 12 repetitions per set or more). During prepuberty, there are no differences between girls and boys with respect to trainability for strength. Boys have a small genetic advantage, which is completely compensated by the developmental advantage of girls.[41] There is no biologic basis for a sex-dependent difference in strength performance. Any difference in the strength between girls and boys, particularly in the shoulders and arms, appears to result from social expectations and gender roles in society.

Puberty

The ability to improve strength increases rapidly during puberty, particularly in boys. The increase in male sexual hormones is significant because of their anabolic (ie, protein-incorporating) component. During maturation, the proportion of muscle in boys increases from 27% to 40% of body mass. With the onset of puberty, the strengths of girls and boys diverge markedly. On average, the strength of girls is 90% that of boys at 11 to 12 years of age, 85% at 13 to 14 years, and 75% at 15 to 16 years. Although this gender difference has a biologic basis, it does not completely account for the differences seen, suggesting continued societal influences.

General strength training is recommended during this phase. Optimal strength and muscular balance is critical for the quickly growing skeleton. Some precautions during strength exercise are still warranted. The epiphyses remain sensitive and liable to injury. Heavy loads, unilateral burdens, or faulty techniques should be avoided to prevent epiphyseal damage.

Early Adulthood

Strength potential is at its highest in the 18- to 30-year period.[42] The competent biologic structures show a state of good adaptability, the joints tolerate high loads, and the social situation makes specific use of strength necessary. Most individuals are actively involved in physical activity without the responsibility of working long hours. During this period, emphasis should be placed on a balanced fitness program for cardiopulmonary fitness, muscle strength, and flexibility.

Middle Age

The decrement of strength during this phase of life must be differentiated according to training activities, gender, and body area. Training for as little as 2 hours or more each week is sufficient to positively influence strength. A small amount of training increases the difference between active and inactive persons with increasing age. Persons from white-collar professions have the same or even more strength than persons from blue-collar professions; leisure time activities account more for existing strength than professional demands.[43]

Advanced Age

The body can adapt to strengthening exercise throughout the lifespan. It is possible to reverse existing muscular weakness in old age.[44] Strength increases result from relatively low stimuli because of the marked atrophy present at the onset of training in many elderly individuals. A study of older men (mean age, 70 years) demonstrated that the training-induced strength gains resulted from neural factors, as indicated by the increases in maximal integrated electromyography (IEMG) in the absence of hypertrophy.[45] Neural factors are a significant mechanism by which older subjects increase strength in the absence of any significant evidence of hypertrophy. In general, fatigability increases with advancing age, and older muscles require a longer period of recovery after strenuous exertion. The rest periods during a training session and adequate intervals between sessions should be extended for elderly persons.

The decrease in muscle performance with advancing age affects men and women differently. The absolute decline in strength is less steep in women than in men. Parts of the body are also affected differently. The arms are more affected than the trunk and legs, probably because of less use of the upper extremities in strength-related activities. Active elderly women surpass inactive men with respect to trunk muscle strength.

Adequate muscle strength helps to prevent or moderate the symptoms of degenerative changes of the joints. Resistive exercise by the elderly should be directed toward the muscles susceptible to atrophic changes.[46] Priority should be given to the deep neck flexors, scapular stabilizers, abdominal muscles, gluteal muscles, and quadriceps. Unjustifiably, little attention is paid to strength of the ventilatory muscles (ie, diaphragm) and pelvic floor muscles. See Chapters 18 through 27 for resistive exercises for the spine, shoulder, arm, hip, knee, and pelvic floor.

With advancing age, the social needs and individual motivation for the use of strength lessen; the atrophy reflects the effects of disuse, not mere age-related changes. The voluntary and deliberate use of the motor system in daily life activities and intentional resistive training are able to counteract the loss of muscle mass with increasing age. The vigorous use of muscles, particularly among old persons, improves their health and sense of well-being.

COGNITIVE ASPECTS OF PERFORMANCE

The cognitive or mental aspects of strength and performance are most easily seen in elite athletes. The use of mental imagery techniques such as visualization and positive self-talk has been supported by sport psychologists and athletes alike. Positive cognitive strategies can enhance strength and performance, and negative strategies may have a negative or negligible impact. A study of different mental preparation techniques (ie, arousal, attention, imagery, self-efficacy, and control-read conditions) showed that preparatory arousal and self-efficacy techniques produced greater posttest strength performance than in the control group.[47] A similar study showed no difference among the mental preparation conditions, but all performed significantly better than a control group.[48]

Some types of mental preparation can have a negligible or negative impact on strength performance. A study of relaxation-visualization training by non–strength-trained men showed poorer knee extensor measures for them than a control group. The investigators suggested that this training diverted their full concentration away from the exercise task.[49] A mental task requiring subjects to imagine situations making them angry or fearful produced increased levels of arousal but no change in strength performance.[50]

A study of the impact of imagery, preparatory arousal, and counting backward on hand grip strength found imagery to enhance grip strength in older and younger subjects.[51] Gould and coworkers[52] found that imagery and preparatory arousal improved strength performance. Different kinds of imagery and their impacts on power and endurance activities (ie, seated shot-put and push-ups to exhaustion) were furthered studied. Results showed that all imagery techniques had a positive impact and that using metaphors was particularly effective in improving power and endurance measures.[53]

A study looking at the knowledge of results of isokinetic peak torque output found that visual knowledge of results provided an important error-correction function. The researchers suggested that this type of training may help patients develop cognitive strategies that can be used to guide performance in clinical and nonclinical settings.[54] Results of all these studies suggest that mental preparation and the current mental state can affect strength performance. This should be considered when performing and interpreting the results of resistive tests.

EFFECTS OF ALCOHOL

The deleterious effects of alcohol abuse on muscle have been well documented.[55] The myopathic changes seen in the alcoholic patient have at times been attributed to malnutrition or disuse. Experiments have demonstrated that, even with nutritional support and prophylactic exercise, normal subjects can develop alcoholic myopathy if they ingest large amounts of ethanol.[56]

Alcoholic myopathy has two clinical phases: an acutely painful presentation that follows "binges" and a chronic phase that consists of morphologic and functional alterations in muscle.[57] Acute alcoholic myopathy has morphologic features, such as fiber necrosis, intracellular edema, hemorrhage, and inflammatory changes, that can be seen under light microscope. Binges by chronic alcoholics can result in an acute myopathy characterized by muscle cramps, muscle weakness, tenderness, myoglobinuria, reduced muscle phosphorylase activity, and decreased lactate response to ischemic exercise. Exercise is contraindicated for persons with acute myopathy and those with myoglobinuria, because it may stress an already compromised system.

Changes seen in chronic alcoholic myopathy include intracellular edema, lipid droplets, excessive glycogen deposition, deranged elements of the sarcoplasmic reticulum, and abnormal mitochondria. Type II fiber atrophy has also been attributed to chronic alcohol abuse.[58] Type II atrophy suggests that alcoholic patients may exhibit specific deficits in muscle performance, such as an inability to generate tension rapidly and to produce power. For many patients, abstinence leads to full recovery of muscle function, but for others, the injury may be more severe and resistant to treatment, and this must be considered as a comorbidity when projecting the prognosis.

EFFECTS OF CORTICOSTEROIDS

The widespread use of oral corticosteroid agents as anti-inflammatory and immunosuppressant agents has led to cases of steroid atrophy.[59] The primary biopsy finding in patients treated with prednisone-like steroids (eg, prednisone, prednisolone, methylprednisolone) is type II fiber atrophy.[59] This reduction is thought to be most pronounced in type IIB fibers[60] and is believed to occur more often in women than men.[61] Corticosteroids are a potent catabolic stimuli, and the atrophy caused by prolonged corticosteroid use occurs as protein degradation exceeds protein synthesis. Goldberg[62] believes that the constant use of the type I fibers during normal voluntary movement provides these fibers with a protective or sparing influence from the catabolic effects of steroids. Exercises recruiting type II muscle fibers may protect them from steroid-induced atrophy. Normal function can be expected to return within 1 year or, more often, within several months after steroid use has stopped.[61]

CAUSES AND EFFECTS OF DECREASED MUSCLE PERFORMANCE

Muscle performance can be impaired for a variety of reasons. Central or peripheral neurologic pathology decreases an individual's ability to effectively recruit and functionally use his muscles. Injury to the muscle from a strain or contusion decreases performance, as does disuse or deconditioning for any reason. Each of these situations necessitates a thorough evaluation to match each problem with the optimal resistive technique. The progression and precautions are different for each situation.

Neurologic Pathology

Individuals with nerve root pathology may present with muscle performance impairments in the nerve root distribution. For example, nerve root compression at the L4–L5 spinal level can produce quadriceps femoris weakness, and nerve root compression at the C5–C6 spinal level can result in deltoid and biceps weakness. Sensory changes usually precede muscle performance changes, but individuals with more severe pathology may have sensory and motor changes. Therapeutic exercise intervention depends on the prognosis for the nerve root involvement. If the changes are relatively recent and resolution of the nerve root compression is expected through conservative or surgical management, preventive and protective measures are taken. Resistive exercise focuses on spine-stabilizing musculature and the peripheral muscles innervated by the spinal segment. Peripherally, resistive exercise maintains what strength the individual has while training synergists to provide functional support. Centrally, resistive exercise trains postural and stabilizing musculature to effectively support the spine. After the mechanical or chemical cause of impaired muscle performance is removed, specific, localized resistive exercise of the involved musculature is often indicated.

Neurologic weakness may result from a peripheral nerve injury. Compromise of the median nerve at the carpal tunnel, the radial nerve at the cubital tunnel, or the common peroneal nerve at the fibular head are examples of such injury. The pattern of sensory loss and weakness depends on which nerve and where along the nerve's course the damage occurs. Some peripheral nerve entrapments have only a motor component, others have only a sensory component, and some are mixed. The innervating motor units influence an individual's ability to generate muscular force. Resistive exercise focuses on strengthening the muscles that are intact and on training synergists to provide functional support. Exercise should try to maintain muscle balance and efficient movement patterns without developing a dominant muscle group that overrides other muscle action. Splinting, bracing, taping, or other supportive measures may be necessary to maintain balance.

Other neurologic conditions include neuromuscular disease such as multiple sclerosis, postpolio syndrome, and Guillain-Barré syndrome, and muscular paralysis or paresis because of spinal cord injury. Resistive exercise programs must consider the prognosis and tailor the exercises appropriately. In situations such as Guillain-Barré syndrome, certain cases of spinal cord injury, and progressive stages of multiple sclerosis, some recovery is expected. Exercise programs focus on maintaining strength in intact musculature and gently strengthening weakened muscles as recovery and remission advances. Care must be taken to avoid fatiguing these weakened muscles during strengthening exercises. Dosage parameters generally include several short exercise sessions of a few repetitions interspersed throughout the day. During quiescent periods of diseases such as multiple sclerosis, a general conditioning program of balanced strengthening and mobility exercises is appropriate. When recovery is not expected, resistive exercise programs emphasize functional strength of remaining musculature. This includes strength for functional activities such as self-care, transfers, and mobility. Care must be taken to avoid overworking these muscles. Unlike persons with full innervation who use their muscles efficiently, the individual with paralysis uses the few innervated muscles they have for nearly all their activities. The potential for overuse injuries is very high.

Muscle Strain

Muscle strain occurs along a continuum from acute macrotraumatic injury to chronic microtraumatic overuse injuries (see Chapter 10). Resistive exercise in the treatment of muscle strain injuries depends on where along this continuum the injury occurs. Resistive exercise that neither overloads nor underloads the tissue is optimal. Determining this resistance dosage is the challenge.

Acute traumatic injuries occur when a muscle is rapidly overloaded or overstretched and the tension generated exceeds the tensile capability of the musculotendinous unit.[63] These injuries occur near the musculotendinous junction and at random areas within the muscle belly. The hamstring muscle is a common site of muscle strain injury. A combination of insufficient strength, reduced extensibility, inadequate warm-up, and fatigue has been implicated in hamstring injuries[64] (see Patient-Related Instruction: Preventing Muscle Strain). Strength, extensibility, and fatigue resistance protect a muscle from strain injury. Eccentric loading is a common mechanism of muscle strain injury, and a muscle prepared for eccentric loading is less likely to sustain an injury. Eccentric loading should be an integral part of any resistance training program. A program to prevent muscle strain injuries should include dynamic resistive exercises with a strong eccentric component, balanced flexibility exercises, an appropriate warm-up before activity, and attention to fatigue levels (see Selected Intervention: Lateral Kicks). The rehabilitation program after injury should focus on these factors.

Muscles may also be injured from chronic overuse. Muscular forearm pain is common in workers doing continuous repetitive elbow, wrist, and hand activities. The iliotibial band and tensor fascia latae muscle are also injured as a result of continuous overuse. A thorough evaluation can determine the source of the overuse problem. The problem may result from too much activity. This happens in the upper extremity during repetitive work or hobbies. The lower extremity can be affected in workers required to stand or walk for extended periods and in recreational distance runners who spend too much time on their feet. In other cases, the overuse is a result of an imbalance that can be corrected with postural or motor program re-education and resistive exercises. For example, as the shoulder muscles fatigue during repetitive work, substitution with distal musculature occurs. Resistive exercise should be directed at the proximal shoulder muscles, followed by the distal muscles. Work site assessment is necessary to prevent a recurrence of the muscle performance impairment. If left untreated, this impairment can quickly lead to disability. The same is true for the overuse problems seen in the lower extremity. For example, strain resulting from muscle dominance overuse is managed by reducing the loads imposed on the strained muscle. When the tensor fascia latae dominates over the iliopsoas during hip flexion and gluteus medius during abduction, the tensor fascia latae is at risk for an overuse strain. Improving the strength and recruitment patterns of the iliopsoas and gluteus medius can reduce the load on the tensor fascia latae and allow it to recover. Postural habits (eg, standing in medial rotation) and movement patterns (eg, hip flexion or abduction with medial rotation) must also be modified to improve recruitment of the underused synergists.

Another subtle form of muscle strain is gradual, continuous overstretching, which occurs when a muscle is continuously placed in a relatively lengthened, tension-producing position. For example, the lower trapezius in a person with forward shoulders is subjected to continuous tension and has adapted to a lengthened state. This overstretch injury results in strain, and the muscle is at risk for two forms of muscle weakness, one from length changes and the other from overstretch strain.

Patient education is a key component of the rehabilitation program in the case of muscle strain from continuous overstretch. In the lower trapezius example, the patient needs to be educated about optimal postural habits to reduce tension on the lower trapezius. Improving postural habits and reducing tension on the lower trapezius may allow it to adapt to a new shortened length and achieve more optimal length-tension relationships.

> ***Patient-Related Instruction***
>
> ### Preventing Muscle Strain
>
> Although some muscle strains are not preventable, precautions can reduce your risk of injury.
>
> 1. Warm-up before a vigorous activity; 5 to 7 minutes of a large muscle group activity such as walking, jogging, or cycling should suffice. This should be enough activity to break a sweat.
> 2. Stretch tight muscles after your general warm-up. Stretch each muscle for 15 to 30 seconds.
> 3. Balance your sports or other leisure activities with strengthening exercises. Your clinician can help you focus on muscles susceptible to injury.
> 4. Avoid fatigue during the activity. Fatigue can increase your risk of injury.

Disuse and Deconditioning

Muscle performance may be impaired because of disuse or deconditioning for a variety of reasons. Illness, surgery, spe-

SELECTED INTERVENTION
Lateral Kicks

See Case Study #1

Although this patient requires comprehensive intervention as described in other chapters, only one exercise related to resistive training is described. This exercise would be used in the late phase of this patient's rehabilitation.

ACTIVITY: Resisted hip abduction and ankle eversion

PURPOSE: To increase the muscle performance of the ankle evertor and hip abductor muscles

STAGE OF MOTOR CONTROL: Controlled mobility

MODE: Resistive band

POSTURE: Standing with one foot on the resistive band and the band around the other foot. A support should be readily available for balance as needed.

MOVEMENT: Standing on the uninjured leg, abduct the hip and evert (pronate) the ankle. Maintain good spinal posture throughout the exercise. Return to the start position.

DOSAGE: Two to three sets per day to form fatigue. If patient does not fatigue by 30 to 40 repetitions, increase the resistance of the band.

EXPLANATION OF PURPOSE OF EXERCISE: This exercise increases muscle performance in the hip abductors and ankle evertors in a coordinated fashion. It may be progressed to a higher speed to challenge stability.

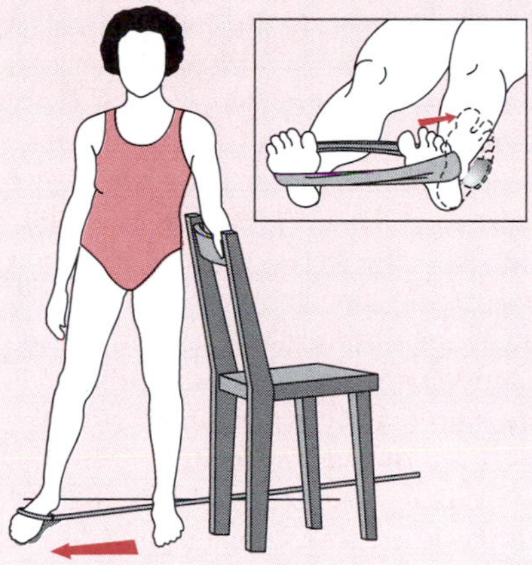

cific physical conditions (eg, pregnancy with twins), or injury may necessitate a period of decreased activity. Subtle muscle imbalances can lead to overuse of one muscle and to disuse and deconditioning of another.

Illness or injury are common causes of deconditioning. For example, illness such as pneumonia or an injury such as a herniated disk can result in a period of decreased activity and subsequent deconditioning. In these situations, total-body deconditioning occurs, and general conditioning is necessary. However, specific exercises also may be necessary to improve muscle performance and prevent secondary impairments. For example, an elderly individual may have relatively asymptomatic osteoarthritis until a bout with pneumonia produces general deconditioning. Subsequently, knee osteoarthritis becomes symptomatic because of impaired muscle performance in the lower extremity muscles involved in gait and other functional activities. Specific resistive exercises to recondition those muscles are necessary to restore this individual's function and prevent further disability.

Reduced activity levels can impair muscle performance in a similar manner. Multiparous pregnancies, exacerbation of a musculoskeletal injury, an episode of colitis, or social factors such as major life changes (eg, job, school, divorce, family illness, death) can reduce activity levels and result in impaired muscle performance. For example, regular exercise may keep a woman's patellofemoral malalignment from becoming symptomatic. When her activity level decreases in the late stages of pregnancy, the combination of decreased activity, weight gain, and hormonal changes produces symptoms at the patellofemoral joint. Selective resistive exercises combined with patient education can prevent this exacerbation. Resistive exercises in the case of overall decreased activity must consider the muscles most likely to be affected, the patient's desired activity level and preference, and any underlying or residual medical conditions.

An often overlooked source of deconditioning or disuse is a subtle muscle imbalance. When activating muscles for a functional movement, the body chooses the most efficient muscular and motor unit activation pattern. Certain motor units in a muscle may be preferentially recruited when a muscle is engaged in a particular task.[65] For example, motor units in the lateral portion of the long head of the biceps are preferentially activated when this muscle is engaged in elbow flexion, whereas motor units in the medial portion are preferentially activated in forearm supination. The recruitment thresholds of motor units in a muscle are also influenced by the type of muscle actions associated with a movement. In elbow flexion, biceps motor units have a lower threshold in slow concentric and eccentric actions than isometric actions; the reverse is true for the brachialis.[66] The recruitment thresholds of motor units of a muscle active in a movement may also be affected by changes in joint angle.[67] Some muscles or portions of a muscle may be overused while other portions are disused, and the resistive rehabilitation program must acknowledge this imbalance. In the previous example, instruction in resisted elbow flexion may exacerbate the imbalance rather than improve muscle performance.

EXAMINATION AND EVALUATION OF MUSCLE PERFORMANCE

Decreases in muscle performance may occur for a number of reasons. A thorough examination is necessary to determine the link between impaired muscle performance and functional limitations or disabilities. After that link is established, the treatment must be matched to the cause of impaired muscle performance. The muscle test is only one small part of the examination process and must be used with additional information (eg, mobility, balance, gait, sensory, reflex) to determine the cause of impaired muscle performance.

The tests and measures recommended by the *Guide to Physical Therapist Practice* (Display 4-2) ensure comprehensive assessment of the patient's impairments, functional limitations, and disability. Within the examination is a subset of measures specific to the performance of the muscle. These tests include an analysis of functional muscle strength, power, or endurance; manual muscle tests; dynamometry; and electrophysiologic testing.

Manual muscle testing is the most fundamental of all strength tests. Length-tension relationships, muscle imbalance, and positional weakness must be considered when choosing manual muscle test positions. Close attention to substitution patterns and testing in a variety of positions minimizes the chance of erroneous results. When used reliably, hand-held dynamometers can provide muscle performance information that is more reliable than that of tests using the traditional criteria of 0 through 5.

Isokinetic dynamometers are commonly used to assess muscle performance. Computerized systems provide tremendous data reduction capabilities. Tests can be performed at a variety of speeds and comparisons made with antagonists, the contralateral limb, normative standards, or previous test results. These tools provide reliable data that can be used to assess progress, as a motivator, or as a criteria for progression to more advanced rehabilitation phases. A variety of muscle actions can be assessed using this equipment.

Dynamic strength can also be determined using the repetition maximum (RM) method; 1 RM is the maximum amount of weight that can be lifted *x* number of times. For example, a 10 RM is the maximum amount of weight that can be lifted 10 times, and a 1 RM is the maximum amount of weight that can be lifted once. The amount of weight that can be lifted for a given number of repetitions can be determined and compared with that for the antagonist, the opposite limb, or to a previous test result.

The magnitude of measured increases in force or torque depends on how similar the test is to the training exercise.[68] For example, if athletes train their legs by doing the squat exercise, the increase in strength measured as maximal squatting is much greater than the strength increase measured in isometric leg press or knee extension tests. This specificity of movement pattern in strength training probably reflects the role of learning and coordination.[69] Improved coordination takes the form of the most efficient activation of all of the involved muscles and the most efficient activation of motor units within each muscle involved. Testing force production in the manner in which the muscle has been trained reflects the morphologic and neurologic adaptations.

DISPLAY 4-2

Tests and Measures to Assess the Patient With Impaired Muscle Performance

- History
- Systems review
- Aerobic capacity and endurance evaluation
- Anthropometric characteristics
- Assistive and adaptive device analysis
- Community and work integration or reintegration
- Environmental, home, and work barriers
- Ergonomics and body mechanics
- Gait, locomotion, and balance
- Joint integrity and mobility
- Muscle performance (including strength, power, and endurance)
- Orthotic, protective, and supportive devices
- Pain
- Posture
- Range of motion (including muscle length)
- Self-care and home management
- Sensory integrity
- Ventilation, respiration, and circulation

THERAPEUTIC EXERCISE INTERVENTION FOR IMPAIRED MUSCLE PERFORMANCE

Physiologic Adaptations to Resistive Exercise

The benefits of resistive exercise extend beyond the obvious improvements in muscle performance to include positive effects on the cardiovascular system, connective tissue, and bone. Moreover, these effects translate into function. Individuals perform their daily activities with more ease because they are functioning at a lower percentage of their maximum capacity. Improved functioning also enhances the patient's sense of well-being and independence.

MUSCLE

The most obvious benefits of resistive training are for the muscular system. Regular resistive exercise is associated with several positive adaptations, most of which are dosage dependent (Table 4-1). The cross-sectional area of the muscle increases as a result of an increase in the myofibrillar volume of individual muscle fibers, fiber splitting, and potentially an increase in the number of muscle fibers. This cross-sectional area increase primarily results from preferential hypertrophy of type II fibers. Changes in the muscle depend on fiber type and the stimulus. Hypertrophy of fast-twitch fibers occurs when all or most of the fibers are being recruited and is considered an adaptation for increased power output. Slow-twitch fibers hypertrophy in response to frequent recruitment. In repetitive, low-intensity activ-

Table 4-1. PHYSIOLOGIC ADAPTATIONS TO RESISTANCE TRAINING.

VARIABLE	RESULT AFTER RESISTANCE TRAINING
Performance	
Muscle strength	Increases
Muscle endurance	Increases for high power output
Aerobic power	No change or increases slightly
Maximal rate of force production	Increases
Vertical jump	Ability increases
Anaerobic power	Increases
Sprint speed	Improves
Muscle Fibers	
Fiber size	Increases
Capillary density	No change or decreases
Mitochondrial density	Decreases
Fast heavy-chain myosin	Amount increases
Enzyme Activity	
Creatine phosphokinase	Increases
Myokinase	Increases
Phosphofructokinase	Increases
Lactate dehydrogenase	No change or variable
Metabolic Energy Stores	
Stored ATP	Increases
Stored creatine phosphate	Increases
Stored glycogen	Increases
Stored triglycerides	May increase
Connective Tissue	
Ligament strength	May increase
Tendon strength	May increase
Collagen content	May increase
Bone density	No change or increase
Body Composition	
Percentage of body fat	Decreases
Fat-free mass	Increases

Adapted from Falkel JE, Cipriani DJ. Physiological principles of resistance training and rehabilitation. In: Zachazewski JE, Magee DJ, Quillen WS, eds. *Athletic Injuries and Rehabilitation.* Philadelphia: WB. Saunders; 1996:211.

ity, fast-twitch fibers are rarely recruited, and these fibers may atrophy while the slow-twitch fibers hypertrophy. A study by Staron and colleagues[37] examined the differences in the proportion of muscle fiber types in distance runners, weight lifters, and sedentary controls. The investigators found the weight lifters had a greater proportion of type IIA fibers and had a greater type IIA fiber area than the controls or distance runners.[70] Specificity of resistive training exists and must be considered when designing a training program.

Other changes occur on cellular and systemic levels. The capillary density is unchanged or decreases, and the mitochondrial density decreases. Some of these changes result from their number relative to total muscle volume. Although protein volume and cross-sectional area increase in response to resistive training, some of the cellular or systemic factors may remain unchanged, giving the perception of a decrease, although the decrease is only relative.

Energy sources necessary to fuel muscle contraction increase after resistive training. In general, levels of creatine phosphate, ATP, myokinase, and phosphofructokinase increase in response to a resistive exercise program.[71–74] Lactate dehydrogenase is variably changed.[72]

Neural adaptations occur with resistive training. Studies have shown increases in the muscle's ability to produce torque and increased neural activation, as measured by electromyography (EMG).[38] Increases in muscle activity were also seen after resistive training that consisted of explosive jumping. Increased EMG values associated with greater power and maximal contraction were attributed to a combination of increased motor unit recruitment and increased firing rate of each unit.[75]

CONNECTIVE TISSUE

Although disuse and inactivity cause atrophy and weakening of connective tissues such as tendon and ligament, physical training can increase the maximum tensile strength and the amount of energy absorbed before failure.[76] Physical activity returns damaged tendons and ligaments to normal tensile strength values faster than complete rest.[77] Physical training, particularly resistive exercise, may alter tendon and ligament structures to make them larger, stronger, and more resistant to injury.

BONE

Weightlessness[78] and immobilization[79] can cause profound loss of bone density and mass. Weight-bearing activities that recruit antigravity muscles can maintain or enhance bone density and mass.[80] Weight training, particularly with a weight-bearing component, can substantially alter bone mineral density. Individuals in sports requiring repeated high-force movements such as weight lifting and throwing events have higher bone densities than distance runners and soccer players or swimmers.[81] Regular tennis players have higher bone density in their dominant forearms, and professional pitchers have greater bone density in the dominant humerus.[82] A 5-month study of weight training compared with jogging found that weight training produced significantly better increases in lumbar bone density than the aerobic exercise.[83]

These studies suggest that regular exercise, specifically exercise such as resistive training, can maintain or improve bone density. Resistive training to improve bone density is important for women of all ages.

CARDIOVASCULAR SYSTEM

Resistive training benefits the cardiovascular system. The idea that strength training causes hypertension is erroneous. Most reports show that highly strength-trained athletes have average or lower than average systolic and diastolic blood pressures.[84] When performed properly and heeding the proper precautions, strength training can have a positive effect on the cardiovascular system.

Increased intrathoracic or intra-abdominal pressures may affect cardiac output and blood pressure during resistive exercise. In the classic model, increased intrathoracic pressures are thought to decrease venous return to the heart and decrease cardiac output. Intrathoracic pressure is inversely related to cardiac output and stroke volume and directly related to systolic and diastolic blood pressure during resistive exercise. Increased intrathoracic pressures may limit venous return and decrease cardiac output while simultaneously causing an accumulation of blood in the systemic circulation that may increase blood pressure. Performing resistive exercises with a Valsalva maneuver, which elevates intrathoracic pressure, leads to a greater blood pressure response than performance of the exercise without a Valsalva maneuver.[85] Instructing the patient to breathe properly during exercise may reduce the increase in blood pressure often seen during exercise.

Increased intramuscular pressure during resistive exercise may result in increased total peripheral resistance and increased blood pressure. Mechanically induced increases in peripheral resistance probably are the cause of higher blood pressures during isometric and concentric exercise compared with pressures during eccentric exercise.[86] Isometric or concentric exercise combined with a Valsalva maneuver can produce the greatest increase in blood pressure. This combination should be avoided, especially by individuals at risk for elevated blood pressure (see the Precautions and Contraindications section).

Resistive exercise does result in a pressor response that affects the cardiovascular system by causing hypertension through exciting the vasoconstrictor center, which leads to increased peripheral resistance. If precautions are taken to ensure proper breathing and avoid isometric contractions in persons at risk for a pressor response, resistive exercise's benefits outweigh the risks. Long-term performance of resistive exercise can result in positive adaptations of the cardiovascular system at rest and during work. Cardiovascular adaptations to resistive training are summarized in Display 4-3.

Activities to Increase Muscle Performance

The specific activities and dosage chosen to improve muscle performance depend on many factors, including the individual's age and medical condition, muscles involved, activity level, goals, and cause of decreased muscle performance. The following sections describe the activities used to increase muscle performance and their relative risks and benefits. The clinician must match the appropriate training mode to the patient's needs.

DISPLAY 4-3
Benefits of Strength Training on the Cardiovascular System

- Decreased heart rate
- Decreased or unchanged systolic blood pressure
- Decreased or unchanged diastolic blood pressure
- Increased or unchanged cardiac output
- Increased or unchanged stroke volume
- Increased or unchanged maximal oxygen consumption
- Decreased or unchanged total cholesterol

ISOMETRIC EXERCISE

Isometric exercise is commonly used to increase muscle performance. Although no joint movement occurs, isometric exercise is functional because it provides a strength base for dynamic exercise and because many postural muscles work primarily in an isometric fashion. Isometric exercise is a valuable rehabilitation tool when joint motion is uncomfortable or contraindicated, during immobilization, or when weakness exists at a specific point in the ROM. Isometric exercise is used as a special technique in proprioceptive neuromuscular facilitation to enhance stability and strengthen muscles in a weak portion of the range. This resistive mode is easy to understand and perform correctly, requires no equipment, and can be performed in almost any setting. Isometric exercise is most effective when individuals are in a low state of training, because the benefits of isometric exercise decrease as the state of training increases. Most gains are made within the first 5 weeks of the onset of training.[87]

Some factors are important in choosing isometric exercise for rehabilitation. Isometric strength is specific to the joint angle. Studies have demonstrated isometric joint angle specificity, noting that strength gained at one joint angle did not predictably carry over to other joint angles.[88] Neuromuscular changes accounted for the joint-angle–dependent effects, and obtaining generalized strength gains required multiple-angle training programs. Whitley[89] found significantly increased strength at all joint angles after 10 weeks of training at specific joint angles. Others have found this general transfer, although only after training was well advanced.[88] In the beginning training phase, the strength gains were transferred only when the muscle was at shorter than resting length.

Because of the angle specificity, multiple-angle isometric training is recommended whenever possible. Isometric contractions should be performed every 15 to 20 degrees throughout the ROM, and each contraction should be held for approximately 6 seconds. The first few seconds of the first maximum contraction appears to trigger the major training effect. After the first few seconds, the ability to maintain a maximal contraction drops off dramatically. The contraction should be held long enough to fully activate all motor units, and it should be repeated frequently throughout the day. Isometric contractions have their greatest effect near maximal contraction, although this may not be possible in many clinical situations.

Isometric exercise is used for purposes other than muscle strength training. One of the benefits of isometric exercise is the ability to perform repetitive submaximal contractions as "reminder" or re-education exercises. Quadriceps sets are used after injury or surgery to maintain patellar mobility and to re-educate the person on how to activate the quadriceps. This prepares the patient for more advanced dynamic activities. Quadriceps sets and gluteal sets are also used to enhance circulation throughout the lower extremity during periods of bed rest.

Caution must be used when prescribing isometric exercise for patients with hypertension or known cardiac disease. Isometric exercise can produce a pressor response, increasing blood pressure. Isometric exercise should be done without breath holding or a Valsalva maneuver. Individuals with hypertension may benefit from simple, repeated contractions held only 1 to 2 seconds (see Self-Management: Cervical Spine Extension).

DYNAMIC EXERCISE

Dynamic resistive exercise can be performed in a variety of modes, postures, and dosages. Isokinetic devices, body weight, resistive bands, free weights, pulleys, and weight machines are a few modes of dynamic resistive exercise (Patient-Related Instruction: Purchasing Resistive Equipment). Manual resistance applied by the clinician, the patient, or a family member is another form of dynamic resistive exercise. As with isometric exercise, each type of dynamic exercise has risks and benefits, and the training mode must be matched to the specific needs of the individual.

Isokinetic Exercise

Isokinetic dynamometers provide maximum resistance through the entire ROM. The first isokinetic dynamometers performed resisted concentric contractions at speeds fixed by the clinician. The dynamometer was passive in that the machine was unable to move independently; the patient was required to move the dynamometer arm. The new isokinetic devices are active computerized training and testing devices that are capable of actively moving the patient's limb for him. These dynamometers provide reciprocal concentric resistance at fixed speeds, and they provide multi-angle isometric resistance, fixed resistance concentric and eccentric contractions, passive motion, and fixed speed concentric and eccentric contractions. The remainder of this discussion focuses on the isokinetic capabilities of these devices.

The major advantage of isokinetic resistive training is its ability to fully activate more muscle fibers for longer periods. Because the machine matches the torque provided by the patient, it "accommodates" the patient's changing abilities throughout the ROM. In contrast, free weights (ie, fixed resistance training) overload only the weakest portion of the range, but the stronger portion (usually the middle third) is not overloaded.

Isokinetic devices allow training at a variety of speeds. The positive effect of fast-speed training on performance is highlighted with isokinetic training. Training at faster speeds can assist the return to functional activities that require less muscle torque development but faster speeds of contraction. Speeds that more closely match the patient's function can be chosen to match functional velocities. Higher speeds can decrease joint compression forces in areas such as the patellofemoral joint, decreasing the pain and discomfort often seen with heavy resistance exercises. Although less torque is generated at high speeds, the decrease in pain and more functional speeds may produce better results.

Studies assessing the speed variable favor slow-speed isokinetic training over fast-speed training for the development of strength.[90] High muscular tension is necessary for generating strength gains and is achieved when the isokinetic speed is slow enough to allow full recruitment and generation of a high resisting force.

Isokinetic resistive training also has disadvantages. These devices are expensive to purchase and maintain. They require trained personnel for setting up patient training programs, testing, and data interpretation. From a biomechanical perspective, most training is done in a single plane, with a fixed axis at a constant velocity in an open kinetic chain. Testing and training in a single plane improve test reproducibility but do not necessarily carry over to function. We rarely move at a constant velocity in functional activities, although this feature provides for maximal loading through the ROM. Newer isokinetic devices have some closed chain components, which have the advantage of testing a functional movement pattern but the disadvantage of being unable to tell where the muscle performance impairment lies.

Weight Machine Exercise

Weight machines are commonly found in rehabilitation clinics and health clubs. Many manufacturers proclaim the

---

Patient-Related Instruction

Purchasing Resistive Equipment

Before purchasing resistive equipment for home use, the following information should be considered:

1. Is the equipment safe? Is it approved by a reputable organization?
2. How easy is the equipment to use? How long will it take to learn how to use it?
3. Is the equipment versatile? Can it be used to train a number of different muscle groups?
4. Will the equipment suit your needs as your training progresses?

Before purchasing equipment, consider joining a health club for a month or two to see:

1. Which equipment you tend to use regularly
2. What features you like about some equipment
3. What features you dislike or seem to be lacking

SELF-MANAGEMENT:

Cervical Spine Extension

Purpose: To strengthen cervical extensors to reduce forward head posture

Position: Lying on your stomach with hands under your forehead and a pillow under your trunk; a small towel roll under your chin may be necessary

Movement technique: Remove your hands from your forehead and hold your head in a proper neutral position.

Repeat: ________ ***times***

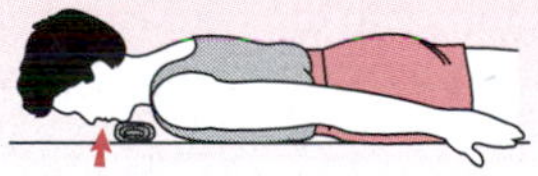

benefits of their particular machines over others. Most of these machines work in a similar fashion, although some differences exist. Historically, most weight machines were designed to isolate a specific muscle group such as the quadriceps or biceps. Some of the newer equipment trains multiple muscle groups in combination patterns such as a leg press or pull-up machine. These machines usually have stacks of plates weighing 5 to 20 pounds each. The weight stack configuration varies with the specific muscle action trained. A pin placed in the weight stack selects the amount of weight to be lifted.

An important weight machine variable is the pulley or cam system used. A simple pulley system provides relatively constant resistance through the ROM. Other machines contain an elliptical cam that varies the resistance through the ROM. The cam is an attempt to account for changes caused by varying length-tension relationships, and the machine is called a variable resistance machine. Less resistance is provided at the beginning and end of the ROM.

Weight machines also differ in their adjustability. Lever arms and seat positions should be adjustable. This ensures the ability to align the joint axis with the axis of the machine and prevent injury from poor posture or exercise mechanics. Stops and range-limiting devices should be available and easily adjustable.

An advantage of weight machines over free weights is safety. Patients are stabilized effectively by the equipment, and the risk of falls or injury due to instability is minimized. It takes less time to learn weight machine exercises. After the adjustments are learned, the equipment is relatively easy to use, and novice weight lifters are less intimidated by the equipment. Weight machines are also relatively time efficient because the machines are already set up. Only a few simple adjustments are necessary, and the patient is ready to begin. Setting up free weights takes more time.

One of the disadvantages of weight machines is their expense. An expensive machine may train only biceps curls, whereas this could be done inexpensively with a couple of free weights and a bar. With the weight machines, the increases in weight are restricted to fixed increments (ie, weight plates). Smaller changes of 1 or 2 pounds are not possible on most machines. Despite the many size adjustments on weight machines, they still do not fit everyone. They also have a fixed, two-dimensional movement pattern. Because the machine guides the patient through the ROM, little proprioception, balance, or coordination is learned from the experience. Most machines are designed to perform bilateral exercise. In some cases, performing unilateral exercise is difficult, if not impossible.

Free-Weight Exercise

Free-weight training is the resistive exercise technique of choice for body builders and power lifters. Free-weight training usually is done with a bar and weight plates, although smaller hand-held weights are available. Resistive bands or tubing is used in a similar fashion to free weights. One benefit of bands over free weights is the ability to position the patient without regard to gravity (see Self-Management: Supine Shoulder Flexion). Free weights and resistive bands have the advantage of movement in a variety of three-dimensional patterns without fixed movement patterns. This allows highly specific training that matches individual needs. For example, resisted lunging patterns forward, backward, laterally, or diagonally can be performed with hand-held resistive bands, free weights, or a bar. These movement patterns can be performed in whatever range is necessary for the individual, rather than in ranges dictated by a weight machine.

Free-weight training allows more discrete increases in resistance, and resistance can differ from one side to the other (see Self-Management: Standing Biceps Curls). For example, reciprocal biceps curls can be performed with 10 pounds on the injured side and 15 pounds on the uninjured side. Incremental increases of 1 to 2 pounds or less are available, allowing a more gradual overload. The free-weight equipment is affordable, and a multitude of exercises can be performed with the same free weights. These exercises include simple strengthening activities and power training techniques.

One of the biggest advantages of free-weight training is the neural component of balance. Compared with the external stabilization provided by a weight machine, the free weight usually has little external stabilization. These exercises require postural muscle stabilization beyond the work required to move the weight. The individual lifting with free weights must understand proper posture and spinal stabilization to prevent injury to the back. The lack of stabilization and free movement also require high levels of balance. The individual must be able to balance a bar with weights at both ends while performing a resistive movement. If balance is a rehabilitation goal, free weight exercise may be indicated.

SELF-MANAGEMENT:
Supine Shoulder Flexion

Purpose: To increase the strength of the shoulder muscles in a gravity-lessened position

Position: Lying on your back with the band tied around your foot or held in your opposite hand

Movement technique:
Level 1: Keeping your elbow bent, lift your arm overhead.
Level 2: Straighten your elbow and lift overhead.
Level 3: Progress to a standing position.

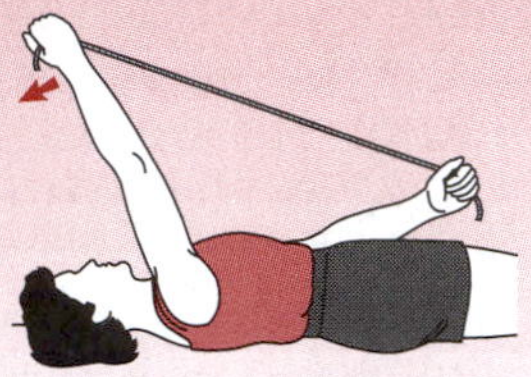

Level 2

SELF-MANAGEMENT: Standing Biceps Curls

Purpose: To strengthen the biceps muscles

Position: Standing position with a weight in each hand

Movement technique: Level 1: Alternately bend and straighten your elbows.

Level 2: Bend and straighten your elbows together; this challenges your back and postural muscles more

Repeat: _______ times

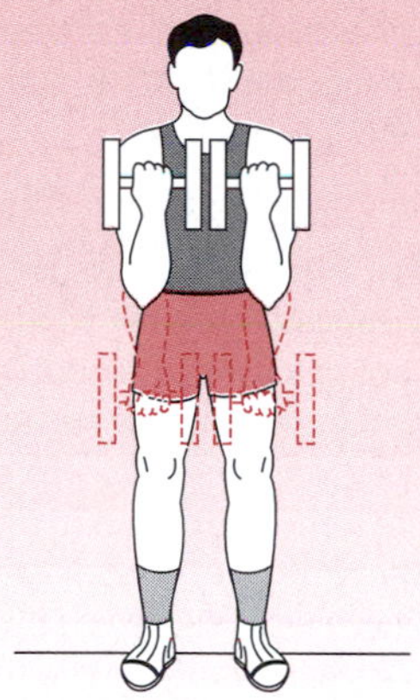

Level 2

The neural demands of free-weight exercise are a disadvantage for some. It takes longer to learn free-weight exercise, because the free-weight tasks usually are more complex than those with weight machines. Free-weight exercise is inherently more unsafe for the same reason. Novice lifters may be at greater risk for injury because of the lack of stabilization (Fig. 4-12). Spotters are necessary for many of the free-weight lifts, increasing the personnel demands of this resistive technique. Because of the time required to load and unload bars, free-weight training is less time efficient.

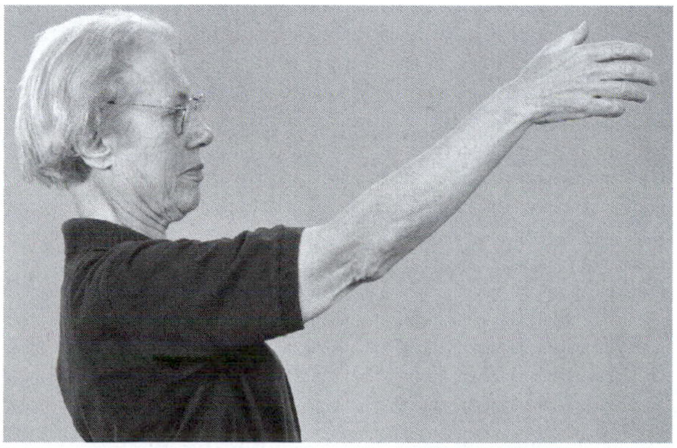

FIGURE 4-12 Lumbar extension is substituted for shoulder flexion.

Safety tips for individuals training with free weights include working with a knowledgeable partner who can spot safely. Collars should always be used to lock the weights on the bar and prevent movement of the plates on the bar. Proper form and technique should be acquired before lifting with any weight.

Plyometric Exercise

Functional activity seldom involves pure forms of isolated isometric, concentric, or eccentric actions, because the body is subjected to impact forces (Fig. 4-13), as in running or jumping, or because some external force, such as gravity, lengthens the muscle. In these movement patterns, the muscles are acting eccentrically and then concentrically. By definition of eccentric action, the muscle must be active during the lengthening phase. The SSC is the combination of an eccentric action followed by a concentric action. Training techniques that employ the SSC are called plyometrics.

Plyometrics are quick, powerful movements that are used to increase the reactivity of the nervous system. Plyometrics enhance work performance by storing elastic energy in the muscle during the stretch phase and reusing it as mechanical work during the concentric phase. Bosco and colleagues[91] found that the amount of elastic energy stored in a muscle during eccentric work determines the recoil of elastic energy during positive work. Part of the developed tension during the stretching phase is taken up by the elastic elements arranged in series with sarcomeres (ie, series elastic component or tendon). This mechanical work is stored in the sarcomere cross-bridges and can be reused during the following positive work if the muscle is contracted immediately after the stretch. The muscle's ability to use the stored energy is determined by the timing of the eccentric and concentric contractions and by the velocity and magnitude of stretch. A quick transition from eccentric to concentric (ie, undamped landings) along with a high-velocity stretch of high magnitude produces the greatest benefits.

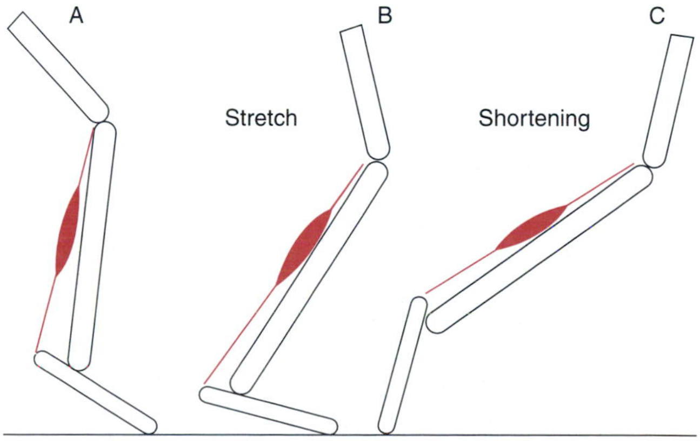

FIGURE 4-13 The stretch-shortening cycle in daily activities. ***(A)*** Before contact the muscles are preactivated ***(A)*** and ready to resist impact, during which time they are stretched ***(B)***. The stretch phase is followed by a shortening (concentric) action ***(C)***. The figure demonstrates the SSC, which is the natural form of the muscle function.

Plyometrics are high-level activities. Because of the stored energy in the series elastic component, the tendon is susceptible to overuse injury when performing plyometric exercises. The individual should be in an advanced training stage before these techniques are employed. In an advanced exercise program, these techniques develop power and speed, the key muscle performance elements of athletics. Jumping from or to different heights, bounding (ie, jumping for distance), progressive throwing programs, and throwing for speed or distance are methods of using SSC for enhancing speed or power performance. Before performing lower extremity plyometrics, the individual must be able to squat his body weight, perform a standing long jump equal to his height, and balance on a single leg with his eyes closed.

Dosage

The exercise dosage can be altered in a variety of ways. Increasing the intensity or amount of weight is the most obvious means. Changing the relationship to gravity, increasing the lever arm length, increasing sets and repetitions, decreasing the rest interval, and increasing the frequency are others. The dosage parameters of intensity, duration, and frequency are related, and all must be considered when designing a resistive exercise program. The resistive exercise must be progressed to a functional activity to carry treatment of an impairment over to a functional situation (Fig. 4-14). The clinician must choose appropriate dosage parameters based on the needs of the patient (Display 4-4).

The most important variables are the amount of tension generated during a training session and specificity for the functional outcome. The other variables, although less important with respect to strength gains, may prevent burnout by offering variety to a training program.

Patients with low levels of function often require resistive exercise prescriptions. Examination of many patients presenting with functional limitations reveals a less than fair grade of muscle strength. Patients with fair and less than fair muscle grades are unable to initiate resistive exercise against gravity with proper recruitment and movement patterns. When resistive exercise is prescribed, the patient is forced to train a faulty movement pattern. For example, a patient may be unable to lift her arm overhead without pain. She is evaluated and is found to have a physical impairment of a muscle strength grade of fair for the lower trapezius and serratus anterior. Her exercise prescription is to dynamically lift a free weight in the sagittal plane through a full arc of motion. Because of the lack of strength of the lower trapezius and serratus anterior, the patient lifts the arm with excessive scapular elevation, recruiting the upper trapezius instead of the preferred scapular upward rotation force couple of the upper, middle, lower trapezius, and serratus an-

DISPLAY 4-4

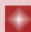

Dosage Variables for Individuals With Muscles of Various Strength Grades

Muscles Fair or Below Progressing to Muscles Above Fair:

1. Gravity lessened or against gravity
2. Active assistive, active, or resisted
3. Range of motion
4. Lever arm length (bent elbow to straight arm)

Muscles Above Fair Strength Grade:

1. Type of contraction (eg, isometric, concentric, eccentric, isokinetic, plyometric)
2. Weight or resistance
3. Sets or repetitions
4. Frequency of training sessions (be cautious of overtraining)
5. Speed of movement (slower speed increases amount of force or torque generated during concentric exercise)
6. Distance (eg, running, jumping, throwing)
7. Rest interval between sets

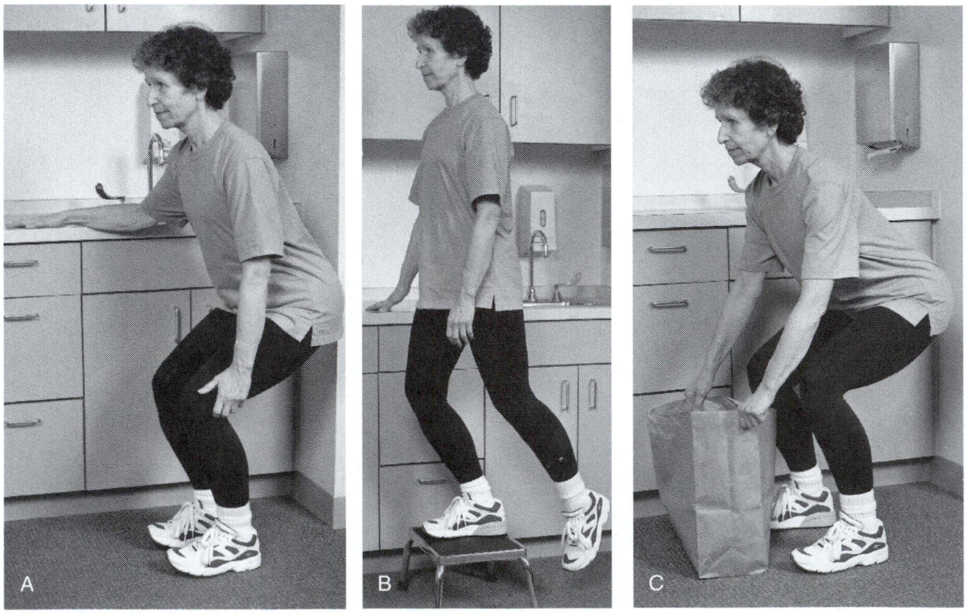

FIGURE 4-14 Progression of exercise. ***(A)*** Squat progressed to ***(B)*** step-up to ***(C)*** squat with a bag of groceries.

terior. This faulty pattern strengthens the upper trapezius and reinforces the faulty osteokinematic motion at the scapulothoracic joint. The patient's functional limitation does not change (ie, still has pain with overhead lifting) even though the straight arm lift gets "stronger" over time.

To resolve the functional limitation of pain with overhead lifting, the impairment of the specific strengths of the lower trapezius and serratus anterior must be addressed. Because these were tested at grades of fair or less than fair, resistive exercise against gravity is an inappropriate initial exercise prescription. The patient must be given an initial exercise program in a gravity-lessened plane for the lower trapezius and serratus (see Self-Management: Serratus Anterior Progression in Chapter 26). Lever arm length and ROM can be altered. To ensure concentric contraction during flexion and eccentric contraction during lowering from flexion (as occurs against gravity), elastic can be used at the appropriate resistance. To ensure that an eccentric contraction of the upward rotators occurs during the lowering phase, care must be taken to ensure resistance is present throughout the entire lowering phase; once resistance is lost, the contraction becomes concentric movement of the scapular rotators downward. After the muscle strength is above a grade of fair, active exercise against gravity can be initiated (eg, bent arm progressed to straight arm) and progressed to resistive exercise against gravity, ensuring that the quality of the movement suggests the proper force couple is being used.

Care must be taken when prescribing exercise for muscles with strength grades of fair or less than fair. Proper positioning in gravity-lessened planes or reduced lever arms or ROM (Fig. 4-15) can provide the appropriate stimulus for increased muscle performance. If the tension is too great for the muscle to overcome, it may become strained, or most likely, the synergists dominate and compromise the quality of the motion.

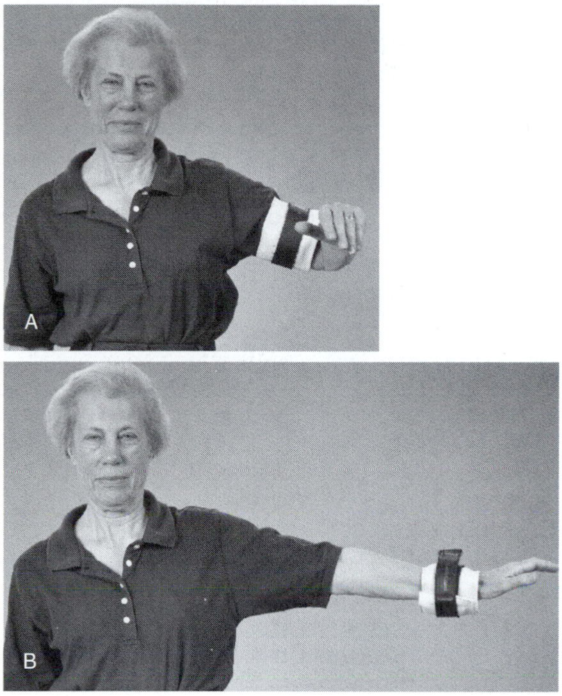

FIGURE 4-15 Use of different lever arms. ***(A)*** Short lever arm with elbow flexed. ***(B)*** Longer lever arm with elbow extended.

INTENSITY

Extensive strength training research has been performed on individuals without injury. Dosage parameters to increase strength began with DeLorme's classic paper in 1945.[92] In it, he reported findings from his therapeutic experiences with more than 300 patients for whom competitive athletic techniques were a part of rehabilitation. He proposed a 10 RM, 10-set regimen. Later, DeLorme and Watkins[35] modified this regimen to a 10 RM, three-set regimen with loads increasing progressively for each set from one half to three fourths to a full 10 RM set. DeLorme called this regimen progressive resistance exercise, a term still used today (Table 4-2). The effectiveness of DeLorme's three-set progressive resistance program has often been examined and has served as a control condition by which to judge the effectiveness of other methods.

In 1951, an alternative to the DeLorme regimen was proposed by Zinovieff[93] at Oxford. He suggested adjusting the intensity of the load to allow for progressive fatigue. This was achieved by selecting an initial load that was just enough to permit each set to be completed. This regimen was called the Oxford technique. McMorris and Elkins[94] compared the DeLorme and Oxford techniques and found the Oxford technique to be slightly better, but the differences were not statistically significant.

The daily adjustable progressive resistive exercise (DAPRE) technique has been proposed as a more adaptable progressive exercise program than the Oxford or DeLorme approaches (see Table 4-2).[95] This program eliminates arbitrary decisions about the frequency and amount of weight increase. The DAPRE program can be used with free weights or with weight machines. A 6 RM is used to establish the initial working weight. Thereafter, weight increases are based on the performance during the previous training session.

Numerous studies have been conducted with various dosages for repetitions, sets, and percent of RM per set. Krusen[96] compared two groups with different progressive resistance exercise programs. One group trained with 25%, 50%, and 75% of the 10 RM for the first, second, and third sets, respectively. The other group trained with 100%, 125%, and 150% of the 5 RM for the first, second, and third sets, respectively. The groups did not differ significantly in strength at the completion of the training program.

Very little stimulus is necessary to make strength gains in the beginner. Ten RM at three sets performed two to three times per week is the typical prescription. However, one set of 10 RM performed two to four times per week is sufficient for strength gains, particularly for the patient with limited time for exercise. Three sets of 10 RM take longer, with minimal improvements in strength beyond one set, and may pose an increased risk for injury. If the patient has the time and is careful with technique, three sets of 10 RM performed three times per week appears to be the optimal stimulus for strength gains.

These guidelines have been based on studies of uninjured subjects. When treating a patient with specific im-

Table 4-2. COMMON STRENGTH TRAINING DOSAGES AND DAILY ADJUSTABLE PROGRESSIVE RESISTIVE EXERCISE PROGRAM AND ADJUSTMENTS

TECHNIQUE	BASE REPETITION MAXIMUM (RM)	SETS	NUMBER OF REPETITIONS
DeLorme	10	1. 50% of 10 RM	10
		2. 75% of 10 RM	10
		3. 100% of 10 RM	10
Oxford	10	1. 100% of 10 RM	10
		2. 75% of 10 RM	10
		3. 50% of 10 RM	10
DAPRE	6	1. 50% of 6 RM	10
		2. 75% of 6 RM	6
		3. 100% of 6 RM	As many as possible
		4. Adjusted weight based on number of reps. performed in set 3	As many as possible; this number of repetitions is used to determine the working weight for the next day

NUMBER OF REPETITIONS PERFORMED IN SET 3*	ADJUSTED WORKING WEIGHT FOR SET 4*	ADJUSTED WORKING WEIGHT FOR NEXT DAY*
0–2	Decrease 5–10 lb and repeat set	Decrease 5–10 lb
3–4	Decrease 0–5 lb	Same weight
5–6	Keep weight the same	Increase 5–10 lb
7–10	Increase 5–19 lb	Increase 5–15 lb
11	Increase 10–15 lb	Increase 10–20 lb

* Adjustments for the Daily Adjustable Progressive Resistive Exercise (DAPRE) program.

pairments, the resistive exercise dosage varies. Exercise should be performed to substitution or form fatigue, the point at which substitution or alterations in form occur.

DURATION

Duration of resistive training can be considered the number of sets or repetitions of a specific exercise session. Because of the close relation to intensity, some aspects of duration were discussed in the previous section. Intensity and duration are inversely related. The greater the intensity, the fewer repetitions are performed. When training at a low RM (near the 1 RM or maximum amount of weight that can be lifted), very few repetitions are performed, and strength gains are the chief goal. When training at 10 RM or higher, many repetitions are performed, and the goals are endurance and other aspects of muscle performance.

Duration also considers the rest interval between sets. Because of the energy systems used in resistance training, rest intervals of 1 to 2 minutes allow adequate recovery for additional exercise, depending on the intensity of the lift. Muscles can be overloaded by decreasing the rest interval between sets.

FREQUENCY

Training frequency depends on the rehabilitation goals. Isometric exercise is performed several times per day, and heavy dynamic exercise may be performed every other day. Frequency of one exercise is related to the exercise goal, intensity, duration, and other exercises in the patient's rehabilitation program. Individuals training for power lifting or body building lift daily or twice daily, whereas individuals in rehabilitation programs may perform resistive exercise three days per week and cardiovascular exercise on alternate days.

Balancing frequency with intensity and duration can be difficult. Study findings[97] can be summarized as follows:

- Performing an exercise between 3 and 9 RM is the most effective number of repetitions for increasing muscle strength.
- Progressive resistive exercise training one time weekly with 1 RM for one set increases strength significantly after the first week of training and each week up to at least the sixth week.
- No particular sequence of progressive resistive exercise training with different percentages of 10 RM is more effective for strength improvement than another, as long as one set of 10 RM is performed during each training session.
- Performing one set of an exercise is less effective for increasing strength than performing two or three sets, and there is some indication that three sets are more effective than two sets.
- The optimal number of training days per week with progressive resistive exercise for improving muscular

strength is unknown. Significant increases have occurred for beginners training 1 to 5 days per week.

- When progressive resistive exercise training uses several different exercises, training 4 or 5 days each week may be less effective for increasing dynamic strength than training two or three times per week. More frequent strength training may prevent sufficient recuperation between training sessions, retarding progress in neuromuscular adaptation and strength development.

DOSAGE FOR THE UNTRAINED INDIVIDUAL

In the beginning stages of a program, maximum lifts should be avoided. Research has unquestionably demonstrated that heavy loads do not produce the greatest force or torque gains,[87] and the individual runs the risk of muscle or joint injury. Beginners should initially attempt to complete 8 to 12 RM. Weight is progressed when 12 repetitions become too easy. If the weight is progressed, but 10 repetitions cannot be accomplished with good form, the weight is too heavy and must be reduced to complete a minimum of eight repetitions with good form. After a few weeks of training, a regimen of 8 to 12 RM performed for one to three sets can be adopted. As the muscle becomes stronger, the weight is adjusted, and a heavier load is attempted. The minimum number of repetitions should be performed at 8 RM with good form. Three training sessions each week, with a day of rest between sessions, is recommended. The day of rest is critical to prevent overtraining.

DOSAGE FOR THE TRAINED INDIVIDUAL

The following techniques are used by coaches and trainers involved in training competitive athletes. They can be used to provide variety, increase resistance, or maximize the workout time in daily workouts. Little or no data support these concepts. They are introduced to familiarize the therapist with the terminology used in training advanced athletes. Clinicians should use good judgment based on scientific principles when using these techniques.

A superset consists of two sets of exercise involving opposing muscles that are performed in sequence without a rest between sets (eg, a biceps curl followed by a triceps extension, rest for 1 to 2 minutes, followed by the remaining sets). Supersets can reduce workout time or allow more exercise to be performed during the same period.

A triset is a group of three exercises, each done after the other with little rest between muscle groups. Trisets can be used to exercise three different muscle groups or three angles of a complex muscle (eg, flat, incline, and decline bench press for the different fiber directions of the pectoralis major).

Pyramid training is a modification of the DeLorme training program. The regimen starts with a high number of repetitions and low weight (to warm-up), but instead of maintaining the repetitions constant and increasing the weight, the repetitions are reduced and weight is increased. After the series is completed, the individual works backward, taking off weight and adding repetitions. The number of repetitions and sets is arbitrarily established as long as the high-repetition, low-weight progression to a heavier-weight, low-repetition regimen is followed (Table 4-3).

A typical split routine consists of a series of exercises that usually emphasize two or three major muscle groups or body parts. This allows the individual to train on 2 consecutive days without overtraining muscle groups, because one muscle group is resting while the other is exercising. Body builders often follow a double-split routine, in which two sessions are performed on each day (Table 4-4).

Matveyev[98] described the basic ideas of periodized training programs. A program is periodized when it is divided into phases, each of which has primary and secondary goals. The program is based on the premise that maximum strength gains are not made by constant heavy training but are made possible by different training cycles or periods. Periodization allows the body to gradually adapt to the stress of exercise. Athletes have found that they can reach maximum performance level at a predesignated time, usually the day of competition.

In his original model, Matveyev[98] suggested the initial phase of a strength-power program (ie, preparation phase) should contain a high volume (ie, many repetitions) with lower intensity (ie, low average weight lifted relative to maximum possible in each movement). As weeks pass, the volume decreases and intensity increases. The resulting higher intensity and lower volume represent the characteristics of a competitive phase of training that leads up to a competition for weight lifters.

Typical high-volume phases (ie, preparation) for weight lifters contain more training sessions per week (6 to 15), more exercises per session (3 to 6), more sets per exercise (4 to 8), and more repetitions per set (4 to 6). Typical high-intensity phases (ie, competition) for weight lifters contain fewer training sessions per week (5 to 12), fewer exercises per workout session (1 to 4), fewer sets per exercise (3 to 5), and fewer repetitions per set (1 to 3). Each phase may be several weeks to several months long. Two or more complete cycles (ie, preparation plus competition) may fit into a training year.

Stone and colleagues[99] proposed and successfully tested a periodized model of strength-power training with sequential phases that change rather drastically. An example is a phase to increase muscle size (five sets of 10 RM in core exercises), a phase to improve specific strength (three to five sets of 3 RM), and a phase to "peak" for competition (one to three sets of one to three repetitions). The use of 10 RM is higher than typically recommended in the early

Table 4-3. SAMPLE PYRAMID TRAINING FOR A SQUAT EXERCISE FOR A HIGHLY TRAINED INDIVIDUAL

SETS	REPETITIONS	WEIGHT
1	12	100
1	8	135
1	6	185
1	4	225
1	2	250
1	1	275

Table 4-4. EXAMPLE OF A SPLIT ROUTINE FOR TOTAL-BODY RESISTIVE TRAINING

FOUR-DAY PROGRAM*	SIX-DAY, TWO SESSIONS PER DAY PROGRAM*
Monday: upper body	Monday AM: chest
Tuesday: lower body	Monday PM: back
Wednesday: rest	Tuesday AM: shoulders
Thursday: upper body	Tuesday PM: upper legs
Friday: lower body	Wednesday AM: triceps
Saturday: rest	Wednesday PM: biceps
Sunday: repeat sequence	Thursday AM: chest
	Thursday PM: back

*Abdominals and calves are exercised each day.

preparation phase but has proved to be successful in a number of studies.[99]

Precautions and Contraindications

When prescribing resistive exercise, certain precautions and contraindications must be considered.

The use of a Valsalva maneuver should be avoided during resistive training, especially by a patient with cardiopulmonary disease or after recent abdominal, intervertebral disk, or eye surgery. Patients must be educated to breathe properly during exercise, typically exhaling on exertion. Isometric exercise should be used with caution by persons at risk for pressor response effects (eg, high blood pressure after an aneurysm).

During resistive training, especially in an untrained state, minor lesions of the muscle structure and inflammation resulting in muscle soreness are common. Soreness may be caused by myofibrillar damage localized to the Z band, membrane damage, or inflammatory processes. The serum or plasma level of creatine kinase is elevated and is considered to be an indicator of muscle damage, because the enzyme is found almost exclusively in muscle tissue. Delayed soreness, clearly linked to eccentric activity, usually peaks about 2 days after exertion. Muscle function deteriorates, and muscle strength may be reduced for a week or more after intensive eccentric exercise. However, an adaptive process reduces the soreness after repeated training sessions.[100] Even during the soreness period, moderate activity is advised, because the adaptation response occurs before full recovery and restoration of muscle function. Patients should be cautioned that eccentric training may lead to muscle soreness 24 to 48 hours after exercise, but that moderate exercise should continue during the recovery period. A somewhat different type of soreness and reduced muscle function may occur during very long and intense exercise bouts. It is probably related to the total metabolic load, not muscle tension development.[100]

Overwork phenomena may exist even at moderate training regimens over an extended period. Overtraining may lead to mood disturbances and reduce the effect of training by a decrease in performance. Fatigue and overtraining should be avoided by patients with metabolic diseases (eg, diabetes, alcoholism), neurologic diseases, or severe degenerative joint diseases because of the risk of further joint damage. Overtraining may be the reason for a lack of progress, decreased performance, or development of joint pain and swelling.

Care should be taken in developing resistive exercise programs for prepubertal and pubertal children and adolescents. Stress of epiphyseal sites should be minimized, and balanced exercise programs should be developed to avoid muscle imbalances that may lead to musculoskeletal pain syndromes later in life.

An absolute contraindication to resistive exercise is acute or chronic myopathy, as occurs in some forms of neuromuscular disease or in acute alcohol myopathy. Resistive exercise in the presence of myopathy may stress and permanently damage an already compromised muscular system.

Scientific knowledge and common sense should be applied in prescribing resistive exercise. Caution should be taken with exercise in the presence of pain, inflammation, and infection. Although resistive exercise may be indicated, the mode and dosage should be carefully chosen.

Key Points

- The term *strength* should be clarified in terms of force, torque, work, and power.
- Muscle actions are static and dynamic. Dynamic actions can be further divided into concentric and eccentric actions.
- The sliding filament theory describes the events that occur during muscle contraction.
- Basic muscle fiber types are slow oxidative, fast glycolytic, and fast oxidative glycolytic.
- Force gradation occurs by rate coding and the size principle.
- Overload training produces changes in the size of the muscle primarily through hypertrophy but also through hyperplasia.
- Muscle strength must be evaluated relative to the muscle's length because of length-tension relationships.
- Pennate muscles are designed for force production, and parallel muscles are best suited for excursion.
- Specificity of training exists, especially relative to training velocity.
- Adaptations to resistive training are partially neurologic in that changes in performance often precede morphologic changes.
- Form fatigue is the point at which the individual must discontinue the exercise or sacrifice exercise form.
- Although dosage and goals differ, resistive training is beneficial from late childhood through old age.
- Impaired muscle performance can result from neurologic pathology, muscle strain, or muscle disuse.
- Adaptations to resistive training extend beyond the muscle to include connective tissues, the cardiovascular system, and bone.
- Dynamic exercise can be performed with a variety of modes, including isokinetic, free weight, resistive bands, weight machines, or body weight.

LAB ACTIVITIES

1. A series of neuromuscular problems is listed from i to x. For each problem, perform the following:
   a. Determine which muscles are involved. List each muscle, origin, insertion, primary and secondary actions (if indicated), and central and peripheral innervation.
   b. Design and perform two exercises for each muscle (group) if the muscle grade was below a fair, and include dosage.
   c. Design and perform two exercises for each muscle (group) if the muscle grade was above a fair. Use a resistive band for one and a free weight for the other, and include dosage.
   d. Progress the exercises in question 1c to two functional activities for the following conditions:
      i. Achilles tendinitis
      ii. Gluteus medius weakness
      iii. Patellar tendinitis
      iv. Hamstring strain
      v. Peroneal nerve palsy (ie, common peroneal nerve) (list muscles innervated)
      vi. Rotator cuff tendinitis
      vii. Long head of biceps tendinitis
      viii. Midscapular pain due to poor posture
      ix. Triceps tendinitis
      x. Lateral and medial epicondylitis
2. Using free weights or a weight machine, determine the 1 RM, 6 RM, and 10 RM for different exercises. Perform Oxford, DeLorme, and DAPRE programs.
3. Pick six muscle groups throughout your body. Design three different exercises for each muscle group. Perform each exercise, and see how they differ. Use a variety of equipment, including resistive bands, handheld weights, bar with weights, body weight, and weight machines.

- Plyometric activities use the stretch-shortening cycle to enhance concentric muscle performance.
- The frequency, intensity, and duration of resistive activity must be balanced to produce gains and prevent injury.

Critical Thinking Questions

1. Consider each of the questions in the Lab Activities in the next section. How would your dosage differ if you were training
   a. For force production
   b. For velocity of movement
   c. For muscle endurance
2. Design a muscle performance maintenance program for a woman confined to bed rest for 3 weeks after an acute lumbar fracture without neurologic involvement.
3. Consider Case Study #5 in Unit 7. Design a comprehensive program to address this patient's muscle performance impairments.

REFERENCES

1. Enoka RM. Force. In: Enoka RM. *Neuromechanical Basis of Kinesiology*. Champaign, IL: Human Kinetics Books; 1988:31–63.
2. Abbott BC, Bigland B, Ritchie JM. The physiological cost of negative work. *J Physiol (Lond)*. 1952;117:380–390.
3. Norman RW, Komi PV. Electromyographic delay in skeletal muscle under normal movement conditions. *Acta Physiol Scand*. 1979;106:241.
4. Komi PV. Stretch-shortening cycle. In: Komi PV, ed. *Strength and Power in Sport*. Oxford: Blackwell Scientific Publications; 1992:169–179.
5. Komi PV. Physiological and biomechanical correlates of muscle function: effects of muscle structure and stretch-shortening cycle on force and speed. In: Terjung RL, ed. *Exercise and Sport Science Reviews*, vol 12. Lexington, MA: Collamore Press; 1984:81–121.
6. Henneman E, Somjen G, Carpenter DO. Functional significance of cell size in spinal motoneuron. *J Neurophysiol*. 1965;28:560–580.
7. Lieber RL. *Skeletal Muscle Structure and Function*. Baltimore: Williams & Wilkins; 1992.
8. Grimby L, Hannerz J. Firing rate and recruitment order of toe extensor motor units in different modes of voluntary contraction. *J Physiol*. 1977;264:865–879.
9. Nardone A, Romano C, Schieppati M. Selective recruitment of high-threshold human motor units during voluntary isotonic lengthening of active muscles. *J Physiol*. 1989;409:451–471.
10. Bell RD, et al. Muscle fiber types and morphometric analysis of skeletal muscle in six year old children. *Med Sci Sports*. 1982;12:28.
11. Saltin B, et al. Fiber types and metabolic potentials of skeletal muscles in sedentary man and endurance runners. *Ann N Y Acad Sci*. 1977;301:3.
12. Campbell CJ, et al. Muscle fiber composition and performance capacities of women. *Med Sci Sports*. 1978;10:151.
13. Billeter R, Hoppeler H. Muscular basis of strength. In: Komi PV, ed. *Strength and Power in Sport*. Oxford: Blackwell Scientific Publications; 1992:39–63.
14. Antonio J, Gonyea WJ. Skeletal muscle fiber hyperplasia. *Med Sci Sports Exerc*. 1993;25:1333–1345.
15. MacDougall DJ. Hypertrophy or hyperplasia. In: Komi PV, ed. *Strength and Power in Sport*. Oxford: Blackwell Scientific Publications; 1992:230–238.
16. Bischof R. Analysis of muscle regeneration using single myofibers in culture. *Med Sci Sports Exerc*. 1989;21(suppl):S163–S172.
17. Schultz E, et al. Absence of exogenous satellite cell contribution to regeneration of frozen skeletal muscle. *J Muscle Res Cell Motil*. 1986;7:361–367.
18. MacDougall JD, et al. Muscle fiber number in biceps brachii in body builders and control subjects. *J Appl Physiol*. 1984;57:1399–1403.
19. Fenn WO, Marsh BS. Muscular force at different speeds of shortening. *J Physiol*. 1935;85:277–297.

20. Tabary JC, Tabary C, Tardieu C, Tardieu G, Goldspink G. Physiological and structural changes in the cat's soleus muscle due to immobilization at different lengths by plaster cast. *J Physiol.* 1972;224:231–244.
21. Oudet CL, Petrovic AG. Regulation of the anatomical length of the lateral pterygoid muscle in the growing rat. *Adv Physiol Sci.* 1981;24:115–121.
22. Kendall HO, Kendall FP, Boynton DA. *Posture and Pain.* Baltimore: Williams & Wilkins; 1952.
23. Williams PE, Goldspink G. Longitudinal growth of striated muscle fibers. *J Cell Sci.* 1971;9:751–767.
24. Herring SW, Grimm AF, Grimm BR. Regulation of sarcomere number in skeletal muscle: a comparison of hypotheses. *Muscle Nerve.* 1984;7:161–173.
25. Kendall FP, McCreary KE, Provance PG. *Muscles Testing and Function.* 4th ed. Baltimore: Williams & Wilkins; 1993.
26. Williams PE, Goldspink G. Changes in sarcomere length and physiological properties in immobilized muscle. *J Anat.* 1978;127:459–468.
27. Josephson RK. Extensive and intensive factors determining the performance of striated muscle. *J Exp Zool.* 1975; 194:135–154.
28. Morrissey MC, Harman EA, Johnson MJ. Resistance training modes: specificity and effectiveness. *Med Sci Sports Exerc.* 1995;27:648–660.
29. Kanehisa H, Miyashita M. Specificity of velocity in strength training. *Eur J Appl Physiol.* 1983;52:104–106.
30. Higbie EJ. Effects of concentric and eccentric isokinetic heavy-resistance training on quadriceps muscle strength, cross-sectional area and neural activation in women. Doctoral Dissertation, University of Georgia; 1994.
31. Weir JP, Housh DJ,Housh TJ, Weir LL. The effect of unilateral concentric weight training and detraining on joint angle specificity, cross-training, and the bilateral deficit. *J Orthop Sports Phys Ther.* 1997;25:264–270.
32. Weir JP, Housh DJ, Housh TJ, Weir LL. The effect of unilateral eccentric weight training and detraining on joint angle specificity, cross-training, and the bilateral deficit. *J Orthop Sports Phys Ther.* 1995;22:207–215.
33. Taniguchi Y. Lateral specificity in resistance training: the effect of bilateral and unilateral training. *Eur J Appl Physiol.* 1997;75:144–150.
34. Wilson GJ, Murphy AJ, Walshe A. The specificity of strength training: the effect of posture. *Eur J Appl Physiol.* 1996;73:346–352.
35. Delorme TL, Watkins AL. *Progressive Resistance Exercise.* New York: Appleton Century; 1951.
36. Moritani T, DeVries HA. Neural factors vs. hypertrophy in time course of muscle strength gain. *Am J Phys Med Rehabil.* 1979;58:115–130.
37. Staron RS, Karapondo DL, Kraemer WJ, et al. Skeletal muscle adaptations during early phase of heavy-resistance training in men and women. *J Appl Physiol* 1994;76:1247–1255.
38. Hakkinen K, Komi PV. Electromyographic changes during strength training and detraining. *Med Sci Sports Exerc.* 1983;15:455–460.
39. Sale D. Neural adaptation to strength training. In: Komi PV. *Strength and Power in Sport.* Oxford: Blackwell Scientific Publications; 1992:249–265.
40. Edman PK. Contractile performance of skeletal muscle fibers. In: *Strength and Power in Sport.* In: Komi PV, ed. Oxford: Blackwell Scientific Publications; 1992:96–114.
41. Crasselt W, Forchel I, Kroll M, Schulz A. *Zum Kinder- und Jugendsport—Realitaten, Wunshe und Tendenzen.* [*Sport of Children and Adolescents—Reality, Expectations, and Tendencies.*] Leipzig: Deutsche Hochschule fur Korperkultur; 1990:327.
42. Hettinger TH. *Isometrisches Muskeltraining.* [*Isometric Muscle Training.*] Stuttgart: George Thieme Verlag; 1968.
43. Yokomizo YI. Measurement of ability of older workers. *Ergonomics.* 1985;28:843–854.
44. Grimby G, Danneskiold-Samse W, Hvid K, Saltin B. Morphology and enzymatic capacity in arm and leg muscles in 78–81-year-old men and women. *Acta Physiol Scand.* 1982;115:125–134.
45. Moritani T. Training adaptations in the muscles of older men. In: Smith EL, Serfass RE, eds. *Exercise and Aging: The Scientific Basis.* New Jersey: Enslow Publishers; 1981: 149–166.
46. Janda V. *Muskelfunktionsdiagnostik.* [*Functional Diagnostic Tests for Muscles.*] Berlin: Verlag Volk & Gesundheit; 1986.
47. Wilkes RL, Summers JJ. Cognitions, mediating variables, and strength performance. *J Sport Psychol.* 1984;6: 351–359.
48. Weinberg R, Jackson A, Seaboune T. The effects of specific vs. nonspecific mental preparation strategies on strength and endurance performance. *J Sport Behav.* 1985;7: 175–180.
49. Tenenbaum G, Bar-Eli M, Hoffman JR, Jablonovski R, Sade S, Shitrit D. The effect of cognitive and somatic psyching-up techniques on isokinetic leg strength performance. *J Strength Condit Res.* 1995;9:3–7.
50. Murphy SM, Woolfolk RL, Budney AJ. The effects of emotive imagery on strength performance. *J Sport Exerc Psychol* 1988;10:334–345.
51. Elko K, Ostrow AC. The effects of three mental preparation strategies on strength performance of young and older adults. *J Sport Behav.* 1992;15:34–41.
52. Gould D, Weinberg R, Jackson A. Mental preparation strategies, cognition and strength performance. *J Sport Psychol.* 1980;2(4):329–339.
53. Gassner GJ. Comparison of three different types of imagery on performance outcome in strength-related tasks with collegiate male athletes. Dissertation thesis, Temple University; 1997.
54. Hobbel SL, Rose DJ. The relative effectiveness of three forms of visual knowledge of results on peak torque output. *J Orthop Sports Phys Ther.* 1993;18:601–608.
55. Rubin E. Alcoholic myopathy in heart and skeletal muscle. *N Engl J Med.* 1979;301:28–33.
56. Song SK, Rubin E. Ethanol produces muscle damage in human volunteers. *Science.* 1972;175:327–328.
57. Rubin E, Perkoff GT, Dioso NM, et al. A spectrum of myopathy associated with alcoholism. *Ann Intern Med.* 1967;67:481–492.
58. Hanid A, Slavin G, Main, et al. Fiber type changes in striated muscle of alcoholics. *J Clin Pathol.* 1981;34:991–995.
59. Mastaglia FL, Argov Z. Drug-induced neuromuscular disorders in man. In: Walton J, ed. *Disorders of Voluntary Muscle.* 4th ed. Edinburgh: Churchill Livingstone; 1981:873–906.
60. Stern LZ, Fagan JM. The endocrine myopathies. In: Vinken PJ, Bruyn GW, Ringel SP, eds. *Handbook of Clinical Neurological Disease of Muscle: Part 2.* Amsterdam: North Holland Publishing; 1979;41:235–238.
61. Bunch TW, Worthingham JW, Combs JJ, et al. Azathioprine with prednisone for polymyositis: a controlled clinical trial. *Ann Intern Med.* 1980;92:356–369.
62. Goldberg AL, Goodman HM. Relationship between cortisone and muscle work in determining muscle size. *J Physiol (Lond).* 1969;200:667–675.
63. Malone TR, Garrett E, Zachazewski JE. Muscle: deformation, injury, repair. In: Zachazewski JE, Magee DJ, Quillen WS, eds. *Athletic Injuries and Rehabilitation.* Philadelphia: WB Saunders; 1996.

64. Worrell TW, Perrin DH. Hamstring muscle injury: The influence of strength, flexibility, warm-up and fatigue. *J Orthop Sports Phys Ther*. 1992;16:12–18.
65. Desmedt JE, Godaux E. Spinal motoneuron recruitment in man: rank deordering with direction but not with speed of voluntary movement. *Science*. 1981;214:933–936.
66. Tax AM, Denier van der Gon JJ, Gielen CAM, Kleyne M. Differences in central control of m. biceps brachii in movement tasks and force tasks. *Exp Brain Res*. 1990;79:138–142.
67. Van Zuylen EJ, Gielen CAM, Denier van der Gon JJ. Coordination and homogenous activation of human arm muscles during isometric torques. *J Neurophys*. 1988;60:1523–1548.
68. Sale DG, MacDougall D. Specificity in strength training: a review for the coach and athlete. *Can J Appl Sports Sci*. 1981;6:87–92.
69. Rutherford OM, Jones DA. The role of learning and coordination in strength training. *Eur J Appl Phys*. 1986;55:100–105.
70. Staron R, Hikida RS, Hagerman FC, Dudley GA, Murray TF. Human muscle skeletal muscle fiber type adaptability to various workloads. *J Histochem Cytochem* 1984;32: 146–152.
71. Costill DC, Daniels J, Evans, Fink W, Krahenbuhl G, Saltin B. Skeletal muscle enzymes and fiber composition in male and female track athletes. *J Appl Physiol*. 1976;40:149–154.
72. Tesch PA, Komi PV, Hakkinen K. Enzymatic adaptations consequent to long term strength training. *Int J Sports Med*. 1987;8(suppl):66–69.
73. MacDougall JD, et al. Mitochondrial volume density in human skeletal muscle following heavy resistance training. *Med Sci Sports*. 1979;11:164–166.
74. Thorstensson A, Spokin B, Karlsson J. Enzyme activities and muscle strength after "sprint training" in man. *Acta Physiol Scand*. 1975;94:313–316.
75. Hakkinen K, Komi PV, Alen M. Effect of explosive type strength training on isometric force and relaxation time, electromyographic and muscle fibre characteristics of leg extensor muscles. *Acta Physiol Scand*. 1985;125:587–600.
76. Stone MH. Implications for connective tissue and bone alterations resulting from resistance exercise training. *Med Sci Sports Exerc*. 1988;20:S162–S168.
77. Tipton CM, Mattes RD, Maynard JA, Carey RA. The influence of physical activity on ligaments and tendons. *Med Sci Sports*. 1975;7:165–175.
78. Vogel JM, Whittle MW. Bone mineral content changes in the Skylab astronauts. *AJR Am J Roentgenol*. 1976;126:1296.
79. Hanson TH, Roos BO, Nachemson A. Development of osteopenia in the fourth lumbar vertebrae during prolonged bed rest after operation for scoliosis. *Acta Orthop Scand*. 1975;46:621–630.
80. White MK, Martin RB, Yeater RA, Butcher RL, Radin EL. The effects of exercise on postmenopausal women. *Int Orthop*. 1984;7:209–214.
81. Nilsson BE, Westlin NE. Bone density in athletes. *Clin Orthop*. 1971;77:179–182.
82. Jones HH, Priest JS, Hayes WC, Tichenor CC, Nagel DA. Humeral hypertrophy in response to exercise. *J Bone Joint Surg Am*. 1977;59:204–208.
83. Lane N, Bevier W, Bouxsein M, Wiswell R, Careter D, Marcus R. Effect of exercise intensity on bone mineral. *Med Sci Sports Exerc*. 1988;20:S51.
84. Fleck SJ. Cardiovascular adaptations to resistance training. *Med Sci Sports Exerc*. 1988;20:S146–S151.
85. Fleck SJ, Henke C, Wilson W. Cardiac MRI of elite junior Olympic weight lifters. *Int J Sports Med*. 1989;10:329–333.
86. Miles DS, Gotshall RW. Impedance cardiography: noninvasive assessment of human central hemodynamics at rest and during exercise. *Exerc Sports Sci Rev*. 1989;17:231–264.
87. Atha J. Strengtheneing muscle. *Exerc Sport Sci Rev*. 1981;9:1–73.
88. Muller EA. Influence of training and of inactivity on muscle strength. *Arch Phys Med Rehabil*. 1970;51:449–462.
89. Whitley JD. The influence of static and dynamic training on angular strength performance. *Ergonomics*. 1967;10:305–310.
90. Gettman LR, Ayres J. Aerobic changes through 10 weeks of slow and fast-speed isokinetic training [abstract]. *Med Sci Sports*. 1978;10:47.
91. Bosco C, Tihany J, Komi PV, Feket G, Apr PL. Store and recoil of elastic energy in slow and fast types of human skeletal muscles. *Acta Physiol Scand*. 1982;116:343–349.
92. DeLorme TL. Restoration of muscle power by heavy resistance exercises. *J Bone Joint Surg Am*. 1945;27:645–667.
93. Zinovieff AN. Heavy resistance exercise: the Oxford technique. *Br J Physiol*. 1951;14:129–132.
94. McMorris RO, Elkins EC. A study of production and evaluation of muscular hypertrophy. *Arch Phys Med Rehabil*. 1954;35:420–426.
95. Knight KL. Knee rehabilitation by the daily adjustable progressive resistive exercise technique. *Am J Sports Med*. 1979;7:336–337.
96. Krusen EM. Functional improvement produced by resistance exercise of the biceps muscles affected by poliomyelitis. *Arch Phys Med*. 1949;30:271–278.
97. Clarke HH. *Muscular strength and endurance in man*. Englewood Cliffs, NJ: Prentice-Hall, Inc.; 1966.
98. Matveyev LP. Periodisienang das Sportlichen Training. Berlin: Beles Wernitz; 1972.
99. Stone M, et al. A hypothetical model for strength training. *J Sports Med Phys Fitness*. 1981;21:342–351.
100. Friden J, Seger J, Sjostrom M, Ekblom B. Adaptive response in human skeletal muscle subjected to prolonged eccentric training. *Int J Sports Med*. 1983;4:177–183.

ADDITIONAL READING

Gans C, Bock WJ. The functional significance of muscle architecture—a theoretical analyses. *Ergeb Anat Entwickel Gesch*. 1965;38:115–142.

CHAPTER 5

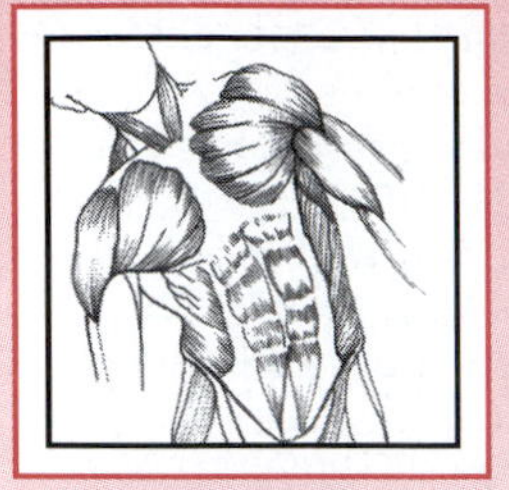

Endurance Impairment

Lori Thein Brody

Endurance is a critical aspect of most peoples' lives. Although some perform work or recreational tasks requiring strength, most people have a greater need for muscular and cardiovascular endurance. Many basic and instrumental activities of daily living (ADLs) require endurance.

Muscular endurance is the ability of a muscle group to perform repeated contractions against a load. These contractions can be isometric, concentric, eccentric, or a combination of these types. For example, the cervical spine muscles need muscular endurance to maintain the head in an erect position. The trunk, hip, or scapular muscles often work isometrically to provide a stable base for a moving leg or arm. The scapulothoracic muscles must possess the endurance to maintain proper upper quarter posture during any upright task. The demand on these muscles is even greater when working over a desk, counter, or work station all day (Fig. 5-1). In addition to the continuous postural muscle challenge, lower extremity muscle endurance is necessary to avoid functional limitations such as the inability to ascend or descend stairs. Stair climbing is a demanding muscular activity. Functional limitations from impaired endurance can lead to disability because of the inability to perform instrumental ADLs (eg, shopping, housework, yard work) or work-related activities (eg, walking mail carrier, night watchman, cashier, firefighter). Limitations in upper extremity muscle endurance can lead to disabilities, particularly when the task requires repetitive upper extremity motion. ADLs such as hair combing and teeth brushing and work such as carpentry and factory labor demand upper extremity muscle endurance.

Cardiovascular endurance is the ability of the cardiovascular system (ie, heart, lungs, and vascular system) to take in, extract, deliver, and use oxygen and to remove waste products. Cardiovascular endurance supports the performance of repetitive activities using large muscle groups for extended periods. For example, cardiovascular endurance is necessary to be able to walk or jog for an extended time without becoming winded. Activities requiring cardiovascular endurance require concurrent muscular endurance, although tasks requiring muscular endurance do not always necessitate cardiovascular endurance. Walking or jogging for an extended period requires adequate endurance of the lower extremity muscles. However, the muscular endurance necessary to maintain the lumbar spine and pelvis in optimal alignment does not require cardiovascular endurance. Some individuals have deficits in cardiovascular and muscular endurance, and this is referred to as deconditioning or a loss of general endurance.

PHYSIOLOGY OF ENDURANCE IMPAIRMENT

Repeated performance of a muscle contraction requires a series of complex activities from the brain to the contractile mechanism. Any step along this path can be a source of impairment. In addition to the physiologic components of this pathway, psychological factors and pain tolerance can affect the ability to perform a repeated activity. Limitations may be found in the musculoskeletal and cardiovascular systems. Muscular limitations may result from the muscle's inability to maintain an isometric contraction (eg, quadriceps femoris during downhill or water skiing) or to contract repeatedly (eg, hiking with a pack).[1] Cardiovascular limitations may result from the inability of the cardiovascular system (eg, excessive fatigue with carrying groceries) or the pulmonary system (eg, becoming winded during a 400-meter dash or ascending the stairs) to continue.

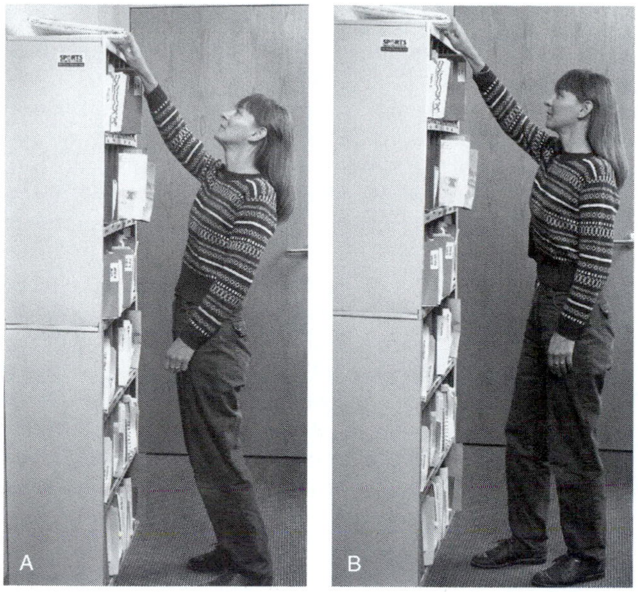

FIGURE 5-1 Individual standing at work station using ***(A)*** poor posture or ***(B)*** good posture.

The physiologic causes of fatigue have been categorized as peripheral and central mechanisms. Central mechanisms are associated with sites found within the central nervous system, and peripheral mechanisms are associated with sites outside the central nervous system[2] (Table 5-1). The differences can be summarized as failure occurring because of electrical excitation (ie, central) or failure within the contractile mechanism itself (ie, peripheral). Peripherally, fatigue can occur as a result of inadequacies of the oxygen transport system or from an inability to use oxygen at the muscular level.[3] Oxygen transportation is impaired by an insufficient capillary system within the muscle, and endurance training can enhance capillary system development. If the exercise intensity exceeds approximately 75% of maximal oxygen uptake, fatigue is likely to occur because of an inadequate capillary supply.[4] Activities requiring higher intramuscular forces, even if rhythmic, interfere with oxygenation. Glycogen stores and the ability to mobilize and transport triglycerides are necessary to prevent fatigue at the muscular level. Endurance adaptations are most likely to occur at the local limb or specific muscle group level, reinforcing the need for specificity of exercise.[5]

Debate continues regarding the role of the central mechanisms in physiologic fatigue. The ability to fully activate a muscle by electrical stimulation even after fatigue and degradation of coordination when fatigued provide support for central fatigue mechanisms. Further evidence includes improvement in force generation when opening the eyes after fatiguing exercise performed with the eyes closed.[6]

Limitations in the ability to take in and use oxygen can arise anywhere in the system. The lungs must be capable of taking in and extracting oxygen and passing the oxygenated blood to the heart. The heart must maintain a cardiac output level adequate to supply the working muscles with oxygenated blood. Limitations can occur in the heart's ability to pump (ie, limitations in heart rate or stroke volume) or peripherally at the muscle cell where oxygen is extracted.

Table 5-1. CHAIN OF EVENTS LEADING TO A MUSCLE CONTRACTION

	CHAIN OF EVENTS LEADING TO A MUSCLE CONTRACTION (ANATOMIC SITES OF FATIGUE)	MECHANISMS INVOLVED IN PROCESSING INFORMATION THROUGH THE CHAIN OF EVENTS (PHYSIOLOGIC PROCESSES RESPONSIBLE FOR FATIGUE)	
Central fatigue	Limbic, premotor, and association cortices ↓	Insufficient motivation or incentive	Processes involved in delivery of sufficient electrical excitation from CNS to muscle
	Sensorimotor cortex ↓	Insufficient cortical motoneuron activation	
	Spinal cord ↓	Depressed alpha motoneuron excitability	
Peripheral fatigue	Peripheral motoneurons ↓	Failure in neural transmission	
	Neuromuscular junction ↓	Failure in neuromuscular transmission	
	Sarcolemma ↓	Depressed muscle membrane excitability	
	Transverse tubules ↓	Failure of muscle action potential propagation	
	Sacroplasmic reticulum ↓	Insufficient release and/or reuptake of Ca^{2+}	Metabolic and enzymatic processes involved in providing sufficient energy for contraction
	Formation of actin-myosin cross-bridges	Failure in excitation-contraction coupling, insufficient energy supplies, inadequate energy supply replenishment, metabolic accumulation	
	Muscle contraction		

From Carrier DP, Nelson RM. *Dynamics of Human Biologic Tissues*. Philadelphia: FA Davis; 1992: 165.

Limitations in cardiovascular and muscular endurance can be treated with appropriate endurance exercise.

MUSCULAR ENDURANCE IMPAIRMENT

Causes and Rehabilitation Indications

Muscle is a plastic tissue that accommodates the stresses placed on it. The muscle can be underloaded or overloaded. Overload is the physiologic stimulus for positive muscular adaptations. Disuse or underuse produces negative changes. Impairment of muscular endurance results when the system is not used, underused, or traumatized.

INJURY

The most apparent cause of muscular endurance impairment is direct injury to the muscle-tendon unit, including the muscle belly, tendon, and bony attachment. In the child or adolescent, avulsion injuries occur to the hamstring muscle origin at the ischial tuberosity. A muscle contusion such as a blow to the quadriceps femoris or biceps brachii causes bleeding and swelling within the muscle. Similar limitations are found with a muscle strain, tear, or tendinitis. Acute muscle or tendon injury from a fall or other trauma also damages the surrounding soft tissues. Damage to the muscle-tendon unit in combination with decreased use because of pain and healing constraints impairs muscular endurance. For example, a fall on an outstretched arm by an elderly person frequently results in a rotator cuff muscle tear. The pain caused by the musculotendinous damage limits use of the arm, and deconditioning of the shoulder girdle muscles results (see Selected Intervention: Isometric Shoulder External Rotation). Other types of trauma such as burns may also directly affect the muscle's endurance.

Injury or surgery at an associated joint can limit muscle use and cause muscular endurance impairment. Secondary muscular changes occur in addition to the primary joint injury. Total joint replacement at the hip or knee, ligament reconstruction, stabilizing procedures, or abrasion arthroplasty limit muscle function. A fall directly on the anterior knee producing patellofemoral injury decreases quadriceps femoris function. The status of the muscle after joint surgery or injury is critical, because it is often the surrounding musculature that provides support to the joint during healing. Rehabilitation procedures should be directed at the joint, the periarticular connective tissues, and the surrounding musculature.

Nonorthopedic trauma or surgery can result in muscular endurance impairment. Generalized trauma after a fall or motor vehicle accident can produce a variety of impairments, including impaired endurance because of decreased activity. Accidents or blunt trauma such as farming acci-

---

SELECTED INTERVENTION
Isometric Shoulder External Rotation

See Case Study #4.

Although this patient requires comprehensive intervention, only one exercise is described:

ACTIVITY: Isometric shoulder external rotation (see the Figure)

PURPOSE: To kinesthetically learn how to fire the shoulder external rotator muscles and to increase strength of the shoulder external rotator muscles

RISK FACTORS: Isometric exercise may be contraindicated for individuals with hypertension

ELEMENTS OF THE MOVEMENT SYSTEM: Base

STAGE OF MOTOR CONTROL: Stability

POSTURE: Exercise can be performed in a variety of positions: sitting, supine, standing

MOVEMENT: The distal forearm should be placed against an immovable object (wall, arm of chair, using contralateral arm, and so on). Attempt to externally rotate the shoulder against the immovable object. A towel or other padding may be used to cushion the distal arm.

SPECIAL CONSIDERATIONS: (1) Ensure that the individual is producing the appropriate level of force. (2) Avoid abduction as a substitution for external rotation.

DOSAGE: Sets of 10 repetitions or repetitions to fatigue are performed several times per day (eg, hourly, each time a new class is started, when answering a phone call).

EXERCISE GRADATION: This exercise can be increased in intensity (pushing with a greater percentage of maximum voluntary contraction) or progressed to isotonic exercise.

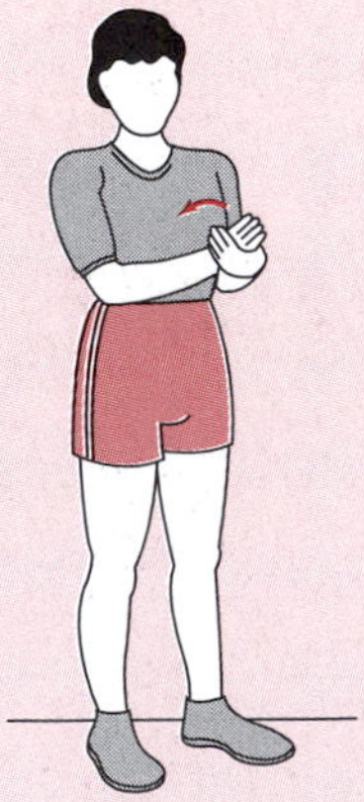

dents or gunshot wounds may damage internal organs. Surgery is followed by a period of decreased activity to allow healing. A mastectomy may produce impairments at the ipsilateral shoulder girdle, and muscular endurance may be impaired after any type of laparoscopy. These conditions result in limitations of cardiovascular and muscular endurance.

OTHER MEDICAL CONDITIONS OR DISEASES

Some medical conditions require a period of bed rest or significantly reduced activity to minimize secondary risks or complications. High-risk births such as multiple births often require a period of bed rest to avoid premature labor. Medical conditions such as pneumonia or unstable hypertension require minimal activity until the condition is under control. Cardiovascular conditions such as myocardial infarction or cerebrovascular accident or pulmonary problems such as atelectasis, unstable emphysema, or chronic obstructive pulmonary disease may necessitate a period of significantly reduced activity. These conditions therefore can cause impairments in cardiovascular and muscular endurance.

Neuromuscular disease such as multiple sclerosis, amyotrophic lateral sclerosis, or myasthenia gravis can profoundly impair muscular endurance. Whether muscular endurance can improve in these situations is questionable, and the prognosis depends on many variables. Any exacerbation of the underlying disease can diminish muscular strength and endurance, some of which may be recoverable during remission.

Individuals with impaired muscular endurance may be candidates for rehabilitation. The relation between the impairment and functional limitations and disability should be determined before initiating treatment. Is the impairment associated with a functional limitation or disability? Is it amenable to physical therapy treatment? If so, treatment should be implemented.

Physiologic Adaptations to Muscular Endurance Training

The muscle's response to endurance training is different from its response to strength training. This response is expected because of the differences in training dosage. Muscular endurance depends on oxidative capacity, and training increases the muscle's metabolic capacity. Muscles trained for endurance demonstrate cells with increased mitochondrial size, number, and enzymatic activity.[7] Increased enzymatic activity allows the muscle to better use the oxygen delivered.

Muscles trained for endurance also demonstrate increased local fuel storage. Glycogen stores may be increased twofold, and when endurance training is combined with appropriate carbohydrate intake, stores may increase as much as threefold.[7] In addition to increasing fuel stores, the endurance-trained muscle also increases fatty acid use and decreases the use of glycogen as a fuel. This alteration allows more exercise before fatigue. Endurance muscle training improves the oxygen delivery system by increasing the local capillary network, producing more capillaries per muscle fiber.[7]

MEASUREMENT OF MUSCULAR ENDURANCE IMPAIRMENT

Measurement of endurance impairment can take several forms and can be direct (ie, muscle biopsy) or indirect (ie, measure of force decrement).[4] Muscular endurance can be evaluated as the ratio of the peak torque generated after some number of repetitions relative to the peak force generated in the first few repetitions.[4] In the clinic, this ratio can be determined isotonically, isokinetically, or isometrically. For example, quadriceps femoris muscle endurance can be estimated isokinetically. The number of repetitions performed before a predetermined decline in torque (eg, 50%) can be recorded and compared with the same activity by the contralateral leg. Isotonically, the amount of weight that can be lifted for a given number of repetitions can be compared with the amount lifted with the contralateral leg. Isometrically, the peak torque before and after fatiguing exercise can be recorded and compared with the same degree of exercise on the contralateral side.

For endurance measures of muscles not amenable to isolated testing (eg, vastus medialis obliquus [VMO], rhomboids, lower trapezius) surface electromyography (SEMG) can provide information about muscle activity. SEMG comparisons of the VMO and the vastus lateralis can provide information about recruitment and relative fatigue in these muscles. This adjunctive method can be used during numerous activities such as stairstepping, bicycling, jogging, weight lifting, or specific rehabilitation exercises. Similarly, SEMG can monitor the lower trapezius during upper extremity activities to ensure proper scapular stabilization. The percentage of time committed to firing the muscle of interest compared with the contralateral side or with an antagonist can be recorded.

Although diminished muscular endurance is considered to be an impairment and is often measured, the functional limitations resulting from the impairment also should be identified and measured. Complaints of muscular fatigue during prolonged activities at work such as repetitive pushing, pulling, or lifting may be quantified. The amount of time, number of repetitions, or frequency or length of rest intervals are objective measures that can be applied to a functional activity. Recreational activities such as time or distance walked or jogged, length of time spent gardening or raking, or number of holes of golf played can quantify functional aspects of endurance impairments.

THERAPEUTIC EXERCISE INTERVENTION FOR MUSCULAR ENDURANCE IMPAIRMENT

The overload principle serves as the foundation of training to increase muscular endurance. Overload can be achieved by manipulating several variables and is discussed more thoroughly in the Exercise Dosage section. However, the overload principle must be considered in concert with pertinent elements of the movement system such as muscle activation patterns, sequencing, and posture. The clinician must ensure that the patient is using proper timing and sequencing and the best posture rather than substituting with synergists as the muscle fatigues (see Selected Intervention: Push-ups With a Plus).

Posture

One purpose of performing muscular endurance exercises is to retrain postural muscles (see Self-Management: Capital Retraction Exercises). If substitution occurs, the individual fails to train the correct muscles (ie, base element), and improper movement patterns are reinforced (ie, modulator and cognitive or affective elements). For example, during step-up exercises, the gluteal muscles can substitute for quadriceps activity by excessive forward lean of the trunk. This posture decreases the flexion moment arm at the knee, minimizing necessary quadriceps activity. Reinforcing improper movement patterns exacerbates the condition rather than increasing endurance of the targeted muscles. Proper muscle firing patterns can be encouraged by use of tactile techniques such as tapping or by the use of SEMG.

Mode

Various training modes can increase muscular endurance, but techniques to increase muscular endurance are more dosage dependent than mode dependent. Any training mode used to increase muscular strength can also be used to increase muscular endurance. Resistive devices such as weight equipment, resistive bands, isokinetic equipment, or the pool can be used (Fig. 5-2). The purpose of the exercise and availability of equipment affect decision making. When trying to isolate specific muscles for endurance training, resistive equipment that provides external stabilization is most effective. When simultaneously training proprioception or stabilization, free weights or body weight can challenge muscular endurance with less muscle isolation (see Self-Management: Split Squats). Eventually, exercise should progress to functional positions and movement patterns to develop the appropriate motor programs.

Movement

The movement chosen is directed at the specific elements of the movement system associated with the impairment or functional limitation. In the early phases, muscle isolation

SELECTED INTERVENTION
Push-ups With a Plus

See Case Study #8.

Although this patient requires comprehensive intervention, only one exercise is described:

ACTIVITY: Push-ups with a plus from the knees

PURPOSE: To strengthen the spine extensor, scapular stabilizers, triceps, and pectoral muscle groups. To teach maintenance of proper posture

RISK FACTORS: None

ELEMENTS OF THE MOVEMENT SYSTEM: Base modulator

STAGE OF MOTOR CONTROL: Controlled mobility

POSTURE: The patient is in a modified push-up position on the knees, with the hands just wider than shoulder width and with the pelvis, spine, and head in proper postural alignment

MOVEMENT: The patient extends the arms until the elbows are fully extended (ie, push-up position) and then performs a scapular protraction (ie, "plus"). The patient then returns to the normal scapular position (reverses the plus) and finally flexes the elbows to return the chest to the floor.

SPECIAL CONSIDERATIONS: (1) Ensure proper posture of the pelvis, preventing excessive hip flexion. (2) Ensure proper lumbar spine posture, maintaining normal lordosis without excessive extension. (3) Ensure proper posture of the cervical spine, avoiding excessive flexion, and proper position of the head on the cervical spine, avoiding excessive extension. (4) Maintain proper scapular stabilization and position on the rib cage, avoiding winging. (5) Activity may be too vigorous for individuals with shoulder pain because of rotator cuff pathology or posterior glenohumeral joint instability or for individuals with low back pain.

DOSAGE: Two to three sets until "form fatigue" or a maximum of 30 repetitions. Exercise is performed twice daily. Speed is slow and controlled.

RATIONALE FOR EXERCISE CHOICE: This exercise increases the dynamic control of the scapula on the thorax, reinforces and teaches the patient about isolated scapular movement and positioning, and increases the strength of the arm, shoulder, scapular, and cervical, thoracic, and lumbar spine muscles.

EXERCISE GRADATION: This exercise can be increased in intensity by moving to a full push-up position from the toes. Increased repetitions or sets of exercise may be added.

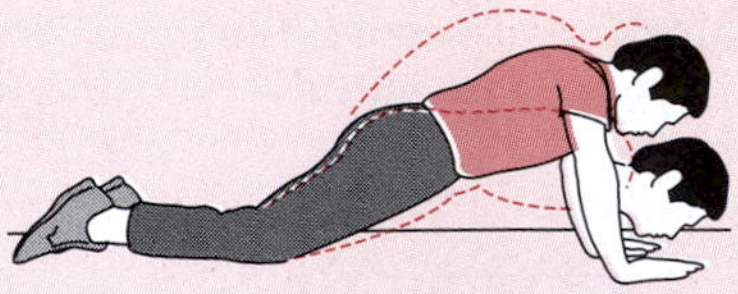

SELF-MANAGEMENT: Capital Retraction Exercises

Purpose: To teach and reinforce proper head and neck posture

Position: Stand or sit up with the shoulders back and the eyes looking straight ahead

Movement technique: Tuck chin in without tipping the head down

Repeat: _______ times

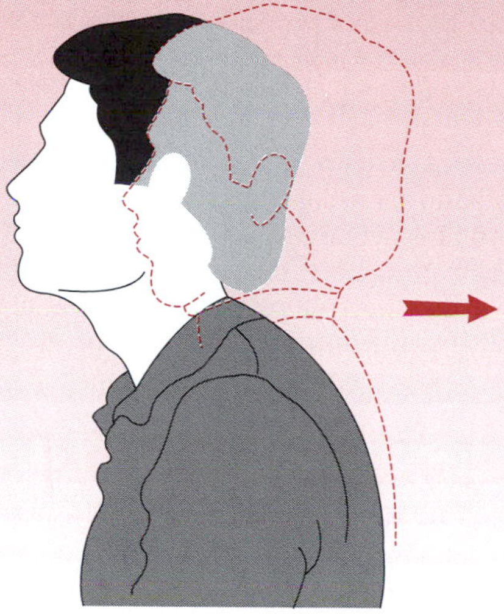

SELF-MANAGEMENT: Split Squats

Purpose: To increase muscle endurance and strength in the leg and hip muscles

Position: Place one foot in front of the other in a wide stance, with weight balanced equally on both feet while keeping an upright posture. The foot of your back leg may be flat on the floor or up on your toes.

Movement technique: Lower yourself part way down until your forward knee is bent about 45 degrees. Be sure your forward leg stays perpendicular to the floor.

Repeat: _______ times

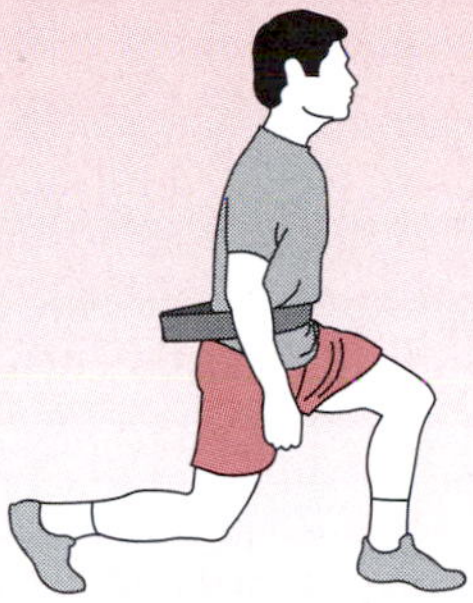

may be necessary to teach the patient how to use the muscle and to increase that muscle's endurance relative to surrounding or opposing musculature. For example, isolated scapular retraction may be trained to increase the endurance of these muscles and to teach the patient about the proper upper quarter posture. The patient may perform scapular retraction while sitting at a desk during the day

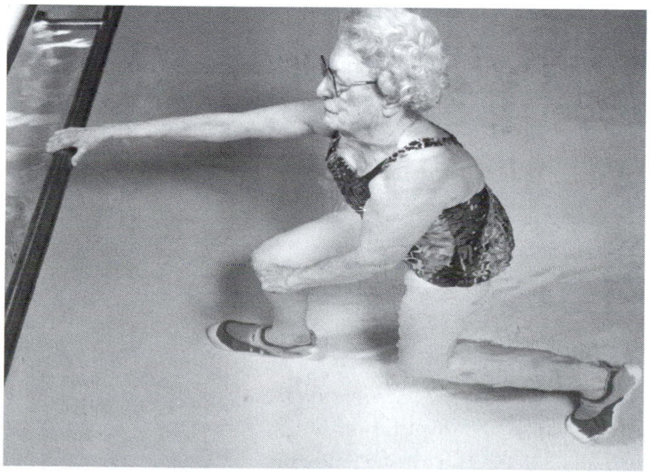

FIGURE 5-2 In-place lunges performed in the pool to train the quadriceps eccentrically while minimizing weight bearing.

(ie, modulator and cognitive or affective elements) and carry out resistive exercises for the rhomboid and trapezius muscles (ie, base and modulator elements) at other times during the day (Fig. 5-3).

In later rehabilitation stages, this same patient can progress to a maintained scapular position while performing functional activities such as computer work, lifting, carrying, and other daily activities. The patient is encouraged to focus on upper quarter posturing before beginning any task. This requires conscious thought initially, but with practice and repetition, the movement should become automatic.

The movement chosen should reflect the physiologic, kinesiologic, and learning factors associated with the patient's impairment or functional limitations. The movement pattern changes throughout the course of rehabilitation as the patient's limitations improve.

Dosage

SEQUENCE

When determining the sequence of exercises, the overall goals should be considered. Most endurance exercise necessitates a warm-up period to prepare the tissues, particularly if resistance is to be used. However, when performing endurance exercises primarily for their learning component (eg, scapular retraction while sitting at a desk), no specific warm-up exercise is necessary. In the latter rehabilitation phases, the patient may perform a warm-up activity, followed by a few repetitions of scapular retraction to reinforce this posture and followed by a resistive activity in

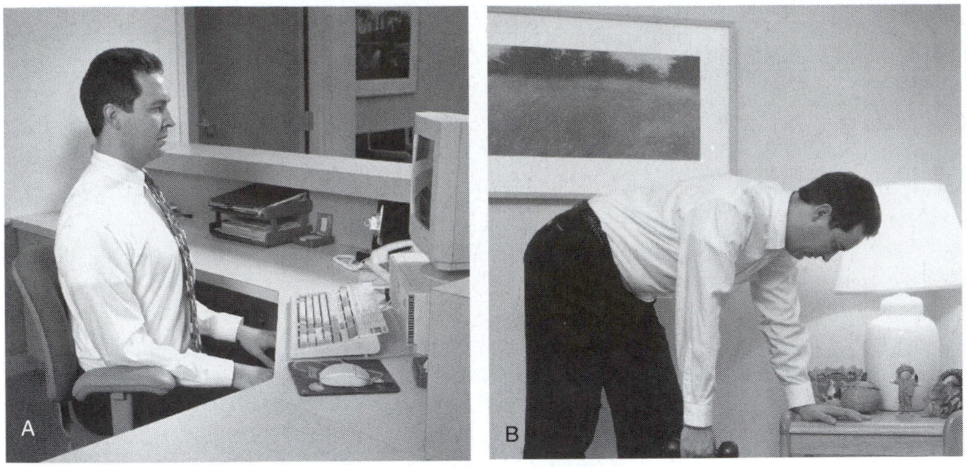

FIGURE 5-3 ***(A)*** Patient sitting at desk performing scapular retraction exercises. ***(B)*** Patient performing resisted scapular retraction with the arm forward flexed.

which scapular retraction is maintained during the activity (see Self-Management: Resisted Flexion Diagonals).

When determining the sequence of exercises, the clinician should remain aware of the effects of fatigue. Fatigue can compromise posture or movement and may result in injury or substitution. For example, fatigue of the VMO while performing quadriceps endurance exercises may not be readily apparent to the patient or clinician. However, use of SEMG, palpation, or close observation skills can alert the individual to these changes. VMO fatigue can lead to poor medial stabilization, patellofemoral pain, and gluteus maximus substitution. Fatigue results in failure to appropriately train the VMO and reinforces inefficient movement patterns by overusing the gluteal muscles.

SELF-MANAGEMENT: *Resisted Flexion Diagonals*

Purpose: To strengthen the muscles used to raise the arm, the shoulder blade muscles, and the back muscles

Position: Standing, with the back straight and gaze straight ahead

Movement technique: Raise the tubing or weight from your opposite thigh to an overhead position. Avoid extending your neck and back as you lift overhead.

Repeat: _______ times

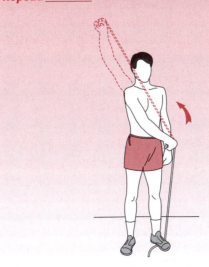

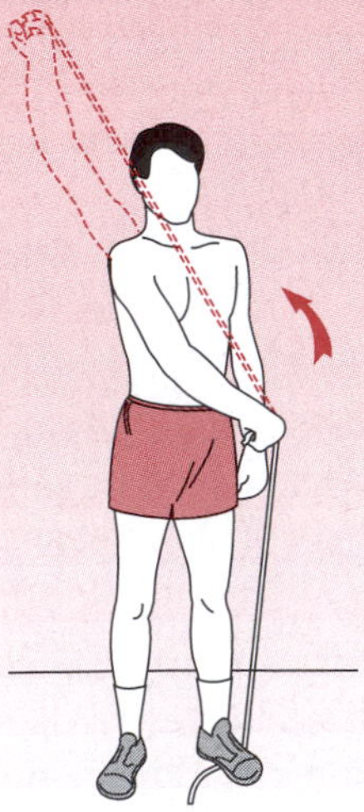

FREQUENCY

The frequency of exercise depends on the goal of the exercise program. Because the intensity of endurance exercises tends to be low, endurance exercise can be performed daily. Some exercises, such as postural reminder activities, are performed frequently throughout the day, but other exercises may be performed only once or twice daily. Exercises should be performed frequently enough to serve as a consistent postural reminder (if the goal is learning factors), which may mean hourly, each time the individual stands up or sits down, or whenever the phone rings. Resistive exercises should be performed with enough frequency, intensity, and duration to produce overload without producing fatigue. Excessive fatigue can result in injury or substitution. The clinician should teach the patient how to recognize this fatigue and how to modify activity.

INTENSITY AND DURATION

After proper firing patterns and postures (ie, modulator elements) have been verified, overload to increase muscular endurance should include increased repetitions or time of activity performance (ie, base elements). High-repetition, low-resistance activity ($\leq$ 25% of maximum voluntary contraction) can produce adaptive changes that increase muscular endurance. For example, continuous, repetitive activities such as running can stimulate adaptive muscle enzyme responses that are intensity and duration specific. For an untrained but active individual, light jogging can increase the muscle content of oxidative enzymes, and an increase in the jogging intensity to 70% or more of maximum oxygen consumption results in much greater adaptations. The effects of prolonged duration on muscle enzyme changes are less clear, with most information extrapolated from rat studies. Dudley and colleagues[8] subjected rats to treadmill running 5 days per week at various durations and intensities (approximately 60% to 115% maximum oxygen consumption). At each intensity, increasing the duration increased the muscle enzyme adaptations up to a plateau at approximately 45 to 60 minutes' duration. The training response varied by fiber type, with an intensity of 80% of maximum oxygen consumption necessary to produce a training response in the fast glycolytic fibers (type IIB). The responses by fiber type appeared to reflect recruitment patterns at different speeds.

When determining the intensity and duration of the exercise, the individual's functional demands should guide exercise prescription. If the goal is to maintain upper quarter posture throughout the day, the intensity is low but the duration is long. If the goal is to maintain adequate VMO firing while carrying a small child intermittently during the day, the intensity should be the person's body weight plus the approximate weight of the child. The exercises (eg, walking, step-ups, lunges) should be performed for a shorter duration than in the previous example.

Muscular Endurance Training by the Young

Muscular endurance training activities are appropriate for adolescents. Whether the goal is rehabilitation from an injury or training as part of a fitness or sports program, this type of training can be healthy for the young individual. Because no maximum or heavy weight lifting is performed, risk of injury is no greater than in the adult population.

Quality and proper performance of exercise are the most important factors. As with strength training by the young person, the goal of endurance training should be learning proper technique, form, and posture. The body weight is used as resistance before any weight training is attempted. Weight machines are appropriate if the equipment can be properly fitted to the young person's size. Like endurance muscle training for the adult, repetitions should be kept high and the resistance low. The exercise session should be supervised by an adult trained in resistive training techniques.

Muscular Endurance Training by the Elderly

Muscular endurance training is particularly beneficial for the elderly, especially in the older woman. Aging is associated with muscle atrophy, declining strength and endurance, decreased exercise recovery capacity, and decreased muscle enzymatic activity.[9] Resistive training can increase muscular strength and endurance in the elderly.[10] Resistive training by elderly women can have a protective effect on bone[11] (Fig. 5-4).

Resistive muscular endurance exercises can be safely initiated in the elderly population. Education regarding proper warm-up, cool-down, and progression techniques is essential, because many elderly individuals have never participated in such programs. Activities using body weight as resistance should be incorporated initially and should remain a large portion of the exercise program (see Self-Management: Abdominal Curls). Exercises should be progressed slowly and may be performed more frequently (up to five times per week) because of the lower intensity. The session duration

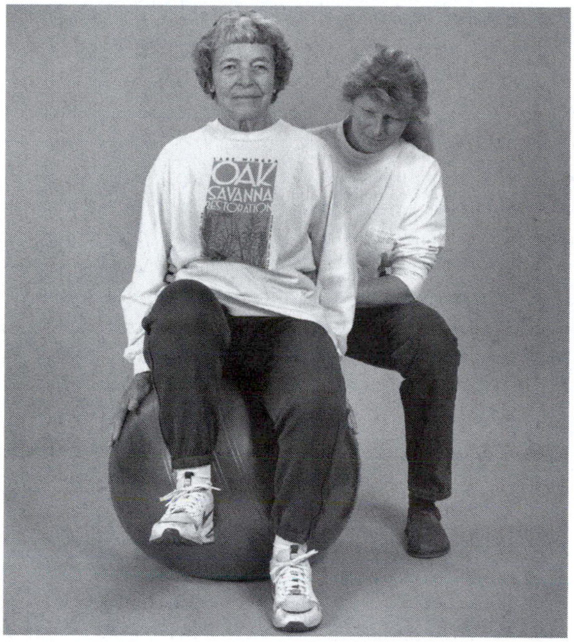

FIGURE 5-4 Weight bearing resistive exercise is particularly beneficial for the elderly female.

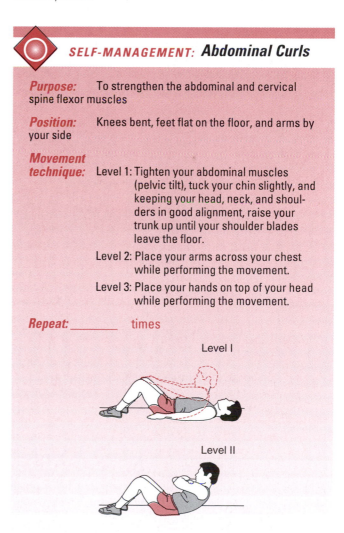

SELF-MANAGEMENT: *Abdominal Curls*

Purpose: To strengthen the abdominal and cervical spine flexor muscles

Position: Knees bent, feet flat on the floor, and arms by your side

Movement technique:
Level 1: Tighten your abdominal muscles (pelvic tilt), tuck your chin slightly, and keeping your head, neck, and shoulders in good alignment, raise your trunk up until your shoulder blades leave the floor.
Level 2: Place your arms across your chest while performing the movement.
Level 3: Place your hands on top of your head while performing the movement.

Repeat: _______ times

Level I

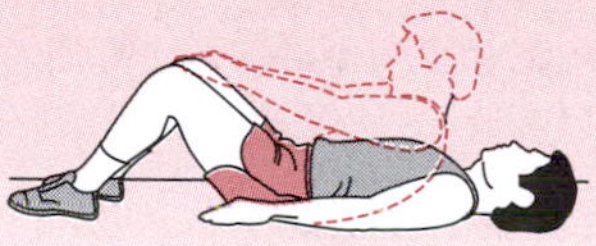

Level II

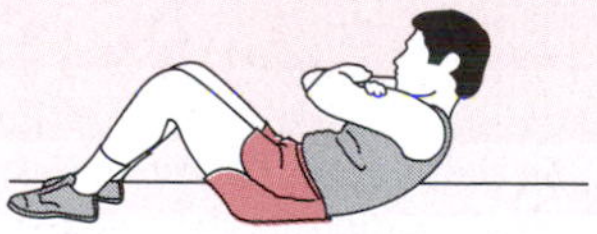

may have to be lengthened because of the lower intensity, or several short sessions may be completed throughout the day.

Precautions and Contraindications

Degenerative joint disease, osteoporosis, diabetes, pregnancy, neuromuscular disease, and other comorbidities should be considered when designing a resistive exercise program. Activities minimizing the risk of injury or extreme fatigue should be emphasized. For example, individuals with degenerative joint disease may focus on non–weight-bearing exercises initially, and those with osteoporosis may emphasize weight-bearing activities (see Selected Intervention: Supine Trunk Stabilization). Pregnant women should avoid positions that place their backs at risk. Those with neuromuscular diseases such as multiple sclerosis should be careful to avoid fatigue.

Active or resistive exercise stresses the cardiovascular system and may be contraindicated for some patients. The patient's physician should be consulted when considering isometric exercise for the individual with hypertension. Resistive exercise is contraindicated for those with unstable cardiac conditions or angina. A complete list of contraindications to exercise in the elderly can be found in Display 5-1.

When active or resistive exercise is prescribed, instruction in proper breathing techniques should be taught as well. Regular inhalation and exhalation without breath holding or a Valsalva maneuver can minimize the cardiac risk.

CARDIOVASCULAR ENDURANCE IMPAIRMENT

Causes and Rehabilitation Indications

Cardiovascular endurance may be limited for several reasons. Injury to the heart, lungs, or vascular system, the primary tissues involved in cardiovascular endurance, may precipitate an impairment or functional limitation. Myocardial infarction, valve replacement, bypass surgery, and various forms of heart disease commonly affect the heart itself. Conditions affecting the pulmonary system such as lung tumors, emphysema, chronic obstructive pulmonary disease, or cystic fibrosis also decrease cardiovascular endurance.

Any medical condition necessitating hospitalization or bed rest results in deconditioning of the cardiovascular system. Surgical procedures for the gallbladder, appendix, uterus, or other internal organs require a period of decreased

SELECTED INTERVENTION
Supine Trunk Stabilization

See Case Study #7.

Although this patient requires comprehensive intervention, only one exercise is described:

ACTIVITY: Supine hand to knee isometrics

PURPOSE: To increase the strength of the abdominal and hip flexor musculature

ELEMENTS OF THE MOVEMENT SYSTEM: Base

STAGE OF MOTOR CONTROL: Mobility and stability

POSTURE: The patient is positioned supine with the knees flexed and the arms at the side.

ASSISTIVE POSITIONING DEVICES: A small towel roll or lumbar pillow may be placed under the lumbar spine to provide additional low back support.

MOVEMENT: A pelvic tilt is performed and maintained while one hip is flexed to 90 degrees. The opposite hand should resist the hip flexion, producing an isometric contraction of the abdominal muscles and hip flexor muscles. Hold the isometric for a count of three while continuing breathing; then lower the leg and arm to the ground and repeat with the opposite arm and leg.

SPECIAL CONSIDERATIONS: (1) Ensure that individuals with low back pain can perform the exercise pain-free. (2) Individuals with hypertension should hold the isometric muscle contraction for only one second. (3) Ensure that proper spinal alignment is maintained throughout the exercise

DOSAGE: Two to three sets of 10 repetitions or to form fatigue, performed two times per day

RATIONALE FOR EXERCISE CHOICE: This exercise requires an active pelvic tilt, abdominal and hip flexor muscle contraction, and shoulder stabilization. This exercise improves hip mobility and trunk and shoulder stability.

EXERCISE GRADATION: This exercise can be increased in intensity (ie, pushing with a greater force or by pushing against both knees simultaneously) or progressed to an upright position.

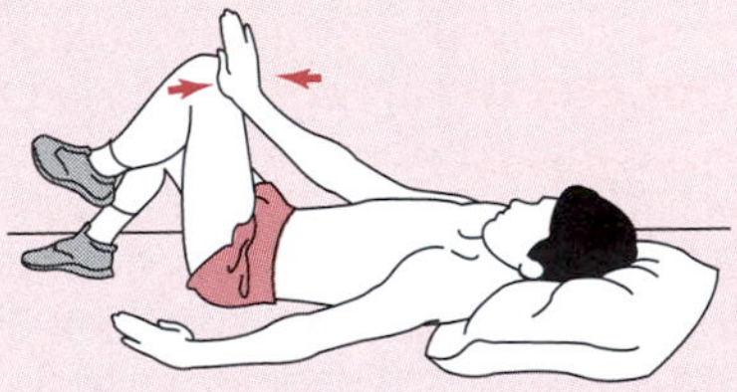

DISPLAY 5-1

Contraindications to Physical Activity by Older Adults

Absolute Contraindications

Severe CAD—unstable angina pectoris and acute myocardial infarction
Decompensated congestive heart failure
Uncontrolled ventricular arrhythmias
Uncontrolled atrial arrhythmias (compromising cardiac function)
Severe valvular heart disease including aortic, pulmonic, and mitral stenosis
Uncontrolled systemic hypertension (eg, > 200/105)
Pulmonary hypertension
Acute myocarditis
Recent pulmonary embolism or deep vein thrombosis

Relative Contraindications

CAD
Congestive heart failure
Significant valvular heart disease
Cardiac arrhythmias including ventricular and atrial arrhythmias and complete heart block
Hypertension
Fixed-rate, permanent pacemaker
Cyanotic congenital heart disease
Congenital anomalies of coronary arteries
Cardiomyopathy including hypertrophic cardiomyopathy and dilated cardiomyopathy
Marfan's syndrome
Peripheral vascular disease
Severe obstructive or restrictive lung disease
Electrolyte abnormalities, especially hypokalemia
Uncontrolled metabolic diseases (eg, diabetes, thyrotoxicosis, myxedema)
Any serious systemic disorder (eg, mononucleosis, hepatitis)
Neuromuscular or musculoskeletal disorders that would make exercise difficult
Marked (gross) obesity
Anemia
Idiopathic long-QT syndrome

CAD, coronary artery disease.
Adapted from Heath GW, Exercise programming for the older adult. In: American College of Sports Medicine: Resource Manual for Guidelines for Exercise Testing and Prescription. *2nd ed. Lea & Febiger; Philadelphia; 1993;419.*

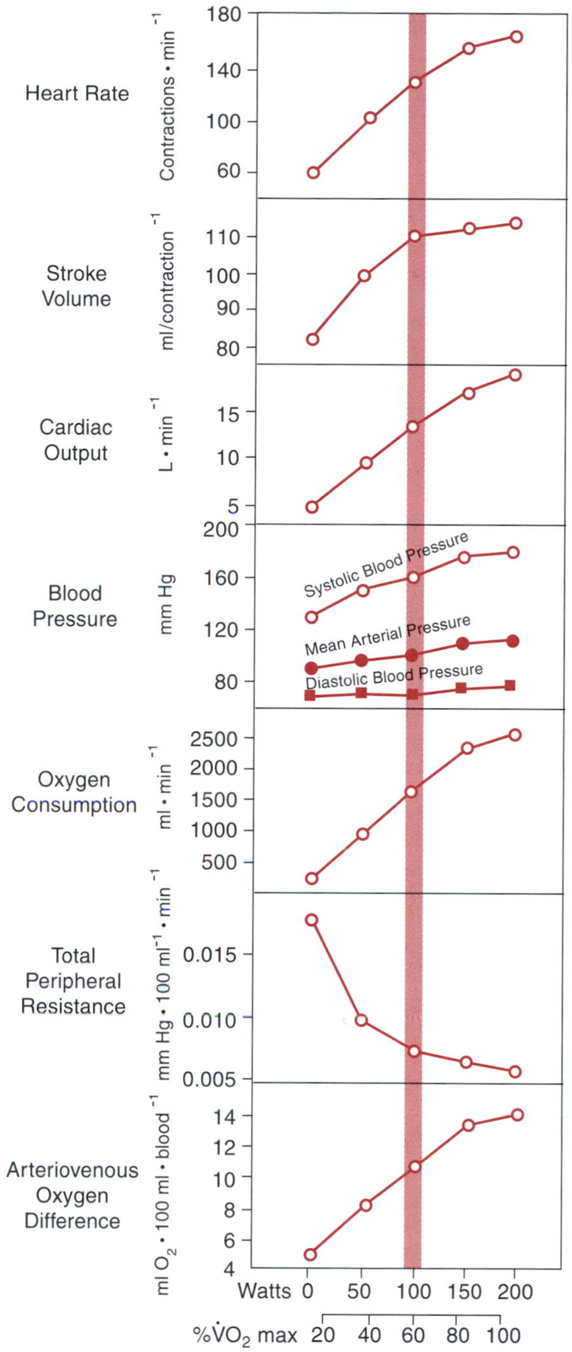

FIGURE 5-5 Acute cardiovascular responses to graded exercise.

activity. Accidents resulting in internal or orthopedic injuries can incapacitate the individual for some time. Medical conditions such as cancer, neuromuscular disease, or cerebrovascular attacks and injuries such as traumatic brain injury or spinal cord injury decrease cardiovascular endurance.

Acute Responses to Cardiovascular Exercise

Cardiovascular changes occur as the body adjusts to a new workload (Fig. 5-5). As the workload increases during the warm-up and training periods, the cardiac output, or the amount of blood pumped by the heart per minute, increases linearly with the workload. Cardiac output is the product of heart rate and stroke volume, or the amount of blood pumped with each heart beat. Stroke volume increases linearly with workload until approximately 50% of maximum oxygen consumption, at which point the stroke volume plateaus.[12] Oxygen consumption, like heart rate, increases linearly with workload.

Total peripheral resistance is the sum of all forces that resist blood flow. Vasodilation of the arterial vascular beds in the active muscles causes a decrease in total peripheral resistance as the workload increases. Systolic blood pressure increases slightly with the initiation of exercise, but diastolic blood pressure remains relatively unchanged. The arteriovenous oxygen difference (a-vO_2) represents the difference in oxygen content of the arterial and venous blood and reflects the oxygen extraction by working muscles. As the workload increases, a-vO_2 increases linearly until maximum oxygen consumption, at which level approximately 85% of oxygen is removed from arterial blood.[12]

Physiologic Adaptations to Cardiovascular Endurance Training

In healthy individuals, cardiovascular training produces profound changes throughout the cardiorespiratory system. The weight and volume of the heart increase with long-term aerobic (ie, with oxygen) training. The left ventricle size is commonly increased in trained individuals.[13] Endurance training improves oxygen delivery, decreases the resting and submaximal heart rates, and increases the stroke volume and total cardiac output. Blood volume is expanded along with increases in plasma volume, total hemoglobin concentration, and peripheral capillary formation. Oxygen use is improved with increases in aerobic enzyme and muscle myoglobin levels. Substrate use is enhanced with increases in fat-mobilizing enzymes and free fatty acid delivery to the muscle. Regular training also reduces systolic and diastolic blood pressure. Regular aerobic training can alter the body composition, reducing body weight by decreasing body fat (see Display 5-2).

MEASUREMENT OF CARDIOVASCULAR ENDURANCE IMPAIRMENT

The gold standard measure for cardiovascular endurance impairments is maximum oxygen consumption (VO_{2MAX}). The VO_{2MAX} is determined directly by a maximum stress test, usually performed on a treadmill. This test can also be performed using a variety of modes, including a bicycle ergometer, swimming flue, cross-country ski track, or rowing ergometer. Although direct testing of maximum oxygen consumption is the most accurate measure, submaximal approximation is frequently performed when the individual should not or cannot be tested maximally. The results of a submaximal test are based on the linear relationship between maximum oxygen consumption and heart rate. However, the confidence intervals around an individual score for submaximal testing are wide, making accurate assessment difficult.[4] Submaximal approximation is valuable when testing the elderly or individuals with a history of cardiac disease. The VO_{2MAX} values predicted from submaximal tests are generally within 10% to 20% of the individual's results for maximal tests.[14]

Oxygen consumption testing may be difficult for the clinician with limited facilities. For a patient with known cardiac disease, the clinician should consult the patient's physician to ensure readiness to undertake a physical exercise program. It is likely that the patient has undergone some stress testing, and this information should be obtained from the physician.

For patients without a history of cardiac disease, simple clinical measures of oxygen consumption are heart rate and perceived exertion. Heart rate rises somewhat linearly with increases in oxygen consumption, and determining a target heart rate using the Karvonen formula can quantify exercise intensity. The Karvonen formula determines a target exercise rate using the heart rate reserve and the age-predicted maximum heart rate. Exercise for cardiovascular endurance should range from 55% to 90% of maximum, but it can vary among patients.[14,15] The lower end of the training zone for an individual working in a 60% to 80% range is determined by this formula:

$$HR_{lower} = HR_{rest} + 0.60(HR_{max} - HR_{rest})$$

in which HR_{rest} is the resting heart rate and HR_{max} is the maximum heart rate, or 220 minus the person's age.

The rate of perceived exertion (RPE) correlates positively with maximum oxygen consumption. Also known as the Borg scale, the original RPE ranged from 6 to 19, but the revised scale ranges from 0 to 10 (Table 5-2). Patients are asked throughout the exercise session to relate the exercise intensity to the sensation they are experiencing. Individuals can be trained to use the RPE as a guideline dur-

DISPLAY 5-2
Physiologic Adaptations to Cardiovascular Endurance Training

Increased heart weight and volume
Increased left ventricle size
Decreased resting and submaximal heart rates
Increased stroke volume
Increased cardiac output
Increased plasma volume
Increased total hemoglobin
Increased peripheral capillary formation
Increased aerobic and fat metabolizing enzymes
Increased free fatty acid delivery
Decreased systolic and diastolic blood pressure
Decreased body fat

Table 5-2. OLD AND REVISED RATE OF PERCEIVED EXERTION SCALES

ORIGINAL SCALE		REVISED SCALE	
6		0	Nothing
7	Very, very light	0.5	Very, very weak
8		1	Very weak
9	Very light	2	Weak
10		3	Moderate
11	Fairly light	4	Somewhat strong
12		5	Strong
13	Somewhat hard	6	
14		7	Very strong
15	Hard	8	
16		9	
17	Very hard	10	Very, very strong; maximal
18			
19	Very, very hard		

ing exercise sessions. Many patients find this easier than trying to count their heart rates during exercise sessions.

The metabolic equivalent (MET) is also used to prescribe activity intensity. A MET is used to estimate the metabolic cost of physical activity relative to that during the resting state. One MET is equal to 3.5 mL of oxygen consumed per kilogram of body weight per minute. In general, walking at 2 miles/hour is the equivalent of approximately 2.0 METs, and walking at 4 miles/hour is the equivalent of approximately 4.6 METs.

THERAPEUTIC EXERCISE INTERVENTION FOR DECREASED CARDIOVASCULAR ENDURANCE

Mode

Several modes of cardiovascular endurance training are available. Any activity that uses large muscle groups and is repetitive is capable of producing the desired changes. Sample activities include walking, jogging, cross-country skiing, bicycling, rope jumping, rowing, swimming, or aerobic dance (see Selected Intervention: Cross-Country Ski Machine). Although lap swimming is the most obvious aquatic cardiovascular exercise, water jogging, cross-country skiing, and water aerobics are also effective aquatic training methods. An upper body ergometer is a good cardiovascular training tool and is especially well-suited for individuals unable to use their legs.

The choice of exercise mode depends on the patient's goals and specific physical condition. Performing an activity that is convenient, comfortable, and enjoyable increases the likelihood of adherence. The amount of impact is also an important consideration when choosing the exercise mode. For the individual with lower extremity degenerative joint disease or the overweight individual, impact activities should be avoided. The pool is a better choice for those who must have weight bearing or impact minimized. Weight bearing can be completely negated by exercising in the deep end of the pool. For those desiring to return to impact activities, gradual impact progression can prepare the body for the demands of this type of

SELECTED INTERVENTION
Cross-Country Ski Machine

See Case Study #10.

Although this patient requires comprehensive intervention, only one exercise is described:

ACTIVITY: Cross-country ski machine

PURPOSE: To increase cardiovascular endurance and musculoskeletal muscle endurance of quadriceps, gluteals, and spine and arm extensors

ELEMENTS OF THE MOVEMENT SYSTEM: Base, support

STAGE OF MOTOR CONTROL: Skill

POSTURE: Standing posture, maintaining proper pelvic and spine posture. Arms are resting on the machine for balance or can participate by performing alternate arm extensions with attached pulleys (with or without resistance)

MOVEMENT: Alternate hip flexion and extension in a walking pattern with minimal knee motion is performed. The patient must be sure to transfer weight completely from leg to leg during the activity, rather than shuffling or sliding the feet while bearing weight bilaterally. The arms can move in an alternate fashion with the legs. Range of motion may be limited by individual needs.

SPECIAL CONSIDERATIONS: (1) All precautions to cardiovascular endurance exercise must be considered. (2) Individuals with balance and coordination difficulty should be assessed for ability to perform the activity safely.

DOSAGE: Ten minutes, adding 5 minutes every three sessions

RATIONALE FOR EXERCISE CHOICE: When the arm movement is included, cross-country skiing is a total body exercise. Aerobic conditioning can be achieved, along with shoulder, trunk, hip, and leg extensor muscle endurance training.

EXERCISE GRADATION: This exercise can be progressed by increasing the frequency, intensity, or duration of activity.

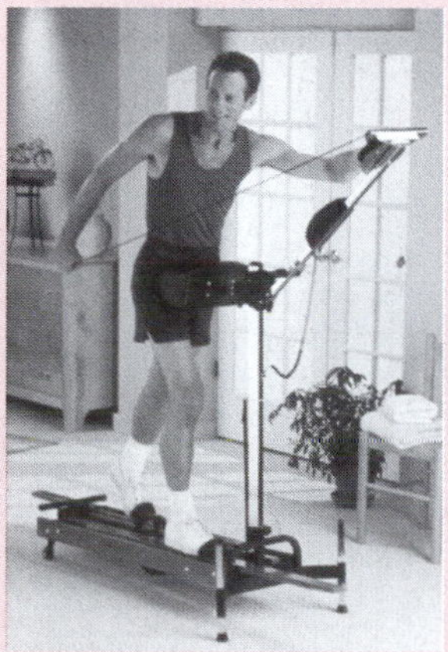

Used with the permission of Nordic Track, Inc., Chaska, Minnesota.

Patient-Related Instruction

Return to Impact Activity

Any return to impact activities such as jogging, impact aerobics, or sports requiring running or jumping should be preceded by impact progression. This approach ensures readiness to return to the activity and decreases the likelihood of setback. Prerequisites for impact progression include the following:

1. Adequate muscle strength and endurance
2. Full range of motion in the joints
3. No swelling

A suggested progression is as follows:

1. Two-footed hopping
2. Alternate-footed hopping
3. Single-footed hopping (optional)
4. Skill drills (optional)

This progression should be implemented as follows:

1. Begin on a low-impact surface (eg, pool, minitramp, shock absorptive floor).
2. Subsequently progress to the terrain you will be using.
3. Begin with 5 minutes, and increase by 2- to 5-minute increments when you are able to complete three consecutive sessions without pain, swelling, or technique compromise.
4. Return to your full activity is determined by the criteria set by your clinician.

loading (Patient-Related Instruction: Return to Impact Activity).

Variety and cross-training in the cardiovascular endurance program are imperative. Alternating modes of activity can alleviate boredom and prevent overuse injuries resulting from repetitive activity. Many individuals have such low muscular endurance that they are incapable of performing the same repetitive activity for more than a few minutes. The activity mode can be changed within the training session and among sessions. Although one individual may bicycle 2 days per week, swim 2 days, and walk 2 days, another may bike, walk, and stairstep for 10 minutes each daily.

Within exercise one mode, several postures or equipment types are available. For example, during bicycling, the trunk posture depends on the goals. Bicycling may be performed on a recumbent bike (Fig. 5-6*A*), with the hips flexed 90 degrees or more and the low back supported, or it may be performed in a upright position with the arms moving (Fig. 5-6*C*) or in forward leaning position (Fig. 5-6*B*). The optimal posture for maximal exercise benefit should be emphasized (Patient-Related Instruction: Bicycling Guidelines).

Dosage

TYPE

The training session itself may be performed using a variety of training techniques, from continuous activity to interval training. Continuous training relies on the aerobic energy system to supply energy for the exercise session and can be carried out for prolonged periods. The individual exercises continuously, without rest, at a steady exercise rate. Although continuous in nature, several different activities can be combined within the same session, such as treadmill and bicycle or swimming and deep-water running.

Interval training incorporates rest sessions between bouts of exercise. When prescribing interval training, the ratio of the rest period to the training period determines the activity intensity and the energy system used. The aerobic energy system is used to a greater extent with longer training intervals and shorter rest periods. The rest periods can be true rest (ie, no activity) or a work-relief interval, during which light activity such as walking may be performed.

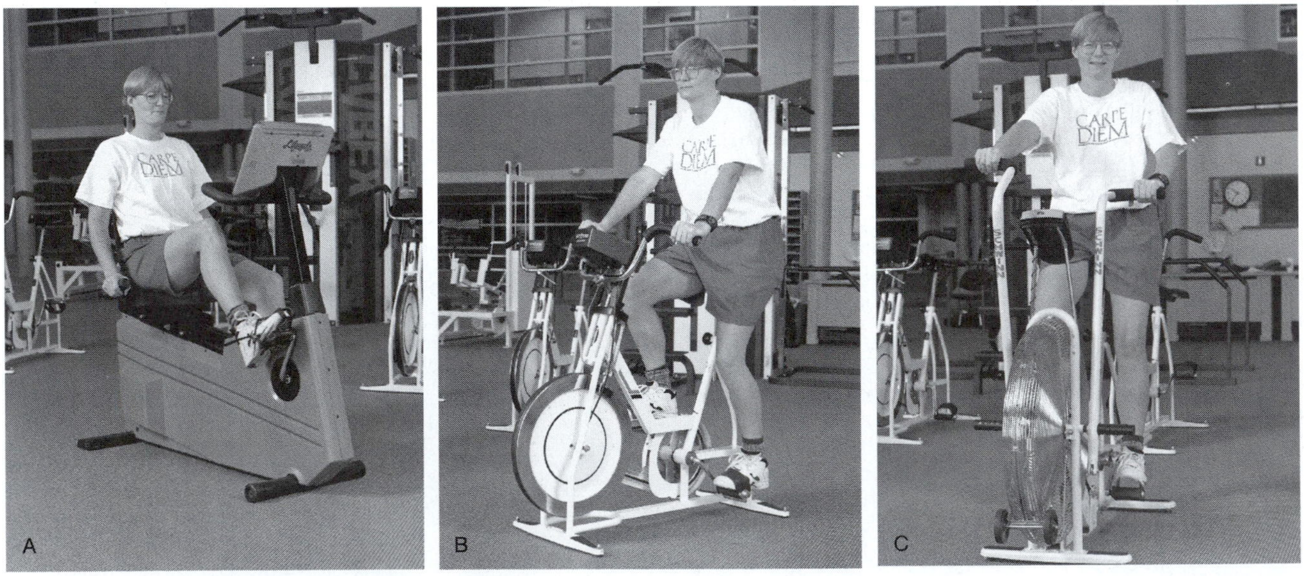

FIGURE 5-6 ***(A)*** Exercise on a semirecumbent bike positions the individual differently from exercise on a traditional bike. ***(B)*** Bicycling in a traditional position places more weight on the upper extremities, challenging the postural muscles more than in a recumbent position. ***(C)*** Exercise on an upright bike with *moving arms* places different loads on the patient.

> **Patient-Related Instruction**
>
> ### Bicycling Guidelines
>
> The following guidelines will keep your bicycling experience healthy and safe:
>
> 1. **Seat height:** The seat should be set so that your knee is slightly bent in the down-most position. If you place your heel on the pedal in the down position, your knee should be perfectly straight. When you place the ball of your foot on the pedal, your knee should be bent at the correct angle.
> 2. **Cadence:** Your pedal cadence should be high, at least 60 rpm or more. Your clinician may have other recommendations, depending on your specific situation.
> 3. **Resistance:** Your resistance should be low enough to allow a higher cadence. Resistance too high can place extra stress on the knee. Keeping the resistance low and the cadence high produces the desired benefits without hurting your knees.
> 4. **Safety:** If riding outside, always wear a helmet, and obey your local bicycle laws.

High-intensity activity usually is combined with longer complete-rest intervals, and low to medium intensities are combined with shorter rest intervals or work-relief intervals.

Circuit training can be continuous or interval. Circuit training is a training technique in which the individual rotates through a series of exercise stations. A variety of upper extremity, lower extremity, core, and cardiovascular training exercises usually are included. The individual performs each station's activity for a specified time (ie, 30 seconds) and then moves on to the next station. The activity choices, activity intensity, and rest between stations determine the energy system used and whether the activity is interval or continuous. This type of training provides the opportunity for a well-balanced exercise program with variety. Many individuals can be trained simultaneously if there are adequate stations (Patient-Related Instruction: Setting Up a Circuit).

> **Patient-Related Instruction**
>
> ### Setting Up a Circuit
>
> Your regular exercise routine can be enhanced and made more enjoyable by breaking up a continuous activity with stations of alternative activities. This can be done outside along a normal walking or running route, or at your indoor exercise location. For example, a walking or jogging program through the neighborhood or on the treadmill can be broken up with the following activities performed at certain intervals throughout the session:
>
> 1. Toe raises
> 2. Abdominal curls
> 3. Push-ups
> 4. Squats
> 5. Dips
> 6. Lunge walks
> 7. Quadriceps, hamstring, and calf stretches

SEQUENCE

Cardiovascular endurance training may be performed as part of a comprehensive rehabilitation program that includes mobility, stretching, and strengthening activities. General warm-up activities should be performed initially, followed by stretching and the cardiovascular training session. The warm-up period should last 5 to 10 minutes to prepare the body for exercise. Large muscle group activity such as walking, calisthenics, or bicycling should be performed with gradually increasing intensity. The warm-up session may be a lower-intensity version of the cardiovascular training activity. Walking at a slower speed for 5 minutes may be used as a warm-up activity for faster walking or jogging. The warm-up activities increase muscle blood flow, muscle temperature, and neural conduction. These changes, along with mental preparedness, can decrease the chances of muscle injury during exercise. After the warm-up, stretching exercises are performed, followed by the more vigorous cardiovascular endurance session. The cardiovascular training session should be concluded with cool-down activities, which often consist of lower-intensity versions of the training session and stretching exercises.

The exercise session should be concluded with a cool-down period of 5 to 10 minutes to allow redistribution of blood flow that has changed with exercise, including prevention of lower extremity pooling of blood by enhancing venous return. Active muscle contraction by continued walking, cycling, or calisthenics at a low level assists in this blood flow redistribution. Stretching should conclude the session to ensure maintenance of the working muscle's optimal length.

FREQUENCY

The frequency of cardiovascular training is related to the patient's goals, the intensity and duration of exercise, and the patient's fitness level. Persons with low exercise tolerance (ie, less than 3 METs) may exercise several times each day at a low intensity. An individual training for long-distance running may run 15 miles on 1 day and rest on the following day. An individual walking 1 mile at a comfortable pace as part of a fitness routine should be able to participate on a daily basis. The exercise program must be viewed in the context of the individual's day. If the patient spends 2 days per week working at a department store where continuous standing and walking are typical, the addition of cardiovascular exercise on that day may result in an overuse injury.

To attain the physiologic benefits of cardiovascular exercise, the activity should be performed at least three to four times per week. This should be a realistic goal for patients who are underconditioned or deconditioned, despite their inability to participate at that level initially. The overload principle should be considered; for the severely deconditioned, only minimal intensity, frequency, or duration are necessary to overload the system. In a highly trained individual, exercise at a greater frequency may be necessary to produce overload, depending on the exercise intensity.

INTENSITY

As with frequency and duration, setting the intensity of exercise should be based on the overload principle and must consider the functional limitations, goals, and fitness level of the individual. In healthy individuals, the training zone necessary to achieve the benefits of cardiovascular exercise is generally 40% to 85% of Vo_{2MAX} or 55% to 90% of HR_{max}.[15] In the pool, the heart rate is decreased when exercising while immersed to the neck because of the Starling reflex and is therefore a poor gauge of workload. The heart rate of deep-water exercise is 17 to 20 beats/minute less than that of the comparable land-based activity.[14]

The exercise intensity can be increased by adding resistance, increasing speed, changing terrain (eg, up hills), removing stabilization, or adding upper extremity activity. The method for increasing intensity is goal specific and may be limited by other medical or physical conditions (eg, rotator cuff tendinitis limiting the use of upper extremities). The intensity necessary to achieve a workload in the target training zone varies among patients and usually correlates with the previously determined conditioning level.

DURATION

Exercise duration can be manipulated to produce overload and a resultant cardiovascular training effect. Duration depends on the frequency, intensity, and the conditioning level of the patient. In general, exercise of greater intensity is performed for a shorter duration, and exercise of lower intensity can be performed for a longer duration. Manipulation of these variables is goal dependent. If the patient is required to perform an activity for a long duration (ie, continuous walking as part of a job or recreation), progression of the rehabilitation program should focus more on increasing the duration and less on increasing the intensity.

The American College of Sports Medicine recommends a duration of 20 to 30 minutes, 3 to 4 days per week, for producing cardiovascular improvements.[15] If the patient is unable to complete this duration of the same activity, alternating activities within the same exercise session can produce the same cardiovascular benefits without injury to the musculoskeletal system. Individuals who are severely deconditioned may need several shorter bouts of exercise during the day to equal a total of 20 minutes of activity daily. This may be achieved by two 10-minute or four 5-minute sessions. The same activity or different activities may be performed in each of these sessions (Patient-Related Instruction: Frequency, Intensity, and Duration).

Cardiovascular Endurance Training by the Young

Adolescents can benefit from cardiovascular exercise. Swimming, bicycling, jogging, and other forms of aerobic exercise can become a part of the person's lifestyle at an early age, thereby establishing healthy habits. The American Academy of Pediatrics Committee on Sports Medicine position statement on long-distance running by children states that this activity is safe as long as the child enjoys the activity and is asymptomatic.[16] The clinician should remember that the young individual is not just a small adult. Youths are susceptible to the same overuse injuries as adults in addition to a variety of overuse problems specific to their age group. The clinician and parents should be aware of the signs and symptoms of overtraining. As for any age group, cardiovascular exercise should be balanced with flexibility and resistive training.

> ***Patient-Related Instruction***
>
> ***Frequency, Intensity, and Duration***
>
> Determining how often (frequency), how hard (intensity), and how long (duration) to exercise can be difficult. These parameters are related and must be balanced to find the right quantity of exercise for you. The following broad guidelines can be refined by your clinician:
>
> 1. **Frequency:** Generally, if you exercise more frequently (more times per day or days per week), the intensity and duration of those sessions must be lower. This allows adequate recovery before the next session. If the intensity and duration are high, you may not be fully recovered before the next session.
> 2. **Intensity:** The more intense the exercise, the shorter is the duration. Intense exercise cannot be sustained very long by most people.
> 3. **Duration:** Exercise that is lower in intensity can be sustained for longer periods. For example, sprinting can be sustained for seconds, but jogging can be sustained for up to several hours. The intensity and duration are inversely related; as one increases, the other must decrease.

Cardiovascular Endurance Training by the Elderly

The effects of cardiovascular endurance training in the elderly include decreased blood pressure, increased high-density lipoprotein cholesterol, improved cardiovascular mortality rates, increased bone density, and maintenance of oxygen consumption values.[17] Endurance training is a safe activity, and as for other populations at risk (eg, the unfit, obese, cardiac patients), it should be implemented slowly. Chosen activities should minimize impact on the joints, emphasizing activities such as water exercise, bicycling, or stair climbing. Exercise should include warm-up and cool-down periods, and the aerobic training session should be at a lower intensity and longer duration than for younger individuals. Recommendations for intensity and duration are 50% to 70% of maximum heart rate for 40 to 50 minutes.[18] Depending on the initial fitness level and previous experience, the elderly individual may be initiated at 35% to 40% of maximum heart rate for 15 to 20 minutes.[18] Recommendations for progression are a duration of 5 minutes and intensity of 5% of HR_{max} every 2 weeks.[18]

Precautions and Contraindications

Endurance exercise places a significant load on the cardiovascular and musculoskeletal systems. Consideration should be given to any injury or disease affecting either of these systems. Individuals with degenerative joint disease should be encouraged to participate in non–weight-bearing exercises such as bicycling and water exercise, and those with low back pain should participate in activities that support or safely strengthen the back (eg, semirecumbant biking, water activities). Individuals with osteoporosis should be encouraged to participate in weight-bearing activities. Positions and postures should be chosen that minimize the risk of fracture.

Compared with other medical comorbidities, cardiovascular disease places the individual participating in cardiovascular exercise at the greatest risk. Individuals with coronary artery disease, previous myocardial infarction, congestive heart failure, hypertension, or valvular heart disease should be closely monitored by their physicians, and exercise should be under the physician's direction. Absolute contraindications to exercise include severe coronary artery disease, uncontrolled ventricular or atrial arrhythmias, uncontrolled hypertension, acute myocarditis, and recent pulmonary embolism or deep vein thrombosis.[19] The individual with uncontrolled diabetes is at risk during exercise and should avoid endurance exercise until the diabetes is controlled (see Display 5-1).

PATIENT EDUCATION

Patient education regarding muscular and cardiovascular endurance training is a critical component of the program. Endurance training should be carried out daily or several times per week, and some of the program may be carried out without the clinician's supervision. Patient education should include the warm-up, training session, and cool-down phases. The patient should be alerted to any signs or symptoms necessitating early cessation of the activity. These symptoms may be musculoskeletal (eg, joint pain, muscle pain, cramps) or cardiovascular (eg, shortness of breath, chest pain, lightheadedness), or they may be specific to the patient's particular problem (ie, reproducing the patient's original symptoms). The patient should be counselled regarding changes in the exercise program based on her fatigue level and other activities that day.

As the patient is prepared for discharge, education regarding a maintenance program is critical to continued adherence with the exercise program. Emphasizing the importance of continued exercise in long-term health maintenance can assist the patient in making exercise a lifelong commitment. Information about safe progression, exercise dosage, and signs and symptoms of overload can assist the patient in making appropriate exercise choices.

Key Points

- Muscular and cardiovascular endurance is necessary for the performance of many basic and instrumental ADLs and for work and leisure activities.
- Cardiovascular endurance requires concurrent muscular endurance to carry out the training activities.
- Endurance training can be performed using a variety of exercise modes and training techniques. Exercise prescription should be based on the individual's needs and interests and on comorbidities affecting exercise participation.
- Low-intensity, long-duration activities train the individual for endurance.
- The endurance training session should begin with general warm-up and end with cool-down activities.

LAB ACTIVITIES

1. Determining muscular endurance:
   a. Isometric approach: Using a hand-held dynamometer, determine the maximum torque produced by the quadriceps femoris. Have the subject ride a bicycle ergometer for 10 minutes at 60 rpm according to the following schedule:
      2 minutes at light resistance
      4 minutes at moderate resistance
      3 minutes at heavy resistance
      1 minute of sprint as fast as possible
      Have the patient dismount from the bike, and retest isometric strength.
   b. Isotonic approach: After a warm-up period, determine the 20-repetition maximum for the anterior deltoid. Have the subject complete an exercise program on the upper body ergometer according to the schedule for question 1a. Determine how many repetitions the individual can complete at the 20-repetition maximum weight.
   c. Isokinetic approach: Determine how many plantar or dorsiflexion repetitions the individual performs at 120 degrees per second before the torque generated decreases to 50% of initial levels. Then take the patient through a velocity spectrum isokinetic training program (ie, 60, 90, 120, 180, 240, 180, 120, 90, and 60 degrees per second), and retest.
2. Cardiovascular measures:
   a. Have the individual lie supine for at least 5 minutes or until heart rate and blood pressure reach steady-state values. Record the resting values.
   b. Have the subject stand rapidly and remain standing with the weight distributed equally on both feet. Record the heart rate and blood pressure immediately on standing and each minute for 3 minutes after standing or until the values reach steady state.
   c. With the subject sitting quietly, record the heart rate and blood pressure.
   d. Have the subject perform the bicycle exercise as outlined in question 1a. Record the blood pressure and heart rate in the last 30 seconds of each stage.
   e. At the conclusion of the exercise session, record the subject's heart rate and blood pressure every minute for 3 minutes or until the values reach steady state.

- Endurance activities should be balanced with appropriate flexibility activities.
- The clinician should be aware of any precautions for or contraindications to endurance exercise.
- Dosage parameters should be adapted to the specific needs of the patient.

Critical Thinking Questions

1. Consider Case Study #1 in Unit 7.
   a. What activities to maintain cardiovascular endurance would you recommend for Lisa as she recovers from her ankle sprain? Be sure to consider the demands of her sport.
   b. What activities would you recommend if she were a long-distance runner? A hockey player? A wrestler?
2. Consider Case Study #3 in Unit 7.
   a. Design a rehabilitation program to improve this journalist's muscular endurance.
   b. Design a rehabilitation program to improve this journalist's cardiovascular endurance.
3. Consider Case Study #8 in Unit 7.
   a. Design a rehabilitation program to address George's postural muscle weakness and fatigue.
   b. Make recommendations for a cardiovascular exercise program, considering George's examination findings and his job.
   c. How would your treatment plan be different if George worked as a long-distance truck driver?

REFERENCES

1. Shephard RJ. Semantic and physiological definitions. In: Shephard RJ, Astrand PO, eds. *Endurance in Sport*. Boston: Blackwell Scientific; 1992.
2. Kukukla CG. Human skeletal muscle fatigue. In: Currier DP, Nelson RM, eds. *Dynamics of Human Biologic Tissues*. Philadelphia: FA Davis; 1992.
3. Fitts RH. Mechanisms of muscular fatigue. In: *American College of Sports Medicine: Resource Manual for Guidelines for Exercise Testing and Prescription*. 2nd ed. Philadelphia: Lea & Febiger; 1993:106–114.
4. Shephard RJ. Maximal oxygen intake. In: Shephard RJ, Astrand PO, eds. *Endurance in Sport*. Boston: Blackwell Scientific; 1992.
5. Ratzin Jackson CG, Dickinson AL. Adaptations of skeletal muscle to strength or endurance training. In: Grana WA, Lombardo JA, Sharkey BJ, Stone JA, eds. *Advances in Sports Medicine and Fitness*. Chicago: Year Book Medical Publishers; 1988.
6. Secher NH. Central nervous influence on fatigue. In: Shephard RJ, Astrand PO, eds. *Endurance in Sport*. Boston: Blackwell Scientific; 1992.
7. Lash JM, Sherman WM. Skeletal muscle function and adaptations to training. In: *American College of Sports Medicine: Resource Manual for Guidelines for Exercise Testing and Prescription*. 2nd ed. Philadelphia: Lea & Febiger; 1993: 93–106.
8. Dudley GA, Abraham WM, Terjung RL. Influence of exercise intensity and duration on biochemical adaptations in skeletal muscle. *J Appl Physiol*. 1982;53:844–850.
9. Bell A. The older athlete. In: Sanders B, ed. *Sports Physical Therapy*. Norwalk, CT: Appleton & Lange; 1990.
10. Grimby G, Aniansson A, Hedberg M, et al. Training can improve muscle strength and endurance in 78–84-year-old men. *J Appl Physiol*. 1992;73:2517–2523.
11. Drinkwater BL. Osteoporosis and the female masters athlete. In: Sutton JR, Brock RM, eds. *Sports Medicine for the Mature Athlete*. Indianapolis: Benchmark Press; 1986.
12. Durstine JL, Pate RR, Branch JD. Cardiorespiratory responses to acute exercise. In: *American College of Sports Medicine: Resource Manual for Guidelines for Exercise Testing and Prescription*. 2nd ed. Philadelphia: Lea & Febiger; 1993:66–74.
13. Foster C. Central circulatory adaptations to exercise training in health and disease. *Clin Sports Med*. 1983;5:589–604.
14. McArdle WD, Katch FI, Katch VL. Exercise Physiology: Energy, Nutrition and Human Performance. 3rd ed. Philadelphia: Lea & Febiger; 1991.
15. American College of Sports Medicine. Position stand: the recommended quantity and quality of exercise for developing and maintaining cardiorespiratory and muscular fitness in healthy adults. *Med Sci Sports Exerc*. 1990;22:265–274.
16. American Academy of Pediatrics Committee on Sports Medicine: Risks in distance running for children. *Pediatrics*. 1990;86:799–800.
17. Pollock ML, Lowenthal DT, Graves JE, Carroll JF. The elderly and endurance training. In: Shephard RJ, Astrand PO, eds. *Endurance in Sport*. Boston: Blackwell Scientific; 1992.
18. Pollock ML, Wilmore J. *Exercise in Health and Disease: Evaluation and Prescription*. 2nd ed. Philadelphia: WB Saunders; 1990.
19. Heath GW. Exercise programming for the older adult. In: *American College of Sports Medicine: Resource Manual for Guidelines for Exercise Testing and Prescription*. 2nd ed. Philadelphia: Lea & Febiger; 1993:418–426.

CHAPTER 6

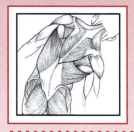

Mobility Impairment

Lori Thein Brody

Most patients with orthopedic conditions need mobility activities during the rehabilitation program. The clinician must provide hands-on rehabilitation techniques and instructions for a home exercise program. The execution of mobility activities is not as difficult as choosing the appropriate level of assistance and ensuring that the patient is performing the exercise with the correct level of assistance. Clear instruction and supervised practice in the clinician's presence can prevent misunderstandings about exercise performance.

Mobility exercises may be initiated early in the rehabilitation program and done throughout the rehabilitation program on a maintenance basis. Some individuals need progressive mobility exercises throughout the rehabilitation course, progressing from passive to active assisted to active range of motion (ROM). The choice of mobility activities depends on the stage of healing, length of immobilization, number and kind of tissues affected, and the specific injury or surgery. Understanding of the effects of decreased mobility and remobilization is the key to making appropriate mobility exercise choices. The clinician also must realize that immobilization is relative; it can be externally imposed by a brace or cast, or the patient may "self-immobilize" by discontinuing the use of the limb.

When considering mobility, the terms arthrokinematic and osteokinematic motion must be differentiated. Arthrokinematic motion refers to movements of the joint surfaces. Roll, spin, and glide are terms used to describe arthrokinematic motion. Arthrokinematic motion is a necessary component of osteokinematic motion, which refers to movement of the bones. Osteokinematic motion is described in terms of planes (eg, elevation in the sagittal plane) or relative movements (eg, flexion, abduction). Mobility can be impaired by alterations in arthrokinematic motion, osteokinematic motion, or both.

Although decreased mobility is the most obvious mobility impairment encountered, the concept of mobility is relative, with the degree of mobility occurring along a continuum. That continuum encompasses hypomobility, or decreased mobility, and hypermobility, or excessive mobility. Hypermobility should not be confused with instability. Instability is an excessive range of osteokinematic or arthrokinematic movement for which there is no protective muscular control.[55] For example, someone may have excessive arthrokinematic anterior, posterior, and inferior glide at the shoulder (ie, hypermobility) that is asymptomatic. Loss of dynamic muscular control at the shoulder produces instability and symptoms.

At the hypomobility end of the continuum, the concepts of contracture and adaptive shortening are important for understanding hypomobility. A contracture is a condition of fixed high resistance to passive stretch of a tissue resulting from fibrosis or shortening of the soft tissues around a joint or of the muscles.[19] Contractures occur after injury, surgery or immobilization, and are the result of the remodeling of dense connective tissue. Immobilization of a tissue in a shortened position results in adaptive shortening, which is shortening of the tissue relative to its normal resting length. Adaptive shortening also can result from holding a limb in a posture that shortens the tissues on one side of the joint. For example, protracting the shoulders in a rounded posture results in adaptive shortening of the pectoral muscles. This shortening can be accompanied by stiffness, or a resistance to passive movement.

Somewhere between the ideas of hypermobility and hypomobility lies the concept of relative flexibility. Relative flexibility considers the comparative mobility at adjacent joints. Movement in the human body takes the path of least resistance. If one segment of the spine is hypomobile because of injury or disease, the segment is stiffer and has more resistance to movement than adjacent joints. When flexion, extension, or rotation is necessary, the adjacent joints produce most of the movement because of the resistance to motion at the hypomobile joint. Likewise, stiffness in the hamstrings is often compensated by lumbar spine motion, placing more load on the spine. Lengthening the hamstrings minimizes the stress placed on the spine and is the basis for hamstring stretching, an approach used by some persons to remedy back pain.

Relative flexibility is not always an impairment. For example, because of its biomechanical and anatomic properties, L5 is more adapted to produce rotation than any other lumbar segment. It is *relatively more flexible* in the direction of rotation. This is a clinical problem (ie, impairment) only if the motion becomes excessive and is not muscularly controlled. This problem may occur because of relative stiffness at other spinal segments (above or below L5) or at the hips. For example, golfing requires a significant amount of total body rotation. If the hips, knees, and feet are relatively more stiff in rotation than the spine, the discrepancy may impose excessive rotation in the spine. If the thoracic spine or upper lumbar segments are stiff in rotation, the difference may impose excessive rotation on the L5 segment. L5 is the site of relative flexibility in the direction of rotation.

PHYSIOLOGY OF NORMAL MOBILITY

Normal mobility, in its broadest definition, includes osteokinematic motion, arthrokinematic motion, and neuromuscular coordination to achieve purposeful movement. Normal mobility requires adequate tissue length to allow full ROM (ie, passive mobility) and the neuromuscular skill to accomplish movement (ie, active mobility).

Structures involved in passive mobility include the joint's articular surfaces and interposed tissues (eg, menisci, labrum, synovial lining), joint capsule, ligaments and tendons (including insertions sites), muscles, bursae, fascia, and skin. Joints must have normal arthrokinematic motion, or the ability of an articular surface to roll, spin, and glide across another. The ability to accomplish active mobility requires an intact, functioning nervous system in addition to the structures necessary to allow passive mobility. Mobility is maintained in most individuals by routine, daily use of their limbs and joints in normal daily activities. However, adaptive shortening can occur in those who spend long periods in single postures (eg, sitting most of the day), and mobility can be lost.

Normal mobility includes adequate joint ROM and muscle ROM. Joint ROM is the quantity of motion available at a joint or series of joints in the case of the spine. In contrast, muscle ROM is the functional excursion of the muscle from its fully lengthened position to its fully shortened position. Examination and treatment techniques for joint ROM impairments and muscle ROM impairments differ.

CAUSES AND EFFECTS OF DECREASED MOBILITY

Individuals can lose mobility at a joint for several reasons. Trauma to soft tissue, bone, or other joint structures can diminish mobility. Operations such as total joint replacements, reconstructions, debridements, arthroplasties, osteotomies, and tendon transfers can reduce mobility, as can surgery for nonorthopedic conditions. Mastectomy or other chest procedures may result in shoulder immobility, and bed rest after cardiac, gynecologic, or other surgical procedures may result in immobility in many joints. Joint disease such as osteoarthritis or rheumatoid arthritis and prolonged immobilization or bed rest for any reason frequently produce immobility. The inability to move a joint because of neuromuscular disease or pain can also result in mobility loss, and pain that inhibits movement can significantly alter mobility.

Immobility at a joint produces a self-perpetuating cycle that can be interrupted by several physical therapy interventions, including ROM modalities, resistive exercises, or mobilizations. Progressive adaptive shortening of the soft tissues occurs as the body responds to decreased loading. This shortening limits mobility and function, reducing the patient's ability to carry out normal activities of daily living, work, or leisure activities. The patient accommodates these limitations by substituting other joints or limbs to achieve functional goals, thereby contributing to the disuse. Pain results from disuse and progressive shortening of the joint capsule (a highly pain sensitive structure), adding to the disuse. Weakness ensues because of changes in the length-tension ratios, furthering the patient's disinclination to use the limb.

Decreased mobility has profound effects on bone and soft tissues, reflecting the body's ability to adapt to various levels of loading. The plastic nature of these tissues works in positive and negative ways. The specific adaptations to imposed demands (SAID) principle is based on Wolff's Law and asserts that tissues remodel in accordance to the stresses placed on them. The effects of overload, or tissue load above its normal usage, and its resulting hypertrophy, the enlargement of a tissue because of an increase in the size of its constituent cells, are well known, but the findings associated with underloading are less well known. Findings such as muscular atrophy, or wasting away of a tissue, and loss of joint motion are evident, but cellular changes, articular cartilage changes, and weakening of ligaments and their insertions are less obvious alterations. The clinician must prevent these effects when possible and consider them when implementing a rehabilitation program.

The following sections review the consequences of immobilization or decreased mobility on various tissues. Generally, the effects reviewed are caused by immobilization of healthy, uninjured tissues (this is how most studies are done). This raises two important issues. First, immobilization usually is initiated in the presence of an injury (although tissue-lengthening procedures are exceptions), and the structural and mechanical properties of the injured tissues probably will be further compromised. The stages of healing can be found in Chapter 10 and should be considered in concert with the immobilization issues. Second, it is tempting to focus only on the injured tissue after immobilization. However, all surrounding tissues also are immobilized, and understanding the immobilization effects on these tissues ensures a safe and effective rehabilitation course.

Effects on Muscle

The atrophying effects of immobilization on muscle have been well documented. These effects are time, muscle composition, and position specific. The longer the immobilization, the greater is the atrophy, with significant structural and functional properties deteriorating during the first week.[41,42] The functional loss is greater than the loss of muscle mass or circumference, probably because of additional neurologic inactivity. Studies of electromyographic activity after immobilization demonstrate a decrease in electrical activity that is disproportionate to the amount of atrophy.[38,49,50] Circumferential measures do not reflect the functional loss; quadriceps changes after 6 weeks of immobilization include a 30% to 40% strength loss, a 20% to 30% cross-sectional area decrease, and a thigh circumference loss of 10% to 20%[5,37,41,42] (Fig. 6-1). Along with muscle fiber atrophy, a concurrent increase in connective tissue occurs that may confound circumferential measures.[84] Moreover, immobility results in a greater deposition of subcutaneous fat, and circumferential measures provide no information about the composition of the underlying tissue.

Muscle composition affects the degree of atrophy. Muscles composed primarily of slow-twitch fibers atrophy to a greater extent than muscles composed primarily of fast-twitch fibers.[50,51] This difference may reflect the use pattern, with the higher-use slow-twitch fibers showing a greater relative decrease. Lieber suggests the most important factors in atrophy from decreased use to be the degree of immobilization (ie, number of joints crossed), followed by the degree of change relative to normal function.[51] For example, calf muscle atrophy is greater when the ankle and knee are immobilized. Atrophy is greater in the soleus (static postural muscle) than the gastrocnemius (relatively lower-use muscle.)

The position of immobilization significantly affects the structural and mechanical properties of muscles. Muscles may be immobilized in a shortened position after injury or surgical repair, as for an Achilles tendon rupture or a rotator cuff tear. Long-term immobilization in a shortened position results in changes in sarcomere length and number as the body attempts to restore the original sarcomere length.[29] Immobilization results in a net loss of sarcomeres, although the remaining sarcomeres are longer. The muscle is stiffer, and less energy is absorbed before failure. A shift to the left in the length-tension ratio occurs. Muscles may also be immobilized in a lengthened position, as in serial casting done to lengthen the muscle. This results in an increase in the number of sarcomeres, with less atrophy occurring than with immobilization in the shortened position. The elastic and connective tissue are reorganized such that the muscle adapts to its new immobilization length.[29,76] The length-tension ratio shifts to the right with immobilization in a lengthened position. The sarcomere changes associated with immobilization take place at the myotendinous junction.

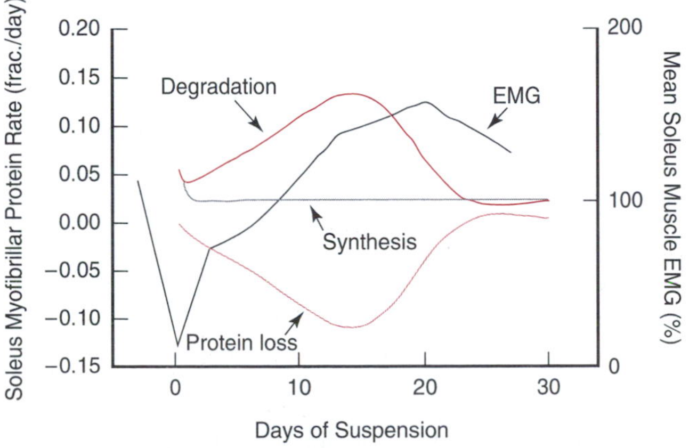

FIGURE 6-1 Time course for muscle mass and protein synthesis and degradation during rat hindlimb unloading. (Adapted from Lieber RL. *Skeletal Muscle Structure and Function.* Baltimore: Williams & Wilkins;1992:240.

Effects on Tendon

Immobilization of any collagenous tissue has significant effects on that tissue, even in the absence of direct injury. Immobilization-related decreases in the size and number of collagen fiber bundles reduce the load tolerance. Decreased water content, decreased total glycosaminoglycans, and increased synthesis (ie, production of a chemical compound) and degradation (ie, breakdown to a less complex compound) of collagen are coupled with profound disorganization of fiber orientation.[78]

The metabolic turnover in tendon is much lower than in muscle, and the tendon is more refractory to immobilization-induced changes. However, the tensile strength, elastic stiffness, and total tissue weight all decrease with immobilization.[41] The collagen fibers become thinner and less organized, and cross-links are reduced.[41,78] Enwemeka[25] studied the effects of various times and positions of cast immobilization on rabbit Achilles tendons. Limbs were immobilized 3 to 8 weeks. Two groups of limbs were placed first in a shortened position and then in a lengthened position for 2 or 4 weeks of the immobilization period. Results demonstrated progressive, profoundly disorganized collagen fibrils, with some sections totally devoid of collagen. By week 8, the cross-sectional area and collagen fibril diameter of immobilized tendons decreased by a 50%. In the two groups that were subsequently immobilized in a lengthened position, a reversal in this progressive decline was observed after 2 weeks. However, this same reversal was not found in the group immobilized in a lengthened position for 4 weeks, suggesting the benefits of the lengthening were negated by or adapted to by the additional immobilization time.

Effects on Ligament and Insertion Sites

Like other primarily collagenous tissues, ligament tissue responds to immobilization at a slower rate than tissues with higher metabolic activity. The total collagen mass decreases in a time-dependent manner, with a concomitant decrease in the ligament's mechanical properties. The ligament's strength and stiffness decrease, and the joint's stiffness increases.[3] This difference probably results from adhesion and pannus formation and from decreased lubrication in the joint.[4] Ligaments devoid of stress demonstrate shortening, as measured by a decrease in the distance between sutures placed in the ligament.[15] The shortening may be an active process; shortening has been inhibited by electrical potentials simulating mechanical loading.

The effects of immobilization and remobilization on the medial collateral ligament (MCL) have been studied extensively. In a classic study, Laros et al. found a significant loss of ligament strength in dogs after as little as 6 weeks immobilization.[45] Woo et al. compared the effects of surgical repair of the MCL followed by 6 weeks of immobilization with the effects of no repair and no immobilization at 6, 12, and 48 weeks postoperatively.[90] At 6 weeks, the varus-valgus instability was similar in the two groups, but by 12 weeks and at 48 weeks, the varus-valgus laxity in the nonrepaired and nonimmobilized group was similar to normal subjects. The tensile properties of this group were also superior to the repaired and immobilized group at all intervals. The mechanical and structural properties of the repaired and immobilized group remained lower than controls and lower than the nonrepaired and nonimmobilized group even at 48 weeks, highlighting the long-term negative effects of this treatment. Noyes[65] studied the effects of an 8-week immobilization on anterior cruciate ligament (ACL) complex failure in primates, finding a 39% decrease in complex load to failure.

The extent of immobilization-induced weakness appears to be time dependent in a nonlinear fashion. Decreases in MCL collagen mass accelerated when immobilization was extended from 9 weeks to 12 weeks.[2,3] Decreased mass is a result of collagen degradation exceeding collagen synthesis. Moreover, this pattern produces a disproportionate quantity of young, immature collagen, laid down in a random, disorganized fashion. The clinician must consider these changes when a joint is immobilized for any reason. Gentle loading, even during the immobilization period, can minimize or negate these changes.

Like other soft tissues, loading is necessary to maintain the integrity of the insertion sites. Loading can include joint motion, muscular action, or weight bearing, providing the clinician with numerous options to maintain the health of this tissue. Because it is more metabolically active than the ligament or tendon, the insertion site can be expected to demonstrate greater changes. The ligament-bone insertion site demonstrates bony resorption and subsequent weakening from immobilization.[46] Noyes et al.[64] studied failure rates of the bone-ACL unit failure in monkeys after 8 weeks of immobilization, finding an increased avulsion rate compared with control values. The researchers thought a loss of cortex at the attachment site was the mechanism of failure. Woo et al.[89] added to this data, suggesting that immobilization has a greater impact on indirect insertion sites (ie, soft tissue junction with bone is more gradual and diffuse) than on direct insertion sites. Subperiosteal resorption of bone accounted for the increased avulsion rate of the femur-MCL-tibia complexes, suggesting that the bone is the weakest portion of the insertion site.

Effects on Articular Cartilage

The harmful effects of immobilization on articular cartilage must be considered by the clinician rehabilitating individuals after injury or surgery. Articular cartilage requires loading to maintain its integrity. Decreased loading and motion leads to degeneration of the articular surface. Immobilization results in increased water content and decreased proteoglycans and alters the proteoglycan organization. These changes precede softening and fragmentation of the chondral surfaces. Decreased proteoglycans (ie, glycoprotein binding materials), may result from increased degradation or decreased synthesis.[11] Subsequent decreases in cartilage stiffness and thickness may make the cartilage more vulnerable to injury. Like a partially torn ligament, loss of matrix proteoglycans places an increased load on the remaining tissue. Progressive deterioration occurs with chondrocyte (ie, mature cartilage cell) loss, collagen fiber splitting, and fibrillation and with subchondral bone sclerosis.[41,42] If immobility continues, bony proliferation results in osteophyte formation. The position of the joint during immobilization also affects the degeneration seen. Knee immobilization in full extension results in irreversible, progressive osteoarthritic joint changes because of the compressive forces between articular surfaces.[1,79,80] These changes are thought to result from the articular hypoxia from decreased synovial fluid, increased compression of the articular surfaces, and increased intra-articular pressure.[40]

Studies of cartilage changes after immobilization in dogs produced decreases in glycosaminoglycan concentrations, cartilage thickness, uronic acid content, and proteoglycan synthesis.[44] The type of fixation affects the stimulus to the articular cartilage. Comparisons of rigid immobilization with external fixation to long leg casting (permitting 8 to 15 degrees of motion) demonstrated more severe proteoglycan loss and prolonged recovery in the joints with rigid fixation.[9] Decreased weight bearing, even in the presence of normal joint motion, appears to be harmful to the articular cartilage.[12,74]

Effects on Bone

Immobilization leads to profound changes in bone, which unchecked can lead to osteoporosis (ie, abnormal decreased density of the bone). Bone resorption (ie, loss of substance) occurs in the early phases, with a decrease in bone mass relative to volume. Bone mineral loss may be as high as 8% per month while on bed rest.[41,42] The total loss is accounted for by approximately a 30% increase in resorption and a 70% decrease in formation.[61] The decreases are most dramatic in the first 6 weeks, followed by a slowing until equilibrium is reached, usually after 5 to 6 months.[61] In trabecular bone, the volumes of haversian canals and resorption areas increase, but the trabecular bone volume decreases.[72] Trabecular bone appears to be more sensitive to loading changes because of its rapid remodeling.[7] In cortical bone, the bone loss occurs more slowly, but over time, it contributes significantly to the fragility associated with immobilization.[41,42,72] Subchondral bone changes are also seen with immobilization, but they appear to be related to alterations in overlying articular cartilage rather than the cancellous bone.[26]

Bone loss depends on the location, normal use patterns, bone composition, and prior status of the bone. Greater loss occurs in weight-bearing bones than in upper extremity bones. For example, bone loss may appear only after 8 months in individuals with upper extremity paralysis.[85] Because of the high turnover rate in children, the effects of immobilization are more profound.

The various mechanical stresses contributing to bone health must be considered in rehabilitation. Bone loss from immobilization must be differentiated from bone loss caused by weight-bearing limitations. Complete bed rest with immobilization or immobilization combined with weight-bearing restrictions has the greatest impact on bone health.[72] Weight bearing and muscular contraction are the two mechanical forces responsible for bone development.[7] Space flight studies of bone loss emphasize the importance of gravity and weight bearing on bone health.[7,59] Studies of individuals immobilized with poliomyelitis, muscular dystrophy, and paraplegia have demonstrated rates of bone loss approaching 1% per week.[72] Muscular pull on the bone can produce a mechanical load to stimulate osteoblast activity. Osteoblast calls are associated with the production of bone. Bone density studies of handicapped, nonambulatory children have demonstrated a 30% deficit in bone density compared with age-matched controls.[63]

MOBILITY EXAMINATION AND EVALUATION

A thorough examination must be performed before choosing a physical therapy intervention. This ensures appropriate indications and goal setting for the specific mobility technique chosen. Moreover, the evaluation, including subjective examination and history taking, informs decisions about exercise dosage, activity type, and elements of the movement system specific to the individual.

The concepts of joint ROM and muscle ROM were clarified earlier. Examination procedures must identify the source of decreased mobility to effectively direct the treatment. Joint ROM is usually measured in the cardinal planes with a goniometer. Goniometric measurements are performed actively or passively, although the reliability of measurement is greater for active measures than for passive measures.[28] Isolated motions such as elbow flexion, knee extension, and ankle dorsiflexion are most commonly measured. Functional goniometric measurements with less stabilization and control can also be taken. Goniometric measurement of forward reach is a common functional assessment. Standards for normal goniometric mobility at each joint are published and provide a guideline for assessing mobility. When assessing joint ROM, the clinician must ensure proper patient positioning to avoid apparent joint motion limitations caused by poor muscle extensibility. For example, hip joint flexion ROM should be performed with the knee flexed to prevent limitations from hamstring excursion (Fig. 6-2). Assessment of joint ROM with a goniometer does not identify the cause of limited motion. Further selective tissue tension tests are necessary.

Muscle ROM is generally assessed using flexibility tests, a few of which are quantified. For example, hamstring extensibility can be assessed goniometrically using the 90–90 straight-leg raise[55] (Fig. 6-3). The Thomas test for hip flexor extensibility and the Bunnel-Littler test for hand intrinsic or joint capsule extensibility are examples of flexibility tests. These tests, when performed correctly, can direct intervention for decreased musculotendinous extensibility as the cause of decreased mobility.

Limitations in arthrokinematic motion decrease a patient's mobility, and increases in arthrokinematic mobility cause hypermobility. Arthrokinematic mobility is assessed through joint play maneuvers. Joint play is the movement of one articular surface on another and is not usually under voluntary control. Joint play is assessed by stabilizing one articular surface (by stabilizing the bone) and applying external pressure on the other to produce movement. For example, applying an anteroposterior glide at the proximal interphalangeal joint of the index finger requires stabilization of the proximal phalanx while the distal phalanx is moved in an anteroposterior direction. In some cases, stabilization of one segment is provided by the surrounding bony and soft tissue structures and the supporting surface. For example, when performing posteroanterior unilateral vertebral pressure, the patient is stabilized in a prone position on the table while unilateral posteroanterior pressure is applied to the transverse process, producing rotation of the vertebral body that should be compared with the contralateral side.[55] Assessment of joint play can identify hypomobile, normal, or hypermobile conditions. These tests direct intervention for increasing capsular mobility, looking

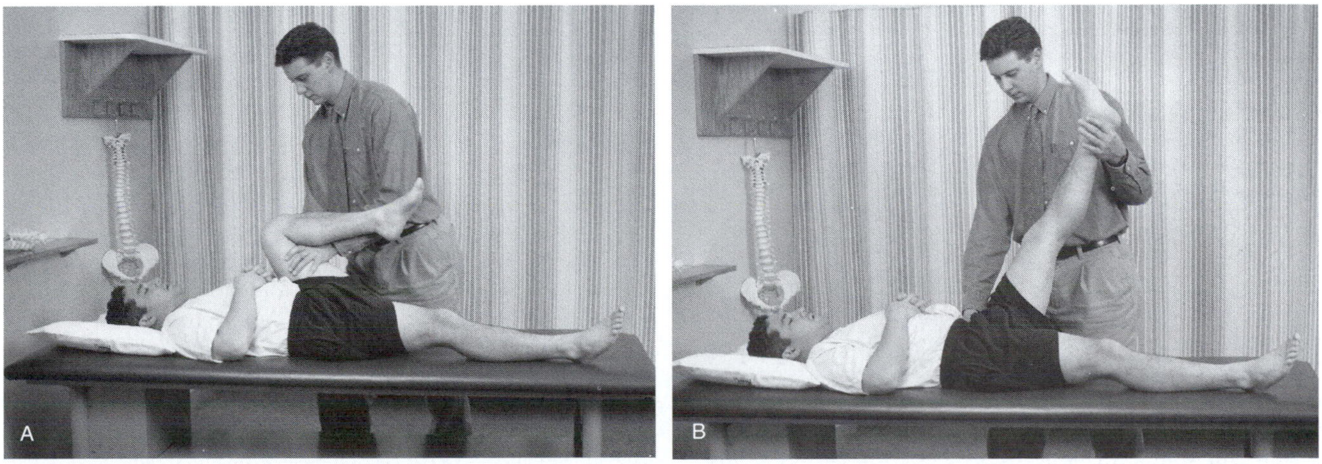

FIGURE 6-2 ***(A)*** Joint range of motion at the hip. The knee is flexed to minimize effects of hamstring tension. ***(B)*** Muscle range of motion for the hamstrings. The same hip flexion activity is done with the knee extended.

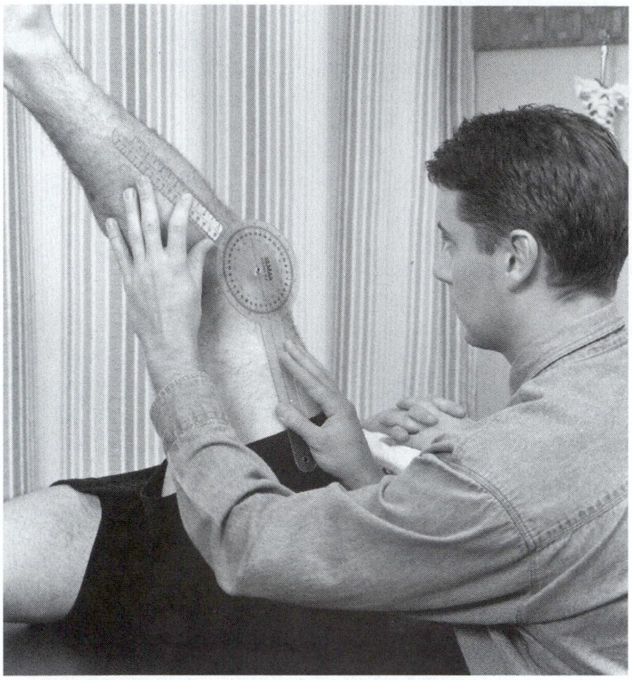

FIGURE 6-3 Assessment of hamstring flexibility goniometrically using the 90–90 straight-leg raise. The hip is flexed to 90 degrees, and the knee gradually extended from flexion to extension. The final angle of knee flexion is measured.

for other sources of mobility loss, or stabilization activities, respectively.

THERAPEUTIC INTERVENTION FOR DECREASED MOBILITY

A variety of interventions are available to treat decreased mobility. After the tissues limiting mobility have been identified, appropriate ROM, stretching, or joint mobilization techniques should be applied. Adjunctive agents enhance the effectiveness of exercise interventions.

Effects of Remobilization

A thorough understanding of the physiologic response to remobilization of immobilized tissues provides the scientific basis for many of the mobility interventions used. Before discussion of specific techniques, the effects of remobilization on collagenous tissues are considered.

EFFECTS ON MUSCLE

Muscular strength deficits after immobilization often require long and tedious rehabilitation for full recovery. However, remobilization studies are lacking, as is a consensus on the parameters for rehabilitation and return to activity. Factors affecting the rate and end point of recovery include predominantly the position and time of immobilization. Lieber immobilized canine quadriceps for 10 weeks, followed by a 4-week remobilization period during which normal activity was permitted.[50] At 4 weeks, a 30% deficit in slow- and fast-twitch muscle fibers remained (Fig. 6-4). Although the atrophy due to immobilization was muscle and fiber specific, the recovery was not. The increased extracellular connective tissue seen after immobilization had returned to normal levels after remobilization, suggesting a decrease in stiffness. The mechanism for fiber regeneration is unclear, although evidence suggests satellite cell activation and myotube formation.[42,49,50]

EFFECTS ON TENDON

Few studies have looked at the effects of remobilization on uninjured, immobilized tendon, but many researchers have examined the results of remobilization after tendon injury with or without repair. Karpakka et al.[43] found that remobilization of rat tendon resulted in acceleration of collagen synthesis. Enwemeka[24,25] studied the remobilization of healing tendon after surgical repair. Limited mechanical stress such as passive mobilization promotes the normal gliding and soft tissue relationships necessary for optimal healing after tendon repair. In a study of Achilles tenotomy in rabbits, the immobilization was removed at 5 days postoperatively, and the tendons were examined at 12, 18, or 21 days postoperatively.[25] Early remobilization was found to significantly improve the tendon's tensile strength and energy absorption capacity over those of immobilized controls at days 12 and 18, and increases in mean cross-sectional area were found at 12 and 21 days. No rerupture was evident,

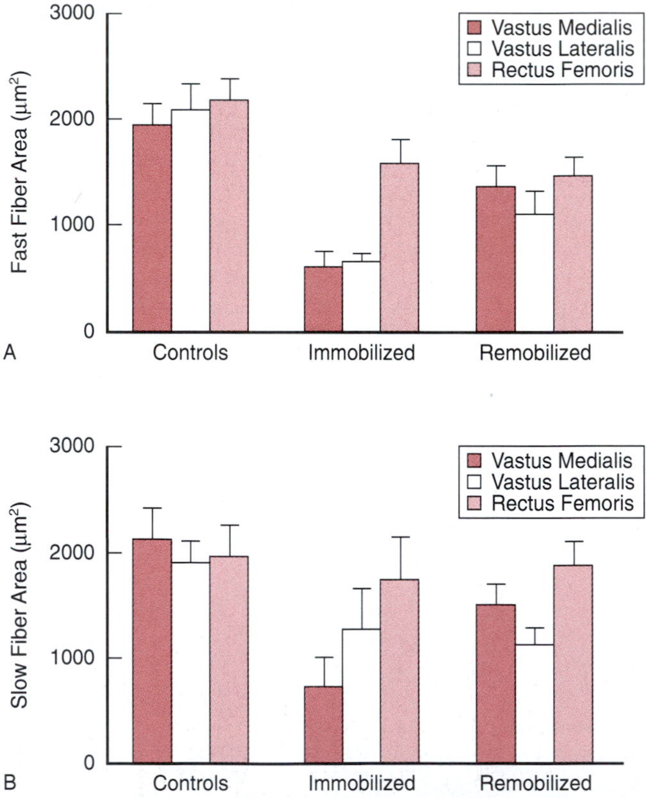

FIGURE 6-4 ***(A)*** Graph of fast fiber area from control, immobilized, and remobilized dog quadriceps muscles. The magnitude of muscle atrophy was muscle-type specific. ***(B)*** Graph of slow fiber area from control and immobilized dog quadripceps muscles. (From Lieber RL. *Skeletal Muscle Structure and Function.* Baltimore: Williams & Wilkins; 1992:219.)

and no differences in tensile strength and energy absorption capacity were found at 21 days postoperatively. The investigator concluded that, despite no differences between the two groups at 21 days, the morbidity associated with immobilization counterbalance the possibility of rerupture.

The effects of remobilization after flexor tendon repair have been systematically studied. Tendons receiving early protected mobilization after repair did not form significant adhesions, nor was there significant repair site deformation.[30–32] The mechanism for improved healing was proposed to be a cellular response from the tendon and epitenon resulting from the mechanical motion. The load at failure of immediately mobilized tendons tested at 3 weeks was found to be twice that of the immobilized tendons. Early mobilization of tendon repairs appears to result in a strong repair without excessive scar formation. The precise parameters for immobilization and remobilization are unknown.[33]

EFFECTS ON LIGAMENT AND INSERTION SITES

Remobilization can restore the mechanical and structural properties of ligament tissues, although the time needed for this reparation has not been established. Because of its low metabolic activity, the remobilization period necessary to restore mechanical properties of the ligament substance generally exceeds the immobilization period. Although the external measures after immobilization may indicate recovery, restoration of the ligament complex mechanical properties lags behind our measurement ability. Clinical examination procedures such as ligament laxity testing, instability testing, and palpation are unlikely to detect residual weakness after immobilization or during the remobilization period. An understanding of the recovery process at the cellular level must guide the rehabilitation program.

Studies of ACL immobilization have found variable results regarding remobilization periods. Larson et al.[46] found that 6 weeks of swimming retraining was needed to restore the separation force and elastic stiffness of the ACL after 4 weeks of immobilization. In contrast, 5 months of reconditioning did not fully restore the ACL failure load after 8 weeks of immobilization.[65] The site of failure returned to control values, with evidence of bone formation at the insertion site. Continued conditioning for 1 year after the immobilization period still left the failure load at 9% less than that of controls. Similar results were observed for energy absorbed to failure.[65]

Insertion sites of ligament and tendon into bone and the myotendinous junction respond favorably to loading after immobilization.[46,65,91] The bone-ligament complex becomes stronger with exercise.[91] Remobilization after immobilization appears to restore the properties of the insertion site and the ligament substance itself at different rates.[52,65] This finding is supported by the study of Woo et al.,[91] who found a return of the mechanical properties of the MCL with 9 weeks of remobilization after 9 weeks of immobilization. However, the structural properties of the bone-ligament complex remained inferior, with failures continuing to occur at the insertion site. The results of these studies and others suggest that changes at the insertion site that occur because of immobilization are reversible with remobilization.[45,46,65,91] The length of remobilization relative to the length of immobilization necessary to restore the original strength levels at the insertion remains undefined. Any lengthy immobilization (6 weeks or longer) appears to require remobilization periods of 4 months or longer to restore the mechanical and structural properties of the tissues. Tissue immobilized for shorter periods probably requires less time to return to preimmobilization levels.

Although the effects of immobilization and the benefits of early remobilization are indisputable, clinicians and researchers are beginning to identify a subgroup of patients who may need to be protected longer. The healing rate and quality of tissue vary along a continuum from stiffness and arthrofibrosis to hyperelasticity. Those presenting with stiffness and decreased motion should be mobilized early, and those with hyperelasticity and hypermobility should be protected longer.

EFFECTS ON ARTICULAR CARTILAGE

Remobilization and prevention of immobilization-associated degeneration can prevent degradation of articular cartilage and progression to osteoarthritis. The response to remobilization depends on the length of immobilization, the associated injury or pathology, the status of the articular cartilage before immobilization, available joint motion, and load distribution. Activity that is too vigorous can harm the joint surface. Activities that maintain loads within the optimal loading zone should be chosen. Signs of overload include pain, swelling, warmth, and tenderness.

Osteoarthritic changes that occur as the result of joint immobilization have poor reparative capabilities. Immobilization for more than 4 weeks probably results in irreversible changes in the articular cartilage, even with remobilization.[12] Articular cartilage changes and connective tissue adhesions after immobilization often persist despite remobilization periods of equal or longer duration.[26] However, these changes may not progress in the presence of appropriate remobilization techniques (ie, avoiding overload), joint stability, equitable load distribution and freedom of motion.[6] Persons with inadequate joint stability may continue to overload their articular cartilage through excessive shearing forces, and those with inequities in load distribution (ie, varus knee) may overload one compartment and underload the other. Both situations can lead to progressive osteoarthritic changes. The individual who lacks full joint motion after immobilization increases loads on the articular cartilage within his limited range. Restoring full active ROM after immobilization is critical for optimizing joint health.

EFFECTS ON BONE

The rate of bone's response to remobilization exceeds that of most other biologic tissues. As with other tissues, the response is related to the metabolic activity of the tissue, and younger persons have greater response rates, probably because of the high rate of bone turnover.[41,42] Although bone may return to normal at a faster rate than soft tissues, the effects of immobilization usually are more profound in bone. In contrast to other tissues, bone changes resulting from immobilization may not be reversible with remobilization.[7,12] Studies of the os calcis of Skylab crew members found decreased bone mineral content 5 years after the flights.[59] Immobilization periods longer than 12 weeks are likely to result in permanent changes, with the recovery period exceeding the immobilization period many times over.[7,12,57]

The outcome of remobilization depends on the bone quality before immobilization and on the immobilization period. Restoration of the mechanical forces on bone (ie, gravity and muscular stress and strain) reverses bone loss. On resumption of weight bearing, trabecular bone increases at about 1% per month and may or may not return to its preimmobilization status.[69]

Elements of the Movement System

Any of the elements of the movement system may contribute to decreased mobility. For example, loss of normal hip extension ROM may contribute to low back pain by transferring the extension mobility requirement from the hip to the low back (ie, relative flexibility). In this case, decreased mobility (ie, impairment) in the hip contributes to low back pain (ie, impairment). The pain arises from compression of the posterior elements of the spine and subsequent inflammation around the nerve roots (ie, pathology) and an inability to sit for long periods (ie, functional limitation). If left untreated, this condition may lead to disability, such as the inability to work at a desk, participate in recreational activities, or sit in car.

In this example, the base elements are the shortened hip flexors and hip joint capsule pulling the pelvis into anterior tilt and the lengthened and weak abdominal muscles that are unable to provide sufficient counterforce. The biomechanical elements are the increased anterior pelvic tilt and increased lumbar lordosis contributing to posterior element compression in the spine. The modulator element is an inability to recruit the abdominal muscles to improve the biomechanical elements. The cognitive or affective element is depression related to chronic low back pain.

The elements of the movement system involved must be prioritized and those elements amenable to physical therapy intervention determined. In this situation, intervention to increase the length of the hip flexors, decrease stiffness in the hip joint capsule, and improve the neuromuscular firing and muscular endurance of the abdominal muscles should be instituted.

Activities to Increase Mobility

A variety of activities are available to the clinician when treating decreased mobility. ROM exercises, stretching, and joint mobilization are the more common interventions applied. ROM activities or joint mobilization can be used to increase joint ROM, and stretching techniques can be used to remedy limitations in muscle ROM. Joint mobilization is considered a manual exercise and therefore is not discussed in this text. Joint mobilization is a technique that preserves or increases arthrokinematic motion. It is a necessary prerequisite for normal osteokinematic mobility. Attempting to perform ROM activities in the absence of normal arthrokinematic motion at the joint surface does not improve the impaired mobility and may increase the patient's symptoms. Self-mobilization activities such as lateral distraction at the glenohumeral joint or long-axis traction at the hip may precede ROM exercises.

When applying interventions to increase mobility, the clinician must consider the continuum of hypomobility to hypermobility and the concept of relative flexibility. Hypomobility can be mistreated if the possibility of adjacent hypermobility is ignored. For example, if a stiff segment exists at L4-L5 and treatment is directed at decreasing stiffness there without stabilizing interventions directed at hypermobile segments above and below, symptoms of instability at these segments may increase. Treatment must include a comprehensive program to improve the mobility at the relatively more stiff segments or regions and to increase the stiffness at the relatively more mobile segment. Because motion always occurs along the path of least resistance, mobility occurs naturally at the stiff segment only if it is of equal mobility or more mobile than other segments. It is important to increase the stiffness at the site of relative flexibility. This is done by improving neuromuscular control, muscle performance capability, and length-tension relationships of the stabilizing muscles around the site of relative flexibility. These techniques are coupled with patient education, postural training, and movement patterns that improve the distribution of mobility.

RANGE OF MOTION

Mobility activities at a joint or series of joints and articulations can offset some of the deleterious effects of immobilization. Movement about a joint, whether passive, active assisted or active, produces a load in the soft tissues. This loading can maintain the integrity of the tendon, ligament and bony attachments, articular cartilage, and muscle. The benefit is determined by the exercise and immobilization parameters and by the status of the tissues before immobilization. Mobility activities are specific exercises or functional activities performed to improve functional ROM about a joint. Mobility activities usually are performed through a joint ROM and can be performed in cardinal planes or in multiple planes using functional movement patterns (eg, reaching, squatting). These activities can be performed actively, passively, or with active assistance.

Passive Range of Motion

Noncontractile tissues potentially limiting passive mobility about a joint include the joint capsule, periarticular connective tissue, and overlying skin. Surgical incisions producing adhesions between the skin and underlying fascial layers limit their ability to glide during joint motion. Shortening, spasm, or contractures of the musculotendinous unit can also limit the passive motion at a joint. Shortening of musculotendinous tissue should be differentiated from stiffness of the connective tissues. Stiffness in soft tissues is felt as an increased resistance to movement and can alter movement patterns passively and actively, resulting in musculoskeletal pain. Bone-on-bone approximation in the presence of degenerative joint disease, loose bodies, and pain can similarly limit passive mobility.

Passive ROM exercises are mobility activities performed without any muscular activation. These exercises are performed within the available ROM. Any overpressure at the end of the range would be categorized as stretching, not passive ROM. Passive ROM and stretching can be combined to increase the ROM about a joint.[27] Passive ROM is applied by some external force, such as the clinician, a family member, the patient himself, or equipment such as a pulley or continuous passive motion device (Fig. 6-5).

Passive ROM is used when active movement may disrupt the healing process, when the patient is physically or cognitively unable to move actively, or when active movement is too painful to perform. Passive movements also are used to teach active or resistive exercises and to produce relaxation. Goals related to the prescription of passive ROM depend on the patient and the setting. In an orthopedic setting, passive ROM is often used to prevent the deleterious effects of immobilization after an injury or surgery. Prevention of joint contractures and soft tissue stiffness or adaptive shortening, maintenance of the normal mobile relationships between soft tissue layers, decreased pain, and enhancement of vascular dynamics and synovial diffusion are goals of passive ROM.[27] These goals are difficult to measure and to document. The clinician must rely on his understanding of the pathologic process to provide the rationale for this intervention. Measurable outcomes related to passive ROM as prevention intervention may include decreased pain, expeditious restoration of motion and strength, and earlier return to function after activity is allowed (see Self-Management: Ankle Passive Range of Motion).

When the patient is comatose, paralyzed, on complete bed rest, wheelchair bound, or cognitively unable to maintain joint ROM, passive ROM is used to achieve the same goals as the orthopedic setting. Because of the long-standing nature of these problems and the profound effects of long-term immobility, prevention assumes even greater importance. The patient usually requires passive ROM exercise two or more times each day, necessitating provision of services by family members or other assistive personnel.

The clinician's skill in performing passive ROM can significantly alter the response. The clinician's handling techniques can affect the patient's comfort and ability to relax during treatment. When active muscle contraction is contraindicated, positioning and handling should allow the patient to fully relax. Any apprehension could result in protective muscle contraction and possible injury. Proper positioning allows adequate stabilization while the clinician's hand control provides stabilization and command of the affected limb. The clinician should use a grip that provides control but considers the patient's condition. Avoiding painful areas or excessively tight grips that produce discomfort assures the patient of the clinician's control. ROM should be performed at a smooth and steady pace, avoiding abrupt movements or excessive speed that may cause protective muscle contraction. The clinician should always monitor the patient's response and be flexible enough to modify the technique when necessary. The hand position, ROM, and speed must be tailored for each patient.

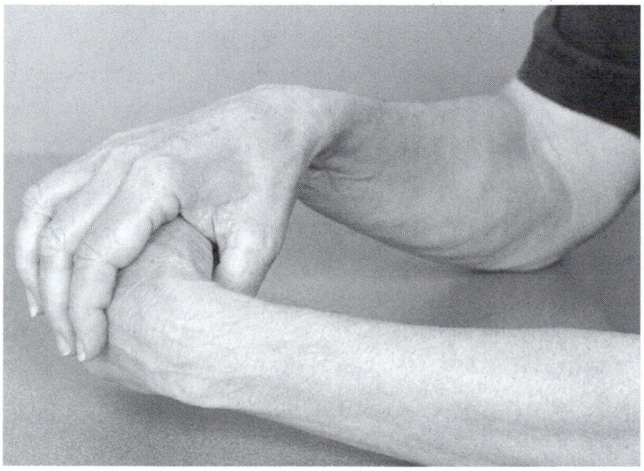

FIGURE 6-5 Self-range activity for wrist flexion.

SELF-MANAGEMENT: Ankle Passive Range of Motion

Purpose: To increase ankle motion in all directions

Position: In a sitting position with the ankle crossed across the knee, with a comfortable grip at the forefoot.

Movement technique: Move the ankle in upward and downward directions. Move the ankle in and out. Stay in a comfortable range of motion. Hold briefly at the end of the range in each direction.

Repetitions:* ______ *times

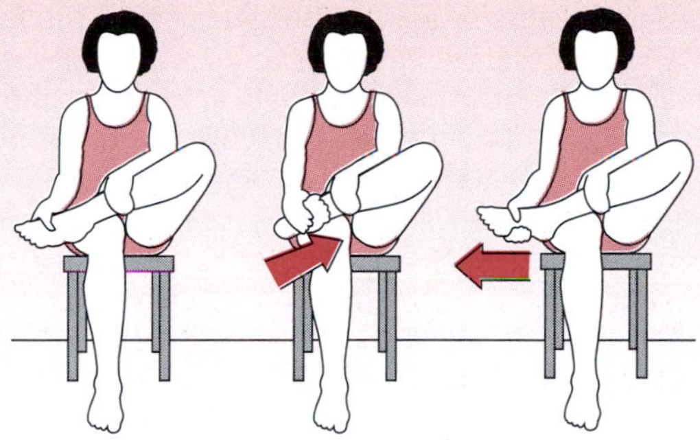

Active Assisted Range of Motion

Active assisted ROM can be defined as mobility activities in which some muscle activation takes place. In this situation, the patient is unable or not allowed to fully activate the muscle. Active assisted ROM is indicated when some muscle activation through the ROM is allowed or desired. Active assisted ROM is frequently used to initiate gentle muscle activity after musculotendinous surgical procedures such as rotator cuff or Achilles tendon repairs. The amount of assistance throughout the ROM may vary. Some individuals may require assistance throughout the entire range, but others may require minimal or no assistance in some ranges while needing nearly maximal assistance in other ranges. This variation may result from a painful arc, limitations imposed by the disease or injury, changing length-tension ratios, or synergist action.

Active assisted exercise is indicated for patients who are unable to complete the ROM actively because of weakness resulting from trauma, neurologic injury, muscular or neuromuscular disease, or pain. The weight of the limb may impede active movement using proper mechanics, and assistance may be provided to ensure proper exercise performance. Some injuries or operations necessitate limitations in active muscle contraction in the early phase of healing (see Self-Management: Knee-to-Chest Stretching).

The expected goals with active assisted ROM intervention are the same as those accomplished with passive ROM. Prevention of the negative effects of immobilization, prevention of joint contractures and soft tissue tightness, decreased pain, and enhancement of vascular dynamics and synovial diffusion can be accomplished with active assisted ROM. The benefits of active muscle contraction extend beyond those of passive ROM. Active muscle contraction significantly enhances circulation. The pull of muscle on its bony attachments is a stimulus for bone activity while maintaining muscle strength. Active muscle contraction also assists in proprioception and kinesthesia, enhancing the individual's awareness of his position in space. Muscle contraction in this situation has little impact on true strength gains, but it teaches the patient how to actively fire the muscle. For example, individuals with rotator cuff injuries require assistance to activate these muscles after injury or surgery (Fig. 6-6). Moreover, active assisted exercise involves the patient in his rehabilitation, rather than acting as the recipient of a passive technique.

Hand placement and cuing when performing active assisted ROM are important for optimal patient participation. When possible, tactile cuing should be on one side of the joint rather than using a grip on the flexor and extensor surfaces. This action cues the patient for the direction of assistance or resistance. This is particularly important when performing a technique such as active assisted ROM when some ranges are assisted but others are not.

SELF-MANAGEMENT: ***Knee-to-Chest Stretching***

Purpose: To increase the mobility of the lumbar spine and hips in flexion

Position: Lying on your back, with your knees bent and feet flat on the floor

Movement technique: Slowly bring one knee to your chest while grasping behind your knee. Bring the second knee to your chest. Hold for 15 to 30 seconds. Slowly lower one leg to the starting position, followed by the other leg.

Repetitions:_______ times

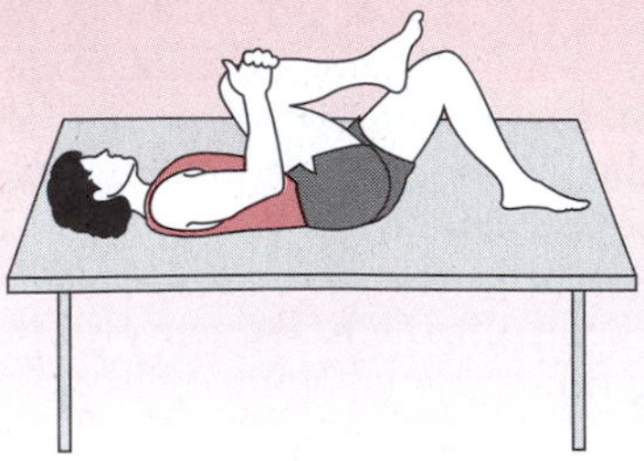

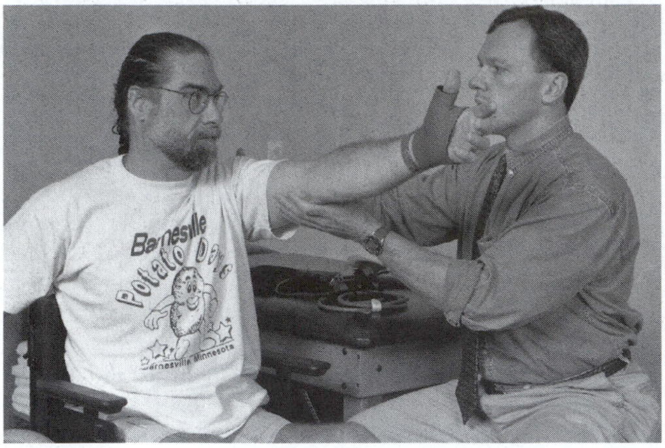

FIGURE 6-6 Active assisted shoulder flexion can be accomplished with assistance from the therapist.

Active Range of Motion

Active mobility can be limited by the same noncontractile and contractile tissues that limit passive mobility. Shortening, stiffness, spasm, or contracture limit the joint's ability to move through a ROM. Additional factors may limit an individual's ability to complete the ROM actively. The strength and endurance of the muscle or muscle group can limit active motion. Strength below a fair (3/5) muscle grade implies an inability to complete the ROM against gravity. Poor neuromuscular coordination and balance, such as the inability to stand on a single leg, may limit active mobility. Strength in an agonist may be adequate to complete the ROM, but antagonist firing because of neurologic pathology or faulty neuromuscular control patterns may limit motion. The patient may lack the ability to complete the ROM with adequate speed or lack agonist or synergist coordination to achieve purposeful movement. Cardiovascular endurance limitations in patients with chronic obstructive pulmonary disease, emphysema, or other cardiovascular conditions can hinder the performance of active exercise.

Active ROM is defined as mobility activities performed by active muscle contraction. These activities can be performed against gravity or in a gravity-minimized position, depending on the individual's strength and the physical therapy goals (Fig. 6-7). Motions in cardinal planes, combination movement patterns, or functional activities such as reaching or combing one's hair are all examples of active ROM. The expected goals or outcomes associated with active ROM intervention include those associated with passive ROM plus the benefits of muscle contraction. These goals parallel those of active assisted ROM, although the results are greater. In addition to the greater strength requirements, active exercise requires more muscle coordination because of the lack of assistance or guidance through the ROM. As with active assisted exercise, the strength gains are minimal in many patients. Only those with fair (3/5) strength or less can be expected to have their strength challenged. However, many patients can expect to be challenged proprioceptively and kinesthetically. For example, after knee injury or surgery, many individuals have difficulty activating the quadriceps femoris. Quadriceps setting exercises show patients how to activate the quadriceps, a pre-

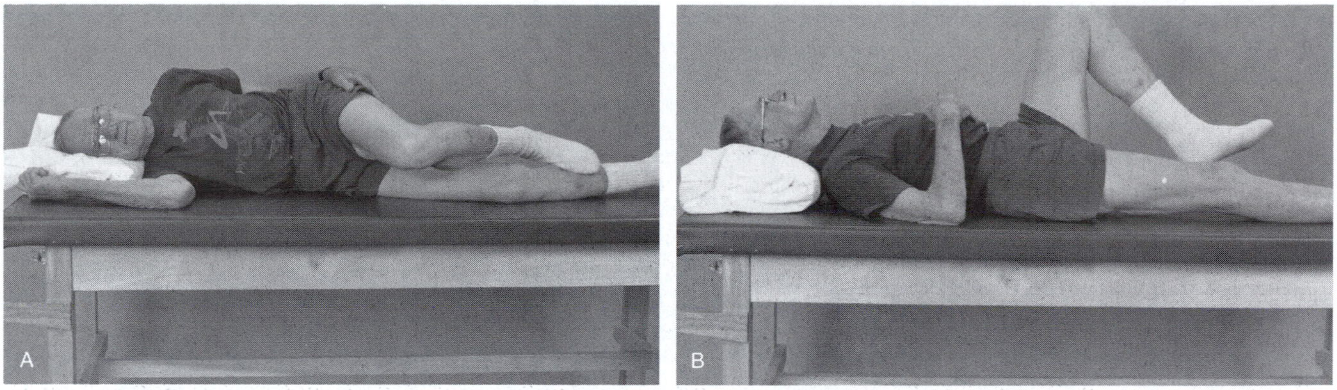

FIGURE 6-7 ***(A)*** Active hip flexion in a gravity minimized position. ***(B)*** Correct performance using proper posture and movement kinematics.

requisite for functional activities. Although little or no tibiofemoral movement occurs, patellofemoral active ROM occurs, with superior glide of the patella on the femur.

Active exercise should follow any passive technique to reinforce proper movement patterns and to overcome maladaptions to tissue stiffness. As new mobility is achieved, active exercise should be used to ensure the ability to use the new range effectively. For example, as hip flexion ROM improves from joint mobilization and stretching techniques, hand-knee rocking can be used to facilitate hip flexion ROM (see Chapter 18, Fig. 18-26). As shoulder flexion mobility increases after stretching exercises, active shoulder flexion exercises should be initiated. Similarly, as knee flexion ROM increases after stretching, active knee flexion should follow (see Self-Management: Active Range of Motion for Shoulder Flexion and Self-Management: Active Knee Flexion). Active exercise enhances the vascular benefits of ROM, with activities such as ankle pumps (ie, repetitive dorsiflexion and plantarflexion) used postoperatively to prevent deep vein thromboses.

Like active assisted ROM, active exercise is indicated when active muscle contraction is desired. Many exercise programs begin with a regimen of active exercise to ensure proper exercise performance before the addition of resistance. In some situations, the weight of the limb alone produces optimal loading and makes a good starting point for the rehabilitation program. After surgery or trauma, passive exercise may be initiated early and then progressed to active assisted and active ROM as healing allows; ultimately, resistive exercise is added. An additional benefit of active exercise is independence. Once instructed by the clinician, the patient is wholly responsible for exercise performance (see Selected Intervention: Active Range of Motion to Improve Mobility).

STRETCHING

Stretching techniques are used to increase the extensibility of the muscle tendon unit and the periarticular connective tissue. Stretching is used to increase flexibility, which depends on joint ROM and soft tissue extensibility. Stretching techniques fall into three broad categories: static stretching, ballistic stretching, and proprioceptive neuromuscular facilitation (PNF) stretching. Specific stretching exercises and methods within these broad categories can increase muscle extensibility and joint ROM.[14,16–18,53,57,62,66,71,75,81,82,95] The clinician must determine which stretching methods and what sequence can best resolve the impairments and functional limitations of each patient.

Static Stretching

DeVries[16–18] is credited with the initial research on the use and efficacy of static stretching and ballistic stretching. Static stretching is a method of stretching in which the muscles and connective tissue being stretched are held in a sta-

SELF-MANAGEMENT: Active Range of Motion for Shoulder Flexion

Purpose: To increase active mobility in a forward and overhead direction

Position: In a sitting or standing position keeping your trunk in good alignment

Movement technique: Reach your arm forward and up overhead. Reach as far overhead as is comfortable.

Repetitions:* _______ *times

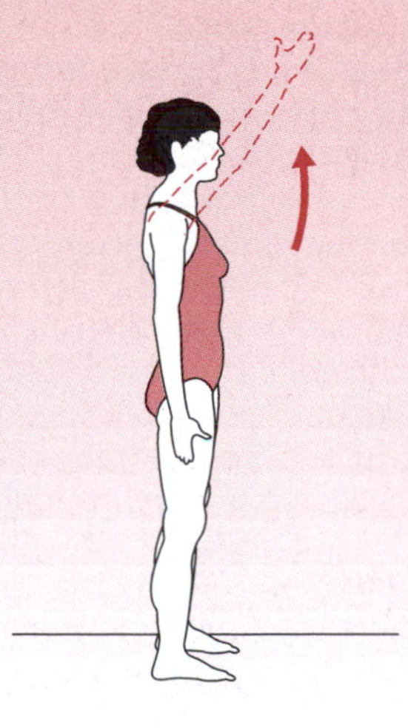

SELF-MANAGEMENT: Active Knee Flexion

Purpose: To increase active range of knee flexion and to initiate muscle activity

Position: Standing on your uninvolved leg on the floor or on a small step, with your involved leg hanging down next to the step, hold onto a stable object for support.

Movement technique: Slowly bend your involved knee up behind you, then lower it slowly and in a controlled fashion. Be sure to keep your knees in line with one another.

Repetitions: _______ **times**

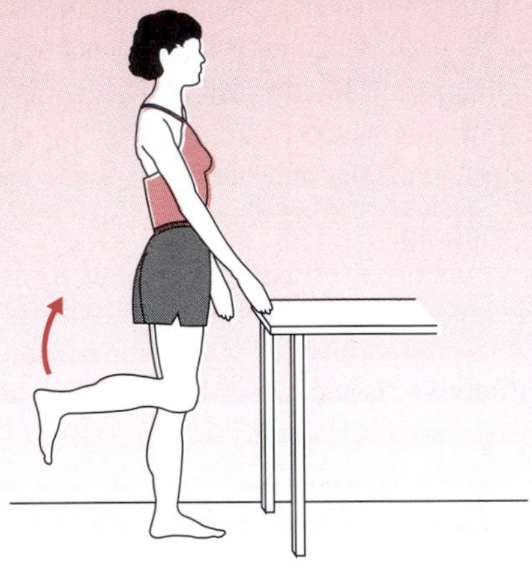

tionary position at their greatest possible length for some period. When using static stretching on a clinical basis, stretches should be held a minimum of 15 to 30 seconds. There does not appear to be any clinical advantage to holding the stretch longer, unless the patient prefers to do so.[8,48,54] Static stretching offers advantages of using less overall force, decreasing the danger of exceeding the tissue extensibility limits, lower energy requirements, and a lower likelihood of muscle soreness.[17] Static stretching also has less effect on the Ia and II spindle afferent fibers than ballistic stretching, which would tend to increase a muscle's resistance to stretch and facilitate the Golgi tendon organ, thereby decreasing the contractile elements' resistance to deformation.

When performing static stretching, the patient is positioned to allow complete relaxation of the muscle to be stretched. This position requires a comfortable, supportive surface. The limb is taken to the point at which a gentle stretching sensation is felt, and the stretch is held for 15 to 30 seconds. The stretch is relaxed and then repeated. Proper limb alignment ensures that the proper tissues are being stretched without causing injury to adjacent structures (see Self-Management: Hip Stretching).

Ballistic Stretching

Ballistic stretching uses quick movements that impose a change in the length of muscle or connective tissue. Initiated by active contraction of the muscles antagonistic to the muscles and connective tissue being stretched, these movements appear to be jerky in nature. Although ballistic stretching has been effective for increasing flexibility in athletes, there may be a greater chance of muscle soreness and injury.[17] Injury may result from excessive uncontrolled forces during ballistic stretching and proposed neurologic inhibitory influences associated with rapid-type stretching.[21–23,62,73,93,94] For these reasons, ballistic stretching should be used only with selected patients, such as individuals preparing for plyometric activities.

The patient performing ballistic stretching should be well stabilized and comfortable. The limb is moved until a gentle stretch is felt, and then gentle "bouncing" at the end range is performed. Care must be taken to avoid ballistic stretching that is too vigorous, because it can produce muscle injury and pain.

Proprioceptive Neuromuscular Facilitation Stretching

PNF stretching techniques have been widely used by the physical therapy community. These techniques seek to capitalize on the use of the neurophysiologic concept of stretch activation. PNF stretching techniques use a contract-relax (CR) sequence, an agonist contraction (AC), or a contract-relax–agonist contraction (CRAC) sequence.[39] Using PNF stretching techniques, the clinician seeks to acti-vate the Golgi tendon organ and inhibit the muscle being stretched or use the principle of reciprocal inhibition.

CR stretching begins like static stretching; the patient is supported, and the limb is brought to the end ROM until gentle stretching is felt. At that point, the muscle being stretched is contracted isometrically against resistance for approximately 2 to 5 seconds and then relaxed. The stretch is then increased, and the procedure is repeated two to four times.

AC stretching uses the principle of reciprocal inhibition. The limb is taken to the position of gentle stretch, and the muscle opposite the muscle being stretched is contracted, facilitating the stretch and inhibiting the muscle undergoing stretch. For example, when stretching the hamstring muscles, a simultaneous contraction of the quadriceps muscles can facilitate the stretch. This contraction is held for 2 to 5 seconds, and the technique repeated two to four times.

CRAC is a technique that combines the CR and AC stretches. The limb is taken to the point of gentle stretch, and a CR sequence is performed (ie, resistance applied against the muscle being stretched). After contracting the muscle being stretched, this muscle is relaxed while the agonist is contracted, facilitating the stretch. For example, when stretching the hamstring muscles, they are brought to a position of stretch. The hamstring muscles are contracted against resistance and then relaxed, and the quadriceps are contracted.

Each of these stretching techniques requires constant communication with the patient to ensure that neither overstretching nor excessive resistance produce muscle injury. These techniques can be performed independently with a family member or alone using a towel or other simple objects to provide resistance or assistance.

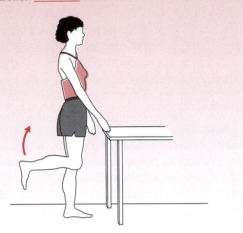

SELECTED INTERVENTION
Active Range of Motion to Improve Mobility

See Case Study #4

ACTIVITY: Wand elevation exercise

PURPOSE: To increase shoulder mobility in abduction, scaption, and flexion

RISK FACTORS: Ensure appropriate stabilization and arthrokinematic motion to prevent substitution

ELEMENTS OF THE MOVEMENT SYSTEM: Biomechanical

STAGE OF MOTOR CONTROL: Mobility

POSTURE: The patient is standing in chest-deep water, with a wand in the hands.

MOVEMENT: The patient allows the buoyancy of the water and the assistance of the uninvolved arm to lift the arm in the frontal, scapular, or sagittal plane. Relaxation of the shoulder muscles allows passive stretch into abduction, scaption, or flexion.

DOSAGE: Sets of 3–5 repetitions with 30-second holding at the end of the range.

RATIONALE FOR EXERCISE CHOICE: This exercise passively assists motion into a functional, frequently limited range. The intensity of stretch is easily modified by changing water depth.

EXERCISE GRADATION: The patient should discontinue use of wand, and progress to active then resisted movements.

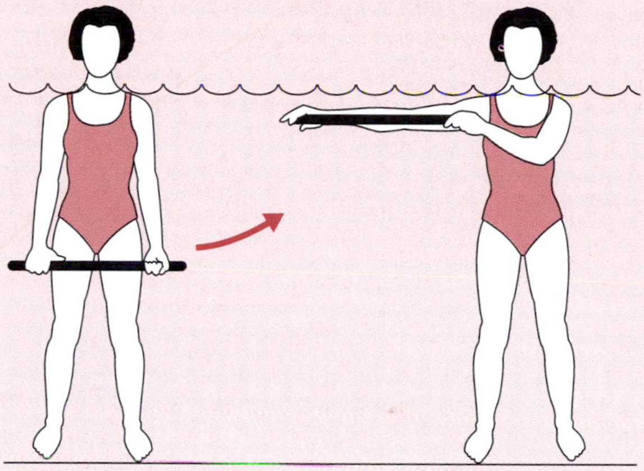

Wand shoulder abduction

SELF-MANAGEMENT: *Hip Stretching*

Purpose: To increase the flexibility of the lateral hip and thigh muscles

Position: Standing with the involved leg out on the surface (eg, table, step) in front of you

Movement technique: Keeping your hips square (do not rotate your hips), bring your leg across in front of you a few inches; next, roll your entire leg in the same direction (across your body). Hold 15–30 seconds.

Repetitions:_______ times

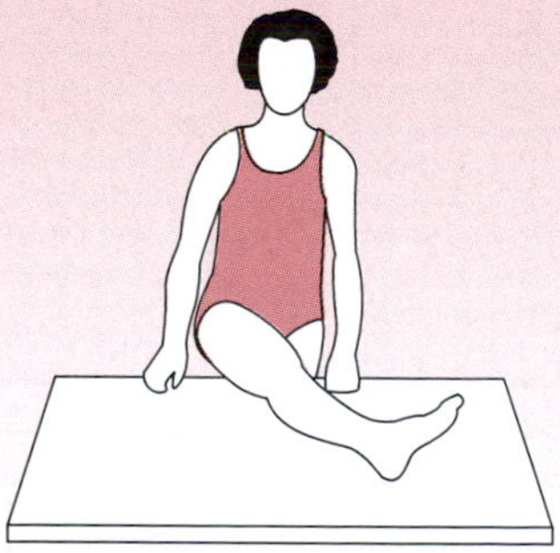

EFFECTS OF STRETCHING

Stretching is one of the most accepted interventions in rehabilitation. Stretching has been studied to determine the effects of different stretching techniques. The effects of stretching are divided into acute effects and chronic effects. Acute effects are the immediate, short-term results of stretching and are the result of elongating the elastic component of the musculotendinous unit (see Chapter 10, Figs. 10-2 through 10-4). The effects of routine stretching exercises are acute in nature. Chronic effects are the long-term results of prolonged stretching and are the result of adding sarcomeres (usually because of immobilization in a lengthened position). Stretching is used to lengthen shortened tissue and to decrease muscle stiffness. Contractile and noncontractile elements of muscle contribute to its resting tension and resistance to elongation.[94] Potential sources of stiffness are adhesions, epimysium, perimysium, endomysium, sarcolemma, contractile elements within the muscle fiber, and associated tendons and their insertions.[94] The relative contribution of the contractile elements to resistance to stretch appears to be velocity related, with increased resistance to stretch occurring at higher velocities.[77] The farther the muscle is stretched, the greater is the relative contribution of noncontractile elements.[94]

There is no agreement about which stretching technique is best.[14,53,57,62,66,71,75,82,95] According to some researchers, PNF techniques may be better than static or ballistic techniques for producing acute, short-term improvements in ROM.

These short-term improvements may result from contraction of antagonistic muscles while performing CRAC stretching, which is based on the principle of reciprocal inhibition.[21–23] Muscle stiffness has been decreased by performing a conditioning isometric or eccentric muscle action.[36] This muscle contraction causes a change in viscosity and resistance to molecular deformation, decreasing stiffness and resistance to stretch. Prestretch conditioning through active or passive movements (ie, passive oscillations or active repetitive eccentric actions) may loosen actin-myosin bonds and increase stretching effectiveness.[39]

Regardless of the type of stretching method used, flexibility gains made may be retained even after the individual has stopped stretching for some time. Zebas and Rivera[95] demonstrated retention of gains from 2 to 4 weeks after the cessation of a 6-week stretching program. Participating in a flexibility exercise program three to five times per week can produce gains. For individuals with significant flexibility deficits, stretching should be part of their daily routine. After the goal is achieved, stretching once each week may be sufficient to maintain gains.

Posture

Posture is a key aspect of any mobility activity performed. The starting and ending positions and the proper posture of associated joints are based on physiologic and kinesiologic factors. Physiologic factors such as the stage of healing affect the starting and ending positions for ROM and the position for stretching. For example, if a patient has just sustained an acute musculotendinous injury, ROM avoids the extreme position of the muscle range that would place too much stretch on the injured tissue.

Kinesiologic factors affecting posture are related to the normal osteokinematics and arthrokinematics at the joint. For example, proper performance of shoulder flexion requires normal arthrokinematic motion at the glenohumeral, sternoclavicular, and acromioclavicular joints and requires normal osteokinematic motion and associated arthrokinematic motion at the scapulothoracic articulation and thoracic spine. If motion is limited at any of these locations, substitution and faulty movement patterns occur. If an individual lacks glenohumeral arthrokinematic motion that limits glenohumeral flexion, scapulothoracic elevation or lumbar spine extension may substitute. Attempts to stretch the shoulder into further flexion can impinge subacromial soft tissues, cause substitution by adjacent joints, or both. The patient can learn an effective substitution pattern that prohibits normalization of movement patterns and the eventual progression to normal arthrokinematic and osteokinematic motion.

Another important kinesiologic factor related to posture is the stabilization of one attachment site of the muscle (usually proximal) or limb during stretching. For example, appropriately stretching the hamstring muscles requires proximal stabilization through proper lumbar and pelvic positions. Failure to stabilize proximally results in lumbar spine flexion, posterior pelvic tilt, and movement of the hamstring origin closer to the insertion, thereby minimizing the stretch. Maintaining correct posture that appropriately stabilizes is essential for effective stretching.

Exercise Mode

The clinician must also decide on the exercise mode. For the individual performing ROM activities, the options depend on whether the exercise is to be performed actively, with assistance, or passively. The stage of healing is the primary physiologic parameter affecting the exercise mode and determines the amount of assistance required. The indications and contraindications for the level of assistance were discussed previously.

After determining the level of assistance necessary, the specific equipment and postures are delineated, with attention focused on kinesiologic factors. Using pulleys to gain shoulder flexion can be helpful if performed properly without scapular or spinal substitution patterns (Fig. 6-8). The same can be said for self-mobilization activities such as stretching the arm forward on a counter (Fig. 6-9).

The exercise chosen should allow full available excursion. Several modes are available for the performance of passive ROM or stretching. Pulleys, continuous passive motion devices, family members, or various household objects such as the floor, counters, or chairs can be used to perform passive ROM. Holding the position at end range adds a stretching component to the passive ROM activity. Passive knee flexion can be easily performed using a towel and a smooth floor, by sitting on a chair, or while in a pool.

The pool can be used to perform ROM exercises with any level of assistance. Passive or active assisted ROM exercises can be performed using buoyancy. Movements toward the surface are assisted by buoyancy, and the assistance level depends on the use of buoyant equipment (Fig. 6-10). Stretching can be performed using equipment or steps, walls, or bars in the pool. The buoyant atmosphere and water's warmth often make stretching more comfortable. Active exercise can be performed by minimizing the effects of buoyancy and viscosity to negate assistance or resistance (see Chapter 17).

Exercise Dosage

The stage of healing (see Chapter 10) and the tissue response to loading relative to the patient's examination findings determine the dosage of mobility exercises. Each patient should be considered on an individual basis, with the dosage matched to the patient's needs. These needs extend beyond the physical impairments to include psychosocial and lifestyle issues.

SEQUENCE

Mobility activities can be performed as part of warm-up exercises before aerobic activity or as a rehabilitative exercise in and of itself. Passive or active assisted ROM is often used to teach active ROM exercises, and active ROM is often used as a teaching tool for resistive exercise. The sequence of exercise depends on the purpose of the ROM activity. ROM exercises as preparation for more difficult exercise should occur before that activity. When mobility exercises are being performed for the benefits of ROM, they should be performed in a sequence of easier to more difficult.

Most exercises performed passively can also be performed actively or actively with some assistance. This makes

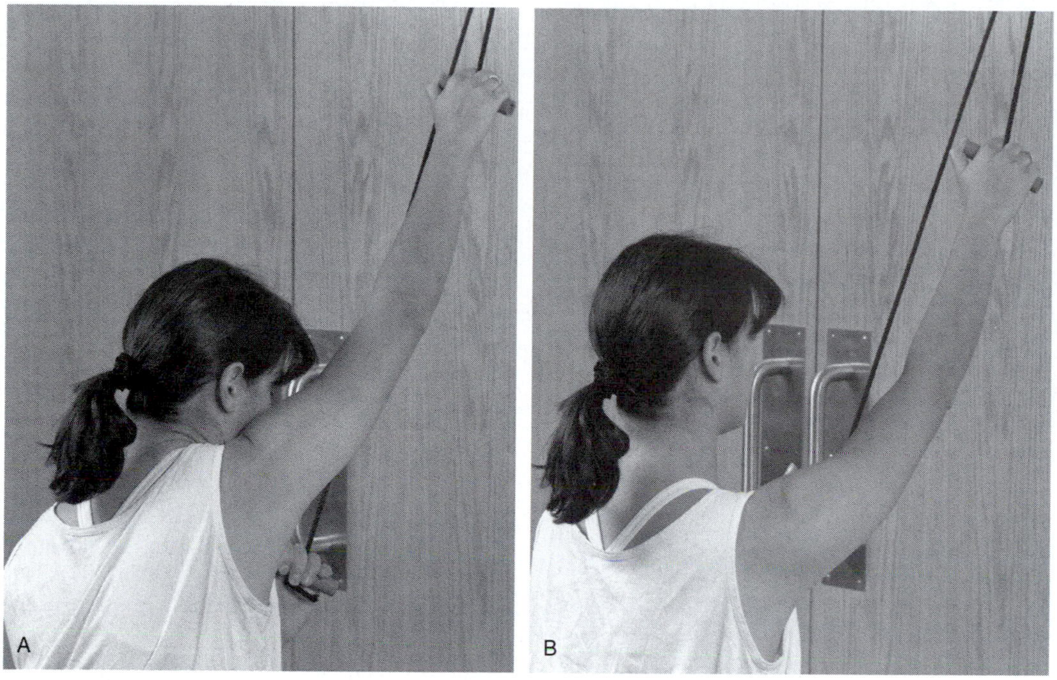

FIGURE 6-8 *(A)* Incorrect performance of shoulder flexion using pulleys. *(B)* Correct performance using proper posture and movement kinematics.

an easy progressive sequence for the patient to follow. For example, a single knee flexion exercise can be easily progressed by changing instructions. Knee flexion with a towel can be actively assisted by using some muscle activity and some passive assistance from the towel (Fig. 6-11). As the patient improves, the same exercise can be performed without assistance. The same is true for shoulder flexion exercises with a pulley or counter; the exercise can be performed with some level of assistance or completely actively.

The concept of active stretching is important when considering sequencing of mobility activities. Active stretching is the use of active movement to stretch the agonist or to use the agonist in its new range. Stretching a short muscle should always be complemented with active stretching by strengthening the opposing muscle in the shortened range. Based on scientific studies of length-tension properties of skeletal muscle, it is hypothesized that a stiff or short soft tissue structure cannot remain lengthened until opposing soft tissue

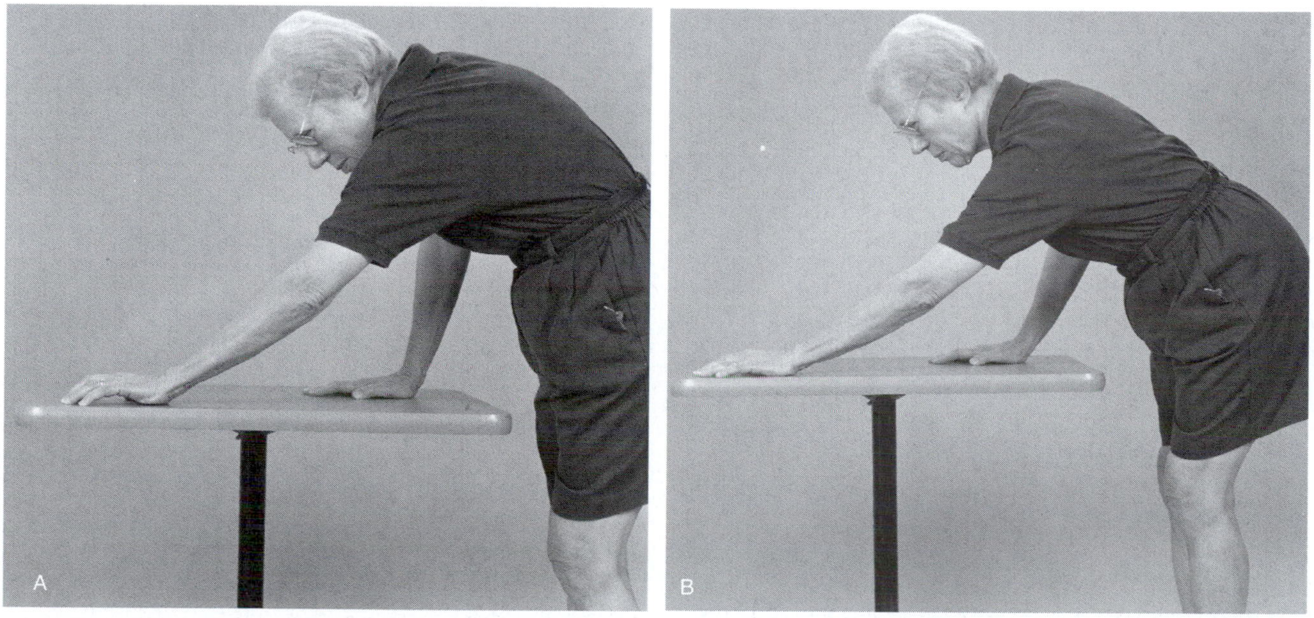

FIGURE 6-9 *(A)* Incorrect performance of passive shoulder flexion on a countertop. *(B)* Correct performance using proper posture and movement kinematics.

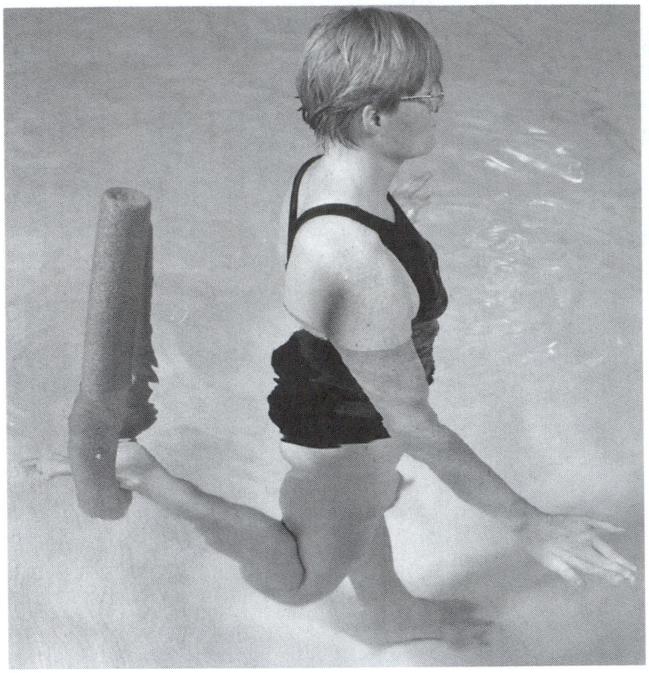

FIGURE 6-10 Knee flexion stretching can be performed in the pool, using buoyant equipment.

structures shorten.[87] The premise behind strengthening the opposing muscle is that its length-tension properties have been disrupted if it has lengthened as a result of the target muscle shortening. It cannot generate tension in the short range as sufficiently as is necessary to oppose the pull of the short muscle. By strengthening the lengthened muscle, particularly in the short range, its length-tension properties can improve, and it can provide a counterbalancing force to the short muscle. Stretching a short muscle can be done passively through a self-stretch or manual stretch, but it should always be accompanied with active stretching through strengthening the opposing muscle in the shortened range.

Active contraction of the antagonist in a shortened position is used to strengthen this muscle while simultaneously actively stretching the agonist. For example, after static stretching of the hamstrings, the patient can extend the knee in a sitting position while the paraspinal muscles stabilize the spine to prevent lumbar flexion. The quadriceps actively stretch the hamstrings into the new range. This repeated activity enhances mobility in the new range. This same sequence concept can be applied throughout the body, as in the treatment of low back and pelvic muscle imbalance. After static stretching of short hip flexor muscles (ensuring appropriate stabilization during this stretching), the patient should extend the hip in a walk stance position while the abdominal muscles stabilize the spine and pelvis (see Self-Management: Active Stretch for the Hip Flexor Muscles).

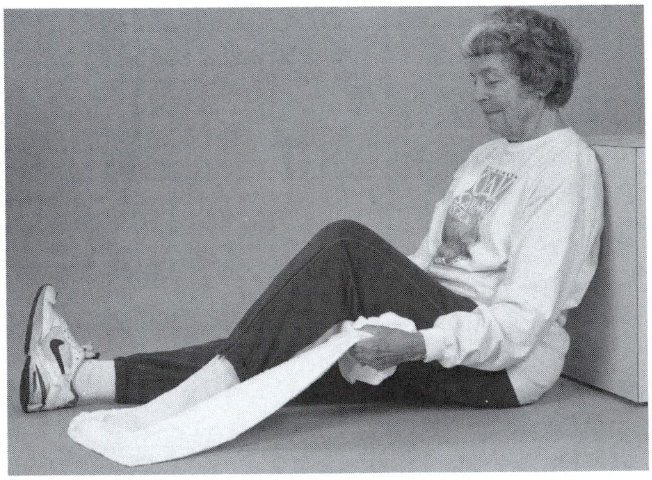

FIGURE 6-11 Active range of motion at the knee using a towel for assistance as needed.

FREQUENCY, INTENSITY, AND DURATION

The frequency of a therapeutic exercise program is often inversely related to the intensity and duration. Exercises of high intensity and duration are performed less frequently and vice versa. ROM activities, because of their purpose and goals, are generally a lower intensity exercise performed for a shorter duration. These exercises can be per-

SELF-MANAGEMENT: Active Stretch for the Hip Flexor Muscles

Purpose: To stretch and use hip flexor muscles in the new range. This activity should follow hip-stretching exercises.

Position: In a stride position, with the leg to be stretched behind and with the opposite foot forward as in taking a step. Be sure to keep the back straight and abdominal muscles tightened.

Movement technique: Shift your weight forward onto your front foot while maintaining proper hip and back position. Hold 15–30 seconds. Be sure that the hip of your back leg is being stretched as shown by the highlighted area in the illustration below.

Repetitions:* _______ *times

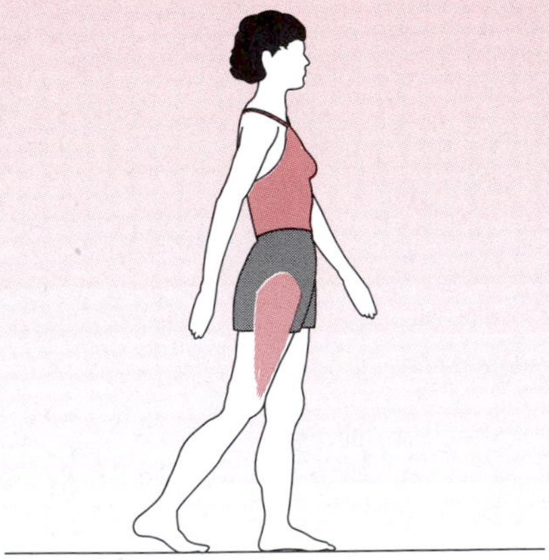

formed more frequently and usually take place in the home or work environment. The clinician should choose exercises that can easily and effectively be performed independently by the patient or with the assistance of a family member.

The exercise frequency is related to the purpose of the exercise, which can be considered relative to physiologic, kinesiologic, or learning factors. Physiologic purposes are those that enhance fluid dynamics, support articular cartilage nutrition, and maintain the integrity of the periarticular connective tissues. Kinesiologic purposes include maintenance of normal arthrokinematic motion and are closely tied to learning factors or choosing the correct motor program. Exercises to teach postural set, appropriate sequencing, and patterning of muscle contraction or to teach a complex motor skill are examples of ROM as a tool for learning.

Exercises performed for physiologic or kinesiologic purposes are performed twice to five or more times each day. The number of times depends on the environment and availability of exercise within that environment. If it is nearly impossible for an individual to perform exercises during the workday, asking him to carry out an exercise program five times each day is unreasonable. Similarly, if the ROM activities require the assistance of another, availability of that help dictates the frequency of the exercise program. As discussed in Chapter 3, exercise prescription should fit within the context of the individual's day.

Exercises performed as learning tools are usually performed more frequently during the day. Examples of these exercises are postural reeducation activities such as scapular retraction and depression, chin tucks while sitting at a desk, and knee extension while driving without posterior pelvic tilt or lumbar flexion (Fig. 6-12). These kinds of exercises are often put "on cue" so that a specific stimulus can elicit the postural response, such as performing postural exercises every time the phone rings, every time a new page is started on a computer document, or every time an instructor poses a question. This type of programming places the exercise in the appropriate functional context, within the environment or situation where the exercise most needs to be performed. With time and repetition, the individual should find that, when the stimulus elicits the response, they are already in the appropriate posture. The intensity of this type of exercise is low, and the frequency is therefore increased.

The number of sets and repetitions depends on the frequency and the number of exercises performed. When several exercises are being performed to maintain ROM during a period of bed rest or in the early healing stages of an injury, the sets and repetitions may be fewer as multiple components of the joint and periarticular connective tissues are being mobilized. Conversely, when only a few exercises can be performed because of healing constraints or other medical conditions, more sets and repetitions of those exercises can be performed. When exercises are being performed frequently throughout the day, fewer sets and repetitions are performed during each session. When active exercise is being used to increase endurance, more repetitions and longer duration rather than greater frequency is the rule. The guiding principle in ROM prescription is understanding the physiologic, kinesiologic, and learning factors associated with each exercise in relation to the patient and exercise goals.

The length of time a stretch must be held to facilitate an increase in muscle flexibility remains a point of disagreement among clinicians. The clinical literature states that stretches should be held for a minimum of 15 to 30 seconds and that there does not appear to be any advantage to holding a stretch longer than that period.[48,54] However, the time that a patient or an athlete wants to hold a stretch may be based on the individual's perceived need or comfort level. When in doubt, a stretch should be held for a longer period rather than a shorter period. Although short-term flexibility improvements can be seen in one stretching session, studies

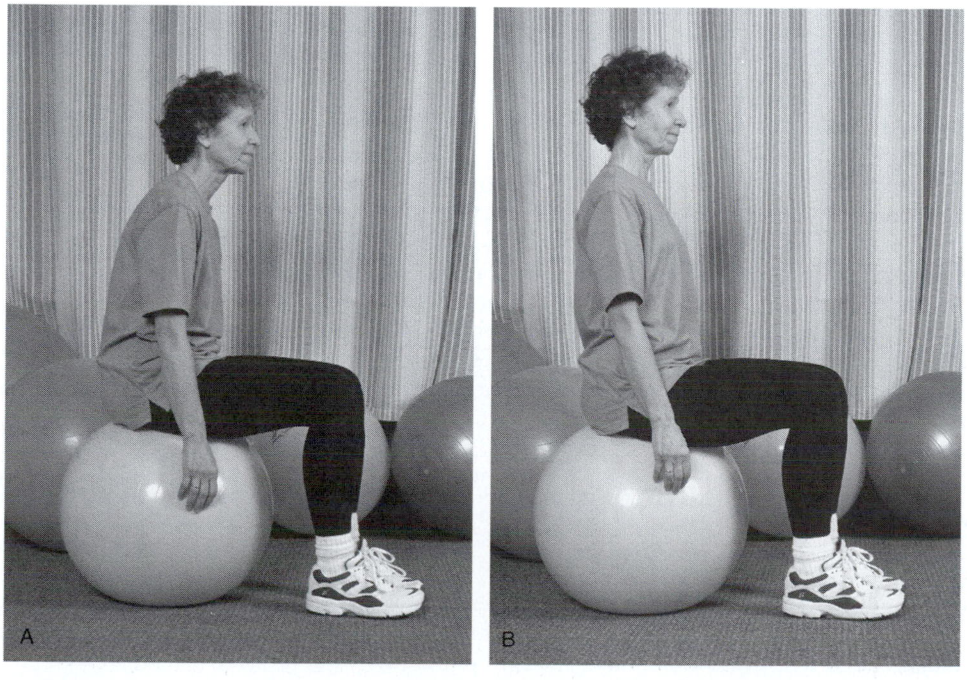

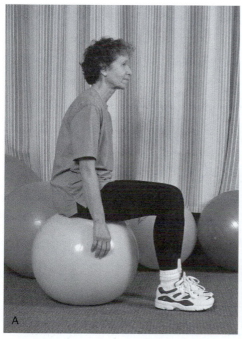

FIGURE 6-12 Chin tucks, pelvic tilts and quadriceps setting can be performed while sitting on an unstable surface. ***(A)*** Poor posture. ***(B)*** Good posture with proper pelvic posture and chin tucks.

on the length of stretching time necessary to effect long-term increases in muscle flexibility are still lacking. The intensity of stretching should be low to medium to prevent reflexive contraction. This contraction occurs in response to discomfort during stretching. The stretch should be comfortable enough to be easily held for 30 seconds.

Precautions and Contraindications

Passive ROM and stretching are not benign processes and are contraindicated when motion could disrupt the healing process. For example, passive motion into full shoulder external rotation may disrupt the healing process after a capsular shift procedure. Passive motion into hip adduction, flexion past 90 degrees, and internal rotation past neutral may result in dislocation of a recent total hip arthroplasty. Caution should be used to ensure that the activity is passive when active muscle contraction is contraindicated, such as after a tendon transfer procedure. The clinician must ensure that the activity is producing *joint* ROM in the case of passive ROM and *muscle* ROM in the case of stretching. Moreover, the speed and patient comfort must be controlled to prevent inadvertent muscle contraction to oppose the passive exercise. Active muscle contraction in response to fear or pain could disrupt the healing process. The clinician must be aware of local anatomy, arthrokinematics, and the effects of passive ROM on these tissues. For example, passive shoulder ROM into full overhead flexion without adequate humeral head depression may compress a recent rotator cuff repair under the coracoacromial arch, producing pain and disrupting the healing process.

As with passive ROM, active assisted ROM is contraindicated when motion or contraction may disrupt the healing process or affect the individual's health status. For example, individuals with unstable cardiac conditions are not candidates for active assisted exercise. When performing exercise with an active component, the clinician must ensure that the type of muscle contraction performed (eg, concentric, eccentric, isometric) is indicated and that the amount of tension generated is appropriate. The indications and contraindications for these contraction types are described in Chapter 4. The clinician should emphasize the importance of muscle relaxation between exercise repetitions to ensure adequate blood flow to the working muscles.

Contraindications and precautions for active ROM are the same as those for active assisted exercise. Muscle contraction that may disrupt the healing process or affect the individual's health status are contraindications to active ROM. The type of muscle contractions being performed should be safe for the specific situation, and the clinician should allow muscle relaxation between repetitions.

CAUSES AND EFFECTS OF HYPERMOBILITY

Although most clinicians are familiar with the treatment of persons with decreased mobility, many patients have problems related to excessive mobility. These impairments and functional limitations often result from the hypermobility. Most individuals do not seek medical attention primarily for possessing excessive mobility about a joint or throughout the body. More frequently, patients seek medical attention for pain, fatigue, or tendinitis that is the result of excessive mobility.

Hypermobility should be differentiated from instability. Hypermobility is excessive laxity or length of a tissue, and instability is an excessive range of movement, osteokinematic or arthrokinematic, for which there is no protective muscular control. Despite hypermobility, the individual may experience no symptoms of instability. For example, individuals with ACL-deficient knees may have measurable anterior laxity (ie, hypermobility) at the tibiofemoral joint with no symptoms of instability. Conversely, individuals may have complaints of instability or "giving way" with no measurable laxity.

Hypermobility can be broadly categorized as excessive joint mobility resulting from trauma or a genetic profile or as excessive tissue length. Hypermobility at a joint caused by traumatic injury can lead to true instability, particularly at the glenohumeral joint, where a traumatic anterior inferior dislocation can result in recurrent dislocation. Similarly, sprains to the lateral ankle ligaments or medial knee ligaments can result in hypermobility and instability. Atraumatic hypermobility is common at the glenohumeral joint; persons with multidirectional instability often seek medical attention for symptoms of rotator cuff tendinitis. At the knee, hypermobility can result in secondary patellofemoral pain. Patients with traumatic or atraumatic hypermobility may seek medical attention for a number of complaints, which may or may not include frank instability.

Hypermobility can develop in response to a relatively less mobile segment or region. In a multijoint system with common movement directions (eg, spine), movement occurs at the segments providing the least resistance. Abnormal or excessive movement is imposed on segments with the least amount of stiffness. With repeated movements over time, the least stiff segments increase in mobility, and the stiffer segments decrease in mobility. A thorough examination, seeking to understand the impairment contributing to the hypermobility, is necessary.

THERAPEUTIC EXERCISE INTERVENTION FOR HYPERMOBILITY

Treatment techniques for hypermobility should be directed at the related impairments and functional limitations and at the underlying causes of hypermobility. For example, a patient with hypermobility at the spinal level probably has pain and decreased mobility. These impairments must be treated along with the underlying hypermobile segment. Although it is important to address the patient's current complaints, failure to recognize hypermobility as the underlying cause ensures the return of symptoms. Hypermobility should be treated only if it is associated with instability or is producing symptoms elsewhere (ie, hypomobile segment) because of relative flexibility.

Elements of the Movement System

The elements of the movement system are important in directing treatment of hypermobility. For example, a patient with spondylolysis at L4 (ie, anatomic impairment) demonstrates faulty dynamic posture with increased lumbar lordosis during movement (ie, impairment). This results in pain (ie, impairment) and an inability to run and jump (ie, functional limitation) and to participate in high school sports (ie, disability).

In this situation, the spondylolysis is the base element, and the faulty dynamic posture is the biomechanical element. The spondylolysis is not amenable to physical therapy intervention, although the biomechanical element must be resolved to allow healing and prevent recurrence of the spondylolysis. The intervention should address the biomechanical element through stabilization exercises and postural exercises to be incorporated into daily activities.

Effects of Stabilization

The concept of stabilization exercises gained popularity in the treatment of conditions of the spine. Stabilization exercises are dynamic activities that attempt to limit and control excessive movement.[69] These exercises do not imply a static position, but rather describe a range of movement (ie, the neutral range) in which hypermobility is controlled. Stabilization activities include mobility exercises for stiff or hypomobile segments, strengthening exercises in the shortened range for hypermobile segments, postural training to ensure movement through a controlled range, and patient education. Supportive devices such as taping or bracing may be necessary initially to keep movement within a range where stability can be maintained. This range is different for every patient and condition. Patient education focuses on helping the patient find the limits of stability and work within those limits.

As mobility exercises to decrease hypomobility and stabilization exercises to increase stiffness improve symptoms, the stability limits increase, allowing the patient to work through a larger ROM. For example, a patient with an L4 spondylolysis may have short hip flexor and lumbar paraspinal muscles in combination with a hypermobile L4 segment. Stabilization focuses on increasing the length of the short muscles through static stretching, followed by active stretching through contraction of the abdominal muscles in a walk stance position. Initially, a stabilization brace may be used during exercise. As mobility of the short muscles and stiffness at the L4 segment improve, the brace can be discontinued and the walk stance position progressed to a lunge position.

Stabilization activities should be chosen based on the direction in which the segment is susceptible to excessive motion, called the direction susceptible to motion (DSM). The DSM can be arthrokinematic or osteokinematic. In the previous example, the DSM is the osteokinematic motion of extension; the spine tends to extend excessively, producing pain. Treatment should focus on training the back to resist extension forces, rather than resisting motion in all directions. For the individual with anterior shoulder instability, the arthrokinematic motion of anterior glide is the symptom-producing hypermobility. Stabilization activities should focus on controlling anterior displacement and on treating the associated impairments.

Stabilization exercises can be performed in a variety of positions and using a range of equipment. When increasing the stability of a hypermobile segment, support (eg, taping, bracing) and strengthening in the short range must be combined with mobility exercises for the hypomobile segment. This approach ensures balance in areas with variable relative flexibility. Gymnastic balls, foam rollers, balance boards, and proprioceptive exercises are effective ways to enhance stability.

Closed-Chain Exercise

Closed-chain exercise has been advocated for those with joint instability or hypermobility. For the lower extremity, exercises such as squats, lunges, or step-ups with the foot fixed are commonly used closed-chain activities. For the upper extremity, any weight-bearing exercise performed in the push-up or modified push-up position is considered to be closed-chain. Weight bearing with the hands against the wall or on a table or countertop is also an effective closed-chain position for the upper extremity. The rationale for this exercise is muscular cocontraction, decreased shear forces, and increased joint compression. Some of this theory is supported by scientific and clinical research.[10,92] Other studies dispute some aspects of this rationale, such as muscular cocontraction with a closed-chain position.[34,35] Particularly for the lower extremity when the foot spends as much time in contact with the floor, use of closed-chain exercise in the case of hypermobility makes good clinical sense. However, for the upper extremity, the closed-chain position is rarely the position of function. The closed-chain position remains an effective position for upper extremity training for individuals with hypermobility, but open-chain stabilization techniques should be incorporated as well. More information on the effects of closed-chain exercise can be found in Chapter 15.

Open-Chain Stabilization

Open-chain stabilization activities are available for the lower and the upper extremities. PNF techniques such as rhythmic stabilization and alternating isometrics can be used effectively to facilitate cocontraction about a joint (see Chapter 14). These techniques are particularly effective in the latter stages of rehabilitation when performed in the position of instability, such as abduction and external rotation for treating anterior glenohumeral instability (Fig. 6-13).

Stabilization exercises for the spine are difficult to categorize, because the spine is often fixed at one end and open at the other end. It is not a true closed or open system. Stabilization exercises for the spine are often initiated in a supine position with abdominal bracing exercises and progressed to sitting and standing positions. A variety of stabilization exercises can be performed on a gymnastics ball, which is an unstable surface, to improve stability within a comfortable range. Sitting, prone, and supine activities combined with arm reaching and leg lifts can be used from early to advanced stages of stabilization training (Fig. 6-14). Many of these same activities can be used to improve stability throughout the upper and lower extremities.

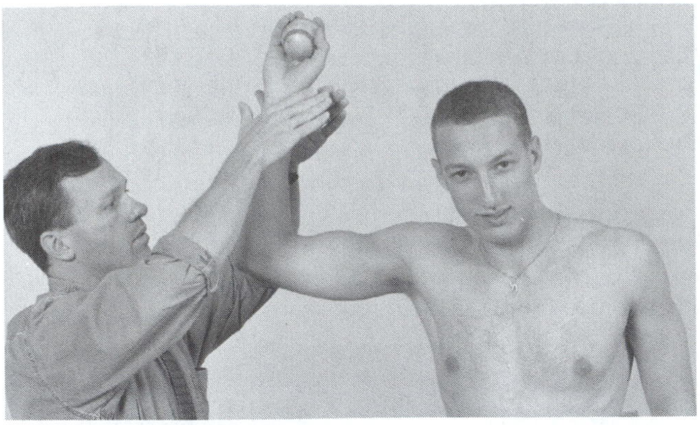

FIGURE 6-13 Rhythmic stabilization performed in a position of apprehension.

Ballistic Exercises

Ballistic exercise has been shown to produce cocontraction about a joint through triphasic muscle activation. High-speed ballistic activities result in different patterns of agonist-antagonist muscle contractions from those of slower activities. Rapid ballistic movements result in synchronous activation of agonists and antagonists.[49,58,86] In contrast, the same movement pattern at a slow speed demonstrates only agonist muscle contraction, with braking provided by passive viscoelastic properties.[49] Although the viscoelastic properties also restrict movement at faster speeds, these properties are inadequate to halt fast movements.[58] These rapid ballistic movement patterns can be used with resistive tubing or inertial exercise equipment (Fig. 6-15).

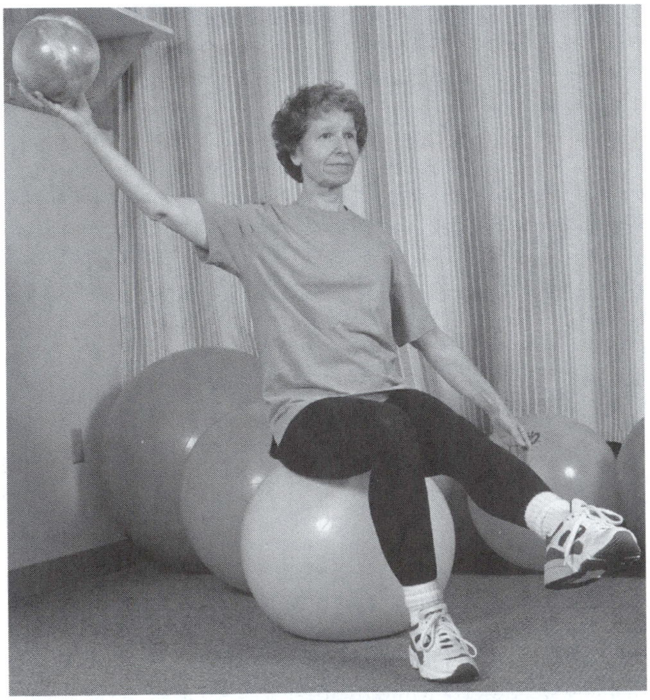

FIGURE 6-14 Sitting on a gymnastics ball while performing simultaneous arm and leg exercises is an example of an advanced spine stabilization exercise.

The amount of antagonist activity needed to halt a movement is related to the velocity of the activity.[58] Subjects were asked to produce fast flexion movements of the thumb and fast extension movements of the elbow over three distances and at a variety of speeds. All movements resulted in biphasic or triphasic muscle contraction. A linear relationship was found between peak velocity and the amount of antagonist activation needed to halt the movement. Movements made through large angles (ie, large amplitude) showed less antagonist activity than those made through small angles at the same speed, and fast, small-amplitude movements demonstrated an earlier onset of antagonist activity. The distance during fast movements is controlled primarily by the first agonist muscle contraction, and increasing antagonist torque is associated with decreasing distance, ultimately controlling the movement time.[86] Producing fast movements requires large agonist torque production, followed by an equally large or larger antagonist torque.

One study concluded that quick movements through small distances result in a large, quick antagonist burst and that slow movements over a long distance result in small and late antagonist bursts.[58] The antagonist burst timing is not specified solely by size; it is also a function of the movement amplitude. Timing and amplitude are regulated by the central nervous system. For example, flexing and extending the hip rapidly through a very small range elicits cocontraction of agonist and antagonist musculature, but flexing and extending slowly through a large range elicits reciprocal activation of the agonists and antagonists. If hip and pelvic stabilization is the goal, small-amplitude, fast movements are more likely to elicit cocontraction than slow, large-amplitude movements.

Another factor that affects antagonist activity is the subject's knowledge of the necessity for such a contraction. On study provided a mechanical stop for preventing further movement in some of elbow flexion and extension tasks.[58] When the subjects knew that the stop was in place, the antagonist burst disappeared after two or three trials. This resulted in a faster movement, suggesting that the antagonist activity brakes and slows the motion. Some cognitive control over the braking mechanism exists.

This research supports the use of rapid, alternating movements, moving quickly through a short distance. Large-amplitude movement does not produce the same muscular coactivation as small-amplitude movement.

Precautions and Contraindications

An important precaution when treating areas of hypermobility is to ensure that areas of relative flexibility are identified. Stretching techniques to improve mobility in a hypomobile area may increase hypermobility in an adjacent area. The clinician must reinforce correct dynamic stabilization to ensure that intervention is isolated to the correct segment. For example, failure to stabilize the pelvis during hip flexor stretching increases lumbar extension, potentially increasing hypermobility in this area.

Any time dynamic stabilization activities are being performed at the limits of stability (eg, resisted shoulder rotation at 90 degrees abduction and full external rotation in a hypermobile shoulder), the clinician must be sure that the

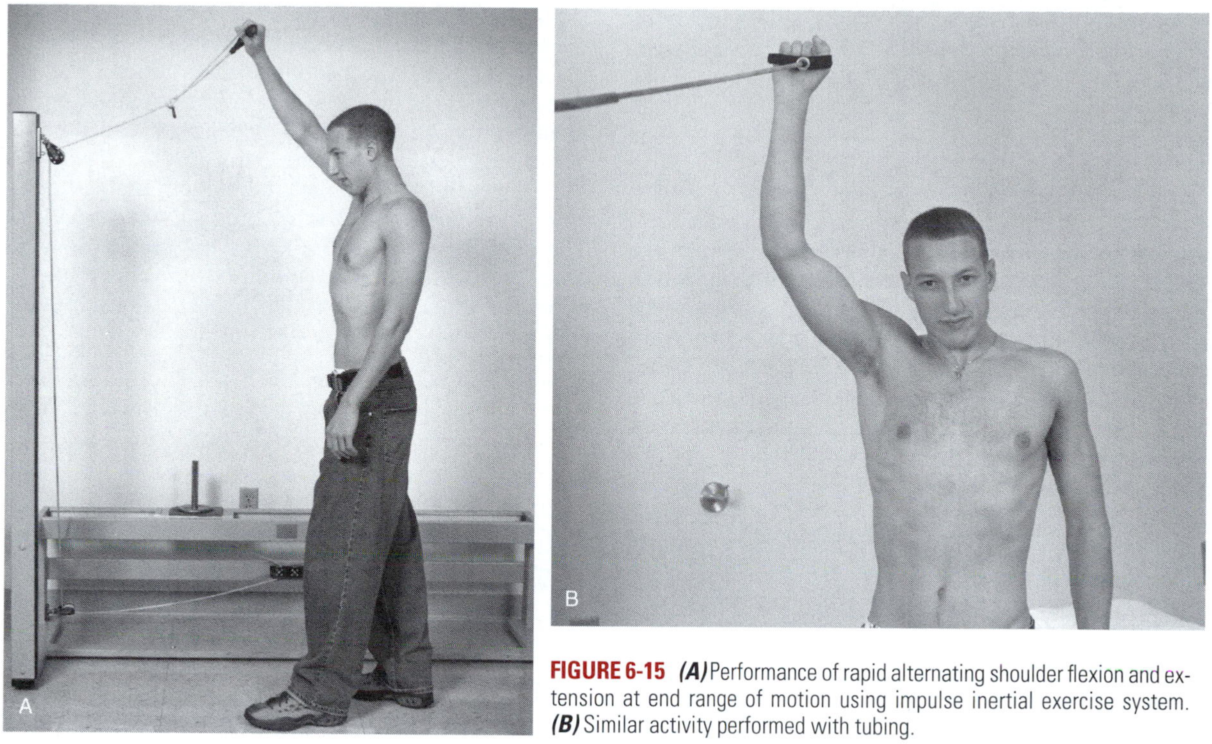

FIGURE 6-15 ***(A)*** Performance of rapid alternating shoulder flexion and extension at end range of motion using impulse inertial exercise system. ***(B)*** Similar activity performed with tubing.

individual has adequate control to prevent instability or dislocation. Activities must be progressed according to the patient's ability to control the limits of stability. Fatigue of dynamic stabilizing musculature places the patient at risk for injury, and the fatigue level should be monitored throughout the exercise session.

ADJUNCTIVE AGENTS

Clinicians often use various treatments or techniques to enhance the effects of another treatment. Forms of tissue heating are the most common adjunctive agents used in combination with ROM exercises to increase mobility. The ability of collagen to be easily and safely deformed or stretched is enhanced by increasing the temperature of the collagen. Because muscle is primarily composed of collagen, the ability of the muscle to be stretched may be enhanced by increasing the temperature of the muscle.[63] The critical temperature for beneficial effects appears to be approximately 39°C or 103°F.[47,67,68,83,84]

Intramuscular temperature may be increased by heating modalities or through exercise. The therapeutic temperature required may be efficiently achieved for the time necessary to complete a flexibility program using a deep-heating modality such as ultrasound.[20,70] Physiologically, the easiest and most appropriate way to increase intramuscular temperature is through the use of exercise. Active, submaximal resistive exercise of the muscle groups to be stretched should be performed before stretching. This type of exercise is capable of producing temperature increases to approximately 39°C after 10 to 15 minutes.

Heating techniques may prepare the tissue for mobility activities by increasing the tissue temperature, promoting relaxation and pain reduction, and increasing the local circulation. Forms of heat other than exercise can be categorized broadly as superficial-heating and deep-heating agents. Although heat can increase local circulation and temperature, it is not a substitute for warm-up exercises before a planned activity. A warm-up exercise such as walking, bicycling, upper body ergometry, or active ROM exercise should take place before any therapeutic ROM activities. This approach increases core temperature and prepares surrounding tissues for the forthcoming activity.

Superficial Heat

The most common superficial heating agents include hot packs, paraffin, and warm whirlpools. These agents primarily increase skin temperature, with little penetration of heat to deeper tissues. Skin temperature increases are the greatest within the first 0.5 cm from the surface, with some increase in muscle temperature at 1 to 2 cm and less heating at 3 cm.[60] To achieve temperature elevations at increasing depths, a treatment time of 15 to 30 minutes is necessary.[60] The depth of penetration is significantly affected by the tissue composition. Areas with less soft tissue heat deeper than areas with greater subcutaneous fat. For example, superficial heat applied to the hands can increase tissue temperature to the joint, but heat applied to the thigh has only shallow penetration.

Hot packs are frequently used over larger surface areas such as the low back, thigh, and knee. Smaller areas such as the hand are more amenable to warm paraffin. The patient usually sits quietly while the treatment is applied. This produces relaxation but may leave the individual unprepared for vigorous exercise. In contrast, a warm whirlpool can provide superficial heating while simultaneously allowing exercise to be performed. Active, passive, or resistive ROM exercises can be performed while in a warm whirlpool, thereby extending the benefits of this heating modality.

Deep Heat

Ultrasound is the most common form of deep heat used in the clinic. The effects of ultrasound are mechanical and thermal, although in this context, the thermal effects are emphasized. The specific effects and depth of penetration are affected by the tissue type, the ultrasound wavelength or frequency, and the intensity and type of wave (ie, continuous or pulsed). Ultrasound has the ability to elevate tissue temperatures to depths of 5 cm or more.[60] The temperature elevation in tissue has been associated with increases in collagen extensibility, changes in nerve conduction velocity, and increases in the pain threshold. Ultrasound intensities necessary to achieve tissue temperatures to a range of 40°C to 45°C range from 1.0 to 2.0 W/cm^2 delivered continuously for 5 to 10 minutes.[60]

Superficial heat such as a hot pack commonly is used in combination with ultrasound to enhance the effects of treatment. The hot pack promotes relaxation and therefore increases the patient's tolerance for stretching, and the deep heat produces changes in the collagen elasticity, preparing it for subsequent stretching.

If extensibility gains are to be maintained after the heat and stretching session, stretching should be performed as the muscle cools to its preheated temperature. Ideally, this new length should be maintained for an extended period after the therapy session. This can be done by the use of splints or continuous passive motion devices.

Key Points

- The effects of immobilization on the injured and uninjured soft tissues are profound. All tissues are affected, including insertion sites and bone.

LAB ACTIVITIES

Perform the following activities with your partner. Not all positions are optimal for performing each of the exercises, but the clinician occasionally is unable to change the patient's position. If not the optimal position, which position would be better and why?

1. With your patient in supine, perform the following:
   a. Passive ROM shoulder flexion
   b. Active assisted ROM shoulder abduction
   c. Passive ROM shoulder internal and external rotation
   d. Contract-relax stretching for pectoralis major
   e. Passive ROM hip and knee flexion
   f. Contract-relax-contract stretching of the hamstring muscles
   g. Passive ROM lumbar flexion
   h. Passive ROM lumbar rotation
2. With your patient sitting, perform the following:
   a. Passive ROM hip internal and external rotation
   b. Active assisted ROM knee extension
   c. Contract-relax stretching hip internal rotator muscles
   d. Active assisted ROM shoulder flexion
   e. Active ROM shoulder abduction
3. With your patient in a sidelying position, perform the following:
   a. Passive ROM shoulder extension
   b. Active assisted ROM shoulder abduction
   c. Contract-relax stretching shoulder internal rotator muscles
   d. Active ROM shoulder flexion
4. With your patient in a prone position, perform the following:
   a. Active assisted ROM elbow extension
   b. Passive ROM hip internal and external rotation
   c. AROM shoulder flexion
   d. Contract-relax stretching hip flexors
   e. Contract-relax-contract stretching for gastrocnemius
   f. Contract-relax-contract stretching for soleus
5. Decide how to best position your patient for the following:
   a. Active ROM shoulder external rotation in a gravity minimized position
   b. Active ROM scapular elevation
   c. Active ROM wrist extension in a gravity-minimized position
   d. Contract-relax stretching of hip adductor muscles
   e. Active ROM shoulder abduction in a gravity-minimized position
   f. Passive ROM cervical rotation
   g. Static stretching of the triceps muscle
6. Choose five of the previous exercises, and write a description of those exercises for a patient in a home exercise program. Include a picture of the exercise.
7. Consider Case Study #6 from Unit 7. Instruct your patient in the first phase of his exercise program. Explain and demonstrate.
8. The clinician is treating a postal worker with rotator cuff tendinitis resulting from hypermobility. This man sorts mail all day at eye level. The rotator cuff tendinitis has resolved with intervention. Instruct this patient in an exercise program to treat the instability. Explain and demonstrate.
9. Instruct a patient in a self-stretching program for the quadriceps, hamstrings, and iliotibial band. Explain and demonstrate three different stretches for each muscle group.

- These effects are the result of the SAID principle; tissue responds to loads placed on them. When underloaded, the tissue weakens.
- The period needed to restore normal structural and mechanical properties to immobilized tissue can be two or more times the immobilization period.
- Joint ROM should be differentiated from muscle ROM. The specific goal dictates the type of mobility activity prescribed.
- A variety of contractile and noncontractile tissues can limit mobility at a joint.
- Passive ROM exercise is a mobility activity performed without muscle contraction. Active assisted ROM is a mobility activity in which some muscle activity takes place, and active ROM exercise uses active muscle contraction to perform the exercise.
- To increase flexibility, static, ballistic, and PNF stretching techniques can be used. The type of stretch chosen depends on the individual's impairments and lifestyle.
- Pulleys, machines, the pool, or objects found in the home or office can be used to perform mobility exercises.
- Mobility exercise prescription depends on the specific goal of the activity and the environment in which it will be performed.
- Hypermobility can be as disabling as hypomobility. Stabilization exercises such as closed-chain and rapidly alternating movements may be incorporated.
- Adjunctive agents such as heat can be used to enhance mobility activities.

Critical Thinking Questions

1. Consider Case Study #2 in Unit 7.
   a. How would you maintain this patient's cardiovascular status while recovering from knee surgery?
   b. Would your treatment differ if she had no other medical complications?
2. Consider Case Study #4 in Unit 7.
   a. How would your treatment differ if the patient was an elderly woman with severe osteoporosis?
   b. How would your treatment differ if the patient was 25 years of age and the joint accessory motion testing result indicated hypermobility?

REFERENCES

1. Akeson WH, Amiel D, Abel MF, Garfin SR, Woo SL-Y. Effects of immobilization on joints. *Clin Orthop*. 1987;219:28–37.
2. Amiel D, von Schroeder H, Akeson WH. The response of ligaments to stress deprivation and stress enhancement: biochemical studies. In: Daniel DD, Akeson WH, O'Conner JJ, eds. *Knee Ligaments: Structure, Function, Injury and Repair*. New York: Raven Press; 1990.
3. Amiel D, Woo SL-Y, Harwood FL, Akeson WH. The effect of immobilization on collagen turnover in connective tissue: a biochemical-biomechanical correlation. *Acta Orthop Scand*. 1982;53:325–332.
4. Andriacchi T, Sabiston P, DeHaven K, et al. Ligament: injury and repair. In: Woo SL-Y, Buckwalter JA, eds. *Injury and Repair of the Musculoskeletal Soft Tissues*. Park Ridge, IL: American Academy of Orthopaedic Surgeons; 1988.
5. Appell HJ. Muscular atrophy following immobilisation: a review. *Sports Med*. 1990;10:42–58.
6. Arnoszky S. *Structure and Function of Articular Cartilage*. Presented at the American Physical Therapy Association Annual Conference; June 12–16, 1993; Cincinnati, OH.
7. Bailey DA, McCulloch RG. Bone tissue and physical activity. *Can J Sport Sci*. 1990;15:229–239.
8. Bandy WD, Irion JM. The effect of time of static stretch on the flexibility of the hamstring muscles. *Phys Ther* 1994; 74:845–852.
9. Behrens F, Kraft EL, Oegema TR Jr. Biochemical changes in articular cartilage after joint immobilization by casting or external fixation. *J Orthop Res*. 1989;7:335–343.
10. Beynnon BD, Fleming BC, Johnson RJ, et al. Anterior cruciate ligament strain behavior during rehabilitation exercises in vivo. *Am J Sports Med*. 1995;23:24–33.
11. Buckwalter JA. Mechanical injuries of articular cartilage. In: Finerman GA, Noyes FR, eds. *Biology and Biomechanics of the Traumatized Synovial Joint: The Knee as Model*. Rosemont, IL: American Academy of Orthopaedic Surgeons; 1992.
12. Burr DB, Frederickson RG, Pavlinch C, Sickles M, Burkart S. Intracast muscle stimulation prevents bone and cartilage deterioration in cast-immobilized rabbits. *Clin Orthop*. 1984; 189:264–278.
13. Condon SA, Hutton RS. Soleus muscle EMG activity and ankle dorsiflexion range of motion from stretching procedures. *Phys Ther*. 1987;67:24–30.
14. Cornelius W, Jackson A. The effects of cryotherapy and PNF on hip extensor flexibility. *J Athletic Training*. 1984; 19:183–184.
15. Dahners LE. Ligament contraction: a correlation with cellularity and actin staining. *Trans Orthop Res Soc*. 1986;11:56–66.
16. deVries HA. Prevention of muscular distress after exercise. *Res Q*. 1961;32:177–185.
17. deVries HA. Evaluation of static stretching procedures for improvement of flexibility. *Res Q*. 1962;33:222–229.
18. deVries HA. The "looseness" factor in speed and oxygen consumption of an anaerobic 100 yard dash. *Res Q*. 1963; 34: 305–313.
19. *Dorland's Illustrated Medical Dictionary*. 26th ed. Philadelphia: WB Saunders; 1981.
20. Draper DO, Ricard MD. Rate of temperature decay in human muscle following 3 MHz ultrasound: the stretching window revealed. *J Athletic Training*. 1996;30:304–307.
21. Entyre BR, Abraham LD. Antagonist muscle activity during stretching: a paradox reassessed. *Med Sci Sports Exerc*. 1988; 20:285–289.
22. Entyre BR, Abraham LD. Ache-reflex changes during static stretching and two variations of proprioceptive neuromuscular facilitation techniques. *Electroencephalogr Clin Neurophysiol*. 1986;63:174–179.
23. Entyre BR, Lee EJ. Chronic and acute flexibility of men and women using three different stretching techniques. *Res Q*. 1988;222:228.
24. Enwemeka CS, Spielholtz NI, Nelson AJ. The effects of early functional activities on experimentally tenotomized Achilles tendons in rats. *Am J Phys Med Rehabil*. 1988;67:264–269.
25. Enwemeka CS. Connective tissue plasticity: ultrastructural, biomechanical and morphometric effects of physical factors on intact and regenerating tendons. *J Orthop Sports Phys Ther*. 1991;14:198–212.
26. Evans EB, Eggers GWN, Butler JK, Blumel J. Experimental immobilization and remobilization of rat knee joint. *J Bone Joint Surg Am*. 1960;42:737–758.

27. Frank C, Akeson WH, Woo SL-Y, Amiel D, Coutts RD. Physiology and therapeutic value of passive joint motion. *Clin Orthop.* 1984;185:113–125.
28. Gajdosik RL, Bohannon RW. Clinical measurement of range of motion. *Phys Ther.* 1987;67:1867–1872.
29. Garrett W, Tidball J. Myotendinous junction: structure, function, and failure. In: Woo SL-Y, Buckwalter JA, eds. *Injury and Repair of the Musculoskeletal Soft Tissues.* Park Ridge, IL: American Academy of Orthopaedic Surgeons; 1988.
30. Gelberman RH, Vande Berg JS, Lundborg GN, et al. Flexor tendon healing and restoration of the gliding surface: an ultrastructural study in dogs. *J Bone Joint Surg Am.* 1983;65:70–80.
31. Gelberman RH, Woo SL-Y, Lothringer K, et al. Effects of early intermittent passive mobilization on healing canine flexor tendons. *J Hand Surg.* 1982;7:170–175.
32. Gelberman RH, Botte MJ, Spiegelman JJ, et al. The excursion and deformation of repaired flexor tendons treated with protected early motion. *J Hand Surg Am.* 1983;11:106–110.
33. Gelberman RH, Goldberg V, Kai-Nan A, Banes. Tendon. In: Woo SL-Y, Buckwalter JA, eds. *Injury and Repair of the Musculoskeletal Soft Tissues.* Park Ridge, IL: American Academy of Orthopaedic Surgeons; 1988.
34. Graham VL, Gehlsen GM, Edwards JA. Electromyographic evaluation of close and open kinetic chain knee rehabilitation exercises. *J Athletic Training.* 1993;28:23–31.
35. Gryzlo SM, Patek RM, Pink M, Perry M. Electromyographic analysis of knee rehabilitation exercises. *J Orthop Sports Phys Ther.* 1994;20:36–43.
36. Hagbarth KE, Hagglund JV, Nordin M, Wallin EU. Thixotropic behaviour of human finger flexor muscles with accompanying changes in spindle and reflex responses to stretch. *J Physiol.* 1985:368:323–342.
37. Haggmark T, Eriksson E. Cylinder or mobile cast brace after knee ligament surgery: a clinical analysis and morphological and enzymatic study of changes in the quadriceps muscle. *Am J Sports Med.* 1979;7:48–56.
38. Hakkinen K, Komi PV. Electromyographic changes during strength training and detraining. *Med Sci Sports Exerc.* 1983; 15:455–460.
39. Hutton RS. Neuromuscular basis of stretching exercises. In: Komi PV, ed. *Strength and Power in Sports.* Boston: Blackwell Scientific; 1992:29–38.
40. Jozsa L, Jarvinen M, Kannus P, Reffy A. Fine structural changes in the articular cartilage of the rat's knee following short-term immobilisation in various positions. *Int Orthop.* 1987;11:129–133.
41. Kannus P, Jozsa L, Renstrom P, Jarvinen M, et al. The effects of training, immobilization and remobilization on musculoskeletal tissue. I. Training and immobilization. *Scand J Med Sci Sports.* 1992;2:100–118.
42. Kannus P, Jozsa L, Renstrom P, et al. The effects of training, immobilization and remobilization on musculoskeletal tissue. II. Remobilization and prevention of immobilization atrophy. *Scand J Med Sci Sports.* 1992;2:164–176.
43. Karpakka J, Vaananen K, Virtanen P, et al. The effects of remobilization and exercise on collagen biosynthesis in rat tendon. *Acta Physiol Scand.* 1990;139:139–145.
44. Kiviranta I, Jurvelin J, Tammi M, et al. Weight bearing controls glycosaminoglycan concentration and articular cartilage thickness in the knee joints of young beagle dogs. *Arthritis Rheum.* 1987;30:801–809.
45. Laros GS, Tipton CM, Cooper RR. Influence of physical activity on ligament insertions in the knees of dogs. *J Bone Joint Surg Am.* 1971;53:275–286.
46. Larsen NP, Forwood MR, Parker AW. Immobilization and retraining of cruciate ligaments in the rat. *Acta Orthop Scand.* 1987;58:260–264.
47. Lehmann JF, Masock AJ, Warren CG, et al. Effect of therapeutic temperatures on tendon extensibility. *Arch Phys Med Rehabil.* 1970;51:481–487.
48. Lentell G, Hetherington T, Eagan J, et al. The use of thermal agents to influence the effectiveness of a low-load prolonged stretch. *J Orthop Sports Phys Ther.* 1992;5:200–207.
49. Lestienne F. Effects of inertial load and velocity on the braking process of voluntary limb movements. *Exp Brain Res.* 1979;35:407–418.
50. Lieber RL, McKee-Woodburn T, Friden J, Gershuni DH. Recovery of the dog quadriceps after ten weeks of immobilization followed by four weeks of remobilization. *J Orthop Res.* 1989;7:408–412.
51. Lieber RL. *Skeletal Muscle Structure and Function.* Baltimore: Williams & Wilkins; 1992.
52. Loitz BL, Frank CB. Biology and mechanics of ligament and ligament healing. *Exerc Sports Sci Rev.* 1993;21:33–64.
53. Loudon KL, Bolier CE, Allison KA, et al. Effects of two stretching methods on the flexibility and retention of flexibility at the ankle joint in runners. *Phys Ther.* 1985;65:698.
54. Madding SW, Wong JG, Hallum A, et al. Effects of duration of passive stretching on hip abduction range of motion. *J Orthop Sports Phys Ther.* 1987;8:409–416.
55. Magee D. *Orthopedic Physical Assessment.* 2nd ed. Philadelphia: WB Saunders; 1992.
56. Maitland GD. *Vertebral Manipulation.* 5th ed. Boston: Butterworth; 1986.
57. Markos PK. Ipsilateral and contralateral effects of proprioceptive neuromuscular facilitation techniques on hip motion and electromyographic activity. *Phys Ther.* 1979;59:1366–1373.
58. Marsden CD, Obeso JA, Rothwell JC. The function of the antagonist muscle during fast limb movements in man. *J Physiol.* 1983;335:1–13.
59. Mazess RB, Whedon GD. Immobilization and bone. *Calcif Tissue Int.* 1983;35:265–267.
60. Michlovitz S, ed. *Thermal Agents in Rehabilitation.* 2nd ed. Philadelphia: FA Davis; 1990.
61. Minaire P. Immobilization osteoporosis: a review. *Rheumatology.* 1989;8(suppl):95–103.
62. Moore M, Hutton R. Electromyographic investigation of muscle stretching techniques. *Med Sci Sports Exerc.* 1980; 12:322–329.
63. Nishiyama S, Kuwahara T, Matsuda I. Decreased bone density in severely handicapped children and adults with reference to influence of limited mobility and anticonvulsant medication. *Eur J Pediatr.* 1986;144:457–463.
64. Noyes FR, DeLucas JL, Torvik PJ. Biomechanics of anterior cruciate ligament failure: an analysis of strain-rate sensitivity and mechanisms of failure in primates. *J Bone Joint Surg Am.* 1974;56:236–253.
65. Noyes FR. Functional properties of knee ligaments and alterations induced by immobilization. *Clin Orthop Relat Res.* 1977;123:210–242.
66. Prentice WE. A comparison of static stretching and PNF stretching for improving hip joint flexibility. *J Athletic Training.* 1983;18:56–59.
67. Rigby JF, Hirai N, Spikes JD, et al. The mechanical properties of rat tail tendon. *J Gen Physiol.* 1959;43:265–283.
68. Rigby JF. The effect of mechanical extension upon the thermal stability of collagen. *Biochem Biophys Acta.* 1964;79:334–363.
69. Robinson R. The new back school prescription: stabilization training, part I. *Occup Med.* 1992;7:17–27.
70. Rose S, Draper DO, Schulties SS, et al. The stretching window part two: rate of thermal decay in deep muscle following 1-MHz ultrasound. *J Athletic Training.* 1996;31:139–143.
71. Sady SP, Wortman M, Blanke D. Flexibility training: Ballistic, static or proprioceptive neuromuscular facilitation? *Arch Phys Med Rehabil.* 1982;63:261–263.

72. Schoutens A, Laurent E, Poortmans JR. Effects of inactivity and exercise on bone. *Sports Med.* 1989;7:71–81.
73. Shindo M, Harayama H, Kondo K, et al. Changes in reciprocal Ia inhibition during voluntary contraction in man. *Exp Brain Res*. 1984;53:400–408.
74. Tammi M, Saamanen A-M, Jauhiainen A, Malminen O, Kiviranta I, Helminen H. Proteoglycan alterations in rabbit knee articular cartilage following physical exercise and immobilization. *Connect Tissue Res*. 1983;11:45–55.
75. Tanigawa MC. Comparison of the hold relax procedure and passive mobilization of increasing muscle length. *Phys Ther*. 1972;52:725–735.
76. Tardieu C, Tabary J-C, Tabary C, et al. Adaptation of connective tissue length to immobilization in the lengthened and shortened positions in cat soleus muscle. *J Physiol*. 1982; 8:214–220.
77. Tillman LJ, Cummings GS. Biologic mechanisms of connective tissue mutability. In: Currier DP, Nelson RM, ed. *Dynamics of Human Biologic Tissues*. Philadelphia: FA Davis; 1992.
78. Tipton CM, Vailas AC, Matthes RD. Experimental studies on the influences of physical activity on ligaments, tendons and joints: a brief review. *Acta Med Scand Suppl*. 1986; 711:157–168.
79. Troyer H. The effect of short-term immobilization on the rabbit knee joint cartilage. *Clin Orthop*. 1975;107:249–257.
80. Videman T. Connective tissue and immobilization. *Clin Orthop*. 1987;221:26–32.
81. Voss DE, Ionta MK, Myers GJ. *Proprioceptive Neuromuscular Facilitation: Patterns and Techniques.* 3rd ed. Philadelphia: JB Lippincott; 1985.
82. Wallin D, Ekblom B, Grahm R, et al. Improvement of muscle flexibility: a comparison between two techniques. *Am J Sports Med*. 1985;13:263–268.
83. Warren CG, Lehmann JF, Koblanski JM, et al. Elongation of rat tail tendon: effect of load and temperature. *Arch Phys Med Rehabil*. 1971;52:465–474.
84. Warren CG, Lehmann JF, Koblanski JM, et al. Heat and stretch procedures: an evaluation using rat tail tendon. *Phys Med Rehabil*. 1976;57:122–126.
85. Whedon GS. Disuse osteoporosis: physiological aspects. *Calcif Tissue Int*. 1984;36S:146–150.
86. Wierzbicka MM, Wiegner AW, Shahani BT. The role of agonist and antagonist in fast arm movements in man. *Exp Brain Res.* 1986;63:331-340.
87. Williams PE, Golkspink G. Changes in sarcomere length and physiological properties in immobilized muscle. *J Anat*. 1978: 127:459–468.
88. Williams PE, Goldspink G. Connective tissue changes in immobilised muscle. *J Anat*. 1984;138:343–350.
89. Woo SL-Y, Gomez MA, Sites TJ, et al. The biomechanical and morphological changes in the medial collateral ligament of the rabbit after immobilization and remobilization. *J Bone Joint Surg Am*. 1987;69:1200–1211.
90. Woo SL-Y, Inoue M, McGurk-Burleson E, et al. Treatment of the medial collateral ligament injury: II. Structure and function of canine knees in response to differing treatment regimens. *Am J Sports Med*. 1987;15:22–29.
91. Woo SL-Y, Maynard J, Butler D, et al. Ligament, tendon and joint capsule insertions into bone. In: Woo SL-Y, Buckwalter JA, eds. *Injury and Repair of the Musculoskeletal Soft Tissues*. Park Ridge, IL: American Academy of Orthopaedic Surgeons; 1988.
92. Yack HJ, Collins CE, Whieldon TJ. Comparison of closed and open kinetic chain exercise in the anterior cruciate ligament-deficient knee. *Am J Sports Med*. 1993;21:49–54.
93. Zachazewski JE. Flexibility for sport. In: Sanders B, ed. *Sports Physical Therapy*. Norwalk, CT: Appleton & Lange; 1990.
94. Zachazewski JE. Improving flexibility. In: Scully RM, Barnes MR, eds. *Physical Therapy*. Philadelphia: J. B. Lippincott; 1989.
95. Zebas CJ, Rivera ML. Retention of flexibility in selected joints after cessation of a stretching exercise program. In: Dotson CO, Humphrey JH, eds.: *Exercise Physiology: Current Selected Research Topics.* New York: AMS Press; 1985.

CHAPTER 7

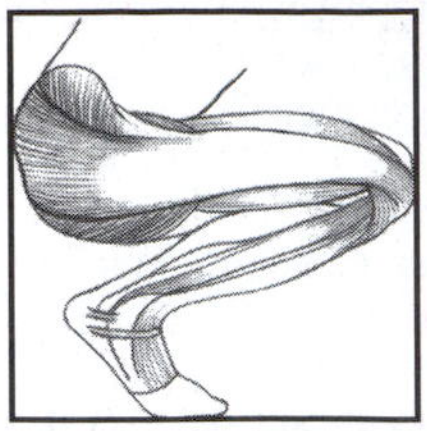

Balance Impairment

Lori Thein Brody

Clinicians recognize the importance of balance in the rehabilitation of patients with a variety of disorders, and balance training is increasingly being integrated into clinical practice.[1–4] Despite the increased clinical application of this training, the definitions of many terms remain unclear. When impaired mobility or muscle performance cannot account for an individual's disability after an injury or surgery, the disability is sometimes attributed to a "lack of proprioception." Neurologic specialists may describe uncoordinated movement in a patient after head injury or stroke. Orthopedic and neurologic clinicians describe increased postural sway and poor balance in elderly patients or patients with osteoarthritis. Sports specialists report that elite athletes lack proprioception or kinesthesia, resulting in injury. Are all of these persons talking about the same thing?

DEFINITIONS

Coordination is the ability to perform smooth, accurate, and controlled movements.[5,6] Coordination is necessary for the execution of fine motor skills such as writing, sewing, dressing, and the manipulation of small objects. Coordination is also necessary when performing gross motor skills such as walking, running, jumping, occupational tasks, and basic and instrumental activities of daily living. Coordinated movements involve proper sequencing and timing of synergistic and reciprocal muscle activity, and they require proximal stability and maintenance of a posture.[5]

The concept of coordination includes balance. *Balance* is the ability to maintain equilibrium or the ability to maintain the center of gravity (COG) over the base of support (BOS).[6] Balance requires the ability to maintain a position, to stabilize during voluntary activities, and to react to external perturbations.[7,8] Despite the simplicity of this definition, the ability to maintain balance involves effective and efficient coordination among multiple sensory, biomechanical, and motor systems. Vestibular dysfunction, visual impairment, or diminished proprioception can impair balance.

Treatment of balance impairment requires a detailed examination to determine the system at fault. *Postural sway* is the normal, continuous shifting of the body's COG over the BOS. When a person is able to keep sway within the *limits of stability*, balance is maintained. When sway exceeds these limits, a corrective strategy is necessary to prevent falling.[9]

BALANCE IN A NORMAL SYSTEM

Identifying causes of and prescribing treatment for balance impairment requires an understanding of the systems engaged in balance control and their normal interactions. These systems provide input into the central nervous system. The information must be processed and an appropriate motor strategy chosen and executed. The systems model of motor control defines postural stability as the ability to maintain the COG within stability limits (ie, boundaries of space).[9,10] These limits are the spatial area in which the individual can maintain equilibrium without changing her BOS. A certain amount of anteroposterior and lateral sway occur while maintaining balance. This sway envelope defines the limits of stability in anterior, posterior, and lateral directions. Normal anteroposterior sway in adults is 12 degrees from the most posterior to the most anterior position.[11] Lateral stability limits vary with foot spacing and height. An average-height adult with 4 inches between the feet can sway approximately 16 degrees from side to side.[11] This stability limit is often characterized by a cone of stability (Fig. 7-1*A* and *B*). As long as the individual's sway envelope stays within the limits of stability, balance is maintained. When the COG is aligned in the middle of the sway envelope, the 12 degrees of anteroposterior sway and 16 degrees of lateral sway can easily occur. If sway exceeds these limits, some strategy must be employed to regain balance. If an individual's COG is aligned more anterior, posterior, or lateral than center, a smaller sway envelop is tolerated before losing balance (see Fig. 7-1*C*).[11]

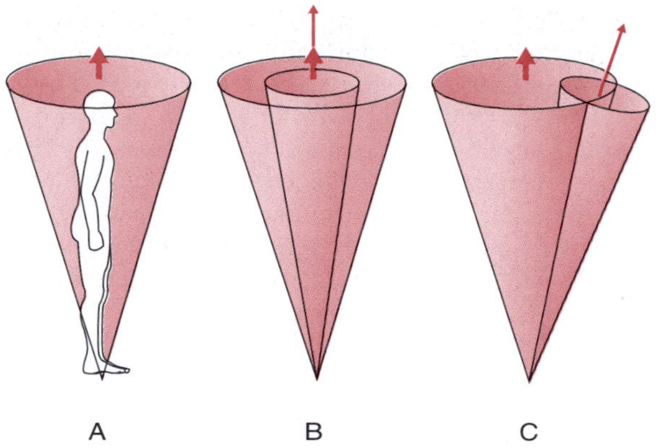

FIGURE 7-1 Relationships of the limits of stability, the sway envelope, and the center of gravity (COG) alignment. ***(A)*** The limits of stability are described by a cone-shaped sway envelope. ***(B)*** When the COG is aligned in the center, the sway envelope remains within the limits of stability. ***(C)*** When the COG is offset, as in a forward leaning posture, the sway envelope exceeds the limits of stability, and a balance restoration strategy must be implemented to regain balance.

Contributions of Sensory Systems

Three sensory systems contribute to the maintenance of upright posture: visual, vestibular, and somatosensory (ie, proprioceptive). They are considered to be the sensory triad of postural control (Fig. 7-2). The systems model suggests interactions among the individual, the environment, and the functional task, with a circular network of subsystems interacting to maintain stability and produce movement.[6] Any of these systems may dominate, and all are context dependent. No single sense directly determines the position of the body's COG; the combined feedback from each system must be integrated. The visual and somatosensory systems gather information from the environment (eg, position relative to other objects, stability of the surface), and the vestibular system provides an internal reference, providing information about the head's orientation in space.[12]

SOMATOSENSORY NEUROPHYSIOLOGY

The somatosensory system contributes to balance by providing information about the relative location of body parts. The term proprioception reflects the static position, and kinesthesia refers to the positions during movement. For example, when a person steps onto a rug that slips beneath her foot, the acceleration of the slipping limb provides the first information to the system.

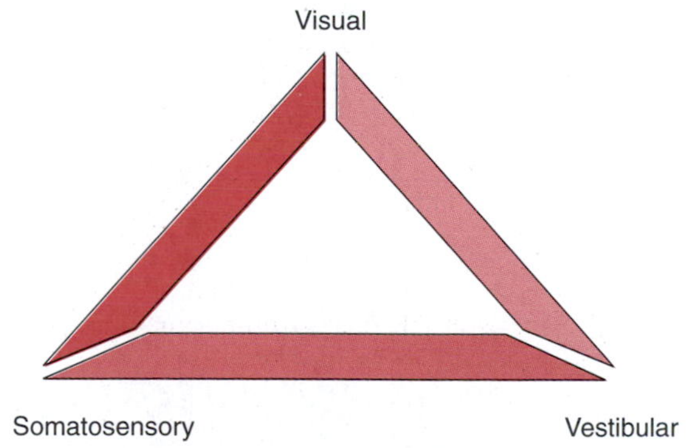

FIGURE 7-2 The triad of balance control.

Information from the somatosensory system arises from peripheral sources such as the muscle, joint capsule, and other soft tissue structures. In the joint capsule, free nerve endings, Ruffini endings, and paciniform corpuscles are found. Ruffini endings are encapsulated endings that respond to passive and active movement.[13] These slowly adapting endings are angle specific and fire continuously as long as the joint is held at a specific angle. Paciniform corpuscles signal joint movement, but they give little information about the final joint position.[13] They are rapidly adapting structures with a low threshold to mechanical stress. These receptors are activated primarily by acceleration and deceleration. The Golgi-Mazzoni corpuscles are slow-adapting receptors, sensitive to joint capsule compression in a plane perpendicular to its surface. The Golgi ligament endings are also slow-adapting receptors that are sensitive to ligament tension or stretch. Free nerve endings are the articular nociceptive system, and they are activated by mechanical deformation or chemical irritation.[14]

Information from these receptors is relayed to the medulla and brain stem through the dorsal column medial-lemniscal pathway.[13] This information assists in coordinating eye, head, and neck movements to stabilize the visual system and in maintaining postures and coordinated movement patterns.[14] Joint afferent information does not contribute to a conscious sense of position.[14,15] This conclusion is based on studies in which local anesthetization of joint tissues failed to reduce joint position awareness and total joint replacement did not diminish joint position sense.[16]

The gamma system may be better suited than the alpha system for delivery of complex information needed for the regulation of movement. The gamma system regulates stiffness in the muscles supporting the joint. By maintaining muscle tone, appropriate posture, and stiffness in the muscles, adjustments in preparation for movement can be made. The joint receptors contribute to the regulation of muscle tone, posture, and stiffness of the muscles around the joint. Stretching the knee ligaments (thereby stimulating joint receptors) increases the firing frequency of primary spindle afferents. The gamma motor system is aided by the joint afferent system and provides position sense and preparatory muscle stiffness adjustments. The joint afferent information assists the muscle spindle afferent fibers during unexpected postural perturbations. The muscle spindle fibers appear best suited for providing joint position sense, and the role of joint afferents may be regulation of muscle stiffness, rather than functioning as mechanical restraints or detectors of motion limits. Intrinsic muscle stiffness is always present and may be the first line of defense against perturbations.

The somatosensory system plays an important role in regulating posture. Information must be detected peripherally and transmitted centrally for processing. The peripheral receptors are an important source of that information.

VISUAL AND VESTIBULAR NEUROPHYSIOLOGY

The visual and vestibular systems contribute significant information about the body's position and movement in space. The visual system provides information about the position of the head relative to the environment and orients the head to maintain level gaze. This system contributes significantly to head and neck posture. The visual system also provides information about the movement of surrounding objects, thereby providing information about the speed of movement. Information entering the visual system travels through the optic nerve to the lateral geniculate nucleus (LGN) of the thalamus to the superior colliculus and through a few fibers to the inferior olivary nuclei. The LGN receives the largest projection and is the first center where information from the retina is represented.[17] From here, neurons project to the primary visual cortex in the occipital lobe (Brodmann's area 17).

The vestibular system provides information on orientation of the head in space and on acceleration. Any movements of the head, including weight shifts to adjust posture, stimulate the vestibular receptors. The vestibular nerve projects to the vestibular nuclei and to the cerebellum. The vestibular nuclei also receive input from other sensory systems, including the visual system. From the vestibular nuclei, two vestibulospinal tracts descend to the spinal cord for postural control.[17] Ascending projections include fibers to control eye movements and fibers to the thalamus. From the thalamus, projections ascend to the head of the caudate nucleus and to the parietal association area, where the information is integrated with other sensory information.

Processing Sensory Information

After information arrives from peripheral receptors, the information must be analyzed. The relative contributions from each system and integration of each system's information are critical. Integration and processing of incoming information occurs in the cerebellum, basal ganglia, and supplementary motor area.[18] The time required to process this information is important, particularly when a quick response is necessary. Generally, the somatosensory system information is processed fastest, followed by the visual and vestibular systems.[18]

Sensory organization is the process of resolving conflicting input; it is necessary because incoming information from a system may be inaccurate. For example, consider sitting stationary on a train in a station when an adjacent train begins moving forward. The visual input is unable to detect whether that train is moving forward or your train is moving backward. The brain must resolve inaccurate input from the visual system with the accurate information from the somatosensory and vestibular systems. Information from the visual system (eg, moving visual fields) and the somatosensory system (eg, moving sidewalks, compliant surfaces) is susceptible to error. If an injury decreases the information processing rate, balance may be impaired. Other systems may adequately compensate for impairments in one system, and this concept is the basis for many treatment programs.

Generating Motor Output

After the sensory information is transmitted centrally, the information is processed, and a response is selected, the response output must be executed. This response programming is influenced by the movement and is the stage most often manipulated in treatment.[19] Complex movements take longer to process and program than simple tasks. Although a multitude of postural responses are available when someone is destabilized, three automatic responses are common. These preprogrammed synergies are the fundamental movement unit engaged when balance is disturbed.[6,9] Rather than determining which muscles to activate and when, the brain only needs to know which synergy to engage, when to engage it, and at what intensity to respond. This is an example of feedforward control, or open loop control. In feedforward control, movement occurs too fast to rely on sensory feedback. Responses are preprogrammed and automatic. In contrast, feedback control, or closed loop control, movement relies on feedback. It is used to learn precision movements. Treatment procedures focus on these preprogrammed synergies to maintain postural control.

Three fundamental movement strategies to maintain equilibrium have been identified: the ankle strategy, the hip strategy, and the stepping strategy.[20] These strategies depend on the intensity of the disruption, the subject's awareness, and the subject's posture at the time of perturbation. The ankle strategy is the most commonly used, particularly when displacements are small. The ankle synergy displaces the COG primarily by rotation about the ankle joint (Fig. 7-3). Posterior displacement of the COG results in dorsiflexion at the ankle, with activation of the gastrocnemius, hamstring, and trunk extensors to slow the backward movement. Anterior displacement of the COG produces plantar flexion, with contraction of the anterior tibialis, quadriceps, and abdominals to control the forward movement. Muscle activation proceeds in a distal to proximal direction.

The hip strategy is employed when ankle motion is limited, when the displacement is greater, or when standing on an unstable surface so that the ankle strategy is not effective. In this case, a posterior displacement of the COG (ie, anterior translation) results in a backward sway with activation of the paraspinal and hamstring muscles (Fig. 7-4). Anterior displacement produces forward sway with contraction of the abdominal and quadriceps muscles. In each case, the muscle activation proceeds from proximal to distal in an attempt to return the COG over the BOS. Little ankle activity occurs in this synergy.

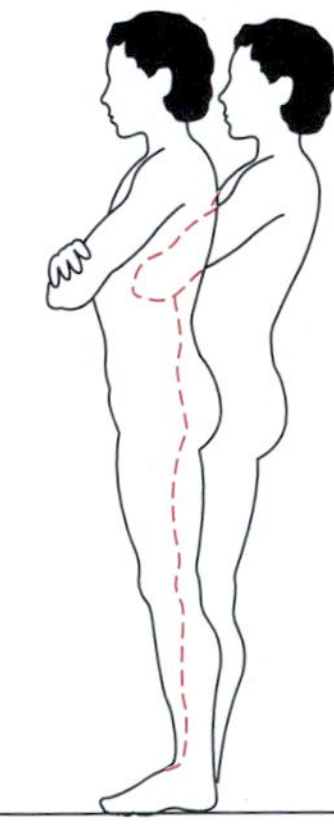

FIGURE 7-3 Ankle strategy in response to small perturbations.

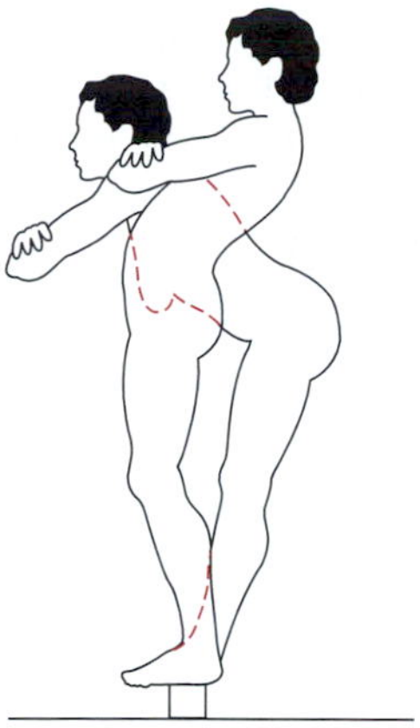

FIGURE 7-4 Hip strategy in response to larger perturbations.

If the displacement is great enough, the stepping strategy may be used, with a forward or backward step elicited to regain postural control. The ankle strategy is used in most cases by healthy persons, with the hip strategy employed in cases of limited ankle movement or greater displacement. However, some persons (eg, the elderly, patients with Parkinson's disease) may use one strategy exclusively or use more than one strategy simultaneously.

Motor Learning

The ankle, hip, and stepping strategies are examples of feedforward control; the response is controlled by motor programs that are preprogrammed collections of motor signals with a goal of achieving a specific task. In the case of balance, the goal is restoring the COG over the BOS. Each of the motor programs contains specific information about the sequencing and timing of muscle activation and postural set. If a movement is performed repeatedly, a pattern is formed that guides future performance of the motor program.

The learner passes through several stages when mastering a new skill. Consider learning a new task such as playing the piano or learning to swim. The first phase is cognitive, in which full attention to the task is necessary to develop gross problem-solving strategies. The second phase is associative, in which further development and refinement of the strategies occur. The movement patterns become more efficient, although still requiring attention to the task. The strategy becomes autonomous, and little cognitive processing is necessary. The goal of training is to get the learner to the autonomous stage so that the movement can occur with little thought. The ability to balance while coordinating other physical and cognitive activities is an example of functioning at the autonomous stage.

Continued practice can move the patient toward the autonomous stage. The early phase of training a new skill requires feedback. The feedback control relies on intrinsic and extrinsic cues to refine the program. As the process moves toward the autonomous level, more feedback should become intrinsic. Cues should rely on joint receptor and muscle spindle feedback, with less feedback from visual and tactile cues. Consider learning to drive from home to work in a new city. In the early stage, concentration on the task is required, and the individual can be overwhelmed with sensory information (eg, other cars, signal lights, commercial signs). As driving this path is repeated, less attention to the task is required, until the drive eventually becomes automatic. Extraneous sensory information can be filtered out and only pertinent information processed. Repeating the pattern progresses it to the automatic stage. However, the patient must continue to learn and adapt to new situations. Continued exposure to new situations such as driving in unfamiliar areas teaches the nervous system how to learn or adapt quickly and effectively to new stimuli and situations.

The same learning process is applied to balance activities. As balancing on a single leg or on a balance board becomes easy, less attention is necessary, and the task becomes automatic. The nervous system must be challenged at a new level. This can be done by changing the surface, BOS, external perturbation, or visual or vestibular input (see Self-Management: Balance Activities in Chapter 22). Continued practice at grossly similar but continuously changing tasks can enhance the patient's ability to adapt to new situations.

CAUSES OF BALANCE IMPAIRMENT

Injury to or disease of any of the structures (eg, eyes, inner ear, peripheral receptors, spinal cord, cerebellum, basal ganglia, cerebrum) involved in the three stages of information processing (ie, sensory input, sensory information processing, and motor output generation) can impair balance. Damage to proprioceptors have been implicated in balance deficits. Injury or pathology of the hip, knee, ankle, and back have been associated with increased postural sway and decreased balance.[15,21–24] The relationship between balance and degenerative disease of the knee joint has been studied, and results showed that the patient group had significantly more postural sway than the control group.[22] Similarly, the relationships among degenerative joint disease, total joint replacement, and balance have been studied.[22,25] Barrack and colleagues[25] studied the effects of degenerative joint disease and total joint replacement on position sense at the knee. The older group had significant decreases in position sense compared with the younger, control group, and an even greater difference was found between age-matched controls and postoperative patients, suggesting declines with age and degenerative joint disease. In patients with knee arthroplasty, no difference was found between the operated and unoperated knees.[25] It is unclear whether the decrease in joint position sense occurs because of changes at the joint or because of the associated decrease in muscle receptor function. Muscle atrophy usually accompanies degenerative joint disease and may account for some of the balance impairment.

Lesions produced by tumors, cerebrovascular accidents, or other insults often produce visual field losses, changing the individual's spatial orientation and altering balance responses. Loss of vision for any of a number of reasons, including aging, can impair balance. Visual losses can often be compensated by input from other sensory systems. Damage to the vestibular system can also cause profound limitations. Viral infections of the vestibular nerve, the aging process, or head injury may damage this system. These individuals experience vertigo, or the feeling of falling or spinning even when stable. Other lesions of the cerebellum, basal ganglia, or supplementary motor area can impair processing of the incoming information. Parkinson's disease, Huntington's disease, and cerebellar tumors affect balance and movement.

Age is a primary consideration in balance impairment. Age appears to affect all aspects of the stability triad (ie, somatosensory, visual, and vestibular) and all three stages of the process (ie, input from periphery, processing information, and generating motor output).[19] Falls by the elderly are of great concern, because the resultant injury and disability are significant. Each year, approximately 30% of persons older than 65 years of age fall, and one half of them fall multiple times.[26] Falls are a leading cause of death of persons older than 75 years of age.[27] Hip fracture-associated mortality is greater for women and has been reported as high as 8% to 18% within the first 2 years after fracture.[27] Falls by the elderly have been attributed to increased postural sway and imbalance and to a decreased ability to balance on a single leg.[7,27–29] Lower maximum walking speed and diminished self-perception of balance have been found in patients with hip fractures.[28] Older individuals have demonstrated larger sway areas than young adults in upright stance and forward lean stance.[30] The elderly are rarely able to complete a test of single-leg stance while blindfolded.[31,32]

The sensory input stage can be affected by losses in proprioception in the elderly. Barrack[25] found a decline in joint proprioception as part of normal aging. This decrease, along with poor vision and impaired vestibular function, predisposes the elderly person to impaired balance and falls.[19] Although declines in sensory input are found with aging, the primary problem appears to occur at the information-processing stage. Information processing can be improved by the use of high-contrast input, for which the difference between the signal and noise is clear. Noisy environments with much visual stimulus from mirrors and windows can make information processing challenging.[19]

After the information is processed and a response is selected, impaired balance can result from weakness, decreased mobility, pain, or impaired posture. The balance strategy chosen will be unsuccessful if the patient lacks the muscle strength or mobility to execute stabilization. Similarly, if the movement is inhibited by pain, the chances of falling are increased. If the patient has a significant posture impairment such as a thoracic kyphosis, the sway envelope is decreased, and the chances of exceeding the limits of stability are increased.

MEASUREMENT OF BALANCE IMPAIRMENT

Evaluation of balance impairment can range from the simple to the complex. Simple clinical measures such as the ability to maintain a single-leg stance with the eyes closed or the Romberg test are commonly used in the clinic. Computerized balance testing systems are increasingly incorporated into the clinical evaluation and treatment. Because balance impairment can arise from many sources, evaluation should differentiate biomechanical, motor, and sensory causes. For example, the clinician commonly attempts to disturb the patient's balance by trying to pushing the subject with instructions such as, "Don't let me push you over." The patient's response is to tighten all muscles in an attempt to resist the clinician's push. This tests the ability to tighten postural muscles, not balance reactions. What determines a positive test, and how would this test subsequently direct treatment? This test, like the single-leg stance and Romberg tests, is a static test, and tells little about the individual's ability to maintain balance while moving. However, this test is a relevant indicator in crowd situations, where a patient may get pushed.

Evaluation of biomechanical causes of imbalance can be readily performed in the clinic. Crutchfield[6] emphasizes the importance of distinguishing among a normal neurologic system working with an abnormal musculoskeletal system, an abnormal neurologic system working with a normal musculoskeletal system, or a combination of both. Joint range of motion, muscle length imbalance, impaired muscle performance, pain, or other postural abnormalities (eg, kyphosis) can contribute to balance impairment. Loss of motion at a joint or series of joints (eg, ankle, knee, and spine), decreased accessory motion, and muscle length imbalance alters posture and movement strategies. Likewise, muscle impairments such as weakness or loss of endurance alters movement strategies. For example, gluteus medius weakness results in a predictable alteration in gait known as a gluteus medius limp (ie, the Trendelenburg sign). Pain often produces changes in movement that, if continued, can produce secondary strength and mobility impairments. Many of these impairments can be assessed using simple clinical measures such as goniometry and manual and functional muscle testing.

Impairment of the sensory system can result in balance impairment. Testing for sensory organization requires more elaborate testing systems such as the visual-conflict dome and rotating platform. The Postural Dyscontrol Test combines and isolates information from the visual, vestibular, and somatosensory systems.[9] Systematically studying the contributions of each of these systems requires different testing situations, including standing with the eyes open on a fixed platform; standing blindfolded on a fixed platform; sway-referenced vision with fixed support; normal vision with sway-referenced support; absent vision with sway-referenced support; and sway-referenced vision and support[11] (Fig. 7-5). The situation with the eyes blindfolded provided information on the contribution of the visual system. In the situation with sway-referenced vision with fixed support, the visual box moved as the subject swayed, presenting a sensory conflict: movement took place, but the eyes did not register movement. Joint receptors sensed the movement, but the eyes did not. The vestibular system provided the resolving information, indicating that movement had taken place. During this testing, normal subjects sway very little.

The situation of normal vision with sway-referenced support presented a different conflict. In this case, the platform was rotated in conjunction with the body sway. The visual system recorded movement, but the joint receptors did not. The vestibular system presented the resolving information. Greater sway occurred in this situation than in the previous three situations. The greatest sway was observed in situations of absent vision with sway-referenced support and of sway-

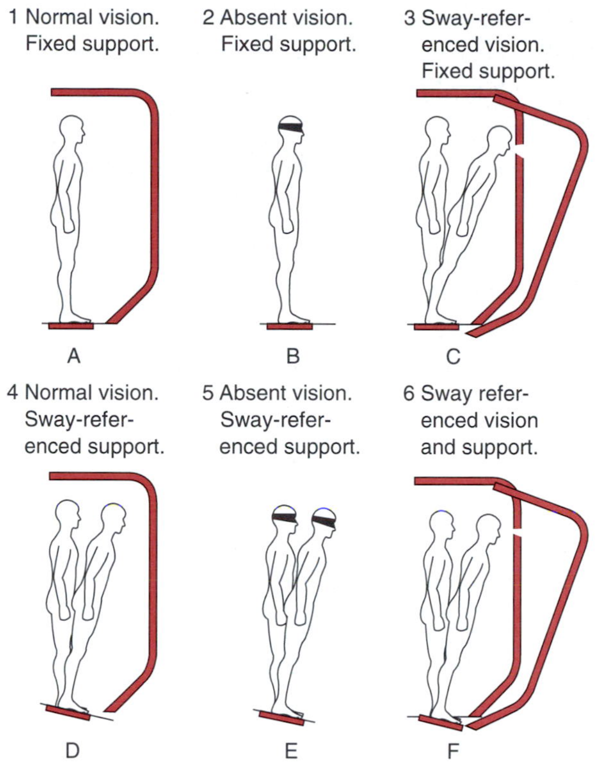

FIGURE 7-5 The six balance testing situations: ***(A)*** standing quietly, eyes open; ***(B)*** standing quietly, with eyes closed; ***(C)*** standing with a visual box, and eyes open; ***(D)*** standing, and body rotates with body sway; ***(E)*** standing, rotating platform, with eyes closed; ***(F)*** standing on a rotating platform with a visual box

referenced vision and support, for which inaccurate information was furnished from more than one source. Blindfolding eliminated visual input, and platform rotation provided inaccurate information to the visual and kinesthetic systems in the situation of absent vision with sway-referenced support, and the rotating platform and visual box provided inaccurate visual and somatosensory information in the situation of sway-referenced vision and support. These tests suggest that individuals rely primarily on the somatosensory system for orientation and postural control and that, when somatosensory and visual information is removed or inaccurate, the vestibular system is left to provide postural control.[6]

Several clinical tests of balance have been developed. The Functional Reach Test, Tinetti's balance and mobility assessment, the Timed Get Up and Go, and Berg Balance Test are used frequently in the clinic to give objective and functional measures of balance.[7,8,33] The Berg Balance Test rates performance from 0 (unable to perform) to 4 (normal) for 14 different tasks. The Berg Balance Test has a 53% sensitivity. Older adults who scored higher on the test were less likely to fall than those who scored below 45 of the 56 points.[34] The Functional Reach Test is an upper extremity balance test that assesses postural adjustments that anticipate upper extremity movement.[33,35] The Timed Get Up and Go Test requires the patient to stand up from sitting in a chair, walk 3 meters, turn around, return to the chair, and sit again.[36] The reliability of this test is high, and it correlates well with the Berg Balance Test.[37] The clinician should choose an evaluation battery that taps the multiple aspects of balance, including sensory, musculoskeletal, and performance factors.

ACTIVITIES FOR TREATING BALANCE IMPAIRMENT

The most important factor in treating balance impairment is determining the cause of the impairment. Repetitive quadriceps strengthening exercises do little to improve balance if the underlying problem is a movement disorder. Conversely, the patient must have adequate strength to maintain balance. Many individuals lack "core" strength, or strength in the trunk and pelvis, which provides a stable base for subsequent movement. A concurrent strength program is often necessary for treating balance impairment. The following treatment suggestions must be matched to the underlying problem and patient.

Mode

A variety of modes can be used to treat balance impairment. Any musculoskeletal cause of impairment, such as weakness, decreased mobility, or pain, should be treated first, with re-evaluation for continued balance impairment after resolution of the musculoskeletal problems. Chapters 4, 6, and 9 provide specific activities to treat these impairments.

Rehabilitation balls, foam rollers, and foam surfaces are often used to provide uneven or unstable surfaces for exercise (Figs. 7-6 and 7-7). Sitting balance, trunk stability, and weight distribution can be trained on a chair, table, or therapeutic ball (see Self-Management: Sitting Balance on a Stable Surface and Self-Management: Sitting Balance on an

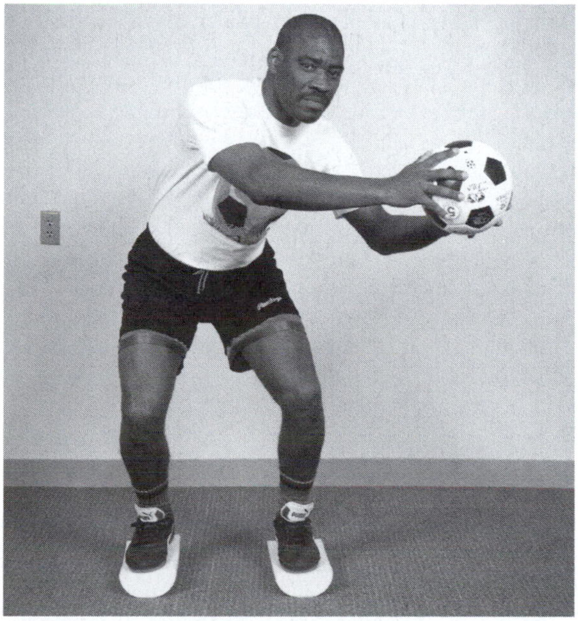

FIGURE 7-6 Foam rollers are used in bilateral stance when the person practices weight shifting while catching a ball.

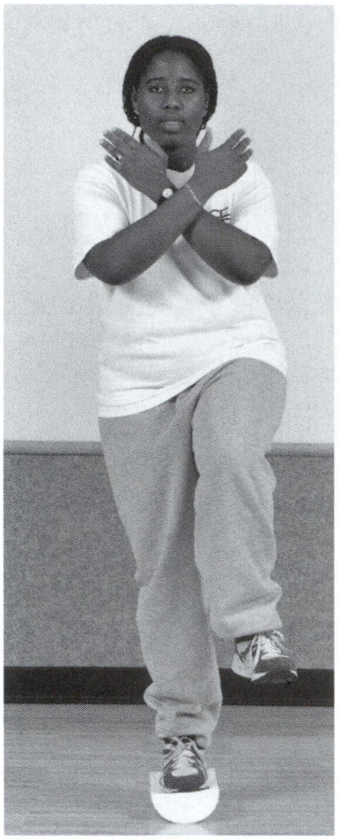

FIGURE 7-7 Tai Chi exercise to improve single leg balance.

Unstable Surface) (Fig. 7-8). Similarly, balance beams, lines drawn on the floor, balance boards, and scales can be used for balance training (Fig.7-9). More sophisticated balance testing and training devices are also available. Any mode used for testing balance can be used for training and is often good for initiating treatment techniques. More challenging surfaces such as a minitramp can also provide a variety of balance experiences (see Self-Management: Minitrampoline Balance). The pool is an ideal place to train balance, because the water's movement causes perturbations, and the water's viscosity slows balance loss, giving individuals more time to respond (see Self-Management: Single-Leg Kicks in Chapter 17).

Learning factors are essential in planning the activity mode for treating balance impairment. Early in the treatment program, simple balance challenges with much external feedback are necessary. This allows the patient to develop gross strategies to manage the perturbation. As the patient learns and develops these gross strategies, increasing the balance challenge while decreasing the external feedback allows internal strategies to develop. In the case of balance training, learning is the ultimate goal.

Posture

Awareness of posture and the position of the body in space is fundamental to balance training. Kinesiologic factors such as achieving and maintaining proper COG control and learning factors such as internalization of balance strategies provide the structural framework for the treatment postures chosen. Mirrors can provide postural feedback

SELF-MANAGEMENT: Sitting Balance on a Stable Surface

Purpose: To increase awareness of and expand stability limits

Movement technique: While sitting on a stable surface such as a chair, practice reaching forward, overhead, and to the side. You may you look in the direction you are reaching or in a different direction, as recommended by your therapist.

Repeat _______ times

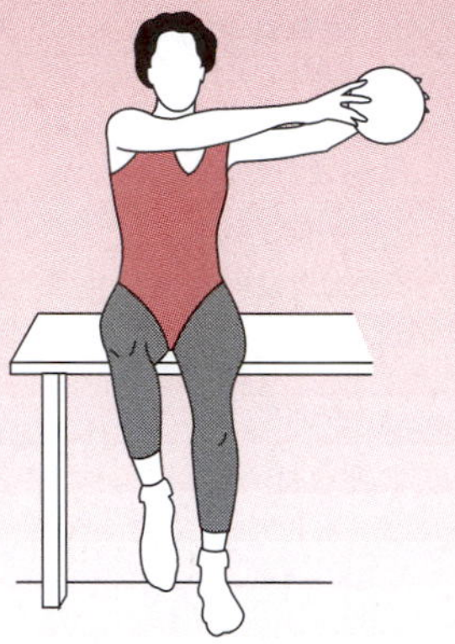

SELF-MANAGEMENT: Sitting Balance on an Unstable Surface

Purpose: To increase postural stability and trunk balance

Movement technique: While sitting on the therapeutic ball, practice reaching forward, overhead, and to the side. You may look in the direction you are reaching or in a different direction, as recommended by your therapist.

Repeat _______ times

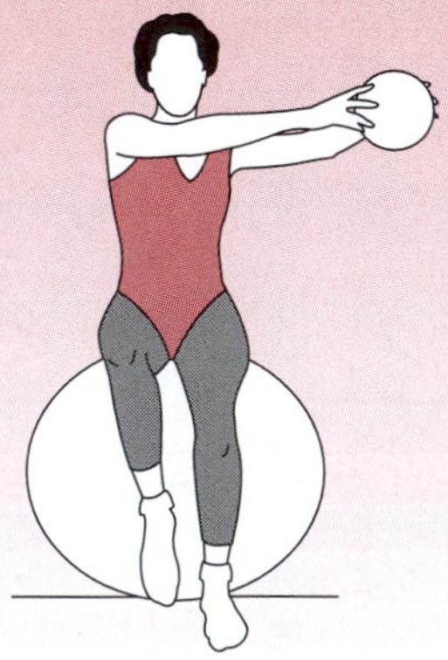

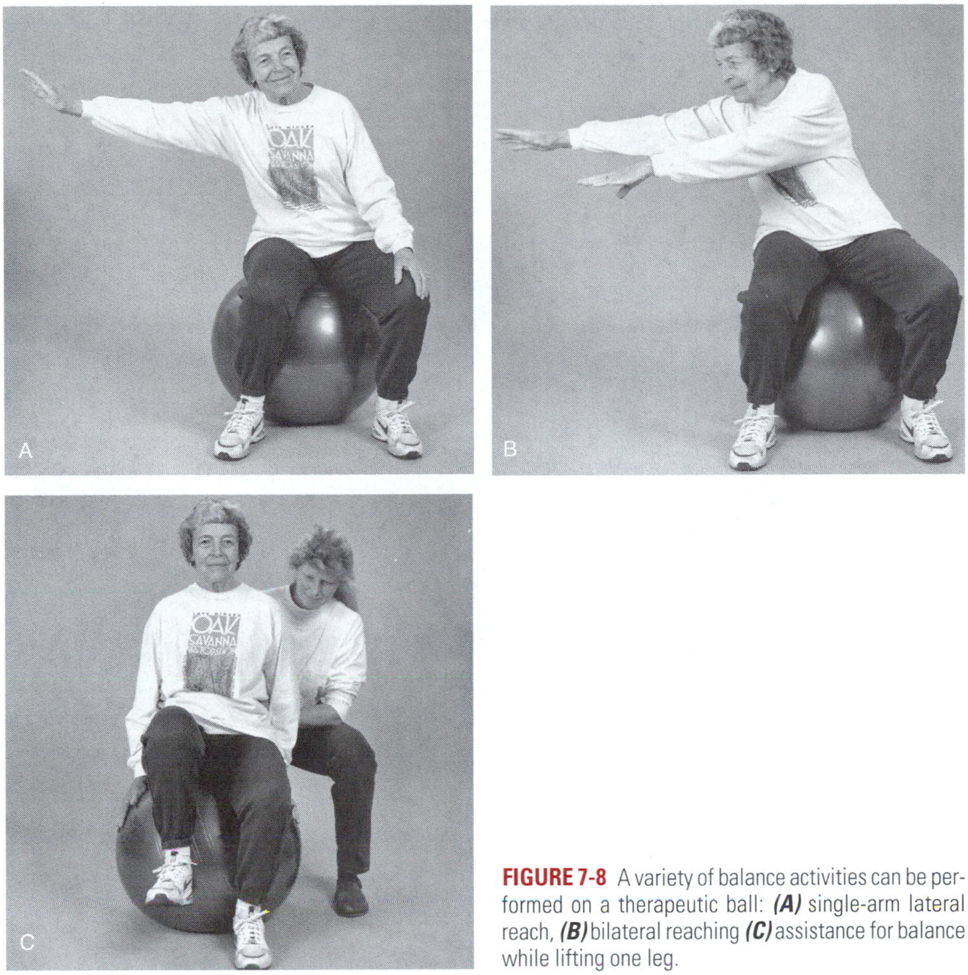

FIGURE 7-8 A variety of balance activities can be performed on a therapeutic ball: ***(A)*** single-arm lateral reach, ***(B)*** bilateral reaching ***(C)*** assistance for balance while lifting one leg.

regardless of the position of exercise. This allows visual feedback (ie, external feedback about position), which must be removed at some point to allow internalization of the balance strategies. For those needing work on core trunk stability first, training may be initiated in a sitting position, which provides an opportunity to develop a sense of trunk posture and equity of weight bearing while sitting. A variety of arm positions, such as forward or lateral reaching, can change the postural challenge. Maintaining equitable weight distribution and trunk posture on an unstable surface such as a therapeutic ball creates an interesting and useful balance challenge.

Static postures such as half kneeling, tall kneeling, and standing are useful positions for training balance, and they can be used in combination with foam surfaces to alter the challenge to the patient. Force platforms or scales may be used while standing to train the individual to distribute weight equally on each lower extremity. More challenging static postures, such as standing heel to toe or a single-leg stance, should be included when the patient is ready. For the athlete, postures encountered in sport should be duplicated and systematically challenged in the clinic. Lunge positions, single-leg stance with a variety of trunk postures, and squat positions are commonly encountered in sport. After stability and optimal posture are achieved in static positions, dynamic movement should be superimposed on the activity (see Selected Intervention: Single Leg Balance on a Foam Roller).

Movement

A variety of movement patterns superimposed on stable postures can increase the balance challenge. Adding anteroposterior and lateral sway assists the patient in determining and increasing her stability limits. This can be performed in a variety of modes (eg, supportive chair, therapeutic ball, foam roll, firm floor, foam pad, balance board, pool) and in a variety of postures (eg, sitting, half kneeling, tall kneeling, standing, single-leg stance). Trunk rotations with the arms in a variety of positions (eg, abducted, forward flexed, arms across chest) with changes in head position (eg, rotated, laterally flexed) to alter vestibular input can be combined in a multitude of ways. Proprioceptive neuromuscular facilitation (PNF) techniques in trunk rotation, called chops and lifts, are excellent dynamic movement patterns. These patterns include arm, trunk, and head rotation, flexion, and extension (see Chapter 14) (Fig. 7-10).

Stepping exercises such as lunges provide an opportunity to control balance as the client first moves outside the stability limit and then restabilizes when her foot hits the

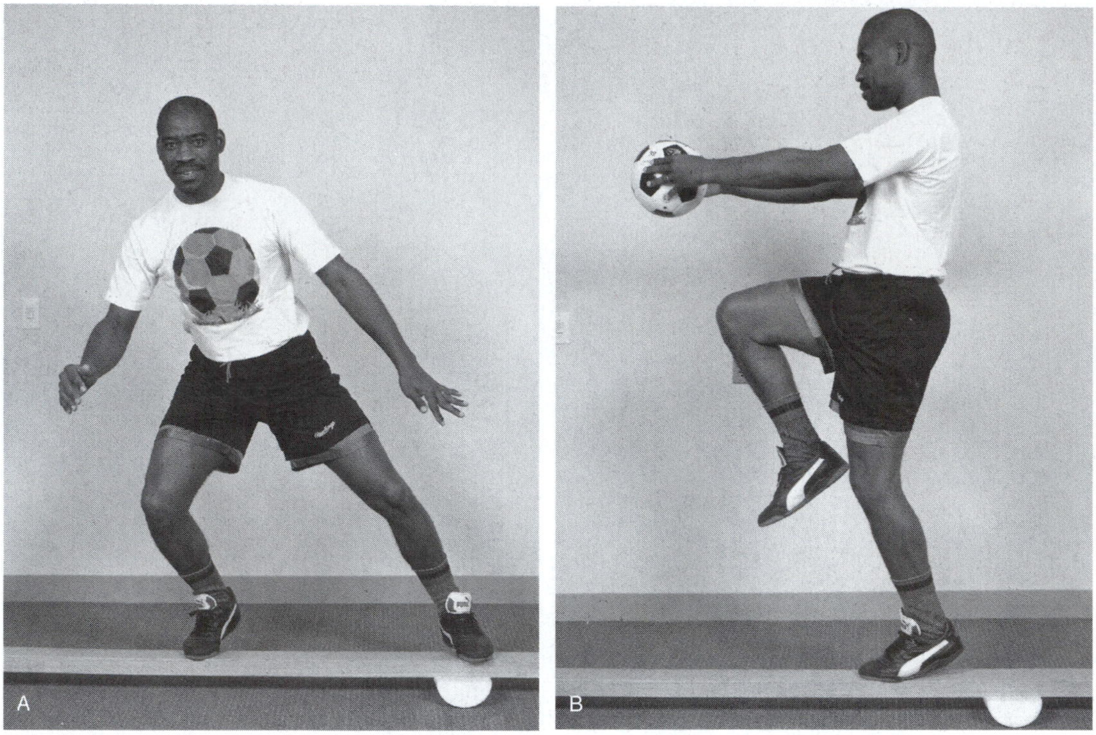

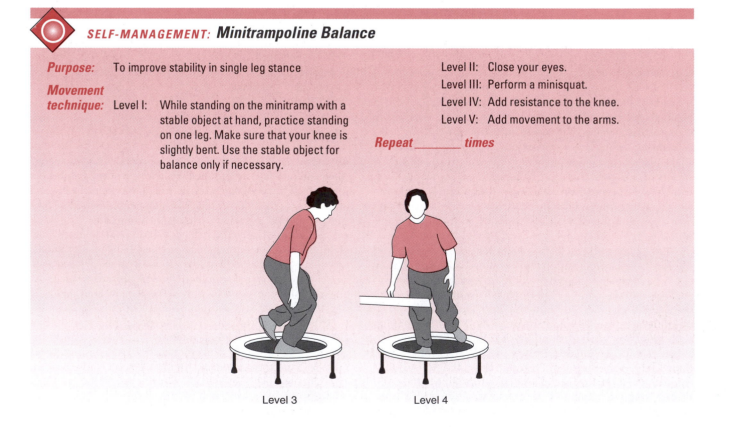

FIGURE 7-9 ***(A)*** Lateral movement on a balance beam on foam rollers. ***(B)*** Adding a soccer ball to drill activities increases the challenge.

SELF-MANAGEMENT: Minitrampoline Balance

Purpose: To improve stability in single leg stance

Movement technique:

Level I: While standing on the minitramp with a stable object at hand, practice standing on one leg. Make sure that your knee is slightly bent. Use the stable object for balance only if necessary.

Level II: Close your eyes.

Level III: Perform a minisquat.

Level IV: Add resistance to the knee.

Level V: Add movement to the arms.

Repeat _______ times

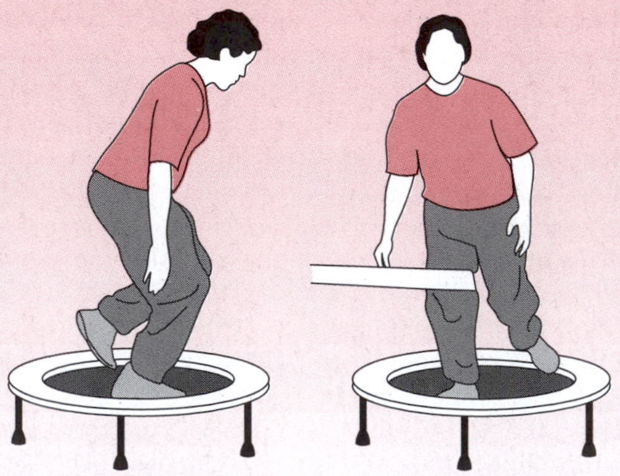

SELECTED INTERVENTION

Single Leg Balance on a Foam Roller

ACTIVITY: Single leg balance on foam roller with added dynamic activity

PURPOSE: To increase stability limits and dynamic balance

PRECAUTIONS: Patient safety: ensure readiness for activity and safeguards in case of balance loss; adequate trunk control

POSTURE: Standing on a foam roller with dynamic control of head, spine, and lower extremity posture

MOVEMENT: Maintain balance while moving a ball into a variety of positions or while playing catch with ball

PROCEDURE: Isometric, concentric and eccentric muscle contractions of the spine extensors, flexors and abdominal oblique muscles. The closed-chain nature of the activity will produce cocontraction of lower extremity musculature including, but not limited to the gastroc-soleus, quadriceps, hamstrings and gluteal muscles.

DOSAGE: Three to six sets of 30-second intervals

FUNCTIONAL MOVEMENT PATTERN TO REINFORCE GOAL OF EXERCISE: A variety of single leg instability situations are encountered in sports. The individual learns to control posture through core muscle contraction while performing a dynamic activity on an unstable surface.

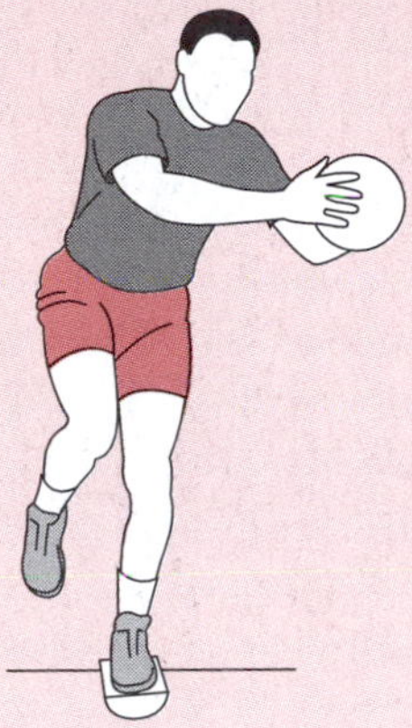

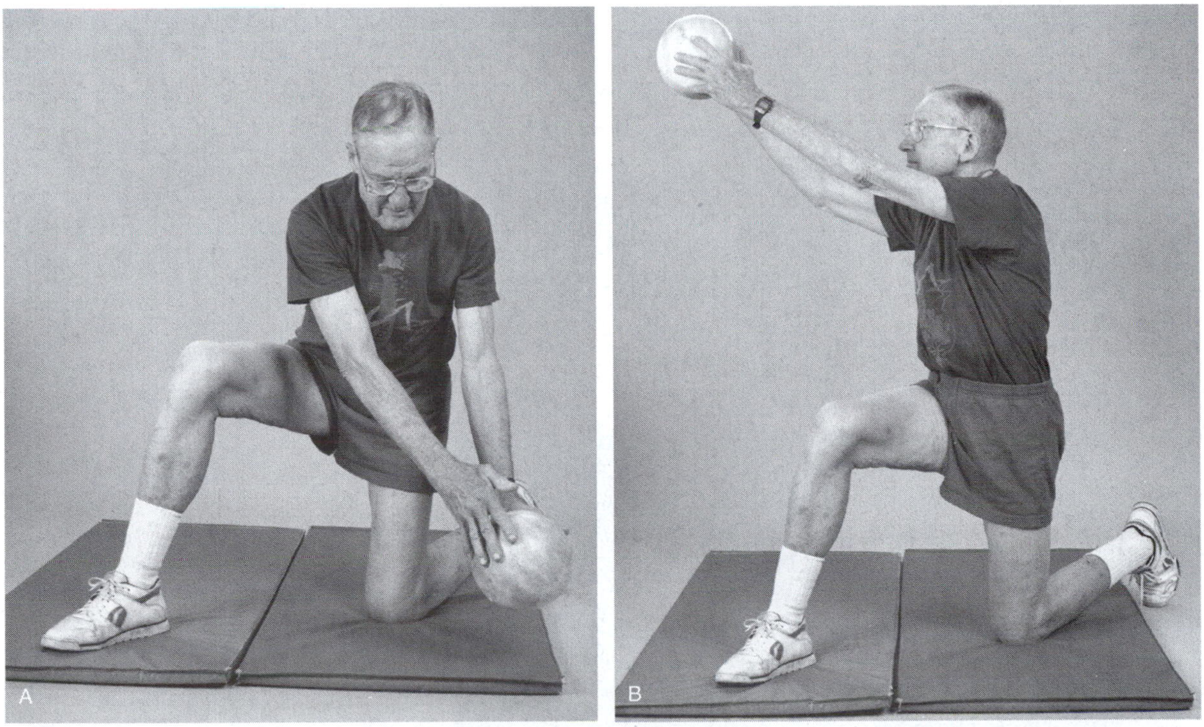

FIGURE 7-10 Proprioceptive neuromuscular facilitations of chop and lift in half-kneeling position: ***(A)*** starting position and ***(B)*** ending position

ground. Starting with small steps and progressing to full lunges (Fig. 7-11) increasingly challenges the patient. Adding a concurrent arm activity can further challenge balance. For example, reciprocally swinging the arms during stepping can make the task easier, but performing a PNF chop or catching a ball can make it more difficult (Fig. 7-12). Completely eliminating the arms for balance by holding them across the chest can make the exercise extremely difficult for a person with poor trunk and hip stability.

More advanced balance and exercises include hopping, skipping, carioka, slide board, and rope jumping (see Self-Management: Slide Board). These exercises can be performed in a variety of patterns, with exaggerated step length or knee lift. Many can be performed backward, with a variety of step techniques incorporated. The "hop and stop" can be performed on a firm surface or a soft surface such as foam or minitramp (Fig. 7-13). The patient is asked to hop single or double footed and to "stick" the landing without losing balance. Exercise equipment such as a stepper can also challenge balance if performed without hand support, backward, or with the eyes closed. For athletes, reproducing movement patterns found in their sports can prepare them for the return to activity. Many traditional sports drills can be modified for use in a clinical setting.

Balance training in the pool provides an ample supply of balance activities. The viscosity and movement of the water constantly challenge balance. Any arm or leg movement can potentially disrupt the patient's balance. For example, performing bilateral shoulder horizontal adduction and abduction results in posterior and anterior displacement of the body, respectively. This activity can be performed with the feet in stride, in normal stance, in a narrowed stance, or in single-leg stance for progressively increasing difficulty (see Self-Management: Shoulder-Level Claps in the Pool).

Dosage

ENVIRONMENT

The environment for balance training depends on the patient's situation. For the frail elderly or those with significant balance impairment, most of the training activity takes place in the clinic. The clinician should supervise for correct posture, avoidance of substitution, proper performance, and safety. Occasionally, some simple activities such as postural awareness exercises may be performed at home in a safe environment.

For athletes or other active individuals with musculoskeletal causes of balance impairments, balance activities may be carried out independently at home, at a local health club, or in a local pool. Safety is the key factor when making choices about the exercise environment. A stable support should always be available for regaining lost balance. This support should be placed such that it does not interfere with the exercise and does not cause injury during an attempt to regain balance.

SEQUENCE

Progression of exercise from simple to complex involves changes in mode, posture, and movement. Advancing from a stable surface to a more unstable surface and from stable posture (eg, sitting) to more unstable posture (eg, single-leg stance) exemplifies appropriate sequencing. For example, performing postural sway in all directions with the arms folded across the chest while sitting on a firm chair is a good precursor to adding arm movements or for performing the same exercise on an unstable therapeutic ball. Closing the eyes is a simple and effective means to increase the difficulty of any exercise.

While standing, starting with simple sway activities that elicit an ankle strategy is an appropriate starting point. Reinforcement of this strategy by verbal or tactile cuing and observation of proper posture and firing patterns prepare

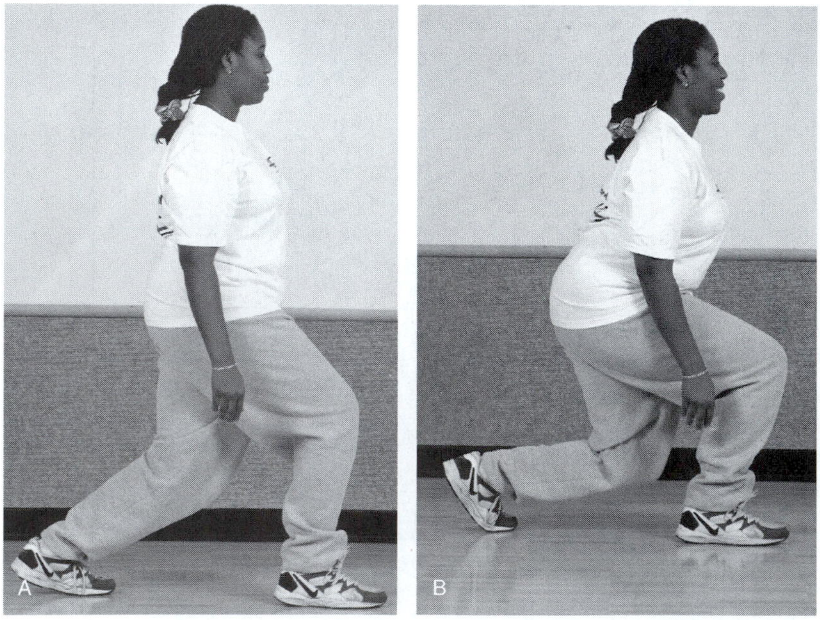

FIGURE 7-11 ***(A)*** Minilunges are progressed to ***(B)*** full lunges.

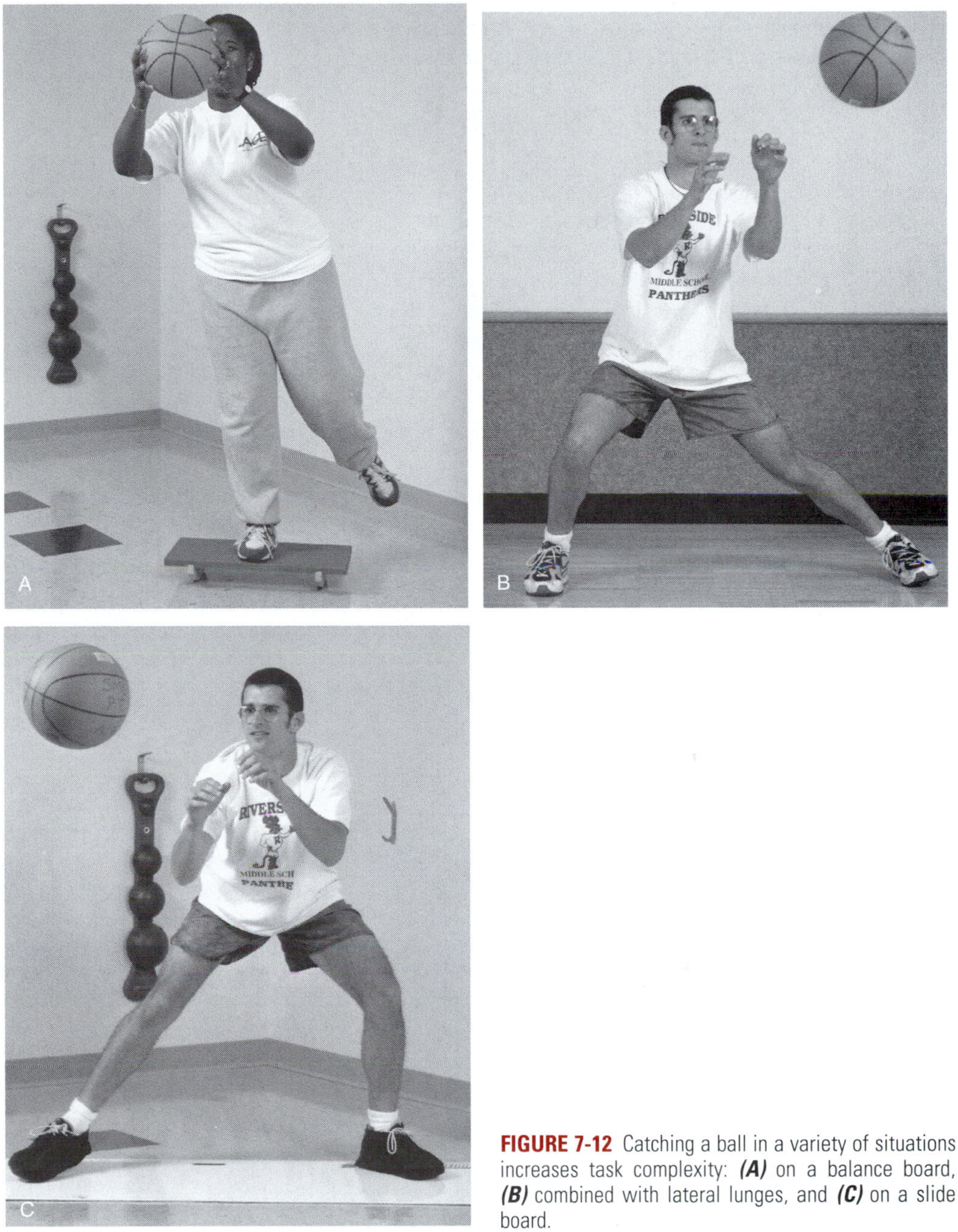

FIGURE 7-12 Catching a ball in a variety of situations increases task complexity: ***(A)*** on a balance board, ***(B)*** combined with lateral lunges, and ***(C)*** on a slide board.

the patient for larger perturbations. The patient is encouraged to gradually increase the stability limits by reaching or swaying farther. Progression to greater disruption of the COG should elicit a hip strategy or a stepping strategy, depending on the intensity of disruption. After these responses are established, progression to more dynamic activities, unstable surfaces, and complex movement patterns should be initiated.

Beginning with simple tasks on a stable surface and moving to progressively more unstable surfaces and complex tasks is the sequence plan, regardless of the age or condition of the patient. For the athlete, progression to a balance board, minitramp, slide board, or computerized balance training system may occur rapidly. Although training the individual in postures or activities encountered in her sport can prepare her for those situations, many unpredictable situations occur, and unpredictable perturbations should be included in the training program to teach the nervous system how to respond to novel situations.

FREQUENCY, INTENSITY, AND DURATION

The dosage parameters of frequency, intensity, and duration of exercise are less of an issue in balance training than in strength exercises. As with any rehabilitation exercise program in which changes in movement patterns or postures are the goal, the more frequently the exercise is performed, the better is the result. Practice increases the like-

SELF-MANAGEMENT: Slide Board

Purpose: To increase balance and coordination during a functional activity

Movement technique:
- Level I: Laterally glide on a slide board.
- Level II: Continuously catch and toss a ball.
- Level III: Increase speed.
- Level IV: Increase the number of balls tossed.

Repeat _______ times

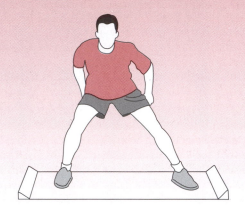

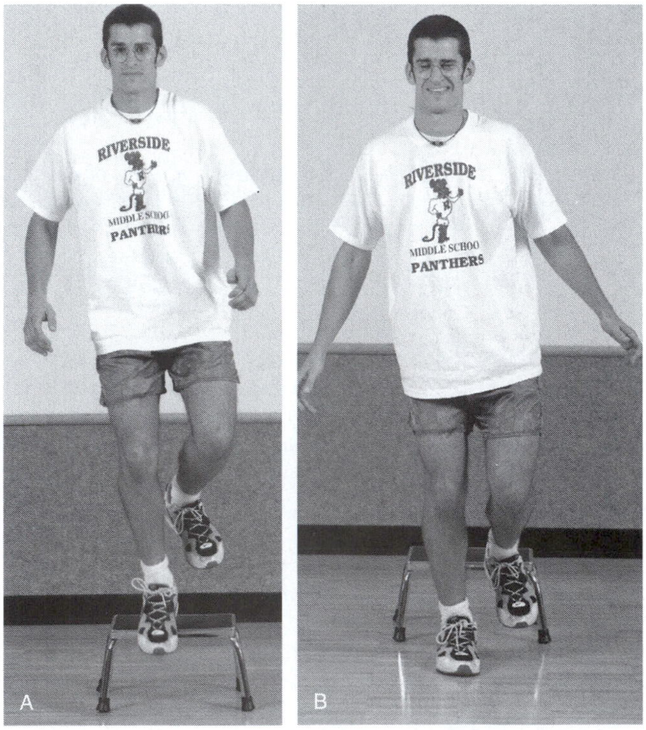

FIGURE 7-13 Hop and stop for dynamic balance. ***(A)*** The patient starts from a small stool, hops down, and ***(B)*** "sticks" the landing.

lihood of the changes becoming a habit. Intensity is generally not prescribed, because no external resistance or load is applied. Duration should be determined by fatigue; the patient should stop the exercise when she is unable to maintain the same level of performance as in the initial repetitions.

Precautions and Contraindications

The most important precaution in balance training is the patient's safety. By definition, balance training challenges the patient's balance. Because the potential for falls is high, the clinician should choose activities that are appropriate for the patient's skill level. A well-performed evaluation and initiation of activities at a lower level than determined by the examination can ensure appropriate exercise choice. It is safer to start the patient with tasks that are simpler and safer and progress to more complex exercises than to misjudge and place the patient in an unsafe situation.

The surrounding environment should have maximum safety as the principal design factor. Eliminating obstacles or unsafe objects from the exercise area and providing additional stabilization for the patient are essential environmental factors. A gait belt, hand contacts from the clinician,

SELF-MANAGEMENT: Shoulder Level Claps in the Pool

Purpose: To increase upper back and chest strength and to challenge balance

Movement technique:
- Level I: While standing in good postural alignment with your arms to the side at shoulder level, bring them forward and back to the starting position.
- Level II: Bring your feet closer together.
- Level III: Stand on a single leg.
- Level IV: Close your eyes
- Level V: Add resistance to the hands.

Repeat _______ times

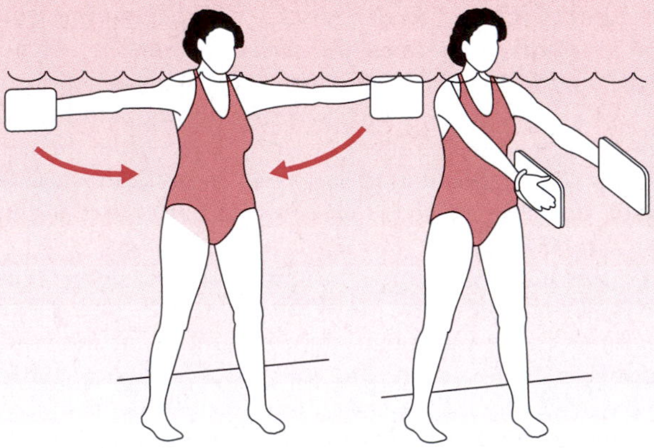

parallel bars, or other stable external objects for the patient to hold should be immediately available.

Balance training is contraindicated for persons who are inherently unsafe in balance-challenged positions. For example, those with cognitive impairments may be unable to understand the purpose and mechanics of the activity.

PATIENT EDUCATION

Patient education is an ongoing process for the patient with balance impairment. Safety is the most important area of education. The individual with significant balance impairment should be counseled regarding use of assistive devices to maintain stability. A walker, one or two crutches, or a cane can widen the BOS, thereby increasing the stability limits. The home should be evaluated for potential balance hazards. Loose rugs, slippery floors or bathtubs, uneven doorway thresholds, and stairs without railings can be hazards. Footwear can affect balance. Shoes that slip on the foot or on the floor or shoes with rubber bottoms that stick on the floor can cause a fall.

The patient should be educated regarding the limits of her balance. Factors include time (eg, walking more than 20 minutes), distance (eg, after walking more than four blocks), time of day (eg, better in the morning than in the evening), and environment (eg, crowds, noise, lights). Understanding the situations that place her at risk can help her make appropriate, safe choices while still participating in desired activities.

The patient should be taught strategies to maximize balance in compromised situations. For reasons beyond their control, patients may find themselves in situations where their balance is at risk. For example, when coming out of a movie, a person may have difficulty adjusting to the light, noise, and crowds in the lobby. Patients should be counseled in strategies to optimize balance, which may include using an assistive device (when the patient normally does not use one), using a friend's arm for balance and escort through the lobby, sitting and planning a path where stable objects may provide some external assistance, or asking someone for assistance.

Key Points

- Balance is one component of coordination, which is a more global concept that includes fine motor skills.
- Aging is associated with balance impairment and places the elderly at risk for falls.
- Some musculoskeletal disorders or injuries are associated with balance impairment. Balance training should be incorporated into the treatment program.
- Balance is a function of the interaction of visual, vestibular, and somatosensory systems.

LAB ACTIVITIES

1. With a partner, perform the following activities. Which balance strategy is elicited and why?
   a. With the patient's feet shoulder width apart, attempt to gently disrupt the patient's balance.
   b. With the patient's feet shoulder width apart, attempt a larger disruption of the patient's balance.
   c. With the patient standing heel to toe, attempt to gently disrupt the patient's balance.
   d. With the patient standing on a balance beam, attempt to gently disrupt the patient's balance.
2. Compare the length of time balance can be maintained in the following situations. Which muscles are working, and how are changes in COG compensated by postural changes? What do the arms attempt to do?
   a. Single-leg stance with eyes open (left and right)
   b. Single-leg stance with eyes closed (left and right)
   c. Single-leg stance, performing tubing-resisted shoulder horizontal abduction
   d. Single-leg stance, performing tubing-resisted shoulder flexion from 120 to 180 degrees of overhead flexion
   e. Single-leg stance, performing tubing-resisted hip extension
   f. Single-leg minisquats with the contralateral knee flexed
   g. Single-leg minisquats with the contralateral knee extended and hip flexed
   h. Single-leg minisquats on a minitramp
   i. Single-leg toe raises from a level surface
   j. Single-leg toe raises from the edge of a step
3. Compare muscle activity in the following situations:
   a. Single-leg minisquats on a minitramp, with tubing around the posterior knee pulling the knee into flexion
   b. Single-leg minisquats on a minitramp, with tubing around the medial knee pulling the hip into abduction
   c. Single-leg minisquats on a minitramp, with tubing around the anterior knee pulling the knee into extension
   d. Single-leg minisquats on a minitramp, with tubing around the lateral knee pulling the hip into adduction
4. Perform the following activities. Which activity is the most challenging to your balance? Your coordination?
   a. Repetitive single-leg hopping with arms free
   b. Repetitive single-leg hopping with arms across the chest
   c. Repetitive single-leg hopping with arms overhead
   d. Rope jumping on alternate feet
   e. Rope jumping on a single foot
   f. Single repetition of a single-leg hop, controlling and stopping the landing as quickly as possible (ie, hop and stop)
   g. Hop and stop on a minitramp

- Ankle strategies are used in response to small perturbations, and hip or stepping strategies are used to counter larger perturbations.
- Measurement of balance impairment should include biomechanical, sensory system, and motor strategy assessments.
- Treatment should be aimed at the cause of the problem, whether biomechanical, sensorimotor, or both.

? Critical Thinking Questions

1. Consider Case Study #1 in Unit 7. Design a progressive balance program for this basketball player. How would your treatment program differ if she were a
   a. Gymnast
   b. Figure skater
   c. Wrestler
   d. Cross-country runner
2. Consider Case Study #5 in Unit 7. Design a progressive balance program for this woman. Include sitting, standing, and transitional postures and movements. What other interventions probably are necessary to improve her balance?
3. What aspects of home design can maximize an individual's independence if balance is impaired?

REFERENCES

1. Swanik CB, Lephart SM, Giannantonio FP, Fu F. Reestablishing proprioception and neuromuscular control in the ACL-injured athlete. *J Sport Rehabil.* 1997;2:182–206.
2. Barrett DS, Cobb AG, Bentley G. Joint proprioception in normal, osteoarthritic, and replaced knees. *J Bone Joint Surg Br.* 1991;73:53–56.
3. Corrigan JP, Cashmen WF, Brady MP. Proprioception in the cruciate deficient knee. *J Bone Joint Surg Br.* 1992;74:247–250.
4. Lamb K, Miller J, Mernadez M. Falls in the elderly: causes and prevention. *Orthop Nurs.* 1987;6:45–49.
5. Schmitz TJ. Coordination assessment. In: O'Sullivan SB, Schmitz TJ, eds. *Physical Rehabilitation: Assessment and Treatment.* Philadelphia: FA Davis; 1994.
6. Crutchfield CA, Shumway-Cook A, Horak FB. Balance and coordination training. In: Scully RM, Barnes MR, eds. *Physical Therapy*. Philadelphia: JB Lippincott; 1989:825–843.
7. Berg KO, Wood-Dauphinee SL, Williams JT, et al. Measuring balance in the elderly: validation of an instrument. *Can J Public Health*. 1992;83:S7–S11.
8. Berg KO, Maki BE, Williams JI, Holliday PJ, Wood-Dauphinee SL. Clinical and laboratory measures of postural balance in an elderly population. *Arch Phys Med Rehabil*. 1992; 73:1073–1080.
9. Shumway-Cook A, Horak RB. Assessing the influence of sensory interaction on balance. *Phys Ther*. 1986;1548–1550.
10. McCollum G, Leen T. Form and exploration of mechanical stability limits in erect stance. *J Motor Behav*. 1989;21:225–238.
11. Nashner LM. Sensory, neuromuscular, and biomechanical contributions to human balance. In: Balance: Proceedings of the American Physical Therapy Association Forum; Nashville, TN, June 13–15, 1989.
12. Nashner LM. Adaptation of human movement to altered environments. *Trends Neurosci.* 1982;5:358–361.
13. Stern EB. The somatosensory systems. In: Cohen H, ed. *Neuroscience for Rehabilitation*. Philadelphia: JB Lippincott; 1993.
14. Rowinski MJ. Afferent neurobiology of the joint. In: Gould JA, Davies GJ, eds. *Orthopaedic and Sports Physical Therapy*. 2nd ed. St. Louis: CV Mosby; 1985.
15. Grigg P. Articular neurophysiology. In: Zachazewski JE, McGee DJ, Quillen WS, eds. *Athletic Injury Rehabilitation*. Philadelphia: WB Saunders; 1996.
16. Grigg P, Finerman GA, Riley LH. Joint-position sense after total hip replacement. *J Bone Joint Surg Am.* 1973;55:1016–1025.
17. Fox CR, Cohen H. The visual and vestibular systems. In: Cohen H, ed. *Neuroscience for Rehabilitation*. Philadelphia: JB Lippincott; 1993.
18. Winstein C, Mitz AR. The motor system II: higher centers. In: Cohen H, ed. *Neuroscience for Rehabilitation*. Philadelphia: JB Lippincott; 1993.
19. Light KE. Information processing for motor performance in aging adults. *Phys Ther*. 1990;70:820–826.
20. Nashner L, McCollum G. The organization of human postural movements: a formal basis and experimental synthesis. *Behav Brain Sci.* 1985;8:135–172.
21. Byl NN, Sinnott PL. Variations in balance and body sway in middle-aged adults *Spine* 1991;16:325–330.
22. Wegener L, Kisner C, Nichols D. Static and dynamic balance responses in persons with bilateral knee osteoarthritis. *J Orthop Sports Phys Ther*. 1997;25:13–18.
23. Freeman M. Instability of the foot after injuries to the lateral ligament of the ankle. *J Bone Joint Surg Br.* 1965;47:669–677.
24. Cornwall M, Murrell P. Postural sway following inversion sprain of the ankle. *J Am Podiatr Med Assoc*. 1991;81:243–247.
25. Barrack RL, Skinner HB, Cook SD, Haddad RJ. Effect of articular disease and total knee arthroplasty on knee joint-position sense. *J Neurophysiol*. 1983;50:684–687.
26. Sattin RW. Falls among older persons: a public health perspective. *Annu Rev Public Health*. 1992;13:489–508.
27. Lichtenstein MJ, Shields SL, Shiavi RG, Burger MC. Exercise and balance in aged women: a pilot controlled clinical trial. *Arch Phys Med Rehabil*. 1989;70:138–143.
28. Jarnlo GB, Thorngren KG. Standing balance in hip fracture patients. *Acta Orthop Scand*. 1991;62:427–434.
29. Bohannon RW, Larkin PA, Cook AC, Gear J, Singer J. Decrease in timed balance test scores with aging. *Phys Ther*. 1984;64:1067–1070.
30. Hasselkus BR, Shambes GM. Aging and postural sway in women. *J Gerontol.* 1975;30:661–667.
31. Ekdahl C, Jarnlo GB, Andersson SI. Standing balance in healthy subjects. *Scand J Rehabil Med*. 1989;21:187–195.
32. Era P, Heikkinen E. Postural sway during standing and unexpected disturbance of balance in random samples of men of different ages. *J Gerontol.* 1984;40:287–295.
33. Duncan PW, Weiner DK, Chandler J, Studenski S. Functional reach: a new clinical measure of balance. *J Gerontol*. 1990;45:M192–M197.
34. Bogle Thorbahn LD, Newton RA. Use of the Berg Balance Test to predict falls in the elderly. *Phys Ther*. 1996;76:576–585.
35. Fishman MN, Colby LA, Sachs LA, Nichols DS. Comparison of upper-extremity balance tasks and force platform testing in persons with hemiparesis. *Phys Ther*. 1997;77:1052–1062.
36. Mathias S, Nayak USL, Isaacs B. Balance in elderly patients: the "get-up and go" test. *Arch Phys Med Rehabil*. 1986;67: 387–389.
37. DiFabio RP, Seay R. Use of the "fast evaluation of mobility, balance and fear" in elderly community dwellers: validity and reliability. *Phys Ther*. 1997;77:904–917.

ADDITIONAL READING

Dietz V, Horstmann GA, Berger W. Significance of proprioceptive mechanisms in the regulation of stance. *Prog Brain Res.* 1989;80:419–423.

Era P, Heikkinen E. Postural sway during standing and unexpected disturbance of balance in random samples of men different ages. *J Gerontol.* 1985;40:287–295.

Hageman RA, Leibowitz JM, Blanke D. Age and gender effects on postural control measures. *Arch Phys Med Rehabil.* 1995; 76:961–965.

Lichtenstein MJ, Shields SL, Shiavi RG, Burger MC. Exercise and balance in aged women: a pilot controlled clinical trial. *Arch Phys Med Rehabil.* 1989;70:138–143.

Province MA, Hadley EC, Hornbrook MC, et al. The effects of exercise on falls in elderly patients. *JAMA.* 1995;273: 1341–1347.

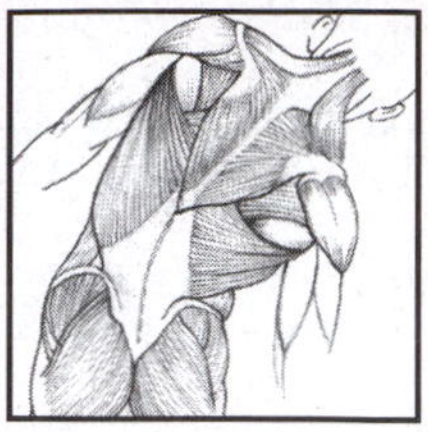

Posture and Movement Impairment

Carrie Hall

Impairments in posture and movement are the bases of many regional neuromusculoskeletal pain syndromes (NMPSs). NMPSs are localized, painful conditions of myofascial, periarticular, articular, or neural tissues. Pain from trauma, such as a fracture or dislocation, or pain caused by systemic disease, such as rheumatoid arthritis or cancer, does not fall into this category. However, impairments of posture and movement can perpetuate the pain resulting from trauma or systemic disease.

Regional NMPSs are often the result of cumulative microtrauma imposed on neuromusculoskeletal tissue. Microtrauma can occur from overuse, which is defined as repetitive, submaximal stress that exceeds the tissue's ability to adapt and repair.[1,2] Overuse can occur during a relatively short period, such as playing the first volleyball game of the season, or over a longer period, such as professional baseball pitching performed every day for many years. Microtrauma also can be caused by movements repeated during activities of daily living (ADLs) with less than optimal starting alignment or faulty osteokinematic motion.

Pain indicates that a mechanical deformation or chemical process has stimulated the nociceptors in the symptomatic structures. However, describing the mechanisms that signal pain is not the same as identifying the cause of pain. The premise of this chapter is that mechanical stress related to sustained faulty postural habits or repeated faulty movement patterns is the primary cause of pain or a primary factor in the recurrence of a painful condition or failure of the condition to resolve. Treatment focuses on correcting the factors predisposing or contributing to the sustained faulty postures or movement. When correction is not possible (eg, anatomic impairments, disease), modification of the posture or movement is indicated. Display 8-1 summarizes the factors influencing impairments of posture and movement.

This chapter defines the terms used in the evaluation and treatment of impairments of posture and movement; provides standards for the techniques used to determine ideal and impaired posture and movement; discusses factors influencing impairments of posture and movement; and outlines the principles of therapeutic exercise prescription for correction of posture and movement impairments.

DEFINITIONS

Posture

Posture is often considered to be a static function rather than being related to movement. However, posture should be considered in the context of the position the body assumes in preparation for the next movement. Traditionally, posture is examined in standing and sitting positions, but posture should be examined in numerous positions, particularly postures in which the patient frequently assumes and positions related to frequently performed movements. For example, standing on one leg is 85% of the gait cycle and therefore should be considered a typical posture to be examined.[3] A useful definition of posture was provided by Posture Committee of the American Academy of Orthopedic Surgeons:

> Posture is usually defined as the relative arrangement of the parts of the body. Good posture is the state of muscular and skeletal balance that protects the supporting structures of the body against injury or progressive deformity irrespective of the attitude (eg, erect, lying, squatting, stooping) in which these structures are working or resting. Under such conditions, the muscles function most efficiently, and the optimum positions are afforded for the thoracic and abdominal organs. Poor posture is a faulty relationship of the various parts of the body, which produces increased strain on the supporting structures and in which there is less efficient balance of the body over its base of support.[4]

An important message of this definition is the link between between posture and neuromusculoskeletal tissues and the link with the organ systems (eg, lungs, abdominal organs, pelvic organs). This definition suggests that, without

DISPLAY 8-1

Factors Influencing Posture and Movement Impairment

- Physiologic impairments.
  - Muscle and fascia length/extensibility
  - Joint mobility
  - Muscle force or torque and endurance capability
  - Patterns of muscle recruitment
  - Timing of muscle activation
  - Balance strategies
  - Pain
- Anatomic impairments (ie, structural scoliosis, hip anteversion, structural limb length discrepancy
- Anthropometric characteristics
- Psychological impairments
- Developmental factors (eg, age)
- Environmental influences
- Disease or pathology

optimal support, organ systems may not function optimally. For example, respiratory insufficiency can result from kyphosis or kyphoscoliosis.[5] These postural faults can reduce mobility of the thorax and thereby increase the work of breathing.[6] Chronically altered respiratory mechanics have been cited as a contributing factor to cardiopulmonary pathology (eg, pulmonary hypertension, right heart failure).[7]

This chapter considers only the upright standing posture. The *standard posture* refers to an ideal posture rather than an average or normal posture. This standard should be used as a basis for comparison; deviations from the standard are called *impairments of posture.*

The terms lordosis, kyphosis, genu recurvatum, genu valgum, genu varum, and pronation denote deviations in alignment with reference to segments of the body. *Lordosis* is an increased anterior curve of the spine, usually of the lumbar spine, but it can affect the thoracic or cervical spine. If used without a modifying word, it refers to lumbar lordosis (Fig. 8-1). *Kyphosis* is an increased posterior curve, usually of the thoracic spine but sometimes of the lumbar spine. If used without a modifying word, the term refers to the thoracic spine (Fig. 8-2).

Anterior pelvic tilt refers to a position in which the vertical plane through the anterior superior iliac spine (ASIS) is anterior to a vertical plane through the symphysis pubis (Fig. 8-3). *Posterior pelvic tilt* refers to a position in which the vertical plane through the ASIS is posterior to a vertical plane through the symphysis pubis.

The normal angle between the tibia and femur in the frontal plane is about 170 to 175 degrees and is called the physiologic valgus angle of the knee.[8] If the valgus angle is less than 165 degrees, *genu valgum* (ie, knock knees) exists.[9] Structural genu valgum can be associated with pronated feet, medially rotated femurs, anteverted hips, and coxa varum (Fig. 8-4*A*) (see Chapter 20). Postural genu valgum results from a combination of lateral rotation of the femurs, supination of the feet, and hyperextension of the knees (see Fig. 8-4*B*).[10] Conversely, if the tibiofemoral angle approaches or exceeds 180 degrees, genu varum (ie, bow legs) exists (Fig. 8-5*A*).[9] Structural genu varum can be associated with coxa valgum (see Chapter 20). Postural genu varum results from a combination of medial rotation of the femurs, pronation of the feet, and hyperextension of the knees (see Fig. 8-5*B*).[10] In the sagittal plane, the tibiofemoral angle should be 180 degrees. If the angle exceeds 180 degrees, *genu recurvatum* (ie, hyperextension) exists (Fig. 8-6).

Scapular adduction is a rest position or movement in which the scapula is positioned or moving toward the vertebral column (Fig. 8-7). *Scapular abduction* is a rest position or movement in which the scapula is positioned or

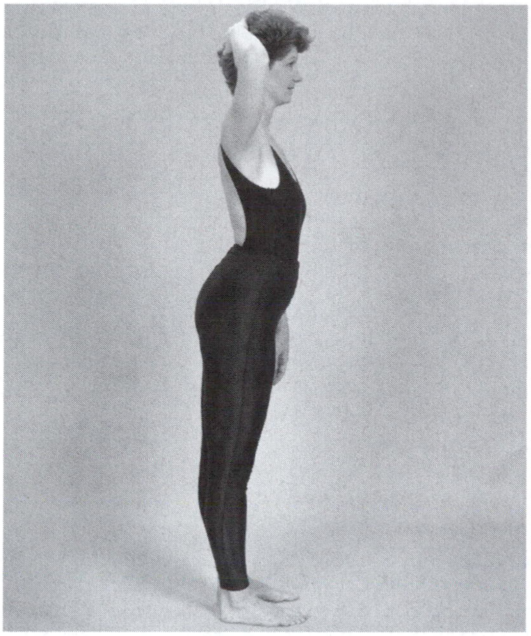

FIGURE 8-1 Marked anterior pelvic tilt and an exaggerated anterior curve of the lumbar spine. This curve is called a lordosis. Note that accompanying the anterior pelvic tilt and lordosis is flexion of the hip joint.

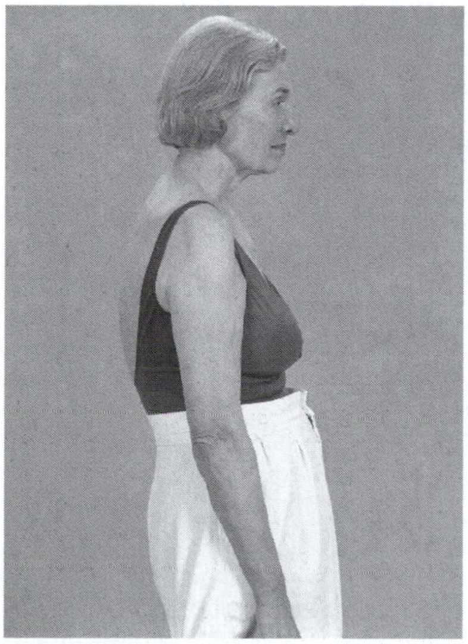

FIGURE 8-2 This person exhibits an exaggeration of the normal posterior curve of the thoracic spine. This is called a kyphosis.

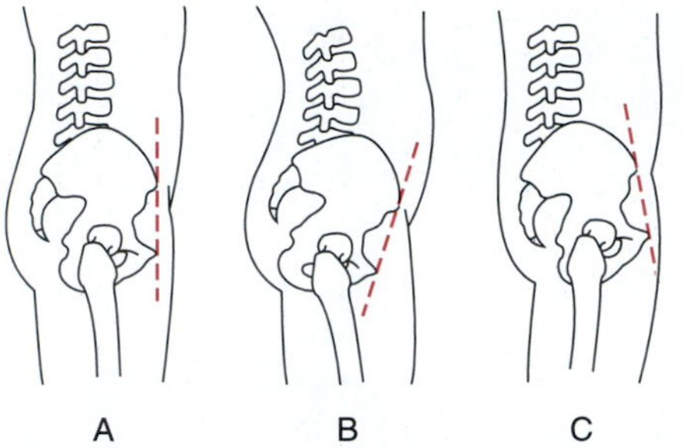

FIGURE 8-3 ***(A)*** The *neutral position* of the pelvis is one in which the anterosuperior iliac spines are in the same transverse plane and in which they and the symphysis are in the same vertical plane. ***(B)*** An *anterior pelvic tilt* is a position of the pelvis in which the vertical plane through the anterosuperior iliac spines are anterior to a vertical plane through the symphysis pubis. ***(C)*** A *posterior pelvic tilt* is a position of the pelvis in which the vertical plane through the anterosuperior iliac spines is posterior to a vertical plane through the symphysis pubis.

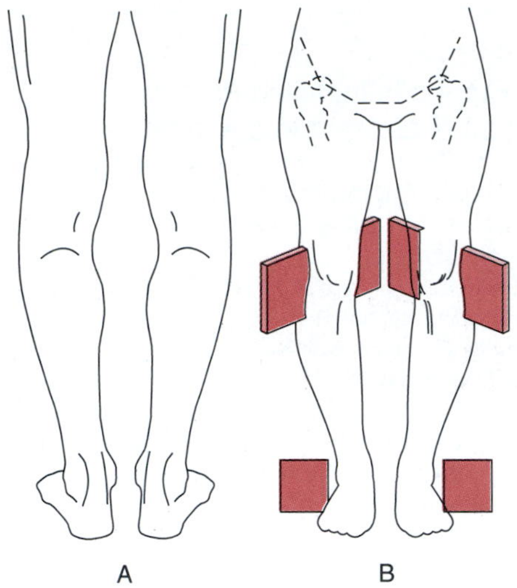

FIGURE 8-5 ***(A)*** Mild degree of structural genu varum, or bow legs. ***(B)*** Postural genu varum results from a combination of medial rotation of the femurs, pronation of the feet, and hyperextension of the knees. When femurs medially rotate, the axis of motion for flexion and extension is oblique to the coronal axis. From this axis, hyperextension occurs in a posterolateral direction, resulting in separation at the knees and apparent bowing of the legs.

moving away from the vertebral column (see Fig. 8-7). The clinician should avoid using "retraction" for scapular adduction and "protraction" for scapular abduction. The arm may be protracted by abduction of the scapula, but the scapula is not protracted; the same concept applies to arm retraction and scapular adduction.

Upward rotation of the scapula is a position or movement about the sagittal axis in which the inferior angle moves laterally and the glenoid fossa moves cranially (see Fig. 8-7). *Downward rotation of the scapula* is a position or movement in which the inferior angle moves medially and the glenoid fossa moves caudally. *Anterior tilt of the scapula* is a position or movement about a frontal axis in which the coracoid process moves in an anterior and caudal direction while the inferior angle moves in a posterior and cranial direction. *Posterior tilt of the scapula* is a position or movement in which the coracoid process moves in a posterior and cranial direction while the inferior angle moves in an anterior and caudal direction (see Fig. 8-7). *Elevation of the scapula* is a position or movement about a vertical axis in which the scapula moves cranially, and *depression of the scapula* is a position or movement in which the scapula moves caudally (see Fig. 8-7). *Winging of the scapula* (ie, medial rotation) is a position or movement about a vertical axis in which the vertebral border of the scapula moves posteriorly and laterally away from the rib cage and the glenoid fossa moves in an anterior and medial direction (see Fig. 8-7). Lateral rotation of the scapula is the converse movement.

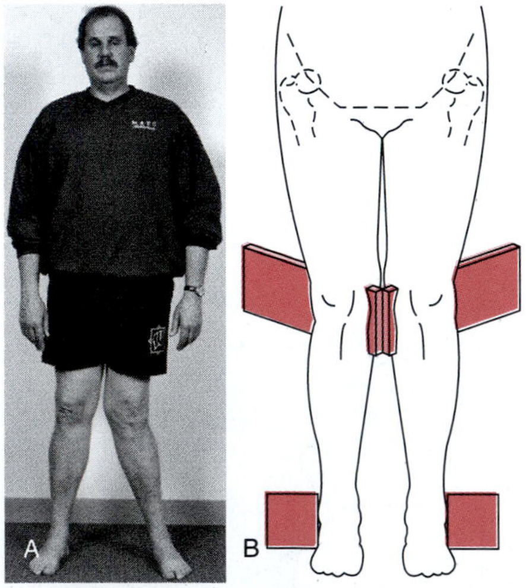

FIGURE 8-4. ***(A)*** This person has marked structural genu valgum, or knock-knees. ***(B)*** Postural genu valgum results from a combination of lateral rotation of the femurs, supination of the feet, and hyperextension of the knees. With lateral rotation, the axis of the knee joint is oblique to the coronal plane, and hyperextension results in adduction at the knees.

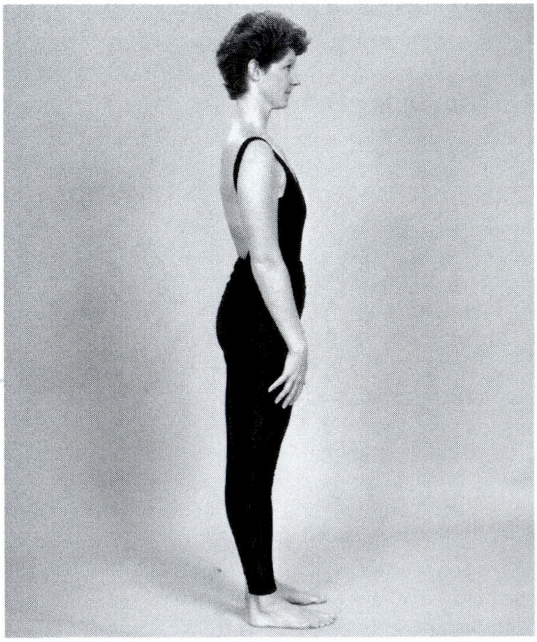

FIGURE 8-6 Moderate genu recurvatum, or hyperextension of the knees.

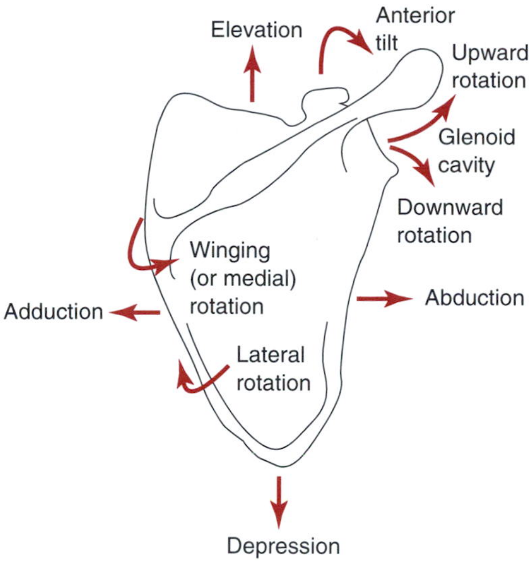

FIGURE 8-7 The positions and movements of the scapula.

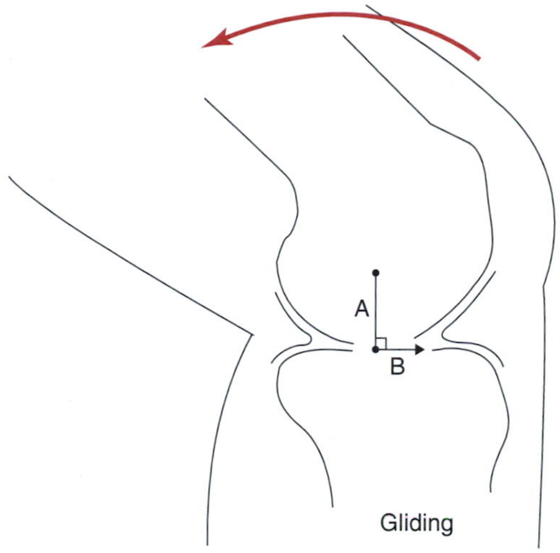

FIGURE 8-8 A normal knee with a line drawn from the instant center of the tibiofemoral joint to the tibiofemoral contact point ***(line A)*** forms a right angle with a line tangential to the tibial surface ***(line B)***. The arrow indicates the direction of displacement of the contact points. Line B is tangential to the tibial surface, indicating that the femur glides on the tibial condyles during flexion-extension motion.

Tautness is defined as muscles or ligaments put on tension. It implies a state in which slack is taken up in the muscles or ligaments. In a *short muscle,* a muscle that is shorter than the kinesiologic standard, the range is limited, and tautness appears before the motion has progressed to the normal limit of joint range. In an *elongated muscle,* a muscle that is longer than the kinesiologic standard, tautness appears after the motion has exceeded the normal joint range. The term tight often is used interchangeably with short or taut, but these terms do not have equivalent meanings. On palpation, a muscle that is short and drawn taut feels tight. A muscle that is elongated and drawn taut also feels tight on palpation. Because the word tight implies that a muscle should be stretched, the terms short and elongated are preferred to describe muscle length to ensure that stretching is applied only to short muscles.

Movement

Evaluating active movement requires precise observation and palpation skills and acute clinical reasoning skills. The focus of active movement assessment is too often on the quantity of osteokinematic range of motion rather than on the quality.

The instant center of rotation describes the relative uniplanar motion of two adjacent segments of a body and the direction of displacement of the contact points between these segments (Fig. 8-8).[11] The instant center of rotation changes over time because of altered joint configurations and external forces. The *path of instantaneous center of rotation* (PICR) is a trace of the sequential instant centers of rotation for a joint in different positions throughout the range of motion in one plane (Fig. 8-9).

Efficiency and longevity of the biomechanical system requires maintenance of precise movement of rotating segments; the PICR must meet a kinesiologic standard.[12] Deviations in the PICR from the ideal for a given joint imply that the arthrokinematic joint motions have become altered, even if the osteokinematic motion is within the normal range. The quality or precision of the osteokinematic motion is affected. Various investigators have shown that PICR deviations provide a noninvasive means of identifying pathomechanics.[13,14] However, because the radiologic methods used to determine the PICR are not available to physical therapists, clinically reliable tools for measuring the PICR need to be established.[12] Precise observation, palpation of osteokinematic movements, palpation or the use of surface electromyography to detect muscle activation patterns during segmental uniplanar and multiplanar movements, and total-body movement patterns are used to qualitatively examine movement. The clinician relies on a thorough knowledge of kinesiology to differentiate ideal from impaired movement patterns.

A major determinant of the PICR during active motion is the muscular force-couple action on the joint. *Force couple* is defined as two forces of equal magnitude but opposite

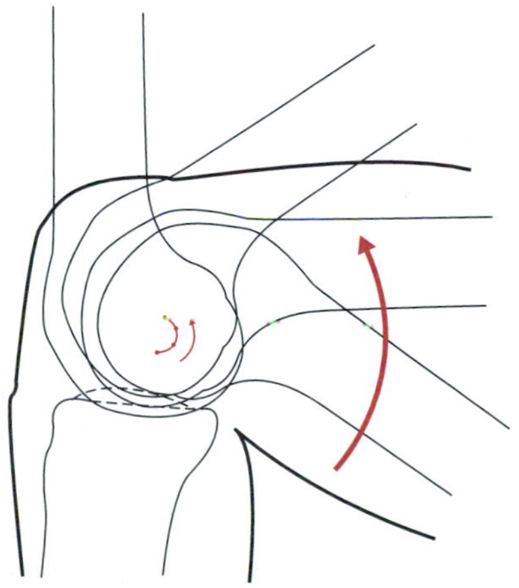

FIGURE 8-9 Semicircular path of instant center of rotation (PICR) for the tibiofemoral joint in a normal knee.

direction with parallel lines of application.[15] The result of the forces is zero, meaning the body is not displaced (ie, the body is in translatory equilibrium). The force couple causes the body to rotate around an axis perpendicular to the plane of the forces (Fig. 8-10).[15] In biomechanics, the instant center of rotation changes as the joint moves; consequently, the force-couple parameters change as the instant center of rotation changes.

Deviation of the PICR from the kinesiologic standard can be an indication of faulty muscle synergy in the force couple. Muscle dominance is defined as one muscle of a synergistic group of muscles that exceeds the action of its counterparts, causing a deviation of the PICR and potential disuse of the other synergists.[12] The factors that affect force-couple balance are discussed later in the chapter.

STANDARD POSTURE

An evaluation of postural faults necessitates a standard by which individual postures can be judged. The standing posture is used as the standard in this chapter and is illustrated from the back and side (Fig. 8-11). In the back view, a line of reference represents a plane that coincides with the midline of the body. It is illustrated as beginning midway between the heels and extending upward to midway between the lower extremities, through the midline of the pelvis, spine, and skull. The right and left halves of the skeletal structures are essentially symmetric. Hypothetically, the two halves of the body are in equilibrium. In the side view, the vertical line of reference represents a plane that divides the body into front and back sections of equal weight. Around this line of reference, the body is hypothetically in a position of equilibrium. The anatomic structures and surface landmarks that coincide with the line of reference for the side view are listed in Table 8-1.

From a mechanical standpoint, it may be logical to assume that a line of gravity should pass through the centers of weight-bearing joints of the body. However, the on-center position is not considered stable, because it can be held only momentarily in the presence of normal external stresses.[16,17] For example, when the center of the knee joint coincides with the line of gravity, there are equal tendencies for the joint to flex and to hyperextend. The slightest force exerted in either direction causes it to move off center. If the body must call on muscular effort at all times to resist knee flexion, muscular effort is unnecessarily expended. To offset this necessity, the line of gravity is considered to be slightly anterior to the joint center. Ligamentous structures and ideal muscle length restrain the knee from moving freely posteriorly. At the hip joint, the same principles apply, but the hip is most stable when the line of gravity is slightly posterior to the center of the joint. The strong ligaments of the hip anteriorly prevent additional hip extension.

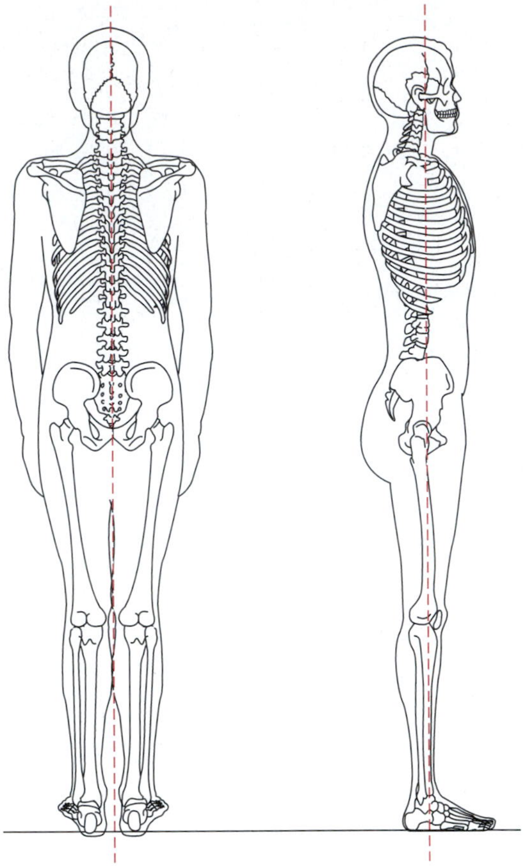

FIGURE 8-11 The back and side views of standard posture. The surface and anatomic landmarks that coincide with these views are listed in Table 8-1.

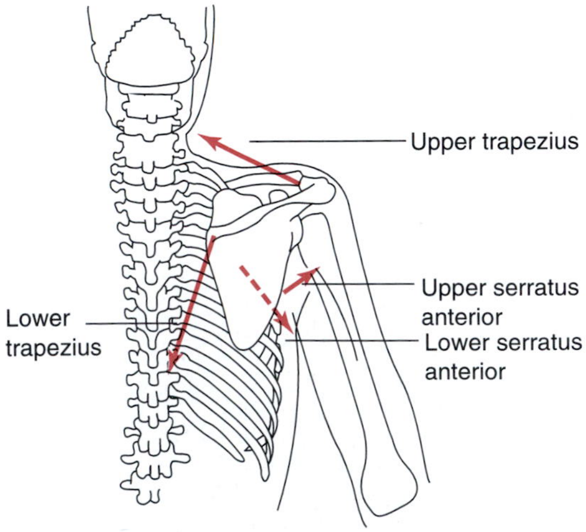

FIGURE 8-10 The action lines of the upper trapezius, lower trapezius, upper serratus anterior, and lower serratus anterior combine in a force-couple action to produce almost pure upward rotation of the scapula.

The pelvis is the link that transmits the weight of the head, arms, and trunk to the lower extremities, and it is considered key to the alignment of the entire lower body. Because of structural variations of the pelvis (ie, women tend to have a shallow pelvis, with the ASIS inferior to the posterior superior iliac spine), it is not appropriate to use an anterior landmark in relation to a posterior landmark. The pelvis is considered to be in a neutral position when the ASIS and the symphysis pubis are in the same vertical plane (see Fig. 8-3*A*). More specific alignment of the upper extremity is summarized in Display 8-2.[18]

Table 8-1. ANATOMIC STRUCTURES AND SURFACE LANDMARKS THAT COINCIDE WITH THE LINE OF REFERENCE FOR THE SIDE VIEW OF POSTURE

ANATOMICAL STRUCTURES	SURFACE LANDMARKS
Through the calcaneocuboid joint	Slightly anterior to the lateral malleolus
Slightly anterior to the center of the knee joint	Slightly anterior to a midline through the knee
Slightly posterior to the center of the hip joint	Through the greater trochanter
Through the sacral promontory	Midway between the back and the abdomen
Through the bodies of the lumbar vertebrae	Midway between the front and back of the chest
Through the dens	Through lobe of the ear
Through the external auditory meatus	
Slightly posterior to the apex of the coronal sutures	

Kendall HO, Kendall FP, Bonyton DA. *Posture and Pain.* Huntington, NY: Robert E. Krieger publishing, 1970.

IDEAL MOVEMENT

The index for optimal movement is the PICR. The ideal PICR for each joint is established by basic kinesiologic principles. The major determinants of the PICR during active motion are

- Osteokinematic and arthrokinematic joint mobility
- Muscular force-couple action on the joint
- Structural, developmental, and environmental influences

DISPLAY 8-2
Alignment of the Upper Extremity

Side view

- Humerus
  No more than one third of the head of the humerus protrudes in front of the acromion.
  Proximal and distal humerus in line vertically
- Scapula
  The inferior pole is held flat against the thorax (if the thorax is in ideal alignment).
  30 degrees anterior to the frontal plane (ie, scapular plane)

Back and front view

- Humerus
  antecubital crease faces anterior, and olecranon faces posterior.
- Forearms
  Palms face the body
- Scapula
  Vertebral borders are about 2 to 2.5 inches from the spine and parallel to the spine.
  The root of the scapula (where the spine of the scapula meets the vertebral border of the scapula) is at the level of T3.
  The vertebral border of the scapula is held against the thorax (if the thorax is in ideal alignment).

EXAMINATION AND EVALUATION

Posture

The lines and points of reference discussed under standard alignment are put to practical use in plumb line tests for postural alignment (Fig. 8-12). A plumb line test is used to determine if the points of reference of the individual being tested are in the same alignment as the corresponding

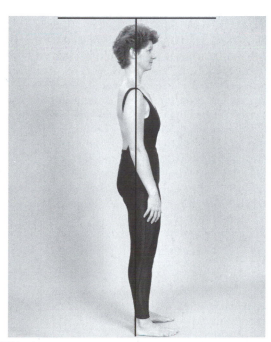

FIGURE 8-12 For the purpose of testing, the client steps up to a suspended plumb line. For the back or front view the subject stands with feet equidistant from the line; for side view, the point just in front of the lateral malleolus is in line with the plumb line. The base points of reference indicated in the illustrations of standard posture are the points with which the plumb line is suspended. The base point should be the fixed reference point, because the base is the only stationary or fixed part of the standing posture.

points in the standard posture. The amount of deviation of the various points of reference from the plumb line reveal the extent to which the subject's alignment is faulty. When deviations from plumb alignment are evaluated, they are described as slight, moderate, or severe. Additional alignment tests can be performed in several positions, such as sitting, recumbency, and single-limb stance. Deviations from acceptable standards can be noted.

Movement

Examination of movement in the clinical setting can be challenging, because sophisticated computerized movement analysis equipment is costly and is not user friendly in the typical physical therapy setting. The clinician must therefore rely on the following test procedures for single-joint movement analysis:

- Palpation skills and precise observation of basic movement patterns at a single joint are used to determine how closely the movement pattern replicates the PICR for a given limb for that movement (eg, observing or palpating the glenohumeral or scapulothoracic joints while raising the arm in flexion; the spine, pelvis, knee, ankle, or foot during standing hip and knee flexion as if to place a foot on a step).
- Palpation or surface electromyography is used to determine the pattern and synchronization of muscle activity for a given movement, which is compared with known kinesiologic standards.

The clinician should rely on the following test procedures for analysis of multiple-segment movement:

- As in gait analysis, break the movement into phases, and look at each segment or component (ie, group of segments) during each phase and relate the segmental movements to the process of movement. For example, the step-up can be broken into a swing and stance phase (Fig. 8-13). Each segment can be analyzed and relationships can be determined. For instance, a hip-hike strategy in the lumbopelvic region is related to insufficient hip and knee flexion and ankle dorsiflexion in the swing phase, and a Trendelenburg position in the stance phase is related to similar abnormal movement patterns (ie, hip adduction occurs in a hip-hike and Trendelenburg movement).
- Similar movement pattern descriptions can be developed for each basic movement required for ADLs (eg, rising from sit to stand, step-down, bed mobility, reaching). By describing movement pattern strategies, the variations in movement patterns and deviations from efficient and healthy patterns can be determined.[12]

Additional examination techniques can offer clues to expected outcomes. By compiling results of additional evaluation techniques, the clinician can hypothesize about what the active movement pattern may look like and what the muscle recruitment patterns may be during a given movement. Re-examination of the movement after additional tests have been performed can enable the clinician to better understand the complexity of movement. Posture assessment and specific muscle length tests also can assist in the evaluation of movement.

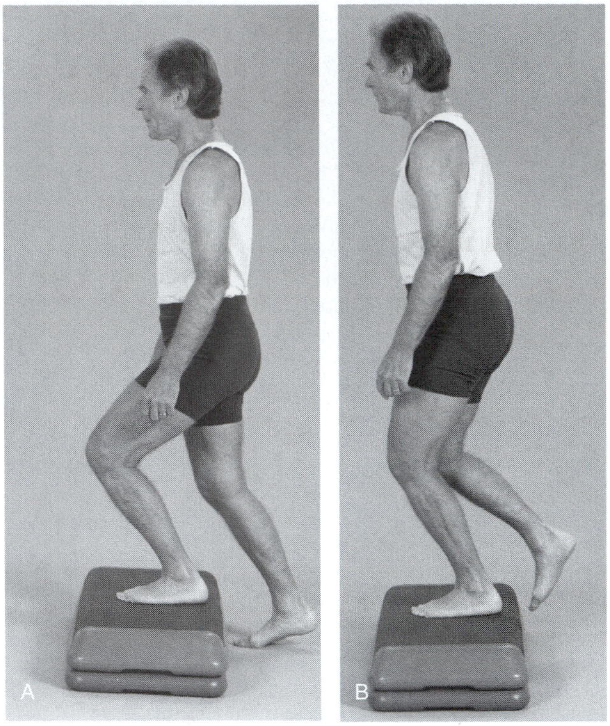

FIGURE 8-13 The step can be broken into two phases. ***(A)*** The swing phase in which the hip and knee are flexed to bring the foot to the surface of the step and ***(B)*** the stance phase in which the body is raised onto the step.

The minimal essential tests of muscle length that should be included in any posture or movement examination of the lower and upper quadrant are listed in Display 8-3. Osteokinematic assessment and arthrokinematic joint mobility testing are available, as is positional strength testing.

DISPLAY 8-3

Essential Muscle Length Tests

Lower Quadrant
- Hamstring: This test should distinguish between the medial and lateral hamstrings.
- Gastrocsoleus: This test, should distinguish between the gastrocnemius and soleus.
- Tensor fascia lata (TFL) and iliotibial band
- Hip flexors: This test should discriminate among the TFL, rectus femoris, and iliopsoas.
- Hip rotators: This test should distinguish between the medial and lateral rotators.

Upper Quadrant
- Teres major and latissimus dorsi
- Rhomboid major and minor and levator scapula
- Pectoralis major
- Pectoralis minor
- Shoulder rotators: This test should distinguish between the medial and lateral rotators.

The minimal essential tests of positional strength that should be included in any posture or movement examination for the trunk, upper quadrant, or lower quadrant are listed in Display 8-4.

FACTORS THAT CONTRIBUTE TO POSTURE AND MOVEMENT IMPAIRMENT

Physiologic impairments such as muscle weakness caused by neurologic pathology, poor endurance caused by cardiopulmonary or neuromuscular disease, or impaired balance caused by vestibular dysfunction can cause posture and movement impairments. However, most posture and movement impairments cannot be traced to specific causes. Habitual postures and repetitive movements often cause physiologic impairments, which perpetuate and contribute to further physiologic impairments, including impaired posture and movement. Many factors influence an individual's posture habits and movement patterns. Understanding these factors can assist the clinician in developing an efficient and effective therapeutic exercise intervention.

Muscle Length

Prolonged posture alterations can result in muscle length changes. The time a muscle spends in the shortened range and the amount a muscle is contracted in the shortened range determines whether it becomes shortened.[20] Conversely, the stimulus for lengthening a muscle is the amount of tension placed on the muscle over a prolonged period.[20] For example, the lower trapezius muscle can experience sustained tension from a short pectoralis minor coupled with gravity and the weight of a limb; these forces act to tilt the scapula anteriorly. The pectoralis minor experiences little to no counterbalancing tension from the lengthened lower trapezius and is assisted by gravity and the weight of the limb to remain in the shortened position. If the pectoralis minor contracts repeatedly in the shortened range (eg, as an accessory muscle of respiration), it can develop adaptive shortening.

Impairment of muscle length is related to movement. Alteration in the muscle length affects the action of the muscular force couple in which the muscle participates, affecting the PICR during active motion.[12] (This is discussed in more detail in the next section.)

Muscle Performance Capability

A long-held belief is that deviations in posture reflect muscle weakness. However, the relationships between postural deviation and muscle strength have been questioned,[21] and the literature instead suggests that the relationship between muscle length and strength may contribute to postural deviation.

Stretch weakness is a term used by Florence Kendall[16] to describe the effect of muscles maintained in an elongated condition beyond neutral physiologic rest position. This definition is based on the results of manual muscle strength testing, at which Kendall is an acknowledged expert.[10] For example, when the shoulders are maintained in a forward position and the scapulae elevated and abducted, the lower and middle trapezius muscles are positioned in an elongated rest position. The manual muscle test[10] would demonstrate weakness (Fig. 8-14). However, the apparent weakness of the posturally lengthened muscle may be an indication of altered length-tension properties such that the elongated muscle cannot produce tension in the shortened range (ie, the manual muscle test position).[20,22,23] Length-tension properties of muscle are also discussed in Chapter 4.

If the elongated middle and lower trapezius muscles are tested in a relatively lengthened range, the force production capability is greater than in the traditional manual muscle test position. This phenomenon can be called a length-associated change.[22] For the muscle to become lengthened, it adds sarcomeres in series and is capable of producing greater peak force than a normal-length or shortened muscle when tested at its optimal length. However, if the lengthened muscle is

DISPLAY 8-4
Essential Positional Strength Tests

Trunk
- Abdominal muscles: separate tests should be performed for the rectus abdominis and internal oblique,[10] external oblique,[12] and if possible, transversus abdominis.[19]

Lower Quadrant
- Illopsoas
- Gluteus medius
- Gluteus maximus
- Hamstrings
- Quadriceps
- Tensor fascia lata

Upper Quadrant
- Serratus anterior
- Upper, middle, and lower trapezius
- Infraspinatus and teres minor
- Subscapularis[12]

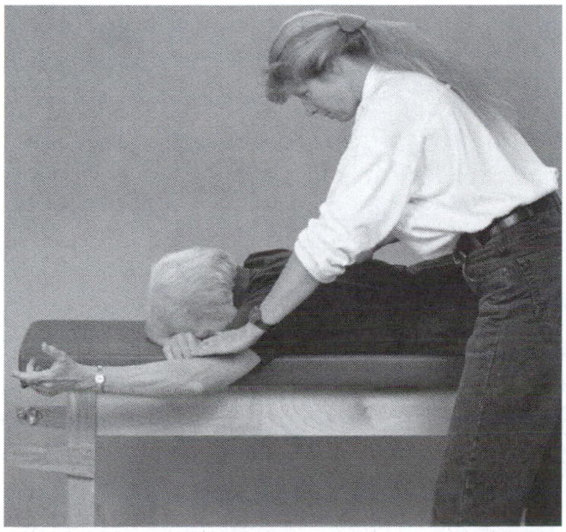

FIGURE 8-14 Manual muscle test position for the lower trapezius. Note that the arm is in elevation, positioning the scapula in upward rotation. The test position for the scapula is upward rotation, adduction, and depression. Failure to hold the test position indicates weakness.

placed in a shortened position for manual muscle test, the filaments would overlap and be less efficient at producing force than a short or normal-length muscle. This is similar to flexing the knee to test the gluteus maximus in hip extension and thereby lessening the contribution of the hamstrings. When testing muscles in the shortened range, a more appropriate description may be positional strength, because it indicates only the force the muscle can create in the short range.[24] One form of stretch weakness may be positional weakness. Testing the muscle at multiple points in the range and comparing findings with those for the opposite extremity (or half of the body when examining axial muscles) can help to differentiate positional weakness from weakness due to strain, disuse, or neurologic involvement. The muscle with associated length changes tests weak in the short range and strong in the lengthened range, whereas the other sources of weakness should test weak throughout the range.

The length-tension properties of the muscle correlate directly with the participation of the muscle in the force couple. The line of pull of its fibers determines the specific function of each muscle. No two muscles in the body have exactly the same line of pull. Whenever muscle weakness exists, the performance of some movement is affected or the stability of some part of the body is impaired. A muscle that becomes elongated over time exhibits positional weakness relative to the same point in the range of normal length or shortened synergists. Compared with its normal-length or shortened synergists, its participation in the force couple is lessened until it can achieve its optimal length-tension relationship. The result is a deviation of the PICR, which may contribute to microtrauma and eventually to macrotrauma, pathology, further impairment, and disability.

A clinical example may illustrate the relationship between length-tension properties and movement. In an individual with a functional limb length discrepancy with a high iliac crest on the right, the right hip is in postural adduction, which places the gluteus medius on stretch. During gait, the gluteus medius participates in the hip abduction force couple to decelerate hip adduction from the initial contact to midstance phase (see Selected Intervention: Prone Hip Abduction). The tensor fascia lata does not necessarily encounter the same stretch stimulus as the gluteus medius when the hip is in postural adduction (particularly the anteromedial fibers) and therefore can create better tension for abduction at initial contact when the hip is in more relative abduction. However, because the tensor fascia lata is also a hip flexor and medial rotator, without strong counterbalance from the gluteus medius (particularly posterior gluteus medius), the PICR of the hip can deviate in the direction of flexion and medial rotation. The overstretched gluteus medius can generate greater counterbalancing tension only after the hip is adducted, flexed, or medially rotated, which places the muscle on stretch. The posturally lengthened muscle affects the force-couple action and ultimately affects active movement patterns.

Endurance

The fatigability of a muscle affects its participation in a force couple, particularly in repeated movements. Muscle fatigue affects movement, but muscle endurance often is not a factor in perpetuating optimal resting alignment; the length of the muscles and periarticular structures support optimal alignment. Little muscle activity is required to maintain a relaxed standing position.[25]

Joint Mobility

The normal limitation of joint motion in certain directions has postural significance in relation to the stability of the body, particularly in standing. For example, dorsiflexion at the ankle with the knee straight is normally about 10 to 15 degrees. This means that when standing barefoot with the feet nearly parallel, the lower leg should not sway anteriorly on the foot more than about 10 degrees. The knee joint has up to 10 degrees of hyperextension. In the standing position, the femur and lower leg relationship should not exceed 10 degrees of postural deviation posteriorly. The hip joint also has about 10 degrees hyperextension, and in standing, the joint motion of the pelvis on the femur is restricted to about 10 degrees of postural deviation anteriorly. Excessive joint mobility can allow proportional postural deviations in the corresponding directions. Joint limitation also can affect postural alignment. Ankle, knee, or hip flexion contractures can cause deviations of posture in the corresponding directions.

A joint can only move through a standard PICR if the joint has the available passive range in osteokinematic and arthrokinematic motions. However, normal passive joint mobility does not guarantee precise PICR during active motion.

Impairments in joint mobility rarely occur in isolation. Active motion is usually affected by a combination of factors such as muscle length, muscle performance, and joint mobility. For example, during active shoulder medial rotation in the prone position with the arm abducted to 90 degrees, the shoulder should medially rotate 70 degrees without an associated anterior glide of the head of the humerus. The active range of motion can be limited by short lateral rotators, stiff periarticular structures (particularly the posterior capsule), and weak medial rotators.

In some cases, the quality of motion is affected. For example, during medial rotation, one deviation of the PICR that may be observed or palpated is an arthrokinetic motion of the head of the humerus gliding excessively anteriorly. This movement may result from one or a combination of factors, such those previously mentioned, combined with specific weakness of the subscapularis; dominance of the pectoralis major, latissimus dorsi, and teres major muscles; and excessive extensibility of the anterior capsule. Joint mobility, whether limited or excessive, can affect active motion, particularly when combined with other physiologic impairments.

Pain

Pain, posture, and movement are inextricably linked. Pain can induce abnormal movement, abnormal movement can induce pain, and it is often difficult to differentiate cause from effect. When a mechanical defect perpetuates the symptom or prevents resolution of the painful condition, the mechanical cause must be diagnosed and treated. Ultimately,

SELECTED INTERVENTION
Prone Hip Abduction

See Case Study #9

Although this patient requires comprehensive intervention, or one exercise is be described:

ACTIVITY: Prone hip abduction through full range of motion

PURPOSE: Strengthen 2+/5 gluteus medius through full range (need to increase the muscle's ability to create tension through full range)

RISK FACTORS: No appreciable risk factors

EFFECT OF PREVIOUS INTERVENTIONS: None

ELEMENTS OF THE MOVEMENT SYSTEM: Base

STAGE OF MOTOR CONTROL: mobility

MODE: resisted exercise in a gravity-lessened position

POSTURE: Beginning and ending position—prone, with a pillow under, stomach, hip slightly laterally rotated, elastic around the ankle (Fig. A)

MOVEMENT: The hip extends just enough to clear from the supporting surface, abducts through the full available range (concentric), rests on the supporting surface, returns to a slightly extended position, and slowly adducts to the starting position (eccentric) (Fig. B).

SPECIAL CONSIDERATIONS: Ensure that the gluteus medius is contracting throughout the entire activity (concentric and eccentric) and that the tensor facia lata (TFL) is maximally relaxed. Ensure that full *end-range* motion is achieved and that the abdominals are stabilizing the spine and pelvis against extension and side-bending forces imposed by motion of the hip. Be sure motion is isolated to the hip and that no motion occurs in the spine.

DOSAGE

SPECIAL CONSIDERATIONS:

- **Anatomical:** Gluteus medius
- **Physiological:** No strain, 2+/5 manual muscle test (MMT) grade
- **Learning capability:** Difficulty isolating gluteus medius over TFL may require tactile facilitation or surface electroyography (SEMG) with biofeedback on gluteus medius for better isolation.
- **Type of Contraction:** Concentric during abduction motion and eccentric during adduction motion
- **Intensity:** Light-resistance elastic tied around the ankle and taut in hip-neutral position
- **Speed of Activity:** moderate on concentric portions; slow on eccentric portion
- **Duration:** To form fatigue for two sets (maximum of 30 repetitions)
- **Frequency:** Daily
- **Environment:** Home
- **Feedback:** Initially tactile facilitation or SEMG with biofeedback, tapered after isolated contraction is achieved

(continued)

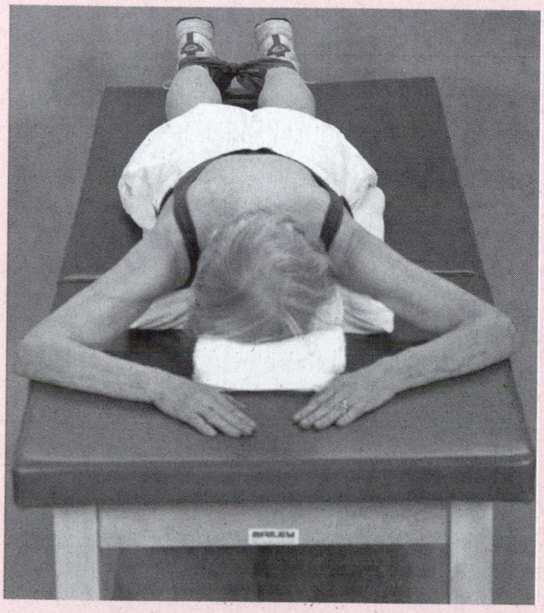

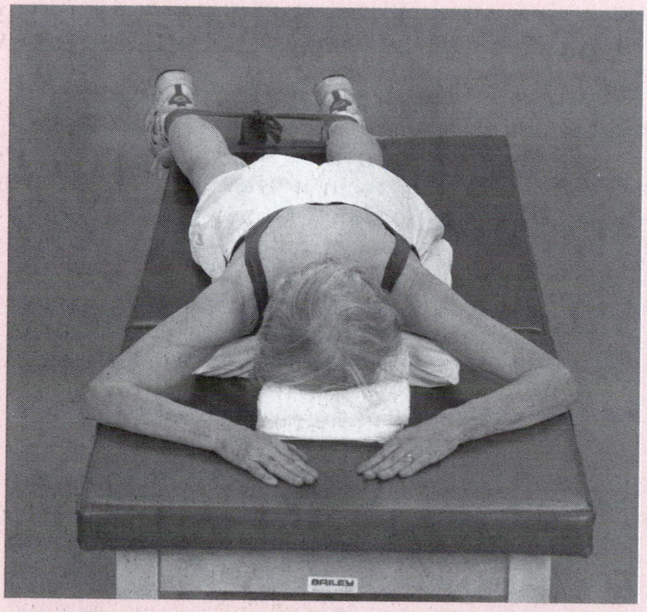

SELECTED INTERVENTION

Prone Hip Abduction *(Continued)*

RATIONALE FOR EXERCISE CHOICE This exercise was chosen to increase the strength of the gluteus medius in isolation from the TFL. Because the MMT grade is 2+/5, a gravity-lessened position was chosen to allow full range of motion. Elastic was used to ensure concentric contraction of the gluteus medius during the abduction motion and eccentric contraction on the return from abduction in a gravity-lessened position. Full range of motion is expected to work on length-tension properties of the gluteus medius (ie, ability to create force throughout the range, including the shortened range).

EXERCISE MODIFICATION/GRADATION: As strength through a full range is developed, the exercise should be progressed to an against-gravity position (ie, sidelying). After a 3+/5 MMT grade is achieved, standing functional activities should be introduced (ie, stability and controlled mobility). After proximal stability and controlled mobility are achieved, the exercise can be progressed to functional gait activities (ie, skill).

Within each activity level, specific dosage parameters can be manipulated to progress the exercise and prepare for gradation to the next level. At each level, care must be taken to ensure synergy between the gluteus medius and TFL in stabilizing the hip in the frontal plane by observing the pelvic and femur positions and preventing anterior pelvic tilt, Trendelenburg gait, or femur medial rotation. In closed chain positions, neutral pelvic, tibial, and foot alignment about all three axis complement the hip position.

FUNCTIONAL MOVEMENT PATTERN TO REINFORCE GOAL OF SPECIFIC EXERCISE:

POSTURE: Educate the patient about asymmetric postures that reinforce a weak, lengthened gluteus medius (ie, standing with weight shifted to the involved side, resulting in a high iliac crest).

MOVEMENT: During gait, think of contracting gluteal musculature at heel strike to prevent a Trendelenburg gait.

the posture habits and movement patterns contributing to the mechanical cause of pain must be modified.

Pain may or may not alter a given posture or movement, depending on the severity of the symptom and the magnitude or intensity of stress imposed by the posture or movement. However, pain that is associated with posture and movement can lead the clinician to an understanding of the kinesiopathologic factors contributing to the pain. For example, if a patient has pain during a medial shoulder rotation movement, such as is used in swimming, it must be determined what impairments are associated with the pain experienced during this movement pattern and how to alter the movement pattern to reduce or eliminate the pain. During movement testing, the movement of the head of the humerus is found to be associated with excessive anterior translation. When the humerus is manually prevented from moving anteriorly during the motion by the clinician, the pain is relieved. The anterior translation can be assumed to be the mechanical cause of the pain. The clinician must perform additional tests to determine the specific impairments that contribute to the anterior displacement of the head of the humerus.

Treatment is based on resolving the impairments associated with the kinesiopathologic pattern. By treating these impairments, the pain often resolves without necessarily requiring direct treatment of the tissue that is the source of pain.

Anatomic Impairments and Anthropometric Characteristics

Anatomic impairments can predispose persons to impairments of posture and movement patterns that can result in NMPSs. Individuals with anatomic impairments (eg, scoliosis, kyphosis from Scheuermann's disease, hip anteversion) are predisposed to develop NMPSs because of altered posture habits and movement patterns. For example, an individual with Scheuermann's disease typically has moderate to marked kyphosis. This patient is prone to increased kyphosis beyond the anatomic impairment because of the effect of gravity and the weight of the upper extremities on the kyphotic posture. Increased thoracic kyphosis can give rise to thoracic, neck, low back, or lower quadrant pain because of compensatory spinal, pelvic, and lower extremity alignments.

The patient may adopt movement patterns that perpetuate the kyphotic posture. For example, during forward bending, instead of initiating the movement with concentric phasic activity from the rectus abdominis and controlling the lowering with eccentric spinal and hip extensors, the bending movement may be produced by tonic concentric rectus abdominis activity and phasic eccentric deceleration from the spinal and hip extensors. The latter movement pattern would contribute to greater kyphotic forces on the thoracic spine than the former pattern. This repetitive movement pattern can lead to neck, thoracic, or lumbar pain because of compensatory neck and lumbar movements resulting from the exaggerated kyphosis.

Anthropometric characteristics can also contribute to impairments of posture and movement. Consider a tall man with broad shoulders and a tall, narrow pelvis. Ideal lumbopelvic rhythm is such that motion at the lumbar spine should be accompanied by motion of the pelvis rotating over the hips.[26] The tall man with broad shoulders and a tall, narrow pelvis has a higher center of mass than an average-height woman with a relatively broader pelvis. When the man bends forward, the fulcrum point is more likely be in the lumbar spine than at the hips because of the high center of mass. The man therefore has a greater tendency to bend with excessive lumbar flexion and limited pelvic rotation (Fig. 8-15). With repeated forward bending using this strategy over a lifetime, the hip joint is at risk for developing hypomobility in the direction of flexion, and the lumbar segments are at risk for becoming hypermobile in the direction of flexion. The hypermobility of the lumbar spine into flexion may be carried through other postures and movement patterns such as sitting, leaning forward in sitting, and the follow-through phase in serving the ball in tennis. Related impairments of muscle length and performance can result from impairments of movement and contribute to perpetuating and further exaggerating faulty movement.

Psychological Impairments

Emotional factors can affect posture and movement. For instance, a person's posture at the funeral of a loved one is different from that at a celebration of a happy occasion. A person with significant negative stresses (eg, divorce, death, illness) occurring simultaneously for long periods may develop profound changes in posture and movement. It is often beyond the scope of physical therapy practice to deal with profound or complex psychological impairments. Nonetheless, the physical therapist must be sensitive to the contribution emotional factors can have on posture and movement. If the physical therapist determines that the emotional state of the patient is inhibiting recovery of the posture or movement impairment, referral to an appropriate mental health practitioner is indicated. Physical therapy intervention may need to stop until the emotional state improves, or it can proceed if it is determined that continued intervention is beneficial to psychological recovery. Improved emotional status often improves posture and movement, and improved posture and movement can improve emotional status, particularly if the emotional status reflected a NMPSs that is resolving with physical therapy intervention.

Developmental Factors

Age affects posture and movement. Children are not expected to conform to an adult standard of posture and movement, primarily because the developing individual exhibits much greater mobility and flexibility than the adult.[16] Developmental deviations appear in many children at about the same age and improve or disappear without any corrective treatment, despite unfavorable environmental influences.[16] However, developmental deviations are perpetuated by habit in some persons. Repeated observation (not a single examination) can determine whether a developmental deviation is being perpetuated by habit. If the condition remains static or if the deviation increases, corrective measures are indicated. A young child (<5 years) is not likely to have habitual faults and can be harmed by corrective measures that are not needed. Any deviations considered severe require immediate attention, regardless of the age of the individual (Fig. 8-16).

Developmental changes occur in the feet, knees hips, pelvis, trunk, and shoulder girdle. Display 8-5 lists the common developmental deviations in children that should gradually diminish as the child reaches adolescence and adulthood.

The aging process can induce many postural and movement changes, primarily because of pathology or disease. The aging process manifests in minor neuromuscular changes, but in the absence of disease, the resulting impairments of posture and movement usually are no more exaggerated than in middle age. Continued attention to posture and movement patterns should minimize the effect of aging in an otherwise healthy individual.

Environmental Factors

The activities in which an individual participates and the surrounding environment may have favorable or adverse effects on posture and movement. The nature of the activities and the time spent doing them and whether the effect of habitual postures and movements during one activity are reinforced or counteracted by habitual positions or repeated movements in other activities determine the overall postural and movement effect. Stresses are put on the basic structures of the human body by increasingly specialized and limited or repetitive activity (eg, working endless hours at a

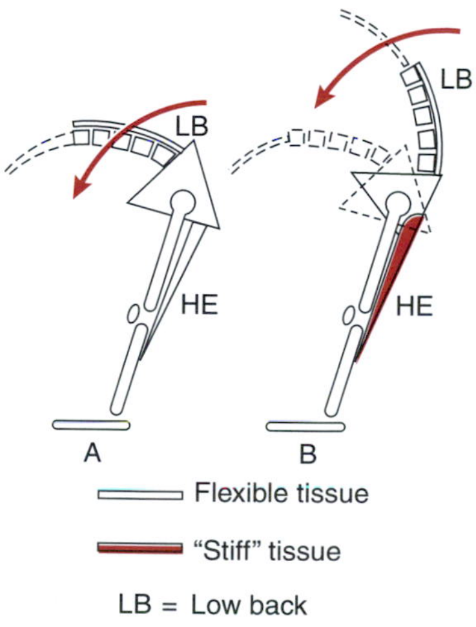

FIGURE 8-15 Faulty lumbopelvic rhythm has less movement of the pelvis relative to the hips. In men, this could result from the anthropometric characteristics of a heavy upper body relative to the lower body.

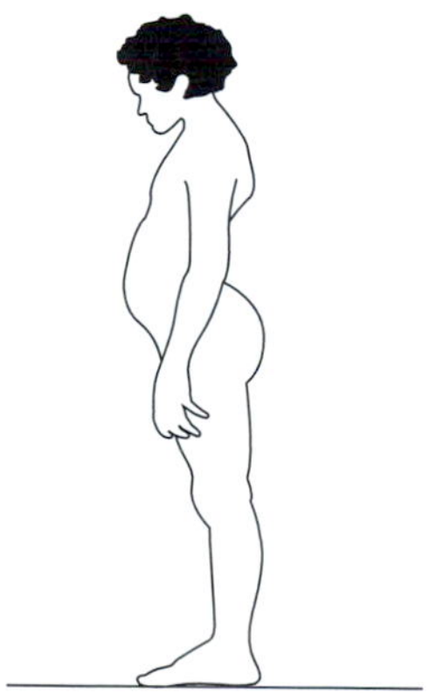

FIGURE 8-16 Severe developmental deviation. This amount of lordosis in an 8-year-old child is considered a severe developmental deviation necessitating intervention. A corset to support the abdomen is needed along with therapeutic exercises.

DISPLAY 8-5
Developmental Deviations in Posture

Feet
- Flat arches are normal in the small child.
- By age 6 or 7, expect good arch formation.

Knees
- Genu valgum is normal in a small child (about 2 inches between ankles is normal for an average-height child).
- By age 6 or 7, genu valgum should be diminished or gone.
- Postural genu varum in the school-age child is not acceptable, and corrective measures should be taken, because it is difficult to change in the young adult.
- Genu varum may be compensatory for genu valgum by hyperextension of the knees.

Hips
- Femur medial rotation is the most common and often result from hip anteversion, foot pronation, knee hyperextension, postural genu varum, and less often, genu valgum. Check for structural sources and treat with the appropriate corrective measures.
- By adolescence, the femur should be in near-neutral alignment.
- Femur lateral rotation is more common in young boys.
- Persistent lateral rotation should be treated, because it can be detrimental in adulthood.

Lumbopelvic Region
- A protruding abdomen is normal for a child.
- By the age of 10 to 12, the abdomen should no longer be protruding.
- Lordosis peaks at age 9 to 10 and should gradually diminish thereafter.
- Handedness patterns emerge in school age children, most commonly with the hip high and shoulder low on the dominant side. This should be monitored if it is borderline or excessive.

Shoulder Girdle
- Scapular tilting is normal in school age children.
- The prominence should diminish as the child approaches adolescence.

From Kendall HO, Kendall FP, Boynton DA. Posture and Pain. *Huntington, NY: Robert E. Krieger Publishing; 1970.*

computer display terminal, going home exhausted, sitting most evenings in a recliner chair in front of a television).

The activities of an individual must be considered as a whole in gauging their postural or movement effects. Concentration on one type of activity can ensure muscle imbalance, but a combination of activities may be almost as unfavorable if each involves the same kind of movement or position. For example, a person working at a video display terminal who engages in piano playing in her leisure time has no real change in the type of activity.

Several environmental factors, such as work stations, beds, pillows, car seats, school chairs and desks, and shoes, influence posture and movement. These environmental influences should be made as favorable as possible. When major adjustments cannot be made, small adjustments often help considerably. A discussion of environmental influences is not complete without reference to body mechanics related to lifting and carrying. These strategies should be examined and favorably modified as much as possible for the individual's circumstances.

INTERVENTION

Healthy, effective, and efficient posture and movement are an integral part of general well-being. Efficiency and longevity of the human biomechanical system requires maintenance of precise movement of the rotating segments. Good posture and movement are fundamental to health of the biomechanical system. Ideally, posture and movement instruction and training should become an integral part of any therapeutic intervention.

Although posture and movement alterations can each be considered as one type of impairment, they cannot be considered in the same way as impairment of muscle performance, muscle endurance, balance, or mobility. Impairment in posture and movement can be the result of many factors, including impairment of muscle performance, muscle endurance, balance, or mobility. To develop an efficient, effective intervention for the treatment of posture and movement impairment, all the functional limitations and the related impairments resulting from and contributing to posture and movement impairments should be understood. The effect of predisposing risk factors, previous interventions, and environmental influences should also be taken into consideration.

This chapter has presented a foundation for developing therapeutic exercise interventions to treat posture and movement impairments. The remainder is devoted to describing therapeutic exercise intervention for posture and movement according to the intervention model described in Chapter 2.

Elements of the Movement System and Other Systems

Any or all elements of the movement system can be involved directly or indirectly in the development of posture and movement impairments and therefore should be dealt with in treatment. Base and biomechanical elements usually require direct intervention for the correction of posture and movement impairments, whereas modulator elements are more critical to movement impairments than posture impairments. Impairments of the cognitive or affective element can limit the progress of an individual with posture or movement impairments. If this is the case, appropriate referral to a mental health practitioner may be required to reach the desired functional outcome. Impairments of the support element can affect posture and movement directly (ie, faulty breathing patterns or reduced energy for movement) or indirectly through oxygen transport deficits in systemic disease that contributes to further faults in posture and movement.[7] Display 8-6 provides examples of impairments of the elements of the movement system associated with posture and movement.

Other bodily systems may be involved directly or indirectly and should be considered if necessary to improve posture or movement. For example, a patient presents with posture and movement impairments about the hip with the comorbidity of urinary incontinence caused by pelvic floor weakness and estrogen depletion. Full correction of posture and movement impairments about the hip may not be achieved without attention to the pelvic floor dysfunction, which is caused by impairments of the musculoskeletal, urogenital, and endocrine systems. The link between the musculoskeletal system and urinary incontinence is discussed in Chapter 19. In this case, without considering the associated urogenital system problems and hormonal imbalance, the pelvic floor problem may not resolve, preventing optimal function of the pelvic floor muscles. Because two of the pelvic floor muscles are also used for hip function (ie, obturator internus and piriformis), dysfunction of the pelvic floor may contribute to posture and movement impairment of the hip, which may contribute to further pelvic floor dysfunction, and so on as the cycle continues. All the systems involved must be addressed to resolve the posture and movement impairment at the hip.

DISPLAY 8-6

Elements of the Movement System and Factors Contributing to Impairment Posture and Movement

Biomechanical Factors
- Anatomic impairments such as scoliosis or hip anteversion
- Physiologic impairments such as postural genu varum
- Anthropometric characteristics

Base
- Overstretched gluteus medius, contributing to high iliac crest and functional limb length discrepancy
- Easily fatigued serratus anterior, contributing to reduced scapular rotation with repetitive overhead activities
- Muscle strain, contributing to reduced activity level and altered movement patterns

Modulator Factors
- Reduced or loss of innervation of the gluteus maximus associated with hip hyperextension
- Tensor facia lata dominance during hip flexion, contributing to hip flexion with medial rotation
- Latent timing of the vastus medialis oblique, contributing to patellofemoral movement impairment

Support Factors
- Inappropriate breathing patterns associated with abnormal rib cage alignment and with rib and thoracic spine movement patterns

Cognitive or Affective Factors
- Depression associated with slumped posture or shuffling gait
- Upright posture associated with feeling proud
- Increased muscle tension associated with stress

Patient-Related Instruction and Adjunctive Interventions

Education regarding attention to postural alignment in frequently held or prolonged occupational or recreational positions is key to optimizing joint position for rest and function and reducing the tension placed on elongated muscles and increasing the tension placed on shortened muscles to restore muscle balance. Photographs of the patient in his typical rest posture and corrected posture can serve as powerful feedback for inducing change. Ergonomic modifications may be necessary to improve the patient's environment. If an on-site visit to the workplace is not feasible, a photograph of the workstation can be analyzed to provide suggestions for change. Other posture habits, including recumbent positions, can be analyzed and suggestions offered. Pillows under the head, under or between the knees, or under the waist in sidelying (Fig. 8-17) can be suggested to offer optimal support to body regions while in recumbent positions. Footwear is another topic about which the physical therapist can provide recommendations (see Chapter 22).

Adjunctive interventions such as supportive devices (eg, corsets, bracing, orthotics, taping) can be used temporarily to assist in creating length-associated and proprioceptive changes or used permanently to provide partial or complete correction of anatomic impairments contributing to posture and movement impairment. For example, taping an be used temporarily in the thoracic region to provide proprioceptive input for a patient about his kyphotic posture (Fig. 8-18). Every time the patient moves into excessive thoracic flexion, the tape serves as a reminder. Conversely, a permanent supportive device such as a corrective orthotic may be necessary to improve alignment throughout the kinetic chain and gait kinetics and kinematics in an individual with structural forefoot varus.

Activity and Dosage

Numerous activities or techniques can be chosen to restore healthy and efficient posture and movement:

- Stretching short muscles, improving extensibility of stiff muscular-fascial tissues
- Strengthening weak and elongated muscles
- Body mechanics and ergonomics training

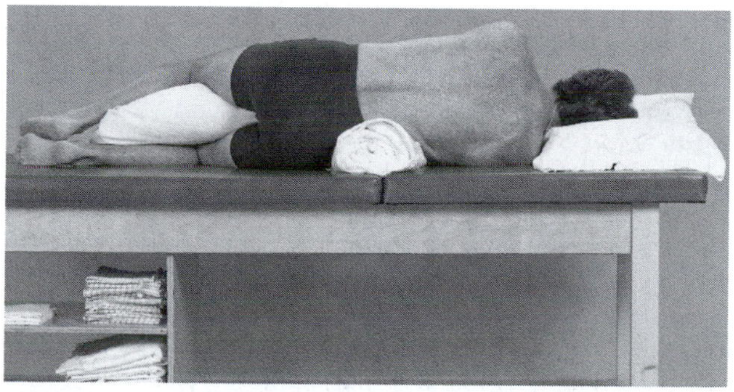

FIGURE 8-17 The use of pillows under the head, under the waist, and between the knees can position the spine in optimal alignment in sidelying.

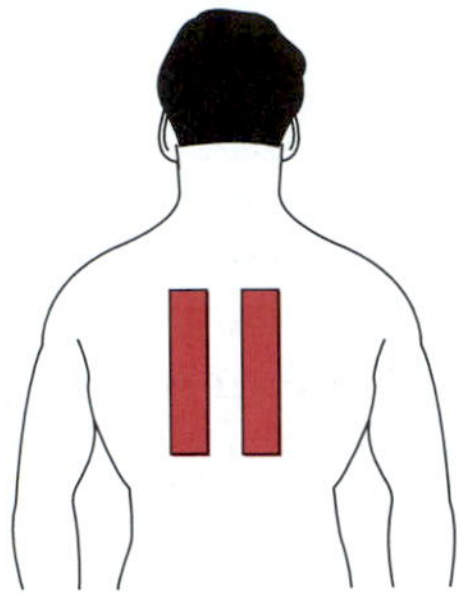

FIGURE 8-18 Taping along the thoracic spine can serve as biofeedback to discourage excessive thoracic flexion. The tape is best applied with the patient in a quadriped position, with the thoracic spine in a flat position.

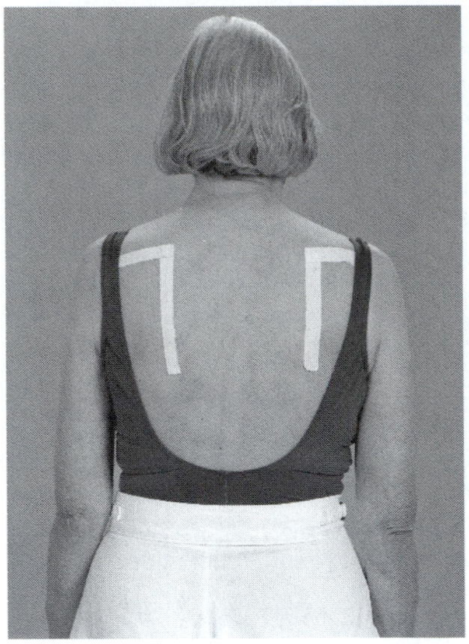

FIGURE 8-19 Although minimal, this figure illustrates abduction and downward rotation of the left scapula relative to the right.

- Neuromuscular re-education
- Breathing exercises
- Aerobic and muscular endurance activities
- Aquatic exercise
- Balance and coordination training
- Posture awareness training
- Movement training
- Developmental activities

Numerous interventions can affect posture and movement. Because posture and movement are components of the intervention model, every activity or technique should promote optimal posture and movement. No activity or technique should compromise kinesiologic standards of posture and movement unless modification is necessary as a result of the condition, such as anatomic impairments or permanent loss of muscle function.

Identifying and prioritizing the elements of the movement system, combined with knowledge of the physiologic status of the component impairments, can help to determine the activities or techniques needed, including the posture, movement, and mode parameters. Dosage parameters depend on the component impairment, stage of motor control, and physiologic status of the tissue being addressed.

To illustrate these points, consider a patient with a mild lower trapezius strain with abducted and downwardly rotated scapulae at rest (Fig. 8-19) and excessive scapular abduction and anterior tilt during horizontal forward reaching activities. Prevention of these impairments is preferable, and there should be careful scrutiny of any posture, activity, or technique that allows overstretching of soft tissues. The ideal length of ligaments and muscles helps to maintain ideal posture alignment with a minimum of muscular effort, and when muscles and ligaments become overstretched, they fail to offer adequate support, the joint exceeds the normal range, and the posture becomes faulty or muscular effort increases to maintain ideal alignment. In this case, it is possible that the lower trapezius is strained by overstretching and that postural and movement patterns perpetuate this condition. Treatment of base and biomechanical elements is indicated.

In addition to posture awareness training and ergonomic modifications to address the biomechanical element, taping can be used to support the scapula in improved alignment (see Chapter 26). This approach also affects the base element by supporting the lower trapezius in the short range, thereby alleviating tension to allow healing and improve length-tension properties.

Combining attention to base and modulator elements is more powerful than focusing on either technique alone. With respect to the base element, the goal is to alter length-tension properties of the lower trapezius. This impairment is often overlooked but is critical to achieving muscle balance to restore healthy and efficient posture and movement. The tendency may be to stretch the opposing short pectoralis minor and major (also contributing to impairment of scapula posture and movement). However, if attention is focused only on stretching the short muscle without shortening the lengthened muscle, equilibrium about the joint can never be achieved. If the hip flexors are stretched in an individual with an anterior pelvic tilt and lordosis without adaptively shortening the abdominal muscles (see Chapter 18), the pelvis does not assume a neutral position in relaxed standing.

One activity that may be useful in this situation is to strengthen the adaptively lengthened muscles in the shortened range. The premise of this intervention strategy is to improve the strength of the lengthened muscle in the short range, where it has the greatest difficulty creating tension. If the focus of the exercise is on strengthening without attention to the ability to create tension in the shortened range, the exercise may reinforce the muscle imbalance by increasing the strength in the lengthened range. Careful decisions must be made regarding the stage of motor control, posture, mode, movement, and dosage parameters to provide the optimal stimulus for strengthening without overloading the target muscle or promoting substitution of a dominant synergist (ie, upper trapezius) or antagonist (ie, pectoralis minor or major). The physiologic status of the tissue (ie, length-associated changes and degree of strain) must be considered when determining each of these parameters.

Stability may be the starting point for the stage of motor control because strengthening is the chosen activity and specificity is critical. Shortening the lever arm and exercising in a gravity-lessened position may be necessary for optimal strengthening (see Fig. 26-26 in Chap. 26). As the muscle becomes stronger in the shortened range, lengthening the lever arm and exercising against gravity can modify the exercise. Submaximal isometric contractions in the short range may be ideal initially, moving toward concentric-eccentric contractions throughout the range as the muscle heals, length-tension properties improve, and muscle performance can substantiate participation in the force couple. After stability is attained, the exercise can be progressed to controlled mobility and skill, with ultimate progression to functional movement patterns involving the total body as the final goal.

Dosage should follow the guidelines for strength training to improve muscle performance capability and generate hypertrophy of the lower trapezius to provide counterbalancing stiffness to the antagonists, the pectoralis major and minor. Eventually, endurance dosage parameters can be applied as more functional movements are incorporated.

Simultaneous stretching of the pectoralis minor and major can be prescribed to augment the improved posture and movement changes. It may also be necessary to address breathing patterns if it is determined that the pectoralis minor is stiff because of overuse as an accessory muscle of respiration. Stretching addresses the base element, and breathing addresses the support element. Both of these interventions can begin at the mobility stage of motor control, progressing somewhat parallel to that for the lower trapezius toward controlled mobility and skill.

Ultimately, the isolated joint function of optimal movements of the scapula must be incorporated into total-body movement patterns (ie, controlled mobility and skill). When this stage is appropriate, movement impairments of related areas may emerge. Perhaps the scapula abducts during horizontal forward movements because of a lack of hip flexion during reaching patterns or a lack of thoracic or hip rotation during cross-body reaching patterns. The related areas may require intervention to restore normal function to the shoulder girdle.

Key Points

- Other physiologic impairments can contribute to and perpetuate impairments in posture and movement.
- Evaluation of posture and movement impairment requires identification of deviations in posture and movement from acceptable standards and assessment of contributing factors such as other physiologic impairments and environmental, structural, developmental, and emotional factors.
- Therapeutic exercise intervention for posture and movement impairment involves prioritization of the elements of the movement system and related impairments, careful determination of the appropriate activities or techniques and stage of motor control, and accurate prescription of dosage parameters for a successful outcome.
- Successful treatment of impaired posture and movement can directly affect the kinesiopathologic pattern responsible for the development, perpetuation, or recurrence of NMPSs.

Critical Thinking Questions

1. How are posture and movement impairments related to NMPSs?
2. Define ideal posture as it relates to surface landmarks from a side view.
3. Consider Case Study #9 in Unit 7.
   a. Given this patient's posture alignment, what muscles would you predict to be too long? What muscles would you predict to be too short?
   b. List the base, modulator, and biomechanical elements of the movement system that contribute to her movement impairment.
   c. Develop an initial list of exercises, posture education, and movement retraining for this patient. Progress one of the listed exercises with respect to the stages of motor control.

LAB ACTIVITIES

1. Assess your laboratory partner's posture from the side and back views. Given your partner's alignment, which muscles would you predict to be too long or short?
2. Design an exercise program that stretches muscles that may be too short and strengthens muscles that are too long.
3. Assess your partner's strategy of rising from sit to stand. Break the movement into component parts. Assess the feet, ankles, knees, hips, pelvis, and lumbar, thoracic, and cervical spine about all three axes of motion during each component of the movement.
4. How would you provide feedback to change your partner's motor control strategy in rising from sit to stand? What verbal, tactile, and visual cues would you provide? What base element impairments may be contributing to the movement impairment?
5. Assess your partner's strategy of balancing on one limb. How does your partner move his center of mass over the base of support? What happens at the foot, knee, hip, pelvis, and spine? Do you think your partner uses a correct strategy? If not, what is faulty? Is one side different from the other? What contributing factors may be responsible for the faulty movement strategy?

REFERENCES

1. Herring SA, Nilson KL. Introduction to overuse injuries. *Clin Sports Med.* 1987;6:225–239.
2. Leadbetter WB. Cell-matrix response in tendon injury. *Clin Sports Med.* 1992;11:533–578.
3. Janda V. On the concept of postural muscles and posture in man. *Aust J Physiother.* 1983;29:83–84.
4. Posture Committee of the American Academy of Orthopedic Surgeons. Posture and its relationship to orthopedic disabilities: a report of the Posture Committee of the American Academy of Orthopedic Surgeons. Evanston, IL: American Academy of Orthopedic Surgeons; 1947:1.
5. Hobson L, Hammon WE. Chest assessment. In: Frownfelter D, ed. *Chest Physical Therapy and Pulmonary Rehabilitation.* St. Louis: Mosby; 1987:147–197.
6. Bates DV. *Respiratory Function in Disease.* 3rd ed. Philadelphia: WB Saunders; 1989.
7. Dean E. Oxygen transport deficits in systemic disease and implications for physical therapy. *Phys Ther.* 1997;77:187–202.
8. Johnson F, Leitl S, Waugh W. The distribution of the load across the knee: a comparison of static and dynamic measurements. *J Bone Joint Surg Br.* 1980;62:3.
9. Norkin C, Levangie P. *Joint Structure and Function.* 2nd ed. Philadelphia: FA Davis; 1992.
10. Kendall FP, McCreary EK, Provance PG. *Muscles Testing and Function.* Baltimore: Williams & Wilkins; 1993.
11. Nordin M, Frankel VH. *Basic Biomechanics of the Musculoskeletal System.* Malvern, PA: Lea & Febiger; 1989.
12. Sahrmann SA. *Diagnosis and Exercise Management of Musculoskeletal Pain Syndromes.* St. Louis: Mosby (in press).
13. Bagg SD, Forest WJ. A biomechanical analysis of scapular rotation during arm abduction in the scapular plane. *Am J Phys Med Rehabil.* 1988;67:238–235.
14. Frankel VH, Burstein AH, Brooks DB. Biomechanics of internal derangement of the knee. *J Bone Joint Surg.* 1971;53: 945–962.
15. Wiktorin CH, Nordin M. *Introduction to Problem Solving in Biomechanics.* Philadelphia: Lea & Febiger; 1982.
16. Kendall HO, Kendall FP, Boynton DA. *Posture and Pain.* Huntington, NY: Robert E. Krieger Publishing; 1970.
17. Steindler A. *Kinesiology of the Human Body Under Normal and Pathological Conditions.* Springfield, IL: Charles C. Thomas; 1955.
18. Sarhmann SA. Diagnosis and treatment of muscle imbalances and associated regional musculoskeletal pain syndromes [course notes]. St. Louis, MO; Washington University, Program in Physical Therapy; 1996.
19. Hodges PW, Richardson CA. Contraction of the abdominal muscles associated with movement of the lower limb. *Phys Ther.* 1997;77:132–144.
20. Williams PE, Goldspink G. Changes in sarcomere length and physiological properties in immobilized muscle. *J Anat.* 1978; 127:459–468.
21. Walker ML, Rothstein JM, Finucane SD, Lamb RL. Relationships between lumbar lordosis, pelvic tilt, and abdominal performance. *Phys Ther.* 1987;67:512–516.
22. Gossman MR, Sahrmann SA, Rose SJ. Review of length-associated changes in muscle, experimental and clinical implications. *Phys Ther.* 1982;62:1799–1808.
23. Tabary JC, Tabury C, Taradiew C, et al. Physiological and structural changes in the cat's soleus muscle due to immobilization at different lengths by plaster casts. *J Physiol.* 1972; 224:231.
24. Goldspink G. Development of muscle. In: Goldspink G, ed. *Growth of Cells in Vertebrate Tissues.* London: Chapman & Hall; 1974:69–99.
25. Basmajian JV, DeLuca CJ. *Muscles Alive.* Baltimore: Williams & Wilkins; 1985.
26. Caillet R. *Low Back Syndrome.* Philadelphia: FA Davis; 1981.

CHAPTER 9

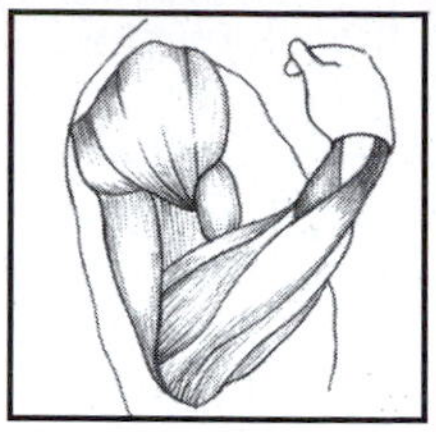

Pain

Lori Thein Brody

Pain is a psychosomatic experience that is affected by cultural, historical, environmental, and social factors. Unlike impairments such as motion or strength loss that can be observed and measured with tools such as goniometers and dynamometers, pain is elusive. Although limited motion produces observable functional limitations or disability, pain produces functional limitations and disability that are not always observable by the outsider. This situation produces anxiety for the patient and can be a source of conflict with spouses, family members, friends, and coworkers. The clinician must recognize the impact of pain on the patient and provide her with strategies to manage the pain.

PHYSIOLOGY OF PAIN

Pain is a complex sensory experience. The physiology of pain is far too complex to be covered in detail in this text. However, a brief overview can give the clinician an understanding of the physiology of pain and the interventions used to treat it.

Sources of Pain

Pain is a component of most musculoskeletal conditions seen in the clinic. Acute pain is associated with muscle strains, tendinitis, contusions, or ligament injuries. Although it is important to acknowledge and treat acute pain, it is usually short lived. Most individuals can tolerate this type of pain because they know that it is temporary. Acute pain is often successfully treated with nonnarcotic analgesics such as nonsteroidal anti-inflammatory drugs (NSAIDs) and modalities such as ice.

Chronic pain is not short lived and produces profound changes in the physical, psychological, and social aspects of the patient's life. Chronic pain typically is a major component of problems such as fibromyalgia, chronic fatigue syndrome, myofascial pain syndrome, rheumatoid arthritis, and low back pain. Physical therapy focuses on treating the pain, the motion and muscle impairments, and the functional limitations and disability that result.

ACUTE PAIN

Acute pain results from microtraumatic or macrotraumatic tissue injury. Microtrauma is defined as a long-standing or recurrent musculoskeletal problem that was not initiated by an acute injury. Macrotrauma is defined as an immediately noticeable injury involving sudden, direct or indirect trauma.[1] Microtrauma is exemplified by the overuse injury in which repetitive activity exceeds the tissue's ability to repair and remodel according to the imposed loads. The athlete playing in a weekend tennis tournament and the worker putting in overtime are prone to microtraumatic injuries. Macrotrauma can produce pain through direct injury of tissues. Joint dislocations injure the joint capsule and periarticular connective tissue, and ligament or tendon injuries damage the respective collagenous tissues. Microtrauma and macrotrauma result in an inflammatory response that secondarily produces pain. Macrotrauma also produces pain directly through damage to the nociceptors.

CHRONIC PAIN

Chronic pain is pain that persists after the noxious stimulus has been removed. It includes persistent pain after healing of an acute injury and pain with no known cause. Chronic pain has strong psychological, emotional, and sociologic effects. Individuals with chronic pain tend to have significant sleep disturbances, depressive symptoms, appetite changes, and decreased activity and socialization.

Theories about the source of chronic pain suggest increased sensitization of nociceptors and spinal level changes that perpetuate positive feedback loops in the pain-spasm cycle.[2] Pain from inflammation in conditions such as osteoarthritis and rheumatoid arthritis sensitizes dorsal horn neurons to the inflammation. After inflammation of a joint or muscle, afferent input to the spinal cord increases the activity of the dorsal horn, spinothalamic tract, and thalamic neurons. The elevated activity increases the frequency of background firing of dorsal horn neurons and increases sensitivity to noxious and non-noxious peripheral stimulation and joint motion. When damage to the central nociceptive system occurs, nonnociceptive afferent activity becomes capable of eliciting pain.[3] Stimuli that were previously innocuous become painful. Moreover, the peripheral receptive field of dorsal horn neurons increases.[4] The pain seems to spread from the originally painful area to adjacent areas. The basis for some of these changes may be an increased sensitization of wide dynamic range (WDR) neurons from nociceptive input, causing them to respond more intensely to more nonnociceptive input and to afferent input from a larger area.[3] The increase in receptive field area, increased background firing, and increased sensitivity to mechanical stimuli after acute or chronic inflammation may set the stage for chronic pain that seems to spread along a limb or to adjacent areas.

REFERRED PAIN

Referred pain is pain felt at a site far distant from the location of the injury or disease. Referred pain is considered to be an error in perception. For example, pain originating from deep visceral tissues may refer to the cutaneous region with the same segmental innervation. Pain originating from the genitourinary system may refer to the low back because of the common T11-L2 segmental origin. Cardiac pain refers to the shoulder because of the common T1-T2 segments. As afferent input from the visceral receptors synapse in the dorsal horn, information is also incoming from skin afferents. Convergence of this incoming information in the dorsal horn results in the sense that the pain is originating from the skin. This same principle underlies the use of electrical stimulation at remote sites to decrease visceral pain.

Pain Pathways

Pain is transmitted from nociceptor and nonnociceptor afferents in the periphery. Nociceptors are defined as pain receptors that transfer impulses to the spinal cord and higher central nervous system (CNS) levels. Nociceptors in the periphery are activated by mechanical stimuli such as strong pressure, irritants such as chemicals (eg, bradykinin, substance P, histamine), or noxious elements such as heat and cold.

Nociceptors in peripheral tissues transmit pain information through A-delta and C fibers. A-delta fibers are small, myelinated fibers carrying information about pain and temperature. The information is carried to the spinal cord at an approximate speed of 15 m/s.[5] The A-delta fibers are most responsive to mechanical stimuli and probably are responsible for the sensation of pain in acute injuries. Type C fibers are slow, unmyelinated fibers carrying information about dull aching or burning pain from polymodal receptors. **Polymodal receptors** are receptors that respond to a variety of stimuli such as temperature and pressure. Type C polymodal fibers are found in the deeper layers of skin and in virtually all other tissues except the nervous system itself. They are also known as "free nerve endings" and are responsive to thermal, chemical, and mechanical stimuli. C fibers probably are responsible for the continued sensation of pain after the noxious stimulus has been removed. Transmission speed to the spinal cord is approximately 1 m/s.

At the spinal cord level, A-delta fibers enter the dorsal roots and ascend and descend several segments before entering the gray matter. These fibers terminate in the substantia gelatinosa on the cells of laminae I and V. The slower C fibers also enter the dorsal root and then enter the gray matter and synapse at the level of entry or ascend or descend a level or two before entering the substantia gelatinosa at laminae II and III. Some processing of information occurs in the spinal cord before the information is transmitted to higher levels.

Three types of interneurons within the dorsal horn are categorized by their response to peripheral stimulation: low-threshold mechanosensitive, responding only to innocuous stimuli such as touching the skin; nociceptive specific, responding only to high-threshold noxious stimuli; and WDR, responding to a wide variety of noxious and non-noxious stimuli. Changes in the firing patterns of the WDR interneurons are suggested as an underlying cause of chronic pain, and convergence of stimuli from various receptors in the dorsal horn is the theoretical basis underlying the gate control theory. This convergence also may be the source of referred pain. Substance P is a neuromodulator shown to be responsible for the transmission of noxious information in the spinal cord.[4]

From the dorsal horn, these signals ascend through the contralateral spinothalamic tract in the ventrolateral white matter of the spinal cord to the ventral posterolateral nucleus of the thalamus. The spinothalamic tract transmits noxious and thermal information. The spinothalamic tract also sends collateral branches to the periadqueductal gray (PAG) nucleus of the brain stem. Synapses in this pathway are morphine sensitive and are an important component of the pain-modulating system. Stimulation of the PAG nucleus has produced analgesia. The thalamus is capable of some conscious awareness of pain before this information reaches the postcentral gyrus of the cerebral cortex.[6] In addition to the spinothalamic tract, some noxious stimuli ascend in the ipsilateral dorsal column of the spinomedullary system.

Descending impulses also influence pain perception. The individual who continues to play sports despite a broken bone or the grandmother who lifts a car to save a child are examples of these descending influences at work. These systems are complex, and the relationships of the system components are being investigated. An overview is given to explain the rationale for some pain control interventions.

Descending pain control occurs through opiate and nonopiate systems. Release of endogenous opiates from the brain stem related to exercise has achieved widespread publicity in the popular press. The "runners high" that occurs with long-distance running has been attributed to the release of β-endorphin and methionine-enkephalin from CNS higher centers. Location of these opiates varies among the periaqueductal gray, hypothalamus, thalamus, substantia gelatinosa, and midbrain structures.[2] Input to the enkephalinergic interneurons in the substantia gelatinosa comes from fibers descending from the midbrain (ie, PAG) that use serotonin as the transmitter. Injection of opiates into the spinal cord inhibits noxious stimulus–elicited dorsal horn neuron activity.[2] Other neurons descending from the midbrain use noradrenaline as their transmitter and provide an analgesic action through direct inhibition of dorsal horn nociceptive neurons, rather than through the enkephalin-ergic interneurons.[5] Continued research in the area of descending influences may provide more effective pain control interventions in the future.

Pain Theory

Melzack and Wall proposed the gate theory of pain in 1965, with revisions added in 1982.[2] This theory replaced previously held pain theories such as the specificity and patterning theories.[2] The cornerstone of the gate theory is the convergence of first-order neurons and associated second-order neurons within the substantia gelatinosa (Fig. 9-1). The system has four components consisting of afferent neurons, internuncial neurons within the substantia gelatinosa, transmission cells (T cells), and descending control from higher centers.[7] The activity of T cells is regulated by the balance of large- and small-diameter fiber input from the periphery and by descending control from higher cells. This balance regulates the transmission of pain information.

The substantia gelatinosa modulates incoming information (ie, regulates position of the gate) presynaptically, before information is passed to second-order neurons. When incoming information increases substantia gelatinosa activity, presynaptic inhibition occurs, closing the gate. Information is not passed from first- to second-order neurons for further transmission to higher centers. If peripheral receptors associated with large-diameter myelinated fibers are stimulated, activity in the substantia gelatinosa may close the gate to the slower C fiber pain information transmission.

This theory provides the rationale for interventions to "close the gate" to pain transmission. Several peripheral stimuli can close the gate to pain. Input from thermal modalities such as heat and cold can successfully decrease pain. When thermal impulses are transmitted, the input can "block" pain transmission from slower fibers at the substantia gelatinosa. Electrical impulses from transcutaneous electrical nerve stimulation (TENS) application can preferentially block pain impulse transmission (discussed in the Adjunctive Therapies section). Exercise can successfully decrease pain by stimulation of joint afferent receptors. These signals travel along A-beta fibers, which have larger diameters and carry information at higher speeds (30 to 70 m/s) than the slower pain fibers. This same mechanical stimulation of peripheral receptors can be achieved through tissue massage. Further revision of the gate theory of pain continues, because descending control from higher centers also influences the transmission of pain information.

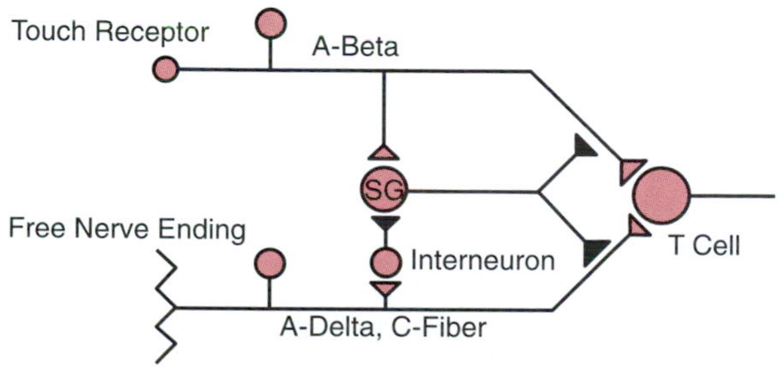

FIGURE 9-1 The gate control theory of paint. T Cells = central transmission cells; SG = substantia gelatinosa.

EXAMINATION OR EVALUATION

A variety of tools help the clinician assess and monitor the patient's pain level. Tools such as the McGill Pain Questionnaire (MPQ) assess affective qualities of pain, and the visual analog scale (VAS) is a nominal scale assessing pain intensity. Because of the multifaceted nature of pain, assessment should include information on the pain's intensity, location, and pattern over a 24-hour period (ie, quantity of pain) and descriptors assessing the affective aspects (ie, quality of pain). The impact of pain (ie, functional limitations and disability) on the patient's life should be determined.

Clinicians perform examinations to determine the source of the patient's pain. This examination directs the subsequent treatment program to the source of pain. Structures within the musculoskeletal system have different levels of pain sensitivity. The periosteum of the bone is a highly pain-sensitive structure, whereas the joint capsule, ligaments, tendons, and muscle are less pain sensitive. Fibrocartilage and articular cartilage are not pain sensitive structures, although injury or damage to these structures can produce a synovitis that results in pain. The clinician should perform an evaluation to determine the source of the pain and to assess the characteristics of that pain.

Pain Scales

The VAS and a 0 (least pain) to 10 (worst pain) scale are used to assess pain intensity. The simplest clinical tool consists of asking the patient to rate her pain on a 0 to 10 scale and recording this in the medical record. Follow-up visits ask the same question to determine the response to treatment. This type of scale has advantages and disadvantages. The clearest advantage is the ease of use. The patient is not burdened with forms to fill out or multiple questions to answer. Language and cultural barriers do not affect the use of this simple scale. The disadvantage is the minimal information acquired with such a tool. Only pain intensity information is gathered. Information regarding the affective aspects of pain, pattern of pain, and the impact of the pain on the patient's life are not included. The patient is likely to remember the previous pain score, which reduces the reliability of this type of measurement. This type of scale presumes equal intervals between each level (ie, the difference between a 1 and a 2 is equal to the difference between a 3 and a 4), and this may not be the case for the patient.

The VAS can be administered in several different forms (Fig. 9-2). A line with words placed at intervals along the line commonly is used. A single word may be used at each end, such as "no pain" and "worst pain," or several words may be placed along the continuum. The more words and lines divide the continuum, the more the patient is likely to recall previous answers. Like the simple 0 to 10 scale, the VAS is easy to administer and is not limited by cultural or language barriers, but it provides a minimal amount of information. When using a VAS, the reliability can be improved by eliminating division marks and only marking both ends of the scale. The patient then places a mark along the scale corresponding to her current pain level. The distance

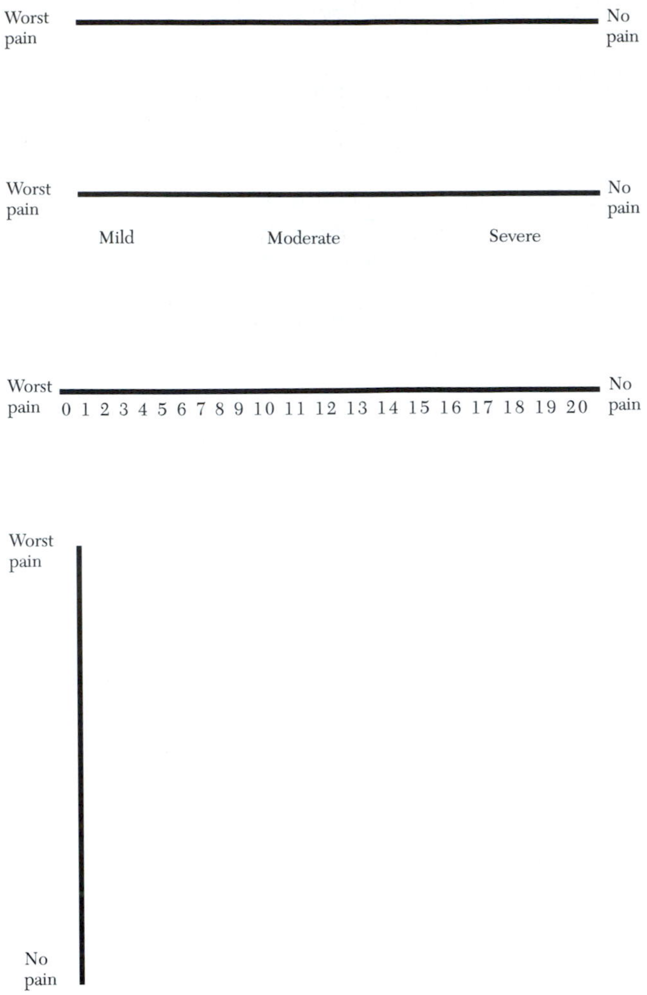

FIGURE 9-2 Variations of a visual analog scale.

from the left or right can be measured to assess progress. The direction of the scale should be altered occasionally. Reversing the "no pain" and "worst pain" sides of the scale or turning the scale from horizontal to vertical can minimize patient recall.[8] These scales should be accompanied by other assessments, including location of pain (using a body diagram) and subjective descriptions of the quality of pain (see Fig. 9-2).

McGill Pain Questionnaire

The MPQ is one of the most widely used tests for the measurement of pain, and several forms of the questionnaire have been developed.[9–11] This pain questionnaire consists primarily of three classes of word descriptors to assess the subjective aspects of pain. The MPQ also contains an intensity score, a body diagram, and an assessment of pain relative to activities and pain patterns. The three major measures are the pain rating index (PRI), the number of words chosen (NWC), and the present pain intensity (PPI).

Part one contains word descriptors classified as three categories (ie, sensory, affective, and evaluative) and 20 subcategories. Subcategories contain two to six words that are qualitatively similar but of increasing intensity. For example, one subcategory assesses the thermal aspects of pain through the descriptors "hot," "burning," "scalding," and "searing." Each word is assigned a numeric value. The patient is allowed to choose only one word from each subcategory and is not required to select an item from every category. The values are summed and the mean determined; the mean is the PRI score. The total number of subcategories selected is summed as the NWC score (Fig. 9-3).

The PPI is determined by use of a five-point scale, asking about the current pain level and the level of pain when it is at its worst and at its best. The PPI is the current pain level.

Part two categorizes the pattern of pain as constant, periodic, or brief and asks about activities that increase or relieve pain. A body diagram allows the patient to mark where the pain is located. The patient marks *E* for external pain and *I* for internal pain and then uses a VAS to document the quantity of pain.

The MPQ better assesses the many dimensions of pain with greater sensitivity than a VAS. The disadvantage is the time required to complete the questionnaire. A short form of the MPQ has been developed to address this issue.

Disability and Health-Related Quality of Life Scales

A variety of tools have been developed to assess pain and the impact of pain and resulting disability on patients' lives. Most tools broadly assess physical, social, and psychological function. Some tools assess health perceptions, satisfaction, and various impairments. Each tool taps these domains in a different way and at a different level. The tool must be matched to the population of interest.

The scales are classified in several ways but are broadly categorized into disease-specific and generic measures. Disease-specific scales are specific to a particular disease and are more responsive to issues of that population. Generic tools are applied across a variety of disease categories; the information has little relevance to a specific disease, and other important issues may not be tapped. However, use of these tools allows comparisons among disease or injury categories.

Commonly used generic tools are the Quality of Well-Being scale (QWB), the Sickness Impact Profile (SIP), the Duke Health Profile (DUKE), and the Short Form-36 (SF-36). The QWB taps six health concepts (ie, physical functioning, mental health including psychological distress, social or role functioning, mobility or travel, and physical or physiologic symptoms), and the SIP measures 12 concepts. Neither of these tools assesses pain directly. The DUKE measures seven health concepts, including self-esteem, health perceptions, and pain. The SF-36 is a derivative of the Medical Outcomes Study-149, a 149-item tool used as a generic assessment. The SF-36 is a 36-item tool measuring seven health concepts, including pain. The clinician must use caution when choosing a generic health assessment tool to ensure that critical parameters are being measured. The tool's range must allow for improvement or decline in the patient's status without exceeding the upper or lower limits of the measure (Fig. 9-4).

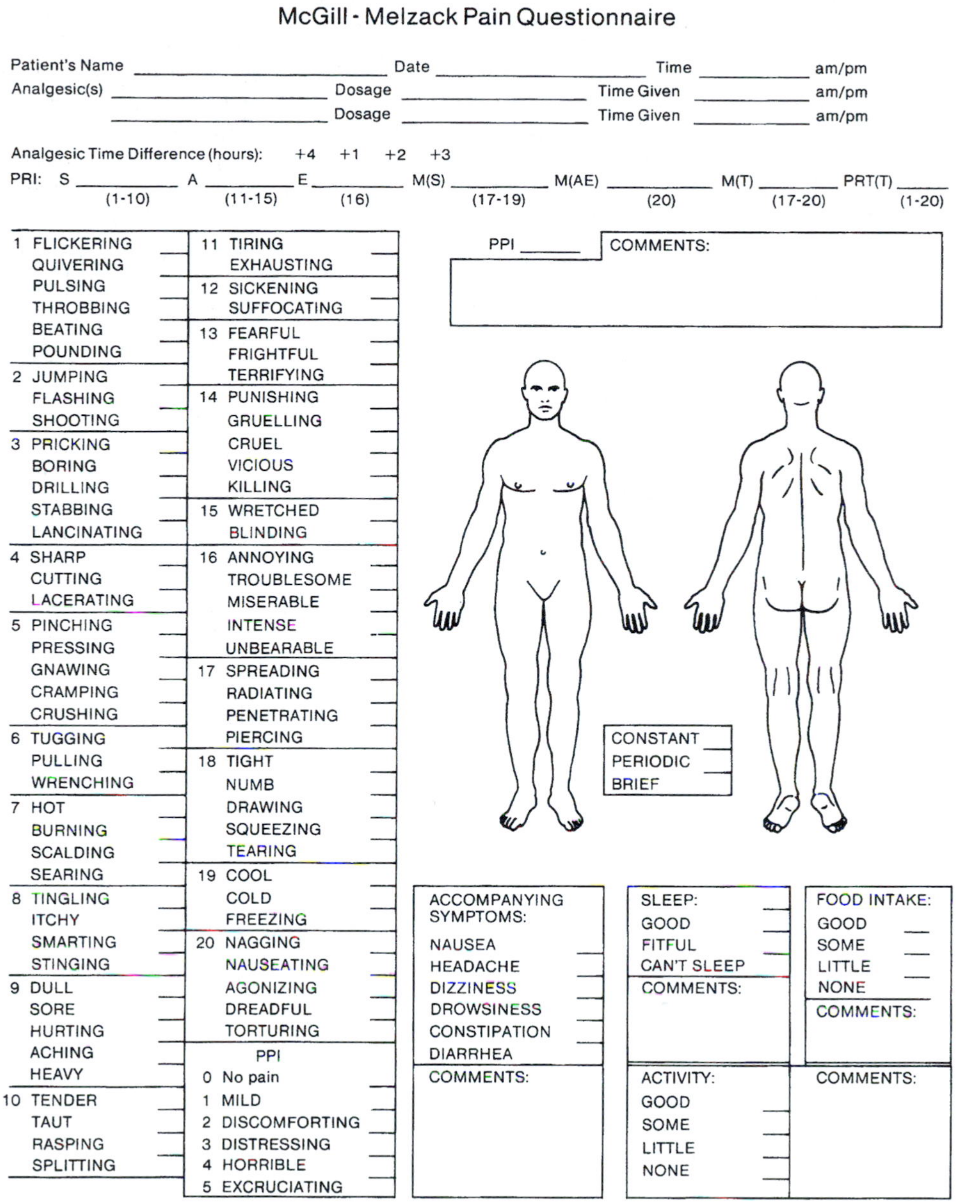

McGill - Melzack Pain Questionnaire

Patient's Name ______ Date ______ Time ______ am/pm
Analgesic(s) ______ Dosage ______ Time Given ______ am/pm
Dosage ______ Time Given ______ am/pm

Analgesic Time Difference (hours): +4 +1 +2 +3

PRI: S ______ (1-10) A ______ (11-15) E ______ (16) M(S) ______ (17-19) M(AE) ______ (20) M(T) ______ (17-20) PRT(T) ______ (1-20)

1 FLICKERING, QUIVERING, PULSING, THROBBING, BEATING, POUNDING
2 JUMPING, FLASHING, SHOOTING
3 PRICKING, BORING, DRILLING, STABBING, LANCINATING
4 SHARP, CUTTING, LACERATING
5 PINCHING, PRESSING, GNAWING, CRAMPING, CRUSHING
6 TUGGING, PULLING, WRENCHING
7 HOT, BURNING, SCALDING, SEARING
8 TINGLING, ITCHY, SMARTING, STINGING
9 DULL, SORE, HURTING, ACHING, HEAVY
10 TENDER, TAUT, RASPING, SPLITTING
11 TIRING, EXHAUSTING
12 SICKENING, SUFFOCATING
13 FEARFUL, FRIGHTFUL, TERRIFYING
14 PUNISHING, GRUELLING, CRUEL, VICIOUS, KILLING
15 WRETCHED, BLINDING
16 ANNOYING, TROUBLESOME, MISERABLE, INTENSE, UNBEARABLE
17 SPREADING, RADIATING, PENETRATING, PIERCING
18 TIGHT, NUMB, DRAWING, SQUEEZING, TEARING
19 COOL, COLD, FREEZING
20 NAGGING, NAUSEATING, AGONIZING, DREADFUL, TORTURING

PPI
0 No pain
1 MILD
2 DISCOMFORTING
3 DISTRESSING
4 HORRIBLE
5 EXCRUCIATING

PPI ______ COMMENTS:

CONSTANT
PERIODIC
BRIEF

ACCOMPANYING SYMPTOMS: NAUSEA, HEADACHE, DIZZINESS, DROWSINESS, CONSTIPATION, DIARRHEA
COMMENTS:

SLEEP: GOOD, FITFUL, CAN'T SLEEP
COMMENTS:

FOOD INTAKE: GOOD, SOME, LITTLE, NONE
COMMENTS:

ACTIVITY: GOOD, SOME, LITTLE, NONE
COMMENTS:

FIGURE 9-3 The McGill-Melzack Pain Questionnaire (From: Melzack, R. The McGill Pain Questionnaire: major properties and sourcing methods. *Pain.* 1975;1: 277–299.)

One way to minimize some of the potential problems associated with generic tools is to use a disease-specific tool. The Oswestry Low Back Disability Questionnaire, the Waddell Disability Index, and the Disability Questionnaire are used for individuals with back pain, and the McMaster-Toronto Arthritis Patient Reference Disability Questionnaire, the Arthritis Impact Measurement Scales (AIMS), the Health Assessment Questionnaire, and the Functional Capacity Questionnaire are used for individuals with arthritis. As with generic tools, disease-specific tools must match the population tested. Reliability of the tool must be determined for the population being evaluated. For example, if the AIMS reliability has been established for Caucasian women who are 65 or older, it is questionable whether this tool can be applied to men between the ages of 40 and 60 (Fig. 9-5).

Generic and disease-specific tools can be administered together to strengthen the information obtained. For example, the SF-36 may be combined with the Oswestry Low Back Disability Questionnaire for individuals with low back pain. A major concern about combination application is the burden placed on the patient who must fill out a number of questionnaires.

TREATMENT OF PAIN IMPAIRMENT

Although many commonalities exist, the approach to treating acute pain differs from the approach to chronic pain. Some combination of exercise and modalities are used; specific choices depend on the patient's circumstances. The treatment program should be tailored to each patient and be responsive to the pain pattern.

(text continues on page 153)

SF-36 HEALTH SURVEY

Instructions: This survey asks for your views about your health. This information will help keep track of how you feel and how well you are able to do your usual activities.

Answer every question by marking the answer as indicated. If you are unsure about how to answer a question, please give the best answer you can.

1. In general, would you say your health is:

(circle one)

Excellent 1
Very good 2
Good 3
Fair 4
Poor 5

2. Compared to one week ago, how would you rate your health in general now?

(circle one)

Much better now then one week ago 1
Somewhat better now than one week ago 2
About the same as one week ago 3
Somewhat worse now than one week ago 4
Much worse than one week ago 5

3. The following items are about activities you might do during a typical day. Does your health now limit you in these activities? If so, how much?

(circle one number on each line)

ACTIVITIES	Yes, Limited A Lot	Yes, Limited A Little	No, Not Limited At All
a. **Vigorous activities** such as running, lifting heavy objects, participating in strenuous sports	1	2	3
b. **Moderate activities**, such as moving a table, pushing a vacuum cleaner, bowling, or playing golf	1	2	3
c. Lifting or carrying groceries	1	2	3
d. Climbing **several** flights of stairs	1	2	3
e. Climbing **one** flight of stairs	1	2	3
f. Bending, kneeling, or stooping	1	2	3
g. Walking **more than a mile**	1	2	3
h. Walking **several blocks**	1	2	3
i. Walking **one block**	1	2	3
j. Bathing or dressing yourself	1	2	3

FIGURE 9-4 The SF-36 assessment tool. (From Medical Outcomes Trust; Boston, MA; 1992.)

4. During the past week, have you had any of the following problems with your work or other regular daily activities as a result of your physical health?

(circle one number on each line)

	Yes	No
a. Cut down on the **amount of time** you spent on work or other activities	1	2
b. **Accomplished less** than you would like	1	2
c. Were limited in the **kind** of work or other activities	1	2
d. Had **difficulty** performing the work or other activities (for example, it took extra effort)	1	2

5. During the past week, have you had the following problems with your work or other regular daily activities as a result of any emotional problems (such as feeling depressed or anxious)?

(circle one number on each line)

	Yes	No
a. Cut down on the **amount of time** you spent on work or other activities	1	2
b. **Accomplished less** than you would like	1	2
c. Didn't do work or other activities as **carefully** as usual	1	2

6. During the past week, to what extent has your physical health or emotional problems interfered with your normal social activities with family, friends, neighbors, or groups?

(circle one)

Not at all 1
Slightly 2
Moderately 3
Quite a bit 4
Extremely 5

7. How much bodily pain have you had during the past week?

(circle one)

None 1
Very mild 2
Mild 3
Moderate 4
Severe 5
Very severe 6

8. During the past week, how much did pain interfere with your normal work (including both work outside the home and housework)?

(circle one)

Not at all 1
A little bit 2
Moderately 3
Quite a bit 4
Extremely 5

FIGURE 9-4 Continued

9. These questions are about how you feel and how things have been with you during the past week. For each question, please give the one answer that comes closest to the way you have been feeling. How much of the time during the past week—

(circle one number on each line)

	All of the Time	Most of the Time	A Good Bit of Time	Some of the Time	Some of the Time	None of the Time
a. Did you feel full of pep?	1	2	3	4	5	6
b. Have you been a nervous person?	1	2	3	4	5	6
c. Have you ever felt so down in the dumps that nothing could cheer you up?	1	2	3	4	5	6
d. Have you felt calm and peaceful?	1	2	3	4	5	6
e. Did you have a lot of energy?	1	2	3	4	5	6
f. Have you felt downhearted and blue?	1	2	3	4	5	6
g. Did you feel worn out?	1	2	3	4	5	6
h. Have you been a happy person?	1	2	3	4	5	6
i. Did you feel tired?	1	2	3	4	5	6

10. During the past week, how much time has your physical health or emotional problems interfered with your social activities (like visiting with friends, relatives, etc.)?

(circle one)

All of the time.. 1

Most of the time.. 2

Some of the time.. 3

A little of the time.. 4

None of the time.. 5

11. How TRUE or FALSE is each of the following statements for you?

(circle one number on each line)

	Definitely True	Mostly True	Don't Know	Mostly False	Definitely False
a. I seem to get sick a little easier than other people?	1	2	3	4	5
b. I am as healthy as anybody I know	1	2	3	4	5
c. I expect my health to get worse	1	2	3	4	5
d. My health is excellent	1	2	3	4	5

FIGURE 9-4 Continued

Health Concepts, Number of Items and Levels, and Summary of Content for Eight SF-36 Scales and the Health Transition Item

Concepts	No. of Items	No. of Levels	Summary of Content
Physical Functioning (PF)	10	21	Extent to which health limits physical activities such as self-care, walking, climbing stairs, bending, lifting, and moderate and vigorous exercises
Role Functioning Physical (RP)	4	5	Extent to which physical health interferes with work or other daily activities, including accomplishing less than wanted, limitations in the kind of activities, or difficulty in performing activities
Bodily Pain (BP)	2	11	Intensity of pain and effect of pain on normal work, both inside and outside the home
General Health (GH)	5	21	Personal evaluation of health, including current health, health outlook, and resistance to illness
Vitality (VT)	4	21	Feeling energetic and full of pep versus feeling tired and worn out
Social Functioning (SF)	2	9	Extent to which physical health or emotional problems interfere with normal social activities
Role Functioning Emotional (RE)	3	4	Extent to which emotional problems interfere with work or other daily activities, including decreased time spent on activities, accomplishing less, and not working as carefully as usual
Mental Health (MH)	5	26	General mental health, including depression, anxiety, behavioral-emotional control, general positive affect
Reported Health Transition (HT)	1	5	Evaluation of current health compared to one year ago

FIGURE 9-4 Continued

Acute Pain

The typical patient with acute pain has recently sustained an injury or undergone a surgical procedure. The pain is related to the acute trauma of an initial injury or an exacerbation of a preexisting injury. This patient may be taking pain medication for a short time after the injury or surgery. This pain is expected to resolve substantially over the course of a few days. Although some residual pain may continue for weeks after the injury or surgery, most pain is expected to resolve with only minimal discomfort remaining.

Acute pain of this type is treated with a combination of medication (ie, prescription or over-the-counter drugs at the patient's discretion), gentle exercise, and ice. Ice is preferred over heat for acute pain because of the acuteness of the injury. Exercise is prescribed based on the specific injury or surgery and is directed at restoring the motion, strength, and function of the injured body part. Rehabilitation of the injured area is the prime focus and provides the framework for exercise prescription. Exercise in this phase is directed toward prevention of injury at adjacent joints because of compensation. Patient education about pain-relieving postures and skills to fulfill the activities of daily living and the instrumental activities of daily living are components of acute pain management (see Patient-Related Instruction: Management of Acute Pain).

Chronic Pain

Treatment of chronic pain requires a team approach because of the multidimensional nature of the pain. Chronic pain is disabling and interferes with all aspects of the person's life. The clinician must work closely with the physician, psychologist, vocational counselor, alternative health care providers, and the patient. In this way, a comprehensive treatment program can be established to ensure all aspects of the pain are being addressed. Therapeutic exercise is a major component of the treatment plan,[12–14] but many adjunctive treatments and alternative therapies are often

INSTRUCTIONS

Check only one box in each section which best applies to you. We realize you may consider that two of the statements in any one section relate to you, but please just mark the box which most closely describes your problem.

SECTION I - PAIN INTENSITY

- ❑ I can tolerate the pain I have without having to use pain killers.
- ❑ The pain is bad but I can manage without taking pain killers.
- ❑ Pain killers give complete relief from pain.
- ❑ Pain killers give moderate relief from pain.
- ❑ Pain killers give very little relief from pain.
- ❑ Pain killers have no effect on the pain and I do not use them.

SECTION II - PERSONAL CARE (Washing, Dressing, Etc.)

- ❑ I can look after myself normally without causing extra pain.
- ❑ I can look after myself normally but it causes pain.
- ❑ It is painful to look after myself and I am slow and careful.
- ❑ I need some help but manage most of my personal care.
- ❑ I need help every day in most aspects of self care.
- ❑ I do not get dressed, wash with difficulty and stay in bed.

SECTION III - LIFTING

- ❑ I can lift heavy weights without extra pain.
- ❑ I can lift heavy weights but it gives extra pain.
- ❑ Pain prevents me from lifting heavy weights off the floor, but I can manage if they are conveniently positioned, e.g., on a table.
- ❑ Pain prevents me from lifting heavy weights, but I can manage light to medium weights if they are conveniently positioned.
- ❑ I can lift only very light weights.
- ❑ I cannot lift or carry anything at all.

SECTION IV - WALKING

- ❑ Pain does not prevent me from walking any distance.
- ❑ Pain prevents me from walking more than 1 mile.
- ❑ Pain prevents me from walking more than 1/2 mile.
- ❑ Pain prevents me from walking more than 1/4 mile.
- ❑ I can only walk using a stick or crutches.
- ❑ I am in bed most of the time and have to crawl to the toilet.

SECTION V - SITTING

- ❑ I can sit in any chair as long as I like.
- ❑ I can only sit in my favorite chair as long as I like.
- ❑ Pain prevents me from sitting for more than 1 hour.
- ❑ Pain prevents me from sitting for more than 30 minutes.
- ❑ Pain prevents me from sitting for more than 10 minutes.
- ❑ Pain prevents me from sitting at all.

FIGURE 9-5 The Oswestry Low Back Disability Questionnaire. (Adapted from Fairbank JCT, Davies JB, Couper J, O'Brien JP. The Oswestry Low Back Pain Disability Questionnaire. *Physiotherapy* 1980:66(8):271–273

SECTION VI - STANDING

- ❑ I can stand as long as I want without extra pain.
- ❑ I can stand as long as I want but it gives me extra pain.
- ❑ Pain prevents me from standing for more than 1 hour.
- ❑ Pain prevents me from standing for more than 30 minutes.
- ❑ Pain prevents me from standing for more than 10 minutes.
- ❑ Pain prevents me from standing at all.

SECTION VII - SLEEPING

- ❑ Pain does not prevent me from sleeping well.
- ❑ I can sleep well only by using tablets.
- ❑ Even when I take tablets I have less than six hours sleep.
- ❑ Even when I take tablets I have less than four hours sleep.
- ❑ Even when I take tablets I have less than two hours sleep.
- ❑ Pain prevents me from sleeping at all.

SECTION VIII - SEX LIFE

- ❑ My sex life is normal and causes no extra pain.
- ❑ My sex life is normal but causes some extra pain.
- ❑ My sex life is nearly normal but is very painful.
- ❑ My sex life is severely restricted by pain.
- ❑ My sex life is nearly absent because of pain.
- ❑ Pain prevents any sex life at all.

SECTION IX - SOCIAL LIFE

- ❑ My social life is normal and gives me no extra pain.
- ❑ My social life is normal but increases the degree of pain.
- ❑ Pain has no significant effect on my social life apart from limiting my more energetic interests, e.g. dancing, etc.
- ❑ Pain has restricted my social life and I do not go out as often.
- ❑ Pain has restricted my social life to my home.
- ❑ I have no social life because of pain.

SECTION X - TRAVELING

- ❑ I can travel anywhere without extra pain.
- ❑ I can travel anywhere but it gives me extra pain.
- ❑ Pain is bad but I manage journeys over two hours.
- ❑ Pain restricts me to journeys of less than one hour.
- ❑ Pain restricts me to short necessary journeys under 30 minutes.
- ❑ Pain prevents me from traveling except to the doctor or hospital.

FOR OFFICE USE
Total Score

Therapist's Signature and Date	Patient's Signature and Date

FIGURE 9-5 Continued

Patient-Related Instruction

Management of Acute Pain

An increase in acute pain is a sign of doing too much. This may disrupt the healing process. In this situation, you should do the following:

1. Find a position of comfort that decreases or eliminates your pain. Your clinician can help you learn what these positions are.
2. Use a pain-relieving treatment such as ice for 10 to 15 minutes every hour.
3. Use an assistive device such as crutches, a cane, or a walker if your leg is involved, a sling or splint for your upper extremity, or a corset for your back. These devices reduce the stress on the injured area.
4. Take your medications as prescribed.

Patient-Related Instruction

Why You Should Exercise When You Have Chronic Pain

You should exercise when you have chronic pain, because exercise can:

1. Improve problems such as inflexibility, loss of mobility, or weakness, which contribute to your pain.
2. Decrease pain by inhibiting transmission of pain impulses.
3. Improve your sleep at night.
4. Control weight gain, which often occurs from inactivity and can have negative physical and psychological consequences.
5. Prevent secondary musculoskeletal complications of pain such as further weakness, immobility, and flexibility at other joints.
6. Prevent secondary cardiovascular changes such as increases in blood pressure, elevated cholesterol levels, or diabetes complications.
7. Enhance your sense of well-being, self-esteem, and accomplishment.

explored by the patient. Herbal remedies, acupuncture, reflexology, and other therapies are often part of a patient's complete treatment program. The clinician must maintain an open dialogue with the patient to ensure a thorough understanding of all therapies occurring simultaneously.

A critical component of chronic pain treatment is a realistic understanding of the goals of the treatment plan. Patient education is a key component; the clinician explains the likely source of pain, activity modifications or postures to minimize pain, and the expected outcomes of intervention. Ultimately, the goal is a return to the highest level of function while managing the pain.

Interventions to inhibit pain input or to facilitate nonpain input are incorporated while simultaneously addressing associated impairments and functional limitations. Therapeutic exercise is used to affect the pain directly through endogenous opiates and indirectly through facilitation of nonpain input and to treat the associated impairments and functional limitations. Exercises chosen may have very different goals. Exercise may be uncomfortable for the individual with chronic pain, and this discomfort may be necessary to achieve pain inhibition through endogenous opiates. This type of intervention requires extensive education regarding the purpose of the exercise and alternative options. It is essential to ensure communication and program adherence.

The goals of the therapeutic exercise program extend beyond treatment of impairments; functional limitations and associated disability related to depression, sleep, and appetite are also of concern. Although simple impairment measures may not change after therapeutic exercise intervention, improvements in sleep patterns, mental state, and appetite may be the first markers of successful intervention (see Patient-Related Instruction: Why You Should Exercise When You Have Chronic Pain).

When designing the therapeutic exercise program, the clinician must consider the current physical and psychological status of the patient and take into account potential secondary problems that must be prevented. The therapeutic exercise program should be directed toward the source of the pain and toward any musculoskeletal impairments or functional limitations and any secondary preventable problems identified during the evaluation process. The elements of the movement system involved in the production of pain should be identified during the evaluation process. The relative contributions of each element to the production of pain should be determined so that treatment procedures may be prioritized (see Selected Intervention: Treatment of the Patient With Fibromyalgia).

ACTIVITY AND MODE

The activity chosen to treat the individual with chronic pain depends on the source of the pain and results of the evaluation process. In addition to the specific interventions chosen to treat the source of the pain, other activities can help the patient.

The patient with chronic low back pain due to a herniated disk should receive treatment specific to the impairments and functional limitations associated with that injury, and several adjunctive measures can be used to treat the associated pain. Individuals in pain, particularly those with chronic pain, are susceptible to changes in posture and movement patterns. These changes can perpetuate the original symptoms or cause secondary impairments or functional limitations. Regardless of the activity chosen, the therapeutic focus should be on awareness and use of proper posture and movement patterns. Movement therapies such as Feldenkrais are helpful in restoring appropriate movement patterns. Total-body movement patterns are often more successful than isolated joint movement when treating individuals with chronic pain. Rhythmic activity of large muscle groups should be the activity of choice. This activity should be balanced with specific exercises to address the impairments and functional limitations (Fig. 9-6).

Diagonal patterns used in proprioceptive neuromuscular facilitation (PNF) techniques (see Chapter 14) are useful for

SELECTED INTERVENTION

Treatment of the Patient With Fibromyalagia

See Case Study #7

Although this patient requires comprehensive intervention, as described in the patient management model, one exercise is described.

ACTIVITY: Hand to knee pushes

PURPOSE: To increase abdominal and hip flexor muscle strength; improve single-leg balance and trunk stability; and increase upper quarter strength through closed chain activity

RISK FACTORS: No appreciable risk factors

ELEMENTS OF THE MOVEMENT SYSTEM: Base

STAGE OF MOTOR CONTROL: Stability

POSTURE: Standing position on a single leg. The opposite hip and knee are flexed to 90 degrees. The opposite hand of the flexed leg pushes isometrically against the movement of hip flexion. A neutral spine is maintained, and concentration on abdominal muscle contraction is emphasized.

MOVEMENT: Isometric contraction of the abdominal, hip flexor, and contralateral upper quarter muscles.

SPECIAL CONSIDERATIONS: Ensure proper posture of the trunk, pelvis, and weight-bearing limb. Cue for an abdominal muscle contraction, using palpation as necessary. This exercise is contraindicated when an isometric muscle contraction is contraindicated.

DOSAGE: Hold contraction for 3–6 seconds at a comfortable intensity that does not cause hip flexor or shoulder fatigue. Repeat on the opposite side.

TYPE OF MUSCLE CONTRACTION: Isometric

Intensity: Submaximal
Duration: Hold for up to 6 seconds
Frequency: During each pool session

RATIONALE FOR EXERCISE CHOICE: This exercise addresses the many components of fibromyalgia, including trunk stability, single-leg stance stability, abdominal muscle endurance, and upper and lower quarter muscle endurance.

EXERCISE GRADATION: This exercise is progressed to greater intensity and more repetitions. More advanced stabilization exercises incorporating upper and lower extremity movements with resistance are then added.

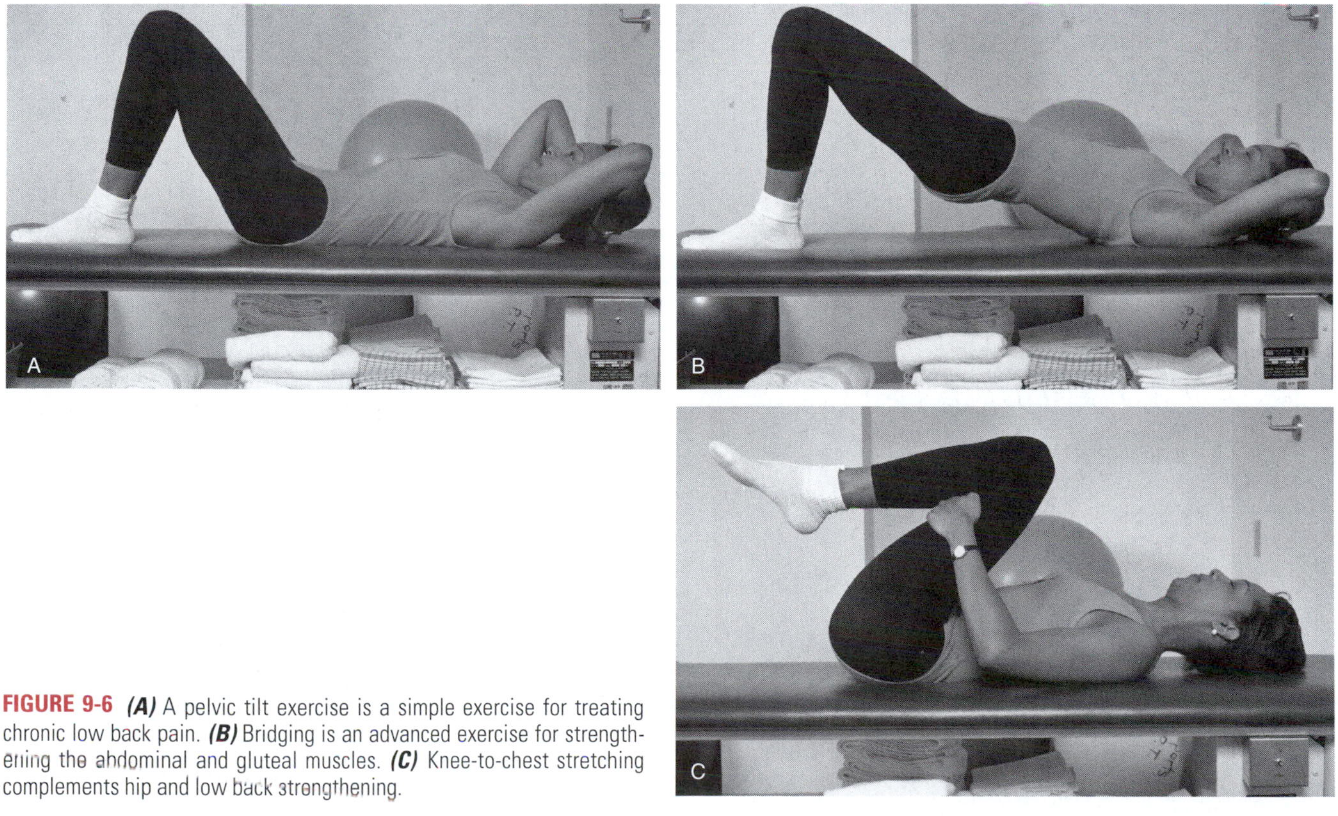

FIGURE 9-6 ***(A)*** A pelvic tilt exercise is a simple exercise for treating chronic low back pain. ***(B)*** Bridging is an advanced exercise for strengthening the abdominal and gluteal muscles. ***(C)*** Knee-to-chest stretching complements hip and low back strengthening.

teaching the patient position and posture awareness while still using multisegmental movement. In addition to assisting in movement awareness, PNF patterns can increase mobility and muscle performance. These patterns can ensure proper muscle recruitment during movement patterns. Substitution patterns often are difficult to observe but are easily palpated during PNF exercises. The posture and movements chosen for PNF should address the specific impairments and functional limitations determined during the evaluation. Bilateral, symmetric patterns are particularly helpful when one side is involved and needs retraining through the uninvolved side. Bilateral patterns that emphasize trunk flexion and extension or rotation and sidebending are effective for normalizing specific movement patterns. The upper extremity diagonal patterns can be performed in a variety of postures and positions, depending on the patient's needs. Upper and lower extremity patterns can be combined for total-body movement patterns. These same patterns can be performed in a pool (see Self-Management: Proprioceptive Neuromuscular Facilitation Postural Technique).

Aerobic exercise is effective for treating chronic pain and is frequently recommended in the treatment of conditions such as fibromyalgia. The pool can be used for aerobic exercise, although consideration must be given to the water's resistance (see Self-Management: Supine Kicking With Optimal Arm Movements and Self-Management: Jumping Jacks). This resistance can produce muscle fatigue before reaching aerobic exercise levels. Walking is a simple form of continuous exercise that can be performed by many persons (Fig. 9-7). Walking is particularly effective because it can be performed for several short bouts several times each day. A stationary bicycle such as a recumbent bike is also an effective tool, although less available. Other exercises enjoyed by the individual, such as aerobic dance, recreational dance, or traditional lap swimming, should be incorporated.

Activities such as yoga, Tai-Chi, or using a therapeutic ball allow a variety of large muscle group activities to be carried out while simultaneously increasing posture awareness (Fig. 9-8). Many of these activities are done in a group setting or individually at home, providing flexibility to suit the needs of each patient (see Self-Management: Yoga Exercise).

SELF-MANAGEMENT: Proprioceptive Neuromuscular Facilitation Postural Technique

Purpose: To improve postural control while moving the arms and sitting on an unstable surface

Position: Sitting on a therapeutic ball, with both feet flat on the floor, grasp wrist or a resistive band with both hands over one shoulder (*A*).

Movement technique:
Level 1: Keeping your arms straight, and rotate your trunk and shoulders down past your opposite hip (*B* and *C*).

Level 2: Increase the resistance.

Level 3: Perform with one foot off the floor.

Repeat _______ times

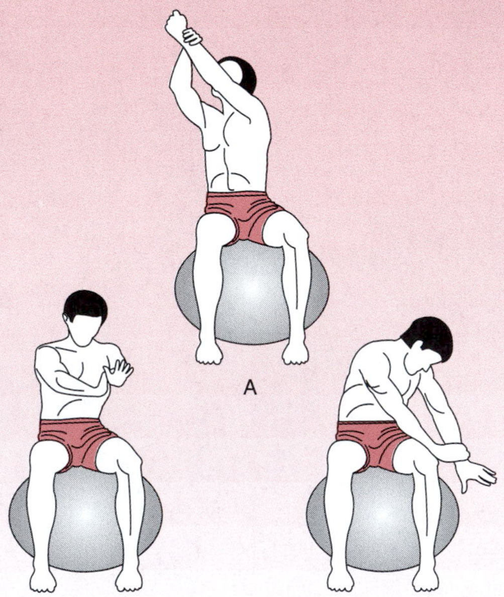

SELF-MANAGEMENT: Supine Kicking With Optional Arm Movements

Purpose: To increase strength and endurance of the neck, trunk, hip, and leg extensor muscles and to increase cardiovascular endurance

Position: Supine with arms in a comfortable position overhead or at the side

Movement technique:
Level 1: Rhythmic, repetitive kicking, keeping knees relatively straight. and kicking from the hips; large or small fins may be used.

Level 2: Add arm movements in an underwater backstroke pattern. Bring arms up along the sides of your body to the shoulders, extend them straight out to the sides, then pull back down toward your sides.

Repeat _______ times

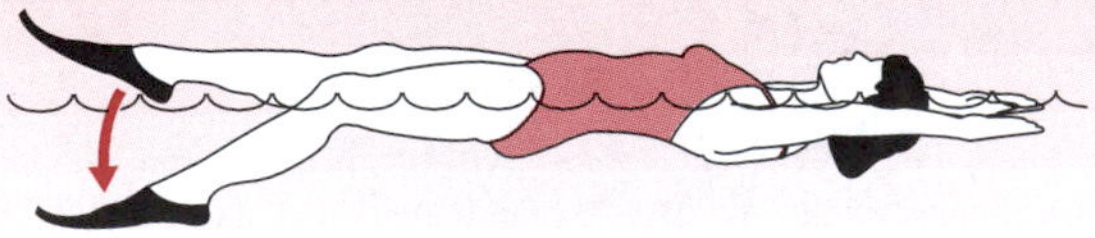

SELF-MANAGEMENT: Jumping Jacks

Purpose: Increase strength in shoulder and hip abductor muscles, initiate gentle impact, and initiate exercise using large muscle groups

Position: Start in chest-deep water, with feet together and arms at sides.

Movement technique: Bring both feet out to the sides while simultaneously bringing arms out to the side. Return to the starting position.

Repeat _______ times

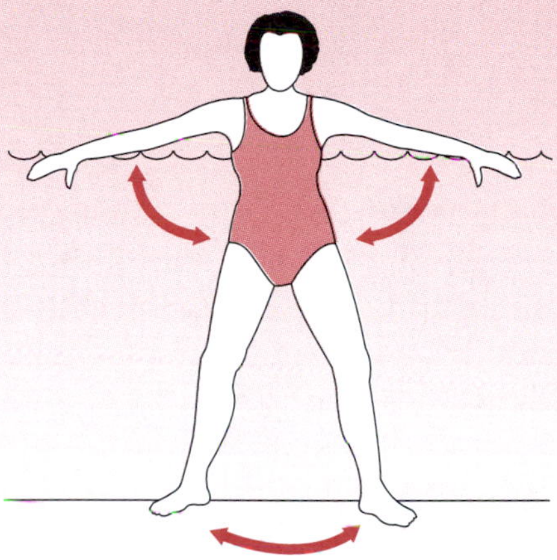

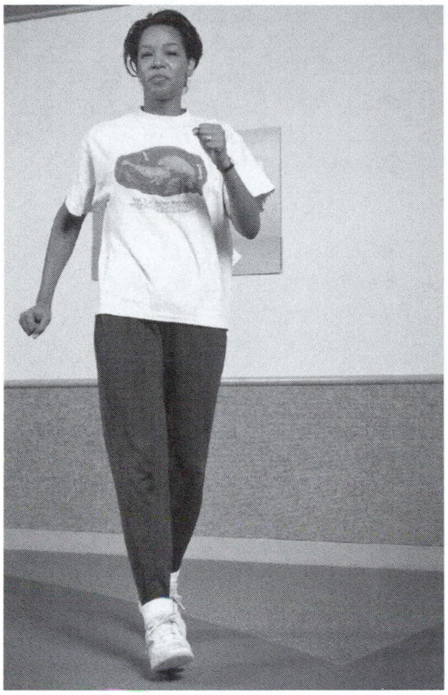

FIGURE 9-7 Walking on a track is a simple, continuous aerobic exercise available to most patients.

The pool is a useful tool in the application of therapeutic exercise for those with chronic pain (see Chapter 17). The advantages include unweighting from the buoyancy and the warmth and contact of the water on the skin. Unweighting the sore limb or painful back allows movement with less pain and provides the opportunity for correct posture and movement patterns during activity or stretching (Fig. 9-9)

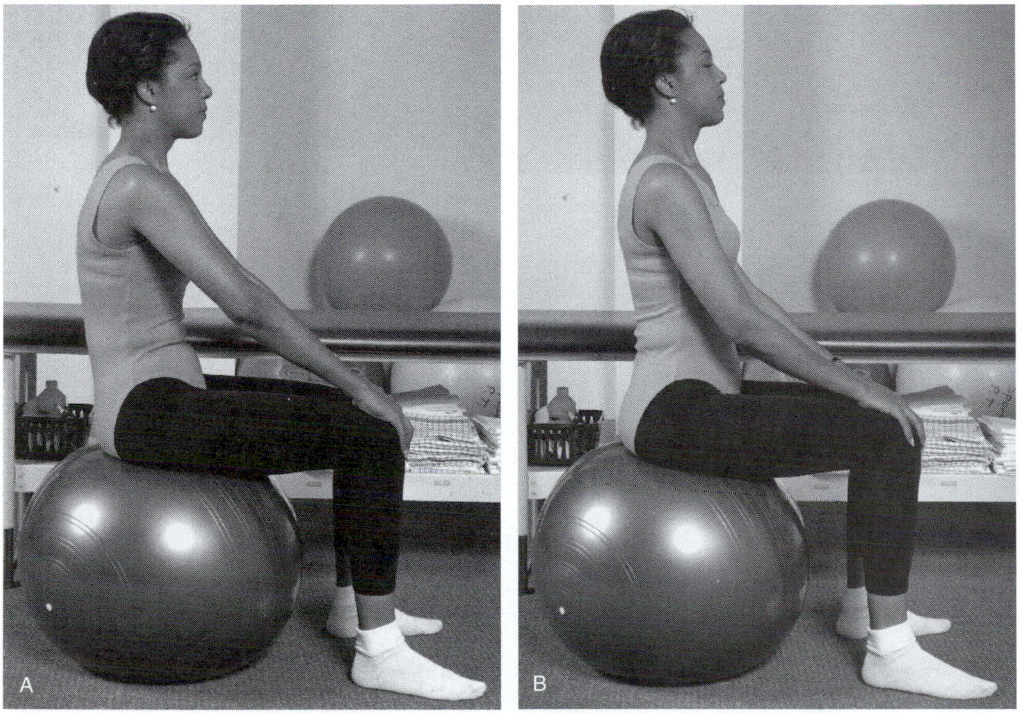

FIGURE 9-8 Therapeutic ball exercises such as pelvic rocking can be performed at home and in the clinic. ***(A)*** Start position. ***(B)*** End position.

SELF-MANAGEMENT: Yoga Exercise

Purpose: To promote relaxation and pain relief and to increase mobility in the low back and hips

Position: Lying supine, with legs elevated on the wall (*A*).

Movement technique: Let the knees and hips bend, sliding the leg down the wall to a comfortable position (*B*). Hold 10 to 15 seconds, and return to the starting position.

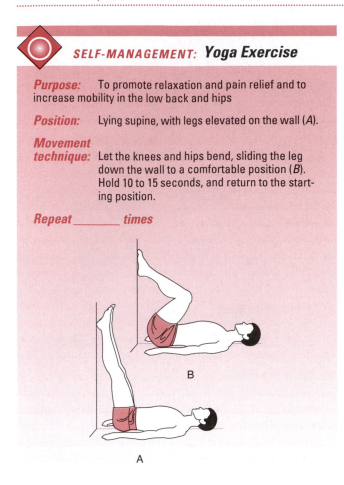

Repeat _______ times

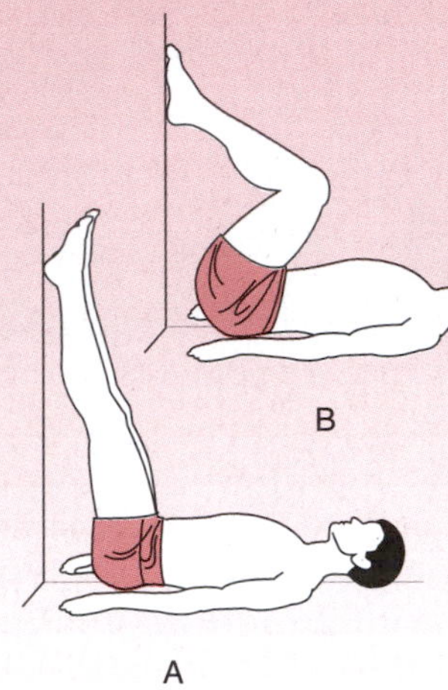

SELF-MANAGEMENT: Hip External Rotation Stretch

Purpose: To increase mobility of the hips

Position: While facing the ladder, set the foot of the hip to be stretched on a step of the ladder. Slide the foot across to the edge of the step. Keeping your foot there, let your knee roll out. Hold for 10 to 15 seconds.

Movement technique: Level 1: Assume the position described above until you feel a gentle stretch in your hip.

Level 2: Assume the position described above until you feel a gentle stretch in your hip. Use your hands to push your knee farther into rotation.

Repeat _______ times

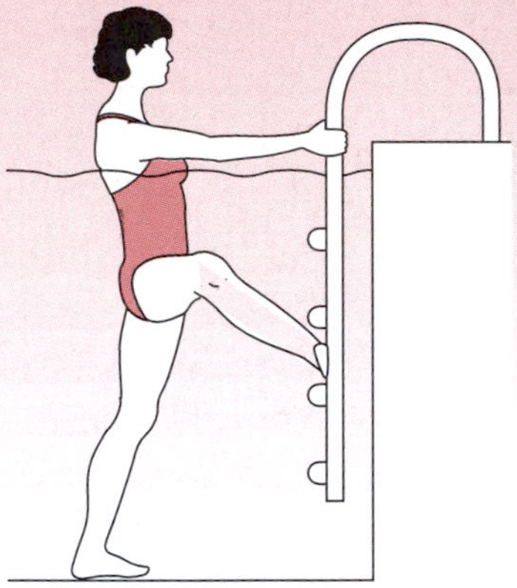

(see Self-Management: Hip External Rotation Stretch; Self-Management: Deep Water March With Barbell; and Self-Management: Alternating Elbow Flexion and Extension). Movements that are too painful to perform on land are performed with greater ease and less pain in the water (Fig. 9-10). The water's warmth and skin contact may function to close the gate to pain at the spinal cord level. A disadvantage of pool use in treating chronic pain is the difficulty in determining proper muscle recruitment and movement patterns. The water's refraction causes distortion, and the clinician cannot observe movement and posture. Actual palpation and tactile cuing in the pool can overcome this problem. A second disadvantage for some individuals with conditions such as fibromyalgia or myofascial pain syndrome is the water's resistance. The viscosity of water provides enough resistance to exacerbate some chronic pain conditions. Positions and movement patterns chosen should minimize resistance caused by turbulence (ie, controlling the speed of movement) and viscosity (ie, minimizing the surface area) (see Self-Management: Water Walking, Forward and Sideways).

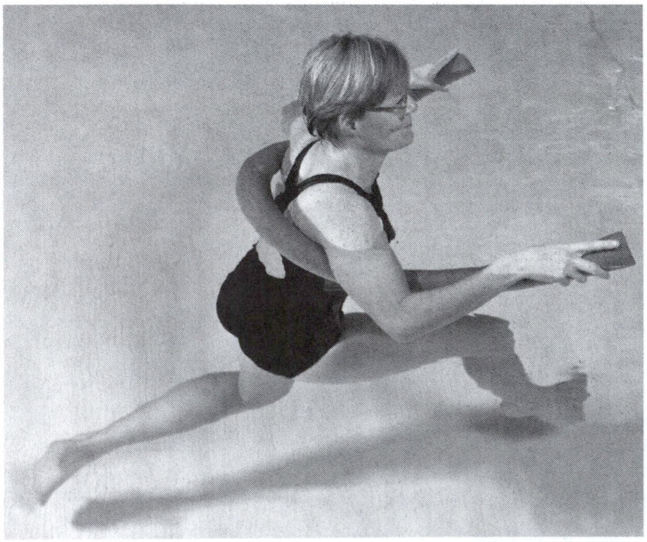

FIGURE 9-9 Deep water bicycling.

EXERCISE DOSAGE

As with the activity chosen, the dosage depends on the specific component of the movement system being treated and the purpose of the exercise, but some generalities about exercise and pain should be considered. The exercise dosage should not increase the pain. The chosen speed, repetitions, intensity, and duration should not increase pain within the

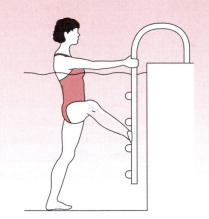

SELF-MANAGEMENT: Deep Water March With Barbell

Purpose: To increase mobility through the low back, hips, and knees

Position: In water depth equal to your height or deeper, use a barbell or other buoyant equipment to support yourself.

Movement technique: Level 1: March in place through a comfortable range of motion at a comfortable speed.

Level 2: Add buoyant equipment to feet and ankles, increase the speed of marching, or do both.

Repeat _______ times

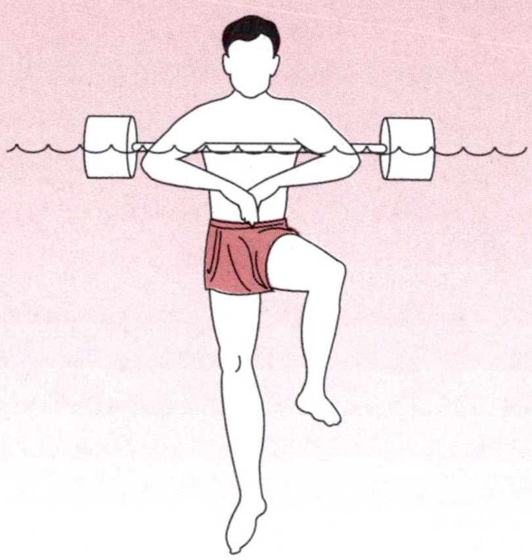

SELF-MANAGEMENT: Alternating Elbow Flexioning Extension

Purpose: To increase mobility in the elbows, increase muscle strength and endurance in the upper extremities, and increase trunk stability

Position: Standing in shoulder-deep water, with your feet in a comfortable stance and arms at the sides

Movement technique: Level 1: Alternately flex and extend the elbows with thumbs pointing up.

Level 2: Turn your palms up.

Level 3: Add gloves or other resistive equipment.

Repeat _______ times

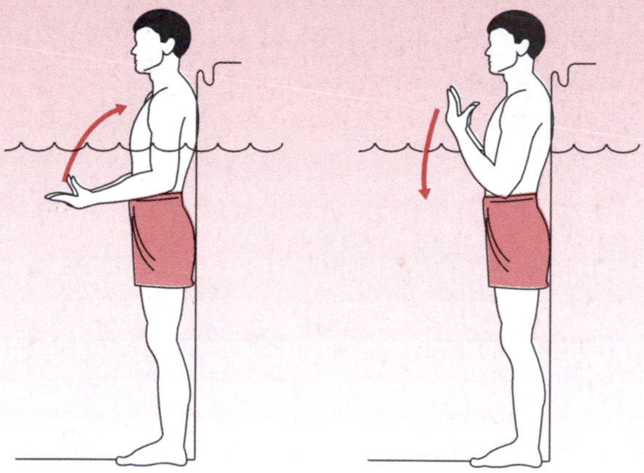

exercise session, nor should symptoms increase after exercise. If the water's resistance is a concern in aquatic exercise, the first session should be kept brief (5 to 7 minutes) to assess the response to this intervention. As tolerance is demonstrated, the intensity or the duration may be increased (see Patient-Related Instruction: How Often and Hard Should You Exercise With Chronic Pain).

The frequency is determined by the activity type and purpose and by the quantity of exercise performed before pain is experienced. For example, if only a few repetitions of activity at a low intensity for a short duration can be performed before experiencing pain, the exercises may be performed with greater frequency. Availability also affects frequency. A pool may not be available more than once each day or even less often. The frequency must be balanced against the intensity and duration of an activity. Some exercise should be performed daily, and matching a land-based exercise program to complement the pool program is necessary.

After the pain-free dosage is determined, the exercise parameters should be progressed to those best suited to treat the patient's underlying pathology, impairment, or functional limitation. The activity should eventually be transferred to a functional progression aimed at returning to previous activity levels.

Adjunctive Agents

Adjunctive agents are essential in the treatment of pain. In the case of chronic pain, more agents are used. The disabling nature of chronic pain leads individuals to seek out any other potentially pain-relieving therapy such as medications, chiropractic, massage therapy, relaxation techniques, biofeedback, and psychological care. Acupuncture, herbal remedies, dietary changes, and a host of other therapies may be employed. Continuous communication with the patient ensures optimal team treatment and avoids conflicting interventions. The clinician must remain open minded and supportive throughout this process as the patient searches for solutions to her pain.

TRANSCUTANEOUS ELECTRICAL NERVE STIMULATION

TENS has been proven useful in the treatment of some types of pain.[15] One mechanism of pain relief with the application of an electric current is based on the gate theory of pain. Application of TENS selectively activates large A-alpha and A-beta fibers, which are stimulated at lower thresholds than the smaller C fibers. These impulses travel to the dorsal horn of the spinal cord, where facilitation of

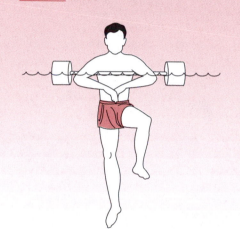

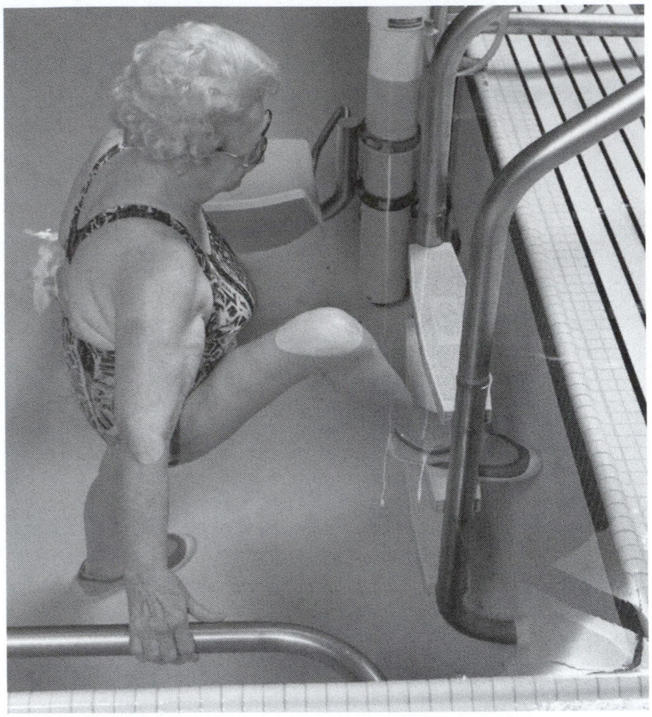

FIGURE 9-10 Knee-to-chest stretching can also be performed comfortably in the pool.

the small interneurons of the substantia gelatinosa inhibit pain transmission through presynaptic inhibition. Activation of these large-diameter fibers closes the gate to small-diameter fiber transmission.

Other theories suggest that TENS may function through antidromic (ie, conducting impulses in a direction opposite to normal) stimulation of afferent neurons. Antidromic stimulation may decrease pain by blocking the nociceptive input to the spinal cord, and it may stimulate release of substance P, resulting in vasodilation. Vasodilation can decrease pain by increasing local circulation, which removes metabolic waste products and supplies oxygenated blood for healing. The increased local circulation may decrease local ischemia enough to decrease pain.[7]

TENS may effect the opiate pain-modulating system. Ascending projections from small-fiber afferents reach the PAG, which is rich with opiates. The PAG provides descending input to the dorsal horn, which probably is opiate mediated. TENS may provide some analgesia through opiate-mediated activation of the brain stem.

The parameters for TENS application are varied. The suggested reading section at the end of the chapter lists references providing such guidelines.

HEAT

Heat is commonly used as a primary or adjunctive agent to decrease pain. Trauma can produce a pain-spasm cycle that activates nociceptors. The nociceptors detect pain that produces reflex muscle activity that, if prolonged, results in muscle ischemia. The ischemia excites muscle nociceptors that perpetuate the muscle spasm. Chemical release at the time of injury or resulting from inflammation can also stimulate nociceptors. Vasoconstriction associated with a sympathetic response or vasoconstriction resulting from muscle spasm can produce pain. The application of heat can decrease pain from any of these sources.

According to the gate theory, heat application can decrease pain directly. Thermal sensations are carried to the dorsal horn of the spinal cord through large-diameter myelinated fibers. These impulses can close the gate, blocking the transmission of pain impulses through small-diameter fibers. The thermal sensations are transmitted to conscious levels preferentially over pain sensations. The increased circulation resulting from heat application decreases pain through two mechanisms. First, pain resulting from ischemia decreases as the local circulation is increased. The increased circulation may break the pain-spasm cycle as pain decreases and the muscle is provided with oxygenated blood. Second, the increased circulation may remove noxious chemicals associated with injury or inflammation, thereby decreasing pain.

SELF-MANAGEMENT: Water Walking, Forward and Sideways

Purpose: To increase mobility throughout the trunk, arms, and legs; increase trunk stability; and increase muscular strength and endurance in the arms, legs, and trunk

Position: Stand in water between waist and shoulder deep; deep water provides more resistance to walking.

Movement technique:
Level 1: Step sideways, raising your arms out to the sides as you step and bringing back down to the sides as you bring your feet together.
Level 2: Walk forward with the opposite arm and leg reaching forward together. Be sure to walk normally using a heel to toe pattern.
Level 3: Add gloves to hands.

Repeat _______ times

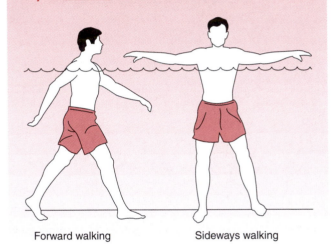

Patient-Related Instruction

How Often and Hard Should You Exercise With Chronic Pain

1. Ideally, you should do something every day, at least once per day. Your clinician can give you further guidelines.
2. Many people do well by performing several short bouts of exercise spread throughout the day. These sessions may be only 5 to 10 minutes long.
3. Any aerobic activity should be continuous, working up to 10 to 20 minutes over time.
4. Stretches should be intense enough to feel a gentle pulling sensation.
5. Other exercises should be performed slowly until slight fatigue is felt or as otherwise instructed by your clinician.
6. If you feel any sharp, stabbing pain or numbness or tingling as a result of the exercise, discontinue the exercise. Use your pain-relieving measures, and tell your clinician.
7. You may feel some discomfort during or for a short time after exercise. This discomfort should not be confused with the pain that brought you to the clinic. Avoid exercises that increase this pain, but you may continue to exercise with some of the discomfort.
8. Ask your clinician if you are unsure about what to feel with your exercise program.

Superficial heat in the form of hot packs is commonly used in the clinic and home to decrease pain and as a precursor to therapeutic exercise. Local heat application increases the extensibility of tissue, preparing it for subsequent exercise. Immersion in a warm pool or whirlpool can also decrease pain, although the water temperature is significantly lower than that of a hot pack because of the size of the area heated. The warmth and buoyancy effects of the water combine to decrease pain sensation. Ultrasound or diathermy can increase the heat's depth of penetration. Any of these modalities can provide valuable assistance in the reduction of pain.

COLD

Cold treatments are commonly used to decrease pain. Cold decreases pain through some of the same mechanisms as heat. Cold sensation is carried to the dorsal horn of the spinal cord through large-diameter afferent fibers and is capable of closing the gate to pain signals through smaller-diameter fibers. The drop in tissue temperature blocks synaptic transmission of any input, rendering the gate inactive. The decrease in pain may help to break the pain-spasm cycle. In acute injury, the vasoconstriction produced by cold may prevent edema that produces pain. Because the application of cold is somewhat noxious, the afferent input to the brain stem through the PAG could cause the release of endorphins at the spinal level; the decrease in pain would be modulated by higher centers.

Cold usually is applied by means of ice in the form of packs, bags, or ice massage. The length of application depends on the size of the area to be cooled, the area of the body to be cooled, the mode of application, local circulation, and patient sensitivity.

MEDICATION

Drug therapy is commonly prescribed for individuals with acute or chronic pain. Many medications are available and act through different mechanisms and at different sites to relieve pain. Medications are administered orally, by intramuscular injection, by injection into other structures, or by intravenous infusion. The dosage necessary to produce analgesia varies among individuals and for various medications.

Acting peripherally, NSAIDs are commonly prescribed. Several chemical classes exist, all of which inhibit the synthesis or release of prostaglandins.[16] Analgesia generally occurs within 24 hours of NSAID administration, and anti-inflammatory responses occur with continued administration. The major side effect of NSAIDs is gastrointestinal upset. Many NSAIDs are enteric coated and long acting, decreasing the frequency of administration. Local injections of anesthetic agents can provide relief from pain in localized areas. Trigger point injections with an anesthetic agent are commonly performed in individuals with chronic pain, particularly pain arising from myofascial tissues.

At the spinal cord and higher levels, a variety of medications can be administered. Antidepressant medications have analgesic effects, and administration may relieve pain at levels below those necessary to achieve antidepressant effects. These medications may be used at levels that have analgesic and antidepressant benefits. At these same levels, muscle relaxants such as benzodiazepines also act as analgesics. Moreover, they help patients relax and sleep, which significantly improves their quality of life. Narcotics acting at opioid receptors are used to treat pain. Morphine and other strong narcotics are commonly used to relieve end-of-life pain and cancer pain.

Some patients receive inadequate pain control from traditional administration methods because of individual differences in absorption and metabolism of drugs or because of fluctuating plasma levels of the drugs or their metabolites. In this situation, patient-controlled analgesia (PCA) may be indicated. The PCA system infuses a drug in a desired location on demand or at a continuous rate.[17] Opioid analgesic drugs such as morphine, meperidine, and hydromorphone are commonly used.[17] In an on-demand system, a small button on the PCA system releases a preset dose of medication. The constant-rate infusion delivers a small but continuous dose to maintain steady plasma levels of the analgesic. A variety of safety features are included in the system. Chronic pain from cancer, surgery, or labor and delivery is a common reason for the use of PCA.

Key Points

- Pain impairment occurs with most musculoskeletal conditions and must be treated as a primary impairment along with any secondary limitations that may result.
- Nociceptors, or pain receptors, transmit impulses from the periphery to the dorsal horn of the spinal cord and higher CNS levels.

- Pain information is transmitted through A-delta and C fibers, which are small, unmyelinated neuronal fibers.
- Information is processed within the spinal cord and then ascends through the contralateral spinothalamic tract to the thalamus.
- The gate theory of pain states that incoming information from nonpain receptors (eg, thermal, mechanical) can close the gate to pain information.
- Chronic pain may result from increased sensitization of nociceptors and spinal level changes that perpetuate positive feedback loops in the pain-spasm cycle.
- Pain can be assessed through direct measurement tools such as the VAS or MPQ questionnaires or through quality of life scales such as the SF-36.
- Descending impulses can influence pain perception through several mechanisms, including endogenous opiates.
- Therapeutic exercise is a cornerstone of treatment for chronic pain. It can remedy pain (through gating mechanisms and descending influences), secondary limitations caused by pain, and associated impairments and functional limitations.
- TENS, heat, cold, and medications are key components of a comprehensive pain treatment program.

? Critical Thinking Questions

1. Consider Case Study #5 in Unit 7.
   a. This patient has pain with standing and walking. What interventions may improve this patient's ability to stand and walk without pain.
   b. This patient has pain with lumbar extension. How does your therapeutic exercise intervention address this problem?
   c. What suggestions can you give this patient to allow her to participate in social activities without pain?
2. Consider Case Study #7 in Unit 7.
   a. Design an exercise program to prevent further decline of her general deconditioning, with consideration of her overall fatigue and daily demands.
   b. Provide this patient with suggestions for energy-reducing measures to allow her to complete daily tasks without increasing pain or fatigue.

REFERENCES

1. Quillen WS, Magee DJ, Zachazewski JE. The process of athletic injury and rehabilitation. In: Zachazewski JE, Magee DJ, Quillen WS, eds. *Athletic Injuries and Rehabilitation.* Philadelphia: WB Saunders; 1996:3–8.
2. Newton RA. Contemporary views on pain and the role played by thermal agents in managing pain symptoms. In: Michlovitz S, ed. *Thermal Agents in Rehabilitation.* 2nd ed. Philadelphia: FA Davis; 1990.
3. Kramis RC, Roberts WJ, Gillette RG. Non-nociceptive aspects of persistent musculoskeletal pain. *J Orthop Sports Phys Ther.* 1996;24:255–267.
4. Sluka KA. Pain mechanisms involved in musculoskeletal disorders. *J Orthop Sports Phys Ther.* 1996;24:240–254.
5. Bowsher D. Nociceptors and peripheral nerve fibres. In: Wells PE, Frampton V, Bowsher D, eds. *Pain Management in Physical Therapy.* Norwalk, CT: Appleton & Lange, 1988.
6. Werner JK. *Neuroscience: A Clinical Perspective.* Philadelphia: WB Saunders; 1980.
7. Hanegan JL. Principles of nociception. In: Gersh MR, ed. *Electrotherapy in Rehabilitation.* Philadelphia: FA Davis; 1992.
8. Scott J, Huskisson EC. Graphic representation of pain. *Pain* 1976;2:175–184.
9. Melzack R. The McGill Pain Questionnaire: major properties and scoring methods. *Pain.* 1975;1:277–299.
10. Melzack R. The short-form McGill Pain Questionnaire. *Pain.* 1987;30:191–197.
11. Melzack R, Katz J, Jeans ME. The role of compensation in chronic pain: Analysis using a new method of scoring the McGill Pain Questionnaire. *Pain.* 1985;23:101–112.
12. Frost H, Klaber Moffett JA, Moser JS, Fairbank JC. Randomised controlled trial for evaluation of fitness programme for patients with chronic low back pain. *BMJ.* 1995;310:151–154.
13. Geiger G, Todd DD, Clark HB, Miller RP, Kori SH. The effects of feedback and contingent reinforcement on the exercise behavior of chronic pain patients. *Pain.* 1992;49: 179–185.
14. Minor MA. Exercise in the management of osteoarthritis of the knee and hip. *Arthritis Care Res.* 1994;7:198–204.
15. Robinson AJ. Transcutaneous electrical nerve stimulation for the control of pain in musculoskeletal disorders. *J Orthop Sports Phys Ther.* 1996;24:208–226.
16. Baxter R. Drug control of pain. In: Wells PE, Frampton V, Bowsher D, eds. *Pain Management in Physical Therapy.* Norwalk, CT: Appleton & Lange; 1988.
17. Nolan MF, Wilson MCB. Patient-controlled analgesia: a method for the controlled self-administration of opioid pain medications. *Phys Ther.* 1995;75:374–379.

UNIT 3

Special Physiologic Considerations in Therapeutic Exercise

CHAPTER 10

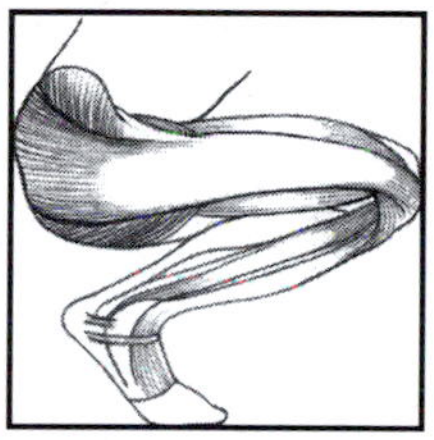

Soft Tissue Injury and Postoperative Treatment

Lori Thein Brody

Some musculoskeletal problems do not resolve with conservative management alone. In these cases, surgical intervention may be necessary to return the patient to optimal function. Frequently, a course of conservative management, including physical therapy, precedes surgery, and follow-up therapy is provided in the postoperative period. This gives the physical therapist the opportunity to participate in the patient's care in two critical perioperative periods.

Many specific physical therapy outcomes can be achieved when the therapist has the opportunity for a preoperative visit. Instruction in the postoperative exercise program occurs at a time when full attention can be given to the rehabilitation program, without the complications of postoperative pain and nausea. Instruction in crutch training, wound care, and use of any immobilization or supportive equipment can take place so the patient is not overburdened with multiple instructions after surgery. Bed mobility, precautions, and contraindications to certain movements should be taught. This visit allows positive interaction and development of a good rapport between the therapist and patient. The importance of adhering to the prescribed exercises in the postoperative program should be emphasized to the patient. Consultation with the patient about expected outcomes and return to function sets up realistic expectations after surgery.

Surgical procedures necessitating rehabilitation can be broadly categorized into soft tissue procedures and bony procedures. Soft tissue procedures are operations primarily directed at the soft tissues, such as tendons, ligaments, or joint capsules. In contrast, bony procedures are operations primarily directed at bone and adjacent tissues. These categories are not exclusive, because surgery often includes soft tissues and bone. However, the primary procedure may affect the soft tissue or bone predominantly, and rehabilitation follows those guidelines. Not all surgical procedures can be discussed here, and as new surgical techniques are employed, the rehabilitation probably will change. The physical therapist should focus on the principles of treating patients with different categories of procedures, rather than on specific diagnosis-based protocols.

PHYSIOLOGY OF CONNECTIVE TISSUE REPAIR

Soft tissues, including ligament, tendon, and other connective tissues, respond to injury in a relatively predictable fashion. The repair process is similar in all connective tissues, although some variability between tissues (eg, bone) exists. Healing is also affected by age, lifestyle, systemic factors (eg, alcohol abuse, smoking, diabetes mellitus, nutritional status, general health) and local factors (eg, degree of injury, mechanical stress, blood supply, edema or infection).[1,2] An understanding of the healing phases helps the clinician choose treatment procedures that are appropriate at various points in the healing process.

Microstructure of Connective Tissues

Tendon, ligament, cartilage, bone, and muscle are some of the major connective tissues in the body. The three main components of connective tissue are fibers (ie, collagen and elastin), ground substance with associated tissue fluid (ie, glycosaminoglycans such as proteoglycans), and cellular substances (ie, fibroblasts, fibrocytes, and cells specific to each connective tissue).[2] The function of the various connective tissues is based on the relative proportions of intracellular and extracellular components such as collagen, elastin, proteoglycans, water, and contractile proteins. At least 15 types of collagen (types I through XV) are known and differ fundamentally in the acid amino sequence of their constituent polypeptide chains (Table 10-1).[3,4]

Water makes up nearly two thirds of the weight of normal ligament, and collagen makes up 70% to 80% of the ligament's dry weight.[5] Nearly 90% of that collagen is type I, and 10% or less is type III collagen. Elastin is found in tiny quantities in ligaments, making up less than 1% to 2% of the total weight. Proteoglycans, another important solid found in ligaments, comprise less than 1% of the ligament's weight, but they are essential because of their water-binding properties.[1]

Tendon is a collection of closely packed collagen fibers that connect muscle to bone. Collagen forms 70% of the dry weight of tendon, and the overall proportions are 30% collagen, 2% elastin, and 68% water.[6] The low proportion of elastin accounts for the low elasticity of tendon. If tendon were more elastic, the tendon would elongate with muscle contraction, rather than transmitting the force to the bone. Muscle contraction would fail to move its insertion toward the origin, and no movement would take place. The structure provides some information about the function of this tissue.

Articular cartilage is composed of similar components, with nearly 80% of its weight from water. The high water content in articular cartilage, as in other viscoelastic tissues, is responsible for the mechanical properties of the tissue. The collagen makeup is primarily type II collagen, with small proportions of other collagen types.[4] Proteoglycans (ie, glycosaminoglycans) are water-loving, or hydrophilic, molecules. Proteoglycans are responsible for the water-binding capabilities of articular cartilage, and proteoglycan loss results in a decreased water content and loss of the tissue's mechanical properties. When a person bears weight on a limb, the compression causes fluid to be squeezed out of the tissue, and unweighting pulls fluid back in because of the hydrophilic nature of the proteoglycans. This action provides nutrition and lubrication for the articular cartilage. Weight bearing is important for the health of articular cartilage. As proteoglycans are lost with degenerative joint disease, the ability to resorb fluid is impaired, decreasing the ability to absorb shock or transmit loads.

Like the soft tissues of the body, bone is composed of solid and fluid components. Organic compounds such as type I collagen and proteoglycans constitute approximately 39% of the total bone volume.[7] Minerals contribute nearly half of the total bone volume, and fluid fills the vascular and cellular spaces comprising the remaining volume. The primary minerals found in bone are calcium hydroxyapatite crystals. These minerals differentiate bone from other connective tissue and provide bone with its distinctive stiffness.

Table 10-1. COLLAGENS OF JOINT TISSUE

TYPE	DISTRIBUTION
I	Bone, ligament, tendon, fibrocartilage, capsule, synovial lining tissues, skin
II	Cartilage, fibrocartilage
III	Blood vessels, synovial lining tissues, skin
IV	Basement membranes
V	Pericellular region of articular cartilage when present,* bone, blood vessels
VI	Nucleus pulposus
VII	Anchoring fibers of various tissues
VIII	Endothelial cells
IX	Cartilage matrix*
X	Hypertrophic and ossified cartilage only
XI	Cartilage matrix*
XII	Tendon, ligament, perichondrium, periosteum
XIII	Skin, tendon

* Small amounts (<20%).

From Walker JM. Cartilage of human joints and related structures. In: Zachazewski JE, Magee DJ, Quillen WS, eds: *Athletic Injuries and Rehabilitation*. WB Saunders; 1996:123.

Response to Loading

When connective tissues are loaded, the amount of force per unit area (ie, stress) can be plotted against the change in length per unit length (ie, strain). From this information, much about the material properties of the tissue can be derived. The relative contributions of composite materials determine the mechanical properties of the specific tissue. However, some general ideas about connective tissues can be determined.

Tensile loads are resisted primarily by the collagen fibrils, which respond first by straightening from their resting crimped state. This straightening requires little force (Fig. 10-1). In the elastic portion of the curve, the collagen fibers respond to the load in a linear fashion up to 4% elongation.[6,8] After the load is removed, the tendon returns to its original length, a characteristic of the elastic range only up to the elastic limit. Beyond this point, removal of the stress does not result in a return to the tissue's original length. If the tissue is elongated beyond approximately 4%, plastic changes begin to occur (ie, plastic range) as the cross-links begin to fail. Permanent deformation is the chief characteristic of the plastic range. After some fibers fail, the load on the remaining fibers is increased, accelerating tissue failure. The yield point is the point at which an increase in strain occurs without an increase in stress; here, the curve plateaus or even dips. The ultimate strength is the greatest load the tissue can tolerate, and rupture strength is the point at which complete failure occurs.

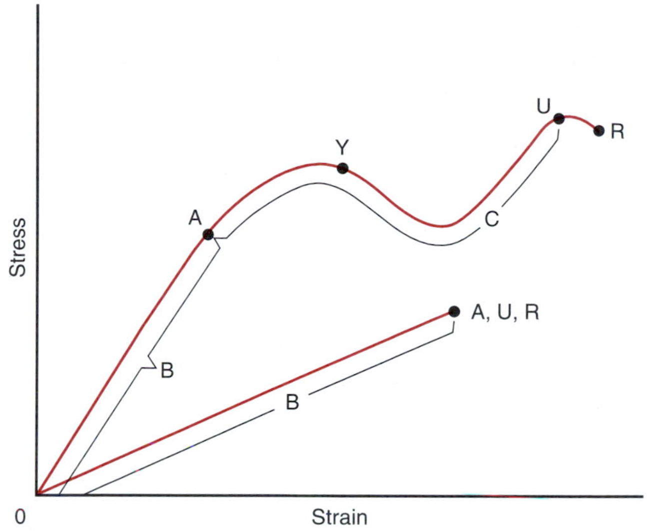

FIGURE 10-1 The stress-strain curve showing the elastic limit (*A*), elastic range (*B*), yield point (*Y*) plastic range (*C*) ultimate strength (*U*), and the rupture strength (*R*). (Adapted from: Cornwall MW. Biomechanics of orthopaedic and sports therapy. In: Malone TR, McPoil T, Nitz AJ, eds. *Orthopedic and Sports Physical Therapy.* 3rd ed. C.V. Mosby, St. Louis: Mosby; 1997:73.

The area under the curve represents the amount of strain energy stored in the tissue during loading. The viscoelastic nature of connective tissue results in an imperfect recovery after deformation, known as hysteresis. This difference between the loading curve and the unloading curve represents energy lost. This energy is lost primarily in the form of heat. A stretched tissue becomes warm in the process.

Other tissue qualities related to the load deformation curve are resilience and toughness. Resilience reflects a material's ability to absorb energy within the elastic range. As a resilient tissue is loaded quickly, work is performed, and energy is absorbed. When the load is removed, the tissue quickly releases energy and returns to its original shape. Toughness is the ability of a material to absorb energy within the plastic range. A critical quality of connective tissues is their ability to absorb energy without rupturing.

A relationship exists between stress and strain called the elastic modulus. The elastic modulus is the ratio of the stress divided by the strain and reflects the amount of stress needed to produce a given strain (ie, deformation). The greater the stress necessary to deform the tissue, the stiffer is the material. For example, bone has a higher elastic modulus than meniscus and deforms less with a given load.

Cyclic loading alters the load deformation curve. Heat accumulates in the area of loading, disrupting the collagen cross-bridges. Cyclic loading produces microstructural damage that accumulates with each loading cycle. Damage accumulates faster at higher intensities of cyclic loading.[9] Failure as a result of cyclic loading, called fatigue failure, is the physiologic basis underlying stress fractures. Endurance limit or fatigue strength is the stress below which fatigue cracks do not begin to form.[9]

Connective tissues also demonstrate viscoelastic properties that provide these tissues with their uniquely mutable characteristics. These properties are creep and relaxation. When a tissue is held with a constant force, it begins

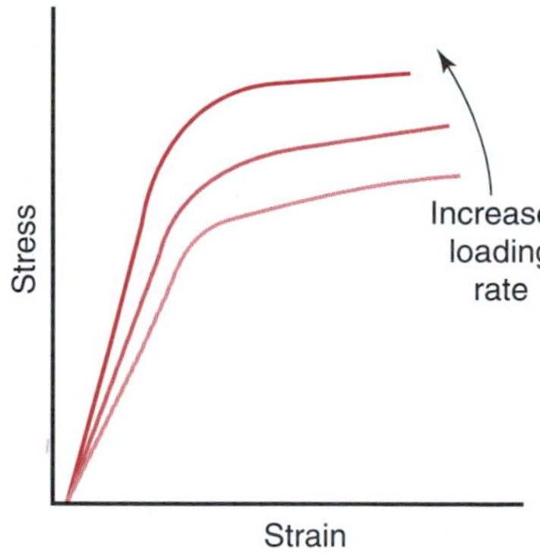

FIGURE 10-2 Three stress-strain curves for cortical bone tissues tested in tension at three different loading rates. As the testing rate increases, the slope (the elastic modulus) of the initial straight line portion increases. (Adapted from Burstein AH, Wright TM., *Fundamentals of Orthopaedic Biomechanics.* Baltimore:Williams & Wilkins; 1994:120.)

to lengthen until equilibrium is reached or until the tissue ruptures, depending on the magnitude of the force. This property is called creep. When a tissue is pulled to a fixed length, a certain force is required. As the tissue is held at this length, the amount of force necessary to maintain that length decreases. This property is called relaxation. These properties allow connective tissues to adapt to and function in a variety of loading conditions without being damaged. Tissues pulled into tension (ie, stretched) lengthen and relax, which provides the rationale for stretching exercises to lengthen shortened soft tissues (Figs. 10-2 through 10-4).

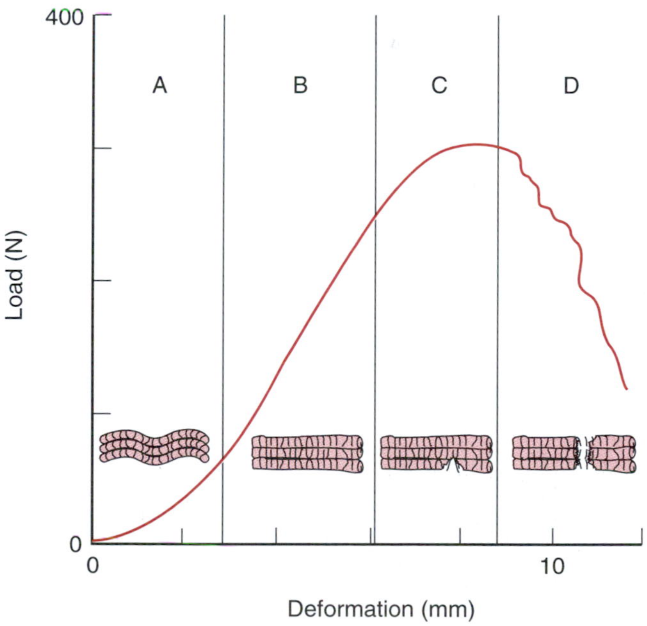

FIGURE 10-3 Stress-strain curve for ligament. As the ligament is distracted, fibers become progressively recruited into tension (*A*) until all the fibers are tight (*B*). The parts of the ligament that are tightened first are likely to be the first to fail (*C*) as the ligament reaches the yield point. Progressive fiber failures quickly results in ligament failure (*D*). (Adapted from Frank CB. Ligament injuries: Pathophysiology and healing. In: Zachazewski JE, Magee DJ, Quillen WS, eds. *Athletic Injuries and Rehabilitation.* Philadelphia:WB Saunders; 1996:15.)

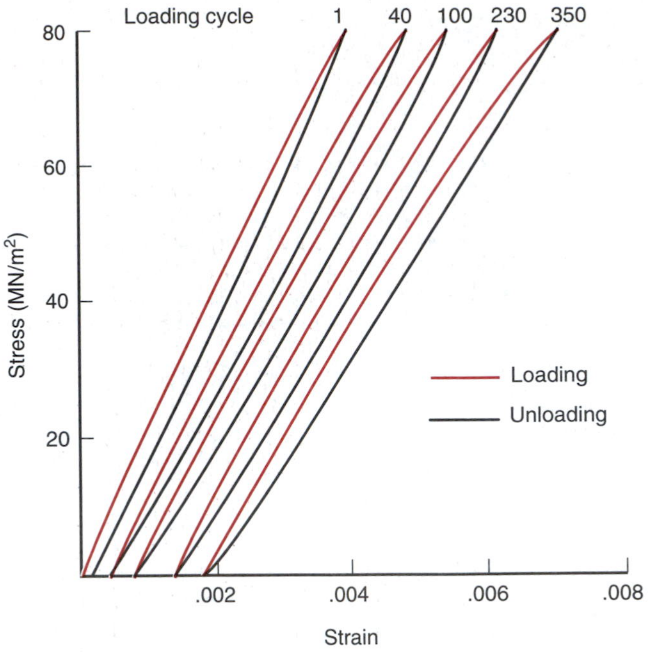

FIGURE 10-4 Effects of cyclic loading. When bone tissue is loaded cyclically to 90% of its tensile yield strength, nonreversible behavior (ie, damage) is seen. By the 350th loading cycle, the elastic modulus has changed appreciably. (Adapted from Burstein AH, Wright TM. *Fundamentals of Orthopaedic Biomechanics.* Baltimore:Williams & Wilkins; 1994:125.)

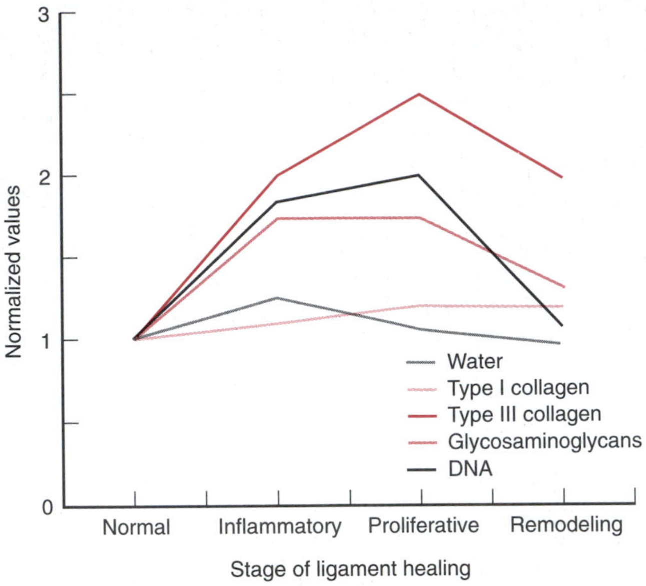

FIGURE 10-5 Changes in components of rabbit medial collateral ligaments at various stages of healing. Values are normalized to that of uninjured ligament (normal = 1). (Adapted from Andriaacchi T, Sabiston P, DeHaven K, Dahners L et al. Ligament: Injury and repair. In: Woo SL-Y, Buckwalter JA, eds. *Injury and Repair of the Musculoskeletal Soft Tissues.* Park Ridge, IL: American Academy of Orthopaedic Surgeons; 1988:115.

Phases of Healing

The clinician must understand the phases of healing to formulate a plan of care matching the tissue's loading capabilities. The phases of healing provide a framework into which the rationale for physical therapy interventions fit. Understanding the healing process gives the clinician the tools to treat a variety of injury and surgical conditions.

PHASE I: INFLAMMATORY RESPONSE

Healing of acute injuries passes through three major phases, beginning with the acute vascular-inflammatory response (Fig. 10-5). When connective tissue is damaged, injured cells in the area release chemical substances (eg, prostaglandins, bradykinin) that initiate the inflammatory response. The gap in the torn tissue is filled with erythrocytes and platelets.[1] Local bleeding is a strong chemotactic stimulus, attracting white blood cells such as neutrophils and mononuclear leukocytes that help rid the site of bacteria and cellular debris through phagocytosis. Concurrently, vasodilation occurs to increase local blood flow while capillary permeability is altered to allow greater exudation of plasma proteins and white blood cells. In this phase, the damaged tissues and microorganisms are removed, fibroblasts are recruited, and some wound strength is provided by the weak hydrogen bonds of collagen fibers.[10] The inflammatory phase is essential in initiating the healing process. This phase is initiated immediately and lasts 3 to 5 days.[10]

Signs and symptoms observed in this phase are pain, warmth, palpable tenderness, and swelling. Pain and tenderness are caused by mechanical and chemical stimulation of nociceptors, and warmth and swelling are caused by acute inflammation. Limitations in joint or muscle range of motion (ROM) from pain or direct tissue damage are likely to occur. ROM testing usually reveals pain before the end of the ROM is reached.

Treatment procedures in this phase are aimed at decreasing pain and tenderness while preventing a progressive chronic inflammation. The mobility and strength of adjacent joints and soft tissues should be maintained while the acutely injured areas are rested (see Patient-Related Instruction: Acute Injury Management).

PHASE II: REPAIR AND REGENERATION

The second phase, lasting from 48 hours to 8 weeks, is the repair-regeneration stage, marked by the presence in tissue of macrophages directing the cascade of events occurring in this proliferative phase. Fibroblasts are actively resorbing

Patient-Related Instruction

Acute Injury Management

Take the following steps when an acute musculoskeletal injury or a flare-up of a pre-existing injury occurs:

1. Ice the area for 10–15 minutes using cold packs or ice. Do this as often as possible throughout the day.
2. If possible, elevate the part to decrease swelling.
3. Apply compression in the form of an elastic sleeve or bandage. Remove the compression at night for sleeping.
4. Use a supportive or assistive device (eg, sling, splint, cane, crutches, walker) to rest the injury.
5. Contact your clinician or physician regarding the need for further evaluation.
6. Resume previous program of care when instructed or able.

collagen and synthesizing new collagen (primarily type III). The new collagen is characterized by small fibrils, disorganized in orientation and deficient in cross-linking.[10] Consequently, the tissue laid down in this phase is susceptible to disruption by overly aggressive activity. As this phase progresses, a gradual decrease in tissue macrophages and fibroblasts occurs, and a grossly visible scar filling the gap can be seen.[11]

The warmth and edema resolves during this phase. Palpable tenderness decreases, and the tissue can withstand gentle loading. Pain is felt concurrent with tissue resistance or stretch of the tissue.

Treatment procedures in this phase include ROM exercises, joint mobilization and scar mobilization to produce a mobile scar. These interventions are most effective during this stage of healing. Gentle resistance may be applied to maintain mobility and strength of the musculotendinous unit.

In bone, osteoclasts perform a function analogous to the macrophages in soft tissue. These cells debride the fracture ends and prepare the area for healing. The infrastructure for healing is assembled, including a capillary structure supporting callus formation. This callus bridges the gap between the fracture ends. Although the bone repair is relatively weak at this point, limited activity is allowed. This loading promotes remodeling and maturation.

PHASE III: REMODELING AND MATURATION

As healing progresses to the third phase, the remodeling-maturation stage, a shift is made to the deposition of type I collagen. This phase is characterized by decreased synthetic activity and cellularity, with increased organization of extracellular matrix. The collagen continues to increase and begins to organize into randomly placed fibrils with stronger covalent bonds. At this point, tension becomes important in providing orientation guidance to the organizing collagen. The new collagen must orient and align along the lines of stress to best accommodate the functional loads required. This tension can be imposed by stretching, active contraction (in the case of the musculotendinous unit), resistive loads, or electrical stimulation. The end of tissue remodeling is unknown and may take months to years for completion.

Like the remodeling-maturation phase in soft tissues, loading is important in the final phase of bone healing. In this phase of bone healing, woven bone (ie, immature bone) is replaced by well-organized lamellar bone. Normal loading is necessary to remodel the bone in accordance to the stresses that it will bear (ie, Wolff's Law). The linkage of electrical charges with mechanical loading is called the piezoelectric effect.[2] Piezoelectric effects in the calcium hydroxyapatite crystals due to loads orient the crystals along lines of stress. In long, weight-bearing bones, activity differs on the concave and convex sides. On the concave side, osteoblasts lay down more bone where bone is subject to compression (ie, negative charge). On the convex side, osteoclasts digest bone that is subject to tension (ie, positive charge). Imposition of normal functional loads are necessary for the final remodeling of bone. Electrical stimulation is used to enhance bone healing using the same piezoelectric effect.

PRINCIPLES OF TREATING CONNECTIVE TISSUE INJURIES

A variety of procedures are available to achieve physical therapy goals. Although detailing every situation the clinician may encounter is difficult, specific principles guide the decision-making process. These principles direct the goal-setting process, providing a framework and rationale for intervention choices.

Restoration of Normal Tissue Relationships

After connective tissue injury, the relationships of a variety of tissues are altered. After injury or immobilization, the tendon may fail to glide smoothly through the tendon sheath, the nerve may be adhered to surrounding tissues, folds of joint capsule may become adhered to one another, or fascial layers may fail to glide on one another. These normal relationships must be restored, or painful and restricted movement may result. Treatments such as active muscle contraction, passive joint motion or mobilization, modality use, or massage restore those relationships. The normal length-tension relationship of the muscle must be recovered to ensure optimal function.

Optimal Loading

After a connective tissue injury, a cascade of events facilitate the body's healing process. If this cascade is interrupted, healing is disrupted, and chronic inflammation may ensue. During each of the healing phases, treatment procedures must be chosen that aid the healing process without disrupting the normal chain of events. This requires optimal loading or choosing a level of loading that neither overloads nor underloads the healing tissue (Fig. 10-6). A thorough understanding of the mechanism of injured tissue loading, including which planes of movement place the greatest loads on the healing tissue, is necessary for the effective application of optimal loads.

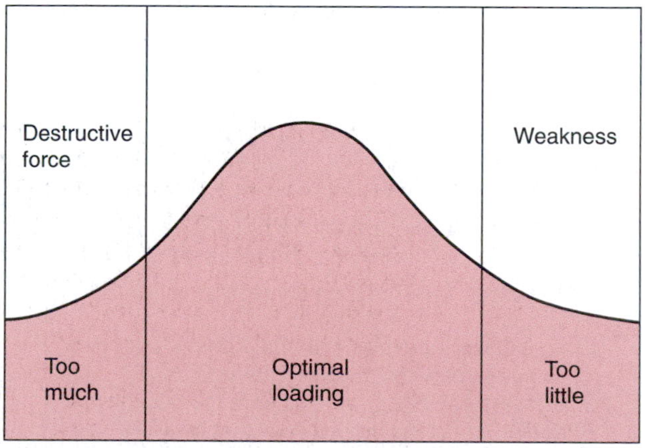

FIGURE 10-6 Optimal loading. Choose a load that neither overloads nor underloads the tissue of interest. (From Porterfield JA, DeRosa C. Mechanical low back pain. Philadelphia: WB Saunders; 1991:13.)

The biomechanical effects of daily activities and therapeutic activities must be considered in the context of the stage of healing, and individual factors such as age, quality of the tissue, nutritional status, and fitness level. A stress that underloads a tissue in the remodeling phase probably overloads the tissue in the inflammatory phase. An exercise that underloads a young athlete after an acute fracture would probably overload an elderly individual after a pathologic fracture. For example, the medial collateral ligament of the knee is loaded most in the frontal plane with the knee near terminal extension. In the acute phase, activities that load the knee in the frontal plane near full knee extension are avoided. However, in the late phases, when remodeling of the ligament is necessary, frontal plane loading is precisely the stimulus needed. Designing the treatment program requires consideration of all of the factors in the intervention model within the injury framework (see Patient-Related Instruction: Signs of Overload).

Specific Adaptations to Imposed Demands

Although the concept of optimal loading guides the *quantity* of activity (eg, volume, intensity), the specific adaptations to imposed demands (SAID) principle expands to include the *type* of activity chosen. The SAID principle is an extension of Wolff's law, which states that a bone remodels according to the stresses that are placed on it. The SAID principle implies that soft tissues remodel according to the stresses imposed on them and is applied when choosing an exercise or activity throughout the stages of healing. Exercise is specific to the posture, mode, movement, exercise type, environment, and intensity used. For example, in the early phase, exercise may be chosen to prepare the quadriceps muscle for weight bearing. The quadriceps muscle contracts eccentrically in a closed chain through the first 15 degrees of knee flexion during the loading response of gait. A closed chain eccentric quadriceps exercise such as a short-arc (0 to 15 degrees) leg press is a better choice than quadriceps setting. This is an example of the SAID principle guiding the activity choice.

The SAID principle also guides exercise prescription parameters. For example, in the late stage of healing, a patient returning to tennis should increase the speed and intensity of his exercise, whereas the patient returning to marathon training should increase the exercise duration. When the stage of healing and optimal loading parameters allow, training should as closely as possible reflect the specific demands of the patient's functional task.

Patient-Related Instruction

Signs of Overload

The following signs and symptoms suggest that exercise or activity is too much and should be decreased or modified:

1. Increased pain that does not resolve within the next 12 hours
2. Pain that is increased over the previous session or comes on earlier in the exercise session
3. Increased swelling, warmth, or redness in the injury area
4. Decreased ability to use the part

Prevention of Complications

The clinician must consider the effects of the connective tissue injury on surrounding tissues. For example, immobilization imposed while a fracture is healing is unhealthy for the joint's articular cartilage, ligaments, and surrounding musculature, although it is necessary for bone repair. Muscle atrophy and weakening of the immobilized ligaments ensue as well. Any available treatment procedures that may minimize these effects should be incorporated. Electrical stimulation or isometric muscle contractions can be used to minimized strength losses in the muscle, tendon, and tendon insertion sites. Active muscle contractions also prevent thrombus formation after surgery. Motion at joints above and below injury sites may preserve some soft tissue relationships and prevent loss of mobility. Weight bearing loads the articular cartilage and lessens changes caused by immobilization.

MANAGEMENT OF SPRAINS, STRAINS, AND CONTUSIONS

Patients with acute soft tissue injuries such as sprains, strains, and contusions are commonly treated by physical therapy clinicians. Management of these injuries is discussed together because of the many similarities, and any differences are highlighted.

Sprain: Injury to Ligament and Capsule

A sprain can be defined as an acute injury to a ligament or joint capsule without dislocation. Sprains generally occur when a joint is extended beyond its normal limit, and the ligament or capsule tissues are stretched or torn beyond their limit. Sprains are common at the ankle (ie, anterior talofibular and calcaneofibular ligaments), knee (ie, medial and lateral collateral ligaments, anterior and posterior cruciate ligaments), wrist, and spine. A sprain may resolve with short-term immobilization, controlled activity, and rehabilitative exercises, but other sprains may require surgery to stabilize the joint.

SPRAIN CLASSIFICATION

Sprain severity occurs along a continuum from microscopic tearing and stretching of ligament or capsule fibers to complete disruption of the ligament. Sprains are classified by severity based on clinical examination or special testing (eg, magnetic resonance imaging, arthrometer testing). Grade I sprains are considered to be mild sprains in which the ligament is stretched, but there is no discontinuity of the ligament. A grade II sprain is considered to be a moderate sprain in which some fibers are stretched and some fibers are torn. This produces some laxity at the joint. A grade III, or severe sprain, is a complete or nearly complete ligament disruption with resultant laxity (Table 10-2).

Table 10-2. CLASSIFICATION OF SPRAIN

GRADE	DESCRIPTION	CHARACTERISTICS
Grade I	Mild	Fibers are stretched without loss of continuity
Grade II	Moderate	Some fibers are stretched, and some are torn. Some laxity observed on examination
Grade III	Severe	Ligament completely or nearly completely torn; laxity results.

From American Academy of Orthopaedic Surgeons. *Athletic Training and Sports Medicine*. Park Ridge, II: American Academy of Orthopaedic Surgeons; 1991.

EXAMINATION AND EVALUATION

Examination techniques for the individual with a ligament sprain include assessment of edema and ecchymosis and assessment of normal movement patterns, such as gait in lower extremity problems and forward reaching in upper extremity injuries. Active and passive ROM, strength testing, and pain assessment provide information regarding impairments associated with the injury. Special tests such as manual or instrumented laxity testing provide a baseline measure of joint laxity (Fig. 10-7). Instability or apprehension testing provide information about the instability associated with that laxity. Palpation identifies the specific location of the primary and any secondary injuries. Joints proximal and distal to the primary joint injury should be evaluated to exclude associated injuries. Functional limitations should be determined, and the relationship between impairments and functional limitations identified.

Strain: Musculotendinous Injury

A strain is an acute injury to the muscle or tendon from an abrupt or excessive muscle contraction. Strains are usually the result of a quick overload to the muscle-tendon unit in which the tension generated exceeds the tissue's capacity. Strains occur when a contracting muscle is excessively or abruptly stretched in the opposite direction. The person who reaches quickly to catch a falling object or the individual who suddenly stops or changes direction when walking or running is susceptible to a muscle strain.

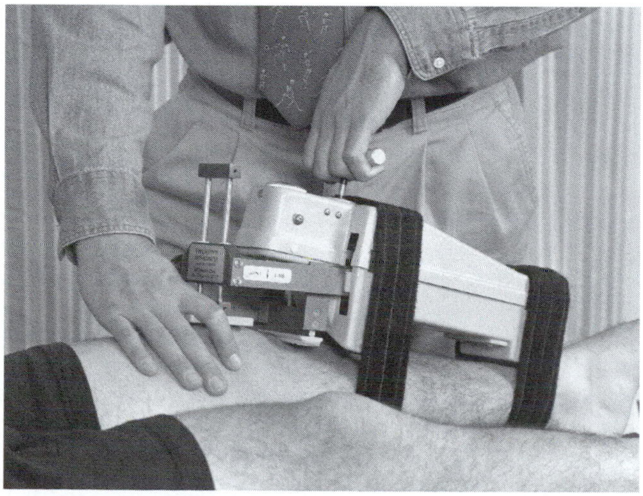

FIGURE 10-7 KT-1000 testing for anterior or posterior cruciate ligament laxity.

Strain injuries are difficult to classify and can be graded as mild, moderate, or severe based on clinical examination findings such as pain, edema, loss of motion, and tenderness. Muscle strains can be complete or incomplete, although complete tears are less common.

Most strain injuries occur at the myotendinous junction.[12] As with many other structures in the body, transitions from one tissue type to another are areas of increased stress and risk of injury. In this case, the transition zone from contractile to noncontractile tissue creates an area of increased stress, susceptible to injury. Structural features of the sarcomeres and connective tissues in this area support the role of load transmission across the musculotendinous junction. Factors that may contribute to muscle strain injuries include poor flexibility, inadequate warm-up exercise, insufficient strength or endurance, and poor coordination.[12]

EXAMINATION AND EVALUATION

A thorough history provides the clinician with clues to the examination of the muscle strain. An abrupt decelerating movement, change of direction, or quick stretch may precipitate a muscle strain. The clinician palpates the location of pain at the musculotendinous junction or along the muscle belly. Muscle injuries can be reproduced clinically by active or resistive contraction of the muscle and by stretching in the opposite direction. For example, a quadriceps strain is reproduced by stretching the knee into flexion and by resisting active knee extension. The muscle may need to be put on stretch during the active or resistive muscle contraction to stress the lesion. Occasionally, localized swelling and warmth may be observed.

Contusion

A contusion occurs as the result of a blow and can occur in any area of the body to a variety of tissues. No break in the skin occurs, although blood vessels below the skin may be injured, causing ecchymosis in the area. If the damage is more extensive and large blood vessels in the area are disrupted, a localized area of blood may accumulate in deeper tissues, forming a hematoma. When a deep tissue hematoma occurs, ecchymosis may or may not be seen on the skin surface. For example, quadriceps femoris contusions frequently result in hematoma formation. This hematoma is easily palpable within the muscle, but it is rarely accompanied by ecchymosis. The severity of this type of injury can be deceptive, and if left untreated, it may progress to myositis ossificans. Myositis ossificans is the formation of heterotopic bone within the muscle. Bleeding in the area of the contusion initiates the inflammatory response and healing process.

EXAMINATION AND EVALUATION

The history of a blow provides the best information for evaluation of a contusion. The size, location, and direction of the blow provide the clinician with valuable clues about the location and extent of soft tissue injuries. After observation and palpation of the area for localized swelling or hematoma, assessment of joint mobility, muscle strength, and mobility and function should follow. A diagnosis and prognosis based on the evaluation guide treatment procedures. Muscle contusions at risk for ectopic bone formation (eg, quadriceps femoris, biceps brachii) are treated more cautiously than simple subcutaneous tissue contusions, and the evaluation process must clarify the extent of tissue involvement.

Application of Treatment Principles

PHASE I

Treatment principles in the early phase include optimal loading and prevention of secondary complications. As the inflammatory response initiates the healing response, an environment conducive to healing must be established. The appropriate balance of rest and loading ensure loads within the optimal loading zone for the patient's age, medical condition, and injury severity. Overload may perpetuate bleeding or the inflammatory response beyond its useful purpose, and underload may result in complications such as motion loss, scar tissue adhesions, or ectopic ossification.

Modality use in this phase primarily includes cryotherapy and compression with elevation to decrease bleeding and swelling. Most injuries allow passive or active ROM in a pain-free range, although exercise may be contraindicated in some cases. Isometric muscle contraction, in the absence of moderate or severe muscle strains, can lessen atrophy and serve as a learning activity, reminding the patient how to contract involved muscles (Fig. 10-8). Because the muscle is the primary tissue involved in a strain, active muscle contraction may be limited or reduced significantly in intensity. When treating lower extremity injuries, assistive devices, immobilizers, and weight-bearing restrictions can maintain tissue loading within the optimal loading zone. Treatments that impose rest or restriction must be balanced with activity that offsets the negative effects of immobility (see Selected Intervention: Isometric Ankle Eversion for the Patient Following Ligament Reconstruction).

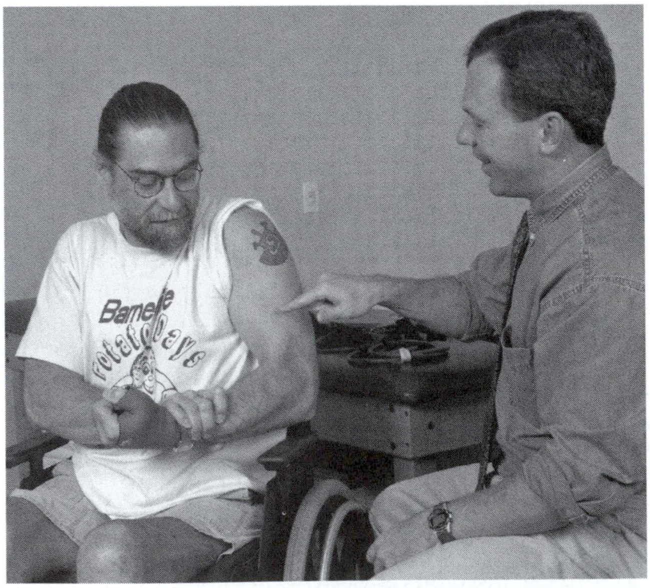

FIGURE 10-8 Clinician instructing patient in isometric biceps curl.

PHASE II

As healing progresses to the repair and regeneration phase, treatment principles focus on restoration of normal tissue relationships, optimal loading, and prevention of complications. Complications in this phase may result from changes in movement patterns to accommodate pain, weakness, or motion loss. These movement pattern changes can create excessive loads on uninjured tissues that can become painful. These changes also become habitual and can be difficult to correct. Examples of these habits are hiking the shoulder (ie, scapular elevation) during forward reaching and ambulating with a flexed knee. Faulty movement patterns are deleterious for the long-term health of the joint and should be corrected as quickly as possible. Complications such as ectopic bone formation can result from improperly treated muscle contusions.

Restoration of normal tissue relationships can prevent these faulty movement patterns by re-establishing joint ROM and muscle length. As healing occurs, connective tissue tends to shorten. Joint mobilization techniques, stretching, postural education exercises, and massage techniques can facilitate restoration of these relationships. Connective tissue massage performed by the patient can increase scar tissue mobility (Fig. 10-9). Active muscle contraction of the muscle opposing the short muscle is an active stretching technique that can restore normal tissue relationships (Fig. 10-10).

Optimal loading concepts provide the framework for exercise parameters. Understanding the effects of muscle contraction and the location and direction of loading on the healing tissue is fundamental to optimally loading the tissue. Loading is important in the repair-regeneration phase, because loads help orient newly forming collagen fibrils along the lines of stress. Excessive loading disrupts the healing process, and underloading results in randomly organized collagen. Weight bearing, active and resistive mobility activities, massage, and functional movement patterns can provide these loads. By the end of this phase, mobility and a strength base should be established.

PHASE III

As the patient returns to activity, the guiding principles are optimal loading and SAID. The type and magnitude of loads encountered in the patient's daily routine, including work and leisure activities, determine the specific rehabilitation activities chosen (Fig. 10-11). The goal in the final phase is to "fine tune" or convert that baseline strength and mobility into functional movement patterns and activities that address the patient's functional limitations and disability. The exercises generally consist of more whole-body patterns and functional activities related to the patient's lifestyle. At the same time, consideration must be given to the status

SELECTED INTERVENTION

Isometric Ankle Eversion for the Patient Following Ligament Reconstruction

See Case Study #1

Although this patient requires comprehensive intervention as described in the patient management model, one specific exercise is described.

ACTIVITY: Isometric ankle eversion

PURPOSE: Increased ability to produce torque in the peroneal muscles without excessively loading the acutely injured tissue

RISK FACTORS: No appreciable risk factors

ELEMENTS OF THE MOVEMENT SYSTEM: Base

STAGE OF MOTOR CONTROL: Mobility

POSTURE: Any comfortable position such as sitting or supine. The lateral border of the foot is stabilized against a stationary object.

MOVEMENT: Patient performs an isometric ankle eversion contraction against a stationary object.

SPECIAL CONSIDERATIONS: Ensure that muscle contraction is at a submaximal level during the acute phase. Maximal muscle contraction can overload recently injured tissues. Be sure eversion is not substituted with tibial external rotation, hip abduction, or external rotation.

DOSAGE

TYPE OF MUSCLE CONTRACTION: Isometric
- **Intensity:** Submaximal
- **Duration:** To fatigue, pain, or 20 repetitions
- **Frequency:** Hourly or as frequently as possible during the day
- **Environment:** Home

RATIONALE FOR EXERCISE CHOICE: This exercise was chosen to begin retraining the peroneal muscles. Isotonic exercises can overload the muscle in the acute phase, but submaximal isometric contraction maintains loading within the optimal loading zone. Gentle isometric activation "reminds" the muscle how to contract, providing a foundation for further strengthening in later phases.

EXERCISE MODIFICATION OR GRADATION: As healing progresses, isometric contractions may be performed at multiple angles. Isometric contractions should be progressed to isotonic exercise through a range of motion. Closed chain exercise should be incorporated as weight bearing allows.

of healing tissue and the loads placed on it with activities chosen. For example, repeatedly throwing a fastball on a repaired elbow medial collateral ligament excessively loads that repair at this point. A graded, progressive functional exercise is necessary to resume activities with such loads (Fig. 10-12).

MANAGEMENT OF FRACTURES

A fracture can be defined as a break in the continuity of the bone.[13] Most fractures are the result of an acute injury (ie, macrotrauma), although stress fractures can occur as

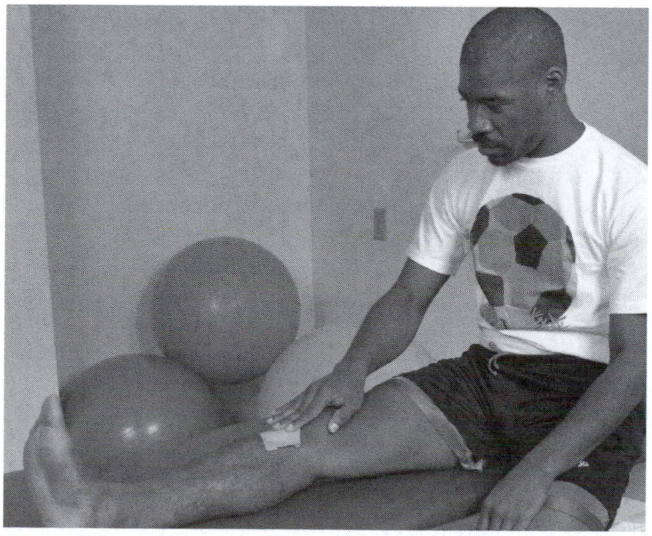

FIGURE 10-9 Scar mobilization performed by the patient.

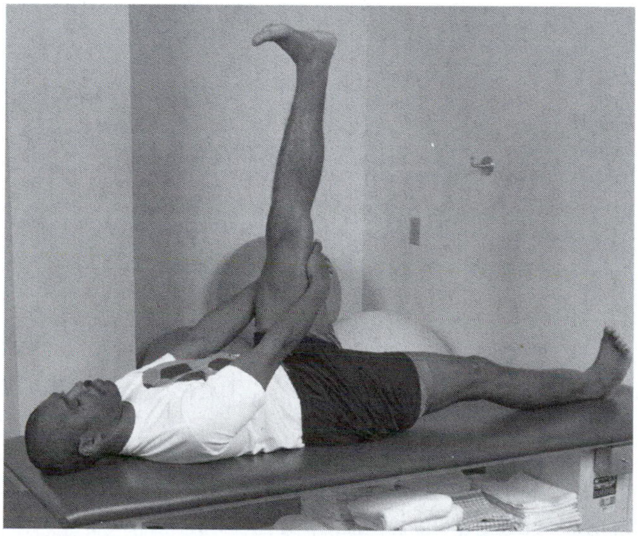

FIGURE 10-10 Active quadriceps contraction facilitating a hamstring stretch.

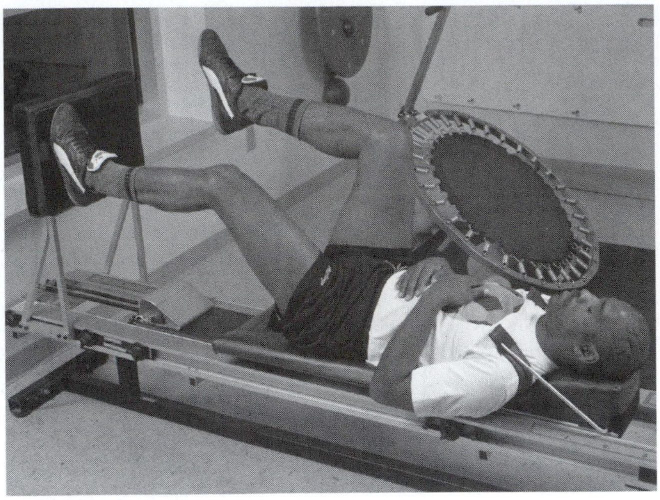

FIGURE 10-11 Example of impact loading in a horizontal position as a transitional activity between strengthening and impact loading in a vertical position.

the result of microtrauma. Fractures are categorized by whether the skin is broken (ie, open or closed), the amount of disruption (ie, displaced or nondisplaced), and the type of fracture (eg, greenstick, comminuted). The type and degree of force required to fracture a bone usually injures the surrounding soft tissue as well. When designing the rehabilitation program, consideration should be given to associated soft tissues that have been injured and subsequently immobilized.

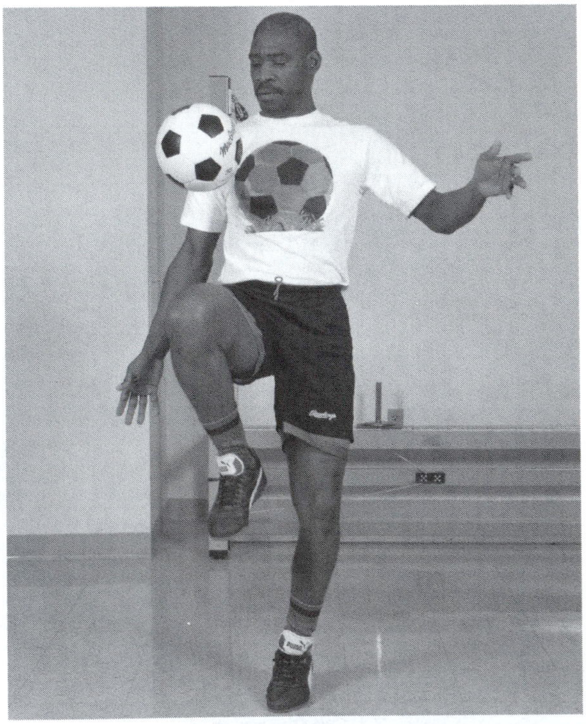

FIGURE 10-12 A soccer drill performed by soccer coach is an example of a graded, progressive study.

Classification of Fractures

Classification is first determined by whether the fractured bone is protruding through the skin. Fractures breaking the skin surface are considered open fractures, and those that do not break the skin are classified as closed fractures. The continuity of the ends of the fracture are then considered. If the bone on all sides of the fracture remain in anatomic alignment, the fracture is considered nondisplaced. Nondisplaced fractures are more difficult to diagnose and require special studies such as radiography to verify. Fractures in which the ends of the bones are not in anatomic alignment with each other are considered displaced fractures.

Fractures are described by the type of break or disruption. A greenstick fracture is an incomplete fracture that occurs in children. It is so named because of its resemblance to a green stick or twig that partially breaks when bent. Epiphyseal fractures also occur in children and are fractures through the growth plate. Salter and Harris[14] subclassified epiphyseal fractures into five different types depending on the extent of fracture affecting the epiphysis and metaphysis. Children are also susceptible to avulsion fractures, in which a tendon or ligament is detached from its attachment by a small piece of bone. Because of the relative strength of the collagenous tissues compared with bone in this population, it is not uncommon to see young persons avulse structures such as anterior cruciate ligaments or the proximal origin of the hamstring muscle from the bony attachments.

Comminuted fractures break into more than two fragments and are often the result of significant trauma, such as a fall or motor vehicle accident. Pathologic fractures occur in damaged or diseased bones, as in the elderly with osteoporosis. These fractures are produced with surprisingly minimal force. Stress fractures are overuse injuries in which the bone's ability to remodel is incapable of keeping up with the breakdown resulting from activity. Stress fractures occur in persons involved in repetitive activities such as running and jumping and in those with decreased bone density.

Application of Treatment Principles

IMMOBILIZED FRACTURES

The fracture site and joints above and below the fracture usually are immobilized for some time to allow healing. For patients with external fixation (eg, cast, splint), physical therapy treatment focuses on rehabilitating the soft tissues that were damaged at the time of fracture and that were subsequently immobilized. The effects of immobilization on soft tissues are described in Chapter 6 and consist of softening of the articular cartilage, shortening and atrophy of musculotendinous units, decreased mobility of the joint capsule and periarticular connective tissues, and decreased circulation. These changes must be considered when initiating rehabilitation after immobilization. Optimal loading and restoration of normal tissue relationships are the goals when rehabilitating patients after fracture immobilization.

Initially, joint mobilization, stretching, and other gentle mobility activities can begin to restore ROM and normal soft tissue relationships without overloading the tissues. Gentle strengthening in the form of isometrics or gentle isotonics stimulates increases in muscle performance. These same activities and controlled weight bearing load articular cartilage to reverse the changes resulting from immobilization. Electrical stimulation or biofeedback may be necessary in treating significant muscle atrophy. As impairments improve, activities to alleviate any remaining functional limitations facilitate the patient's return to work, leisure, and community activities.

SURGICALLY STABILIZED FRACTURES

Fractures of the hip and femur are examples of fractures that are frequently treated with surgical stabilization. The lengthy immobilization and significant lifestyle restrictions make conservative treatment of some fractures unrealistic. Open reduction and internal fixation (ORIF) provides immediate fixation of the fracture without the deleterious effects of immobilization.

When treating the individual who underwent surgical fixation of an acute fracture, treatment principles in the early phase focus on recovery from the trauma of the original injury and the trauma of surgery. The principles are the same as those for treating soft tissue strains, sprains, and contusions while also addressing postfracture and postoperative pain. When choosing exercises, the clinician must also consider the effects of the magnitude and direction of loading on the fracture site. The stability of the fracture and fixation guide exercise choice, and this information should be obtained from the chart or from the physician. For example, a patient with a fixated patellar fracture may avoid weight bearing to prevent distraction loads at the fixation site, but a patient with a fixated tibia fracture may be allowed to bear weight as tolerated to compress the fracture. Activities that address impairments and functional limitations while keeping loads within the optimal loading zone can then be safely chosen.

STRESS FRACTURES

Stress fractures are a type of overuse injury in which the osteoblastic activity cannot keep pace with osteoclastic activity. This occurs when repetitive loading without adequate recovery is imposed. The metatarsal bones, tibia, and spine are common sites of stress fractures.

The most important aspect of stress fracture care is decreasing loading to allow healing to occur. This may range from leisure activity limitation to short-term immobilization. During this phase, rehabilitation procedures include treating any impairment of mobility, muscle balance, or movement patterns that may have predisposed the individual to a stress fracture. If decreased bone mineral density is suspected as an underlying problem, education or referral for proper evaluation and testing should be instituted.

After loading at the fracture is allowed, determination of the optimal loading zone is imperative. The patient must learn which exercise or work parameters (eg, intensity, repetitions, duration, frequency) keep him within the optimal loading zone. Activities chosen should duplicate the activities to which the patient will be returning. If possible, the activity should be used as a component of the rehabilitation program. The functional activity, whether work, leisure, or recreational activities, should be used as the measure of progress, and full return can be allowed when the fracture has healed and is no longer painful to load.

MANAGEMENT OF TENDINITIS AND TENDON INJURIES

Tendon failure can occur as a result of macrotrauma or microtrauma. Tendons are able to withstand high loads, but if these loads become repetitive, injury may result. Injury occurs on a microscopic or macroscopic level, with damage to the structural proteins and the blood supply. Adequate time must be allowed for healing to take place, or tendinitis will develop. As the understanding of tendinitis has progressed, new classification schemes of tendon injury have been developed. In addition to the global categories of acute and chronic, tendon injuries have been subclassified as paratenonitis, tendinosis, tendinitis, and paratenonitis with tendinosis.[15] Each of these subcategories has treatment ramifications.

Classification of Tendon Injuries

Acute injuries occur as a result of sudden injury, often decelerating in nature, and they are followed by a lengthy but predictable outcome.[15] Loads during normal activities generally do not exceed 25% of the tendon's ultimate tensile strength.[16,17] However, loads during high-level activities, such as kicking, have been found to exceed this average level. For example, loads estimated in a weight lifter at the time of patellar tendon rupture were 17 times body weight.[18] Most acute injuries occur at the musculotendinous junction and result in a profound inflammatory reaction.[19] This reaction initiates the phases of healing outlined previously.

Microtrauma without adequate recovery time can also result in injury to the tendon. Paratenonitis is an inflammation of the outer layer of the tendon (ie, paratenon), whether lined with synovium or not.[15,20] Histologically, inflammatory cells are found in the paratenon or peritendinous areolar tissues, and clinically, the cardinal signs of inflammation such as pain, crepitation, swelling, and palpable tenderness occur. Treatment procedures, including anti-inflammatory measures, are indicated.

Tendinosis is an intratendinous degeneration without an inflammatory response. It is generally caused by atrophy from aging, microtrauma, or vascular trauma. Histologic findings include fiber disorientation, hypocellularity, scattered vascular ingrowth, and occasional necrosis or calcification.[15,20] Because there is no inflammatory response, none of the cardinal signs of inflammation is present, and anti-inflammatory measures are ineffective. A nodule may be palpable but nontender. Tendinosis may also occur with paratenonitis, in which paratenon inflammation accompanies intratendinous degeneration. Symptoms in this case may be confusing, combining signs of inflammation with a palpable tendon nodule. Histologically, scattered vascular ingrowth may be present, although no true intratendinous inflammation exists.

The term tendinitis is used to describe a tendon strain or tear and is defined as symptomatic degeneration of the tendon with vascular disruption and an inflammatory repair response.[15,20] Histologically, tendinitis is classified into three subgroups, each with different findings, from purely inflammation to inflammation superimposed on pre-existing degeneration to calcification and tendinosis changes in chronic conditions. The chronic stage is further categorized:

1. Interstitial microinjury
2. Central tendon necrosis
3. Frank partial rupture
4. Acute complete rupture[15]

The symptoms in this group are proportional to the vascular disruption or atrophy and can be inflammatory, depending on the duration (Table 10-3).

Examination and Evaluation

In examining the individual with a tendon injury, history and subjective symptoms are of primary importance because of the differences in classification and treatment. The global classification of acute versus chronic injury is usually easily clarified by injury profile, but distinguishing between various types of chronic injuries can be more difficult. The events leading up to the onset of pain in the chronic case are significant in that the predisposing factors may be identified. Modifying the components that may have contributed to the problem is essential to recovery. Training errors, inappropriate equipment, environmental factors, excessive fatigue, or an apparently small injury without adequate recovery can precipitate tendon injury. Work or training restrictions, or modification of the home or work environment may be necessary to give the body an adequate opportunity for recovery (Fig. 10-13).

Physical examination follows traditional orthopaedic assessment procedures and includes observation, ROM, resistive testing, and special tests. The clinician must observe for any structural abnormality that may have predisposed the patient to tendinitis. Selective tissue tension testing to determine the tissue at fault and muscle testing to assess length and functional muscle imbalances provide the clinician with underlying factors to be addressed in rehabilitation. Palpation skills to determine the precise areas of tenderness isolate the tendon injury's location. Any nodules, palpable defects (in acute trauma), and crepitus should be documented, because this provides the therapist with valuable information for classification.

Treatment Principles and Procedures

Treatment of tendinopathies is based on the specific tendon injury, framed within the context of the tendon's role in function. Restoring the tendon to optimal length, cellularity, and ability to withstand loads is fundamental to complete rehabilitation. The optimal loading zone is the foundation principle for choosing loading techniques. Education about outside activities that maximize symptom resolution

Table 10-3. CLASSIFICATION TERMINOLOGY OF TENDON INJURY

NEW	OLD	DEFINITION	HISTOLOGICAL FINDINGS	CLINICAL SIGNS AND SYMPTOMS
Paratenonitis	Tenosynovitis, tenovaginitis, peritendinitis	An inflammation of only the paratenon, lined by synovium or not	Inflammatory cells in paratenon or peritendinious areolar tissue	Cardinal inflammatory signs: swelling, pain, crepitus, local tenderness, warmth, dysfunction
Paratenonitis with tendinosis	Tendinitis	Paratenon inflammation associated with intratendinosis degeneration	Same as above, with loss of tendon collagen, fiber disorientation, scattered vascular ingrowth, but no prominent intratendinous inflammation	Same as above, with often palpable tendon nodule, swelling, and inflammatory signs
Tendinosis	Tendinitis	Intratendinous degeneration due to atrophy (aging, microtrauma, vascular compromise)	Noninflammatory intratendinous collagen degeneration with fiber disorientation, hypocellularity, scattered vascular ingrowth occasional local necrosis,or calcification	Often palpable tendon that is *asymptomatic;* no swelling of tendon sheath
Tendinitis	Tendon strain or tear	Symptomatic degeneration of the tendon with vascular disruption and inflammatory repair response	Three recognized subgroups; each displays variable histology, from pure inflammation to inflammation superimposed on preexisting degeneration in chronic conditions: 1. acute 2. subacute 3. chronic	Symptoms are inflammatory and proportional to vascular disruption, hematoma, or atrophy-related cell necrosis. Symptom duration defines each group: 1. <2 wk 2. 4–6 wk 3. 6 wk

From American Academy of Orthopaedic Surgeons. *Athletic Training and Sports Medicine.* Park Ridge, Il: American Academy of Orthopaedic Surgeons; 1991.

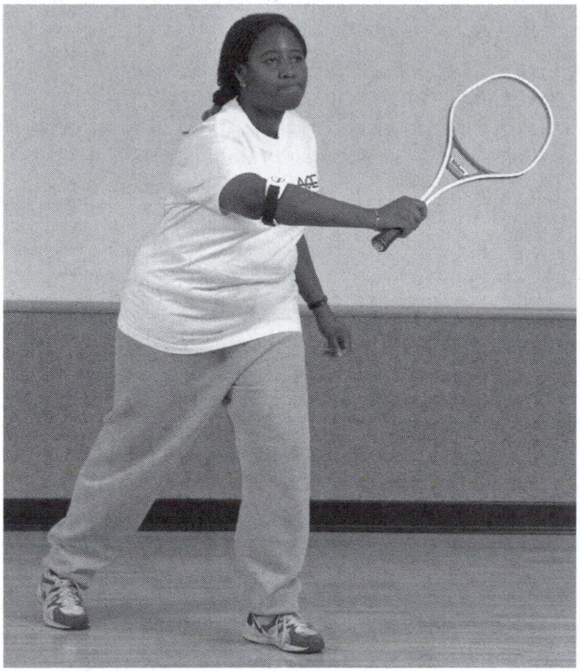

FIGURE 10-13 A tennis elbow strap can be used to decrease loads on the wrist extensor musculature during drills.

and minimize harmful effects is essential in the long-term care of tendinopathies. Rehabilitation should be of appropriate intensity, frequency, and duration such that, when combined with essential activities of daily living, it keeps loading within the optimal loading zone.

When inflammation is a component of the tendinopathy, anti-inflammatory measures are helpful. Physical agents such as ultrasound and cold packs, as well as electrotherapeutic modalities such as electrical muscle stimulation and iontophoresis, can reduce inflammation. Other physical agents or modalities can reduce the pain associated with inflammation, allowing greater participation in the therapeutic exercise program.

Stretching should be incorporated if muscle length is inadequate for the demands placed on the musculotendinous unit. In cases of recovery from an acute tendon injury, stretching is critical for restoring the normal length of the tissue. Moreover, stretching is a stimulus in the early healing stages for the proper alignment of healing collagen. In healing tissue, gentle stretching to provide a stimulus for fiber orientation without disruption of the immature collagen facilitates the remodeling process. In the chronic tendon injury, stretching increases the tissue's resting length, allowing loading through a greater range and force dispersion over a larger surface area. Changes in resting length may affect the muscle spindle, altering its sensitivity and resultant muscle stiffness. Like resistive exercise, stretching should be prescribed according to intensity, frequency, and duration parameters. Too often, these prescriptive factors are neglected, leading to overload.

Eccentric muscle contractions have been implicated in the development of tendinopathies. Eccentric contractions allow the series elastic component (SEC) to contribute to force production. Tendon is considered to form part of the SEC.[8] Other connective tissue proteins in parallel with the muscle fiber are thought to contribute to force production. Eccentric contractions usually precede concentric contractions in activities such as jumping, allowing the SEC to contribute to force production. The force generated in the tissue during eccentric contractions depends on the velocity of the stretch, the distance moved, and the amount of load placed on the tissue (eg, body weight, external loads). These parameters are used in the rehabilitation of tendon injuries.

Curwin and Stanish[8] outlined a progressive resistive exercise program in an attempt to strengthen the tendon tissue. Because eccentric muscle contractions allow the SEC to contribute to force production and because eccentric muscle contractions are frequently associated with the development of tendinopathies, this muscle contraction type is emphasized. Before an effective eccentric contraction can be performed, the individual must first be able to isometrically hold at the starting position. The first appropriate resistive exercise may be a submaximal isometric contraction. As the individual progresses, an eccentric program is initiated, with a progression of speed built into the program. The exercise session begins and ends with stretching, with a resistive eccentric program performed slowly for the first 2 days, progressed to a moderate speed for 3 days, and then to a fast speed for 2 days. The resistance is then increased, and the speed progression instituted again. This program is easily performed at home, and intensity, frequency, and duration are clearly outlined to prevent overload (Fig. 10-14).

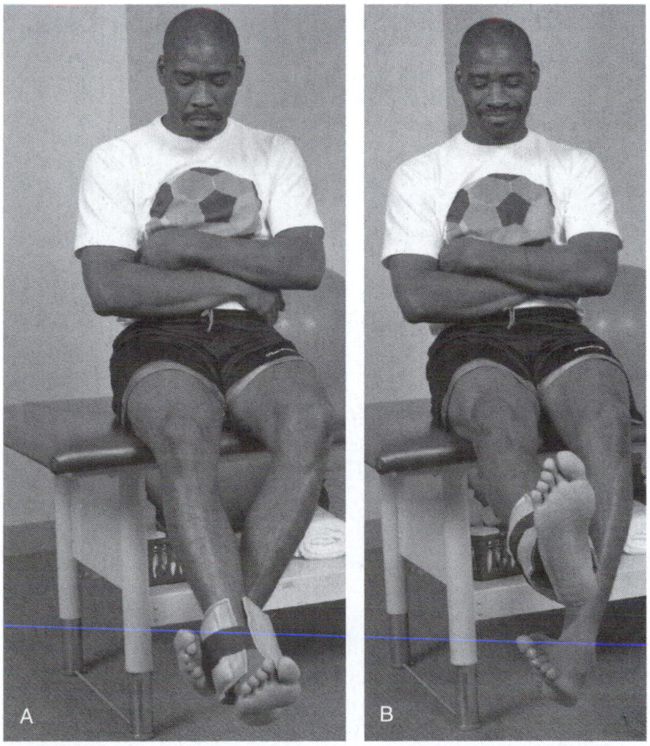

FIGURE 10-14 Eccentric quadriceps work with an ankle weight is performed by the patient. ***(A)*** Uninvolved leg lifts the relaxed involved leg. ***(B)*** Uninvolved leg is then lowered eccentrically by the involved leg.

As with any soft tissue injury, rehabilitation activities must mimic the demands placed on those tissues on return to activity. The prescription parameters are framed around the functional outcome. For the individual returning to a work, leisure, or home environment that places him at risk for reinjury, appropriate modifications to the environment or to the individual (eg, technique, adaptive or supportive devices) must be made as part of the prevention and long-term care program.

MANAGEMENT OF CARTILAGE INJURY

Classification of Cartilage Injury

Damage to the articular cartilage can occur from mechanical injury or from other nonmechanical trauma. Nonmechanical traumas include infection, inflammatory conditions or prolonged joint immobilization and can result in loss of proteoglycans. Proteoglycan degradation or suppression of synthesis from these conditions results in articular cartilage damage that may be irreversible. Mechanical damage to the articular cartilage (ie, chondral injury) or to the articular cartilage and underlying bone (ie, osteochondral injury) can happen as a result of blunt trauma, frictional abrasion, or excessive weight-bearing forces.[21] Knee hyperextension injuries or ankle rotational injuries can result in chondral or osteochondral injuries in addition to ligamentous injuries.

In addition to classification by cause of damage (mechanical or nonmechanical), articular cartilage injury is classified by whether it is partial or full thickness and by the size of the lesion. Depth and diameter of the lesion also have implications for treatment, and classification systems for these lesions have been developed.

Examination and Evaluation

Important clinical information relative to rehabilitation includes the cause of the damage (ie, mechanical or nonmechanical), area of damage (eg, weight-bearing surface), classification of damage, and other factors that may affect health of the articular cartilage, such as general health, lifestyle factors, body weight, joint alignment, and stability. If surgery was performed, the status of the articular cartilage and the associated soft tissues should be available in the chart. Patient goals should be determined and a realistic prognosis determined based on available information. For example, an individual with an articular cartilage lesion on the weight-bearing surface of the medial femoral condyle in a varus-aligned anterior cruciate ligament–deficient knee will have difficulty when returned to high-demand cutting sports.

Other assessment procedures of merit include posture, ROM, strength, and stability examinations. Assessment of swelling and pain influences intervention choices and progression of the treatment program. A swollen and sore knee indicates that the joint is inflamed, which is unhealthy for the articular cartilage. Resolution of the swelling and inflammation as quickly as possible is imperative for the joint's health.

Treatment Principles

Minimum requirements for healthy articular cartilage are freedom of motion, equitable load distribution, and stability.[22] Treatment focused on restoration of motion as a primary goal should be initiated. The aggressiveness of other interventions such as strengthening exercises is dictated by the other factors and the medical treatment. The articular cartilage has a better chance of recovery after injury or surgery in the presence of equal load distribution (ie, medial and lateral compartments) and joint stability. A knee with significant varus or valgus alignment excessively loads the medial and lateral compartments, respectively. This loading is the rationale for tibial osteotomy procedures, which attempt to balance load distribution medially and laterally. An unstable knee (anterior or posterior cruciate deficient) also places greater loads on the articular cartilage, and rehabilitation after articular cartilage injury or surgery in an unstable knee must proceed cautiously.

Restoration of motion in a compromised joint allows loads to be distributed across a greater joint surface area, decreasing peak focal loads. Mobility activities enhance fluid dynamics in the joint, assisting with lubrication and nutrition of the joint. Active and passive ROM activities are important for the recovery of articular cartilage lesions.

In addition to the restoration of motion, normalization of gait and increased muscle performance decreases loads on the articular cartilage. Effective eccentric muscle forces during the loading response of gait can minimize articular cartilage and subchondral bone loads. Strengthening activities play an important role in the protection of articular cartilage.

SURGICAL REHABILITATION

Soft Tissue Procedures

A multitude of soft tissue procedures are routinely performed by surgeons and include transfer, reattachment or realignment of tendons, ligament reconstructions, capsular tightening, debridement and synovectomy procedures, and stabilization techniques. Regardless of the specific procedure, the therapist must consider the stages of healing and the effects of immobilization and remobilization on soft tissue. In addition to the specific tissues involved in the surgery, the clinician must consider adjacent tissues that may be affected indirectly by the surgery. These tissues may include supporting musculature, tissues at adjacent joints, articular cartilage, and associated joint structures.

Some soft tissue procedures often require a longer recovery period than bony procedures because of the difficulty in obtaining fixation in soft tissue. Capsular reefing or tightening surgeries in which soft tissue is sutured to soft tissue or tendon transfer or repair procedures in which soft tissue is attached to bone require adequate healing time to ensure fixation. Most important, the clinician should understand the surgical procedure and communicate with the surgeon to ensure optimal rehabilitation for the patient.

The goals of therapeutic exercise in the perioperative period are to restore motion, strength, and function and to reduce pain. The principles of optimal loading and SAID provide the framework for intervention choices. Be sure to observe for and educate the patient about potential postoperative complications such as infection or deep vein thrombosis. Prevention of these complications by early detection minimizes the risk of and protracted course of care associated with these problems. The rehabilitation program should include exercises and modality treatments to be performed at home to reinforce self-management of the condition.

LIGAMENT RECONSTRUCTIONS

The most common sites of ligament reconstructions are the ulnar collateral ligament at the elbow, the lateral ankle ligaments, and the anterior and posterior cruciate (ACL, PCL) and medial collateral ligaments (MCL) of the knee. Ligament reconstruction should not be confused with a primary ligament repair. Ligament reconstructions generally use other tissues (eg, tendon) to create a new ligament, rather than repairing the original ligament. Communication with the surgeon regarding the specifics of the procedure provides the clinician with information critical to proper patient care.

Not all individuals with ligament injuries are candidates for reconstructive procedures. Ample evidence exists supporting the conservative management of knee MCL injuries in the presence of an intact ACL. Many individuals are able to return to their previous activity levels after ACL injury without surgical reconstruction. Decisions regarding the appropriateness of reconstructive procedures are based on the patient's activity level, his clinical signs and symptoms, and the natural history of the injury.

The postoperative rehabilitation course after ligament reconstructions depends on factors such as the graft material, fixation, quality of the tissue, status of the joint surfaces, comorbidities, and associated injuries. In the knee, bone-patellar and tendon-bone ACL reconstructions have solid, bone-to-bone fixation, whereas use of hamstring or iliotibial band tissues may have soft tissue fixation. Frequently, associated injuries or procedures affect the rehabilitation (eg, meniscus injury or repair, ulnar nerve transposition). Comorbidities such as diabetes or degenerative joint disease may alter the typical postoperative procedures by accelerating some aspects (eg, mobility), but in other cases, it may slow down elements of the rehabilitation program (eg, weight bearing). Every individual should be considered in light of the specific situation.

Impairments after ligament reconstructive surgeries include loss of mobility and strength, pain, and swelling. Weight bearing and all weight-bearing activities are impaired after lower extremity procedures. These impairments may result in functional limitations, including inability to perform activities of daily living such as bathing, dressing, and household chores or an inability to participate in leisure activities. Associated disabilities may include an inability to fulfill expected roles as worker, student, or spouse (see Selected Intervention: Quadriceps Setting for the Patient With a Knee Injury).

SELECTED INTERVENTION
Quadriceps Setting for the Patient With a Knee Injury

See Case Study #6

Although this patient requires comprehensive intervention as described in the patient management model, one specific exercise is described.

ACTIVITY: Quadriceps setting

PURPOSE: To increase superior glide of the patella, to teach activation of the quadriceps, and to maintain or increase strength in the quadriceps muscle

RISK FACTORS: No appreciable risk factors

ELEMENTS OF THE MOVEMENT SYSTEM: Biomechanical and neuromuscular

STAGE OF MOTOR CONTROL: Mobility

POSTURE: A variety of positions such as long sit, supine, or standing. The knee is fully extended.

MOVEMENT: Isometric contraction of the quadriceps muscle

SPECIAL CONSIDERATIONS: Ensure normal tracking of the patella. Avoid substitution with hip extensor musculature. Check quadriceps muscle contraction by attempting to mobilize the patella. With an effective quadriceps set, the patella should not be mobile.

DOSAGE

TYPE OF MUSCLE CONTRACTION: Isometric
- **Intensity:** Submaximal to maximal
- **Duration:** Hold for up to 6 seconds for up to 30 repetitions
- **Frequency:** Hourly or as frequently as possible

RATIONALE FOR EXERCISE CHOICE: Quadriceps setting is a key exercise to maintain the health of the extensor mechanism. This activity lubricates the patellofemoral joint, increases superior glide of the patella (necessary for full knee extension), and increases or maintains quadriceps muscle strength. Full knee extension with quadriceps activation is necessary for a normal gait.

EXERCISE GRADATION: Quadriceps setting is a foundation exercise that serves as a precursor to other exercises. This activity is progressed to more difficult exercises that require quadriceps muscle activation (ie, any closed chain exercise).

TENDON SURGERY

Surgery to repair or transfer tendons is commonly performed in orthopedics. Whether a tendon has been torn acutely or has undergone a degenerative process over a protracted period, surgery to repair or debride the injury can maximize the outcome. Common areas of tendon surgery include the tendons of the hand and the rotator cuff, and Achilles and patellar tendons. Like ligament injuries, not all tendon ruptures need to be treated surgically. Many individuals return to a high level of function despite an unrepaired rotator cuff tear or conservative management of an Achilles tendon rupture.

The specific rehabilitation program depends to a great extent on the location and function of the musculotendinous unit, the location and extent of damage within the musculotendinous unit, the quality of the tissue, and the ability of the surgeon to effectively repair the damage. Areas of poor blood supply, inferior tissue quality, extensive damage, or comorbidities can deleteriously affect the surgical outcome. The clinician must communicate with the physician to ensure an understanding of the quality of the surgical repair to avoid overtreating or undertreating the patient.

Key issues after a tendon injury are the prevention of mobility impairment without overloading the tendon repair and prevention of excessive atrophy. Immobilization results in loss of normal tendon gliding within the tendon sheath and the associated soft tissue and joint adhesions because of the restrictions placed on muscle-tendon stretch and contraction. Unlike ligament reconstruction surgery, after which strengthening exercises can be initiated early, these same exercises may overload the repaired tendon.

DEBRIDEMENT

Surgical debridement is performed alone or combined with other procedures at a number at joints. Debridement refers to the removal of tissue from an area until healthy tissue is exposed. The purpose is to remove potential sources of pain or irritation and, in some cases, to stimulate a healing response. For example, in osteoarthritic knees, debridement may remove osteophytes and loose bodies, shave or trim areas of roughened articular cartilage, and trim or remove areas of torn meniscus. When performing a ligament reconstruction, the remains of the torn ligament are debrided before the reconstruction is performed, and the torn ends of a tendon are debrided before tendon repair.

Because of the variety of situations in which this procedure is used, rehabilitation is dictated by the primary procedure. Rehabilitation after debridement that accompanies tendon or ligament repair follows the repair guidelines. Debridement performed primarily (eg, arthritis) is guided by the underlying pathology. Understanding the extent of debridement and the status of the joint (eg, location, extent, and depth of articular cartilage changes, meniscus tears) ensures appropriate pacing of the rehabilitation program.

SYNOVECTOMY

Synovectomy, the removal of the synovial lining of the joint, is a procedure performed primarily in the case of rheumatoid arthritis and other diseases such as pigmented villonodular synovitis. The purpose of synovectomy in the case of rheumatoid arthritis is to remove the inflamed synovium and thereby relieve pain and swelling and perhaps retard the progressive joint destruction associated with chronic inflammation.[23] This procedure is performed only after conservative measures to control the pain and swelling have failed.

Rehabilitation after synovectomy is guided by the primary pathology, such as rheumatoid arthritis. Because this procedure has been performed as a last resort to control pain and swelling, every effort should be made during rehabilitation to restore motion and strength without increasing pain or swelling. These two factors guide the pace of the rehabilitation program and provide the clinician with the parameters for optimal loading.

DECOMPRESSION

Decompression procedures are used to relieve pressure in an area and are commonly performed at the shoulder to reduce pressure on the subacromial soft tissues and in the spine to reduce pressure on the spinal cord. Surgery in the wrist to relieve pressure in the carpal tunnel and fasciotomies in the leg to reduce compartment pressures may be considered forms of decompression. The excessive pressure in these areas may result from bony or soft tissue architecture, and decompression involves the release or removal of these soft tissues and shaving or removal of bony sources of pressure.

Rehabilitation after a decompression is guided by the primary pathology and the status of the tissues decompressed, which depends on the amount and duration of compression and on the type of tissue compressed. For example, if excessive pressure on a nerve has caused neurologic changes, rehabilitation focuses on recovery of nerve function. If pressure has caused poor muscle function (eg, rotator cuff), rehabilitation focuses on recovery of muscle function. As rehabilitation progresses, avoid using activities or positions that may excessively compress the tissue just decompressed.

SOFT TISSUE STABILIZATION AND REALIGNMENT PROCEDURES

Soft tissue stabilization procedures are performed in the case of joint instability due to capsular laxity. This procedure is performed most frequently to correct an unstable shoulder and may be combined with other stabilization procedures (eg, bony stabilization). A variety of surgical techniques can stabilize a joint with capsular laxity. Likewise, soft tissue realignment procedures are performed to redirect the pull of soft tissues that may or may not be the result of instability. For example, proximal patellar realignment is used to enhance the effective pull of the vastus medialis obliques on the patella. Regardless of the procedure, the fixation usually is soft tissue to soft tissue, without bony stability.

Because of the lack of rigid fixation and length of time necessary for soft tissue to heal, the loads placed on the repair site are controlled for some time after stabilization. For example, when stabilizing the shoulder for anterior inferior glenohumeral instability, external rotation is limited for a short time after surgery to allow the anterior capsule to heal. Because the repaired tissue is noncontractile, muscle activation is usually allowed early in rehabilitation, as long as ROM precautions are considered. As rehabilitation progresses into the range that stresses the repaired tissue, be alert for signs of progressive loosening of the repair, such as complaints of slipping or instability. Mobility recovery should be full, without the return of instability symptoms.

MENSICAL AND LABRAL REPAIRS

The meniscus of the knee and the labrum of the shoulder are two common sites of fibrocartilage repair. Tears of the glenoid labrum are more difficult to identify, and repair techniques lag behind those for the menisci. Repair of torn menisci of the knee is commonly performed alone or in combination with other procedures such as ACL reconstruction. In the knee in particular, the repair is of a soft tissue with an inferior blood supply. Healing may be enhanced by associated procedures to increase the blood supply to the area.

Important issues during rehabilitation include understanding the loads placed on the repair when the joint is in a variety of positions. These positions should be avoided in the early stages when the repair is still fragile. For example, full knee flexion in weight bearing is limited for several weeks after meniscal repair, because this position places high loads on the meniscus. Full overhead positions may be avoided early after labral repairs in the superior zone. Communicate with the surgeon regarding the location and extent of tissue repair.

Bony Procedures

Rehabilitation is often necessary after bony surgical procedures to restore motion at adjacent joints, strengthen related soft tissues and increase general endurance. Some interventions have a direct effect on the bone and can enhance the healing process. The specific procedure, tissue damage, and patient's general health, balanced with the optimal loading and SAID principles, guide intervention choices.

ABRASION CHONDROPLASTY

Abrasion chondroplasty is a procedure performed alone or in combination with other procedures in cases of articular cartilage lesions. This procedure is performed most commonly at the knee, where articular cartilage lesions may result from degenerative joint disease or acute injury. These lesions produce impairments such as pain, swelling, and motion loss, as well as functional limitations such as the inability to walk distances, stand for long periods, or negotiate stairs. After other conservative measures have failed to resolve impairments and functional limitations, surgery to debride the joint and stimulate healing may be performed. In this situation, a variety of techniques (eg, burring, punctating, shaving) may be used to smooth a roughened area and cause localized bleeding. The surgical "roughening" is only deep enough to create bleeding in the eroded area. This stimulates a healing response and local fibrocartilage ingrowth. Unfortunately, the mechanical properties of the replacement fibrocartilage are significantly inferior to the original tissue.

Rehabilitation after abrasion chondroplasty varies with the extent and location of the articular cartilage lesion. Large lesions on weight-bearing surfaces have a poorer prognosis than small lesions on nonweight-bearing surfaces. The joint with extra loads from excessive body weight, malalignment, or instability is likely to require a longer rehabilitation course, with a greater likelihood of overloading the new fibrocartilage. These individuals may have weight-bearing and exercise limitations for up to 8 weeks after surgery. Restoration of motion and strength as quickly as possible without disrupting the healing process provides the best opportunity for healing of this fresh injury (Fig. 10-15).

OPEN REDUCTION AND INTERNAL FIXATION

ORIF of a fracture is commonly performed when closed reduction is impossible or when fracture healing would be protracted if treated without fixation. Goals of ORIF are to stabilize a fracture while allowing early motion and activity, to decrease the chances of nonunion, and to decrease the effects of immobilization on the limb. Surgical fixation may use plates, screws, wires, or other forms of hardware to stabilize the bone and fragments. In most situations, the hardware is left in permanently, although it may be removed if superficial location causes discomfort.

Rehabilitation after ORIF is directed at any impairments or functional limitations associated with the injury. Any force great enough to fracture a bone is likely to have produced some local soft tissue damage, which must be treated as well. Restrictions (eg, weight bearing, motion) are specific to the location and severity of the fracture and to the extent of associated soft tissue injury. In general, surgical fixation stabilizes the fracture, and treatment focuses on associated soft tissue damage and restoration of full function.

FUSION

Fusion is the operative formation of an ankylosis or arthrodesis.[24] Fusions are performed most commonly in the spine, although some joints in the extremities are fused. Spinal fusions are used to treat problems such as instability, facet pain, and disk disease. Glenohumeral joints are fused in cases of severe pain, especially in the presence of neurologic injury (eg, axillary nerve, long thoracic nerve) that severely restricts functional use of the arm. Knee joints are fused when severe arthritis produces pain and disability and total joint replacement is not a treatment option. Fusions about the ankle are used to treat hindfoot pain and arthritis.

The postoperative rehabilitation program must consider the mechanical changes that occur as a result of the fusion. Because mobility is limited at a joint (or series of joint in the spine), adjacent joints compensate to restore the presurgical mobility. How effectively these joints compensate or overcompensate has a profound impact on the result. If the

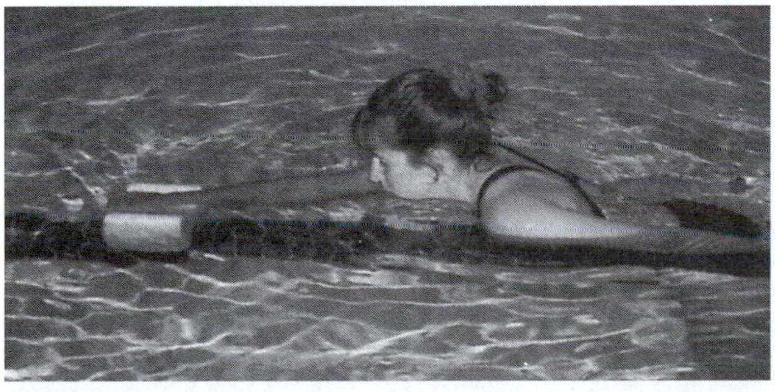

FIGURE 10-15 Using activities in a gravity-minimized environment can progressively load the lower extremly.

hip and ankle are unable to adequately compensate for a fused knee, the patient has difficulty getting in and out of a car, a chair, and on and off the floor. Because the spine is a series of joints, adjacent segments can often compensate for fusion at one or more levels. However, adjacent segments may become hypermobile in response to the fusion, creating pain above or below the fusion. An important aspect of postoperative rehabilitation is focused on the adjacent joints and procedures necessary to ensure the long-term health of these joints. The muscles must be retrained to function in a new movement pattern.

OSTEOTOMY

Osteotomy, the surgical cutting of a bone, is a procedure performed to correct bony alignment. This procedure is performed most commonly at the knee to correct excessive genu varus or valgus. Excessive varus or valgus places increased loads on the medial and lateral compartments of the knee, respectively. This may result in degeneration of the articular cartilage in that compartment. The purpose of performing an osteotomy is to redistribute weight off the compromised compartment and to disperse the load over a larger area. To correct for excessive varus, a high tibial osteotomy (or valgus osteotomy) is performed at the proximal tibia. To correct for excessive valgus, a distal femoral osteotomy is performed. These procedures remove a wedge of bone from the respective site, and the "fracture" is fixated with hardware.

Rehabilitation focuses on the precipitating issues that led to surgery (usually degenerative joint disease) and the preservation or restoration of motion and strength. An important consideration is the change in loading patterns on the articular cartilage. One compartment that has been excessively loaded will have decreased loading, and the other compartment that has been underloaded will have increased loading. How well a compartment adapts to the increased load depends on many factors. The health of the articular cartilage in this compartment is probably the most important factor. Weight bearing and weight-bearing activities may have to be restricted until the joint can adapt to this change.

JOINT ARTHROPLASTY

Joint replacement surgery is performed to remedy significant degenerative joint disease after other conservative or surgical measures have been exhausted. Joint replacement is performed in many joints, including the hip, knee, shoulder, elbow, wrist, and hand. The chief goal of joint arthroplasty is pain relief. Generally, the clinician cannot expect increased joint motion, strength, or function other than that resulting from a decrease in a patient's pain.

Joint replacement is categorized by component design (ie, constrained, unconstrained, or semiconstrained), fixation (ie, cement or cementless), and materials (ie, cobalt-chrome alloy, titanium alloy, or high-density polyethylene). A *constrained* design allows motion in only one plane, and an *unconstrained* design allows motion in any axis. A *semiconstrained* allows full motion in one plane and some motion in other planes. Fixation is achieved with cement or with some type of biologic fixative. Biologic fixation may include a porous coat or similar surfaces that allows bony ingrowth into open areas on the surface. Recovery of components with this type of fixation are difficult in the patient in need of revision arthroplasty. Materials usually are a combination of metals and plastic.

Rehabilitation issues are joint and prosthesis specific. In general, restoration of motion, strength, and function and consideration of the underlying cause of the surgery constitute the rehabilitation framework. Consideration must also be given to the adjacent joints, which may be compromised by the same disease process and the excessive loads placed on them in the perioperative period. After recovery from the operation, the patient generally feels much better than before the surgery, with less pain in the affected joint. Education regarding the long-term health of the joint replacement and the adjacent joints is a large component of the patient care program.

Key Points

- The composition and structure of connective tissues provide information about each tissue's mechanical properties and function.
- The unique viscoelastic characteristics of connective tissues are the result of their fluid and solid constituent materials.
- When connective tissues are loaded, the stress (ie, force per unit area relative to the strain) or change in the length per unit length provides information about the tissue's ability to withstand loads.
- The viscoelastic properties of relaxation, creep, and hysteresis are the physiologic basis for changes seen with stretching.
- The stages of healing along with knowledge of the specific injury provide the clinician with guidelines for intervention selection throughout the episode of care.
- Restoration of normal tissue relationships, optimal loading, the SAID principle, and prevention of secondary complications are broad rehabilitation principles that guide treatment.
- Acute soft tissue injuries such as sprains, strains, and contusions necessitate early intervention to avoid secondary complications.
- Management of tendon injuries and prognosis varies according to the injury classification.
- Interventions used in the treatment of bony or surgical procedures should have a solid foundation in basic science and require an understanding of the anatomy and kinesiology of the area.

Critical Thinking Questions

1. Consider Case Study #2 in Unit 7, before her total knee replacement surgery. Presume she came to your clinic 2 years earlier in an attempt to delay surgery. At that time, her motion was decreased by 15%, and her overall strength was decreased by 20%. Describe her exercise program. Provide the rationale for restoration of her joint motion and strength in the case of osteoarthritis of the knee.

LAB ACTIVITIES

1. A patient comes to the clinic Monday morning with acute Achilles tendinitis after a weekend tennis tournament.
   a. Instruct your patient in a home exercise program, including dosage, to be performed until he returns in 4 days.
   b. Explain to your patient about adjunctive agents and give any special instructions.
2. The patient returns 4 days later and is in a subacute phase of injury.
   a. Demonstrate five stretching techniques for the Achilles tendon.
   b. Instruct the patient in a home stretching program, including dosage.
   c. Demonstrate three ways to strengthen this muscle group, including dosage, using
      i. Concentric only
      ii. Isometric only
      iii. Eccentric only
3. This patient has improved with the exercise program and desires to return to basketball. Demonstrate the final phase of the rehabilitation program to prepare the patient for this activity.
4. Instruct each of the following patients in five exercises to increase knee flexion mobility:
   a. A 19-year-old student 2 weeks after a grade II medial collateral ligament sprain of the right knee with a 0- to 90-degree ROM
   b. A 75-year-old woman who is unable to get up and down off the floor 2 weeks after a total right knee replacement with a 0- to 60-degree ROM

2. The patient in the first question is given a home exercise program to carry out for 2 weeks, after which she returns to the clinic for reevaluation and progression. Explain to this patient how to differentiate the discomfort associated with some exercise from pain that may be related to harming her knee.
3. Why are repeated eccentric muscle contractions associated with tendinitis?
4. If eccentric muscle contractions contribute to tendinitis, why are they used to treat tendinitis?
5. Consider Case Study #6 in Unit 7. How would your acute-phase mobility program differ if the patient
   a. Was generally hypermobile, demonstrating elbow hyperextension, knee recurvatum, and thumb to volar forearm?
   b. Was generally hypomobile, with a history of excessive scar formation?

REFERENCES

1. Frank C, Woo S-L, Andriacchi T. Brand R, et al. Normal ligament: Structure, function and composition. In: Woo SL-Y, Buckwalter JA (eds): *Injury and Repair of the Musculoskeletal Soft Tissues*. Park Ridge, IL: American Academy of Orthopaedic Surgeons; 1988:45–101.
2. Riegger-Krugh C. Bone. In: Malone TR, McPoil T, Nitz AJ, eds. *Orthopaedic and Sports Physical Therapy*. 3rd ed. St. Louis: Mosby; 1997.
3. Walter JB. *Principles of Disease*. 2nd ed. Philadelphia: WB Saunders; 1982.
4. Walker JM. Cartilage of human joints and related structures. In: Zachazewski JE, Magee DJ, Quillen WS, eds. *Athletic Injuries and Rehabilitation*. Philadelphia: WB Saunders; 1996.
5. Woo SL-Y, Maynard J, Butler D, Lyon R, et al. Ligament, tendon and joint capsule insertions into bone. In: Woo SL-Y, Buckwalter JA, eds. *Injury and Repair of the Musculoskeletal Soft Tissues*. Park Ridge, IL: American Academy of Orthopaedic Surgeons; 1988:133–167.
6. O'Brien M. Functional anatomy and physiology of tendons. *Clin Sports Med*. 1992;11:505–520.
7. Loitz-Ramage B, Zernicke RF. Bone biology and mechanics. In: Zachazewski JE, Magee DJ, Quillen WS, eds. *Athletic Injuries and Rehabilitation*. Philadelphia: WB Saunders; 1996.
8. Curwin S, Stanish WD. *Tendinitis: Its Etiology and Treatment*. Lexington, MA: DC Heath; 1984.
9. Burstein AH, Wright TM. *Fundamentals of Orthopaedic Biomechanics*. Baltimore: Williams & Wilkins; 1994.
10. Leadbetter WB. An introduction to sports-induced soft-tissue inflammation. In: Leadbetter WB, Buckwalter JA, Gordon SL, eds. *Sports-Induced Inflammation*. Park Ridge, IL: American Academy of Orthopaedic Surgeons; 1990;3–24.
11. Andriaacchi T, Sabiston P, DeHaven K, Dahners L, et al. Ligament: injury and repair. In: Woo SL-Y, Buckwalter JA, eds. *Injury and Repair of the Musculoskeletal Soft Tissues*. Park Ridge, IL: American Academy of Orthopaedic Surgeons; 1988:103–132.
12. Malone TR, Garrett WE, Zachazewski JE. Muscle: deformation, injury, repair. In: Zachazewski JE, Magee DJ, Quillen WS, eds. *Athletic Injuries and Rehabilitation*. Philadelphia: WB Saunders; 1997:71–91.
13. American Academy of Orthopedic Surgeons. *Athletic Training and Sports Medicine*. Park Ridge, IL: American Academy of Orthopedic Surgeons; 1991.
14. Salter RB. *Textbook of Disorders and Injuries of the Musculoskeletal System*. 2nd ed. Baltimore: Williams & Wilkins; 1983.
15. Leadbetter WB. Cell-matrix response in tendon injury. *Clin Sports Med*. 1992;11:533–578.
16. Elliot DH. Structure and function of mammalian tendon. *Biol Rev*. 1965;40:392–421.
17. Walker LB, Harris EH, Benedict JV. Stress-strain relationships in human plantaris tendon: a preliminary study. *Med Elect Biol Eng*. 1964;2:31–38.
18. Zernicke RF, Garhammer J, Jobe FW. Human patellar tendon rupture. *J Bone Joint Surg Am*. 1977;59:179–183.

19. Nicholas JA. Clinical observations on sports-induced soft-tissue injuries. In: Leadbetter WB, Buckwalter JA, Gordon SL, eds. *Sports-Induced Inflammation*. Park Ridge, IL: American Academy of Orthopaedic Surgeons; 1990; 129–148.
20. Clancy WJ. Tendon trauma and overuse injuries. In: Leadbetter WB, Buckwalter JA, Gordon SL, eds. *Sports-Induced Inflammation*. Park Ridge, IL: American Academy of Orthopaedic Surgeons; 1990;609–618.
21. Buckwalter J, Rosenberg L, Coutts R, et al. Articular cartilage: injury and repair. In: Woo SL-Y, Buckwalter JA, eds. *Injury and Repair of the Musculoskeletal Soft Tissues*. Park Ridge, IL: American Academy of Orthopaedic Surgeons; 1988: 465–482.
22. Arnoczky S, Adams M, DeHaven K, Eyre D, Mow V. Meniscus. In: Woo SL-Y, Buckwalter JA, eds. *Injury and Repair of the Musculoskeletal Soft Tissues*. Park Ridge, IL: American Academy of Orthopaedic Surgeons; 1988:465–482.
23. Insall JN. *Surgery of the Knee*. New York: Churchill Livingstone; 1984.
24. *Dorland's Illustrated Medical Dictionary*, 26th ed. Philadelphia: WB Saunders; 1981.

CHAPTER 11

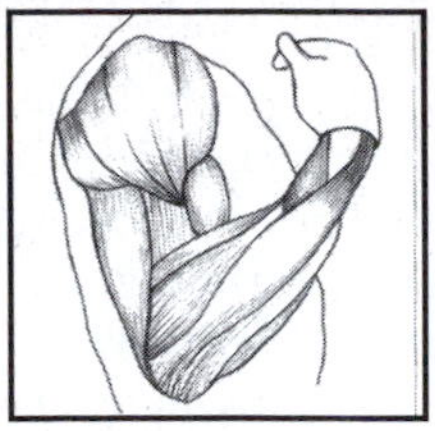

Therapeutic Exercise for Arthritis

Kimberly Bennett

About 40 million people in the United States have some form of arthritis.[1] The economic impact of arthritis is significant. Studies carried out between 1960 and 1982 showed that direct medical costs and lost wages represented slightly less than 1% of the gross national product, with wage loss representing 38% to 50% of this total.[2] Hidden in these numbers are the personal effects of rheumatic diseases on the affected individuals and their families and employers. Pain and decreased ability to function influence parenting and spousal roles, community involvement, and work performance. All of these issues can affect self-image, esteem, and the quality of life. Declines in strength, cardiovascular endurance, range of motion (ROM), and flexibility are well documented in juvenile and adult arthritic populations.[3–11] These factors underlie the extent of physical fitness in an individual, and physical fitness can be a critical indicator of the capacity to function.[12]

Previous treatment strategies, especially for the treatment of inflamed joints, favored rest. However, several recent studies showed that rheumatic patients who participated in regular exercise programs experienced increased flexibility, strength, cardiovascular status, and in some cases, functioning and that they were able to do this without apparent joint aggravation.[13–16] The study results suggest that rehabilitation programs for rheumatic patients should include ROM, isometric, isotonic, and aerobic exercise to decrease joint pain and to increase muscle function, strength, flexibility, and cardiovascular conditioning.

Although exercise appears to be an important intervention tool, the clinician and the patient should have a clear understanding of the role of exercise in the treatment of arthritis. Exercise cannot cure arthritis.[17] It is a powerful tool for maximizing function and for controlling the emotional, physical, and societal losses associated with the disease. It is ultimately a tool that can affect the quality of life. A carefully prescribed therapeutic exercise program with an emphasis on patient-related instruction can achieve several goals:

- Slow or reverse the body's response to joint pathology by increasing flexibility, strength, and endurance and by decreasing pain
- Directly address impairments, functional limitations, and disabilities resulting from arthritis
- Lead to overall improved health status as an effect of cardiovascular, strengthening, ROM, and stretching exercises

REVIEW OF PERTINENT ANATOMY AND KINESIOLOGY

Synovial joints are the primary sites of arthritis. Their dysfunction can affect the ability of the entire organism to function. In a normal synovial joint (Fig. 11-1), ligaments, muscles, tendons, capsule, cartilage, and subchondral and trabecular bone provide stabilizing, shock-transmitting, and shock-absorbing structures to cope with the considerable stress on the joint that occurs with movement and weight bearing. For example, in running, the tibiofemoral joint experiences forces 2.5 to 3 times body weight.[18] In deep knee bends, the patellofemoral joint experiences forces 10 times body weight.[19]

Stabilizing forces are provided by balanced alignment of soft tissue, including muscle, ligament, and tendon around the joint; by the congruity of the joint surfaces in their contact with one another; and by the surface tension provided by synovial fluid in the joint. Another protective component is the shock-absorbing and shock-transmitting properties of articular cartilage and of subchondral and trabecular bone. The neuromuscular system plays an important role as well. Stretching slightly stretched muscle absorbs energy and spreads force temporally and spatially across the articular surface (ie, compare jumping off a height with locked knees and with flexible, slightly bent knees). This mechanism requires an intact neuromuscular reflex arc and good joint proprioception.[20]

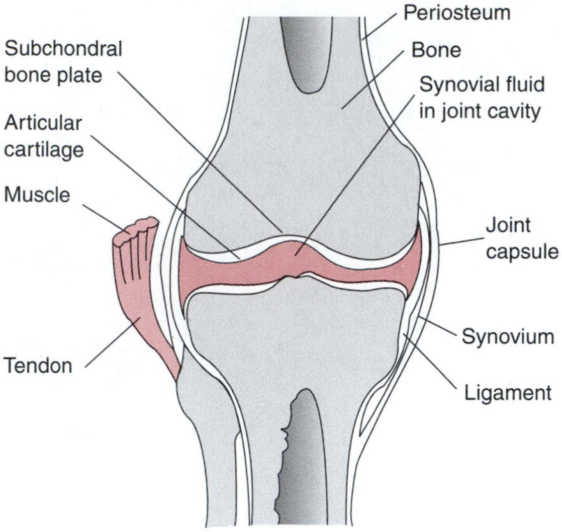

FIGURE 11-1 Normal joint function depends on the integrity of all the joint structures. (Adapted from AHPA Arthritis Teaching Slide Collection. American College of Rheumatology, Atlanta, Georgia.)

PATHOLOGY

An important principle of therapeutic intervention is that treatment should be aimed at the underlying causes of the disease, rather than the symptoms. This approach necessitates an understanding of the pathology and its relation to broader functional effects.

For osteoarthritis and rheumatoid arthritis, treatment plans should be designed based on a knowledge of the pathologic processes of the diseases. This knowledge guides the choice of interventions, observation of precautions, and formulation of rational goals. Understanding the relation of this pathology to broader functional effects facilitates design of a program that can address the deficits.

Arthritis literally means joint inflammation, but there are approximately 120 different forms of arthritis (inflammatory and noninflammatory, affecting not only joints but soft tissue). Osteoarthritis and rheumatoid arthritis, two of the most common forms of arthritis, are discussed in this chapter. Because these two diseases have distinctly different pathologic mechanisms, some of the exercise design considerations vary.

Osteoarthritis represents a type of nonsystemic, mostly noninflammatory, localized pathology. Rheumatoid arthritis is a systemic, inflammatory disease that usually involves multiple joints and often affects organ systems. Understanding the basic processes involved in these forms of arthritis can help the physical therapist in designing appropriate treatment plans, and the same principles of degenerative and inflammatory processes are encountered in the less common forms of arthritis. Effects of the two diseases on joints and related structures are listed in Table 11-1.

Table 11-1. EFFECTS OF OSTEOARTHRITIS AND RHEUMATOID ARTHRITIS ON JOINT STRUCTURE AND FUNCTION

STRUCTURE	FUNCTION	EFFECTS OF OSTEOARTHRITIS	EFFECTS OF RHEUMATOID ARTHRITIS
Cartilage	Shock absorption, joint congruence	Thickening to softening to thinning to loss	Erosion of cartilage
Synovium	Secretes synovial fluid for nutrition of cartilage, lubrication, and stability	Secondary involvement occasionally	Microvascular lining cells activated to start inflammatory process, pannus formation
Ligaments	Stability, reinforce capsule and limit movement, guide movement	Abnormal joint alignment stresses	Erosion weakens
Muscles	Reinforce joint capsule, reflex joint protection, move joints	Immobility shortens, pain causes guarding and reflex inhibition leading to weakness	Joint deformity interferes with peak torque generation; immobility shortens; myositis weakens; pain and effusion cause guarding and reflex inhibition leads to weakness.
Bone	Structural support	Subchondral bone remodeling changes shock absorbing properties, joint margin spurring leads to bony blockade and pain	Erosion leads to joint deformity, bony blockade, pain
Extraarticular system		Increased energy expenditure from abnormal movement patterns	Myositis Anemia Sleep disruption Fatigue Increased energy expenditure due to abnormal movement patterns

Osteoarthritis

ETIOLOGY

Osteoarthritis is defined as a degenerative joint disease characterized by the breakdown of articular cartilage under a load and by bony hypertrophy leading to joint margin bone spur formation (ie, spurring). It can be caused by excessive loading of normal cartilage (ie, one large or many small forces) or the application of reasonable loads to abnormal cartilage. Abnormal cartilage may be of genetically poor quality or may result from the body's attempt to repair normal cartilage that has been damaged.[19] Osteoarthritis can be idiopathic, but there are several predisposing factors, including obesity, trauma, hypermobility, overuse, infection, inflammation (including rheumatoid arthritis), and genetic factors.[19,21] Incidence is highly correlated with aging; the disease affects about 50% of those older than 65 and 80% of those older than 75.[19]

CLINICAL MANIFESTATIONS

Osteoarthritis typically affects weight-bearing joints, including metatarsophalangeal joints, hips, knees, spine, and the first metacarpophalangeal, first carpometacarpal, and proximal interphalangeal joints (ie, Bouchard's nodes) and distal interphalangeal joints (ie, Heberden's nodes). The disease is usually unilateral, often affecting only one joint compartment, and has no direct systemic effects.

The pathologic changes of osteoarthritis reflect damage to the articular cartilage and the joint's reaction to that damage. Cartilage damage is accompanied by decreased shock-transmitting and shock-absorbing capacities of subchondral and trabecular bone, which diminish the joint's ability to withstand loading forces. This condition further stresses the articular cartilage, resulting in cartilage failure and chondrocyte death. Tissue damage leads to proteolytic enzyme release and low-grade synovial inflammation. If chronic, inflammation can lead to fibrosis of the joint capsule, limiting movement and adding to joint pathology (see Chapter 21). Hypertrophic bone formation at joint margins (ie, marginal spurring), often asymmetrically within the joint, leads to joint deformity and pain (Fig. 11-2).

Extraarticular soft tissue structures are affected by asymmetric joint deformity. Uneven pull on muscles and ligaments can lead to shortening of structures on one side and lengthening on the other, further changing normal joint alignment. The muscle length imbalances lead to strength changes and force couple imbalances, which can damage the joint by altering active joint mechanics.

A common example of this imbalance is seen in the osteoarthritic knee. Lateral compartment cartilage loss results in a valgus deformity of the knee, which stretches muscles and ligaments medially and shortens soft tissue structures laterally. In addition to affecting alignment of the knee and weight bearing through the joint, the deformity changes the mechanical advantage of medial and lateral muscle groups and the stability of the joint as stretched ligaments become lax. Joint pain and swelling, together with splinting and guarding, can lead to muscle disuse atrophy and loss of this important component of the shock-absorbing system.

Although cartilage failure may be the primary event in osteoarthritis, the disease can be regarded as failure of the entire joint complex. Cartilage failure disrupts the protective system of the joint, which compounds the effects of the initial cartilage damage in an ongoing process. The overall effect of the disease is rarely confined to the involved joint.[22] Minor[22] cites studies of patients with osteoarthritis in the lower limb that showed joints adjacent to the affected joint can have limitations in ROM and strength and that contralateral joints also can be affected in ROM and in functional use. In attempting to improve overall function, the exercise program should focus on impairments at the affected joint and on secondary impairments and functional limitations at associated joints caused by the primary impairments and by inactivity.

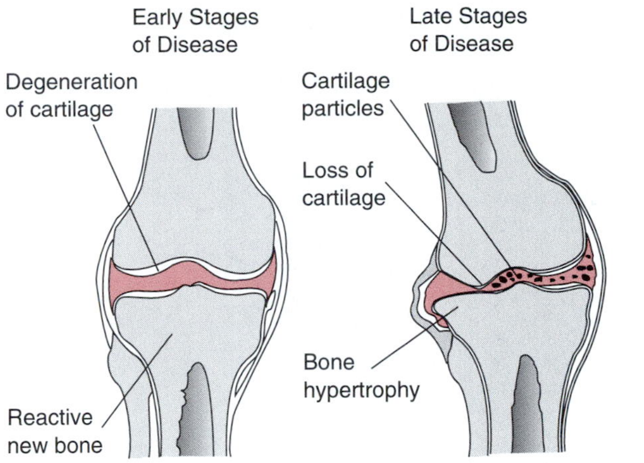

FIGURE 11-2 Osteoarthritis starts with asymmetric cartilage loss, which leads to abnormal forces on the joint. Soft tissue imbalance, joint malalignment, and bony hypertropy can result. Inflammation is not the major component of the osteoarthritis process (Adapted from AHPA Arthritis Teaching Slide Collection. American College of Rheumatology, Atlanta, Georgia).

Rheumatoid Arthritis

ETIOLOGY

Rheumatoid arthritis is a disease characterized by chronic, erosive synovitis. Immunologic events are triggered when synovial vascular lining cells are "activated" by some process not yet understood, causing the transformation of synovial membrane cells. These cells proliferate, resulting in thickening and inflammation of the synovial membrane. The new cell layers become an invasive, fibroblast-like cell mass called pannus, which is capable of eroding cartilage and bone. Synovial fluid accumulates, and the joint swells, distending the capsule, pulling on its periosteal attachment, and causing pain and potential rupture. Ligaments and muscles around the inflamed joint are also subject to weakening and potential rupture.

CLINICAL MANIFESTATIONS

Loss of cartilage and bone integrity, soft tissue disruption, and swelling lead to joint dysfunction as they do in osteoarthritis, but often the deformities are more severe, and usually the entire joint is affected rather than just one joint compartment (Fig. 11-3). As the disease becomes more chronic, it symmetrically affects joints. The joints of the hands, wrists, elbows, shoulders, feet, ankles, and cervical

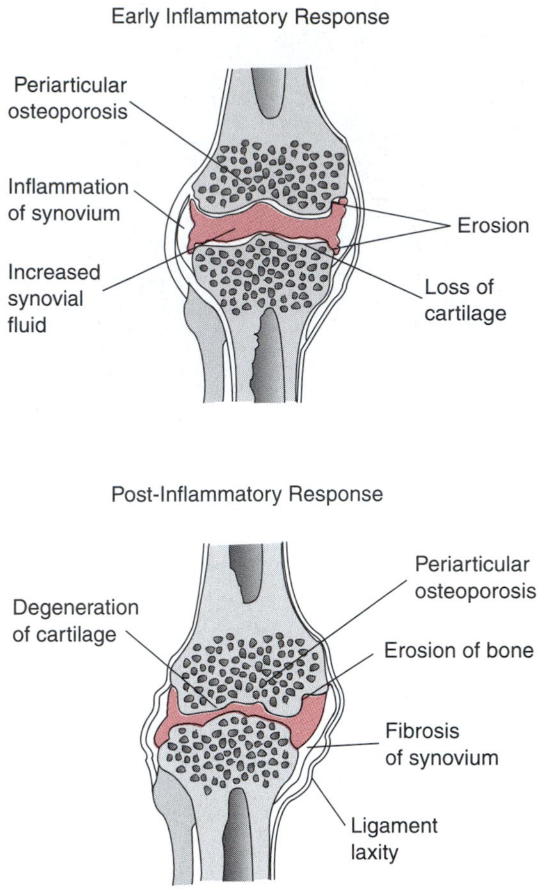

FIGURE 11-3 Early inflammatory joint response to rheumatoid arthritis includes pannus formation and erosion of cartilage and bone. Post-inflammatory irreversible joint changes include destruction of cartilage, bone, and soft tissues and fibrosis of the joint capsule. Damage affects joint alignment, stability, and range of motion. (Adapted from AHPA Arthritis Teaching Slide Collection. American College of Rheumatology, Atlanta, Georgia.)

spine are most likely to be affected. The joint changes are usually reversible if the disease remits within 1 year and no structural deformity has occurred. Early intervention with an emphasis on education regarding joint protection strategies is important. Irreversible changes usually occur between the first and second year in more chronic forms of rheumatoid arthritis.[23]

Unlike osteoarthritis, rheumatoid arthritis has systemic effects such as fatigue, malaise, anemia, and sleep disorders (ie, pain and abnormal sleep cycles). Organ systems, including lungs and the cardiovascular system, may also be affected. Medications used to treat rheumatoid arthritis may contribute to myositis, gastrointestinal distress, and sleep disruption. These systemic effects should be considered in designing exercise programs for the patient with rheumatoid arthritis.[23,24]

PHASES OF RHEUMATOID ARTHRITIS

The course of rheumatoid arthritis is variable and characterized by exacerbations (ie, flares) and remissions. The patient with rheumatoid arthritis may experience an exacerbation and remission with no further occurrence, exacerbations and remissions that gradually decrease over time, or a fast-progressing disease state with few remissions. During a flare, joints are hot and swollen, morning stiffness is present and often lasts longer than 60 minutes, and systemic effects may be more obvious. This is considered an acute phase of the disease. As the pain, swelling, systemic effects, and morning stiffness decrease, the disease state is considered to be subacute. Between exacerbations, the disease state is considered chronic.

The clinician needs to consider the phase of rheumatoid arthritis when designing an exercise program. However, prolonged inflammation during the acute stage contributes to difficulty in determining the phase of the disease. After prolonged inflammation, synovial membranes fibrose, decreasing the vasculature such that joints may not appear hot and swollen. These are referred to as burned-out joints. Although it may appear that the disease has gone into remission (ie, the subacute or chronic phase) and has ceased to damage the joint, the joint destruction and systemic effects continue,[23] and the disease state remains active.

Because symptoms wax and wane, the type and intensity of appropriate exercise also vary. The clinician must consider the phase of rheumatoid arthritis when designing an exercise program, and the patient must be taught to modify the program to match the phase of their illness. Various classifications have been useful in guiding exercise prescription and in teaching patients to monitor and appropriately modify their home programs and activities of daily living (ADLs). In the classification of functional status proposed by the American College of Rheumatology, patients are divided into four groups based on their ability to perform self-care, vocational activities, and avocational activities (Display 11-1). Most exercise program studies that looked at exercise effects considered patients in functional class I, II, and occasionally, III.

Another classification scheme that may guide the therapist in exercise program design examines the radiologic and clinical evidence of disease progression (Display 11-2). Exercise should be tailored to impairments at each stage. The degree of activity of the inflammatory event should espe-

DISPLAY 11-1
Classification of Functional Status of Rheumatoid Arthritis Patients*

Class I: Completely able to perform usual activities of daily living (self-care, vocational, and avocational)*
Class II: Able to perform usual self-care and vocational activities, but limited in avocational activities
Class III: Able to perform usual self-care activities, but limited in vocational and avocational activities
Class IV: Limited in ability to perform usual self-care, vocational, and avocational activities

**Usual self-care activities include dressing, feeding, bathing, grooming, and toileting. Avocational (recreation, leisure) and vocational (work, school, homemaking) activities are patient desired and age and sex specific.*
From Hochberg MC, Chang RW, Dwosh I, et al. The American College of Rheumatology 1991 revised criteria for the classification of global functional status inrheumatoid arthritis. Arthritis Rheum *1992;35:498–502.*

DISPLAY 11-2.
Classification of Progression of Rheumatoid Arthritis

Stage I, Early

*1. No destructive changes on roentgenographic examination
2. Roentgenologic evidence of osteoporosis may be present

Stage II, Moderate

*1. Roentgenologic evidence of osteoporosis, with or without slight subchondral bone destruction; slight cartilage destruction may be present
*2. No joint deformities, although limitation of joint mobility may be present
3. Adjacent muscle atrophy
4. Extra-articular soft tissue lesions, such as nodules and tenosynovitis may be present

Stage III, Severe

*1. Roentgenologic evidence of cartilage and bone destruction in addition to osteoporosis
*2. Joint deformity, such as subluxation, ulnar deviation, or hyperextension, without fibrous or bony ankylosis
3. Extensive muscle atrophy
4. Extra-articular soft tissue lesions, such as nodules and tenosynovitis may be present

Stage IV, Terminal

*1. Fibrous or bony ankylosis
2. Criteria of stage III

**The criteria prefaced by an asterisk are those that must be present to permit classification of a patient in any particular stage or grade.*
From Schumaker HR Jr, ed. Primer on the Rheumatic Diseases. *10th ed. Atlanta: Arthritis Foundation; 1993:188–190.*

cially be taken into account. It is also necessary to accommodate or anticipate joint structural integrity problems so that the affected joint is not unduly stressed. A clearer picture of the joint pathology being addressed allows a safer and more specific exercise design.

Clinical Implications of Pathophysiology

Display 11-2 summarizes the effects of osteoarthritis and rheumatoid arthritis on joint and extra-articular structures and function. In addition to the local pathologic changes caused by these diseases, the resulting pain and effusion trigger protective and reflex spasm and immobility. Immobility leads to further muscle atrophy and loss of normal protective reflex responses.[18,25,26] Immobility combined with non-weight bearing has been shown in animal models to contribute to cartilage breakdown, aggravating the condition.[27,28] Diminished joint complex integrity can also lead to movement patterns that are energy inefficient, limiting activity. When a joint is abnormally aligned, muscles can no longer generate peak force, contributing to strength deficits. For these reasons and because of the effects of low-dose steroids on muscle[29] and the destructive effect of myositis in rheumatoid arthritis, muscles often atrophy significantly. Type II fiber deficits occur in rheumatoid arthritis and osteoarthritis patients,[30,31] and isometric strength deficits have been reported for these patients compared with controls.[8,15,26,32] These impairments underlie the development of functional deficits as patients find it more difficult, painful, and less efficient to move. Exercise correctly prescribed can address impairments and functional deficits.

EXERCISE RECOMMENDATIONS FOR PREVENTION AND WELLNESS

There is no direct way to prevent rheumatoid arthritis, but the literature suggests that certain controllable factors (eg, obesity, trauma, hypermobility, inflammation) correlate with the development of osteoarthritis. Maintaining appropriate body weight, sustaining good postural alignment, developing good muscular strength and length, and correctly using joints in ADLs may be logical and desirable for joint protection, but they are no guarantee against the development of osteoarthritis, which has a genetic basis in some persons.

The main goal of treatment is to limit the progression of the arthritic damage at the affected joint and the joints showing adaptive changes to pathology at the primary joint. Intervention includes assessing and treating impairments and functional losses.

In osteoarthritis, the goal of treatment is to decrease inflammation, to restore normal joint flexibility, and to reestablish balance between muscle length and strength around the joint. Any adaptive changes caused in joints proximal, distal, or contralateral to the affected joint must also be addressed. Performance of basic functional tasks (eg, sit to stand to sit, balance, timed walking, performance of household, vocational and recreational activities) and optimization of cardiovascular fitness are the tasks of an exercise program designed for a patient with osteoarthritis.

For patients with rheumatoid arthritis, exercise program considerations are largely those outlined for osteoarthritis, but because of the variability of its course and because of the possible systemic involvement of the disease, careful monitoring by the physical therapist and the patient is necessary. Patients must be taught to recognize symptom development and the stage of the illness and to modify activity appropriately.

THERAPEUTIC EXERCISE INTERVENTION FOR COMMON IMPAIRMENTS

The patient with arthritis typically presents with pain, mobility impairment, imbalances in muscle length and movement patterns contributing to impaired muscle performance, and cardiovascular endurance impairment. These factors should be evaluated bilaterally throughout the entire extremity joint chain and the trunk. It is equally important to look at functional movement patterns, including gait, stairs, sit to stand to sit, and manipulation of tools when hands are involved.

The exercise program must carry the effects of therapy beyond treatment of a localized joint problem to issues of function in an attempt to reverse the disablement process. In planning an exercise regimen, the impairment at the affected joint and secondary impairments and functional limitations must be addressed. Limitations may occur along a continuum of function, ranging from deficits in high-level athletic performance to an inability to perform self-care activities.

The aims of treatment are to decrease impairment while improving function. Functional improvement includes performance of ADLs and improved muscle and cardiovascular conditioning. Functional activities should be incorporated into the exercise routine to ensure that functional skills are mastered and carried into daily life in an attempt to reverse the disablement process. Joints should be protected during exercise and during functional activities.

Pain

Therapeutic exercise is not usually prescribed specifically for treating pain related to arthritis, because such interventions often exacerbate the symptoms. However, it is important to address pain and minimize pain during therapeutic intervention, because pain may lead to other impairments. Joint pain and swelling resulting from osteoarthritis and rheumatoid arthritis, together with splinting or guarding, can inhibit periarticular muscle function and lead to disuse atrophy, suppress the normal protective reflex response, and cause further cartilage breakdown.[18,25–28] These changes can lead to inefficient movement patterns, thereby decreasing cardiovascular endurance and further limiting activity. The changes may also disrupt the soft tissue balance around the joint, affecting its stability, alignment, and active motion. When a joint is abnormally aligned, muscles can no longer generate peak force, contributing to strength deficits.

The use of exercise to restore muscle balance and joint range for cardiovascular conditioning and to improve functional status was associated with no increase in pain in some studies on the effect of exercise on arthritis[13,16] and with a decrease in pain in others.[14,15] Patients typically present with some degree of pain in the affected joints, which may prevent exercise to the full extent possible or signal the presence of an inflammatory process. In either case, helping to control the pain during and after exercise can maximize possible exertion and help to control inflammatory processes.

Thermal modalities and electrical stimulation to control pain can be applied in conjunction with exercise in the clinic. When possible, the patient should be taught to apply them at home and be instructed about sources for these modalities. The patient should learn how to apply these treatments, because the chronic condition mandates a continued need for them, at least episodically. Heat application to muscles may be appropriate for the rheumatoid arthritis patient before exercise. Ice applied to joints after exercise may also be appropriate for the osteoarthritis patient and for the rheumatoid arthritis patient, if tolerated. Transcutaneous nerve stimulation (TNS) may be useful in conjunction with other modalities in managing pain. TNS should be used with caution with exercise, because it could mask symptoms of overexertion. It has been suggested that regular exercise be scheduled for late morning or early afternoon, especially for rheumatoid arthritis patients with stiffness early in the day and fatigue later in the day.[33]

Mobility Impairment

Osteoarthritis and rheumatoid arthritis often contribute to mobility impairment. ROM can be diminished by several factors:

- Stiffness and shortening of muscles or tendons from spasm, guarding, or habitual postures
- Capsular stiffness or contracture
- Loss of joint congruity because of bony deformity

A thorough musculoskeletal evaluation should indicate which of these factors are present.

Cartilage maintenance depends in part on joint movement.[27,28] Passive, active, and active assisted ROM exercises are designed to ensure that affected joints move through the full range available to them.

Passive ROM is rarely necessary, except in cases of acute joint exacerbation and of severe muscle weakness and inflammation in rheumatoid arthritis. These patients probably are in functional status classes III and IV and often need to be at rest. To avoid contracture and to ensure maintenance of full ROM, one or two repetitions of gentle passive movement through full available range each day is required. Repetitive passive ROM movements may increase joint inflammation.[33] For patients with rheumatoid arthritis who are in functional status classes I and II or who have osteoarthritis, active ROM exercises should be performed daily for affected joints.

When weakness prevents the patient from attaining full ROM, assistance from another person or another limb may be required to achieve full available range. Typically, patients start with one to five repetitions and progress to 10 each day.

When muscle shortening is the cause of range limitations, passive stretch controlled by the patient or clinician may be provided as long as the joint is stable. Considerations outlined in Chapter 6 regarding stabilization of proximal and distal attachment sites to avoid stressing joints above and below the target muscle are especially important in this population. In rheumatoid arthritis patients for whom the integrity of muscle, tendon, or ligament is in question (especially in smaller joints), *gentle* active ROM exercises are preferable. As a safety measure, it is important that the arthritic patient be safely positioned while performing active ROM exercises to ensure they do not fall, lose control of a limb, or apply more force than is intended (Fig. 11-4).

Ligament laxity can occur in the cervical spine of rheumatoid arthritis patients, and special considerations, especially for stretching exercise, apply. A more detailed

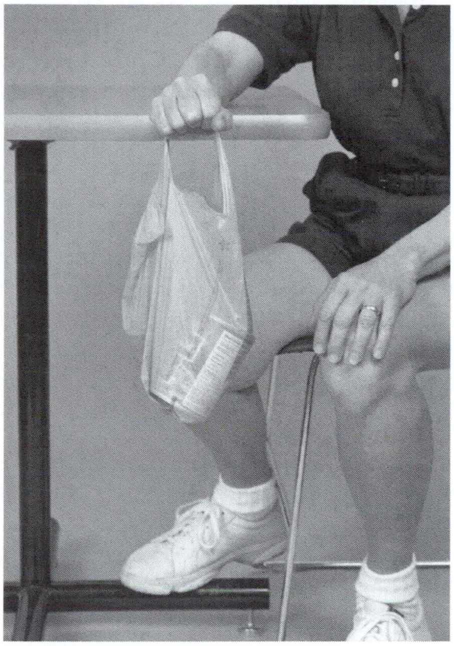

FIGURE 11-4 The patient performs an active range of motion exercise (wrist extension) with her arm and wrist firmly stabilized on the table for safety.

description of these precautions is given in the section on Precautions During Strengthening Exercises When Ligament or Capsular Laxity Exists.

Rheumatoid arthritis patients with prolonged morning stiffness or osteoarthritis patients with the brief stiffness (<0.5 hour) common in the morning may benefit from instruction in a ROM and stretching routine targeting the stiff areas. This exercise can be done before retiring at night, in the morning after a warm shower, or during both periods.

Instruction of the patient in self-mobilization techniques as part of a home exercise program may be useful in cases of osteoarthritis in which capsular restriction limits movement but no acute joint irritation or bony block exists[20] (see Self-Management: Self-Mobilization of the Shoulder Joint). Capsular stiffness in rheumatoid arthritis patients often results from joint distention, and further distractive forces on this inflamed and often weakened tissue should be avoided. When stability is good, passive application of grade 1 oscillations by a skilled therapist to relax periarticular spasm before passive or active ROM activities may be beneficial (see Chapter 21).

Impaired Muscle Performance

Strengthening of weakened muscles is an important part of regaining muscle balance around the joint. It can be done isometrically, isotonically, or isokinetically (see Chapter 4). Each form of exercise has its place in rehabilitation of the arthritic joint, depending on the state of the joint. Isokinetic equipment is most readily available in a clinical setting and is not likely to be practical for independent exercise programs; it is not discussed here.

SELF-MANAGEMENT: Self-Mobilization of the Shoulder Joint

Purpose: To stretch the tight capsule and muscles around the shoulder, which are limiting movement

Position: Sit on a straight-back chair as shown, with a folded towel padding your arm.

Movement technique: Let your arm hang down.

Grasp it just above the elbow.

Repeat a gentle, rhythmic series of downward tugs, trying to keep your shoulder muscles relaxed.

Repeat: _______ **times**

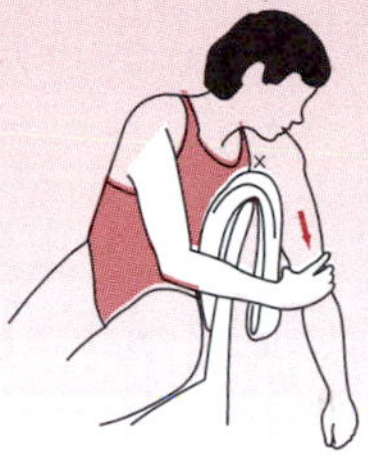

ISOMETRIC EXERCISE

Isometric exercise is most appropriate for acute flares in osteoarthritis and rheumatoid arthritis, but precautions to avoid increased intra-articular flares should be observed.

Rheumatoid Arthritis

Patients suffering acute exacerbations of rheumatoid arthritis are primarily at rest, are positioned to prevent deformity, and may have one or two daily applications of passive ROM applied to large joints and active ROM applied to small joints. In this stage, the prevention of muscle atrophy is important. Muscle strength declines 3% each week in a patient at rest.[34] Because it appears that isometric contractions are associated with the least joint shear and intra-articular pressure increases,[35] this form of exercise is often prescribed in the acute and subacute phases of disease (Fig. 11-5). A single isometric contraction at two thirds of maximal effort, which is held for 6 seconds, increases strength in a normal person; three maximal contractions, with 20-second rest periods, performed three times each week increase strength in rheumatoid arthritis patients.[33,36] However, one drawback is that maximal isometric contraction raises blood pressure.

As a means of increasing muscle strength without raising blood pressure significantly, Gerber and Hicks[37] described a program of brief isometric exercise (BRIME) of one to six isometric contractions, held for 3 to 6 seconds, with 20-second rests between contractions (see Self-Management: Brief Isometric Exercise—Isometric Quadriceps Contraction).

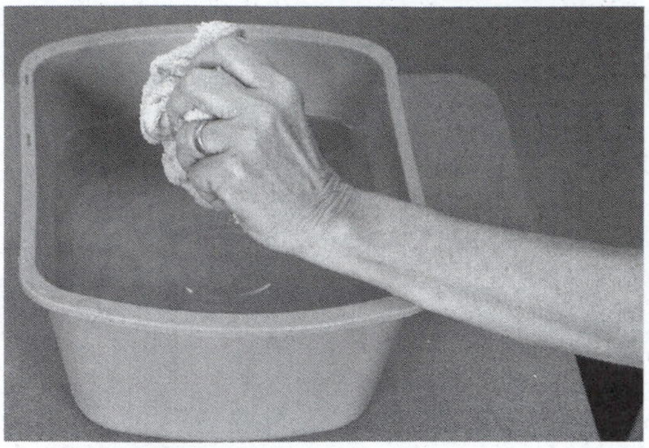

FIGURE 11-5 Squeezing a wet towel is an example of an isometric exercise that can strengthen an arthritic hand. The patient avoids movement into painful ranges or applying pain-causing pressure. Using warm water soothes joints.

Isometric contractions performed at one joint angle only strengthen the muscle at that angle selectively.[38] For this reason, repetitions at various angles may be desirable. During an acute exacerbation of arthritis, it may be necessary to limit contraction to one joint angle to avoid stressing the joint.

Osteoarthritis

In the osteoarthritic joint that is acutely painful, especially if there is significant inflammation and swelling, intra-articular pressure and shear should be limited while preventing muscle atrophy. Isometric contractions are often the exercise of choice in this stage. The same considerations apply as for the patient with rheumatoid arthritis. Brief intense isometric exercises are appropriate when controlling blood pressure is an issue (see Selected Intervention: Hand-to-Knee Pushes).

For the patient with an acute arthritic joint, the home program should start with five repetitions of 6-second contractions and assessment of the response. The patient can gradually increase repetitions to two sets of 15 if symptoms are not exacerbated. As acute pain, swelling, and inflammation resolve, movement into an isotonic routine is appropriate.

SELF-MANAGEMENT: *Brief Isometric Exercise—Isometric Quadriceps Contraction*

Purpose: To maintain or slightly increase strength of quadriceps muscles during acute knee joint inflammation when the joint is otherwise held at rest and to avoid increasing blood pressure when this is a consideration

Position: Sit with the back supported or in a supine position; bend one knee and straighten the other.

Movement technique:

Tighten the quadriceps of the straight leg.

Hold 3 to 6 seconds.

Rest 20 seconds

Repeat: _______ times

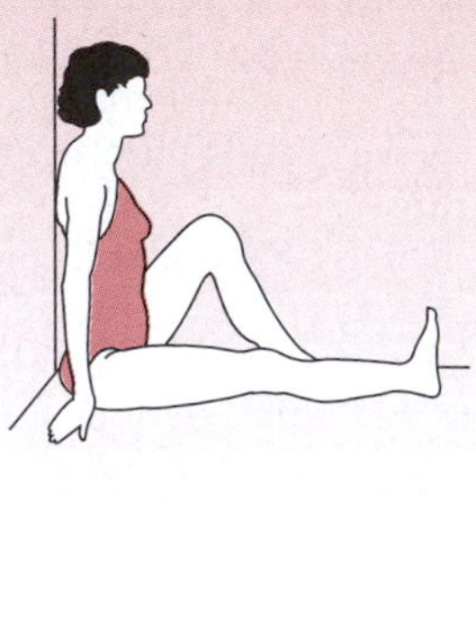

DYNAMIC TRAINING

Dynamic muscle strengthening occurs when muscles contract as they shorten (ie, concentric contractions) or lengthen (ie, eccentric contractions), resulting in movement of the joint they cross. The advantages of dynamic exercise include increased movement of the joint, resulting in maintenance of capsular, ligament, and muscular flexibility and increased cartilage nutrition. Muscle strengthening occurs in all the joint ranges achieved during the exercise and results in a functionally more efficient muscle joint complex. Joint stress and intra-articular pressure are higher than with isometric exercise.[35] Dynamic training is therefore appropriate for chronic, subacute rheumatoid arthritis patients of class I and II and for most patients with osteoarthritis.

In prescribing an exercise regimen, the use of low resistance and high repetition (to fatigue) in a motion arc that does not irritate the joint is preferred to high-load, low-repetition routines in which increased joint loading may cause joint inflammation.[33]

The use of free weights, machines, resistance tubing, and body weight in closed chain activities can be appropriate ways to apply resistance, but their limitations and advantages must be considered in relation to the individual needs of the patient. For example, resistance tubing is less likely to get out of control and torque a joint out of alignment than a free weight, but tubing resistance increases when it is stretched, just as end range movement is achieved and the exercising muscle is out of range of its mechanical advantage. Used correctly, machines offer the advantage of stabilizing the body and exercised joint but rarely offer a low enough resistance to allow a very deconditioned patient to use them. Closed chain exercises, which can range from minisquats to single-leg squat reaches, offer functional movement patterns for retraining activities (eg, sit to stand to sit, stair walking, normal gait). Without an assistive device, however, closed kinetic chain activities apply the patient's weight to an affected lower extremity joint and often require some sophistication in balance. The choice of resistance modality depends on the patient's presentation and the goal of treatment.

In general, start with low enough weight to allow three sets of 10 repetitions, with rest between sets and no resulting joint pain or swelling. The patient should gradually progress to 30 repetitions without rest and without symptom exacerbation and then increase the resistance and start the protocol again.

SELECTED INTERVENTION:
Hand-to-Knee Pushes

See Case Study #11

Although this patient requires comprehensive intervention as described in other chapters, only one exercise will be described. This exercise would be used in the early to intermediate phases of this patient's rehabilitation.

ACTIVITY: Standing hand-to-knee pushes

Purpose: To increase the muscle performance of the hip abductor (stance limb) and abdominal muscles

Stage of motor control: Stability

Mode: Aquatic environment

Posture: Standing on one leg with your back against a wall, maintaining a proper lumbar alignment by pelvic tilting. Bend the opposite knee and flex the hip to approximately 90 degrees.

Movement: With the hand opposite your flexed hip, press isometrically against your knee. Maintain good spinal posture throughout the exercise. Hold for a count of three. Return to the start position.

DOSAGE: 5 to 7 repetitions with each knee, 2 to 3 sets to form fatigue.

EXPLANATION OF PURPOSE OF EXERCISE: Hip abductors on the stance limb are trained to maintain transverse plane pelvic position, while the abdominals work to maintain pelvic tilt against the isometric exercise. This exercise is performed in the upright position to enhance carryover to daily activities, but is performed in a gravity lessened environment to reduce weight bearing on the single stance limb.

Cardiovascular Endurance Impairment

The effects of osteoarthritis and rheumatoid arthritis on joint structure can lead to a loss of functional movement patterns and affect cardiovascular fitness. Patients affected with either disease have decreased cardiovascular endurance, strength, walking time, and total work capacity compared with controls.[6,15,16,32]

Addressing the cardiovascular endurance impairment of arthritic patients has several benefits, including improved cardiorespiratory status and endurance,[38] improved sense of well-being,[13,39] and improved walk distance.[14] Cardiovascular training should be a major part of therapy programs for osteoarthritis patients and chronic functional class I and II (possibly class III) rheumatoid arthritis patients.

Cardiovascular programs for patients with osteoarthritis or rheumatoid arthritis of weight-bearing joints need to be designed to minimize joints stress and shock, to encourage calcium uptake into bone, and to account for any balance difficulties. Several options are available, but adherence to a program is likely to be better when patients are able to pursue activities they find pleasurable.[40] Patient input into this aspect of the program design is important.

Water is a good medium for exercise. One study demonstrated positive effects on pain, muscle strength, flexibility, depression, and anxiety.[13] Water provides a means of unloading joints; in waist-level water, the body weight is 50% of that on land, and in neck-level water, the body weight is 10%.[41] Water provides a medium that can resist or facilitate movement:

- It allows performance of movement patterns that may not be possible on land because of balance or strength deficits.
- It can relax muscles.
- It can modify pain perception through sensory stimulation.

Aquatic therapy can facilitate social interaction in class settings or during family recreation. This aspect may be an added benefit for a population that may be socially limited from active participation in physical activities.

Cardiovascular work can come from walking in the shallow end of a pool, from the use of a foam noodle or float belt (eg, an Aquajogger, which allows walking or running in deeper water), water exercise classes, or swimming (Fig. 11-6). Swimming is best done by skilled persons with good form so that abnormal movement patterns of the back, neck, and shoulders are prevented. Use of a snorkel and swim mask can be beneficial for patients with cervical spine disorders.

Pool temperatures should be 82°F to 86°F for active exercise or 92°F to 98°F for pain relief and gentle ROM activities.[41] Local Arthritis Foundation offices can provide a list of regional pools that meet their requirements, including temperature and accessibility. The Arthritis Foundation also sponsors water exercise classes taught by certified instructors. These classes are available to arthritis patients for a nominal fee.

Stationary or recreational bicycling is another form of low-impact exercise that can improve strength and cardiovascular conditioning. Bicycling is more effective than brisk walking or swimming for weight loss by obese patients needing to decrease the load on weight-bearing joints.[42] In a excellent article on the use of biking in arthritis programs, Namey[43] discusses frame types, fit, and progression of exercise programs. He suggests an upright position on the bike with handle bars that are flat or that curve upward. He

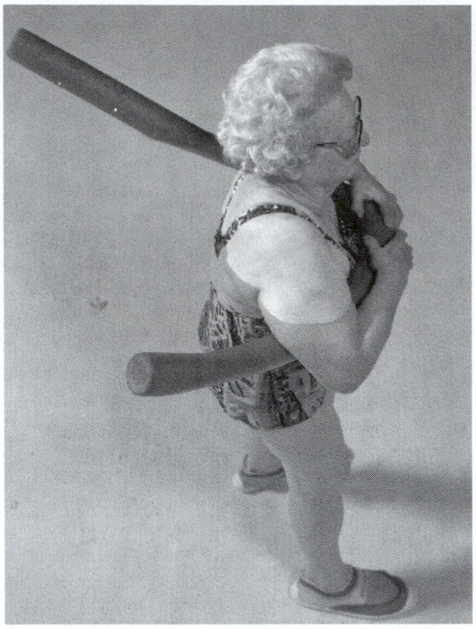

FIGURE 11-6 Walking in shallow water with a foam noodle allows the patient to improve cardiovascular endurance while unweighting arthritic joints. The deeper the water, the more unweighting.

suggests that the seat should be high enough to allow the rider to have only a very mild bend in the knee at the bottom of the pedal stroke. It is worthwhile to have the rider take the bike to a bike store so that frame adjustments can be made for correct length from trunk to handlebars and for correct seat horizontal alignment (ie, angled to allow neutral lumbar alignment unless the patient has a posterior element problem requiring lumbar flexion). Initial outings should be on level, low-traffic streets or trails, and they should be well within the ability of the rider in terms of strength and endurance. A helmet is a must.

A walking program can improve cardiovascular endurance. Several studies have shown additional benefits of a walking program for arthritic patients, including reduction of pain, increase in flexibility and strength, and improvement of function.[13,14] Assessment for balance safety and current levels of function combined with advice regarding supportive footwear, acceptable walking surfaces, and progression of activities are necessary. Most neighborhoods have high school tracks that make an ideal exercise arena because of shock-absorbing level surfaces, easily calibrated distances, freedom from traffic hazards, and easy accessibility to a car to return home when the person becomes fatigued. Many shopping malls make their hallways available before hours for mall walking. This is ideal in bad weather or as a social opportunity, and it provides frequent opportunities for resting if necessary. In both settings, it is safer to use headphones for music or inspirational tapes than in public traffic areas, where the patient must attend to vehicular traffic. This form of exercise, however, is not without risk, because falls are always possible.[14]

The use of treadmills, cross-country ski machines, or rebounders (ie, minitrampolines) offers options for low-impact, weight-bearing activity. This equipment requires more agility, balance, and coordination than outdoor or mall walking. Whichever form of exercise is chosen, cross-training can prevent boredom, stimulate different muscle groups, and alternate joint stress from session to session.

To modify exertion during training sessions, patients should be taught to monitor their heart rates or reliably apply the Borg perceived exertion rating technique[44] (see Chapter 5). They must also know their training parameters. Based on results of a study on aerobic exercise by rheumatoid arthritis and osteoarthritis patients, Minor[6] suggested that disease-related cellular changes in the muscle tissue of rheumatoid arthritis patients might contribute to low aerobic capacity. At similar prescribed heart rates, a patient with rheumatoid arthritis might be working at a higher percentage of aerobic capacity than a patient with osteoarthritis. Both patients, however, might be working at a higher capacity than a younger or more fit individual. Minor[6] pointed out that high-intensity exercise is neither required nor appropriate for effective conditioning of deconditioned subjects.

Another useful form of monitoring for patients with rheumatic disease is the training index. Originally developed by Hagberg[45] for determining minimal beneficial cardiovascular fitness levels in cardiac patients, this tool was adapted by Burkhardt and Clark for use in a rheumatic population. In this technique, the pulse during exercise is divided by the maximum heart rate (ie, 220 minus the person's age) and multiplied by the number of minutes of exercise to yield the training index for that session of exercise. At the end of a week of exercise, daily training index values are added to give the total for the week. The recommended number of units is 42 to 90 per week to maintain cardiovascular fitness. This is a useful monitoring tool for tracking the level of activity and to coach patients in pacing exercise when needed (see Patient-Related Instruction: Determining the Training Index to Track the Level of Exertion).

The training index can have motivational value because it can serve as a tangible sign of progress. Tracking the training index may be especially motivating for patients who view aerobic exercise primarily as a means to weight loss, which is generally slower than most persons need for positive reinforcement. The training index may also be useful for motivating patients who are at a very low level of activity, because they can see evidence of accumulated effort over time in a quantified manner. Introducing the training index in conjunction with a discussion of the benefits of aerobic exercise may be one more way to help the patient remain motivated.

Whatever form of cardiovascular exercise is chosen, it should be fun and satisfying for the patient. This is an important link in maintaining or regaining function, because the more closely training fits with patient goals, the more effective it is.

Special Considerations in Exercise Prescription and Modification

The impairments common to the arthritic patient can pose specific challenges in designing a safe, effective exercise routine. The possibility of joint inflammation, laxity, and

Patient-Related Instruction

Determining the Training Index to Track the Level Of Exertion

This is a simple way for you to keep track of how much exercise you are doing and whether you are (1) progressing in the amount you are doing and (2) whether you are gradually reaching a level of exertion that helps your heart and lungs stay healthy. Always pay attention to your symptoms, and modify exercise appropriately. Remember, every little bit you do adds up!

Your training index (TI) goal is 42 to 90 each week. As time goes on, this number may rise. You and your therapist will discuss this.

Max Heart Rate (MHR) = 220 minus your age.
Intensity = pulse with exercise divided by MHR.

Example: A 40-year-old woman who exercises 3 times each week:

- Session 1: pulse = 100 for 10 min of exercise
- Session 2: pulse = 110 for 15 min of exercise
- Session 3: pulse = 110 for 20 min of exercise

Her MHR = 220 − 40 = 180.

- Session 1: 100/180 = 0.55; 0.55 × 10 min = 5.5
- Session 2: 110/180 = 0.61; 0.61 × 15 min = 9.2
- Session 3: 110/180 = 0.61. 0.61 × 20 min = 12.2

Her total TI = 26.9

deformity in rheumatoid and osteoarthritis and of systemic effects in rheumatoid arthritis necessitate precautions during exercise. Pain in both conditions can interfere with function and therapeutic exercise, and it must be dealt with.

All positive findings from the initial evaluation should be considered when identifying the specific impairments to be addressed with exercise. These findings guide decisions about the prescription variables and necessary precautions and may suggest other options:

- Protect joints during strengthening when ligament or capsular laxity exists.
- Restore muscle balance when splinting, postural habit, or pain inhibition has selectively weakened muscle groups around one or more joints.
- Normalize specific joint movement patterns.
- Restore functional activities.
- Treat pain during and after exercise.

Take into account systemic variables such as fatigue levels, irritability of joints, and cardiovascular fitness, especially in the rheumatoid arthritis patient.

PRECAUTIONS DURING STRENGTHENING EXERCISES WHEN LIGAMENT OR CAPSULAR LAXITY EXISTS

Joint instability caused by ligament laxity, muscle atrophy, or bony joint deformity can affect arthritic joints (see Figs. 11-2 and 11-3) and must be assessed during evaluation. Muscle strengthening around these joints can increase stability without external support, but it is undesirable to load these joints in a way that aggravates the instability. For example, in medial or lateral collateral ligament laxity of the knee, dynamic abductor or adductor strengthening without increased joint stress may be performed by placing the weight proximal to the knee joint rather than at the ankle. Other protective approaches may include bracing of the knee during exercise or the use of a closed chain pattern if proximal muscles are adequate to stabilize the knee in good alignment and the loading forces are tolerated by the joint.

In the small joints of the hand and foot, ligament laxity caused by the erosive effects of rheumatoid arthritis or asymmetric joint deformity from cartilage destruction and marginal spurring resulting from osteoarthritis need to be considered as carefully in exercise prescription as they are in instructions for joint protection during ADLs. The use of ring and wrist splints and foot orthotics helps stabilize and align joints in neutral positions under stress (Fig. 11-7).

Ligament integrity during ROM activities is a crucial safety issue for the upper cervical spine. Rheumatoid arthritis can affect the ligaments of the upper cervical spine and middle spine segments (ie, C5 and C6 areas) and can cause erosion of the dens.[23] Any patient presenting with upper cervical spine instability or long tract signs should be referred to the physician for consideration of immobilization. Patients with a history of rheumatoid arthritis who do not have objective signs of cervical instability should be warned that any cervical spine ROM exercise that results in upper extremity pain or paresthesia or dizziness should be discontinued and that they should consult their physicians.[46]

Joint protection can be approached through mechanisms that unload the joint, attenuate shock, and maximize neutral joint alignment. In addition to use of splints and braces, the following approaches may be implemented to decrease joint forces:

- Unweighting joints through the use of assistive devices (eg, in hip osteoarthritis, use of a cane on the contralateral side to reduce joint reaction forces as much as 50%)[47]

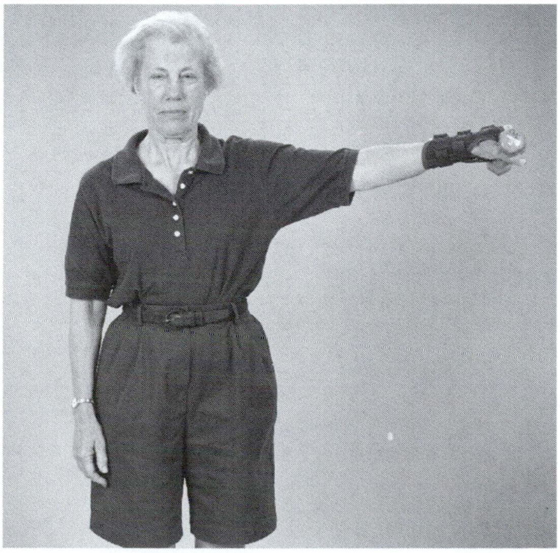

FIGURE 11-7 The patient uses a wrist brace to stabilize joints during exercise.

- Attenuating shock forces in weight-bearing joints (eg, viscoelastic insoles decreased impact vibration by 42% in tibias of experimental subjects)[48]
- Using a water medium[41] or unloading equipment in a clinic setting[49]

Weight reduction is an important goal of exercise for patients with pathologic joints and is often a major goal of exercise programs. The Framingham studies indicated that obesity was a major predictor of the development of osteoarthritis[50] and that loss of as little as 10 pounds decreased the risk of developing knee osteoarthritis by 50% in women.[51] Reduction of joint loading forces by weight loss decreases one of the stresses acting on the joint. Strengthening and recovery of joint reflex mechanisms offers increased joint protection, and normalizing joint alignment to as nearly neutral as possible distributes forces more symmetrically through the joints.[19]

Choosing exercise equipment that does not stress joints (eg, cuff weights for upper extremity strengthening rather than free weights when there is wrist or finger joint instability), that can be of low enough resistance to ensure control of the joint by the patient (ie, some machines do not start at a low enough weight setting for deconditioned individuals), and that encourages movement in physiologic patterns (eg, shoulder abductor strengthening in shoulder external rotation) contributes to patient safety during exercise. By understanding the factors necessary for good joint health, the therapist is able to design an exercise program that protects the unhealthy joint from forces it is unable to resist while helping the patient achieve muscle balance around the affected joint in an effort to improve joint physiology.

RESTORING MUSCLE BALANCE

Disuse atrophy from guarding, pain inhibition, or postural habit can be addressed with ROM and strengthening exercise for patients with osteoarthritis, chronic rheumatoid arthritis, and to some extent, subacute rheumatoid arthritis. These conditions lead to muscle imbalances that can initially limit joint range and lead to joint contractures and muscle weakness affecting the entire limb and eventually affecting the whole body. The therapist must be aware of the muscle groups most typically affected by osteoarthritis and rheumatoid arthritis in specific joints. Muscle shortening leads to weakness and joint malalignment. For example, in hip osteoarthritis, hip flexor shortening and hip flexor and extensor weakness are common (Table 11-2).

Table 11-2. COMMON PATTERNS OF JOINT RESTRICTION IN OSTEOARTHRITIS AND RHEUMATOID ARTHRITIS

JOINT	RESTRICTION	STRETCH	STRENGTHEN
Hip (OA/RA)	• All planes, especially internal rotation and extension	• Flexors • Extensors • Internal and external rotators • Tensor fascia lata	• Abductors • Extensors
Knee (OA/RA)	• Extension	• Hamstrings (quadriceps)	• Quadriceps
Ankle and foot (RA)	• Ankle dorsiflexion • MTP flexion • PIP extension	• Ankle dorsiflexors and plantarflexors • Tarsal invertors and evertors • Toe flexors and extensors	• Toe extensors and flexors • Tibialis posterior
Shoulder (RA)	• Abduction • Flexion • External rotation	• Careful in deranged joints • PROM, AAROM, AROM	• Abductors • External and internal rotators • Biceps • Triceps
Elbow (RA)	• Extension lost early	• Careful in deranged joints • PROM, AAROM, AROM	• Biceps • Triceps
Hand and wrist (RA)	• MCP extension • Wrist extension • First web space	• Careful in deranged joints • ROM wrist daily • Stretch wrist flexors and extensors, forearm pronators and supinators, hand intrinsics	• Finger extensors • Wrist extensors

AAROM, active assisted range of motion; AROM, active range of motion; MCP, metacarpophalangeal joint; MTP, metatarsophalangeal joint; OA, osteoarthritis; PIP, proximal interphalangeal joint; PROM, passive range of motion; RA, rheumatoid arthritis; ROM, range of motion.

Data from Hicks JE. Exercise in patients with inflammatory arthritis and connective tissue disease. *Rheum Dis Clin North Am.* 1990;16:845–870 and from Moskowitz RW, Goldberg VM. Osteoarthritis: clinical features and treatment. In: Schumaker HR Jr, ed. *Primer on the Rheumatic Diseases.* 10th ed. Atlanta: Arthritis Foundation; 1993:188–190.

To modify the processes leading to muscle atrophy, a combination of medications (for pain and reduction of inflammation), therapeutic modalities, posture and body mechanics instruction, external bracing, and other support devices are often necessary. For example, a patient with osteoarthritis of the hip may be requested to temporarily use a cane to unload the painful joint; instructed in stretching of hip flexors and strengthening of weak hip abductors and extensors; educated in correct rest postures and lower extremity alignment with walking; and undergo joint mobilization to restore capsular mobility.

RESTORING FUNCTIONAL ACTIVITIES

The closed chain activities often used in strengthening programs may be introduced through functional activities such as walking, stair climbing, sit to stand, bending, and squatting. Inclusion of these activities in the strengthening routine provides the clinician with an opportunity to confront safety issues (eg, balance, body mechanics) while addressing daily activities. Bracing, assistive devices, and exercise intensity also should be considered.

Functional use of hand joints may have to be restored in osteoarthritis and rheumatoid arthritis patients. Interventions to improve functioning include bracing, medication, therapeutic modalities, ROM, strengthening, and especially the use of adaptive equipment. Functional use of pens, kitchen utensils, levers, and buttons (including keyboards) provide opportunities for a combination of strengthening and safe functional training (Fig. 11-8).

NORMALIZING SPECIFIC JOINT MOVEMENT PATTERNS

Observation of the functional use of affected joints (ie, primary sites of disease and those with adaptive responses) indicates where abnormal movement patterns exist. Abnormal movement patterns can result from irreversible joint surface deformity or erosion of the capsule or ligaments. External support in the form of bracing or splinting may be required. Abnormal movements also can be caused by muscle imbalance around joints earlier in the course of disease or in joints undergoing adaptive response to disease in a removed joint. Assessment of muscle balance between synergist and agonist or antagonist muscles (eg, in the hip between iliotibial band and iliopsoas, in the shoulder between the deltoid and rotator cuff muscles) may be useful for designing a program aimed at restoring a muscle balance that allows the joint to function as close to the kinesiologic standard as possible. This approach decreases the energy required to function and contributes to healthier joint alignment.

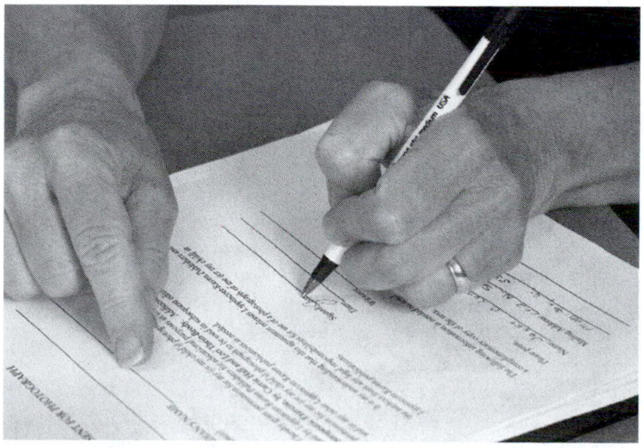

FIGURE 11-8 It is important to incorporate functional activities into the treatment plan. Here, the patient with arthritic fingers practices writing skills.

EXERCISE MODIFICATION IN RESPONSE TO PAIN AND FATIGUE

Systemic deconditioning, muscle and joint irritability, and possibly anemia characterizes patients with inflammatory arthritis. Evaluation of the patient's response to treatment allows appropriate and timely modification of the exercise prescription. Irreversible changes such as cartilage loss, bony deformity, or ligament laxity, together with systemic symptoms such as fatigue or reduced cardiovascular capacity, require modification of exercise to avoid aggravation of joint irritation or undue fatigue. In the past, exercises that increased pain for longer than 2 hours after exercise were modified. It is now accepted that any exercise that increases joint pain should be modified or avoided.[46] The patient should be taught to differentiate between muscle reaction to exercise and joint pain. Undue fatigue after exercise in deconditioned osteoarthritis and rheumatoid arthritis patients and in rheumatoid arthritis patients who may be functioning at a lower aerobic capacity indicates a need to further modify the exercise prescription. Compliance with exercise programs increases when exertion and pain are within acceptable limits for the patient.[17,33,40] The patient's reaction to exercise should be carefully monitored, and self-monitoring skills should be taught as part of the therapy program.

PACING TREATMENT

A patient with more advanced or complicated arthritis may have a team consisting of a rheumatologist, orthopedic surgeon, psychologist, vocational counselor, orthotist, nurse, podiatrist, nutritionist, occupational therapist, and physical therapist. Demands made on the patient's time, energy, and financial resources by individual team members must be considered. Duplication of services should be avoided, whereas teamwork to provide positive functional outcomes should be practiced.

PATIENT EDUCATION

Chronically affected patients should be educated about their conditions during treatment and given self-help literature and information about community resources such as the Arthritis Foundation. Some treatments may be appropriately applied by family members or caregivers, and their involvement in treatment sessions to learn these techniques and to ask questions can be an efficient use of treatment time.

Working with patients with arthritis can be an exciting challenge to the physical therapist. This is a chance to apply the principles of exercise prescription in a situation demanding knowledge of joint and muscle pathology, the ability to do careful and complete assessment, the ingenuity to modify treatments to fit the determined requirements, and the ability to motivate patient cooperation. The benefit to the patient of this successful process can be an improvement in the quality of her life.

Key Points

- Exercise can address impairments that lead to functional deficits in patients with rheumatoid arthritis and osteoarthritis and has a positive effect on their quality of life.
- The stability and mobility of a normal diarthrodial joint depend on the integrity of its anatomic parts. The disease processes of osteoarthritis and rheumatoid arthritis attack these anatomic parts and affect join integrity and function.
- The pathology of one diarthrodial joint in a kinetic chain can adversely affect joints proximal and distal in that same chain and the contralateral joints. Exercise prescription should consider these joints when assessment indicates the need.
- Pain is a common impairment in patients with osteoarthritis or rheumatoid arthritis. Management of pain with therapeutic modalities, safe alignment, bracing, and pacing is a necessary component of exercise prescription.
- Joint movement is necessary for maintaining joint health. Passive, active assisted, and active ROM exercises are appropriate, and the choice depends on the severity of involvement of the joint.
- Isometric exercise is useful in maintaining strength of the muscles around an affected joint. It can be done without aggravating an inflamed joint and without raising blood pressure in patients when this is a consideration by using BRIMEs.
- Dynamic training offers the advantage of strengthening periarticular musculature through full join range and increasing cartilage nutrition. Certain precautions must be followed, especially in strengthening muscles around unstable joints.
- Cardiovascular conditioning is frequently necessary for patients with osteoarthritis or rheumatoid arthritis. It has a positive effect on the quality of life. Following specified guidelines, it is possible to prescribe exercise that does not aggravate existing joint pathology.
- Because of inflammation and joint instability, exercise prescription must include special precautions such as joint bracing, nonjarring movements, conjunctive therapeutic modality use, and pacing.
- Patients' adherence to an exercise program often depends on their belief in the program and on sharing common goals with the therapist. For this reason, the therapist must be aware of patients' beliefs and goals during the treatment program.

Critical Thinking Questions

1. In Case Study #3 (see Unit 7), decide which joints should be addressed in a rehabilitation program.
2. Formulate an exercise prescription for the patient's right hip, including exercise type, intensity, progression parameters, precautions, and adaptation.
3. Decide which outcome measures would indicate that the patient had reached her goals and which would indicate she had reached goals you feel are important. Are there disparities you may have to reconcile?

REFERENCES

1. Yelin E, Felts W. A summary of the impact of the musculoskeletal conditions in the United States. *Arthritis Rheum.* 1990;33:750–755.
2. Yelin E. Economic impact of arthritis. In: Schumacher HR Jr, ed. *Primer on the Rheumatic Diseases.* 10th ed. Atlanta: Arthritis Foundation; 1993:322–323.
3. Ekdahl C, Eberhardt K, Andersson SI, Svensson B. Assessing disability in patients with rheumatoid arthritis: use of a Swedish version of the Stanford Health Assessment Questionnaire. *Scand J Rheumatol.* 1988;17:263–271.
4. Ekblom B, Lovgren O, Alderin M, Fridstrom M, Satterstrom G. Physical performance in patients with rheumatoid arthritis. *Scand J Rheumatol.* 1974;3:121–125.
5. Ekdahl C, Broman G. Muscle strength, endurance, and aerobic capacity in rheumatoid arthritis: a comparative study with healthy subjects. *Ann Rheum Dis.* 1992;51:35–40.
6. Minor MA, Hewett JE, Webel RR, Dreisinger TE, Kay DR. Exercise tolerance and disease related measures in patients with rheumatoid arthritis and osteoarthritis. *J Rheumatol.* 1988;15:905–911.
7. Messier SP, Loeser RF, Hoover JL, Semble EL, Wise CM. Osteoarthritis of the knee: effects on gait, strength, and flexibility. *Arch Phys Med Rehabil.* 1992;73:29–36.
8. Nordesjo LO, Nordgren B, Wigren A, Kolstad K. Isometric strength and endurance in patients with severe rheumatoid arthritis or osteoarthritis in the knee joints. *Scand J Rheumatol.* 1983;12:152–156.
9. Klepper SE, Darbee J, Effgen SK, Singsen BH. Physical fitness levels in children with polyarticular juvenile rheumatoid arthritis. *Arthritis Care Res.* 1992;5:93–100.
10. Gianini MJ, Protas EJ. Comparison of peak isometric knee extensor torque in children with and without juvenile rheumatoid arthritis. *Arthritis Care Res.* 1993;6:82–88.
11. Gianini MJ, Protas EJ. Aerobic capacity in juvenile rheumatoid arthritis patients and healthy children. *Arthritis Care Res.* 1991;4:131–135.
12. Burckhardt C, Moncur C, Minor MA. Exercise tests as outcome measures. *Arthritis Care Res.* 1994;7:169–175.
13. Minor MA, Hewett JE, Webel RR, Anderson SK, Kay DR. Efficacy of physical conditioning exercises in patients with rheumatoid arthritis and osteoarthritis. *Arthritis Rheum.* 1989;32:1396–1405.
14. Kovar PA, Allegrante JP, MacKenzie CR, Peterson MGE, Gutin B, Charlson ME. Supervised fitness walking in patients with osteoarthritis of the knee. *Ann Intern Med.* 1992;116:529–534.
15. Fisher NM, Pendergast DR, Gresham GE, Calkins E. Muscle rehabilitation: its effect on muscular and functional per-

formance of patients with knee osteoarthritis. *Arch Phys Med Rehabil.* 1991;72:367–374.
16. Stenstrom C. Therapeutic exercise in rheumatoid arthritis. *Arthritis Care Res.* 1994;7:190–197.
17. Bunning RD, Materson RS. A rational program of exercise for patients with osteoarthritis. *Semin Arthritis Rheum.* 1991; 21(suppl 2):33–43.
18. Allen ME. Arthritis and adaptive walking and running. *Rheum Dis Clin North Am.* 1990;16:887–914.
19. Brandt KD, Slemenda CW. Osteoarthritis epidemiology, pathology and pathogenesis. In: Schumacher HR Jr, ed. *Primer on the Rheumatic Diseases.* 10th ed. Atlanta: Arthritis Foundation; 1993:184–187.
20. Kessler RM, Hertling D. *Management of Common Musculoskeletal Disorders.* Philadelphia: Harper & Row; 1983: 10–50.
21. Mease P. Rheumatologic issues. In: Agostini R, Titus S, eds. *Medical and Orthopedic Issues of Active and Athletic Women.* Philadelphia: Hanley & Belfus; 1994:230–246.
22. Minor MA. Exercise in the management of osteoarthritis of the knee and hip. *Arthritis Care Res.* 1994;7:198–204.
23. Anderson RJ. Rheumatoid arthritis clinical features and laboratory. In: Schumacher HR Jr, ed. *Primer on the Rheumatic Diseases.* 10th ed. Atlanta: Arthritis Foundation; 1993:90–95.
24. Gerber L. Rehabilitation of patients with rheumatic diseases. In: Schumacher HR Jr, ed. *Primer on the Rheumatic Diseases.* 10th ed. Atlanta: Arthritis Foundation; 1993:90–95.
25. Jokl P. Prevention of disuse muscle atrophy in chronic arthritides. *Rheum Dis Clin North Am.* 1990;16:837–844.
26. Fahrer H, Rentsch HU, Gerber NJ, et al. Knee effusion and reflex inhibition of the quadriceps. *J Bone Joint Surg Br.* 1988;70:635.
27. Bland JH, Cooper SM. Osteoarthritis: a review of the cell biology involved and evidence for reversibility. Management rationally related to known genesis and pathophysiology. *Semin Arthritis Rheum.* 1984;14:106–132.
28. Roy S. Ultrastructure of articular cartilage in experimental immobilization. *Ann Rheum Dis.* 1970;29:634–642.
29. Danneskiold-Samsoe B, Grimby G. The relationship between the leg muscle strength and physical capacity in patients with rheumatoid arthritis with reference to the influence of corticosteroids. *Clin Rheumatol.* 1986;5:468–474.
30. Edstrom L, Nordemar R. Differential changes in type I and type II muscle fibers in rheumatoid arthritis. *Scand J Rheumatol.* 1974;3:155–160.
31. Sirca A, Susec-Michiel M. Selective type II fiber muscular atrophy in patients with osteoarthritis of the hip. *J Neurol Sci.* 1980;44:149–159.
32. Lankhorst GJ, van de Stadt RJ, Van der Korst JK. The relationship of functional capacity, pain and isometric and isokinetic torque in osteoarthrosis of the knee. *Scand J Rehabil Med.* 1985;17:167–172.
33. Hicks JE. Exercise in patients with inflammatory arthritis and connective tissue disease. *Rheum Dis Clin North Am.* 1990; 16:845–870.
34. Muller EA. Influence of training and of inactivity on muscle strength. *Arch Phys Med Rehabil.* 1970;51:449–462.
35. Jayson MIV, Dixon SJ. Intra-articular pressure in rheumatoid arthritis of the knee. Part III: pressure changes during joint use. *Ann Rheum Dis.* 1970;29:401–408.
36. Machover S, Sapecky AJ. Effect of isometric exercise on the quadriceps muscle in patients with rheumatoid arthritis. *Arch Phys Med Rehabil.* 1966;47:737–741.
37. Gerber L, Hicks J. Exercise in the rheumatic diseases. In: Basmajian, ed. *Therapeutic Exercise.* Baltimore: Williams & Wilkins; 1990:333.
38. McCubbin JA. Resistance exercise training for persons with arthritis. *Rheum Dis Clin North Am.* 1990;16:931–943.
39. Danneskiold-Samsoe K, Lyngberg K, Risum T, et al. The effect of water exercise therapy given to patients with rheumatoid arthritis. *Scand J Rehabil Med.* 1987;19:31–35.
40. Jensen GM, Lorish CD. Promoting patient cooperation with exercise programs. *Arthritis Care Res.* 1994;7:181–189.
41. McNeal RL. Aquatic therapy for patients with rheumatic disease. *Rheum Dis Clin North Am.* 1990;16:915–929.
42. Gwinup G. Weight loss without dietary restriction: efficacy of different forms of aerobic exercise. *Am J Sports Med.* 1987; 15:275–279.
43. Namey TC. Adaptive bicycling. *Rheum Dis Clin North Am.* 1990;16:871–886.
44. Borg GAV. Psychophysical basis of perceived exertion. *Med Sci Sports Exerc.* 1980;14:377–381.
45. Hagberg JM. Central and peripheral adaptations to training in patients with coronary artery disease. *Biochem Exerc.* 1986;16:267–277.
46. Lorig K, Fries JF. *The Arthritis Help Book.* 4th ed. Reading, MA: Addison-Wesley; 1995:124.
47. Neumann DA. Biomechanical analysis of selected principles of hip joint protection. *Arthritis Care Res.* 1989;2:146–155.
48. Voloshin A, Wosk J. Influence of artificial shock absorbers on human gait. *Clin Orthop Rel Res.* 1981;160:52–56.
49. Essenberg VJ Jr, Tollan M. Etiology and treatment of fibromyalgia syndrome. *Orthop Phys Ther Clin North Am.* 1995; 4:443–457.
50. Felson DT, Anderson JJ, Naimark A, et al. Obesity and knee osteoarthritis the Framingham study. *Ann Intern Med.* 1988; 109:18–24.
51. Felson DT, Zhang Y, Anthony JM, Naimark A, Anderson JJ. Weight loss reduces the risk for symptomatic knee osteoarthritis in women. *Ann Intern Med.* 1992;117:535–539.
52. Moskowitz RW, Goldberg VM. Osteoarthritis: clinical features and treatment. In: Schumaker HR Jr, ed. *Primer on the Rheumatic Diseases.* 10th ed. Atlanta: Arthritis Foundation; 1993:188–190.

CHAPTER 12

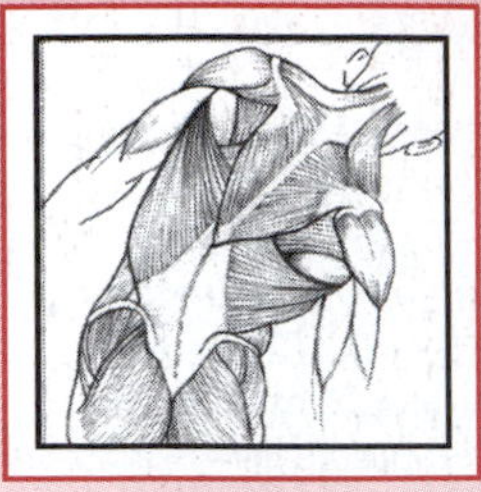

Therapeutic Exercise for Fibromyalgia Syndrome and Chronic Fatigue Syndrome

Kimberly Bennett

Patients with fibromyalgia syndrome (FMS) or chronic fatigue syndrome (CFS) are being increasingly recognized clinically. Significant impairments exist in patients with FMS, including widespread pain,[1] decreased joint range of motion,[2] and impaired respiratory[3] and cardiovascular status.[4] Patients frequently decrease work hours and change tasks,[5] and they develop significant conflicts about life roles.[6] Twenty-five percent of CFS patients are bedridden or unable to work.[7] These disabilities have negative economic and quality of life effects. Patients with FMS and CFS symptoms are being seen increasingly in the physical therapy clinic because carefully prescribed exercise appears to be one of a few interventions of value.[8–11]

PATHOLOGY

The causes of FMS and CFS are not clear despite research looking at many different physiologic systems for evidence of involvement. Central neurologic and peripheral causes have been hypothesized to underlie these conditions, and these concepts provide the basis for treatment strategies. However, because the causes remain unclear, treatment is largely empiric, targeting known symptoms and depending on outcome studies for validation.

Fibromyalgia Syndrome

The cause of fibromyalgia is uncertain. FMS is characterized by widespread body pain, fatigue, and morning stiffness. FMS tends predominately to affect females (80% to 90% of patients). Patients typically are between 20 and 60 years of age,[12] though there have been reports of children being affected.[13,14] Persons with FMS are estimated to comprise about 5% of the patients seen in general medical practices and up to 15% of the patients in general rheumatology practices.[12]

ETIOLOGY

One of the characteristics of FMS is the absence of consistent, positive laboratory findings.[1] Because its symptoms mimic those of other diseases (eg, other rheumatic diseases, multiple sclerosis, malignancies, hypothyroidism, anemia), a thorough medical evaluation is necessary to exclude other possible causes of the presenting complaints.[15] Onset of FMS can be insidious; it may occur after a viral infection[16–18] or trauma.[17–19] It also may be related to stress[20]; sleep disruption such as occurs in sleep apnea, sleep myoclonus, and alpha-delta sleep[21,22]; or be related to central nervous system (CNS) mechanisms.[23]

Many researchers have attempted to identify the causative factors of FMS, but the pathomechanics remain elusive. Historical references to FMS-like symptoms are found as far back as Hippocrates.[24,25] Straus[25] cites the treatise of an 18th century physician who describes such a disorder found predominately "among women . . . who are sedentary and studious," and that he felt was "precipitated by antecedent causes including grief and intense thoughts." In the 1800s and early 1900s, muscle inflammation (giving rise to the term *fibrositis*) was considered a cause. The term fibrositis has generally been disregarded based on the lack of histologic evidence of inflammation in the muscles of FMS patients.[26,27] Later research on the possible causes of FMS has focused on peripheral (muscle physiology) and central (CNS function) phenomena.

Peripheral Origin

Aggressive exercise is not well tolerated by FMS patients and often results in increased perception of pain and fatigue.[28–31] Muscle adaptation to decreased activity has been hypothesized to be at least partially responsible for the adverse reaction to overexertion, and muscle morphology and physiology in FMS patients have been investigated.[32] No muscle morphologic changes specific to FMS have been found.[27] In a very few muscle samples, evidence suggesting a mitochondrial disorder and possibly microcirculation compromise was documented, but these changes were not widespread in the muscle.[26,33–35] Neither muscle energy metabolism[36,37] nor enzyme levels[29] vary from those of controls. Reports of decreased exercise-induced muscle blood flow in FMS patients[38] were not, however, accompanied by the expected decrease in capillary density that this finding suggested.[34] It is not clear whether localized metabolic or morphologic changes in muscle can account for the pain and fatigue associated with FMS.

Epidural blockade does reduce FMS tender points,[39] and there is evidence of increased nociceptor reactivity in FMS patients,[40] which suggests that the pain may be of peripheral origin. Muscles of FMS patients do not show a drop in surface electromyographic activity during short pauses between muscle contractions, which may be a response to perceived pain and fatigue.[41] Studies found that patients with FMS or CFS do not sustain repeated muscle contractions at the same intensity as controls.[42,43,47] Other studies show that they do.[44,45] However, when electrical stimulation of muscles accompanied repeated contractions, the contraction intensity and duration matched those of controls.[46] This finding suggests that the muscle itself is capable of normal work but that there may be a central mechanism limiting that work by producing symptoms of FMS and CFS, which the patient interprets as pain and fatigue.

Central Nervous System Origin

Pain modulation may be disrupted in FMS at the spinal cord level or in higher CNS centers. Although endorphin levels have been found to be normal,[48,49] lowered levels of serum tryptophan[50] and elevated levels of substance P[51] may amplify pain perception.

Pituitary hormone secretion changes have been found in FMS patients.[52–54] Growth hormone is adversely affected by sleep deprivation.[55] The production of an FMS-like state in healthy volunteers through alpha-delta sleep induction[56] may point to a role for abnormal growth hormone secretion in FMS symptom production.[32]

Another hypothesis in which CNS regulation is proposed to be aberrant suggests that the level where control is lost is the limbic system. This area affects sensory gating and processing of sensory input.[57] Autonomic nervous system dysfunction has also been suggested by the results of several studies.[29,58] Stress and anxiety associated with FMS would be expected to increase sympathetic tone, but the expected commensurate increase in plasma and urinary catecholamines were not found.[59]

A hypothesis unifying many of the theories about FMS pathophysiology has been proposed by Yunus.[23] This model emphasizes the possible role of neurohormonal dysfunction resulting in aberrant central pain mechanisms, which are proposed to lead to fatigue, depression, anxiety, and mental stress, further altering sympathetic activity and amplifying pain perception. He also suggests that physical deconditioning, trauma, spinal stress from poor posture, and environmental stimuli may further amplify pain.

SIGNS AND SYMPTOMS

FMS is a chronic condition in which symptoms wax and wane but are typically unrelenting. In addition to pain and fatigue, this population experiences lowered respiratory function,[3] joint range, and muscle endurance and has strength impairments[2,60] and below average cardiovascular fitness levels.[4]

FMS is listed in the American College of Rheumatology (ACR) classification of rheumatic disease as an extra-articular disorder. In a multicenter study,[1] which established the 1990 ACR criteria for definition of FMS, the most common symptoms of FMS patients were fatigue, sleep disturbance, and morning stiffness (73% to 85% of patients). Pain all over, paresthesia, headache, and anxiety affected 45% to 69% of patients. Less common, but still significantly more frequent than in controls, were findings of irritable bowel syndrome, sicca syndrome (ie, dry eyes and mouth), and Raynaud's phenomenon (<35%). In this same study, factors found to affect the musculoskeletal symptoms of FMS patients included cold, poor sleep, anxiety, humidity, stress, fatigue, weather changes, and warmth, as they did to a lesser degree in control subjects.

The diagnostic criteria for FMS were developed from this study (Display 12-1). The diagnosis is based on finding at least 11 of 18 tender points (Fig. 12-1) in the presence of widespread pain (ie, pain in all four quadrants of the body,

DISPLAY 12-1

Classification of Fibromyalgia

1. History of widespread pain.

   Definition. Pain is considered widespread when all of the following are present: pain in the left side of the body, pain in the right of the body, pain above the waist, and pain below the waist. In addition, axial skeletal pain (cervical spine or anterior chest or thoracic spine or low back) must be present. In this definition, shoulder and buttock pain is considered as pain for each involved side. Low back pain is considered lower segment pain.

2. Pain in 11 of 18 tender point sites on digital palpation.

   Definition. Pain on digital palpation must be present in at least 11 of the following 18 tender point sites:

   Occiput: bilateral, at the suboccipital muscle insertions
   Low cervical: bilateral, at the anterior aspects of the intertransverse spaces at C5–C7
   Trapezius: bilateral, at the midpoint of the upper border
   Supraspinatus: bilateral, at origins, above the scapula spine near the medial border
   Second rib: bilateral, at the second costochondral junction, just lateral to the junctions on upper surfaces
   Lateral epicondyle: bilateral, 2 cm distal to the epicondyles
   Gluteal: bilateral, in upper outer quadrants of buttocks in the anterior fold of muscle
   Greater trochanter: bilateral, posterior to the trochanteric prominence
   Knee: bilateral, at the medial fat pad proximal to the joint line

Digital palpation should be performed with an approximate force of 4 kg. For a tender point to be considered "positive," the subject must state that the palpation was painful. *Tender* is not to be considered *painful.*

** For classification purposes, patients are said to have fibromyalgia if both criteria are satisfied. Widespread pain must have been present: for at least 3 months. A second clinical disorder does not exclude the diagnosis of fibromyalgia.*
From Wolfe F, Smythe HA, Yunus MB, et al. The American College of Rheumatology 1990 criteria for the classification of fibromyalgia. Arthritis Rheum. 1990;33:160–172.

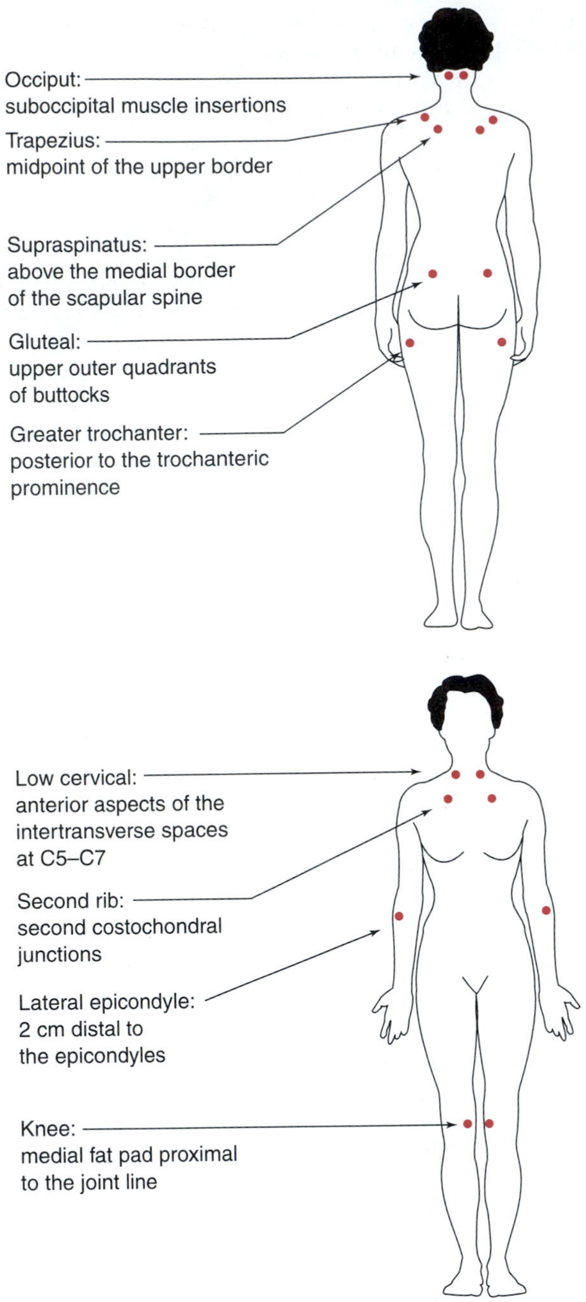

FIGURE 12-1 Location of 18 tender points.

including at least part of the axial skeleton) persisting for at least 3 months' duration. Tender points were defined as anatomically discrete and reproducible areas of heightened pain perception in FMS patients.

FUNCTIONAL LIMITATIONS

Several studies have examined the effect of FMS on everyday life. Fifty-five percent of working patients were found to have changed work tasks and to work shorter hours than before the illness. Motor tasks were reported as being more difficult to perform than before FMS onset, and 67% reported no or short pain-free periods.[5]

The lack of objective findings in light of the patients' perception of their illness is stressful, leading to feelings of rejection and of being misunderstood or disbelieved. These feelings compromise the patient's ability to deal with the illness. Daily routines are disrupted, conflicts about life roles emerge and lead to further stress, and loss of physical fitness and loss of future opportunities occur. Patients need early and adequate information, along with acknowledgement of the conditions to minimize psychosocial consequences.[6]

Chronic Fatigue Syndrome

Chronic fatigue syndrome (CFS) is characterized by profound fatigue. Descriptions of similar illnesses are found throughout the medical literature.[24,25] These disorders include neurasthenia, myalgic encephalomyelitis, and chronic Epstein-Barr virus infection (ie, "yuppie flu"). With an estimated incidence of 0.1%, CFS is much less prevalent than in FMS, and studies suggest that CFS affects both sexes and occurs across almost all races and ethnic groups.[61]

ETIOLOGY

Various studies have looked for the causes of CFS. Immune system changes have been reported in CFS patients. Early reports of viral markers have not been confirmed in later studies. The Epstein-Barr virus is not thought to be a causative agent in CFS onset, though some viral trigger may be involved.[62] Neuroendocrine changes, especially in hypothalamic hormone production or release of corticotrophin-releasing hormone, have been found.[63] CFS does not appear to be a form of depression, because neurohormonal and sleep cycle findings characteristic of depression are not found in CFS patients, though illness-related depression may occur, as it does in FMS.[61] Up to 70% of CFS patients simultaneously present with FMS.[64]

SIGNS AND SYMPTOMS

The onset of CSF is typically sudden, and the fatigue is profound. Twenty-five percent of CFS patients are bedridden or unable to work, and 33% can work only part time.[7] CFS patients may tolerate exertion at first, but 6 to 24 hours later, symptoms often increase. This must be considered by the clinician when designing and teaching an exercise program.

In 1994, the Centers for Disease Control and Prevention (CDC) published a working case definition of chronic fatigue syndrome[65] (Display 12-2). Unexplained, debilitating fatigue of at least 6 months' duration that is unalleviated by rest and four of eight listed symptoms are required for case definition. Symptoms include impairment in memory or concentration, sore throat, tender cervical or axillary lymph nodes, muscular pain, multijoint noninflammatory arthralgia, new or different headaches, nonrefreshing sleep, and prolonged (at least 24 hours) generalized fatigue after previously tolerated exercise.

Among the eight symptoms detailed by the CDC, sleep disruption is reported by about 95% of CFS patients. Other common complaints include neurocognitive difficulties,

DISPLAY 12-2
The Centers for Disease Control and Prevention Working Case Definition of Chronic Fatigue Syndrome

Fatigue criteria and four of eight symptom criteria must be present to fulfill the case definition.

Fatigue criteria

1. Persistent or relapsing fatigue that
   a. Has been clinically evaluated
   b. Is of definite onset
   c. Is not the result of exertion
   d. Results in substantial reduction in activity
2. Other conditions that explain the fatigue have been excluded, including:
   a. Active medical conditions (eg, untreated hypothyroidism)
   b. Previously diagnosed medical condition whose resolution has not been clinically documented (eg, treated malignancies)
   c. Past or present psychotic or melancholic depression, bipolar disorder, schizophrenia, delusional disorders, dementia, anorexia nervosa, bulimia
   d. Alcohol or substance abuse within 2 years of the onset of fatigue or anytime thereafter.

Symptom criteria

Persistent or recurrent symptoms lasting more than 6 consecutive months:

1. Self-reported impairment in short-term memory or concentration, which causes substantial reduction of occupational, educational, social, or personal activities
2. Sore throat
3. Tender posterior cervical, anterior cervical, or axillary lymphnode pain
4. Muscle pain
5. Multijoint noninflammatory arthralgias
6. New or different headaches
7. Unrefreshing sleep
8. Prolonged (at least 24 hours) generalized fatigue after previously tolerable levels of exercise

From Buchwald D. Fibromyalgia and chronic fatigue syndrome. Similarities and differences. Rheum Dis Clin North Am. *1996;22:219–243.*

muscle weakness, frequent need for naps, dizziness, shortness of breath, and adverse responses to stress.[7]

EXERCISE RECOMMENDATION FOR PREVENTION AND WELLNESS

Because the causes of FMS and CFS are unknown, it is difficult to know how to prevent the onset of these conditions other than to encourage a life of balanced activity, rest, and stress management and to encourage family practitioners to regard evidence of imbalances in these areas or of sleep disorders as worthy of early intervention. After FMS and CFS are present, an exercise routine in conjunction with pharmacologic and psychologic interventions seems to be the most effective treatment strategy.

THERAPEUTIC EXERCISE INTERVENTIONS FOR COMMON IMPAIRMENTS

Clinical manifestations of FMS and CFS include evidence of impairments that affect functioning. Studies carried out over the past 10 years[8–10,66–70] and reviews of treatment approaches for FMS and CFS[11,61,71] support the need for multidisciplinary intervention in the treatment of these impairments. Pharmacology, psychotherapy, and education, and physical medicine (including exercise and manual therapy) are used and are largely empiric with ongoing outcome studies. Pharmacologic and psychotherapeutic approaches are discussed with adjunctive interventions.

Physical medicine is an important part of treatment for patients with FMS or CFS. Evidence of deconditioning,[4] lowered respiratory function,[3] decreased joint range, depleted muscle endurance, and reduced muscle performance[2,60] has been found in these patients. Abnormal joint alignment and posture may contribute to peripheral stresses and amplify pain.[10,11,23] Deconditioning may make muscle more vulnerable to physiologic changes (hypothesized by some researchers to underlie peripheral pain[26,32]) and affect neurohormonal regulation.[8,23] Stress is an exacerbating factor for some patients with these conditions. Careful prescription of an exercise program depends on significant findings during the initial evaluation. The clinician working with a FMS or CFS patient should assess posture, strength, joint play, and cardiovascular conditioning to design a treatment program.

Therapeutic exercise can address four main areas of impairment:

1. Stress
2. Impaired posture and mobility
3. Impaired muscle performance
4. Impaired cardiovascular endurance

Techniques used to address impairments in one area may also be useful in treating impairments in other areas. It is important to introduce exercise slowly, progressing intensity and duration as symptoms allow. The regimen depends on good communication between the clinician and patient. The order in which exercise is introduced and impairments are addressed generally follows the order of impairments outlined previously. The exercises used to treat each impairment are increasingly stressful and can be better monitored if this order is followed (Table 12-1).

Therapeutic intervention for a structured return to physical activity is suggested for CFS patients because complete inactivity appears to promote fatigue.[61] Although little literature exists on the effect of exercise for CFS,[35] one study showed improvement in global self-assessment scores for CSF patients after aerobic exercise training.[70] Treatment of FMS-like symptoms of CFS could follow the FMS protocols suggested in the next sections, and physical symptom exacerbation should guide progression of the program.

Table 12-1. EXERCISE FOR FIBROMYALGIA PATIENTS

EARLY PHASE (WEEK 1)	MIDPHASE (WEEK 2)	LATE PHASE
Goal: stress and pain management	Goal: Musculoskeletal balance	Goal: Maintenance
Relaxation Progressive relaxation Autogenic deep breathing Visualization	Fluromethane spray and stretch Self-mobilizations Neuromuscular techniques: hold and relax, contract and relax	Stretch, cont.
Deep breathing	Strain-counterstrain	Musculoskeletal balanace, cont.
Stretch	Muscle system balance (Sahrman)	General strength: resistance tubing, machines, closed chain eccentric exercise
	Neutral spine (± tubing)	Aerobic exercise: non–weight-bearing to weight-bearing and nonjarring activities (ski machine, seated stationary bike, treadmill) and water exercises (aerobics, flotation belt)
	Closed chain eccentric exercise	
	Early aerobic exercise: supine bike, unloading equipment, easy exercises in water	

Stress

If the evaluation indicates a need for stress management, it should be initiated in the early phase of treatment, probably within the first or second visit. Stress management may include an exercise program with relaxation, deep breathing, and stretch exercises. These are unlikely to be stressful to most patients and usually provide benefits that are immediately obvious and typically pleasurable. This approach can provide a positive introduction to the benefits of exercise and offer an opportunity to demonstrate that exercise does not have to mean maximal exertion to be beneficial. Progressive relaxation, autogenic deep breathing, and visualization exercises (see Chapter 25) can be taught, or tapes can be made available to patients for use at home.

Instruction in diaphragmatic and lateral costal expansion breathing (see Chapter 25) can help respiratory function and is a good adjunct to any treatment requiring soft tissue or joint mobilization of the thoracic cage. Approaches such as Aston patterning and Feldenkrais (see Chapter 16) or use of biofeedback (see Chapter 4) also can be considered.

General stretching following accepted guidelines (see Chapter 6) can be prescribed if no joint instability has been found. It is often necessary to make the patient aware of the distinction between stretch and pain, which can be difficult when generalized pain and aching is chronic and patients have learned to disregard these signals. Limiting stretches to specific areas of restriction ensures a more manageable program, modeling the concept of pacing and prioritizing for the patient.

In introducing these exercises, it may be useful to suggest that the patient choose a pleasurable place at a time when interruptions are minimal. Enjoyable background music can be played. Defining this experience to the patient as a pleasurable and relaxing one that can have a positive impact on symptoms of FMS allows clinicians to reinforce success through an achievable task, builds patient confidence in the use of exercise therapeutically, and may help modify unrealistic beliefs about exercise.

Posture and Mobility Impairment

Because of fatigue and pain, many FMS and CFS patients are leading sedentary lives, often in poorly supported, prolonged postures of rest. This can lead to habitual joint malalignment with resultant length and strength impairments of the muscles around the joints, muscle deconditioning, and abnormal movement patterns in the joints. Biomechanical faults in joint alignment may lead to joint discomfort, abnormal muscle holding patterns, tender points (see Fig. 12-1), and areas of fibrositic density and tenderness in muscle bellies and musculotendinous junctions.[11] All of these impairments may contribute to FMS pain.[11,23]

A careful initial evaluation can reveal the problems for which exercise-based treatment can be of benefit. Interventions for musculoskeletal imbalances should be initiated in the middle phase of treatment, after the early phase is incorporated into the routine and tolerated. Soft tissue and joint mobilization techniques for these areas should be supported by specific, moderate exercises designed to strengthen and stretch affected muscles. Several techniques can be taught as independent exercises so that the patient can self-treat, and these techniques are considered in the Adjunctive Physical Therapy Interventions section.

The Sahrman approach to muscle balance in joint or movement dysfunction (see Chapter 4) appears to be an especially effective and well-tolerated approach to treating FMS patients. These exercises are specific and can be progressed slowly, allowing pacing and monitoring of symptoms, ideally short of causing overexertion flares. Most do not require resistance equipment and are easily related to functional tasks (eg, reaching overhead without shoulder or back pain, standing without back or hip pain).

Stabilization exercises for trunk and proximal limb girdle muscles are useful when muscle weakness or joint hypermobility impairments exist and proximal control during functional tasks with the limbs is compromised. This is especially true for spinal segmental dysfunction. An approach that has been nonstressful for patients is the use of graded-resistance tubing attached to the wall or door, with the performance of extremity proprioceptive neuromuscular facilitation diagonals while neutral trunk alignment is maintained during resisted limb movements (Fig. 12-2). This exercise can be progressed in difficulty by adding movement of the entire body (eg, lunging) against resistance while holding a neutral alignment.

Eccentric control is an important part of functional activity, introducing control and balance to movement patterns, and one that is frequently lost in deconditioned patients. Closed-chain activities and movement therapies, including tai chi chuan, are exercise strategies that may help restore periarticular muscle balance and function and stimulate vestibular balance (Fig. 12-3). Introduction of these strategies should be slow, probably after successful introduction of concentric forms of exercise, and always according to the patient's tolerance and carefully monitored for progression of intensity, duration, and frequency.

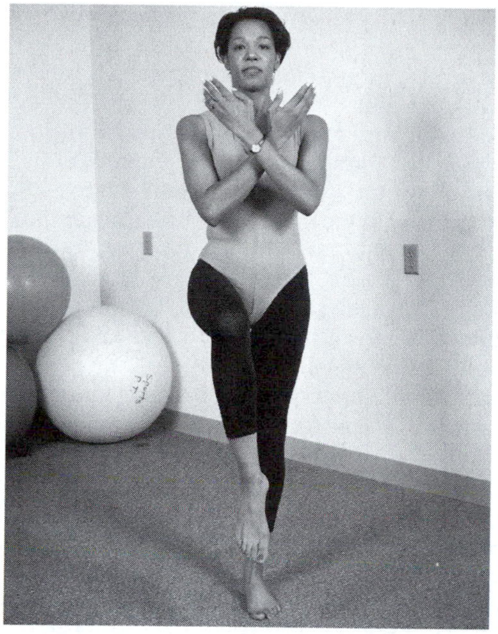

FIGURE 12-3 Tai Chi is an excellent exercise strategy to help restore control and balance to the movement patterns of deconditioned patients. The teacher should have experience working with patients with joint problems or chronic illness.

Impaired Muscle Performance

Muscle performance in FMS patients declines compared with controls. This loss does not appear to result from metabolic or morphologic changes in the muscle of FMS patients; it is caused by some change in central control. Perception of pain and fatigue may limit production of muscle contraction force and eventually affect functional activities of the patient because of resulting deconditioning. When insignificant muscle imbalances are found or are being successfully addressed, patients can begin to direct their energy toward general strengthening routines for conditioning, especially if this goal is a priority for them. Strength training is initiated in the middle phase of treatment and for maintenance purposes. There is no evidence that increasing general strength levels affects FMS symptoms.

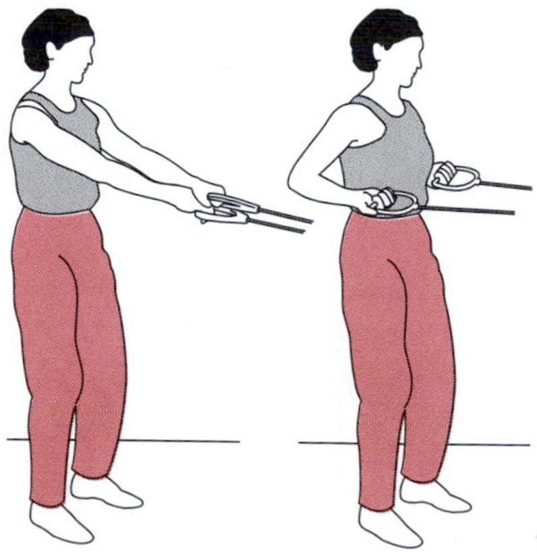

FIGURE 12-2 The use of graded-resistance tubing attached to the wall, with performance of upper extremity proprioceptive neuromuscular facilitation diagonals provides a nonstressful stabilization exercise. ***(A)*** Holding onto the tubing, the patient crosses her wrists with her palms facing downward. ***(B)*** Maintaining her hand at waist level, the patient bends her elbows as she turns her palms upward.

The same conditions apply to exercise prescription for general strengthening as apply to treatment of specific movement faults. The program should start with low-resistance and low-repetition work, avoid static holding, monitor symptoms, and progress slowly. Allowing the patient to choose the form of exercise may increase enjoyment and compliance. Exercise can be isometric or isotonic. If isometric activities are chosen, avoidance of prolonged static holding is important. Contractions should not be held longer than 3 to 5 seconds, with three to six repetitions of the exercise performed three times each week, a level that has been demonstrated to increase periarticular muscle strength.[72]

In dynamic exercise, slow movement through full range with return to the lengthened range allows a slight muscle stretch between contractions. Resistance tubing and, further into the program, resistance machines, which are designed to provide good body alignment and smooth resistance, seem preferable to free weights, perhaps because they allow more complete muscle relaxation between repetitions than free weights, which depend on static muscle contraction of the forearm and fingers. Closed chain, lengthening exercises of the Pilates type (a form of exercise developed and used with dancers, emphasizing strength and flexibility over bulking) are useful when the patient is ready for active movement. If no prior weight training has been done by the patient, calibrating the response by starting with three to five repetitions of three to five exercises at the lightest weight and monitoring the response over 24 to 48 hours can provide the baseline of the patient's tolerance. Patience is important in introducing exercise to decrease setbacks.

Cardiovascular Endurance Impairment

Because aerobic exercise may have a positive effect on some of the impairments seen in FMS patients, including endurance, pain, and flexibility, it should be introduced as soon as possible. Initially, only a few minutes of the activity should be allowed (2 to 5 minutes, unless the patient is already active for longer periods without symptom flares). This allows the gradual build up of tolerance. By the late phase of rehabilitation, the patient may be ready to work on elevation of the heart rate to 50% to 60% of the maximum heart rate. Monitoring techniques including the training index and pulse determination; use of the perceived exertion scale[73] should be discussed so pacing and progress can be monitored. The patient should keep a record of exertion and symptoms to facilitate this assessment.

During the first session, it may be a good idea to make a contract with the patient to start pre-aerobic activities of daily walking, even if only one half of a block. For the patient who is able to walk more than one fourth of a mile, a high school track offers several advantages. Typically, it has a shock-absorbing surface; it is a safe place to use headphones without worrying about traffic, which may make it more enjoyable; accurate distance estimates are possible so progress in distance and rate can be tracked; and the patient who fatigues part way through can usually walk back to a car rather than all the way home or ask someone to come for him. It is important to consider the patient's interests and goals in designing a walking program and in suggesting a particular environment. Initially, the rate of walking should be slow and comfortable until tolerable levels, without a flare of symptoms, can be established.

Another approach to introducing exercise gently is to have the patient lie behind a stationary bike supported in a spinal-neutral position with the feet on the pedals of the bike (Fig. 12-4). During the first session, the patient should pedal about 2 to 3 minutes; 1 to 2 minutes can be added each session (at first not more than once a day) until, by the late phase of treatment, the patient may reach 15 minutes. At this point, the patient probably can tolerate sitting on the bike seat to pedal, but time should be decreased to 7 to 10 minutes and slowly advanced until the patient reaches 20 to 25 minutes. After this level is reached, it should be possible to allow the patient to choose some other form of nonjarring aerobic exercise that is personally enjoyable.

In some clinics, unweighting equipment (eg, harness) is available and has been used successfully in introducing patients to aerobic exercise[74] (Fig. 12-5). Water exercise is another form of reduced weight-bearing exercise. The patient can walk in the shallow end, move rhythmically, or participate in exercise classes. Community pool programs, such as the ones offered by the Arthritis Foundation and the YMCA, have instructors trained to work with persons with various disabilities. These programs have the added benefit of social contact. For some FMS patients, socializing has been markedly decreased because of fatigue and pain. The Arthritis Foundation has a list of pools with this program in many areas, and having this list in the clinic for patients may help them initiate contact.

Nonjarring sources of aerobic exercise for slightly more advanced patients may include a treadmill, ski machine, seated push-pull arm and leg machines, and minitramp. For patients who enjoy the water or who were avid runners, there are specially designed flotation belts that allow the user to walk or jog in the deep end of the pool and that some FMS patients tolerate well after they learn pacing techniques.

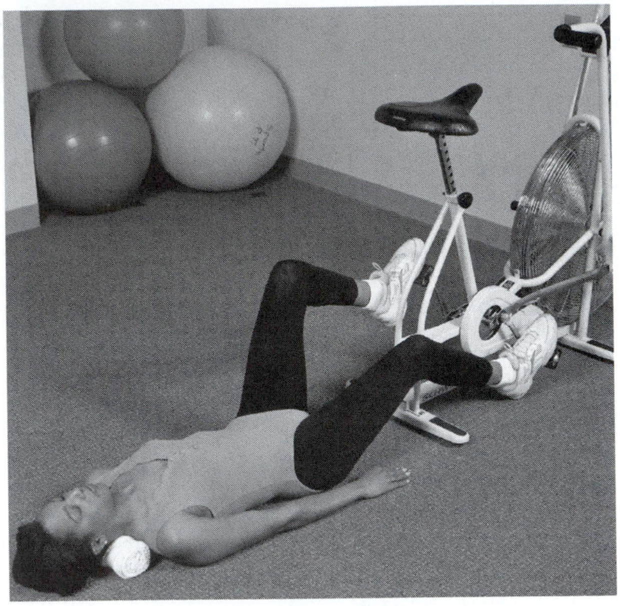

FIGURE 12-4 For FMS or CFS patients, it is important to introduce exercise gently. Exercise phase cardiovascular training can begin with the patient lying on the floor behind a stationary bicycle. The patient should pedal for approximately 2 to 3 minutes in the first training session. By late phase of treatment the patient may have progressed to 15 minutes of cycling while lying on the floor.

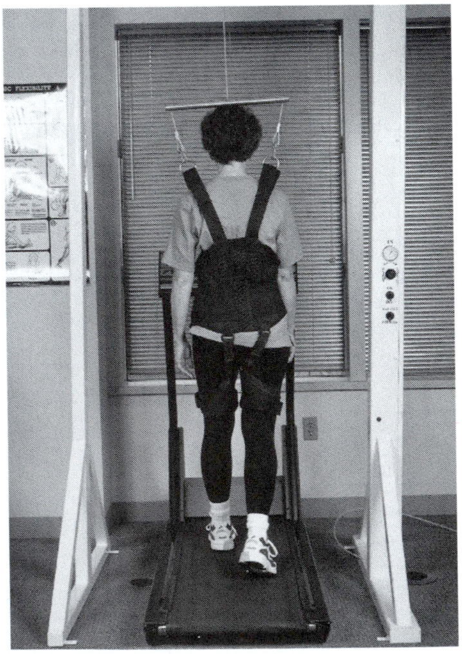

FIGURE 12-5 Unweighting equipment supports part of the patient's body weight. This decreases joint stress and body weight resistance, enabling the patient to do cardiovascular exercise with less physiologic stress.

In several studies of the effects of aerobic exercise on FMS, the first 10 to 12 weeks were problematic for musculoskeletal symptom flares and for adherence.[8,75] More gradual introduction of aerobic exercise may solve some of this problem, and the knowledge that this is a common finding may help the clinician and the patient persevere beyond this point in conditioning.

In introducing aerobic exercise routines, the therapist should let the patient know that continuous monitoring and pacing are important. During periods of symptom flares, the patient should be encouraged to modify exercise intensity appropriately. It is easy for patients to become discouraged and stop a program. Their records and the encouragement of the clinician may help them push through this difficult time and allow them to comply with what appears to be one of a few treatment approaches with a positive impact on FMS.

Special Considerations in Exercise Prescription

Exercise can be a two-edged sword for patients with FMS or CFS. Overexertion can lead to a relapse or exacerbation of symptoms.[8,35,66,69,75] Because most persons with FMS or CFS have experienced this phenomenon, they may resist the idea of exercise, and adherence to an exercise program may be difficult.

ADHERENCE

In an excellent paper that reviews factors influencing patient adherence to an exercise routine, Jensen and Lorish[76] highlight the importance of the patient's beliefs about the nature of the disease and the benefits of exercise. They point out that the process of negotiating for mutual therapeutic goals is an important part of treatment. Although the therapist may be modeling goals on a pathophysiologic concept of the disability, the patient's view is probably different. The patient's view is shaped by his perception of the disability and its effects, what he perceives to be helpful, and treatment goals and activities that are important personally. The therapist has the opportunity to influence these beliefs and positively affect treatment and adherence with the program through a process of mutual information sharing, listening, trust building, and negotiation.

Adherence with exercise programs may be problematic. FMS and CFS patients may feel as if their energy reserves are nearly depleted and may want to avoid exercise. Patients may fear exercise based on past experience with exacerbations after overexertion. As more is being learned about the treatment of these conditions, patients may seek exercise prescription based on the encouragement of their physician or knowledge gained from support groups, literature, or word of mouth. Patients may hope for the clinician to reconcile the apparent discrepancy between their experiences and what they are told is helpful, making it easier for the clinician to convince the patient about the benefits of exercise.

One function of the initial assessment is to provide the opportunity for exchange of information. Another is to set mutual goals. During the assessment, the clinician should listen to and attempt to understand the patient's point of view. In this way, the patient can develop confidence in being part of a team. These are important processes in promoting the patient's adherence to an exercise program (see Chapter 3).

CLARITY OF INSTRUCTION

Mental fog and poor memory are frequent complaints of FMS and CFS patients. Clear written and drawn instructions should be given the patient, and the patient's performance of the exercise based on these instructions should be reviewed periodically. A checklist of all prescribed exercises may be useful for selected patients.

PACING

Pacing is crucial for patients who are chronically fatigued.[77] For many persons, exercise conjures up images of a well-known athletic clothing company's famous exhortation to "just do it." This is one patient belief that may be useful to explore. A patient may fear that exercise means jogging for 3 miles. For people who have been active exercisers before the onset of the disease, the inability to meet this expectation may be a source of grief or frustration. The concept of therapeutic exercise and the importance of pacing needs to be carefully explained.

Another frequently encountered expectation is that exercise can help control weight. It is common for weight gain to occur with these conditions, partially because of inactivity and the effects of some medications. It is important for the patient to understand that therapeutic exercise must be slowly introduced to monitor reactions and to teach pacing. The initial disparity of goals may lead to nonadherence to the program, whereas a clearer mutual understanding of goals may prevent frustration.

Most patients have experienced symptom flares with overexertion. Initiating an exercise routine requires starting slowly, with few repetitions (three to five may be enough the first time), light resistance (none to very minimal), and a limited number of exercises (usually, three is enough). Feedback 24 to 48 hours after exercise is necessary for pacing the progression of the program. Sometimes, a patient who is progressing the intensity and duration of an activity, has a setback unrelated to exercise, and needs to temporarily drop back to earlier levels of performance. Recognition and applause from the patient and the clinician for efforts to pace and avoid overexertion and avoid flares helps in redefining the value of exercise for the patient.

The training index is one form of monitoring that can be used to help the patient in pacing. The training index was originally introduced for use with cardiac patients by Hagberg[78] and modified by Clark[79] for use with FMS patients. This is a quantitative measure of exertion based on simple calculations using pulse rate and the duration of exercise. The training index provides target values for basic cardiovascular fitness, which may be used by patients to track their progress toward these goals (see Patient-Related Instruction: Determining the Training Index to Track the Level of Exertion in Chapter 11). Some patients may find it helpful to keep a diary of daily activities to monitor possible correlations between symptoms and activity levels, and this may also be a useful pacing tool.

CONSIDERATIONS IN THE APPLICATION OF EXERCISE

Empiric findings suggest that exercise approaches requiring high numbers of repetitions or static holding should be avoided by FMS patients. Exacerbations of FMS were triggered in one study that looked at the effects of repetitive dynamic muscle contraction and sustained static muscle contractions in FMS patients and in sedentary, healthy control subjects. It was found that, 24 hours after exercise, exercise-induced extremity pain had not returned to pre-exercise levels in FMS patients.[31]

In the past, eccentric exercise was avoided by FMS patients because muscle pain in FMS was believed to be caused by unrepaired muscle fiber damage with exercise and because normal muscle eccentric exercise was known to create more muscle damage.[79] However, evidence suggests that FMS patients are not more susceptible to activity-induced muscle damage than healthy subjects.[36] In one study in which exercise-induced pain was monitored in FMS patients, insignificant differences in self-assessed pain were found in response to concentric and eccentric forms of exercise.[75] Unfortunately, the avoidance of eccentric exercise has become a "rule" for many FMS patients, and the therapist may need to be ready to discuss its importance if the patient is concerned.

ADJUNCTIVE INTERVENTION

Treatment of FMS and CFS typically is multidisciplinary, and the therapist should be aware of other intervention strategies that are being used. The list of caregivers for a FMS or CFS patient may include an internist, rheumatologist, acupuncturist, occupational therapist, massage therapist, naturopath, psychologist, biofeedback therapist, and physical therapist. Planning an exercise routine for a fatigued patient who is seeing multiple practitioners requires care, consideration, and communication. In the physical therapy clinic, interventions adjunctive to exercise are useful.

Pharmacologic and Psychological Intervention

Pharmacologic therapy is based on findings of neurohormonal alterations and sleep disruption in CFS and FMS and on treating associated symptoms (eg, fever in CFS, muscle pain and gastrointestinal irritation in CFS and FMS). Low-dose tricyclic medications, which in much larger doses act as antidepressants, may be beneficial in addressing pain and sleep disruption. Selective serotonin-uptake inhibitors may help the fatigue component.[71] Buchwald[61] points to anecdotal reports of antiviral and immunomodulating drugs in the treatment of CFS. Simms[71] offers a complete review of the pharmacologic treatment of FMS.

The association of pain, fatigue, and disordered sleep of FMS and CFS with psychological status is controversial.[24,80–82] This controversy is stressful for many patients.[6] As Hendriksson's studies point out, the effects of these chronic, long-term conditions can be profound.[5,6] Aside from the question of any possible causal relationship between psychopathology and CFS or FMS, various types of psychotherapeutic and educational interventions aimed at teaching coping strategies and at adjustment to lifestyle changes have been found to be beneficial.

One study[83] showed a 63% rate of return to work by CFS patients after 1 year of cognitive behavioral therapy, and a study by Buckelew and coworkers[84] correlated higher self-efficacy with less pain and impairment in physical activities for FMS patients. Self-efficacy can be defined as a belief that one can successfully do a thing. Self-efficacy has been shown to impact behavior, motivation, thoughts and emotions.[84] A meditation-based stress-reduction program was also shown to be effective in improving physical symptoms.[85] Because CFS and FMS may be long-term, life-changing conditions, individual and group psychotherapy may be beneficial. In a review of programs using education for self-management of FMS, Burkhardt and Bjelle[86] concluded that self-efficacy and life quality can be enhanced for patients who undergo even short-term intensive treatment, with improvement lasting beyond the end of the program. Several organizations sponsor support groups and education classes throughout the United States and Canada (see Patient-Related Instruction: Organizations for Information About Fibromyalgia Syndrome and Chronic Fatigue Syndrome).

Adjunctive Physical Therapy Interventions

The use of ice, heat, and electrical stimulation to modify the pain of FMS and CFS may help with general patient comfort and with adapting to the effects of exercise. It is important to teach patients to apply the therapeutic modality so they can use it independently in coping with these conditions.

Patient-Related Instruction

Organizations for Information About Fibromyalgia Syndrome and Chronic Fatigue Syndrome

For information about fibromyalgia or chronic fatigue syndrome, contact one of these organizations:

- Arthritis Foundation is an excellent source of information, has support groups, and provides leadership training. Phone numbers of local chapters can be found in phone books.
- Fibromyalgia Alliance of America provides patient information and support group resources.

  FMAA
  P.O. Box 21990
  Columbus, OH 43221-0990
  (614) 457-4222

- Chronic Fatigue Immune Deficiency Syndrome Association of America, Inc. provides patient information, support group resources, and data on research, treatment, and conferences.

  CFIDS Assoc.
  P.O. Box 220398
  Charlotte, NC 28222-0398
  800-848-7373

SELF-MANAGEMENT: Neuromuscular Relaxation of Suboccipital Muscles

Purpose: To restore normal length to one group of suboccipital muscles and to decrease craniovertebral compression and possibly relieve headache

Position: Lie on your back with your knees bent and neck supported on a small pillow or towel roll.

Movement technique: Gently tuck your chin without lifting your head.

Hold for 6 seconds.

Relax.

Repeat: _______ **times**

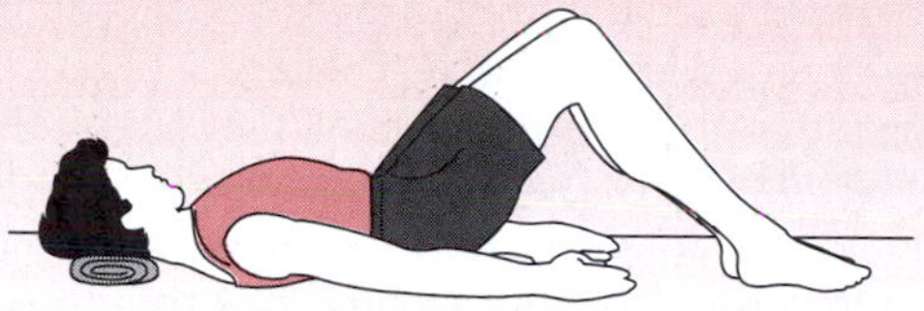

SELF-MANAGEMENT: Neuromuscular Relaxation of a Second Set of Suboccipital Muscles

Purpose: To restore normal length to a second set of suboccipital muscles and to decrease craniovertebral compression and possibly relieve headache

Position: Lie on your back with your knees bent and neck supported on a small pillow or towel roll.

Movement technique: Glide your head to the right without bending your neck.

With one finger tip on the bone behind your right ear, gently push your head to the right, but resist isometrically with your neck muscles.

Hold for 6 seconds.

Repeat on the opposite side.

Repeat: _______ **times**

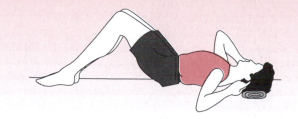

SELF-MANAGEMENT: Neuromuscular Relaxation of a Third Set of Suboccipital Muscles

Purpose: To restore normal length to a third set of suboccipital muscles and to decrease craniovertebral compression and possibly relieve headache

Position: Lie on your back with your knees bent and neck supported on a small pillow or towel roll.

Movement technique: Lift your chin about one-eight inch, so your head tips back.

Bring your right ear toward your right shoulder one-eight inch, so your head tips to the right.

Turn your head one-eight inch to the right, so your heads rotates to the right.

With one fingertip on the right temple, gently push your head back to the left, but your neck muscles resist so no motion occurs.

Repeat: _______ **times on each side (do not alternate)**

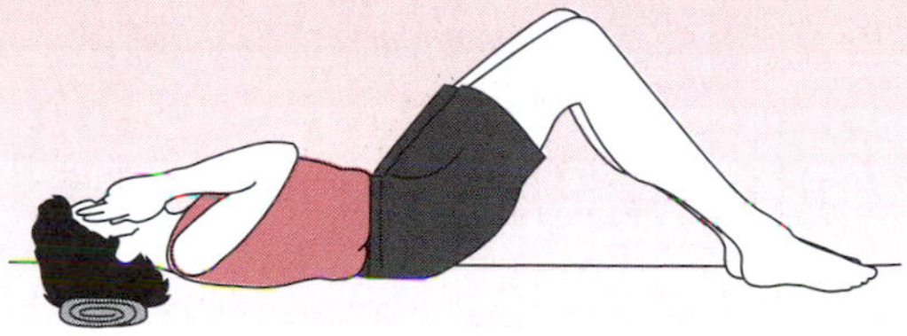

Moist heating packs (rice bags that can be made for less than a dollar and heated in the microwave), ice cups or probes and ice packs, and fluoromethane spray and stretch are all effective treatments. Their use is covered in an excellent self-help book by Penner.[87]

Alpha Stim (form of microcurrent stimulation) is approved for use in helping with sleep and pain. It tends to be tolerated well by CFS and FMS patients compared with transcutaneous nerve stimulation.

Temporomandibular joint, shoulder, craniovertebral joints, rib, lumbar spine, and patellofemoral pain resulting from joint malalignment, headache, and periarticular spasm are encountered by FMS and CFS patients. It is important to teach these patients self-mobilization or neuromuscular techniques to use in conjunction with exercise aimed at balancing the muscles around the affected joints (see Self-Management: Neuromuscular Relaxation of Suboccipital Muscles; Self-Management: Neuromuscular Relaxation of a Second Set of Suboccipital Muscles; Self-Management: Neuromuscular Relaxation of a Third Set of Suboccipital Muscles; and Self-Management: Neuromuscular Relaxation of Tight Rib Joints). This helps to make them independent in coping with the effects of their conditions and may help them progress in their strengthening routines because they are less interrupted by pain.

SELF-MANAGEMENT: Neuromuscular Relaxation of Tight Rib Joints

Purpose: To decrease tightness at the rib joints and decrease posterior costovertebral pain

Position: With help of your therapist or once you are experienced, push on the rib in the front that corresponds with the level of pain on the back.

Even though this might not have seemed painful to you until you touched it, it will almost feel like a red-hot type of pain if it is the correct level. The place you push in front is on the same side as the back pain and near where the rib attaches to the sternum.

After you have located the spot, place the fist of the same-side hand flat against the spot.

Press the opposite hand on top of your fist; your elbow on the side of the pain sticks out.

Movement technique: Stand next to a wall or have a partner gently resist that elbow as it starts to elevate from your side.

Hold for a slow count of 6. *Be very gentle with resistance.*

Repeat:_______ times

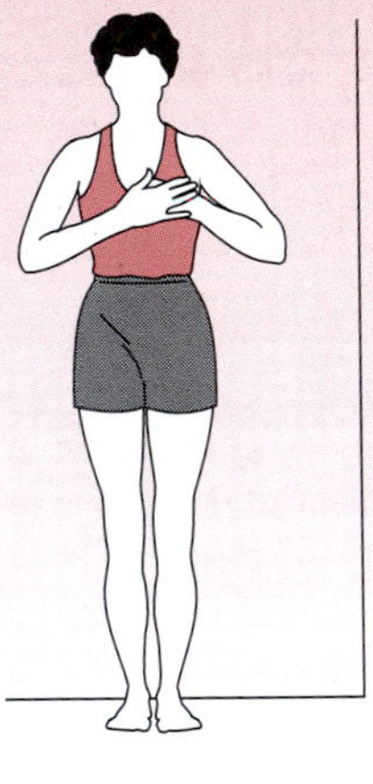

Key Points

- FMS and CFS are increasingly recognized in clinic patient populations, have widespread effects, and limit functioning.
- The cause of FMS is unclear; CFS may be viral in origin.
- Exercise appears to be one of a few effective treatments for FMS and possibly for CFS.
- Because of the fatigue and ease of symptom exacerbation with exertion, exercise prescription must be done carefully and thoughtfully, tracking responses continuously.
- Exercise for the treatment of FMS and CFS can be expected to address stress, posture, and mobility impairments; impaired muscle performance; and cardiovascular endurance.
- Exercise should be introduced slowly and progressed from exercises likely to lead to success to those that may be more stressful. Relaxation, breathing, stretching exercises, and gentle, limited walking exercises can progress to strengthening and to slowly progressing aerobic exercises.
- Physical therapy treatments should always attempt to model the concepts of pacing and limiting overexertion and overcommitment as they apply to daily activities of the patient and in therapeutic exercise.
- The physical therapist should attempt to encourage good communication and establish mutually acceptable goals in an attempt to contribute to the patient's adherence to the exercise program.
- Aerobic exercise should be progressed slowly, be nonjarring, and be pleasurable if possible.
- During physical therapy treatment, patients often are undergoing adjunctive treatments from other medical disciplines, which may stress them in terms of energy, time, and money. The therapist should be aware of the other commitments and help the patient prioritize realistically.
- The use of physical agents for pain control should be taught as self-treatment techniques, because using clinic time for their application may not be the best use of the patient's resources.
- Patients should be taught appropriate self-mobilization or neuromuscular techniques to cope with chronic biomechanical faults so that they have tools to manage their condition independently.

Critical Thinking Questions

1. Outline the questions you would ask in the subjective portion of an evaluation of a patient with FMS. Be sure you cover the areas of their presentation that may affect development of the condition and that may contribute to its exacerbation.
2. What physical tests and measurements would you perform in the objective portion of the evaluation?
3. What forms of exercise would you need to introduce over time to the patient with FMS?
4. List the order in which you would probably introduce the various types of exercise over the course of treatment of the FMS patient.
5. Discuss special considerations for introducing exercise.
6. List the functional goals of physical therapy treatment that would be appropriate for this clinical population.

REFERENCES

1. Wolfe F, Smythe HA, Yunus MB, et al. The American College of Rheumatology 1990 criteria for the classification of fibromyalgia. *Arthritis Rheum.* 1990;33:160–172.
2. Mannerkorpi K, Burckhardt CS, Bjelle A. Physical performance characteristics of women with FM. *Arthritis Care Res.* 1994;7:123–129.
3. Lurie M, Caidahl K, Johansson G, Bake B. Respiratory function in chronic primary fibromyalgia. *Scand J Rehabil Med.* 1990;22:151–155.

4. Bennett RM, Clark SR, Goldberg L, et al. Aerobic fitness in patients with fibrositis. *Arthritis Rheum*. 1989;32:454–460.
5. Henriksson C, Gundmark I, Bengtsson A, Ek AC. Living with fibromyalgia. *Clin J Pain*. 1992;8:138–144.
6. Henriksson CM. Living with continuous muscular pain—patient perspectives. *Scand J Caring Sci*. 1995;9:67–76.
7. Komaroff AL, Buchwald D. Symptoms and signs of CFS. *Rev Infect Dis*. 1991;13(suppl 1):S8–S11.
8. McCain GA, Bell DA, Mai FM, Halliday P. A controlled study of the effects of a supervised cardiovascular fitness training program on the manifestations of primary fibromyalgia. *Arthritis Rheum*. 1988;31:1135–1141.
9. Burkhardt CS, Mannerkorpi K, Hedenberg L, Bjelle A. A randomized controlled clinical trial of education and physical training for women with fibromyalgia. *J Rheumatol*. 1994;21: 714–720.
10. Goldman JA, Hypermobility and deconditioning: important links to fibromyalgia/fibrositis. *South Med J*. 1991;84: 1192–1196.
11. Rosen NB. Physical medicine and rehabilitation approaches to the management of myofascial pain and fibromyalgia syndromes. *Baillieres Clin Rheumatol* 1994;8:881–916.
12. Wolfe F. Fibromyalgia: the clinical syndrome. *Rheum Dis Clin North Am*. 1989;15:1–17.
13. Romano TJ. Fibromyalgia in children: diagnosis and treatment. *W V Med J* 1991;87:112–114.
14. Gedalia A, Press J, Klein M, Buskila D. Joint hypermobility and fibromyalgia in school children. *Ann Rheum Dis*. 1993;52: 494–496.
15. Freundlich B, Leventhal L. The fibromyalgia syndrome. In: Schumacher HR, ed. *Primer on the Rheumatic Diseases*. 10th ed. Atlanta: Arthritis Foundation; 1993:247–248.
16. Moldofsky H. Fibromyalgia, sleep disorder and chronic fatigue syndrome. *Ciba Found Symp*. 1993;173:262–271.
17. Greenfield S, Fitzcharles MA, Esdaile JM. Reactive fibromyalgia syndrome. *Arthritis Rheum*. 1992;35:678–681.
18. Buchwald D, Goldenberg DC, Sullivan JL, et al. The "chronic active Epstein-Barr virus infection" syndrome and primary fibromyalgia. *Arthritis Rheum*. 1987;30;1132–1136.
19. Romano TJ. Clinical experiences with posttraumatic fibromyalgia syndrome. *W V Med J*. 1990;86:198–202.
20. Dailey PA, Bishop GD, Russell IJ, Fletcher EM. Psychological stress and the fibrositis/fibromyalgia syndrome. *J Rheumatol*. 1990;17:1380–1385.
21. Moldofsky H. Sleep and fibrositis syndrome. *Rheum Dis Clin North Am*. 1989;15:90–103.
22. Branco J, Atalaia A, Paiva T. Sleep cycles and alpha delta sleep in fibromyalgia syndrome. *J Rheumatol* 1994;21: 1113–1117.
23. Yunus MB. Towards a model of pathophysiology of fibromyalgia: aberrant central pain mechanisms with peripheral modulation. *J Rheumatol*. 1992;19:846–849.
24. Powers R. Fibromyalgia: an age-old malady begging for respect. *J Intern Med*. 1993;8:93–105.
25. Straus SE. History of chronic fatigue syndrome. *Rev Infect Dis*. 1991;13(suppl 1):S2–S7.
26. Henriksson KG, Chronic muscular pain: aetiology and pathogenesis. *Ballieres Clin Rheumatol*. 1994;8:703–719.
27. Yunus MB, Kalyan-Raman UP. Muscle biopsy findings in primary fibromyalgia and other forms of nonarticular rheumatism. *Rheum Dis Clin North Am*. 1989;15:115–133.
28. Bengtsson A, Henriksson KG, Jorfeldt L, Kagedahl B, Lennmarken C, Lindstrom F. Primary fibromyalgia: a clinical and laboratory study of 55 patients. *Scand J Rheumatol*. 1986;15: 340–347.
29. vanDenderen JC, Boersma JW, Zeinstra P, Hollander AP, van Neerbos BR. Physiological effects of exhaustive physical exercise in primary fibromyalgia syndrome (PFS): is PFS a disorder of neuroendocrine reactivity? *Scand J Rheumatol*. 1992;21:35–37.
30. Yunus M, Masi AT, Calabro JJ, Miller KA, Feigenbaum SL. Primary fibromyalgia (fibrositis): clinical study of 50 patients with matched normal controls. *Semin Arthritis Rheum*. 1981; 11:151–171.
31. Mengshoel AM, Vollestadt NK, Forre O. Pain and fatigue induced by exercise in fibromyalgia patients and sedentary healthy subjects. *Clin Exp Rheumatol*. 1995;13:477–482.
32. Bennett RM, Jacobsen S. Muscle function and origin of pain in fibromyalgia. *Baillieres Clin Rheumatol*. 1994;8:721–746.
33. Henriksson KG, Bengtsson A, Larsson J. Muscle biopsy findings of possible diagnostic importance in primary fibromyalgia. *Lancet*. 1982;2:1395.
34. Bengtsson A, Henriksson KG, Larsson J. Muscle biopsy in primary fibromyalgia: light microscopical and histochemical findings. *Scand J Rheumatol*. 1986;15:1–6.
35. McCully K, Sisto SA, Natelson BH. Use of exercise for treatment of chronic fatigue syndrome. *Sports Med*. 1996;21:35–48.
36. Jubrias SA, Bennett RM, Klug G. Increased incidence of a resonance in the phosphodiesterase region of ^{31}P nuclear magnetic resonance spectra in the skeletal muscle of fibromyalgia patients. *Arthritis Rheum*. 1994;37:801–807.
37. Simms RW, Roy SH, Hrovat M, et at. Lack of association between fibromyalgia and abnormalities in muscle energy metabolism. *Arthritis Rheum*. 1994;37:794–800.
38. Bennett RM, Clark SR, Goldberg et al. Aerobic fitness in patients with fibrositis: a controlled study of respiratory gas exchange and 133 xenon clearance from exercising muscle. *Arthritis Rheum*. 1989;32:454–460.
39. Bengtsson A, Bengtsson M, Jorfeldt L. Diagnostic epidural opioid blockade in primary fibromyalgia at rest and during exercise. pain. 1989;39:171–180.
40. Littlejohn GO, Weinstein L, Helme RD. Increased neurogenic inflammation in fibrositis syndrome. *J Rheumatol*. 1987; 14:1022–1025.
41. Elert J, Rantapaa-Dahlqvist SB, Henriksson-Larsen K, Gerdle B. Increased EMG activity during short pauses in patients with primary fibromyalgia. *Scand J Rheumatol*. 1989; 18:321–323.
42. Lindh M, Johansson G, Hedberg M, et al. Studies on maximal voluntary contraction in patients with fibromyalgia. *Arch Phys Med Rehabil*. 1994;75:1217–22.
43. Mengshoel AM, Forre O, Komnaes HB. Muscle strength and aerobic capacity in primary fibromyalgia. *Clin Exp Rheumatol*. 1990;8:475–479.
44. Lloyd AP, Hales JP, Gandevia SL. Muscle strength, endurance and recovery in the post-infection fatigue syndrome. *J Neurol Neurosurg Psychiatry*. 1988;51:1316–1322.
45. Stokes MJ, Cooper RG, Edwards RH. Normal muscle strength and fatigability in patients with effort syndromes. *BMJ* 1988; 297:1014–1017.
46. Kent-Braun J, Sharma KR, Weiner MW, et al. Central basis of muscle fatigue in chronic fatigue syndrome. *Neurology*. 1993;43:125–131.
47. Rutherford OM, White PD. Human quadriceps strength and fatigability in patients with post viral fatigue. *J Neurol Neurosurg Psychiatry*. 1991;54:961–964.
48. Yunus MB, Denko CW, Masi AT. Serum beta endorphin in primary fibromyalgia syndrome: a controlled study. *J Rheumatol*. 1986;13:183–186.
49. Vaeroy H, Helle R, Forre O, et al. Cerebrospinal fluid levels of beta-endorphin in patients with fibromyalgia (fibrositis syndrome). *J Rheumatol*. 1988;15:1804–1806.
50. Russell IJ, Michalek JE, Vipraio GA, et al. Platelet 3-H-imipramine uptake receptor density and serum serotonin levels in patients with fibromyalgia/fibrositis syndrome. *J Rheumatol*. 1992;19:104–109.

51. Vaeroy H, Helle R, Forre O, Kass E, Terenius L. Elevated CSF levels of substance P and high incidence of Raynaud phenomenon in patients with fibromyalgia new features for diagnosis. *Pain.* 1988;32:21–26.
52. McCain GA, Tilbe KS. Diurnal hormone variations in fibromyalgia syndrome: a comparison with rheumatoid arthritis. *J Rheumatol.* 1989;16(suppl 19):154–157.
53. Neeck G, Riedel W. Thyroid function in patients with fibromyalgia syndrome. *J Rheumatol.* 1992;19:1120–1122.
54. Bennett RM, Clark SR, Campbell SM, Burkhardt CS. Somatomedin-C levels in patients with fibromyalgia syndrome: a possible link between sleep and muscle pain. *Arthritis Rheum.* 1992;35:1113–1116.
55. Davidson JR, Moldosfsky H, Lue FA. Growth hormone and cortisol secretion in relation to sleep and wakefulness. *J Psychiatry Neurosci.* 1991;16:96–102.
56. Moldofsky H, Scarisbrick P. Induction of neurasthenic musculoskeletal pain syndrome by selective sleep stage deprivation. *Psychosom Med.* 1976;38:35–44.
57. Goldstein JA. Fibromyalgia syndrome: a pain modulation disorder related to altered limbic function? *Ballieres Clin Rheumatol.* 1994;8:777–800.
58. Vaeroy H, Qiao ZG, Morkrid L, Forre O. Altered sympathetic nervous system response in patients with fibromyalgia (fibrositis syndrome). *J Rheumatol.* 1989;16:1460–1465.
59. Yunus MB, Dailey JW, Aldag JC, Masi AT, Jobe PC. Plasma and urinary catecholamines in primary fibromyalgia: a controlled study. *J Rheumatol.* 1992;19:95–97.
60. Jacobsen S, Danneskiold-Samsoe B. Inter-relationships between clinical parameters and muscle function in patients with primary fibromyalgia. *Clin Exp Rheumatol.* 1989;7: 493–498.
61. Buchwald D. Fibromyalgia and chronic fatigue syndrome. Similarities and differences. *Rheum Dis Clin North Am.* 1996; 22:219–243.
62. Buchwald D, Komaroff AL. Review of laboratory findings for patients with CFS. *Rev Infect Dis.* 1991;13(suppl 1): S12–S18.
63. Demitrak MA, Dale JK, Straus SE, et al. Evidence for impaired activation of the hypothalamic-pituitary-adrenal axis with chronic fatigue syndrome. *J Clin Endocrinol Metab.* 1991; 73:1224–1234.
64. Goldenberg DL, Simms RW, Geiger A, Komaroff A. High frequency of FM in patients with CF seen in a primary care practice. *Arthritis Rheum.* 1990;33:381–387.
65. Fukuda K, International Chronic Fatigue Syndrome Study Group. The chronic fatigue syndrome: a comprehensive approach to its definition and study. *Ann Intern Med.* 1994;121: 953–958.
66. Nichols DS, Glenn TM. Effects of aerobic exercise on pain perception, affect and level of disability in individuals with FM. *Phys Ther.* 1994;74:327–332.
67. Isomeri R, Mikkelsson M, Latikka P. Effects of amitriptyline and cardiovascular fitness training on the pain of fibromyalgia patients. *Scand J Rheumatol.* 1992; (suppl 94):47.
68. Burckhardt CS, Clark SR, Campbell SM, O'Reilly CA, Wien AW, Bennett RM. Multidisciplinary treatment of fibromyalgia. *Scand J Rheumatol.* 1992; (suppl 94):51.
69. Martin L, Nutting A, Macintosh BR, Edworthy SM, Butterwick D, Cook J. An exercise program in the treatment of fibromyalgia. *J Rheumatol.* 1996;23:1050–1053.
70. Fulcher KY, White PD. Randomised controlled trial of graded exercise in patients with the chronic fatigue syndrome. *BMJ.* 1997;314:1647–1652.
71. Simms RW. Controlled trials of therapy in FMS. *Baillieres Clin Rheumatol.* 1994;8:917–934.
72. Hicks JE. Exercise in patients with inflammatory arthritis and connective tissue disease. *Rheum Dis Clin North Am.* 1990; 16:845–870.
73. Borg GAV. Psychophysical basis of perceived exertion. *Med Sci Sports Exerc.* 1980;14:377–381.
74. Essenberg VJ Jr, Tollan MF. Etiology and treatment of fibromyalgia syndrome. *Orthop Phys Ther Clin North Am.* 1995;4: 443–457.
75. Mengshoel AM, Komnaes HB, Forre O. The effect of 20 weeks of physical fitness training in female patients with fibromyalgia. *Clin Exp Rheumatol.* 1992;10:345–349.
76. Jensen GM, Lorish CD. Promoting patient cooperation with exercise programs. *Arthritis Care Res.* 1994;7:181–189.
77. Lorig K, Fries HF. *The Arthritis Helpbook.* 4th ed. Reading, MA: Addison-Wesley; 1995.
78. Hagberg JM. Central and peripheral adaptations to training in patients with coronary artery disease. *Biochem Exerc.* 1986; 16:267–277.
79. Clark SR. Prescribing Exercise for fibromyalgia patients. *Arthritis Care Res.* 1994;7:221–225.
80. Goldenberg DL. Psychological symptoms and psychiatric diagnosis in patients with fibromyalgia. *J Rheumatol.* 1989;16 (suppl 19):127–130.
81. Goldenberg DL. Psychologic studies in fibrositis. *Am J Med.* 1986;81:67–70.
82. Yunus MB, Ahles TA, Aldag JC, Masi AT. Relationship of clinical features with psychological status in primary fibromyalgia. *Arthritis Rheum.* 1991;34:15–21.
83. Sharpe M, Hawton K, Simkin S, et al. Cognitive behaviour therapy for the CFS: a random controlled trial. *BMJ.* 1996; 312:22–26.
84. Buckelew SP, Murray SE, Hewett JE, Johnson J, Huyser B. Self-efficacy, pain, and physical activity among FM subjects. *Arthritis Care Res.* 1995;8:43–50.
85. Kaplan H, Goldenberg DL, Galvin-Nadeau M. The impact of a meditation-based stress reduction program on fibromyalgia. *Gen Hosp Psychiatry.* 1993;15:284–289.
86. Burkhardt CS, Bjelle A. Education programs for fibromyalgia patients: description and evaluation. *Baillieres Clin Rheumatol.* 1994;8:935–955.
87. Penner B. *Managing Fibromyalgia: A Six-Week Course on Self-Care.* Helena, MT: Capital Physical Therapy, 1997.

CHAPTER 13

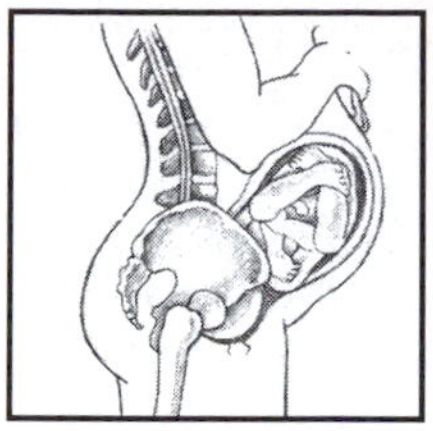

Therapeutic Exercise in Obstetrics

M.J. Strauhal

From the moment of conception, pregnancy profoundly alters a woman's physiology. Every system in her body changes during the childbearing year to provide for the diverse needs of fetal growth and development, meet the metabolic demands of pregnancy, and protect her normal physiologic functioning.[1–4] By considering these changes, the physical therapist can carefully implement a therapeutic exercise program that is safe for the mother and fetus. Therapeutic exercise may be prescribed to pregnant women for several reasons:

- Primary conditions unrelated to pregnancy
- Impairments related to the physiologic changes of pregnancy, such as back pain, faulty posture, or leg cramps
- Physical and psychological benefits
- Preventative measures (Display 13-1)

Women are usually healthy and highly motivated at this time of their lives, and the physical therapist has the opportunity to introduce important lifestyle changes. Therapeutic exercise during this phase in life can play an important role in immediate intervention and in prevention of dysfunction and disease in the future.

PHYSIOLOGIC CHANGES

Physiologic changes related to pregnancy include significant alterations in the maternal endocrine, cardiovascular, respiratory, and musculoskeletal systems.

Endocrine System

The endocrine system orchestrates the hormones that mediate changes in soft tissue and smooth muscle. Various levels of relaxin, estrogen, and progesterone cause fluid retention, growth of uterine and breast tissue, greater extensibility and pliability of ligaments and joints, and a reduction in smooth muscle tone. Hormonal changes and structural adaptations alter gastrointestinal function.[3] Nausea, vomiting, changes in appetite, constipation, heartburn, and abdominal pain may interfere with a pregnant woman's ability and motivation to perform an exercise program.

The thyroid gland enlarges moderately during pregnancy because of hyperplasia of the glandular tissue and increased vascularity.[3] The basal metabolic rate increases during a normal pregnancy by as much as 15% to 30% by term (ie, birth occurring between 38 and 42 weeks of gestation).[1–5] The pregnant woman requires approximately 300 kilocalories more per day to meet this increased metabolic need.[1,2,4] Metabolic need is increased further (up to 500 kcal per day) in pregnant women who regularly exercise and with lactation (ie, secretion of milk by the breasts).[1,2,6,7]

The thermoregulatory abilities of the body are affected by endocrine changes. Increased metabolism results in excess heat that is dissipated by peripheral vasodilation and acceleration of sweat gland activity. The pregnant woman may experience heat intolerance and many complain of fatigue after only minimal exertion.

GESTATIONAL DIABETES MELLITUS

The pancreas adapts to the increased nutrient demands of the mother and fetus. There is a progressive rise in insulin levels during pregnancy into the third trimester. The rise in the serum insulin level, which peaks at about 32 weeks' gestation, is a result of pancreatic islet hypertrophy.[6] Specific hormones promote maternal glucose production or decreased peripheral use of glucose to provide more full fuel for the fetus.[6] Approximately 1% to 12% of pregnant women experience a failure of the pancreas to secrete insulin in sufficient quantity to take care of this glucose or they experience a failure of the body to properly use insulin, resulting in hyperglycemia (ie, high blood sugar).[8,9] This is called gestational diabetes mellitus (GDM) and is considered the most common medical complication of pregnancy.[6]

> **DISPLAY 13-1**
> **Possible Benefits of Prenatal Exercise**
>
> - Preservation or increase of maternal metabolic and cardiopulmonary capacities (fitness)
> - Facilitation of labor, endurance for labor and delivery, possible decreased perception of pain, and improved relaxation
> - Promotion of faster recovery from labor
> - Promotion of good posture and body mechanics
> - Prevention of injury and protection of connective tissue at risk because of laxity
> - Prevention of low back pain, diastasis recti, and urinary incontinence
> - Psychological benefits—improved mood, body image, and self-esteem and reduction of postpartum depression
> - Assistance in the management of gestational diabetes
> - Prevention of excessive weight gain
> - Improvement of muscle tone
> - Decreased risk of venous stasis, deep vein thrombosis, varicose veins, edema, and leg cramps
> - Decreased risk of bone loss because of high circulating estrogen levels
> - Reduction of postdate deliveries
>
> *Data from references 5, 6, 31, 40, and 49.*

The highest prevalence of GDM occurs at 24 to 48 weeks' gestation.[2] All pregnant women should be screened for diabetes, because it can occur even when no risk factors or symptoms are present. Management consists of diet, careful monitoring of glucose levels, and possibly insulin therapy.[6]

Because cardiovascular conditioning exercise facilitates glucose use and reduces the amount of insulin needed to keep blood glucose levels normal, it may play an important role in the management of GDM.[6,10–19] One study documented that women with GDM training with arm ergometry lowered levels of glycemia better than with dietary changes alone.[15,16]

Further research is needed, because some studies show that prolonged strenuous exercise may induce hypoglycemia (ie, low blood sugar) faster in the pregnant than in the nonpregnant woman. Hypoglycemia means that levels of glucose in the bloodstream are too low to meet the body's energy needs. In pregnancy, hypoglycemia may develop in women whose bodies cannot adjust to the increased glucose requirements of the fetus, with or without exercise.[20] Some pregnant women feel better when they eat frequent, small, high-protein meals with an emphasis on complex carbohydrates (ie, whole grains, fruits, and vegetables) rather than simple sugars (ie, sweets).[21]

Whether or not maternal glucose control improves, exercising three to four times each week for 30 minutes does improve cardiorespiratory fitness in pregnant women with GDM.[11] Because overt diabetes mellitus develops in 50% or more of women with GDM, they are at greater risk for cardiovascular complications.[6] Pregnancy provides an excellent opportunity to educate these patients, instruct them in an exercise program, and stress the importance of continuing exercise after delivery.

Cardiovascular System

Maternal hemodynamic changes include a blood volume increase of 30% to 50% that peaks in the middle of the third trimester.[3,6,22] The increase in maternal blood volume varies with the size of the fetus and with multiple fetuses (eg, twins, triplets).[6] In normal pregnancy, one sixth of the total maternal blood volume is within the uterine vascular system.[3]

ANEMIA

Hemoglobin levels fall progressively because of a greater increase in plasma than of red blood cells.[1,2,4–6] A deficiency in red blood cells, hemoglobin, or both is called anemia and during pregnancy has been called physiologic dilutional anemia (ie, 15% below nonpregnant levels).[6] Many cases of anemia are caused by iron deficiency, because the body uses iron to produce hemoglobin. In pregnancy, iron stores are heavily called on to increase blood volume and to provide hemoglobin for the placenta and fetus.[23–25] Women are usually prescribed supplemental iron to prevent anemia during pregnancy and during breast-feeding. Symptoms of mild iron deficiency may be experienced early in pregnancy and include fatigue, lightheadedness, and decreased tolerance for exercise.

Hemoglobin concentration determines the oxygen-carrying capacity of the blood. The amount of oxygen transferred across the placenta is influenced by maternal and fetal hemoglobin concentrations.[6] The relative difference between red blood cell volume and plasma volume does not interfere with oxygen distribution to various organs during pregnancy as might be expected. Changes in cardiac output, stroke volume, and heart rate contribute to an increase in oxygen distribution.[6] When a pregnant woman exercises, many of the variables that determine the transfer of oxygen across the placenta are affected. In animal studies, some of the physiologic effects of exercise augment oxygenation, and there appears to be a balanced net effect. Further research is needed to confirm these effects.[6]

Contributing to oxygen distribution is an increase in cardiac output by 30% to 50% and an increase in resting pulse by 8 beats per minute (bpm) in the early weeks of pregnancy to a plateau of about 20 bpm at 32 weeks.[1–3,6] During normal pregnancy, cardiac output is influenced by increased maternal weight, basal metabolic rate, and blood volume and by decreased arterial blood pressure and vascular resistance.

Hormonal changes influence the decrease in total systemic vascular resistance by 25% and in total peripheral vascular resistance by 30%. This helps to balance the change in cardiac output and produces an arterial blood pressure decrease of 5 to 10 mm Hg for the duration of the pregnancy.[1,2,4,5] Peripheral vasodilation keeps the blood pressure within normal limits despite the increase in blood volume during pregnancy.[3]

SUPINE HYPOTENSIVE SYNDROME

Body position also influences hemodynamic changes. As pregnancy progresses, supine hypotension or inferior vena cava syndrome may develop when the backlying position is assumed.[26] The aorta and inferior vena cava may be occluded by the increased weight and size of the uterus (usually after the fourth month of pregnancy). The obstruction of venous return and subsequent hemodynamic adjustments from aortic compression decrease cardiac output.[1–4] Research suggests a variety of factors involved in determining the possible severity and significance of supine hypotensive syndrome (SHS).[26] Signs and symptoms of SHS are presented in Table 13-1. Because physical therapists treat and prescribe exercises in the supine position, they must have a thorough understanding of SHS and the rationale behind position changes. This knowledge can help to reduce the alarm and paranoia occasionally associated with SHS.

Some women are asymptomatic during documented severe supine hypotension (arterial pressure of 80/40 mm Hg) or report symptoms before or after the hypotensive episode. The variability in signs and symptoms may reflect different degrees of reflex autonomic activation.[26] As many as 60% of women may experience symptoms at some time during pregnancy, but the incidence of true SHS is about 8%, with risk peaking at 38 weeks' gestation.[26] Cappe and Surks[27] estimated the incidence of severe cases of SHS to be less than 1% of the 2000 women they studied. Other studies report that there is sufficient uteroplacental perfusion even if aortocaval circulation is diminished over time.[27] An important indicator of risk is a history of recently experienced symptoms, such as an increase in maternal heart rate and decrease in pulse pressure in the supine position.

The earliest sign of impending SHS is an increase in maternal heart rate and a decrease in pulse pressure. Spontaneous recovery usually occurs with a change in maternal position, even if very slight.[3,4,26] Maximum venous return and cardiac output are obtained in the left lateral recumbent position, but the right lateral recumbent position also reduces symptoms.[1,2,4,26]

SHS is confined almost exclusively to the supine position, although anatomic anomalies (eg, bicornuate uterus, which has two horns or horn-shaped branches) may predispose a small number of women to symptoms in sidelying positions. Prolonged and motionless standing also can occlude the inferior vena cava and the pelvic veins during pregnancy, decreasing cardiac output, increasing venous pressure, and contributing to edema and varicosities in the lower extremities.[3]

Awareness of hemodynamic changes and SHS becomes important to the physical therapist when performing manual therapy techniques or prescribing exercises that require supine positioning or prolonged standing. Accommodating a more upright or sidelying position (especially in the third trimester) or frequent position changes may be appropriate when working with patients at risk for SHS. Suggestions for position changes include placing a small wedge or pillow under the right hip in supine, raising the head and shoulders 20 to 30 degrees, semisitting, prone (on a special support or with use of pillows or wedge to decrease abdominal compression and ensure patient comfort), or quadruped (ie, all-fours position). Changing positions from lying to upright should be done cautiously to decrease symptoms of orthostatic hypotension. Symptoms have disappeared with manual displacement of the uterus to the left or with lifting of the uterus in supine.[26] Conversely, SHS has been induced by abdominal pressure, which should be considered when positioning a patient in prone or when prescribing a maternal external support that may put pressure on the abdomen.[26] The physical therapist should encourage the pregnant woman to shift positions frequently during exercise, work, and treatment to avoid stasis and hypotension. Because supine positioning during labor has been associated with a lower fetal oxygen saturation, position changes apply to the laboring woman as well.[28]

Respiratory System

The respiratory system also adapts to the many changes of pregnancy. Hormonal changes produce increased mucus in the respiratory tract with associated increases in sinus and cold-like symptoms.[1,4] The upper respiratory tract may become predisposed to coughing and sneezing, increasing the likelihood of stress urinary incontinence in the pregnant woman with weak pelvic floor and abdominal muscles. The

Table 13-1. SUPINE HYPOTENSIVE SYNDROME

SIGNS	SYMPTOMS	SIGNS IN SEVERE CASES
Pallor or cyanosis	Faintness	Unconsciousness
Muscle twitching	Dizziness	Incontinence
Shortness of breath	Restlessness	Impalpable pulses
Hyperpnea	Nausea and vomiting	A lifeless appearance
Yawning	Chest and abdominal discomfort or pain	Convulsions
Diaphoresis	Visual disturbances	Cheyne-Stokes respiration
Cold, clammy skin	Numbness or paresthesias in the limbs	
A wild expression	Headache	
Syncope	Cold legs	
	Weakness	
	Tinnitus	
	Fatigue	
	Desire to flex hips and knees	
	Anguish	

Data from references 26 and 27.

lower urinary tract itself undergoes hormonal changes that also make incontinence more likely during pregnancy.[1–4]

The diaphragm is displaced upward by about 4 cm, but diaphragmatic excursion is increased.[1,2,4,6] An increased pulmonary ventilation rate (ie, the total exchange of air in the lungs measured in liters per minute) during pregnancy is achieved by the woman breathing more deeply, increasing tidal volume (ie, the amount of gases exchanged with each breath).[1–3,6] The respiratory rate increases only slightly (approximately 2 bpm), but there is an associated increase in respiratory minute volume, which is the amount of air inspired in 1 minute.[1–4,6] Lung compliance increases, and airway resistance decreases from the relaxing effect of progesterone on smooth muscles.[6] This has been referred to as *hyperventilation of pregnancy*. Although arterial blood gases reflect an increase in oxygen and a decrease in carbon monoxide, causing mild respiratory alkalosis, this is not true hyperventilation. This mild maternal alkalosis promotes placental gas exchange and prevents fetal acidosis.[6] It may be perceived as dyspnea at rest and during exercise or as a decrease in the tolerance for exercise and exertion. In early pregnancy, it is unrelated to the encroachment of the uterus on the diaphragm. Later, as the lower costal girth is increased, greater breathing movement takes place at the middle costal and apical regions compared with the abdomen.[29]

Pregnancy is characterized by a 10% to 20% increase in oxygen consumption that, combined with a reduction in functional residual capacity, results in a lower oxygen reserve.[6,30] Exercise produces an increased demand for oxygen and risks the possibility of blood flow being shunted from the uterus to the active skeletal muscles, although research has not proved this to be true.[6] Some studies show this increase in oxygen demand to be more dramatic during weight-bearing exercises, which are more energy costly in pregnancy because of the extra body weight.[6,31] With increasing body weight, more oxygen is required to exercise, and a woman reaches her maximal exercise capacity at a lower level of work.[31] Maximal exercise capacity of most pregnant women declines by approximately 20% to 25% in the second and third trimesters of pregnancy.[6] Pregnant women should be advised to decrease workloads later in pregnancy, when fetal demand is at its greatest.[29]

Musculoskeletal System

The physical therapist is perhaps best suited to deal with the multiple musculoskeletal changes that occur in response to pregnancy. Many of these changes may make the childbearing woman more vulnerable to pain and injury.[32] Although the physiologic and morphologic changes in pregnancy are normal, symptoms should not be considered normal despite the fact that they are common.

Optimal weight gain by the mother during pregnancy is important to pregnancy outcome,[1–4] but a wide range in weight gain is compatible with good clinical outcomes. The pattern of weight gain may also have important implications. Birth weight of the infant parallels maternal weight gain, and overweight and underweight women face increased risks during pregnancy. There are potential hazards for the mother and the infant when weight gain is restricted, and exercise should not be used to decrease weight. An average weight gain of 12.5 kg (27.5 lb) is usually recommended during pregnancy, but the desirable range is related to prepregnancy weight status. The American College of Obstetricians and Gynecologists (ACOG) supports the guidelines established by the National Academy of Science that recommend a weight gain of 12.5 to 18 kg (27.5 to 40 lb) for underweight women, 11.5 to 16 kg (25 to 35 lb) for normal-weight women, and 7 to 11.5 kg (15 to 25 lb) for overweight women.[1] These figures are based on prepregnancy body mass index (ie, weight in kilograms divided by the square of the height in meters).

The uterus and its contents, increases in blood volume and extracellular fluid, and an increase in breast tissue contribute to weight gain during pregnancy.[1,2] The nonpregnant uterus is approximately 6.5 cm long, 4 cm wide, and 2.5 cm deep and weighs 50 to 70 g.[1–3,31] By term, the uterus has dramatically increased to 32 cm long, 24 cm wide, and 22 cm deep and weighs about 1100 g.[1–4] By the end of 12 weeks, the uterus becomes too large to remain wholly within the pelvis and becomes an abdominal organ.[1–3] It enlarges more rapidly in length than in width. This gradual increase in size and weight causes an upward and forward shift in the woman's center of gravity. The result may be a progressive increase in lumbar lordosis and compensatory thoracic kyphosis. Enlarging breasts gaining up to 500 mg each add to this tendency.[31] As the shoulders become rounded, the head shifts forward, and the posterior neck muscle activity increases to support the head. Posterior suboccipitals may increase activity, extending the head on the neck to maintain eyes horizontal (ie, optical righting reflex). Scapular adductors and upward rotators may undergo stretch weakness.

The subcostal angle of the thorax increases from approximately 68 degrees in early pregnancy to approximately 103 degrees in late pregnancy.[1–4,6] Expansion of the rib cage and the upward pressure of the enlarging uterus produces up to 4 cm of elevation of the diaphragm.[1–4] Chest circumference increases by 5 to 7 cm. In the last trimester, the trunk may rotate to the right as the growing uterus rotates to the right on its long axis. This dextrorotation most likely occurs because of the position of the rectosigmoid (ie, lower portion of the sigmoid colon and upper portion of the rectum) on the left side of the pelvis.[1,2,6] Rotation to the left, or levorotation, is rare.

Changes in hormones contribute to joint laxity and subsequent hypermobility. Changes occur in the foot and ankle. A drop in the arches and increased pronation are usually apparent during pregnancy. Poor foot alignment affects the mechanics of the lower kinetic chain. Unlike other joints in the body that return to their normal prepregnancy position, the foot may not.[3] The postpartum woman may notice a permanent increase in shoe size. Because laxity and weight gain change foot biomechanics, pregnant women should be advised regarding proper footwear and possibly orthotics for support (see Chapter 22).

Postural changes in response to pregnancy can be further exaggerated by work, activities of daily living (ADLs), recreation, and exercise. Hormonal changes facilitating ligamentous laxity, softening of cartilage, and proliferation of synovium also influence postural changes and possibly contribute to injuries during more strenuous movement. Because these mechanical changes may aggravate preexisting conditions, it must not be assumed that a pregnant woman's complaints of aches and pains are always a result of the pregnancy.

THERAPEUTIC EXERCISE PRESCRIPTION

Every pregnant woman adapts differently to the physiologic changes of pregnancy. Age, level of fitness, past and current exercise history, and concurrent adaptations to the changes of pregnancy must be considered when the physical therapist designs a therapeutic exercise program for the childbearing client.

Research[32] focused on physical activity in the workplace has identified four physical stressors that are associated with an increased incidence of prematurity and low birth weight, both factors of poor pregnancy outcome: quiet standing, long hours, protracted ambulation, and heavy lifting. It is believed that these activities cause intermittent but protracted reductions in uterine blood flow. Research focused on recreational exercise during pregnancy has not identified similar associations but rather indicated an overall positive impact on pregnancy outcome.[33,34] The interaction between the physiologic adaptations to exercise and pregnancy appear to improve maternal cardiovascular reserve, maternal heat dissipation, placental growth, and functional capacity.[33] Women who engage in active exercise during pregnancy have fewer of the common discomforts associated with pregnancy, such as swelling, leg cramps, fatigue, and shortness of breath.[35,36] Some studies have shown a reduction in the duration of labor and incidence of obstetric complications during delivery associated with maternal exercise.[37–39]

Although there is a limited scope of applied research on the effects of pregnancy on exercise and exertion, enough data have been produced to support the claim that moderate exercise, carefully prescribed and monitored, during pregnancy is safe for the mother and the fetus.[5,6,22,33–48] However, concerns about exercise during pregnancy exist (Table 13-2). Although many of these concerns are not substantiated by research, the guidelines for exercise err on the side of conservative management, because human studies are not ethically possible. Precautions and contraindications should be considered, and prudent guidelines should be followed in the initiation of an exercise program for a pregnant woman.

Precautions and Contraindications

Pregnant and postpartum women should be advised to seek the approval of their health care providers (eg, physician, midwife) before engaging in an exercise program. They should be screened for contraindications or risk factors for adverse maternal or perinatal outcome. Displays 13-2 and 13-3 detail the absolute and relative contraindications to exercise in pregnancy. Limitations or modifications of the exercise program may be recommended at any time during the pregnancy.[5,6,31,40] For example, a pregnant woman with pre-existing pulmonary disease may be able to exercise, but her intensity level may vary as pregnancy-induced changes affect the respiratory system.

Exercise Guidelines

ACOG[7] and the Melpomene Institute for Women's Health Research[49] have published guidelines for exercise during pregnancy and after delivery (Displays 13-4 and 13-5). ACOG recommends that women who are accustomed to aerobic exercise before pregnancy continue but cautions against starting a new aerobic exercise program (other than walking) or intensifying training levels.[7] A gentle-paced water aerobics class may be appropriate for the beginner. Exercise in water offers several physiologic advantages to the pregnant woman.[50,51] The hydrostatic force of water, proportional to the depth of immersion, produces an increase in central blood volume by pushing extravascular fluid (edema) into the vascular spaces. This may lead to increased uterine blood flow and keeps the maternal heart rate and blood pressure lower than with land exercise. The buoyancy of water is supportive, and water is thermoregulating.[50–52]

The guidelines offered here are for the general population.[3,6,7,31,40,49,53–55] These differ from those given to the elite

Table 13-2. EXERCISE RISKS DURING PREGNANCY

MATERNAL	FETAL
Hypoglycemia	Hypoxia—possibility that blood flow will be shunted from the uterus in favor of exercising muscles
Chronic fatigue	Distress
Musculoskeletal injury from repetitive mechanical stress, changes in balance, and soft tissue laxity	Intrauterine growth retardation from alterations in energy and fat metabolism
Cardiovascular complications	Malformations
Spontaneous abortion	Hyperthermia secondary to maternal hyperthermia, increasing risk of neural tube defects and preterm labor
Preterm labor	Prematurity
	Reduced birth weight

Data from references 5–7, 31, 40, and 49.

DISPLAY 13-2

Absolute Contraindications to Exercise During Pregnancy

1. Pregnancy-induced hypertension (BP >140/90 mm Hg)
2. Diagnosed cardiac disease (ischemic, valvular, rheumatic, or congestive heart failure)
3. Premature rupture of membranes (ie, risk of prolapsed cord)
4. Placental abruption
5. History of preterm labor during current pregnancy (initiation of labor before the 37th week)
6. History of recurrent miscarriage (no exercise in first trimester, but may be able to exercise after that)
7. Persistent vaginal bleeding
8. Fetal distress
9. Intrauterine growth retardation
10. Incompetent cervix
11. Placenta previa (ie, partial or complete covering of the cervix by the placenta)
12. Thrombophlebitis or pulmonary embolism
13. Acute infection
14. Preeclampsia or toxemia (ie, hypertension with proteinuria or edema) and eclampsia (ie, hypertension, proteinuria, and edema associated with convulsions and possible loss of consciousness and cardiac arrest)
15. Polyhydramnios (ie, amniotic fluid volume >2000 ml)
16. Oligohydramnios (ie, abnormally low amount of amniotic fluid)
17. Severe isoimmunization
18. No prenatal care

Data from references 6, 7, 40, and 73.

DISPLAY 13-3

Relative Contraindications or Limitations to Exercise During Pregnancy

1. Diabetes
2. Anemia or other blood disorder
3. Thyroid disease
4. Dilated cervix
5. History of preterm labor during previous pregnancy
6. Uterine contractions that last several hours after exercise
7. Sedentary lifestyle
8. Extreme obesity or underweight (including eating disorders, poor nutrition, and inadequate weight gain)
9. Overheating—high maternal core temperature may be associated with abnormal fetal development (teratogenesis) in the first trimester
   - Swimming pool temperatures should not exceed 85–90°F (29.4–32.2°C)
   - Avoid Jacuzzi temperatures above 101°F (38.5°C)
   - Avoid exercising in hot, humid weather or with fever
10. Breech presentation during the third trimester
11. Multiple gestation
12. Pulmonary disease (eg, exercise-induced asthma, chronic obstructive pulmonary disease)
13. Peripheral vascular disease
14. Hypoglycemia
15. Cardiac arrhythmias or palpitations
16. Pain of any kind with exercise
17. Musculoskeletal conditions (eg, diastasis recti, pubic symphysis separation, sacroiliac dysfunction)
18. Medication that alters maternal metabolism or cardiopulmonary capacity
19. Smoking, alcohol, recreational drug, and caffeine consumption

Data from references 6, 7, 40, and 49.

or professional athlete, whose risks and precautions are similar but whose training level may be more intense if closely supervised.[6,34,56,57] Several activities should be discouraged or avoided during pregnancy.[5,6,31,40] The pregnant woman should be dissuaded from participating in competitive or contact sports, and activities that have the potential for high-velocity impact that may cause abdominal trauma should be discouraged:

- Horseback riding
- Snow and water skiing
- Snow boarding
- Ice skating
- Diving
- Bungee jumping
- Heavy weight lifting
- High-resistance activities

Hyperbaric conditions, as in scuba diving, and activities that may promote extreme Valsalva maneuvers, as in weight lifting, should be avoided. The pregnant woman should not partake in activities that pose an increased risk to damage of joints, ligaments, and disks secondary to hormonal changes (eg, positions in which free weights may put joints into traction or stress the ligaments.) The shift in the center of gravity along with increasing weight gain puts the pregnant woman at a higher risk for injury in sports that require balance and agility.[49] The pregnant woman should avoid activities and exercises in which loss of balance is increased (eg, mountain climbing, gymnastics, downhill skiing, sliding into base), especially in the third trimester. Caution should be used when exercising at high altitudes during pregnancy.[58]

EXERCISE INTENSITY

Exercise prescription regarding target heart rate or workout intensity, duration, and frequency during pregnancy remains controversial. There are drawbacks with using the target heart rate formula for the aerobic portion of an exercise session during pregnancy.[6,22,40] It usually is expressed as 60% to 90% of an individual's age-predicted maximum heart rate. Wisewell et al.[6] reported that the maximum heart rate in pregnant women is lower than this estimated value. In pregnancy, the maternal resting heart rate is elevated over nonpregnant values by 15 to 20 bpm.[4,6] Mitral valve prolapse occurs more frequently during pregnancy and may be aggravated by heart rates above 140 bpm.[6,40] With this in mind, recommendations for the general population include the reduction of exercise intensity during pregnancy by approximately 25%. A maximal heart rate of

DISPLAY 13-4

General Exercise Guidelines

- Exercise regularly, at least three times per week.
- Avoid ballistic movement, rapid changes in direction, and exercises that require extremes of joint motion.
- Include warm-ups and cool downs.
- Avoid an anaerobic (breathless) pace.
- Strenuous activity should not exceed 30 minutes; 15- to 20-minute intervals are recommended to decrease the risk of hyperthermia. Ketosis and hypoglycemia are more likely to occur with prolonged strenuous exercise.
- Discourage vigorous exercise or exertion in high heat and humidity, with high pollution levels, and during febrile illness.
- Frequent change of positions may be required to avoid supine hypotensive syndrome, but be careful of sudden changes in posture to reduce possible orthostatic hypotension.
- Avoid prolonged periods of standing, especially in the third trimester.
- Modify the intensity of exercise according to symptoms and stage of pregnancy.
- Do not exercise to exhaustion or undue fatigue. Adequate rest is important. Rest after exercise in the left lateral recumbent position for maximum cardiac output. *Exercising to the point of fatigue or exhaustion may compromise the function of the uterus, with a detrimental effect on the fetus.*
- Maintain metabolic homeostasis by adequate caloric intake. Increase to 300 kcal/day for pregnancy alone, 500 kcal/day more for exercising during pregnancy, and 500 kcal/day more for lactation (may vary based on prepregnancy weight).
- Fluids should be taken before, after, and possibly during exercise to avoid dehydration.
- Avoid gastrointestinal discomfort by eating at least 1½ hours before an exercise workout.
- "No pain, no gain" does not apply to exercise during pregnancy.
- Low-resistance and high-repetition exercise is recommended. Avoid Valsalva maneuvers and encourage proper breathing during exercise.
- Maternal adaptations favor non–weight-bearing exercise instead of weight-bearing exercise.
- Postpartum progression into prepregnancy exercise routines should be gradual.
- Stop exercise or activity if unusual symptoms occur (see Display 13-5).

Data from references 1 through 7 and 49.

60% to 75% is considered safe: a maximum maternal heart rate of 140 bpm for those just starting an exercise program and 160 bpm if previously exercising.[6,40]

Exercise intensity may also be determined by the degree of respiratory distress or rate of perceived exertion.[6] These levels correlate with maximal heart rate percentages:

Light: 40% to 50% of heart rate maximum
Moderate: 51% to 65% of heart rate maximum
Heavy: 66% to 80% of heart rate maximum

Conversing with ease during exercise indicates that the woman is exercising at the light to moderate intensity that is optimal for pregnancy.[6]

DISPLAY 13-5

Signs and Symptoms That Signal the Patient to Stop Exercise and Contact Her Physician

1. Pain of any kind
2. Vaginal bleeding
3. Uterine contractions that persist at 15-minute intervals or more frequently and are not affected by rest or change of position
4. Persistent dizziness, numbness, tingling
5. Visual disturbance
6. Faintness
7. Shortness of breath
8. Heart palpitations or tachycardia
9. Persistent nausea and vomiting
10. Leaking amniotic fluid
11. Decreased fetal activity
12. Generalized edema (rule out preeclampsia)
13. Headache (rule out hypertension)
14. Calf pain or swelling (rule out thrombophlebitis)

Data from references 1 through 7 and 49.

Endurance exercises have the additional benefit for pregnant women of preparing them for the increased exertion of labor and delivery. With the fluctuation in the hormonal milieu, aerobic exercise is an excellent mood elevator. However, if the key postural muscles, especially those of the pelvic floor, are weak, aerobic exercise can be detrimental because of the added stress to those structures. Water aerobics or bicycling are appropriate forms of cardiovascular fitness that may decrease stress on these structures and vulnerable joints.[50,51]

ADJUNCTIVE INTERVENTIONS

Pregnancy restricts the use of many modalities, especially ones that increase body heat. This is especially important over the abdomen or uterus.

Hot packs are generally safe to use on the back, neck, and extremities. Ultrasound may be considered at sites away from the uterus, especially when treating nonpregnancy related concerns (eg, whiplash, peripheral joint or muscular injury).[59] Continuous shortwave or microwave diathermy should not be applied to the low back, abdominal, or pelvic regions of the pregnant woman because of the possible thermal effect on the fetus.[59–61] This finding has only been documented in pregnant laboratory animals, and for obvious reasons, the approach has not been tested on pregnant women.

Ice, when properly applied, should be encouraged for muscular and joint pain and inflammation during pregnancy. Electrical stimulation is contraindicated during pregnancy, except for the use of transcutaneous electrical stimulation (TENS) during labor and delivery. Manual therapy and muscle energy techniques should be used with caution because of soft tissue laxity. Heavy traction techniques and vigorous manipulations with pregnant patients should be avoided.[31]

THERAPEUTIC EXERCISE INTERVENTION FOR COMMON MUSCULOSKELETAL IMPAIRMENTS

Focusing on the balance of muscle length and strength in key postural muscles in pregnant and postpartum women is extremely important. These muscles are most affected by the biomechanical changes of pregnancy. Stretch weakness arising from the typical kyphotic-lordotic posture can be prevented by addressing the posterior neck muscles, the middle and lower trapezius muscles, the lower abdominals, hip extensors, and the pelvic floor. Adaptive shortening is common in the anterior shoulder muscles, lumbar paraspinals, and hip flexors. Appropriate active and passive stretches should be prescribed for these areas. Lumbar, sacroiliac, and pubic symphysis problems may be greatly relieved by lumbopelvic stabilization exercises and by the use of external supports during pregnancy.

Normal Antepartum Women

For the pregnant woman, postural awareness is vital when considering accommodations resulting from the shift in the center of gravity, weight gain, and possible joint hypermobility. Frequent attention to cervical retraction (ie, chin tucks), scapular adduction and upward rotation (ie, forward arm lift against a wall), abdominal facilitation (ie, posterior pelvic tilts), and patellofemoral function (ie, small knee bends to decrease knee hyperextension and associated femoral internal rotation) are effective in reducing stretch weakness and adaptive shortening (Fig. 13-1). Postural faults may be perpetuated into the postpartum period, especially when caring for the new infant. Proper body mechanics and joint protection should be stressed to decrease abnormal forces on joints that are at increased risk of injury because of hormonally induced laxity.

Sample musculoskeletal evaluations that incorporate adaptations for manual muscle testing and limit the number of body position changes for the pregnant client can be found in *Obstetric and Gynecologic Care in Physical Therapy*[30] and *Clinics in Physical Therapy: Obstetric and Gynecologic Physical Therapy*.[31]

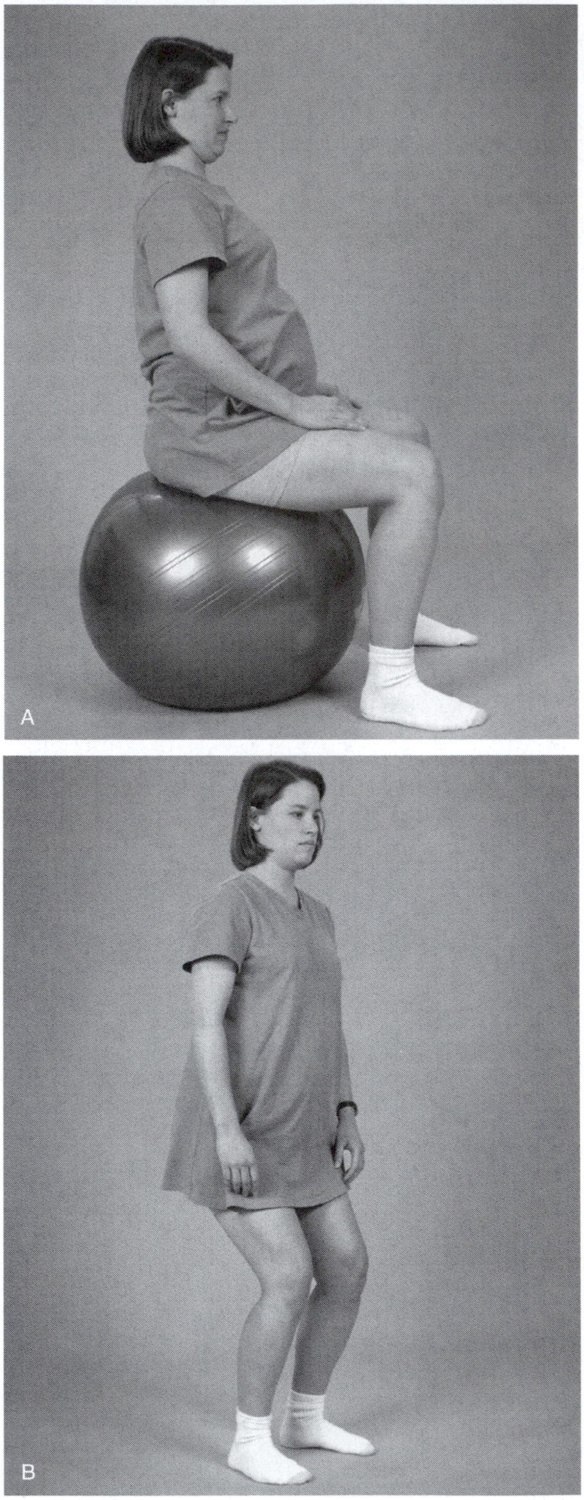

FIGURE 13-1 The pregnant women is performing ***(A)*** chin tucks and ***(B)*** small knee bends to minimize stretch weakness and adaptive shortening.

ABDOMINAL IMPAIRMENT

Goals for performing abdominal exercises during pregnancy include improvement of muscle balance and posture, support of the growing uterus, stabilization of the trunk, and maintenance of function for more rapid recovery after delivery. Most pregnant women can perform supine position abdominal exercises with frequent position changes. Exercises such as bent knee fallouts and progressive leg slides are appropriate as long as the neutral spine position is maintained (see Chapter 18). Posterior pelvic tilts can be performed in a variety of positions, including supine, to reduce low back pain from an excessive lordosis while actively stretching the low back extensors and strengthening the abdominals. Bilateral straight-leg raising and leg-lowering exercises should be avoided during pregnancy because of the vulnerability of the vertebral joints and excessive pull on an overstretched abdomen. When the women has SHS, the supine position should be avoided, and the use of sidelying, sitting, standing, and quadruped positions can be creatively used to train the patient in abdominal facilitation and neutral spine. The quadruped position is excellent for performing concentric and eccentric contractions of the abdominal muscles (see Self-Management: Quadruped Abdominal Exercise).

SELF-MANAGEMENT: Quadruped Abdominal Exercise

Purpose: To train the patient in abdominal facilitation when backlying is uncomfortable or not possible (eg, supine hypotensive syndrome)

Position: On hands and knees

Movement technique:
1. Concentric contraction
   a. Inhale, allowing the abdomen to expand.
   b. While exhaling slowly, pull tummy in and push lower back up. Tuck chin down.
2. Eccentric contraction
   a. Slowly relax your tummy, and return to the starting position

Repeat _______ times

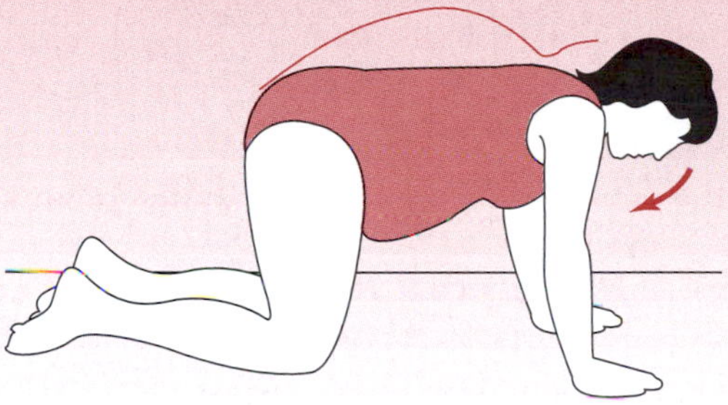

Diastasis Recti

Modifications to exercise for abdominal muscles are necessary for a women with diastasis recti.[62–64] In standing, the abdominal wall supports the uterus and maintains its longitudinal axis in relation to the axis of the pelvis.[2] The muscles of the abdomen that must lengthen to accommodate the enlarging uterus and growing fetus in pregnancy are the external and internal obliques, transversus abdominis, and rectus abdominis. The linea alba is formed by the crossing fibers of the aponeuroses of these muscles, making a tendinous seam from the sternum to the symphysis pubis. Hormonal changes and the increasing mechanical stress placed on these structures during pregnancy may result in a painless separation of the linea alba.[31] The rectus muscles separate in the midline, creating a diastasis recti.

The rectus muscles are normally about 2 cm apart above the umbilicus and are in contact with each other below the umbilicus. A separation greater than this is considered to be a diastasis recti.[31,62–64] If severe, the anterior uterine wall may be covered by only skin, fascia, and peritoneum. If extreme, the gravid uterus drops below the level of the pelvic inlet when the woman stands. The pelvic inlet is bound posteriorly by the body of the first sacral vertebra (promontory), laterally by the linea terminalis, and anteriorly by the horizontal rami of the pubic bones and symphysis pubis.[2] Descent of the fetal head below this point is called *engagement* and occurs normally during the last few weeks of pregnancy or during labor. Upright exercise should be restricted if engagement occurs at any other time during the pregnancy.[2]

The presence of a diastasis recti potentially reduces the ability of the abdominal wall muscles to contribute to their role in trunk motion, trunk stability, pelvic alignment, support of pelvic viscera, and by way of increasing intra-abdominal pressure, forced expiration, defecation, urination, vomiting, and the second stage of labor (ie, pushing).[31] Weak abdominals, with or without a diastasis, contribute to excessive lordosis and the characteristic "waddle" gait of pregnancy. Checking for a diastasis recti should be done beginning in the second trimester and continuing throughout the rest of the pregnancy and into the postpartum phase. To evaluate the abdominal wall for a diastasis, the pregnant woman should lie in the supine hooklying position. With chin tucked and arms extended to the knees, she should raise her head and shoulders until the scapulae clear the surface. The therapist checks for a central bulge in the abdomen and, with fingers placed cephalocaudally, measures the amount of separation between the rectus muscles 2 inches above, 2 inches below, and at the level of the umbilicus.[31,63] Each finger represents approximately 1 cm (Fig. 13-2).

A diastasis correction exercise can be performed to maintain alignment and discourage further separation. This is performed with the woman in the supine hooklying if she tolerates backlying (ie, exclude SHS). With arms crisscrossed over the abdomen, the patient manually approximates the recti muscles toward midline, performs a posterior pelvic tilt, and slowly exhales while lifting her head. The scapulae should clear the surface[64] (see Self-Management: Correction of Diastasis Recti). Exhalation prevents an increase in intra-abdominal pressure.[31] The additional support of a large sheet folded lengthwise under the patient's back may be helpful as pregnancy progresses. The two ends of the sheet are brought up and crisscrossed over the abdomen to simulate support of the abdominal wall. The patient can grip each end of the sheet and pull outward to support the recti muscles toward the midline (see modification in Self-Management: Correction of Diastasis Recti). If diastasis is detected, patients are usually encouraged to avoid unsupported curl-ups, trunk rotation exercises, and sitting straight up from a supine position (ie, jackknifing), because these activities may encourage further separation.

As an adjunct to therapeutic exercise, an external support in the form of an abdominal binder, lumbopelvic support, or sacroiliac belt can assist the patient in achieving improved body mechanics and postural alignment. When a diastasis is present, the external support helps to re-establish and maintain normal alignment of the abdominal wall and support the gravid uterus to prevent further stretch weakness. These supports are worn during upright exercises and ADLs.

PELVIC FLOOR IMPAIRMENTS

The pelvic floor muscle may undergo stretch weakness from the long-standing pressure of the growing uterus. Hormonally softened tissue further complicates the increased load

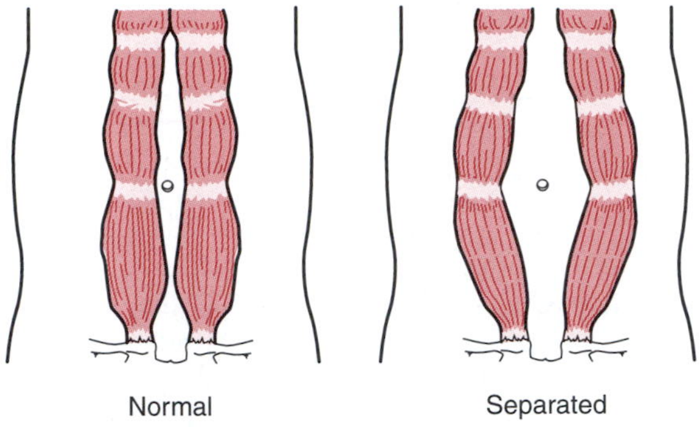

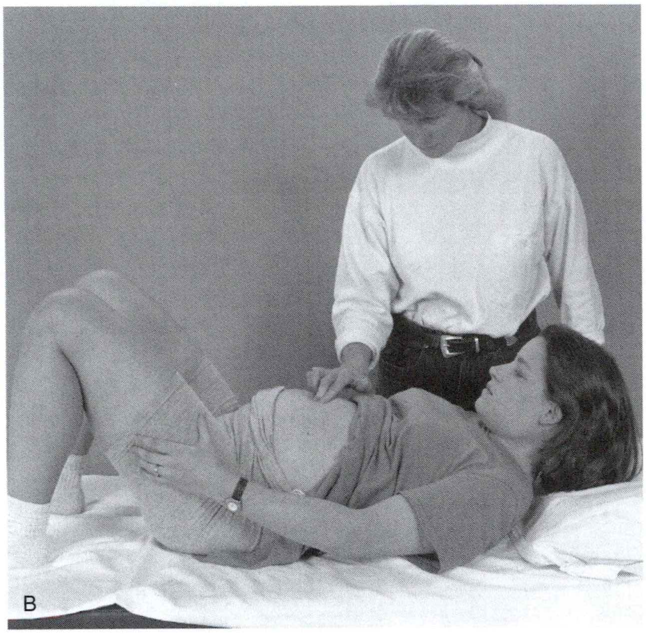

FIGURE 13-2 ***(A)*** Comparison of a normal abdomen with a diastasis recti abdominis. ***(B)*** The therapist checks for a central bulge in the abdomen and measures the amount of separation between the rectus muscles.

SELF-MANAGEMENT: Correction of Diastasis Recti

Purpose: To correct a diastasis recti and improve the length-tension relationship of abdominals (rectus abdominis)

Position: Backlying with knees bent and feet flat. Cross hands over the midline.

Movement technique:
1. Inhale.
2. As you exhale, rock your pelvis back, flattening your lower back.
3. Tuck your chin, and slowly raise your head off the surface while pulling the belly muscle toward the midline.
4. Slowly lower the head and relax.

Repeat _______ times

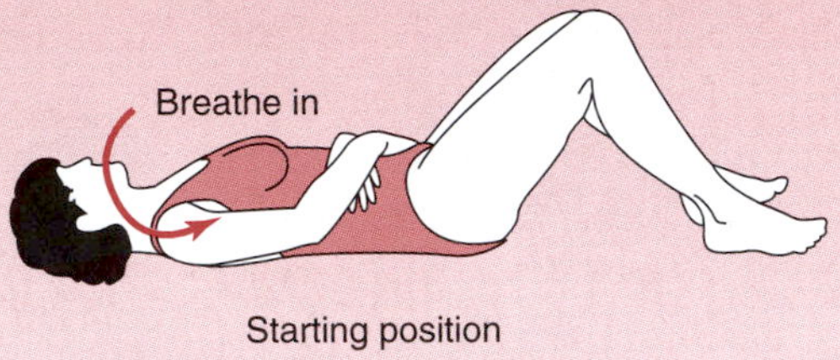

Starting position

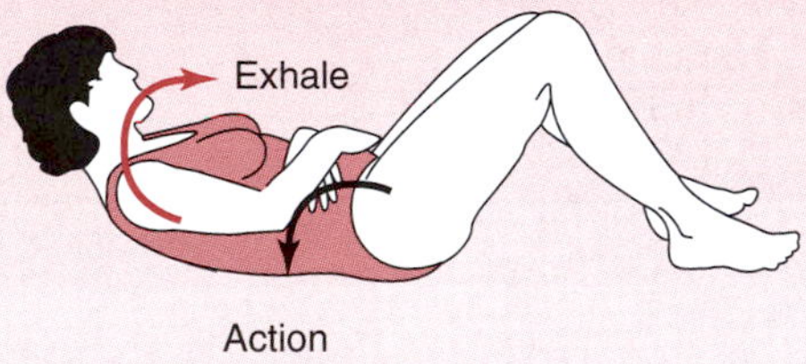

Action

Modification: Fold sheet lengthwise under your low back. Cross sheet over the midline, holding the opposite ends in each hand. As you tuck your chin and slowly raise your head, pull outward on the ends of the sheet. As you lower your head and relax, release your grip on the sheet.

on the pelvic floor. A vaginal birth or a lengthy and unproductive second stage of labor (ie, pushing phase) before cesarean section poses its problems for a vulnerable pelvic floor. There is the potential for direct trauma to the muscles with an episiotomy (ie, incision in the pelvic floor made during childbirth to enlarge the vaginal opening and allow faster delivery), tears, or lacerations. Pudendal or obturator nerve stretch injuries may occur.

The importance of pelvic floor muscle strength cannot be overemphasized, because these muscles affect bladder, bowel, and sexual function and are supportive and sphincteric in nature. They play a role in supporting the internal organs (eg, rectum, vagina, uterus) by preventing downward displacement (ie, prolapse or pelvic relaxation). Pregnancy and postpartum pelvic floor dysfunction may manifest as pelvic organ prolapse; urinary or fecal incontinence; pelvic pain from muscle spasm, painful episiotomy, or tears; or joint malalignment (ie, sacrococcygeal involvement). A strong, coordinated pelvic floor may demonstrate improved control and relaxation during the second stage of delivery and in the postpartum recovery. Attention to the pelvic floor muscles should occur early in the pregnancy and should continue throughout the duration of the pregnancy and postpartum phase for vaginal and cesarean section births[31,64] (see Chapter 19).

If there is coccyx pain and an associated pelvic floor tension myalgia, pelvic floor relaxation or "inversed command" must be emphasized.[65] The patient is instructed to place her hand over the anal cleft, placing the middle finger in the cleft and the other fingers on the buttocks. As she pretends to "pass gas" gently without straining or bearing down, she should feel the anal cleft bulge out against the middle finger.[66] This is pelvic floor relaxation, and the exercise should be practiced several times each day to recall the sensation.

The use of a donut cushion or sitting with layers of towels under the thighs may be useful in keeping pressure off the coccyx.[31,66]

If focal irritability is experienced over the sacrococcygeal joint, direct mobilization of this articulation may be performed to reduce pain.[67] This technique also is appropriate for a subluxed coccyx after childbirth.[30] Dysfunction of L5-S1 segment may refer symptoms to the sacrococcygeal joint.

LOW BACK AND PELVIS PAIN

Approximately 50% of women experience low back pain with pregnancy.[4,6,29] It may occur at any time throughout the pregnancy but most commonly occurs between the fourth and seventh months.[29] Back pain can have many causes:

- Biomechanical strain from weight gain, increased spinal loading, and pressure from the uterus or fetus
- Postural changes, such as an increased lumbar lordosis creating increased stress on the facet joints, posterior ligaments, and intervertebral disks
- Postural changes that aggravate pre-existing spondylolisthesis, degenerative facet joint disease, and lateral stenosis
- Ligamentous laxity affecting the sacroiliac joints, pubic symphysis, and sacrococcygeal joint
- Weakening of the abdominal and pelvic floor muscles

Patients may need to be advised to adjust their exercise habits as the pregnancy progresses. Low back pain and other pregnancy-related discomforts may be minimized by reducing the duration and intensity levels of exercises.[6,49]

Postural Changes

Excessive lumbar lordosis may result from the pregnancy, or pregnancy may aggravate a preexisting lordosis problem. Ideal postural alignment, as defined by Kendall,[68] involves a minimal amount of stress and strain and is conducive to maximal efficiency of the body (see Chapter 8). In a lateral view, normal curves of the spine consist of a slight anterior convexity in the cervical region, slight posterior convexity in the thoracic region, and slight anterior convexity in the lumbar region. The pelvis is in a *neutral position,* meaning that the bony prominence at the front of the pelvis (ie, the anterior superior iliac spines and the pubic symphysis) are in the same vertical plane.[68]

During pregnancy, the center of gravity shifts anteriorly with a resulting anterior rotation of the ilium. This accentuates and increases the normal anterior curve of the lumbar region, creating an excessive lordosis (Fig. 13-3) (see Patient-Related Instruction: Postural Correction). Muscle weakness due to stretch in the abdominal muscles and the hip extensor muscles results in poor control of the pelvis (in this case, an anteriorly tilted pelvis).

Frequent posterior pelvic tilting in various positions enhances muscular control and strength and the postural awareness required throughout the day to relieve pain and fatigue in the low back. Caution should be exerted when performing hip extension in the quadruped position. The lower extremity should be raised carefully and within physiologic range to avoid hyperextension in the lumbar spine.

An increased lordosis at the thoracolumbar junction may cause mechanical stress on the muscles and ligaments, producing foraminal narrowing. The result may be radicular irritation manifesting as pain along the course of the iliohypogastric and ilioinguinal nerves anteriorly and posteriorly—a common referral source of pain for prepartum and postpartum women.[31] Radicular symptoms may also be experienced in the upper extremities, chest, and neck because of a compensatory thoracic kyphosis and increased cervical lordosis. Changes in the transverse diameter of the chest may mechanically aggravate pre-existing costovertebral or thoracic joint dysfunction.

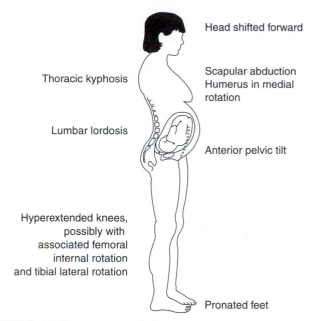

FIGURE 13-3 Incorrect posture during pregnancy.

Forward arm lifts while standing against the wall (see Chapter 26) facilitate muscle balance and postural awareness and lift the rib cage off the uterus. This exercise also supports the thoracic curve and helps to prevent thoracic kyphosis, which may develop during pregnancy and the postpartum period. Performing this exercise frequently throughout the day can reduce postural pain and discomfort. Another useful exercise to improve posture during pregnancy is a wall abdominal isometric (Fig. 13-4). This exercise helps to maintain tone in the abdominal region and normal length of hip flexors, both of which support the lumbar curve and pelvic position. Frequent changes of position, proper posture, and body mechanics during daily activities at home and at work apply to the pregnant woman and the nonpregnant woman (see Chapter 18).

Sacroiliac Pain

Pain in the sacroiliac joints may occur very early in pregnancy, possibly because of circulating hormones. Although the lumbar spine and the hip may refer pain into the sacroiliac region, a variety of alterations in the sacroiliac joint configuration and movement may produce impairment and functional limitations. Manual therapy techniques may be used to reduce asymmetry and abnormal motion. Muscle imbalances in the major muscles influencing ileal rotation (ie, iliopsoas, quadriceps, and hamstring muscle groups) must be addressed. Stretching techniques must be performed

Patient-Related Instruction

Postural Correction

To correct posture during pregnancy, follow the steps below. Perform these steps simultaneously as often as you can—at least six times per day. Try them during different daily activities such as brushing your teeth, washing the dishes, or standing in line. Maintain them while performing exercises in the standing position.

1. Elongate the neck by drawing the chin back and keeping eyes level.
2. Lift your breastbone, ribs, and head without arching your lower back, as though you are trying to be taller. Breathe normally; do not hold your breath.
3. Pull your lower abdominal muscles in by pulling your belly button toward your spine. The pelvis should be in neutral position.
4. Unlock your knees, squeeze your buttock muscles to separate your knees, and turn your thighs slightly outward so that the kneecaps face the middle of your feet.
5. Pull "up and in" with the pelvic floor muscles.
6. Shift your weight slightly so half of your weight is on your heels and half is on the balls of your feet. Slightly lift the arches of your feet without rolling out on the sides of your feet.

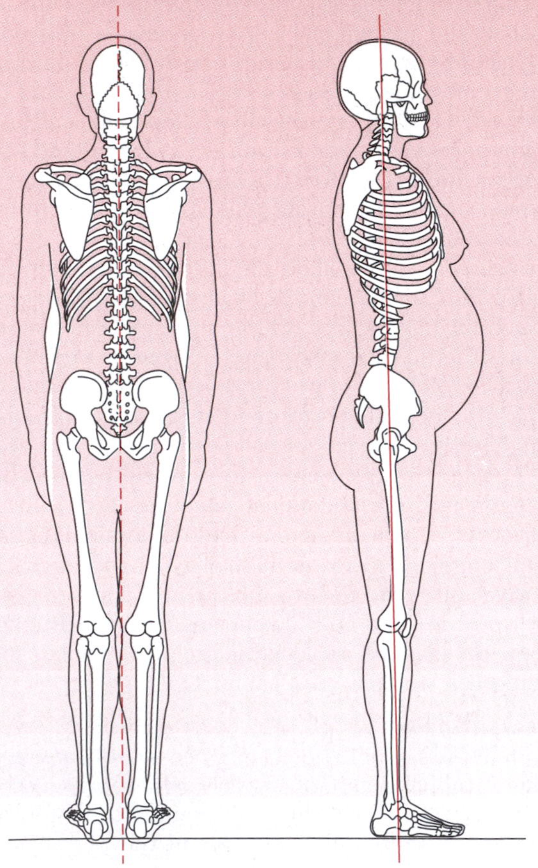

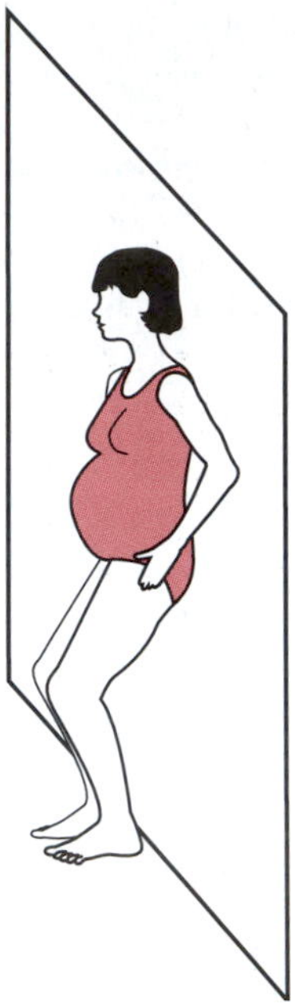

FIGURE 13-4 Wall abdominal isometrics. Standing with feet about 3 inches from the wall, bend hips and knees to put hip flexors on slack. Pull belly button in toward the spine. Slowly straighten hips and knees while keeping low back in neutral (not flat back) position. Stop when low back moves into extension.

gently and cautiously because of possible joint instability. Hip abduction in any position should be performed cautiously to avoid compressing the sacroiliac joint. Equal weight bearing through both lower extremities is encouraged in standing exercises instead of single lower extremity weight bearing to avoid aggravating the sacroiliac joints.

Pubic Symphysis Pain

The pubic symphysis is the only bony junction in what Noble calls the "vulnerable midline."[64] This area includes the abdominal and pelvic floor muscles that are connected in midline by a tendinous seam. There is marked widening of the pubic symphysis by 28 to 32 weeks of gestation, from approximately 4 to 7 mm.[1] This widening facilitates vaginal delivery but can lead to pelvic discomfort and gait unsteadiness in late pregnancy. Wide leg motions or reciprocal movement of the lower extremities such as stair climbing or turning in bed may cause pain in a lax pubic symphysis. If such pain occurs, leg exercises may need to be eliminated until the joint is stabilized by manual therapy techniques. Vigorous stretching of the hip adductor muscles should be avoided, because this exercise may result in pubic symphysis separation.[69] An external support or belt may be appropriately applied to enhance stabilization of this region.

Round Ligaments

The round ligaments are two rounded cords that run from the superior angle of the uterus on either side to the labia majora. During pregnancy, these ligaments must stretch with the growing uterus and may intermittently spasm, causing sharp pain in the groin. This is especially true with sudden position changes. Gentle side stretching in tailor or regular sitting positions with arms overhead may relieve this discomfort (Fig. 13-5). This stretch may also help relieve heartburn and the feeling of shortness of breath as it lifts the rib cage upward and away from the pelvis.

NERVE COMPRESSION SYNDROMES

Nerve compression syndromes may arise during pregnancy because of fluid retention, edema, soft tissue laxity, and exaggerated postural changes.

Intercostal Neuralgia

Intercostal neuralgia is the term used to describe unilateral, intermittent pain in the rib cage or chest from flaring of the rib cage. Exercises to relieve this discomfort include spinal elongation with arms overhead in supine, sitting, or standing positions and trunk side bending away from the pain.

Thoracic Outlet Syndrome

If muscle support is inadequate, spinal curves may become more pronounced as the center of gravity changes and the woman gains weight, especially in the breasts. The forward head and shoulder posture may lead to thoracic outlet syndrome, with compromise of the brachial plexus and subclavian vessels. Strengthening of the upper back and scapular muscles and lengthening of the pectorals may assist in relieving symptoms. Support for the upper back and breasts in the form of a good brassiere and manufactured supports may be appropriate to decrease the load.[68] This is especially important after delivery for the nursing mother.

A variant of thoracic outlet syndrome called *acroparesthesia* occurs when the neurovascular bundle becomes stretched over the first rib, which may be elevated in pregnancy. The woman may complain of pain, numbness, and tingling in the hand and forearm.[31]

Carpal Tunnel Syndrome

Carpal tunnel syndrome of pregnancy usually disappears after delivery but may persist or develop in the postpartum phase if the woman is breast-feeding. It is addressed much the same as in the nonpregnant client, with a decrease in hand and wrist flexion activities, night use of resting splints, and exercises to keep fingers mobile and improve movement of fluids. Unlike patients with cumulative trauma-type carpal tunnel syndrome, pregnant and breast-feeding clients typically have bilateral symptoms.

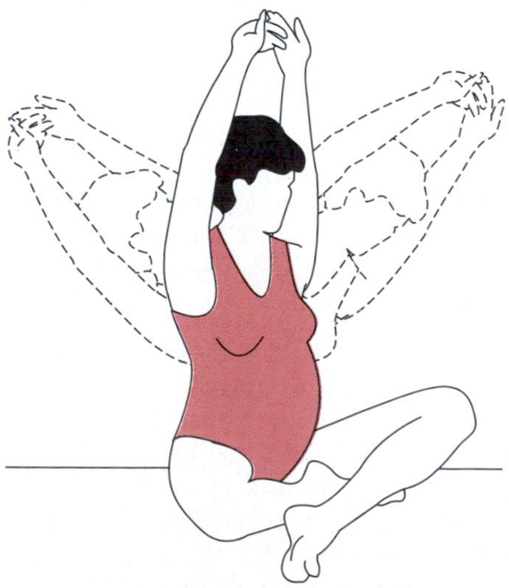

FIGURE 13-5 Gentle side stretching in tailor sitting.

Lateral Femoral Cutaneous Nerve Entrapment

Lateral femoral cutaneous nerve entrapment (ie, meralgia paresthetica) occurs in pregnancy when the nerve is compressed as it emerges from the pelvis at the inguinal ligament adjacent to the anterior superior iliac spine or where branches enter the tensor fascia lata. Adequate length is needed in the tensor fascia lata, iliopsoas, and rectus femoris muscles. Exercises to balance the hip muscles may be appropriate (see Chapter 20). Lying on the unaffected side draws the uterus away from the compressed area. Soft tissue techniques may be helpful.

Tarsal Tunnel Syndrome

Tarsal tunnel syndrome (ie, posterior tibial nerve compression) occurs with edema in the tarsal tunnel just posterior to the medial malleolus. Compression of the posterior tibial nerve produces numbness and tingling in the medial aspect of the foot and possibly weakness of the flexor muscles of the toes.[6] Elevation and active foot and ankle exercises help to decrease edema and relieve compression. A posterior splint may be used to immobilize the ankle at night.

Peroneal Nerve Compression

The peroneal nerves wrap around the neck of the fibula and supply the muscles that dorsiflex the ankle. Prolonged squatting may compress these nerves and cause foot drop.[6] Pregnant women should be discouraged from prolonged squatting during exercise and during delivery.

OTHER IMPAIRMENTS

Other impairments that may result from pregnancy include temporomandibular joint (TMJ) dysfunction, patellofemoral dysfunction, joint discomfort or dysfunction, and varicosis. Exercise interventions are presented in other chapters for some of these impairments, but guidelines for pregnancy should be carefully followed.

Temporomandibular Joint Dysfunction

TMJ dysfunction may be related to pregnancy. TMJ dysfunction is caused by hypermobility resulting from increased laxity or may appear after delivery because of excessive tension in the face during the "pushing" phase of delivery[30] (see Chapter 23).

Patellofemoral Dysfunction

Patellofemoral dysfunction and pain may occur from the added stress of weight gain and fluid retention, especially with preexisting muscle weakness. Knee hyperextension and foot pronation are common in pregnancy, possibly because of the change in the center of gravity. This results in additional stress on the knees. Kinematic studies show that patellofemoral force increases by 83% in a pregnant woman rising from a chair without the use of her upper extremities.[6] Enlargement of the uterus causes a reduction in hip flexion and repositions the center of mass farther from the axis of rotation. Greater muscular effort is therefore required.

This muscular effort is reduced if the pregnant woman uses her arms to rise from a chair or avoids low seating (see Chapter 21).

Joint Discomfort or Dysfunction

Weight gain in pregnancy increases stress in weight-bearing joints, causing discomfort in normal joints or potentially increasing dysfunction in joints with pre-existing arthritis or instability. Stair climbing produces forces of three to five times the body weight in the hip and knee joints. In a woman who increases her weight by 20% in pregnancy, forces on her weight-bearing joints may increase by 100%[31] (see Chapters 20 and 21).

Varicosis

Venous pressure in the lower body increases with advancing pregnancy. Venous distention and stasis contribute to varicosities of the lower extremities and vulvar region.[4] Frequent foot and ankle exercises help to alleviate edema and muscle cramps, especially if the patient is sedentary or sits on the job. They also help reduce the likelihood of lower extremity deep venous thrombosis (DVT). Patients should be advised to elevate the lower extremities higher than the heart to assist venous circulation (Fig. 13-6). The quadruped position reduces stress on the lower extremity vascular structures, and sidelying positions decrease compression of the inferior vena cava. Because long periods of static standing increase compressive forces of the weight of the fetus on the vascular system, the patient should sit instead of stand when she has the option. Immersion in water has been shown to mobilize extravascular fluid and reduce edema.[70] Compression stockings should be considered.

High-Risk Antepartum Patients

When the outcome of pregnancy is adversely affected by maternal or fetal factors, the pregnancy is identified as high risk.[71,72] Bed rest is used in nearly 20% of all pregnancies to treat a wide variety of conditions. Bed rest may be prescribed when a pregnancy becomes complicated at conception when pre-existing maternal disease such as heart disease is present or as the pregnancy advances. It is estimated that approximately one of four complicated pregnancies leads to the birth of a premature baby.[73]

The detrimental effects of inactivity in the form of bed rest vary according to the duration of bed rest, the patient's prior state of health and conditioning, and activity performed during bed rest. Much has been written about the effects of bed rest, many of which occur within the first 3 days. These effects include decreased work capacity, orthostatic hypotension, increased urine calcium (possibly leading to bone loss), and increased risk of DVT. The theoretical basis for bed rest during a high-risk pregnancy is to promote uterine and placental blood flow and to reduce gravitational forces that may stimulate cervical effacement (ie, obliteration of the cervix in labor, when only the thin external os remains) and dilation.[74–77] The left lateral recumbent or Trendelenburg position may be recommended. Bathroom privileges may be restricted. Typically, these patients report musculoskeletal, cardiovascular, and psychosocial complaints.

Even modest activity can reduce detrimental effects of bed rest.[71,72] Therapeutic exercises for this patient population focus on several features:

- Improvement of circulation
- Promotion of relaxation
- Avoidance of increased intra-abdominal pressure by minimizing abdominal contractions during exercise, basic ADLs, bed mobility, transfers, and self-care
- Avoidance of Valsalva maneuvers
- Prevention of decreased muscle tone and deconditioning effects
- Prevention of musculoskeletal discomfort

Activity guidelines for the high-risk antepartum patient are outlined in Display 13-6. Contraindications include increased bleeding, contractions, blood pressure, or leakage of amniotic fluid; exacerbation of the condition (depends on the diagnosis); unstable conditions; and extreme cases when the patient should not move more than needed for basic care.

CIRCULATION EXERCISES

Supine or sidelying circulation exercises should be done every waking hour. If allowed, these exercises may be performed while sitting at the edge of the bed. This reduces the likelihood of lower extremity DVT. Ankle pumps and circles improve circulation by facilitating a pumping action in the muscles of the lower extremities. Gentle lower extremity isometrics may also help. However, the therapist must be extremely careful that the patient avoids increasing intra-abdominal pressure or blood pressure. Examples of lower extremity isometrics include quadriceps, gluteal, and adductor muscle exercises. Unilateral heel slides may be performed if abdominal contractions are avoided.

RELAXATION EXERCISES

There are several ways of instructing relaxation exercises.[29,30,64] Two methods of relaxation require conscious recognition and release of muscle tension. The Mitchell method involves contraction of the opposing muscle groups to release stress-induced tension in muscles.[78] The Jacobson method, also known as progressive relaxation, involves alternately contracting and relaxing muscle groups progressively throughout the body.[79]

Visualization techniques or meditation may be helpful as a way to withdraw from the stress-producing situation tem-

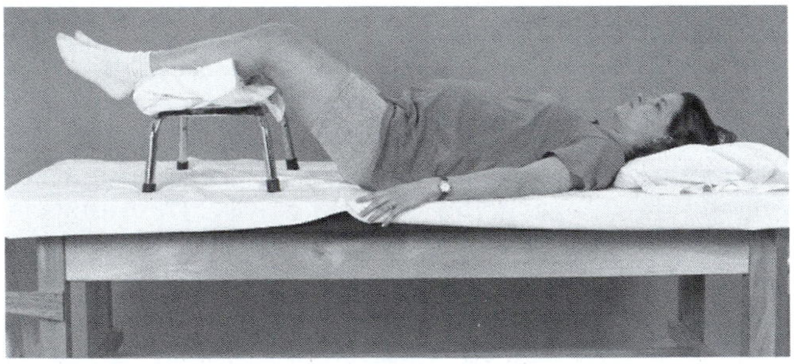

FIGURE 13-6 Elevation of feet to reduce varicosis. *Note:* The feet are higher than the heart to assist venous circulation.

DISPLAY 13-6

Activity Guidelines for the High-Risk Antepartum Patient

1. Obtain approval from the health care provider before any exercise.
2. Tell the patient not to lift legs against gravity (including kicking off covers). Lower extremity movement may increase symptoms (eg, increased bleeding, contractions, blood pressure, leakage of amniotic fluid). If symptoms increase, lower extremity exercises should be deferred first. Active assisted or passive range of motion exercises for the lower extremities may be appropriate.
3. Do not perform resisted lower extremity exercise.
4. Do unilateral exercises, except for ankles and wrists, to avoid stabilization by abdominals.
5. Progress the number of exercises and repetitions gradually.
6. Do not overdo. Exercises may become more difficult as pregnancy progresses and fatigue increases or when medicated with tocolytics medications used to stop or control preterm labor. You may need to modify exercises if tocolytics increase fatigue or give the patient the "jitters." Timing exercise further from dosage time is helpful.
7. *Avoidance of abdominal contractions* during exercise is necessary to help eliminate expulsion forces and uterine irritability, especially with preterm labor.
8. Avoid Valsalva maneuvers. Valsalva maneuvers are bearing-down efforts accompanied by holding the breath without exhalation (closed glottis). This increases the intraabdominal pressure and pressure on the uterus. Valsalva maneuvers may be performed by a patient with abnormal respiratory rate and rhythm and may or may not include an abdominal contraction. A Valsalva maneuver must be avoided during bed mobility, transfers, exercises, or bowel movements to avoid irritating the uterus. The therapist instructs the patient to exhale on any effort.
9. Comfort measures include body mechanics and positioning in bed to support the spine and abdomen in proper alignment. In sidelying, pillows between the legs, under the abdomen, and behind the back and shoulders may be helpful. Frequent changes of position should be encouraged.
10. If symptoms increase with bed rest exercises, stop and report to the physician.

porarily. Diaphragmatic breathing and body awareness during exercises or ADLs also improve relaxation.[64]

Biofeedback and stretching are more active forms of relaxation. The patient is required to be mentally attentive to purposefully reduce a state of tension and recognize a state of relaxation.

GENERAL STRENGTHENING AND TONING EXERCISES

General strengthening and toning exercises help prevent or reduce decreased muscle tone and the deconditioning effects of bed rest. Frequent position changes in bed should be encouraged to avoid SHS and prevent musculoskeletal discomfort. Discomfort may be experienced because of static positioning, joint stiffness, and decreased circulation. These strengthening and toning exercises can be done in the supine position:

- Neck rotation and side bending
- Gentle isometric neck extension into a pillow
- Shoulder presses down and back into a pillow
- Unilateral heel slides, hip internal rotation and external rotation, hip abduction and adduction, and terminal knee extension off a pillow
- Graded pelvic floor contractions if performed correctly (without abdominals or breath holding)

These strengthening and toning exercises can be done in the sidelying position:

- Unilateral shoulder circles (downward and backward), arm circles, hand and wrist active range of motion, knee extension with hip flexed, partial knee to chest, hip external rotation
- Unilateral resistive band (or light weights) for upper extremities only: biceps curl, triceps press, shoulder press, diagonal lift, shoulder extension, and horizontal abduction and adduction (avoid proprioceptive neuromuscular facilitation pattern D_2 upper extremity extension with or without resistive band because it facilitates the abdominals)
- Graded pelvic floor contractions

The support of a spouse, family, and friends can greatly reduce the anxiety and stress the high-risk antepartum patient may experience. Bed rest places the patient in the difficult position of limiting simple ADLs and limiting her roles as mother (if she has other children), spouse, and provider (unless she can work from her bed). The physiologic effects of stress can take its toll, and the patient and caregivers must understand the rationale for bed rest and importance of therapeutic exercise to enhance fetal and maternal outcomes. Most patients are home for this bed rest, although some women are hospitalized. A home visit to teach the patient and family proper exercise performance may be appropriate (see Self-Management: Sidelying Exercises for the Patient on Bed Rest and Patient-Related Instruction: Bed Mobility).

One study reported noncompliance of 33.8% for bed rest in the high-risk antepartum women they studied.[80] Reasons for noncompliance included not feeling ill, child care responsibilities, household demands, lack of support, having to work, and discomfort while on bed rest. Pregnancy outcomes were similar for women who did and did not adhere to bed rest recommendations. Further research is needed to address the validity of the practice of bed rest as treatment for high-risk pregnancies.[80–84]

Because many high-risk pregnancies end in cesarean section deliveries, it may be an appropriate time to prepare the patient for cesarean recovery and rehabilitation.

Postpartum Women

When a woman has maintained good physical condition during pregnancy, her postpartum fitness is improved. If labor and delivery are uncomplicated, exercise can usually

SELF-MANAGEMENT: Sidelying Exercises for the Patient on Bed Rest

Purpose: To maintain strength of the lower extremities while on bed rest restrictions

Position: Sidelying. Place a pillow below your head and between your knees.

Movement technique:

1. Knee extension with hip flexed. Begin with the hip partially flexed. Bend and straighten the knee as shown in Figure *A*.
2. Knee extension with hip extended. Begin with the hip in a straight position. Bend and straighten the knee as shown in Figure *B*.
3. Knee-to-chest exercise. Slowly draw knee up to the chest and then slide it back down as shown in Figure *C*.

Precaution: Stop exercising if contractions or pain are experienced.

Repeat _______ times

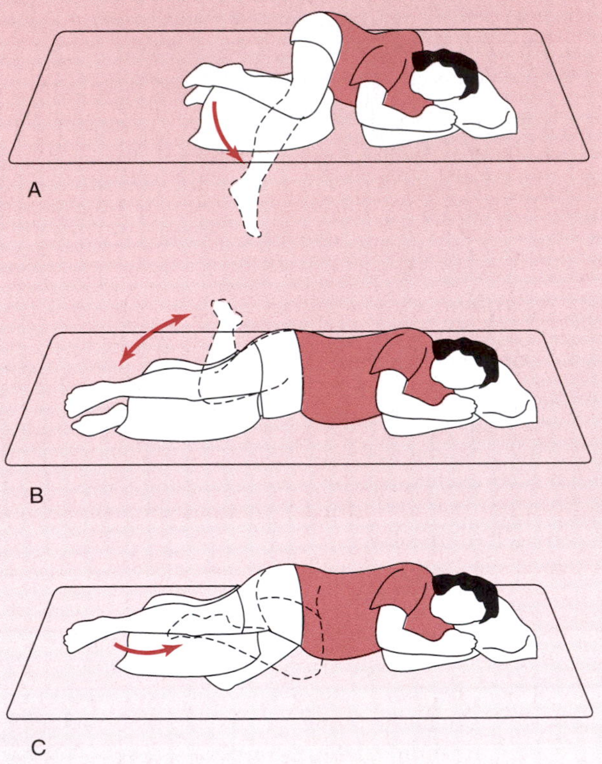

(A) Knee extension with hip flexed. ***(B)*** Knee extension with hip extended. ***(C)*** Knee to chest.

Patient-Related Instruction

Bed Mobility

For moving from side to side:

1. Keep your head on the pillow.
2. Roll like a log.

For moving from lying to sitting using the "bedrest pushup".

1. Roll to one side.
2. Keeping your back straight, use your arms to push up to sitting while you swing your legs over the edge of the bed.
3. Reverse to lie back down.

Be sure to breath and keep your stomach muscles relaxed. This helps avoid Valsalva maneuvers. Never jackknife to sit.

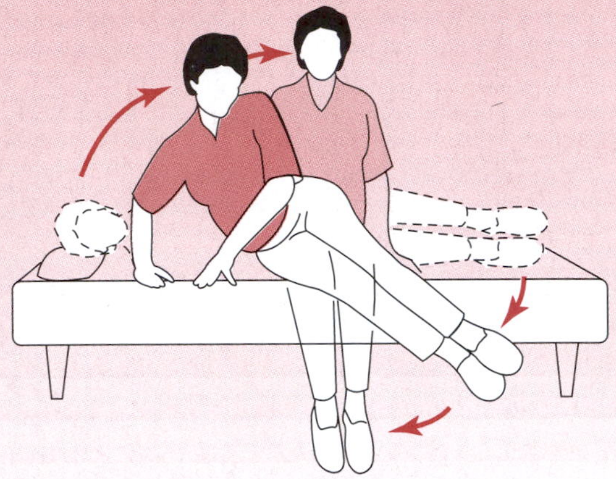

Bed-rest pushup

be resumed before the 6-week checkup.[31] Return to exercise should be gradual and based on her comfort level. Postpartum exercise guidelines are listed in Display 13-7.

Postpartum exercise is vital for restoration of normal muscle function. Pelvic floor and abdominal contractions could be started within the first 24 hours after delivery to restore tone.

Although pregnancy itself may be a factor in the development of lumbar disk disease, second-stage labor may markedly increase intradiskal pressure.[31] A disk protrusion may develop, or a preexisting protrusion may be exacerbated. This is treated with posture, body mechanics, exercise, manual therapies, and modalities as in the general population but keeping in mind that hormonal changes persist for several weeks after delivery.

Even if a rectus diastasis was not present during pregnancy, a separation could have developed during the second stage of labor. A diastasis does not always resolve spontaneously after delivery and may persist well into the postpartum phase. It should be evaluated and reduced before aggressive abdominal strengthening begins. However, isometric activation and facilitation of these muscles in various positions is appropriate. Remind the patient that these muscles may not provide adequate support initially for the trunk and low back, which are more vulnerable to injury. In some cases, the temporary use of an abdominal binder is advisable.

Pelvic floor contractions immediately after delivery are essential in restoring muscle tone, reducing edema, facilitating circulation, and relieving pain, especially if an episiotomy has been performed or the perineum was torn. The

DISPLAY 13-7

Postpartum Exercise Guidelines

1. Gradually return to exercise but exercise regularly (3 times/wk). The process of reversal to the prepregnant state is thought to take 6 to 8 weeks (although the anatomic effects of relaxin may persist as long as 12 weeks).
2. Correct anemia before engaging in moderately strenuous activities. Stop exercising if vaginal bleeding increases or bright red blood appears.
3. Avoid moderately strenuous activities if excessive vaginal bleeding occurs or soreness of an episiotomy persists.
4. Avoid exercises that raise the hips and pelvis above the chest, such as bridging, knee-chest positions, and inverted postures, until postpartum bleeding has stopped completely. These positions put the body at risk for a rare but fatal air embolism through the vagina.
5. Avoid ballistic movements, extreme stretching, and heavy weight lifting for 12 weeks or longer if joint laxity persists.
6. Use the same precautions as in pregnancy to prevent musculoskeletal injury, for approximately 12 weeks.
7. Provide good support to the breasts during exercise, especially if nursing. Nursing mothers should feed the infant before exercising to avoid discomfort.
8. Target heart rates and limits should be established in consultation with a physician and may be based on the fitness level during and before pregnancy.

Data from references 6, 31, 40, 64, 85, and 86.

perineum comprises the pelvic floor and associated structures occupying the pelvic outlet; the area is bound anteriorly by the pubic symphysis, laterally by the ischial tuberosities, and posteriorly by the coccyx. The patient should be instructed to contract or "brace" the pelvic floor muscles with coughing, sneezing, or laughing; avoid Valsalva maneuvers when lifting the infant; and initially support the sutured perineum manually during defecation.

If muscle tension in the pelvic floor is increased as a result of pain from an infected or poorly healed episiotomy or tear, the inversed command may be initiated. Modalities in the form of superficial heat, ultrasound, ice, TENS, and perineal massage may help to reduce discomfort.[29]

Pelvic floor strengthening should continue in the postpartum phase and beyond to restore muscle tone and to enhance normal bowel, bladder, and sexual function. The supportive function of the pelvic floor is additionally challenged by lifting and carrying the infant and various pieces of child care equipment (eg, stroller, infant seat, diaper bag) (see Chapter 19).

The patient must accommodate to multiple body changes that occur rapidly. Weight loss and a change in the center of gravity produce postural readjustments. Ligaments and connective tissue may remain under hormonal influence for up to 12 weeks.[6] The key muscles to address with exercise are the same as those conditioned prenatally.

If the mother is breast-feeding, the neck and upper back muscles are affected by the increased weight of the lactating breasts and by the positions assumed by the mother during nursing. Exercises that improve postural awareness and the length-tension properties of the posterior neck muscles and scapular muscles such as the lower and middle trapezius are appropriate (see Chapter 26). Certain exercises may be uncomfortable for a nursing mother to perform because of breast tenderness (eg, prone positioning). Attention should be paid to sitting posture and positioning of the baby during breast-feeding. The breast-feeding mother requires adequate caloric intake, fluids, and plenty of rest to produce milk for lactation.

A transient depression (ie, postpartum depression or postpartum blues) may occur because of physiologic readjustments and endocrine upheaval. New responsibilities as a parent may be overwhelming. These may initially interfere with exercise performance but should level out within a few days to weeks. Support and involvement of the spouse and family members can make a difference in the new mother's desire to exercise after delivery. Group classes for postpartum exercise encourage mothers to exchange experiences and work thorough problems together. Many classes incorporate exercises that include the infant and the mother.

Cesarean Recovery

A cesarean section (ie, C-section) is the surgical delivery of the baby through the wall of the abdomen and the uterus after a horizontal (most preferred in the United States) or vertical incision has been made. The horizontal, or transverse, incision extends from side to side, just above the pubic hairline. This incision is preferred because there is less blood loss, it heals with a stronger scar, and is less likely to result in complications in a subsequent vaginal delivery.[1–4,87] Vertical incisions are sometimes needed because of certain positions of the baby or placenta.

The rate for cesarean births in the United States is approximately 10% to 25%.[87] About 25% to 30% of these are performed because the pregnant woman has had a previous cesarean section.[88] Most women are being encouraged to try a vaginal birth after cesarean (VBAC) delivery. Reasons to consider VBAC are less risk, shorter recovery time, and more involvement in the birth process.[88,89]

The cesarean procedure may be planned for reasons such as placenta previa (ie, placement of the placenta below the fetus and over part or all of the cervix), breech presentation (ie, presentation of the buttocks or feet of the fetus in the birth canal), or maternal illness or for emergent for reasons such as fetal distress (ie, condition of fetal difficulty in utero detected by electronic fetal monitoring and fetal scalp sampling), prolapse of the umbilical cord, or failure to progress in labor. In childbirth classes, all women should be prepared for the possibility of a cesarean section birth. Some health care facilities have group classes before delivery for planned cesarean section patients. This class provides an excellent opportunity to educate and instruct patients in recovery after the procedure. They experience many of the same physical discomforts associated with major abdominal surgery but have the additional responsibility of caring for the newborn.

Exercises may begin within 24 hours after delivery but should be graded and based on the patient's comfort level.[64,90] Breathing exercises are important to keep lungs clear of mucus. Coughing may be painful, and "huffing" (by pulling the abdominals up and in) is recommended while splinting the incision. Pelvic rocking or bridging with a gentle twist from side to side may assist in alleviating discomfort from decreased intestinal motility. Lower extremity exercises help prevent DVT and orthostatic hypotension before early ambulation. Despite the absence of a vaginal delivery, the pelvic floor has undergone dramatic changes during the pregnancy, or there may have been a lengthy and unproductive trial of pushing. Pelvic floor exercises should be continued or initiated immediately. Gentle activity of the abdominal muscles stimulates healing of the incision and facilitates the return of muscle tone.

Progress with abdominal exercises as tone increases and tissues tolerate added stress. Scar mobilization after sutures are removed (usually 3 to 6 days) or as comfort allows further assists proper healing and reduces adhesion formation. Postpartum precautions and exercises apply, but exercise is progressed more slowly. Attention to balanced upright posture is important, because pain and discomfort at the incision may prompt a protective flexed posture. TENS may be helpful in alleviating incisional pain.

EXERCISE CLASSES

Prenatal wellness can be greatly enhanced by prenatal exercise classes. Physical therapists' understanding of the musculoskeletal system make them ideal instructors. An individual approach and the focus on essential muscles affected by pregnancy make these classes different from other community-based classes. Special certification is not required to teach classes, but special continuing education in this area is recommended.

Prenatal exercise classes should address the physiologic changes that occur during pregnancy and the therapeutic exercises that prepare the body for these changes. Compliance with exercise is enhanced when clients understand that musculoskeletal dysfunction and associated discomfort may be prevented. Many women return to these classes after delivery for continued socialization and support.

Key Points

- The many physiological changes that occur during pregnancy affect a woman's ability and motivation to exercise.
- By following precautions, contraindications, and guidelines, a safe therapeutic exercise program may be established for pregnant women.
- Exercise during pregnancy has many benefits and may prevent or assist in the treatment of common impairments.
- Therapeutic exercise during pregnancy focuses on key postural muscles most affected by the biomechanical changes of pregnancy.
- A high-risk pregnancy may require bed rest; however, specific exercises may be performed and are beneficial.
- Therapeutic exercise is beneficial for postpartum recovery, even if a cesarean section has been performed.

Critical Thinking Questions

1. The pregnant woman is positioned in supine for a manual therapy technique. Her face begins to lose color, and she complains of faintness.
   a. Should you continue with the technique but move very gently?
   b. Should you offer the patient a glass of water?
   c. Should you have her lie on her side until the symptoms resolve?
   d. Would you proceed with the technique after the symptoms resolved?
   e. What are some possible position changes you could make other than sidelying that could alleviate symptoms?
   f. Can you treat the patient in positions other than supine?
2. A 32-year-old woman, 6 weeks after delivery of her second child, experienced severe lower quadrant pain while lifting a stroller into the trunk of her car.
   a. List possible causes for her pain.
   b. What specific muscle groups would you assess, and what treatment options would you consider?
3. The pregnant patient is being instructed in an exercise program to improve her posture. She begins to experience contractions.
   a. Should you stop the exercise and send the patient home?
   b. Should you have the patient lie in left lateral recumbent position until the contractions stop? Would you then proceed?
   c. Should you call the patient's doctor immediately?
   d. What is your advice to the patient regarding performance of her exercise program?
4. With a partner, demonstrate evaluation of the abdominals for a diastasis recti and the appropriate corrective exercise. Discuss other treatment options for a diastasis recti and the advice you would give to the postpartum patient with a diastasis recti regarding basic ADLs.
5. Discuss possible reasons for a pregnancy becoming high risk. Demonstrate exercises that could be taught to a pregnant woman on bed rest.

REFERENCES

1. Cunningham FG, MacDonald PC, Gant NF, et al. *Williams Obstetrics*. 20th ed. Stanford, CT: Appleton & Lange; 1997.
2. Cunningham FG, MacDonald PC, Gant NF. *Williams Obstetrics*. 18th ed. Norwalk, CT: Appleton & Lange; 1989.
3. Bobak IM, Jensen MD, Zalar MK. *Maternity and Gynecologic Care*. 4th ed. St. Louis: CV Mosby; 1989.
4. Scott JR, DiSaia PJ, Hammond CB, Spellacy WN, eds. *Danforth's Obstetrics and Gynecology*. 7th ed. Philadelphia: J.B. Lippincott; 1994.
5. Wolfe LA, Amey MC, McGrath MJ. Exercise and pregnancy. In: Torg JS, Separd RJ, eds. *Current Therapy in Sports Medicine*. 3rd ed. St. Louis: Mosby; 1995:550–555.
6. Artal Mittelmark R, Wisewell RA, Drinkwater BL, eds. *Exercise in Pregnancy*. 2nd ed. Baltimore: Williams & Wilkins; 1991.

7. American College of Obstetricians and Gynecologists. Exercise during pregnancy and the postpartum period. *ACOG Technical Bull.* 1994;189.
8. Avery MD, Rossi MA, Gestational diabetes. *J Nurse Midwife.* 1994;39:95–195, 35–85.
9. Weller KA. *Diagnosis and Management of Gestational Diabetes. Am Fam Physician.* 1996;53:2053–2057, 2061–2062.
10. Bung P, Artal R. Gestational diabetes and exercise: a survey. *Semin Perinatol.* 1996;20:628–333.
11. Avery MD, Leon AS, Kopher RA. Effects of a partially home-based exercise program for women with gestational diabetes. *Obstet Gynecol.* 1997;89:10–15.
12. Jovanovic-Peterson L, Peterson CM. Exercise and the nutritional management of diabetes during pregnancy. *Obstet Gynecol Clin North Am.* 1996;23:75–86.
13. Jackson P, Bash DM. Management of the uncomplicated pregnant diabetic client in the ambulatory setting. *Nurse Pract.* 1994;19:64–73.
14. Bung P, Artal R, Khodiguian N, Kjos S. Exercise in gestational diabetes: an optional therapeutic approach? *Diabetes.* 1991; 40(suppl 2):182–185.
15. Jovanovic-Peterson L, Peterson CM. Is exercise safe or useful for gestational diabetic women? *Diabetes.* 1991;40(suppl 2): 179–181.
16. Jovanovic-Peterson L, Durak E, Peterson CM. Randomized trial of diet versus diet plus cardiovascular conditioning on glucose levels in gestational diabetes. *Am J Obstet Gynecol.* 1990;162:754–756.
17. Horton ES. Exercise in the treatment of NIDDM: applications for GDM? *Diabetes.* 1991;40(suppl 2):175–178.
18. Bung P, Bung C, Artal R, Khodiguian N, Fallenstein F, Spatling L. Therapeutic exercise for insulin requiring gestational diabetics: effects on the fetus—results of a randomized prospective longitudinal study. *J Perinat Med.* 1993;21:125–137.
19. Winn HN, Reece EA. Interrelationship between insulin, dietary fiber, and exercise in the management of pregnant diabetics. *Obstet Gynecol Surv.* 1989;44:703–710.
20. Field JB. Exercise and deficient carbohydrate storage and intake as causes of hypoglycemia. *Endocrinol Metab Clin North Am.* 1989;18:155–161.
21. Carlson KJ, Eisenstat ST, Zipporyn T, eds. *The Harvard Guide to Women's Health.* Cambridge, MA: Harvard University Press; 1996.
22. Shangold M, Mirkin G, eds. *Women and Exercise: Physiology and Sports Medicine.* Philadelphia: FA Davis; 1994.
23. Lops VR, Hunter LP, Dixon LR. Anemia in pregnancy. *Am Fam Physician.* 1995;51:1189–1197.
24. Engstrom JL, Sittler CP. Nurse-midwifery management of iron-deficiency anemia during pregnancy. *J Nurse Midwife.* 1994;39:205–345.
25. Scholl TO, Hediger ML. Anemia and Iron-Deficiency Anemia: Complication of Data on Pregnancy Outcome. *Am J Clin Nutr.* 1994;59:4925–5005.
26. Kinsella SM, Lohmann G. Supine hypotensive syndrome. *Am J Obstet Gynecol.* 1994;83:774–787.
27. Kotila PM, Lee SN. *Effects of Supine Position During Pregnancy on the Fetal Heart Rate.* Forest Grove, OR: Pacific University; 1994. Thesis.
28. Carbonne B, Benachi A, Leeque ML, Cabrol D, Papiernik E. Maternal positions during labor: effects on fetal oxygen saturation measured by pulse oximetry. *Obstet Gynecol.* 1996;88: 797–800.
29. Polden M, Mantle J. *Physiotherapy in Obstetrics and Gynecology.* Oxford: Butterworth-Heinemann; 1990.
30. O'Connor LJ, Gourley RJ. *Obstetric and Gynecologic Care in Physical Therapy.* Thorofare, NJ: Slack; 1990.
31. Wilder E, ed. *Clinics in Physical Therapy,* vol. 20. *Obstetric and Gynecologic Physical Therapy.* New York: Churchill Livingstone; 1988.
32. Heckman JD, Sassard R. Musculoskeletal Considerations in Pregnancy. *J Bone Joint Surg Am.* 1994;76:1720–1730.
33. Clapp JF. Pregnancy outcome: physical activities inside versus outside the workplace. *Semin Perionatol.* 1996;20: 70–76.
34. Clapp JF. A clinical approach to exercise during pregnancy. *Clin Sports Med.* 1994;13:443–458.
35. Horns PN, Ratcliffe LP, Leggett JC, Swanson MS. Pregnancy outcomes among active and sedentary primiparous women. *J Obstet Gynecol Neonat Nurs.* 1996; 25:49–54.
36. Sternfeld B, Quesenberry CP Jr, Eskenazi B, Newman LA. Exercise during pregnancy and pregnancy outcome. *Med Sci Sports Exerc.* 1995;27:634–640.
37. Botkins C, Driscoll CE. Maternal aerobic exercise: newborn effects. *Fam Pract Res J.* 1991;11:387–393.
38. Clapp JF 3rd. The course of labor after endurance exercise during pregnancy. *Am J Obstet Gynecol.* 1990;163:1799–1805.
39. Beckmann CR, Beckmann CA. Effects of a structured antepartum exercise program on pregnancy and labor outcome in primiparas. *J Reprod Med.* 1990;35:704–709.
40. Kulpa P. Exercise during pregnancy and postpartum. In: Agostini R, ed. *Medical and Orthopedic Issues of Active Athletic Women.* Philadelphia: Hanley & Belfus; 1994.
41. Wolfe LA, Walker RM, Bonen A, McGrath MJ. Effects of pregnancy and chronic exercise on respiratory responses to graded exercise. *J Appl Physiol.* 1994;76:1928–1936.
42. Zeanah M, Schlosser SP. Adherence to ACOG guidelines on exercise during pregnancy: effect on pregnancy outcome. *J Obstet Gynecol Neonat Nurs.* 1993;22:329–335.
43. McMurray RG, Mottola MF, Wolfe LA, Artal R, Millar L, Pivarnik JM. Recent advances in understanding maternal and fetal responses to exercise. *Med Sci Sports Exerc.* 1993;25: 1305–1321.
44. Wolfe LA, Mottola MF. Aerobic exercise in pregnancy: an update. *Can J Appl Physiol.* 1993;18:119–147.
45. Clapp JF 3rd. Exercise and fetal health. *J Dev Physiol.* 1991; 15:9–14.
46. Sady SP, Carpenter MW. Aerobic exercise during pregnancy: special considerations. *Sports Med.* 1989;7:357–375.
47. Clapp JF 3rd. The effects of maternal exercise on early pregnancy outcome. *Am J Obstet Gynecol.* 1989;161:1453–1457.
48. Hall DC, Kaufmann DA. Effects of aerobic and strength conditioning on pregnancy outcomes. *Am J Obstet Gynecol.* 1987;157:1199–1203.
49. The Melpomene Institute for Women's Health Research. *The Bodywise Woman.* New York: Prentice Hall Press; 1990.
50. Ruoti RG, Morris DM, Cole AJ. *Aquatics Rehabilitation.* Philadelphia: Lippincott-Raven Publishers; 1997.
51. Katz VL. Water exercise in pregnancy. *Semin Perinatol.* 1996; 20:285–291.
52. McMurray RG, Katz VL. Thermoregulation in pregnancy. *Sports Med.* 1990;10:146–158.
53. Bell R, O'Neill M. Exercise and pregnancy: a review. *Birth.* 1994;21:85–95.
54. Yeo S. Exercise guidelines for pregnant women. *Image J Nurs Sch.* 1994;26:265–270.
55. Treyder SC. Exercising while pregnant. *J Orthop Sports Phys Ther.* 1989;10:358–365.
56. Hale RW, Milne L. The elite athlete and exercise in pregnancy. *Semin Perinatol.* 1996;20:277–284.
57. Wiswell RA. Applications of methods and techniques in the study of aerobic fitness during pregnancy. *Semin Perinatol.* 1996;20:213–221.

58. Huch K. Physical activity at altitude in pregnancy. *Semin Perinatol.* 1996;20:304–314.
59. Michlovitz SL, ed. *Thermal Agents in Rehabilitation.* 2nd ed. Philadelphia: FA Davis; 1990.
60. Edwards MJ. Congenital defects in guinea pigs: prenatal retardation of brain growth of guinea pigs following hyperthermia during gestation. *Teratology.* 1969;2:329.
61. Smith DW, Clarren SK, Harvey MAS. Hyperthermia as a possible teratogenic agent. *J Pediatr.* 1978;92:878.
62. Boissannault J, Blaschak M. Incidence of diastasis recti abdominis during the childbearing years. *Phys Ther.* 1988;68:1082.
63. Bursch S. Interrater reliability of diastasis recti abdominis measurement. *Phys Ther.* 1987;67:1077.
64. Noble E. *Essential Exercises for the Childbearing Years.* Harwich, MA: New Life Images; 1995.
65. Sinaki M, Merrit JL, Stillwell GK. Tension myalgia of the pelvic floor. *Mayo Clin Proc.* 1977;52:717–722.
66. Mayo Clinic. *Home Instructions for Relief of Pelvic Floor Pain.* Rochester, MN: Mayo Foundation for Medical Education and Research; 1989.
67. Hansen K. Sacrococcygeal instability in pregnancy. *Obstet Gynecol Phys Ther.* 1993;17:5–7.
68. Kendall FP, McCreary EK, Provance PG. *Muscles Testing and Function.* Baltimore: Williams & Wilkins; 1993.
69. Callahan J. Separation of the symphysis pubis. *Am J Obstet Gynecol.* 1953;66:281–293.
70. Katz VL, Ryder RM, Cefalo RC, Carmichael SC, Goolsby R. A comparison of bed rest and immersion for treating the edema of pregnancy. *Obstet Gynecol.* 1990;75:147–151.
71. Pipp LM. The exercise dilemma: considerations and guidelines for treatment of the high risk obstetric patient. *J Obstet Gynecol Phys Ther.* 1989;13:10–12.
72. Frahm J, Davis Y, Welch RA. Physical therapy management of the high risk antepartum patient: physical and occupational therapy treatment objectives and program, part III. *Clin Manage Phys Ther.* 1989;9:28–33.
73. Gilbert ES, Harmann JS. *Manual of High Risk Pregnancy and Delivery.* St. Louis: Mosby; 1993.
74. Goldenberg RL, Cliver SP, Bronstein J, et al. Bed rest in Pregnancy. *Obstet Gynecol.* 1994;84:131.
75. Maloni JA, Kasper CE. Physical and psychosocial effects of antepartum hospital bed rest: a review of the literature. *Image J Nurs Sch.* 1991;23:187–192.
76. Maloni JA, Chance B, Zhang C, et al. Physical and psychosocial side effects of antepartum hospital bed rest. *Nurs Res.* 1993;42:197–203.
77. Maloni JA. Home care of the high-risk pregnant woman requiring bed rest. *J Obstet Gynecol Neonat Nurs.* 1994;23:696–706.
78. Mitchell L. *Simple Relaxation.* 2nd ed. London: John Murray; 1987.
79. Jacobson E. *Progressive Relaxation.* Chicago: University of Chicago Press; 1938.
80. Josten LE, Savik K, Mullett SE, et al. Bed rest compliance for women with pregnancy problems. *Birth.* 1995;22:1–12.
81. Schroeder CA. Women's experience of bed rest in high-risk pregnancy. *Image J Nurs Sch.* 1996;28:253–258.
82. Maloni JA. Bed rest and high-risk pregnancy: differentiating the effects of diagnosis, setting, and treatment. *Nurs Clin North Am.* 1996;31:313–325.
83. Smithing RT, Wiley MD. Bedrest not necessarily an effective intervention in pregnancy. *Nurse Pract Am J Primary Health Care.* 1994;19:15.
84. Bogen JT, Gitlin LN, Cornman-Levy D. Bedrest treatment in high-risk pregnancy: implications for physical therapy. Platform Presentation at the American Physical Therapy Association Combined Sections Meeting; February, 1997; Dallas, Texas.
85. Knee-chest exercises and maternal death [comments]. *Med J Aust.* 1973;1:1127.
86. Nelson P. Pulmonary gas embolism in pregnancy and the puerperium. *Obstet Gynecol Surv.* 1960;15:449–481.
87. American College of Obstetricians and Gynecologists. *Cesarean Birth.* ACOG patient education pamphlet AP06. Washington, DC: American College of Obstetricians and Gynecologists; 1983.
88. American College of Obstetricians and Gynecologists. *Vaginal Birth After Cesarean Delivery.* ACOG patient education pamphlet AP070. Washington, DC: American College of Obstetricians and Gynecologists; 1990.
89. Rangelli D, Hayes SH. Vaginal birth after cesarean: the role of the physical therapist. *J Obstet Gynecol Phys Ther.* 1995;19:10–13.
90. Gent D, Gottlieb K. Cesarean rehabilitation. *Clin Manage Phys Ther.* 1985;5:14–19.

RECOMMENDED READING

Myers RS, ed. *Saunders Manual of Physical Therapy Practice*, chapters 22 and 23. Philadelphia: WB Saunders; 1995.

Nobel E. *Essential Exercises for the Childbearing Year.* 4th ed. Harwich, MA: New Life Images; 1995.

Nobel E. *Marie Osmond's Exercises for Mothers-To-Be.* New York: New American Library; 1985.

Nobel E. *Marie Osmond's Exercises for Mothers and Babies.* New York: New American Library; 1985.

Pauls JA. *Therapeutic Approaches to Women's Health.* Gaithersburg, MD: Aspen Publishers; 1995.

Simkin P, Whalley J, Kepler A. *Pregnancy, Child Birth and the Newborn: The Complete Guide.* Deephaven, MN: Meadowbrook Press; 1991.

RESOURCES

American College of Obstetricians and Gynecologists (ACOG), 409 12th Street, SW, Washington, DC 20024-2188; (202) 638-5577.

American College of Sports Medicine, P.O. Box 1440, Indianapolis, IN 46206; (317) 637-9200.

American Physical Therapy Association, Section on Women's Health, P.O. Box 327, Alexandria, VA 22313; (800) 999-2782 ext. 3237.

Melpomene Institute for Women's Health Research, 1010 University Avenue, St. Paul, MN 55104; (612) 642-1951.

UNIT 4

Methods of Therapeutic Exercise Intervention

CHAPTER 14

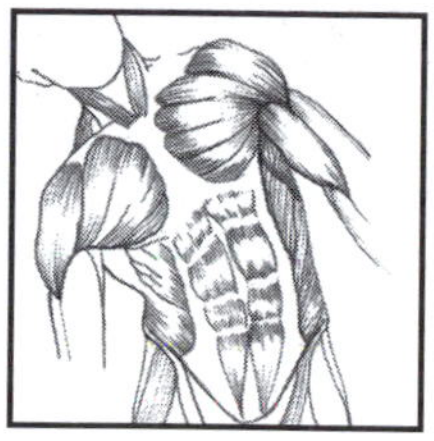

Proprioceptive Neuromuscular Facilitation

Chuck Hanson

In the late 1940s, Dr. Herman Kabat, a neurophysiologist and physician at the University of Minnesota, began to analyze the work of Sister Elizabeth Kenny and her treatment approach for patients with anterior poliomyelitis. Dr. Kabat found that the Kenny method was lacking in neurophysiologic principles. He then looked to classic research in neurophysiology for the basis of his treatment approach to neurologic disability. He coupled the work of Sir Charles Sherrington regarding facilitation and facilitation patterns of the nervous system with his own observations of functional human movement, as witnessed in sports and the work of Sister Kenny. These building blocks became the foundation for what is now internationally recognized as proprioceptive neuromuscular facilitation (PNF).[1–4]

Maggie Knott, a young, ambitious physical therapist, helped to further develop Dr. Kabat's basic patterns and principles. Together, Maggie Knott and Dr. Kabat created the basis of the handling skills, techniques, and principles that are applied widely today. Maggie Knott is recognized as a pioneer in manual therapy. By the early 1950s, Dorothy Voss, director of physical therapy at George Washington University Hospital in Washington, DC, joined Maggie Knott. Dorothy Voss contributed her skills and background in therapeutic exercise and motor learning theory to the basic patterns and handling skills in place at that time.[1–4] The collaboration of these two extraordinary therapists and the basic work of Dr. Kabat created this functional approach to therapeutic exercise and rehabilitation.

The purpose of this chapter is to present a foundation in the practical application of PNF. Practice suggestions accompany each section to transform written concepts into manual experience. As with all manual techniques, PNF is only as powerful as the skill with which it is applied. Intensive practice is essential for best results.

DEFINITION AND GOALS

PNF is best defined by first defining the individual terms. *Proprioceptive* refers to stimuli aroused within an organism through the movement of its tissues.[5] *Neuromuscular* pertains to the nerves and muscles. *Facilitation* is the hastening of any natural process. This results from reducing nerve resistance through one stimulus, allowing a second stimulus to more easily evoke a response. As a whole, PNF is defined as methods of promoting or hastening the response of the neuromuscular mechanism through stimulation of the proprioceptor.[1]

PNF is initiated when a deficient neuromuscular mechanism results in altered or inefficient patterns of motion or posture. There may be several goals of PNF treatment. One major goal is to restore or enhance postural responses or normal patterns of motion. Specific demands are used to facilitate a direct effect on the target muscle group or an indirect effect on the synergists or antagonists of the target group.

BASIC NEUROPHYSIOLOGIC PRINCIPLES OF PROPRIOCEPTIVE NEUROMUSCULAR FACILITATION

Muscular Activity

Muscle groups are classified as agonists, antagonists, neutralizers, supporters, and fixators. Within a movement pattern, several muscle groups may work in synergy to create a specific movement. Agonists work to produce movement, whereas antagonists relax to allow movement to occur. Neutralizers inhibit a muscle from performing more than one action. Supporting muscles stabilize the trunk and proximal extremities, and fixators hold bones steady.[6]

Muscle contractions are classified as dynamic (ie, isotonic) or static (ie, isometric). With isotonic contractions, the intention of the patient is to move; with isometric contractions, the intention is to hold a position or stabilize. Dynamic contractions are concentric (ie, active shortening of a muscle), eccentric (ie, active lengthening of a muscle), or maintained isotonic (a PNF term) in which the patient's intention is to move, but no motion occurs. Static contractions are those in which no motion occurs.[3] For a fuller discussion of muscular activity, see Chapter 4.

Diagonals of Movement

Three planes of movement occur simultaneously during normal-functioning motor activity. Because of the agonist-antagonist relationship of the nervous system, each component is associated with an antagonistic motion:

- Flexion versus extension
- Abduction versus adduction in the extremities and lateral movement in the trunk
- Internal rotation versus external rotation

Combinations of these components work together to produce the *diagonals of movement* (ie, innate path in which maximal response of the trunk and extremities can be facilitated).[1,2,3,7–9] There are two diagonals of movement for each major body part: the head, neck, and upper trunk; the lower trunk; the upper extremities; and the lower extremities (Table 14-1). Although the diagonals of movement have been isolated for ease of description, the diagonal patterns of the head, neck, and trunk occur simultaneously with the diagonal patterns of the extremities.

Normal coordinated patterns of motion, which facilitate the strongest output, are diagonal in direction with spiral components. These patterns reflect the functional relationship of the trunk and extremities in sports and work activities (Fig. 14-1).[4] While looking at the component motions in a diagonal sit-up exercise, try to observe or "feel" the spiral, diagonal movement pattern of the body. As the arms move diagonally across toward the right knee, the trunk begins to flex, rotate, and sidebend.

Diagonals of movement are useful during treatment. The therapist may rely on these normal functional movement patterns to identify quality of contractions, range of motion (ROM), and functional impairments or limitations. Altered movement patterns may be modified through the use of patterns of facilitation, which are discussed in the Treatment Implementation section.

Motor Development

PNF is based on 11 basic principles drawn from the fields of neurophysiology, motor learning, and motor behavior.[1] These principles have been relied on to guide the direction of the patient-therapist interaction, setting the tone and character of the approach. Current neurophysiology theories reflect a different model of central nervous system control than that used to develop PNF.[10,11] The 11 original principles are summarized in Display 14-1 to provide a historical perspective and to promote a basic understanding of the theory behind PNF.

EXAMINATION AND EVALUATION

Success in physical therapy is measured by improving physical function. A thorough subjective and objective examination or evaluation enables the therapist to diagnose impairments and functional limitations. During the examination, the patient's capabilities are assessed in the following areas:

Mobility impairment
- Mobility: The ability to initiate and stop movement on command
- Controlled mobility: Proper timing and balanced recruitment of trunk and proximal or distal extremity muscle groups to allow for smooth and coordinated movement in functional ranges of motion
- Joint and soft tissue ROM: Sufficient joint and soft tissue ROM in the trunk and extremities for functional activities

Force or torque impairment
- Tone: Sufficient postural tone to provide stability in the trunk and proximal limb segments, but not so extreme as to prevent smooth, coordinated purposeful movement (see Chapter 4)
- Recruitment: Sufficient motor unit recruitment occurring during functional activity.

Endurance impairment
- Adequate cardiovascular conditioning, attention span, and neuromuscular force potential to complete repetitive or sequenced activity

Balance and coordination impairment
- Presence of proper balance, righting, and equilibrium reactions
- Proper proximal to distal timing
- Able to start, stop, accelerate, decelerate, or reverse motion as necessary to perform skillful functions

Posture and movement impairment
- Stability: Adequate trunk stability to maintain postures
- Bed mobility, transfers, and gait: Equilibrium and righting reactions to allow for transition between postures, including advanced developmental postures in which the center of gravity is displaced higher or over

Table 14-1. DIAGONALS OF MOVEMENT

DIAGONAL PATTERN | **ILLUSTRATION**

Head and Neck

A: flexion with rotation to right (D fl, R)
B: extension with rotation to left (D ex, L)

A
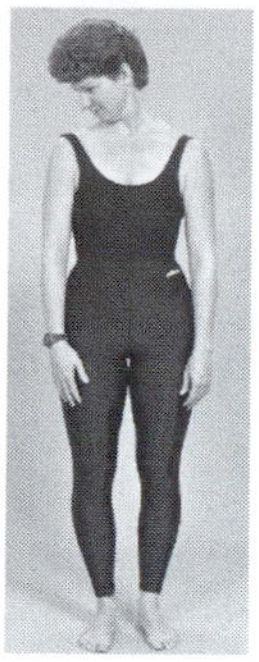

B
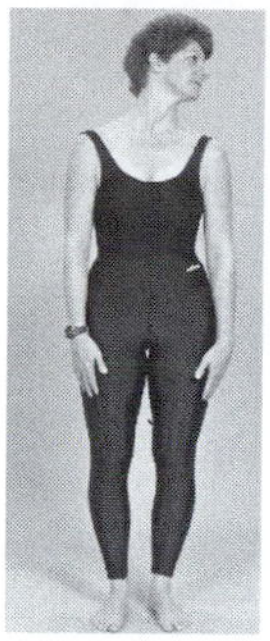

A: flexion with rotation to left (D fl, L)
B: extension with rotation to right (D ex, R)

A
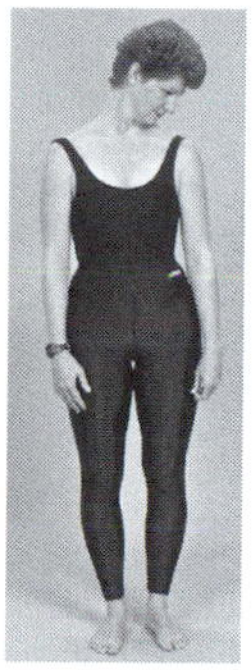

B
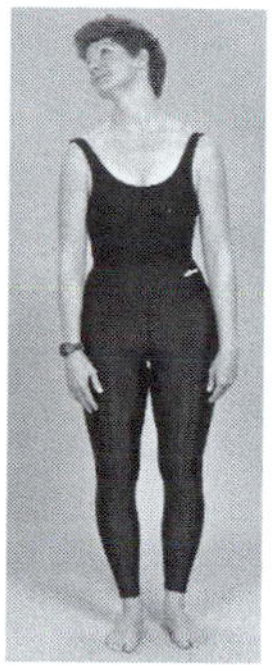

Upper Trunk

A: flexion with rotation to right (D fl, R)
B: extension with rotation to left (D ex, L)

A
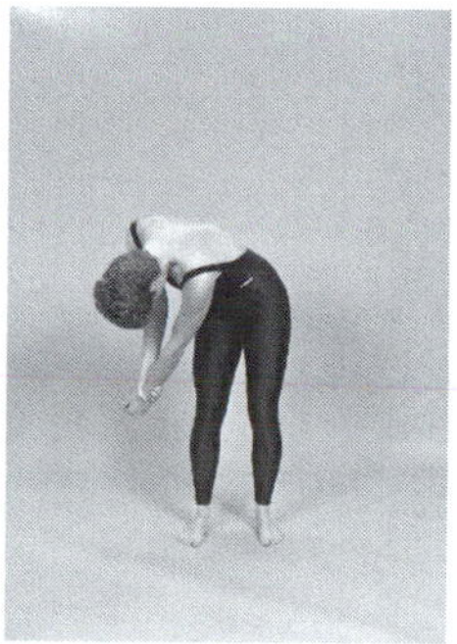

B
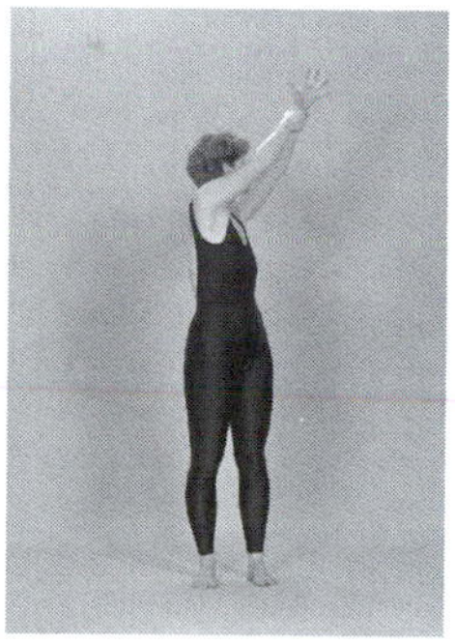

A: flexion with rotation to left (D fl, L)
B: extension with rotation to right (D ex, R)

A
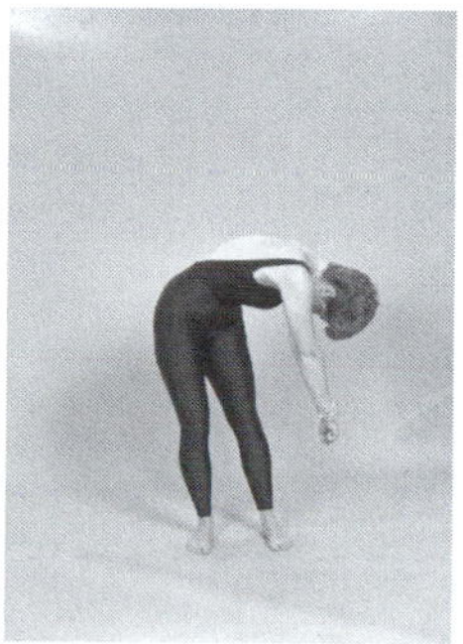

B
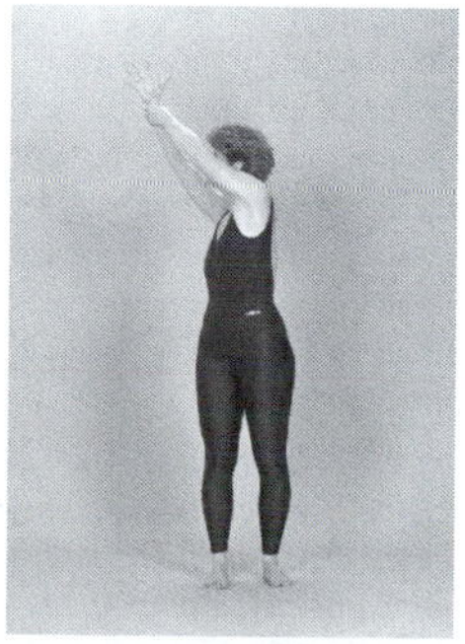

(continued)

Table 14-1. DIAGONALS OF MOVEMENT *(continued)*

DIAGONAL PATTERN	ILLUSTRATION	
Upper Extremities A: flexion-adduction-external rotation (D1 fl) B: extension-abduction-internal rotation (D1 ex)	A 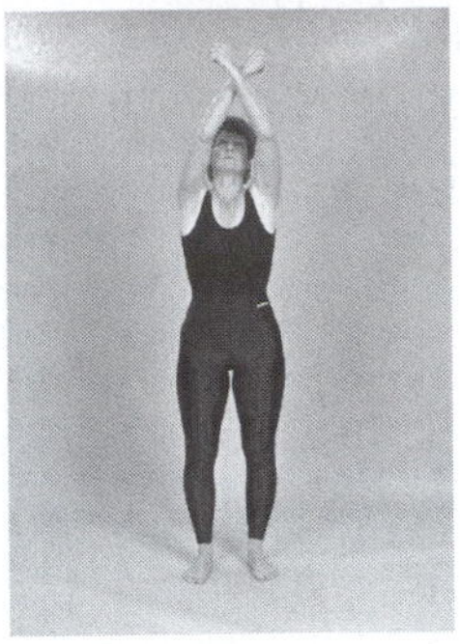	B 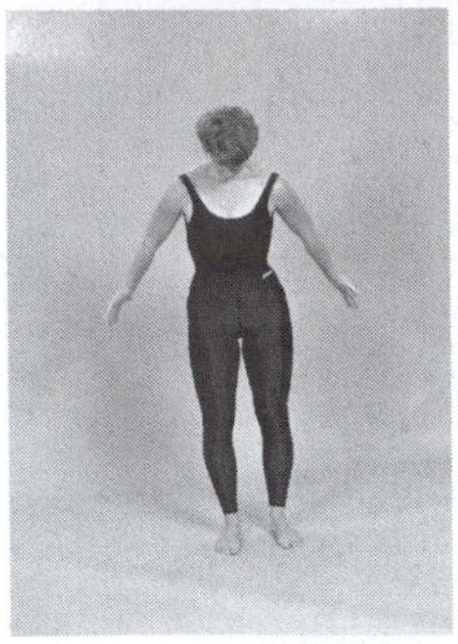
A: flexion-abduction-external rotation (D2 fl) B: extension-adduction-internal rotation (D2 ex)	A 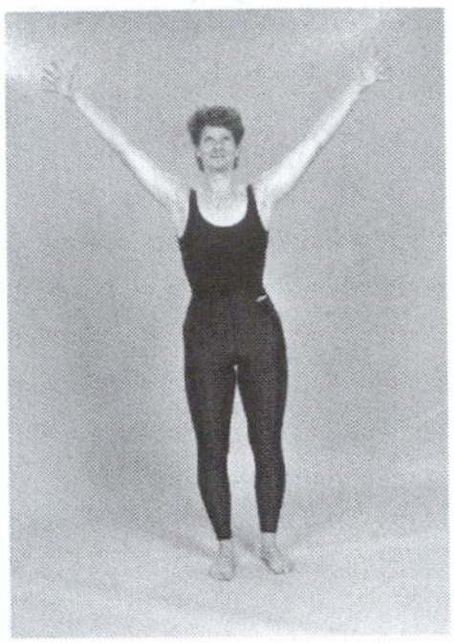	B 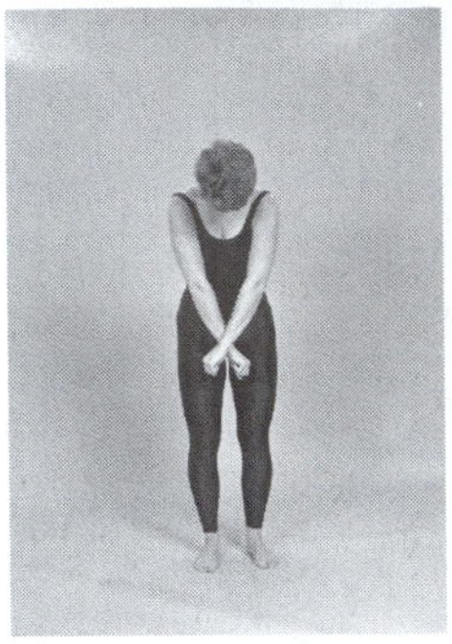
Lower Extremities A: flexion-adduction-external rotation (D1 fl) B: extension-abduction-internal rotation (D1 ex)	A 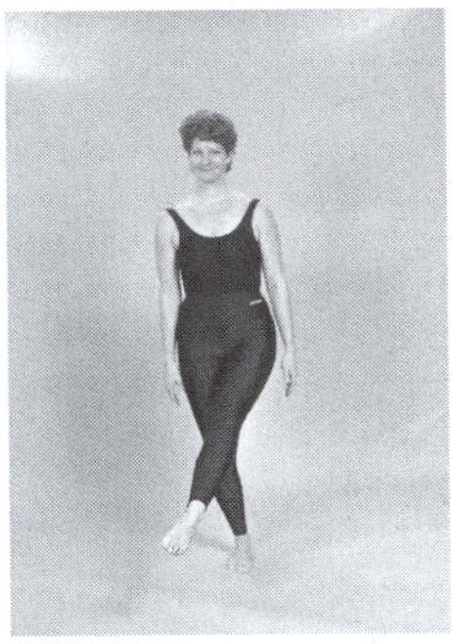	B 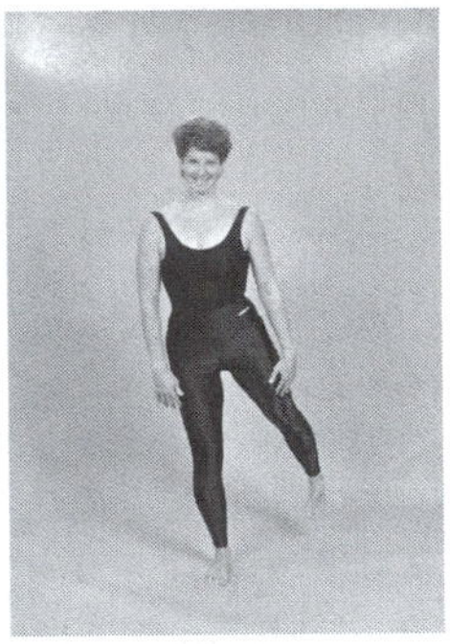
A: flexion-abduction-external rotation (D2 fl) B: extension-adduction-internal rotation (D2 ex)	A 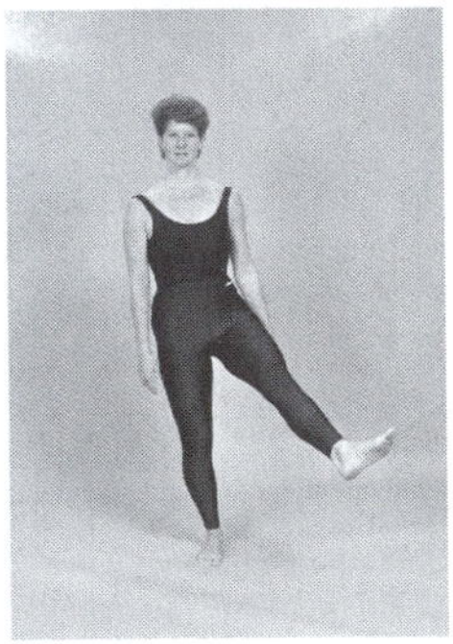	B 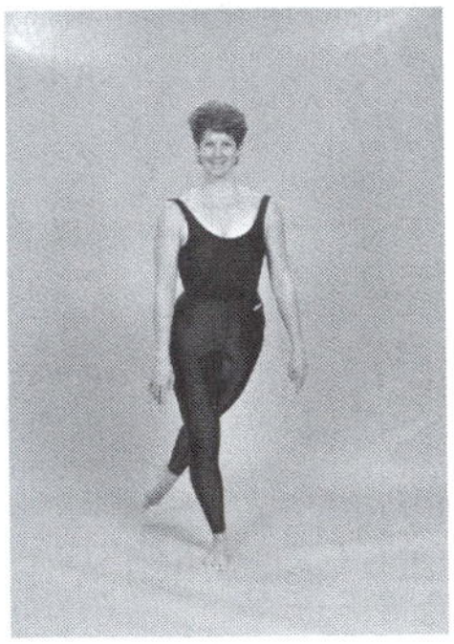

With flexion goes external rotation, supination, and wrist radial deviation.
With extension goes internal rotation, pronation, and wrist ulnar deviation.
With abduction goes wrist extension.
With adduction goes wrist flexion.
With wrist extension goes finger extension.
With wrist flexion goes finger flexion.
With abduction goes internal rotation and foot eversion.
With adduction goes external rotation and foot inversion.
With hip flexion goes foot dorsiflexion.
With hip extension goes foot plantarflexion.
With plantarflexion goes toe flexion.
With dorsiflexion goes toe extension.

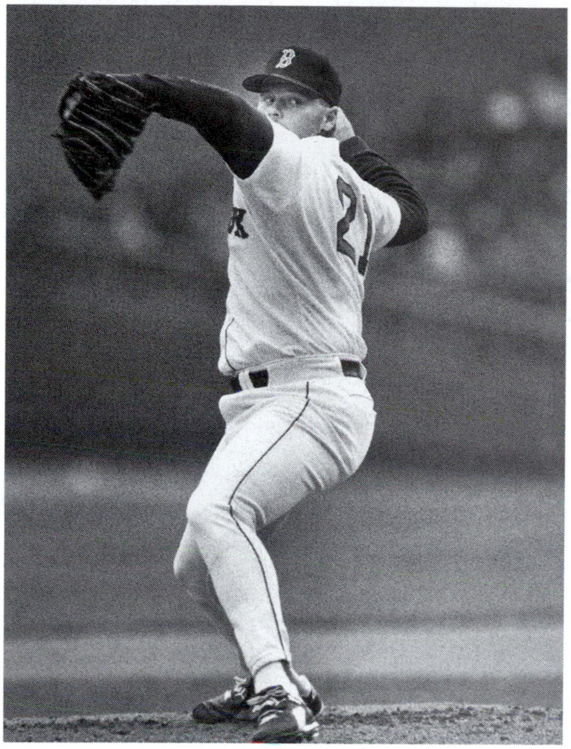

FIGURE 14-1 A baseball pitch exemplifies the spiral, diagonal movement pattern of the body. (© Stock Boston/Peter Southwick.)

a smaller base of support and moves through a larger excursion

Pain

- Pain as an inhibitor: Must consider tactile sensitivity, joint or soft tissue ROM, and weight-bearing tolerance

A customized treatment plan maximizes the patient's strengths and minimizes his weaknesses. Through examination and evaluation, the therapist must judge what postures, contacts, cues, and goals are most effective. The evaluation should therefore take into account several factors:

- The patient's short-term and long-term goals
- The patient's receptive potential for language, vision, and manual contacts to promote appropriate cuing
- The patient's strengths (eg, what the patient does well; which body half, quadrant extremity or joint is most sound, strong, and usable for irradiation; at which developmental level the patient has a spectrum of neuromuscular capabilities to practice transitions; what motivates the patient, such as sports participation or task completion without assistance)
- The patient's weaknesses (eg, postures that cause the patient difficulty in functioning because of mechanical disadvantage, incoordination, or excessively high postural tone; body parts that are less functional or painful)

Because treatment is dynamic, requiring continuous reassessment of results and restructuring of inputs, goals, and tasks, this examination or evaluation process is ongoing.

DISPLAY 14-1

Principles of Proprioceptive Neuromuscular Facilitation

1. **All human beings have potentials that are not fully developed.** Motor activity is limited to the individual's physical ability and inherent and previously learned neuromuscular responses. However, the normal person has a vast and untapped neuromuscular potential, which may be developed through environmental influences and voluntary decisions or tapped during stressful episodes. Based on this philosophy, the therapist always strives to treat function, motivate the patient to achieve higher levels, and uses the patient's strengths to minimize his weaknesses.
2. **Normal motor development proceeds in a cervocaudal and proximodistal direction:*** Development of motion occurs first in the head and neck, then in the trunk, and finally in the extremities. Motion develops from proximal points to distal points. During treatment, the head and neck are treated first because they influence the movement pattern of the body. Next, the trunk is treated, because it provides the foundation of function. After adequate control of the head, neck, and trunk is established, fine motor skills may be developed.
3. **Early motor behavior is dominated by reflex activity. Mature motor behavior is reinforced or supported by postural reflex mechanisms.** During treatment, reflexes may be facilitated to support weak muscles by choosing a specific developmental posture, initiating part of a functional activity or pattern, or involving the head and trunk with extremity patterns.
4. **The growth of motor behavior has cyclic trends as evidenced by shifts between flexors and extensor dominance.** During functional activity, movements alternate between flexion and extension. This reciprocal relationship leads to stability and balance of postures. In treatment, the reciprocal relationship of flexors and extensors may be facilitated to reestablish stability and balance.
5. **Goal-directed activity is made up of reversing movements.** Normal movements are rhythmic and reversing. Reversing movements establish an equilibrium among activities and establish a balance and interaction between antagonist. Treatment must facilitate movement in both directions to enhance functioning.
6. **Normal movement and posture depend on "synergism" and a balanced interaction of antagonists.** Functional movement relies on a balance of reflex activity, flexor-extensor dominance, and reversing movements. During treatment, imbalances among these factors are corrected to restore normal patterns of motion and postural responses. This may be achieved by performing transitions between postures (eg, rolling reversals, supine to or from sitting, performing reciprocal or reversing patterns).
7. **Developing motor behavior is expressed in an orderly sequence of total patterns of movement and posture.** Motor behavior develops in a specific sequence. During development, early-milestones provide the basis for more complex function. Motor behavior progresses in an orderly fashion from mobility to stability to controlled mobility and into skill or function, creating a diverse repertoire of motor behavior. Combined movements of the neck, trunk, and extremities also progress in a specified sequence (Fig. 14-2). Treatment must progress in a similar fashion. More fundamental developmental levels often are used initially to emphasize proximal stability, enhance

(continued)

DISPLAY 14-1 (Continued)
Principles of Proprioceptive Neuromuscular Facilitation

balance, and encourage a greater sense of security. As success is achieved, the sophistication of the task is progressed within the same developmental level or to a more advanced developmental posture.

8. **Normal motor development has an orderly sequence but lacks a step by step quality (overlapping results).*** Although development of motor behavior is sequential, one activity is not perfected before another more advanced activity is initiated; overlapping occurs. In treatment, this overlapping may be used to facilitate progress. More difficult activities may be performed at lower developmental postures, whereas easier tasks may be performed at more advanced developmental postures.
9. **Improvement of motor ability depends on motor learning:** Motor learning is enhanced through the use of multisensory inputs. Auditory, visual, and tactile stimuli are used to progress learning. Visual cues help coordinate and guide movement. Various tones of auditory cues may influence muscle reaction. Verbal cues influence the quality of the patient's response. Tactile cues may provide direction and encouragement. Treatment that uses these multisensory inputs may optimize learning opportunities, thereby maximizing the patient's progress toward more complete functional ability.
10. **Frequency of stimulation and repetition of activity are used to promote and retain motor learning and for the development of strength and endurance.** The motor learning process requires repetition or practice of the task to be learned. Therapeutic tasks need to offer *transfer appropriate processing,* the process of putting the learner into a problem-solving mode most comparable with later performance. In this way, learning is enhanced through repetitive tasks, and through a repetitive therapeutic exercise program. Variations of repetitive exercises may include retrieval of a certain motor sequence, performance of a particular action in a variety of environmental contexts, and performance of an anticipatory mode of control as opposed to a reactive mode of control
11. **Goal-directed activities coupled with techniques of facilitation are used to hasten learning of total patterns of walking and self-care activities.** Realistic functional goals are continually set for the patient throughout treatment. The patient's goals are included in decision making to establish a closer bond for meeting a common target. Activities that have meaning for the patient are more effectively integrated into motor learning.

**Current thought contradicts these two principles. Although true for infants, studies have found that adults do not necessarily follow these patterns.*

Combined Movements of Paired Extremities

Symmetrical: perform like movements at the same time
Asymmetrical: perform movements toward one side at the same time
Reciprocal: perform movements in opposite direction at the same time

Combined Movements of Upper and Lower Extremities

Ipsilateral: extremities of same side move in same direction at same time
Contralateral: extremities of opposite sides move in same direction at same time
Diagonal reciprocal: contralateral extremities move in same direction at same time while opposite contralateral extremities move in opposite direction

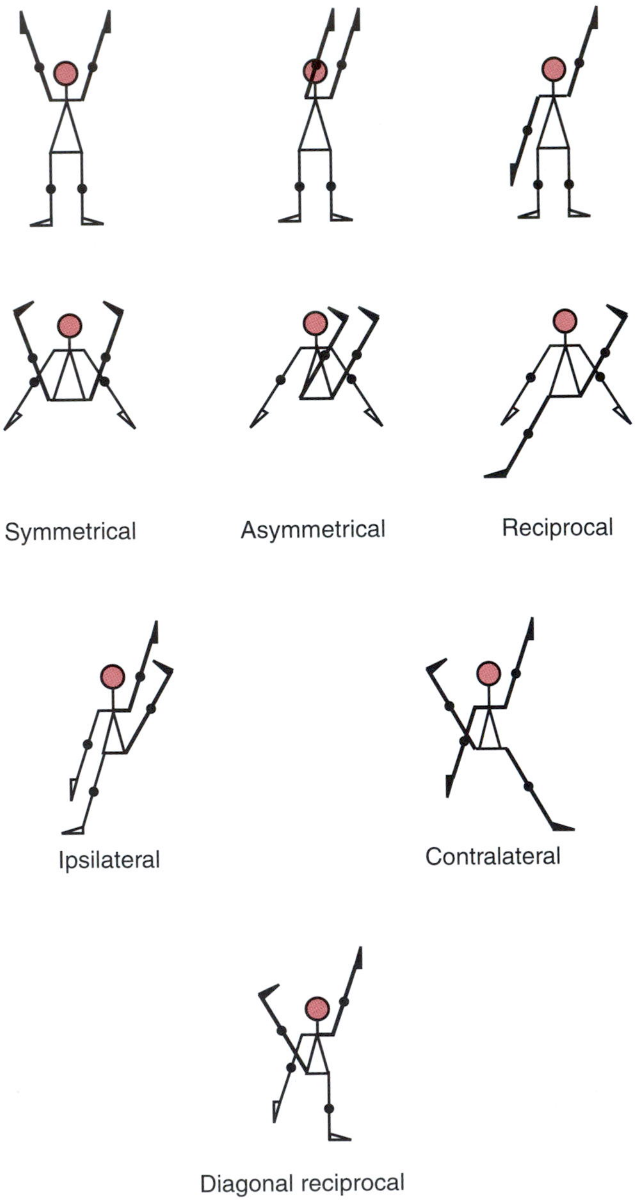

FIGURE 14-2 Interaction of segments

TREATMENT IMPLEMENTATION

Functional capabilities are described as a product of environmental, social, psychological, medical, and physical factors.[7] Treatment interventions that address the proper impairment may include these features:

- Modification of the environment
- Education and compensation for the impairment

- Treatment directed at changing the individual's neuromuscular capabilities

PNF is an invaluable tool in this final strategy. Successful implementation depends on the therapist's thorough understanding of the principles of anatomy, biomechanics, exercise philosophies, and theories of motor control and motor learning. The therapist can then choose to apply the patterns of facilitation, procedures, and techniques of facilitation. The *patterns of facilitation*, the most familiar hallmark of PNF, provide the framework for educating movement. The *procedures* define the methods of manual handling and facilitating inputs. The *techniques of facilitation* are applied to the agonist-antagonist muscle groups to address particular neuromuscular impairment. Display 14-2 summarizes the PNF treatment process.

Patterns of Facilitation

Knowledge of the normal functional movement patterns of the body allows the therapist to identify altered patterns of motion. During treatment, the therapist may cue and resist the spiral, diagonal patterns of the neck, trunk, or extremities (ie, the diagonals of movement) to promote a maximal response from muscle groups and to move the patient toward functional gains. Voss[1] and Adler[3] have thoroughly described this approach. Patterns of facilitation are manually resistive exercises that create the diagonals of movement by coupling pairs of antagonistic patterns, providing a path for reversing motions and using the agonist-antagonist relationship of the nervous system as techniques are applied. Figure 14-3 illustrates a sample pattern of facilitation. Voss et al.[1] have provided a pictorial description of the various patterns of facilitation.

DISPLAY 14-2

Proprioceptive Neuromuscular Facilitation Treatment Planning Process

1. **Diagnose impairment or functional limitation.** Based on a thorough subjective and objective evaluation, diagnose impairments and functional limitations. Set short- and long-term goals.
2. **Choose the pattern or function.** Make a decision about whether to treat the functional limitation directly (eg, through resisted gait, bed mobility) or to identify a component impairment that, when addressed, will result in greater gains toward the functional goal.
3. **Choose the task.** The task needs to be "transfer appropriate." Make a decision to have the patient perform one of the following:
   - The full pattern or function
   - A "part task" or limited range pattern, which is a natural subset or portion of the targeted task
   - An "adaptive training" task, in which an easier version of the targeted function is performed
4. **Apply a technique:** Choose a technique to target the observed impairment or functional limitation. Apply the technique to the movement pattern.
5. **Reevaluate responses and adjust inputs.** As the patient's response is observed, the facilatory inputs are adjusted to maximize their effect. Varying the task also has proven to be beneficial to learning. This can be achieved by changing the developmental level of the task to progress its difficulty. Another task, which addresses the same or another related impairment, may also be chosen.
6. **Integrate into function.** The final step is to integrate the gains from the technique into function. Whether a stretching, strengthening, or coordinating task has been performed, give the patient a chance to use the gains in a functional manner.

Procedures

PNF is a manual therapy approach to functional rehabilitation with specific guidelines regarding the procedures of patient handling.[1–3] Basic procedures of facilitation include body positioning and mechanics, manual contacts, manual and maximal resistance, irradiation, verbal and visual cuing, traction an approximation, stretch, and timing.

BODY POSITIONING AND MECHANICS

Be positioned "in the diagonal" or treatment plane whenever possible[12] (Fig. 14-4). Shoulders and hips face toward the direction of movement. Having your forearms in this plane is especially important. This positioning provides the best mechanics for manual cuing. The desired effects of manual contacts and resistance may be altered by even a slight deviation from this position.

MANUAL CONTACTS

The therapist uses contacts overlying the agonist muscle group to strengthen contractions or direct movement. Research indicates that the afferent input of contact over a muscle group is facilitating to that muscle through a polysynaptic pathway.[13] Movement requires a dynamic response from the trunk and proximal and distal limb segments in synergy; therefore, manual contacts can be applied to any of these areas to provide facilitation. To provide the contact, the therapist often uses the lumbrical grip (Fig. 14-5), a hallmark of PNF. This aides in keeping contacts and cues unidirectional.

The point of manual contact is slightly different in each individual because of variations in anatomic structure and neuromuscular control. The therapist needs to identify the specific point of manual contact. This location is the point at which a maximal response in the correct direction is facilitated. The manual contacts used to facilitate these individual patterns vary in treatment, depending on the desired movement response and need for emphasis in the facilitation. The contacts need to provide the patient with a sense of security and the therapist with proper leverage to apply appropriate resistance and cuing throughout the desired movement.

The therapist may plan for a direct effect, contacting the target group, or an indirect effect, contacting the synergist or antagonists to the targeted group. The therapist then may apply the proper inputs for the desired response.[3] There are other variations:

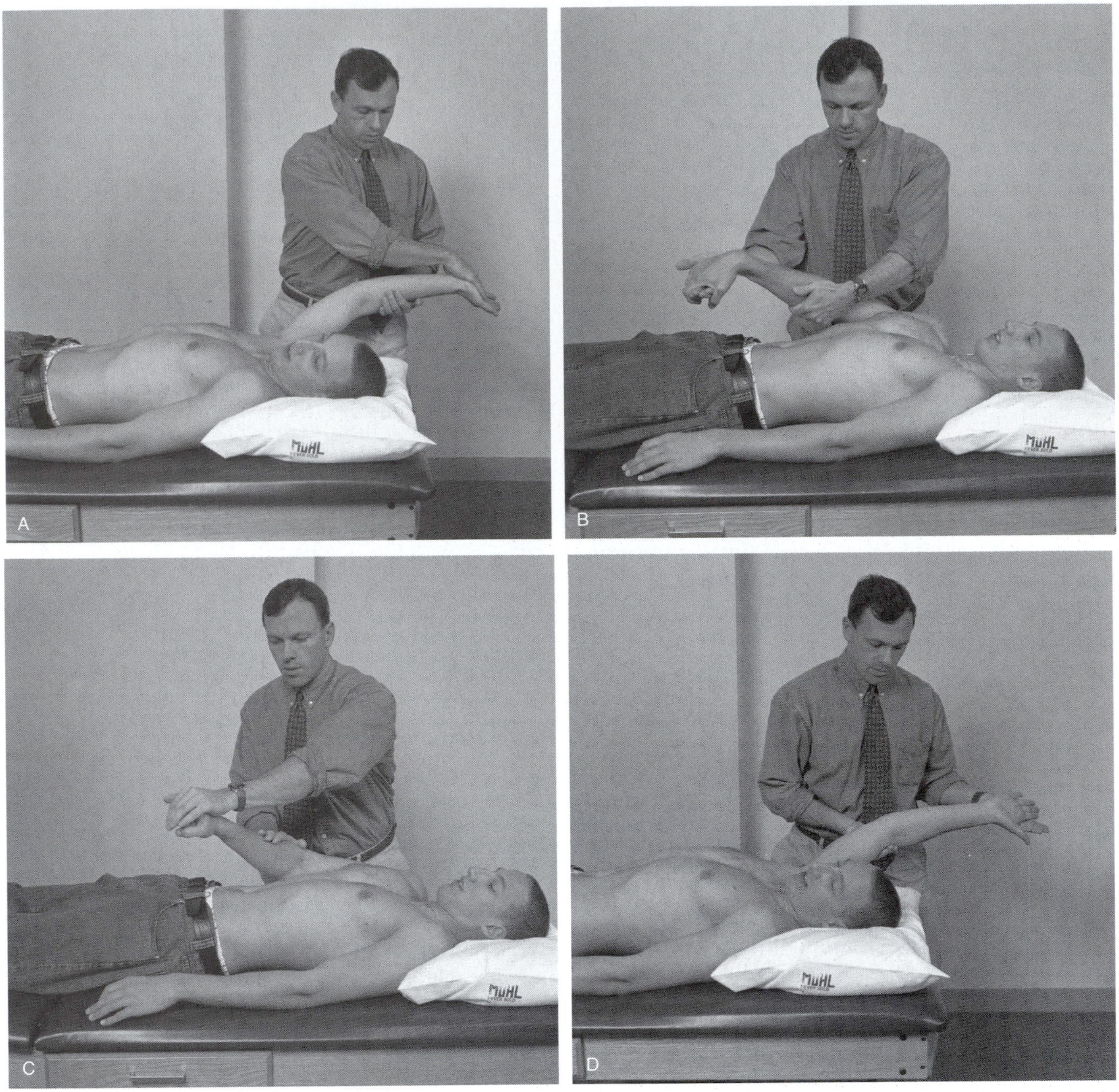

FIGURE 14-3 Pattern of facilation: ***(A)*** starting point for D2EX pattern with elbow straight. ***(B)*** Ending point for D2EX pattern with elbow straight. ***(C)*** Starting point for D2FL pattern with elbow straight. ***(D)*** Ending point for D2FL pattern with elbow straight. Note that the starting point or "lengthened range" for one pattern in the diagonal is the end point or "shortened range" for the antagonist pattern. A practical tip for finding the correct manual contacts and body mechanics for the therapist is to start by positioning the patient at end range of the pattern to be performed, making certain your handholds will be effective at that point and to "wind up" the extremity to the lengthened range.

- ROM within a pattern
- Speed of contraction
- Type of muscle contraction
- Number of repetitions
- Direction and quantity of resistance for emphasis[1–3]

MANUAL AND MAXIMAL RESISTANCE

A classic therapeutic exercise principle, demonstrated by Delorme,[13] is that resistance to motion enhances muscle activation. In PNF, the direction, quality, and quantity of resistance is adjusted to prompt a smooth and coordinated response, whether for stability (ie, holds) or for ease, smoothness, and pace of movement. The resistance should be appropriate to prompt proper irradiation and facilitate function. The amount of resistance applied to a dynamic (isotonic) contraction should be no greater than the resistance that allows full ROM to occur. For a static (isometric) contraction, the therapist should gradually build to the greatest amount of resistance tolerated without defeating or breaking the patient's hold.[1]

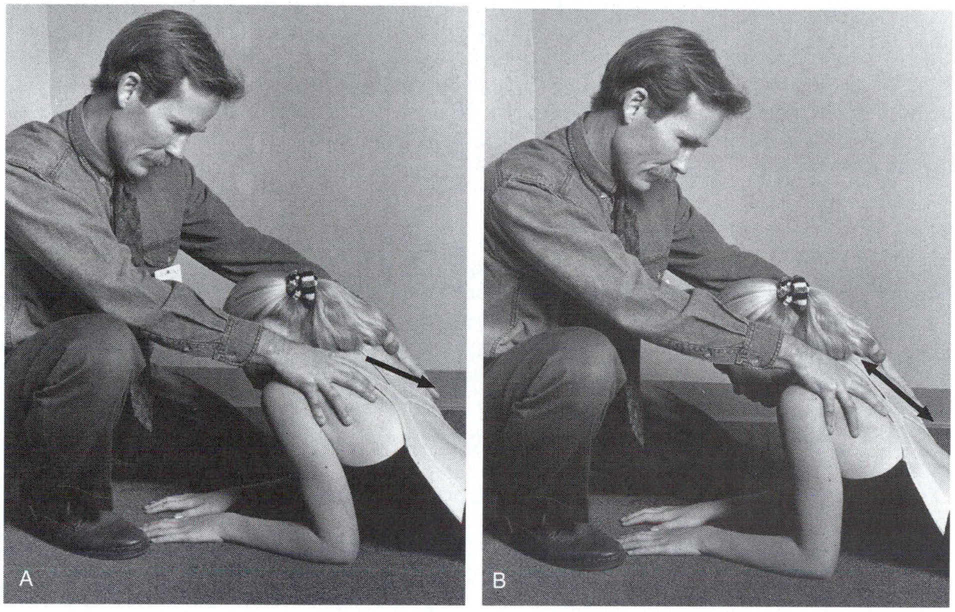

FIGURE 14-4 Therapist positioned in the diagonal or treatment plane, with the forearms, shoulders and hips facing toward the direction of movement.

When applying resistance, consider the treatment goal:

- Power or endurance
- Quality of movement
- Presence of spasticity

IRRADIATION

Irradiation, also called overflow, is the spread of energy from the prime agonist to complementary agonists and antagonists within a pattern.[14] Irradiation can occur from proximal to distal muscle groups, distal to proximal, upper trunk to lower trunk (and vice versa), and from one extremity to another. Weaker muscle groups benefit from the irradiation they gain while working in synergy with stronger, more normal partners.[9,15] PNF is based on the belief that contacting and applying the proper inputs to the synergists or antagonists of a target group is more effective than conventional resistance exercises, which target a single muscle group.

The therapist may stimulate irradiation through the use of resistance. According to Sherrington, the response can be excitatory or inhibitory.[16] The increase in effort to overcome resistance changes the excitation of motor neurons. As motor neurons respond, it is thought that they create a spread of energy from the agonists to "coagonists" at distant sites to assist with task completion. As the amplitude of the agonist contraction increases, antagonists that are usually reciprocally inhibited at low levels of resistance may become facilitated in cocontraction.[17] Another explanation is that excitation in stabilizers or fixators enhances the biomechanical advantage of the agonist group.[18–20]

The therapist learning the PNF approach is often instructed to "treat the good extremity first," creating an irradiation pattern from the contralateral side and a motor template for the desired task. Combined movements of extremity patterns have predictable irradiation patterns within an intact nervous system; Figure 14-2 reviews combined movement patterns. The bilateral combinations of extremity motion have different effects on the trunk. Symmetric movements promote trunk flexion or extension, whereas reciprocal movements promote trunk rotation. Asymmetric movements combine trunk flexion or extension with rotation and lateral bending. Cross-diagonals use opposite limb movements to produce a stabilizing force in the trunk.[21] The therapist can selectively choose the appropriate type of pattern or movement to elicit the desired response from the trunk for a function.

VERBAL CUING

The timing and tone of verbal cues are chosen carefully by the therapist and are a hallmark of PNF. Effective verbal cues coordinate the therapist's efforts with the patient's. Cues should be clear, concise, and appropriate to the patient's individual needs and comprehension.[1–3] Commands frequently start off by detailing a particular patient response ("lift your toes and pull up and across") and then change to more simple cues for subsequent repetitions ("and pull; good . . . again").

Verbal cuing during treatment becomes goal dependent. A skilled therapist uses a quiet voice to promote concentration or inhibit hypertonus and a progressively louder voice

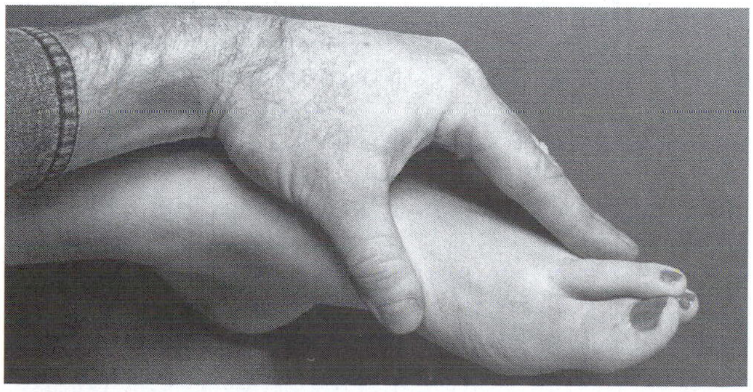

FIGURE 14-5 The lumbrical grip.

to encourage greater recruitment or progressively greater ROM in a task or pattern. Cues can also prompt the initiation of movement ("squeeze and pull up and across"), the timing of reversals or reciprocal movements ("push and pull and push . . ."), or remind the patient of a functional task that facilitates an established motor pattern or engram ("reach to touch my face").

APPROXIMATION AND TRACTION

Handling techniques are designed to maximize the output or response by the patient. Approximation (ie, compression), as evidenced in weight-bearing joints, stimulates receptors to facilitate cocontraction and stability around the joint.[22] The effects of approximations are employed by the therapist through the use of weight-bearing developmental postures or by adding manual force into gravity.

For example, a young athlete with a recent medial meniscus strain has difficulty with vastus medialis oblique recruitment during straight-leg raises. By coupling light compression through the knee with the limb in an unlocked extended position with verbal cues to "hold," cocontraction of vastus medialis oblique and hamstrings can be facilitated. This can be an effective technique in which full weight in gravity creates pain and inhibition.

Traction separates joint surfaces, provides a stretch stimulus, and enhances movement by elongating the adjacent muscles.[17] Commonly used with pulling movements, traction can be used selectively in the presence of pain to inhibit excessive compression. For example, physiologic mobilization in grades I and II of spinal joints are traditionally suggested to inhibit pain.[23] If mild distraction is added, the amplitude of such mobilizations can frequently be increased, enriching mechanoreceptor stimulation and hastening progression toward functional ranges of motion in treatment.

STRETCH

Whenever appropriate, the therapist promotes reflexive activity that is facilitating. Stretch is frequently performed at the starting position of a pattern or movement (ie, lengthened range) and produces further muscle elongation. The resulting reflex activation is then synchronized with volitional effort through verbal cues ("pull").

Resistance through the entire available range provides continued stretch through tension. Stretch can be repeated at the start of the range or superimposed during a pattern to redirect or strengthen a patient's response.[1–3] Because the muscle spindle is sensitive to microns of motion, be careful to keep the amplitude and vigor of the stretch stimulus appropriate. To rely on this reflex response, the targeted muscle group must possess tone at rest and not be flaccid.

TIMING

Timing describes the sequencing of motion. Normal timing requires proper coordination and proportional contribution from proximal and distal muscle groups.

Timing for emphasis suggests that, to facilitate an enhanced muscular response, the therapist can intentionally interrupt the normal timing sequence at specific points in the ROM and apply specific contacts to promote an optimal response.[1–3]

Techniques of Facilitation

With its basis in the neurophysiologic work of Sherrington,[17] the PNF techniques of facilitation were developed to tap into the "circuitry" of the nervous system. Whether applied to formal patterns or to functional movement, reflex responses and the predictable patterns of facilitation and inhibition are skillfully manipulated by the therapist. These techniques are based on Sherrington's principles of

- Irradiation: Energy is channeled from stronger to weaker muscle groups or patterns.
- Successive induction: An increased response of the agonist results after contraction of its antagonist.
- Reciprocal innervation: Facilitation of the agonist results in simultaneous inhibition of the antagonists.[17]

These techniques are proving to be valuable adjuncts in other treatment approaches such as joint mobilization, myofascial release, and stabilization exercises. They are being adapted also in aquatics, sports medicine, and other therapeutic environments. The techniques include[3]

- Rhythmic initiation
- Repeated stretch and repeated contractions
- Reversals of antagonists: dynamic reversals, stabilizing reversals, rhythmic stabilization
- Hold and relax
- Contract and relax
- Combination of isotonics

Techniques directed at facilitating the agonist muscle group follow the next few sections. Information regarding the basic goals of the techniques are accompanied by a clinical example of how it may be put to use. Each example contains a description of how to use patient positioning, verbal commands, manual contacts, stretch, repetition, and timing and how to make conscious choices to maximally facilitate the desired outcome.

RHYTHMIC INITIATION

The goal of rhythmic initiation is to improve the ability of the target agonist to direct and begin movement. By starting with passive movement in a chosen direction or pattern, encouraging gradual patient participation, and resisting the patient as performance improves, the therapist can cue the direction, rate, and sense of the movement while building motor output. In many cases, this approach also promotes a reflexive relaxation response.

In deciding on the ROM in an exercise, the therapist must decide if the full or a partial range of a pattern or task is to be attempted to maximally facilitate the agonist. By this repetitive approach, a weak or paralyzed patient initiates rolling by "pumping up" the nervous system. Do not be overly concerned with the detail of the pattern if the functional goal is being achieved with good quality.

Rhythmic initiation also helps set a selected rate of movement. This application is particularly helpful with patients who suffer from rigidity (eg, parkinsonism) or severe spasticity. For example, standing behind a subject holding two canes, it is possible to facilitate upper trunk rotation by grasping the canes and facilitating arm swing. Try this before and then during walking, and remember the power of verbal cuing ("reach, and reach, and reach, . . . and reach!"). Display 14-3 provides a sample exercise that uses rhythmic initiation. Rhythmic initiation may be used to

- Initiate movement
- Define the direction or pattern of movement
- Set the appropriate rate of movement
- Improve coordination and sense of motion
- Promote general relaxation

REPEATED CONTRACTIONS

Temporal and spatial summation are key to facilitation and movement reeducation. Spatial summation results from overlapping multiple facilitating inputs simultaneously to promote excitation of a maximal response (ie, positioning, contracts, resistance, stretch, and verbal cuing). In temporal summation, facilitation occurs by grouping repeated inputs close together in time to promote the desired response.[16]

The technique of repeated contractions repeatedly elongates the agonist muscle groups to reintroduce reflexive output. The therapist must resist the response to stretch. The timing of the verbal cues is also critical to success.

When the therapist's stretch occurs in the fully lengthened range, the technique is called repeated stretch. When the restretch occurs within the active ROM, it is called repeated contractions. When performed midrange, this technique can help to redirect the patient's movement pattern. As new range is achieved, the therapist may want to facilitate a stabilizing dynamic (isotonic) contraction by adding slight approximation and telling the patient to "hold." The technique can commence again after the hold with a restretch. Display 14-4 provides a sample exercise that uses repeated contractions. Repeated contractions may be used to

- Help to initiate movement
- Strengthen the agonist movement pattern from lengthened range
- Strengthen the agonist movement pattern from within the available active ROM
- Redirect motion within a pattern or task

REVERSALS OF ANTAGONISTS

Reversing movement patterns that afford the body balance and postural stability is key to many functional

DISPLAY 14-3
Sample Exercise Using Rhythmic Initiation

Goal

Joe Newman complains of shoulder pain while throwing a ball. The goal of treatment may be to improve the following:

1. Faulty timing of trunk or scapula (proximal) and extremity (distal) motions
2. A flat plane of arm motion during delivery
3. Poor follow through

Implementation

- Standing slightly to the right of Joe, a right-handed thrower, start your re-education with your right hand cuing his right hand and your left hand on his right anterior shoulder.
- With a cue of "Let me move you," demonstrate passively the desired diagonal path, directing the motion of the limb and trunk in an efficient pattern.
- Focus on the elements of range for follow through, staying in the upright path and keeping appropriate timing of the proximal and distal components.
- Repeating your passive movement pattern, instruct Joe and his proprioceptors about your desired results.
- Next, ask Joe, "Help me a little."
- Maintain the timing, range, and path while transitioning to active assistive movement.
- Redirect the timing, path, or range if Joe's efforts do not match yours.
- As Joe responds appropriately, add resistance and say, "Now pull down and across, and again!"
- Progressively build your resistance to reinforce the weight shift, the trunk flexion with rotation, and proper contributions of the proximal and distal components.
- Try to maintain appropriate resistance throughout the movement.

DISPLAY 14-4
Sample Exercise Using Repeated Contractions

Goal

Anna Lewis presents with glenohumeral dysfunction. Scapular stabilizer weakness has been identified by many researchers as a deficiency contributing to glenohumeral dysfunction. The goal of treatment in this example is to initiate lower trapezius function from the lengthened range.

Implementation

- Try starting with the prone-on-elbows position.
- Stand or kneel in front of Anna, placing your hands over the inferior half of each scapula, below the scapular spine.
- Passively pull or glide the left scapula into elevation, elongating the scapula depressors.
- With a gentle additional stretch and coupled cue ("Pull!"), stretch the lower trapezius, and resist its reflexive response as soon as it is felt.
- As you feel the resisted response start to wane, immediately restretch to the lengthened range and repeat the cue ("Pull again!").
- This input can be repeated as long as it proves effective in increasing muscle recruitment. Repetitions can be dosed to increase strength and endurance.
- Follow-up with a functional motion requiring the lower trapezius to function as a stabilizer and use of manual cues to maximize its response, are recommended.

DISPLAY 14-5
Sample Exercise Using Dynamic Reversals of Antagonists

Goal

Bob Desmond has trouble rolling in bed. He is recovering from a mild stroke and has difficulty with coordination and fine motor control in his right upper extremity. The goal is to improve independence in rolling to the left in bed and proximal control of the right upper quadrant to increase upper extremity function.

Implementation

For a better understanding of this example, refer to Figure 14-6.

- Biomechanically, rolling from supine to prone typically requires head and upper trunk flexion, with rotation in the direction of the roll. From sidelying left, for example, the motion of the head and right scapula to the left can be resisted as the patient initiates rolling. (Contacts: The therapist's right hand is over the anterior deltoid and humeral head. The left hand contact cnsists of fingertip pressure over the left brow, with the fingers pointing in the direction of the roll to gently cue neck flexion and rotation.)
- The cue is "Tuck your chin and roll left!" This midrange starting position is selected to benefit from the effects of gravity and decrease the inhibitory effects of tonic reflexes from the supine position.
- As the power begins to fade, release the scapular contact while still cuing at the head.
- By placing the right palm over the supraspinatus fossa and posterior aspect of the acromion process, a gentle stretch can be applied to the scapula, accompanied by a succinct verbal cue to "Push back and roll . . . look at me!"
- As the reversal of the roll begins to take shape, seize the opportunity to quickly and accurately replace the left (head) hand to resist neck extension and rotation or side bending right as its power builds. This placement should be posterolateral to the crown of the head.
- As the roll returns the patient to sidelying, switch your "scapular" hand again to the position over the anterior deltoid, restretching into a relative position of posterior elevation (the lengthened range for any motion is the shortened range of its antagonist). Light traction applied through the movement can help to "jumpstart" the agonist group.
- Repeat the process, attempting to build the range and strength of the roll to the left.
- Take care to select the optimal point for cue reversals. Effective stretch and secure contacts are key elements of facilitation.

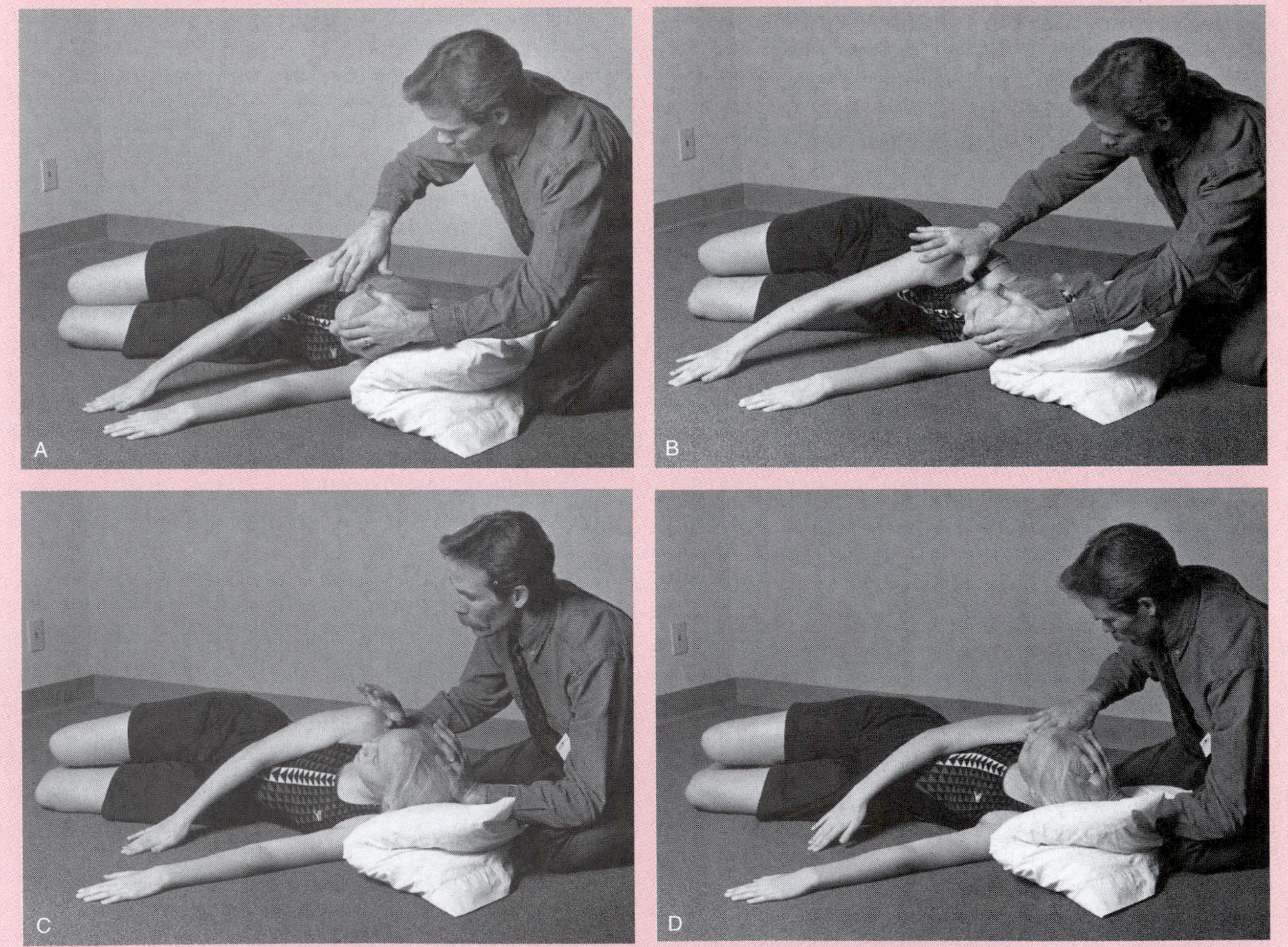

FIGURE 14-6 ***(A)*** Reversing patterns of neck flexion with scapular anterior depression. ***(B)*** Transition between motions. Here the therapist's forehead contact continues to facilitate rolling towards prone, while the other hand is positioned on the scapula to reverse into rolling toward supine. ***(C)*** Neck extension with scapular posterior elevation. ***(D)*** Preparing to reverse motion, note change in scapular contact.

tasks. The reciprocal activity of the limbs in the swing compared with stance phases of walking (ie, flexion adduction [swing] and extension abduction [stance]) demonstrate this. Additional examples include sawing, chopping wood, rowing a boat, running, and grasping and releasing objects.

The principle of successive induction provides that the agonist is facilitated after contraction of the antagonist.[16] To promote facilitation of the agonist, a better balance between the agonist and its antagonist is needed. To facilitate static and dynamic postural balance, reciprocal movements of the antagonistic groups are facilitated with static (isometric) or dynamic (isotonic) contractions. When movement is the intention, dynamic reversals of antagonists use push-pull–type dynamic (isotonic) contractions. Holds can also be added as appropriate ("push, now pull, now push, and hold that push"); this is a dynamic reversal hold. By using alternating dynamic (isotonic) contractions, during which the therapist's resistance prevents the motion, stabilizing reversals are performed.[3] The patient's intention in this case is to move only if static (isometric) contractions are used; stability is the focal goal. The technique is called rhythmic stabilization.

Dynamic Reversals of Antagonists

Reciprocal or reversing motions are enhanced by the technique of dynamic reversals. In this technique, dynamic (isotonic) contractions of antagonistic movements are facilitated reciprocally in a range appropriate to the goal of the exercise. The movements can be cued to increase range as strength and control improve or scaled down through repeated reversals to enhance stability.

These techniques can be applied to the activities of daily living, self-care activities, and isolated patterns of movement. Rolling is an example of one such application. Although the specific impairments limiting the ability to roll may vary, the therapist may use reversals in rolling to maximize independence. Display 14-5 provides a sample exercise that uses dynamic reversals of antagonists. Dynamic reversals are used to

- Increase active ROM
- Improve strength in the available ROM
- Improve balance and coordination of antagonists
- Improve endurance of antagonistic patterns

Stabilizing Reversals

Balance and stability are enhanced by stabilizing reversals. This is achieved by applying alternating resistance to an agonist–antagonist pair and seeking a maximal dynamic (isotonic) contraction. The therapist grades the resistance to facilitate a unidirectional hold, preventing the patient's attempts to move. This technique is similar in many ways to rhythmic stabilization, but it can also be used when a patient is unable to perform a true static (isometric) contraction.

This technique facilitates stability in a new or difficult ROM. During a treatment session in which the patient transfers to a new posture, range, or weight-bearing status, the implementation of stabilizing reversals may prove valuable to integrate the new abilities into function. Display 14-6 provides a sample exercise that uses stabilizing reversals of antagonists. Stabilizing reversals are used to

- Improve balance and stability
- Improve strength
- Integrate a new posture or ROM into function

> **DISPLAY 14-6**
> **Sample Exercise Using Stabilizing Reversals**
>
> **Goal**
> William Tavish, age 68, is status post total hip arthroplasty. The goal of treatment is to improve decreased range of motion (ROM) in hip extension and lack of stability in late stance phase of gait.
>
> **Implementation**
> - While in the parallel bars, have William stand in a staggered stance position with the involved extremity a small distance ahead. His hands should be on the bars and open, not grasping.
> - You can effectively resist the forward weight shift to the involved leg by a manual contact at the pelvic crest, with pressure aimed downward toward the heels. Your verbal cues are, "Push into my hands. Stand tall!"
> - After William has come as far forward as his hip joint flexibility and hip, and trunk strength allows, tell him to "Keep pushing your hips here; don't let me push you back!"
> - Build your resistance to recruit gluteals and trunk extensors, watching for excessive lordosis.
> - Then, release one of your hands from the pelvis and place it over the patient's scapula on the same side to resist the trunk from behind. "Now, don't let me pull you forward!"
> - After he responds to the new resistance, you can change the second hand to the posterior surface of the trunk with a pelvic or scapular contact, whichever gives you the best stabilizing response.
> - Continue sequencing the reversals as you build the patient's balance and stability in this late stance position.
> - When used after joint mobilization and muscle stretching techniques, this technique is effective in integrating the new ROM into function.

Rhythmic Stabilization

Cocontraction of antagonists is the goal of rhythmic stabilization. The technique can be performed at any point in a given ROM. The keys are to slowly build resistance; make smooth, coordinated transitions between antagonists; and ensure that the resistance promotes stability and does not break the patient's hold. Rhythmic stabilization is used to

- Improve strength of antagonists
- Improve balance of antagonists
- Improve stability
- Increase active and passive ROM following the technique
- Decrease pain by reflexive relaxation

Display 14-7 provides a sample exercise that uses rhythmic stabilization.

DISPLAY 14-7

Sample Exercise Using Rhythmic Stabilization

Goal

Elizabeth Curtis became a C5 quadriplegic after a spinal fracture sustained in a motor vehicle accident. She has fair balance in long sitting. The goal is to improve trunk control and upper extremity strength while increasing stability in long sitting.

Implementation

An excellent strategy in rehabilitation is to try to treat the patient in his position of function. Compared with the able-bodied population, a person with a spinal cord injury often spends more time in long sitting (for dressing, bed mobility and transfers).

- Kneel behind Elizabeth, who is positioned in long sitting, with arms extended.
- Allow Elizabeth to chose a hand position forward of or behind the greater trochanter, whichever promotes the best stability to start.
- Place one of your hands anteriorly over the humeral head and the other over the scapular spine on the other shoulder.
- Add a bit of approximation through both hands to promote stability.
- Slowly build your resistance with appropriate vigor at each hand to promote a maximal response. "Hold; don't let me twist you!" is your cue.
- While maintaining your contact at the weaker side, reverse the contact at the free hand and start to build the new direction of resistance there. Be certain to maintain the hold through the transition: "Keep holding." Your intonation should be encouraging but not excitatory, which may break the hold.
- Reverse the second hand, gradually decreasing its input before removing it and then gradually rebuilding its input as it shares the manual cuing in the new combination. Simultaneous switching of both hands often causes the hold to be lost. Take care to keep the manual contacts pure and unidirectional from each hand.
- By altering Elizabeth's hand position after initial success with this technique, it is possible to progress the difficulty of this exercise and further integrate the sitting balance into function.
- By having Elizabeth lift an arm and continue to stabilize, progression can be made up the developmental ladder and toward greater functional independence.

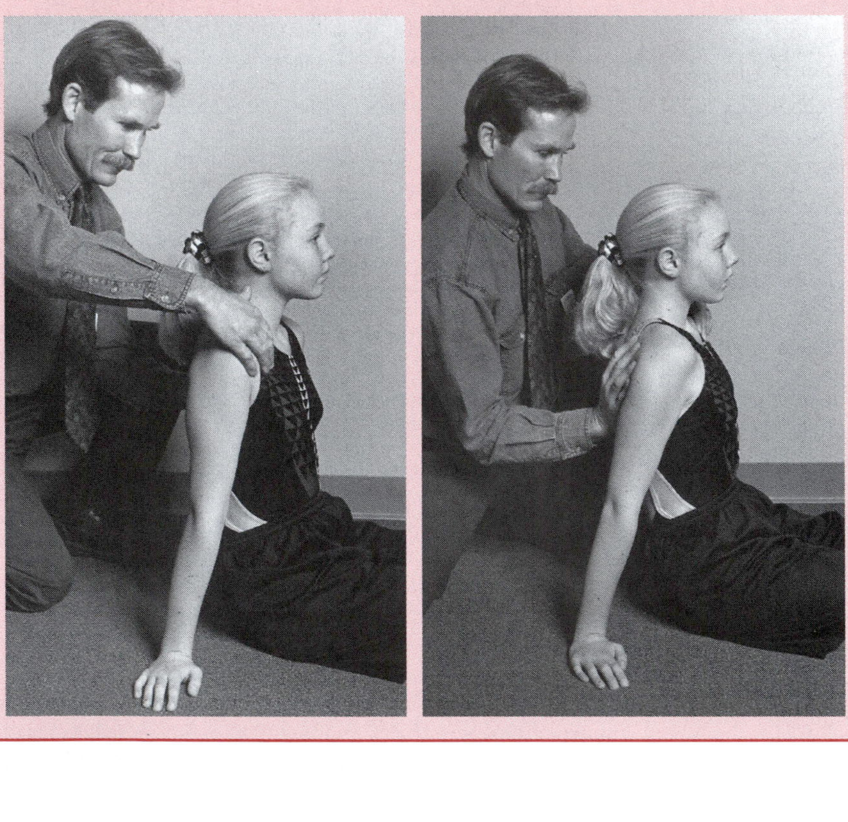

FIGURE 14-7 Example of rhythmic stabilization performed in long sitting. Therapist slowly changes resistance from flexor to extensor surface while maintaining resistance on opposite side.

HOLD AND RELAX

Reflex relaxation is the goal of the hold and relax technique. Relaxation may allow an increase in passive ROM and may help to decrease pain related to excessive tension. Sherrington's concepts of reciprocal innervation and successive induction call for inhibition of the antagonist during an agonist contraction and inhibition of a muscle group immediately after its contraction.[16] By using this phenomenon, the hold–relax and contract-relax techniques are valuable adjuncts to muscle stretching.

In the hold–relax technique, after reaching the end range of the agonist pattern, a "hold" (static) contraction is performed against gradually building resistance. The goal is a maximum pain-free response. After the ensuing *relax phase,* the new agonist range is achieved, and the process is repeated. This technique is helpful when the patient is experiencing pain. In facilitating the *hold phase,* take care to avoid pain and not break the patient's holding contraction.

Relaxation techniques are effective when used in conjunction with formal joint mobilization and manual therapy.[23] Display 14-8 demonstrates the use of the hold-relax technique with a common manual therapy technique. Hold and relax may be used to

- Improve passive ROM
- Provide relaxation
- Reduce pain

CONTRACT AND RELAX

The goal of the contract–relax technique is relaxation of the antagonist to a desired motion. A dynamic (isotonic) contraction of the antagonist is performed, allowing only the rotation component to occur against maximal resistance. After the contract phase, ask the patient to relax; the passive motion into the agonist pattern is achieved. As with the hold–relax technique, a key component in integrating the new range is resistance of the agonist after the relaxation phase.

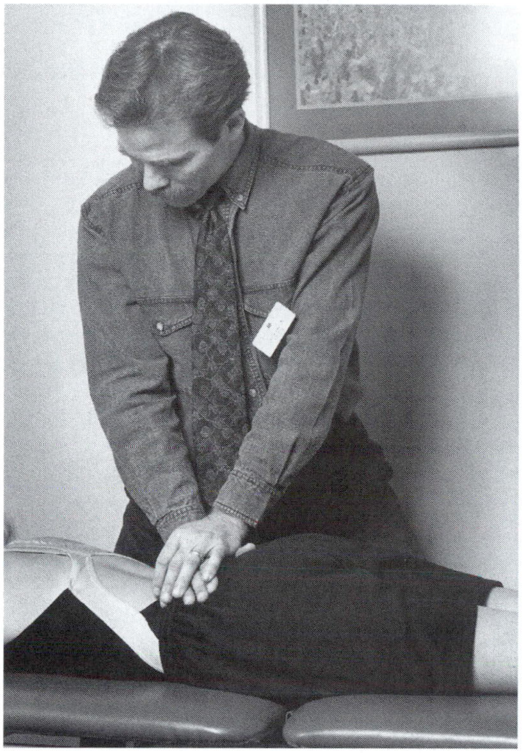

FIGURE 14-8 Example of posterior to anterior mobilization of L5 on the sacrum using hold-relax.

DISPLAY 14-8

Sample Exercise Using the Hold–Relax Technique

Goal

Mary Brown presents with a diagnosis of lumbar sprain, which occurred as a result of a lower back injury 3 weeks ago. Your objective tests include active range of motion assessment, palpation, a neurologic examination and passive intervertebral motion testing. You determine that Mary has pain with passive extension mobilization in prone and flexion in sidelying, with the focus on the dysfunction and pain at the L5-S1 segment. Mary has been unable to make headway with the lumbar flexion exercises prescribed by the physician, and says, "I'm just too tense and in too much pain." The goal is to mobilize the L5-S1 segment to promote relaxation, reduce the pain, and improve spinal mobility.

Implementation

- You position Mary in a prone position with a pillow under the abdomen to maintain the lumbar spine in a neutral position.
- You notice that a grade I P/A (posterior to anterior) glide of L5 is pain-free, and you can increase it to a slightly larger excursion, but less than 50% of normal accessory range.
- You maintain your pressure just below the pain threshold and tell Mary, "Hold." The goal is for Mary to try to isometrically tighten or cocontract, avoiding pain.
- After about a 6-second hold, you tell Mary, "Take a deep breath . . ., and relax."
- As the patient exhales, you can perform P/A mobilization in the new pain-free range of L5 on the sacrum (Fig. 14-8).
- Repeat this process to increase the pain-free range of motion.
- This passive technique should be followed by an agonist contraction to integrate the new pain-free range. In this case, a gluteal set or bridging will irradiate to the lumbar extensor and provide this integration function.

Many acquired orthopedic conditions surface as a result of muscle imbalances.[24,28] Therapeutic intervention with these problems must focus on re-establishing a balance between agonists and antagonists and re-educate their recruitment patterns in function. This is accomplished by shortening the lengthened group and lengthening the shortened group. Display 14-9 provides a sample exercise that uses contract and relax. The contract-relax technique is used to

- Improve passive ROM
- Provide relaxation

COMBINATION OF ISOTONICS

The techniques of rhythmic initiation and repeated stretch are designed to facilitate the concentric component motion of a given movement pattern. However, many activities require a mix of concentric, eccentric, and maintained dynamic (isotonic) contractions. The goal of a combination of isotonics is to integrate the movement by varying the type of agonist contraction required for function. It is solely an agonist–direction technique, but like all other techniques, it is rarely used alone during treatment (see Self-Management: Bridging Sequence). Display 14-10 provides a sample exercise that uses a combination of isotonics. The combination of isotonicsis used to

- Integrate the components of dynamic (isotonic) contractions, concentric, eccentric and maintained
- Increase strength of agonist

DISPLAY 14-9

Sample Exercise Using the Contract–Relax Technique

Goal

Holly Carson presents with chronic plantar fasciitis, which presents a challenge in controlling the inflammatory process and modifying pathomechanics. Physical therapy treatment usually involves antiinflammatory modalities, control of forces borne on the fascia, and stretching exercises. Myofascial release can be used effectively as an adjunct in this process. Muscle biasing results in part from stimulation of stretch receptors situated in the fascia. Releasing undo tension in that tissue can amplify the effects of selected therapeutic exercises by speeding tissue adaptation. Myofascial release to the plantar flexor or long toe flexor groups can be used during stretching and in conjunction with postural and gait retraining exercises to establish better muscle balance in the limb.

Implementation

- Ask Holly to lie prone on a treatment table with her toes approximately 6 inches past the table edge.
- Stand at the foot of the table with the plantar aspect of the Holly's foot resting against your thigh. By rocking forward, Holly's ankle can be brought into graded dorsiflexion.
- To perform the myofascial technique, place both hands palm down on the distal calf, near the end of the Achilles tendon.
- Leaning from the trunk and using a stacked lumbrical grip, exert deep pressure into the posterior calf and apply a massage stroke, moving proximally.
- Progress very slowly, as if moving a wave of tissue in front of your finger pressure.
- When a thickening or increased tension in the contractile elements of the calf is noted, exert mild dorsiflexion by leaning forward from your lower trunk. At the point where moderate passive tension is noted, tell the patient, "Push your foot into my thigh; keep pushing . . . and relax."
- The contraction phase should last about 3 to 6 seconds.
- As the relaxation response is noted, pick up the slack created in the fascial tissue and the ankle dorsiflexion (Fig. 14-9). Commonly, extreme tightness can be noted in the region of the musculotendinous junction of the gastrocnemius.
- After a set of multiple repetitions (10 to 15), tell the patient, "Now, push your heel at me!" This integrates the new range of motion with an agonist contraction to the end range. Try to resist a sustained hold at maximum stretch.
- Followup should include closed-chain exercises that encourage talocrural dorsiflexion while controlling pronation.

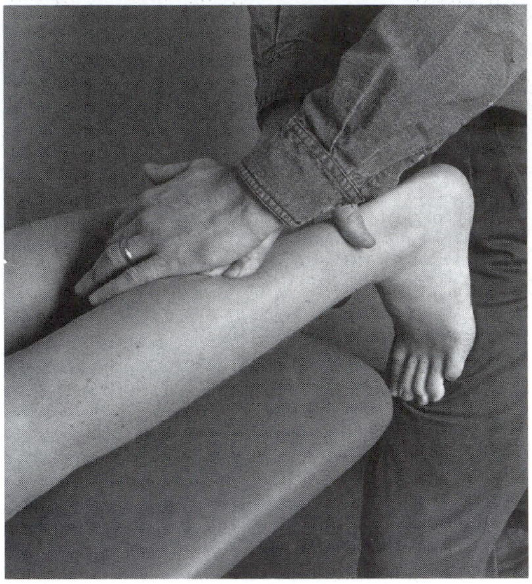

FIGURE 14-9 Coupling contract–relax with myofascial release.

- Increase active ROM
- Teach functional control

PATIENT EDUCATION

From the initial interaction with the patient, the therapist must be working toward independence and the development of an effective home program of care. Provide education and training directly to the patient or to family members and aides. When carried over to the home, manual handling and exercise techniques progress and prolong the

SELF-MANAGEMENT: *Bridging Sequence*

Purpose: To strengthen the gluteal muscles and lower trunk, while maintaining a neutral position of the lower back.

Position: Start by lying on your back with knees bent and feet flat, shoulder-width apart.

Movement Technique: Lift the pelvis off the floor by tightening the buttock muscles.

Raise to a comfortable height, being sure not to arch the lower back.

Hold this position 2 to 3 seconds.

Slowly lower halfway down, again holding this new position for 2 to 3 seconds.

Return to the "up" position, again focusing on preventing the arching tendency of the lower back.

For greater strength demands, try the same motion while holding a resistance band (supplied) across the pelvis during the exercise (see diagram). Be certain to monitor the position of the lower back during the exercise to prevent arching and pain. Progress to higher raises of the hips only as your strength and flexibility allow.

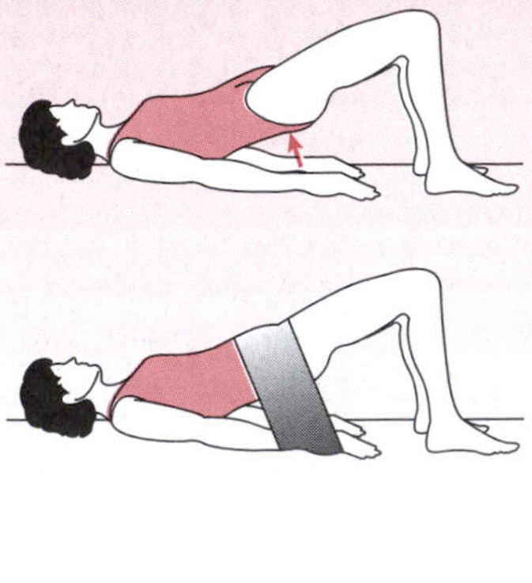

LAB ACTIVITIES

Rhythmic Stabilization

1. Start with your partner seated on the edge of his chair and with his feet on the floor. In this exercise, manually challenging your partner's sitting balance,
   a. Try resisting at one shoulder and then both.
   b. Resist at the pelvis; then try the head. Try a combination.
   c. Try varying the rate at which you apply resistance.
   d. Try resisting in the sagittal plane and then on a diagonal.
   e. Resist at both shoulders pushing from the front. Resist at both shoulders pulling from the rear. Try pulling with one and pushing with the other.
   f. Try adding approximation through the shoulders. Then try traction at the shoulders as if lifting the scapulae.

1. Which rate of resistance application facilitated strength and stability?
2. Which muscles were recruited from resistance at the different locations, with the different combinations?
3. Did straight or diagonal resistance promote the greatest recruitment of strength and stability?
4. What influences did anterior, posterior, and anterior-posterior pressures provide?
5. What happened by adding traction and approximation?

Irradiation

1. Start with your partner supine, close to you on the right side of a high treatment table.
   a. Resist your partner's right hip flexion and adduction through active ROM. Your left hand is on your partner's thigh and your right hand on the dorsum of his foot.
   b. Have your partner roll to sidelying, and repeat the movement.
   c. Repeat the sidelying task with your partner holding on to the far side of the table.
   d. Let your partner place the sole of his left foot against your thigh or pelvis for stability and have him repeat the resisted movement.

1. In which position could your partner tolerate the greatest resistance? Why?
2. In what part of the full ROM did your partner tolerate the strongest resistance? Why?
3. What influence did holding the table provide? What about placing your partner's opposite foot against you?
4. What happens in your partner's strongest part of the range if you focus your resistance on the dorsiflexing foot? What if the focus is on the hip flexing?

Have your partner practice rolling from sidelying toward prone to his left on a treatment table or mat. Next, make him work a bit harder to roll by holding back over his anterior right shoulder. You should be positioned in line with the rolling motion of his shoulders.

- As your partner rolls into gravity what happens to his ability to overcome your resistance?
- What do you notice happening if you exert strong resistance against your partner's shoulders rolling forward? Do other areas come in more strongly in an attempt to succeed in overcoming your resistance?
- What happens if you exert strong resistance as your partner tries to initiate rolling from the supine position toward prone?
- Notice the effect on your partner's ability if you change your position relative to his shoulders. Try changing the direction of your resistance off of your partner's line of movement. What happens to his strength?

PNF Approach

1. List the advantages of PNF as a therapeutic exercise approach.
2. List the disadvantages of PNF as a therapeutic exercise approach.

Patient Problem

A 30-year-old man has complaints of chronic shoulder pain. His diagnosis is impingement syndrome. Your findings include

- Painful arc from 90 to 110 degrees of flexion
- PROM limited to 125 degrees abduction
- Fair middle and lower trapezius strength
- Functionally unable to undress overhead
- Unable to sleep on the shoulder at night because of pain

Goals: scapulothoracic stability, glenohumeral mobility, functional needs for dressing, positioning for improved sleep at night, and decreased pain.

Devise a treatment plan or progression, including your response

- Treatment postures with their rationale
- Techniques of facilitation to be applied
- Which pattern or movement
- Range to be emphasized

Techniques

Which techniques would you consider if your patient demonstrates poor stance stability because of

1. Tight hip flexors
2. Weak gluteals
3. Hip pain
4. Ataxia

Demonstrate your choices of treatment postures, techniques, and handling skills with a laboratory partner. Discuss your thoughts.

DISPLAY 14-10

Sample Exercise Using a Combination of Isotonics

Goal

Tom Dewey is a 64-year-old man who fell 12 weeks ago and sustained a fracture to the right proximal femur. He currently shows decreased stance stability on the right in gait and some difficulty with coming to stand from lower chairs and the commode. The goal of treatment is to improve lower extremity strength, independence with sit to stand from low surfaces, and stance stability in gait.

Implementation

Bridging is a bilateral, symmetric, lower extremity pattern, typically incorporating hip extension, abduction, and knee extension. The most effective manual contact to resist bridging is over the anterior rim of the iliac crest, adjacent to the anterior superior iliac spine.

- The initial phase of the bridge is concentric, and the cues are a light manual stretch into further hip flexion while vocalizing, "Push up into my hands."
- As the maximum response begins to taper, change the cue: "Keep it there. Don't let me push you down!" The intention of the patient is to continue pushing up against a true hold.
- If you feel restretching from this hip-extended position could yield further facilitation, coordinate a manual cue with "Push some more, and again!"
- To control the eccentric phase, continue the resistance, and say to the patient, "Make me work to push you down . . . slowly."
- The sequence of the combination is determined by the output of the patient and your specific goals. The sequence could be bridge–side shift right–slowly lower–bridge–side shift left to center–slowly lower–bridge–side shift left–slowly lower, and so on. In this particular pattern, the goals may be
  1. Increased endurance (16 to 20 repetitions, less strenuous holds and combinations)
  2. Improved hip extension range of motion (few repetitions with multiple repeated contractions; holds at maximum range)
  3. Improved bed mobility (add a side scoot to the task)

benefits of clinical care, joint and soft-tissue mobility, strengthening, improved stability, and safety in self-care and activities of daily living.

Carefully choose exercise postures to challenge strength and stability at a level appropriate for the patient. Resistance is provided by gravity, manually, by adding free weights, or by using resistive tubing or bands. The quantity of resistance, range and rate of movement, repetitions and sets, and duration of the exercise session are dosed to meet the patient's physical and medical profile. Creative home programs combine specific patterns to isolate impairments with progression into functional tasks to promote transfer processing toward function. Techniques such as contract and relax, reversals of antagonists, and adding holds can be used to enhance more basic movement patterns.

Key Points

- PNF is a manual therapy approach that applies postures, movement patterns, contacts, cues, and goals, all of which are maximally facilitating.
- Treatment is based on improving function and using functions that are possible to reach those that are attainable as goals.
- PNF is not a treatment per se; it is a philosophy that lends itself to use as an adjunct to other treatment approaches in most therapeutic environments.

Critical Thinking Questions

1. Consider Case Study #8 in Unit 7. Describe PNF techniques indicated to improve this patient's
   a. Scapula posture
   b. Cervical spine mobility
   c. Lengthened rhomboids and lower trapezius
   d. Abdominal weakness
2. Consider Case Study #5 in Unit 7. Describe PNF techniques indicated to improve this patient's
   a. Standing balance
   b. Balance during gait
   c. Trunk posture during gait

REFERENCES

1. Voss D, Ionta M, Myers B. *Proprioceptive Neuromuscular Facilitation, Patterns and Techniques*. 3rd ed. Philadelphia: Harper & Row; 1985.
2. Knott M, Voss D. *Proprioceptive Neuromuscular Facilitation, Patterns and Techniques*. 2nd ed. Philadelphia: Harper & Row; 1968.
3. Adler S, Beckers D, Buck M. *PNF in Practice: An Illustrated Guide*. New York: Springer-Verlag; 1993.
4. Murphy W. *Healing the Generations: A History of Physical Therapy and the American Physical Therapy Association*. Lyme, CT: Greenwich Publishing Group; 1995:165–168.
5. *Webster's Collegiate Dictionary*. 10th ed. Springfield, MA: Merriam Webster; 1995.
6. Roberts S, Falkenberg S. *Biomechanics: Problem Solving for Functional Activity*. St. Louis: Mosby–Year Book; 1992.
7. Sullivan PE, Markos PD. *Clinical Decision Making in Therapeutic Exercise*. Norwalk, CT: Appleton & Lange; 1994.
8. Sullivan PE, Markos PD. *An Integrated Approach to Therapeutic Exercise: Theory and Clinical Application*. Reston, VA: Reston Publishing; 1982.
9. Kabat H. Studies on neuromuscular dysfunction, XI: new principles on neuromuscular reeducation. *Permanente Found Med Bull*. 1947:5:111–123.
10. Umphred D. *Neurological Rehabilitation*. 3rd ed. St Louis: Mosby, 1995.
11. Shumway-Cook A, Woolacott M. *Motor Control: Theory and Practical Application*. Baltimore: Williams & Wilkins; 1995.
12. Mangold ML, Harper L. Proprioceptive neuromuscular facilitation residency program. Vallejo, CA, January 1981.
13. Delorme TL, Watkins AL. Techniques of progressive resistive exercise. *Arch Phys Med*. 1948:29: 263.
14. Knutsson E. Proprioceptive neuromuscular facilitation. *Scand J Rehab Med Suppl*. 1980:7:106–112.

15. Hildebrandt FA. Application of the overload principle to muscle training in man. *Arch Phys Med Rehabil*. 1958:37:278–283.
16. Sherrington C. *The integrative action of the nervous system*. 2nd ed. New Haven, CT: Yale University Press; 1947.
17. Loofburrow GN, Gellhorn E. Proprioceptively induced reflex patterns. *Am J Physiol*. 1948:154:433–438.
18. Hellebrandt FA, Parrish AM, Houtz SJ. Cross education, the influence of unilateral exercise of the contralateral limb. *Arch Phys Med*. 1947:28:76–85.
19. Markos PD. Ipsilateral and contralateral effects of proprioceptive neuromuscular facilitation techniques on hip motion and electromyographic activity. *Phys Ther*. 1979:59:1366–1373.
20. Pink M. Contralateral effects of upper extremity proprioceptive neuromuscular facilitation patterns. *Phys Ther*. 1981:61: 1158–1162.
21. Winstein CJ. Designing practice for motor learning: clinical implications. *Proceedings of the II STEP Conference*, Norman, OK; 1990. Alexandria, VA: Foundation for Physical Therapy; 1991:65–76.
22. Wyke BD. Articular neurology: a review. *Physiotherapy*. 1972: 58:94–99.
23. Maitland GD. *Vertebral Manipulation*. 5th ed. London: Butterworths; 1986.
24. Sahrmann SA. *Diagnosis and Treatment of Muscle Imbalances and Musculoskeletal Pain Syndromes.* Course handout 1994. Washington University Program in Physical Therapy, St. Louis, MO.
25. Davies GJ, Dickoff-Hoffman S. Neuromuscular testing and rehabilitation of the shoulder complex. *Journal of Orthopedic and Sports Physical Therapy.* 1993;18:449–458.
26. Jobe FW, Pink M. Classification and treatment of shoulder dysfunction in the overhead athlete. *Journal of Orthopedic and Sports Physical Therapy.* 1993;18:427–432.
27. Wilk KE, Arriga C. Current concept in the rehabilitation of the athletic shoulder. *Journal of Orthopedic and Sports Physical Therapy.* 1993;18:365–378.
28. Kendall HO, Kendall FP, Boyton DA. *Posture and Pain*. Baltimore: Williams & Wilkins, 1952.

CHAPTER 15

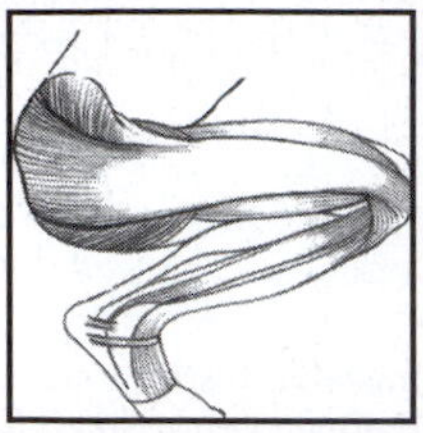

Closed Kinetic Chain Training

Susan Lefever-Button

Historically, the concepts and principles involving the disciplines of human kinesiology and the biomechanics of movement have been inextricably woven into the study of mechanical engineering, and understanding engineering concepts is essential in the study of human kinesiology. The kinetic chain concept originated in 1955, when Steindler[1] used mechanical engineering theories of closed kinematic and link concepts to describe human kinesiology. In the link concept, rigid overlapping segments are connected in a series by movable joints. This system allows for predictable movement of one joint based on the movement of the other joints and is considered a closed kinematic chain.[2,3] In the lower extremity of the human body, each bony segment can be viewed as a rigid link; bones of the foot, lower leg, thigh, and pelvis are seen as rigid links. Similarly, the subtalar, talocrural, tibiofemoral, and hip synovial joints act as the connecting joints.

Applying these concepts to human movement, Steindler[1] observed that two types of kinetic chains exist, depending on the loading of the "terminal joint." Steindler[1] classified these as an open kinetic chain (OKC) and a closed kinetic chain (CKC). He observed that muscle recruitment and joint motions were different when the foot or hand was free to move or met considerable resistance.[1] An OKC was described when the end segment is free to move.[1] Examples include the hip flexion of the swing limb during walking or waving the hand. In a CKC, "the terminal joints meet considerable external resistance which prohibits or restrains its free motion."[1] Examples include descending stairs or using the upper extremity during crutch walking.

The use of CKC exercises in rehabilitation began in the 1980s, when physicians began looking for safe ways to rehabilitate the quadriceps mechanism in patients after anterior cruciate ligament (ACL) reconstruction. During the 1960s and 1970s,[4,5] documentation in the biomechanics literature demonstrated an increase in the anterior shear forces during the last 30 degrees of OKC knee extension. Numerous researchers[6–10] thought that this increase in anterior shear placed a detrimental strain on the healing graft that could compromise the surgical result.

Using cadaveric experiments, Grood and associates[8] documented increased anterior tibial translation with OKC knee extension and subsequently suggested exercising in an upright posture to use the "forces of weight bearing" to minimize anterior tibial translation. Increased joint compressive forces, improved joint congruency, and muscular cocontraction are enhanced in a weight-bearing position.

Henning and colleagues[9] supported this hypothesis by the findings of an in vivo ACL strain study. By placing a strain gauge in the ACL of two volunteers, the amount of strain across the ACL was measured during various exercises, including isometric knee extension at 0 and 22 degrees and such daily activities as walking and stationary biking. It was found that isometric knee extension at 0 and 22 degrees placed more strain on the ACL than walking or stationary biking.

Although most of the scientific literature concerning CKC activities is focused on quadriceps rehabilitation after ACL reconstruction, contrasting research by Hungerford and Barry[11] evaluated patellofemoral contact pressure areas during OKC and CKC exercises. The investigators believed an OKC extension exercise, performed in the 0- to 30-degree range of knee flexion, resulted in high patellofemoral contact pressures because of the decreasing patellofemoral contact area with an increasing length of the moment arm as the limb assumed a more horizontal position. This same exercise performed in an upright CKC position resulted in a reduction of the force on the patellofemoral joint. As the limb position became more vertical, an increase in the patellofemoral contact area occurred with a decrease in the length of the moment arm.[11]

DEFINITIONS AND GOALS

CKC training is a method of exercise in which the end segment is fixed and "meets considerable external resistance, which prohibits or restrains its free motion."[1] This approach results in a predictable pattern of movement of the joints in the chain. For example, performing the CKC activity of sitting results in a predictable pattern of movement of the hip, knee, and ankle joints. Hip flexion depends on the amount of ankle joint dorsiflexion and knee joint flexion. The predominant muscle activity in this example is eccentric contraction of the hip and knee extensors. An example of CKC activity for the upper extremity is using the upper extremity to perform a wheelchair to bed transfer.

Open kinetic training is a method of exercise in which the end segment is free to move.[1] The movement of one joint does not result in a predictable movement pattern of any of the other joints in the chain. Examples include kicking a ball or reaching overhead to retrieve an object. The goal of CKC exercise is to use the forces of weight bearing and the effect of gravity to simulate functional activities, ultimately enabling patients to return to their usual environments and perform activities safely.

The following characteristics are common to CKC activities:

- Interdependence of joint motion (ie, knee flexion depends on ankle joint dorsiflexion)
- Motion occurring proximal and distal to the axis of the joint in a predictable fashion (eg, knee flexion is accompanied by hip flexion, internal rotation, and adduction and by ankle joint dorsiflexion and internal tibial rotation)
- Recruitment of muscle contractions that are predominantly eccentric, with dynamic muscular stabilization in the form of cocontraction
- Greater joint compressive forces resulting in decreased shearing
- Stabilization afforded by joint congruency
- Normal posture (weight bearing) and muscle contractions
- Enhanced proprioception because of the increased number of stimulated mechanoreceptors

The following are characteristics common to OKC activities:

- Independence of joint motion (eg, knee flexion is independent of ankle joint position)
- Motion occurring distal to the axis of the joint (eg, knee flexion results with motion of only the lower leg)
- Muscle contractions that are predominantly concentric
- Greater distraction and rotary forces
- Stabilization afforded by outside means
- Activation of mechanoreceptors limited to the moving joint and surrounding structures

All exercises cannot be classified as purely open chain or closed chain. A few investigators have tried additional classification schemes to add clarity to choosing appropriate exercises. Gray[12] and Panaviello[13] think the body weight must be supported and the end segment fixed to be classified as a CKC activity.

Palmitier[14] recommends thinking in terms of joint isolation exercises and kinetic chain exercises. Joint isolation exercises involve activities designed for only one joint. The motion produced by these exercises occurs only distal to the axis of the joint. These exercises do not take into consideration or depend on the position of other joints within the same limb. Examples include prone knee flexion or seated knee extension exercises. Alternatively, kinetic chain exercises involve the entire segment. The motion produced by muscular contraction occurs proximal and distal to the axis of the joint. Kinetic chain exercises depend on the position and motion of the all the joints linked in series.[14] Wall squats are an example of kinetic chain exercise.

Dillman and associates[15] also proposed an alternative classification system based on the biomechanics of the exercise—the mobility of the distal segment and the application of an external load. The researchers referred to the distal segment as the boundary. The boundary condition may be fixed or movable. An external load may or may not be present at the distal segment. They suggest the following classification: fixed boundary with an external load (FEL), movable boundary with an external load (MEL), and movable boundary no load (MNL). FEL corresponds to a CKC exercise, and MNL responds to OKC exercises. The MEL is a partially closed system.

Wilk and colleagues[3] presented a kinetic chain continuum, on which an exercise such as an isometric squat is at the extreme end of the CKC spectrum. A movement in which no body part was attached to the ground, as in a jumping, is at the extreme end of the OKC spectrum. Exercises are placed along the continuum relative to the status of the end segment and amount of external load. Squats and step-ups are closer to the CKC end, and seated leg extensions are closer to the OKC end.[3]

When choosing rehabilitative activities, it is important to consider the type of muscle contractions and joint motions necessary for the patient to achieve her optimum function. Different types of muscle contractions and joint motions occur during different types of kinetic chain exercises. For example, stationary cycling employs the use of a CKC movement; the foot is fixed to a pedal, and the foot meets resistance, but the foot is free to move, resulting in a predominance of concentric type of muscle contraction.[16,17] In this case, the proximal segment is fixed, and the distal segment is moving. Knee extension occurs as the medial aspect if the tibia moves anteriorly and laterally on a relatively fixed femur. Additional examples of similar types of CKC exercises using concentric muscle contraction of the hip and knee extensors include the use of a stair-climbing machine and knee extension using the seated leg press.

The CKC activity of descending stairs results in a fixed distal segment with the proximal segment moving. Knee extension is the result of the medial aspect of the femur moving posteriorly and medially over a relatively fixed tibia. The muscle action is eccentric contraction of the hip and knee flexors. When analyzing functional activities such as walking, descending stairs, or sitting, determining the type of muscle contractions and joint motions necessary to complete the task should help guide the decision-making process about the type of kinetic chain exercise to prescribe.

All closed chain exercises are not functional. Similarly, all open chain exercises should not be dismissed because they are non–weight-bearing activities.[2] A more pragmatic approach to choosing rehabilitation activities should be investigated; it is sometimes appropriate during rehabilitation to prescribe nonfunction CKC exercises. For example, consider a patient who is unable to stand from a seated position.

The patient presents with concentric quadriceps and hip extensor muscle weakness, mild knee joint anterior laxity, moderate tibiofemoral arthritis, and limited ankle dorsiflexion. Exercise should include stationary cycling because it requires concentric quadriceps, and hip extensor muscle contraction affords joint stability, decreases joint compressive forces, and allows the ankle to move freely. Consider another patient who presents with left arm hemiplegia and with a subluxated humeral head with anterior ligamentous laxity, poor stability of the humeral head in the glenoid fossa, poor scapulothoracic rhythm, and altered kinesthesia. Exercise should include upper extremity weight bearing with weight shifting to improve stability and enhance kinesthesia.

OKC exercises performed at the appropriate time and combined with CKC exercises performed according to the patient's needs and goals provide an integrated, comprehensive rehabilitation program.[18–20]

BASIC PHYSIOLOGIC PRINCIPLES OF CLOSED KINETIC CHAIN TRAINING

Muscular Contraction

CKC exercises stimulate muscular cocontractions, joint approximation, and joint congruency, thereby providing dynamic stabilization and postural holding around the joint.[21,22] Stability is enhanced in a weight-bearing position.[3–7] For example, weight-bearing activities decrease the amount of anterior shear across the ACL.[5–9,17] These activities stimulate cocontraction of the hamstring musculature, providing dynamic stabilization that results in improved postural holding and additional support for the joint.[14,23,24]

Biomechanical Factors

Biomechanical factors contributing to joint stability are accomplished through the geometry of the joint surfaces, joint approximation, and stimulation of joint receptors. The geometry of the joint surfaces appears to aid in the decrease of anterior tibial displacement in the loaded joint.[24,25] Controlling anterior tibial displacement has been accomplished in cadaveric studies by loading the knee joint.[25,26] CKC activities increase ankle joint approximation, enhancing joint congruency and contributing to joint stability.[27]

Additional support for using CKC exercises in rehabilitation is provided by the constant remodeling of tissues.[2] Wolff's law states that bone remodels according to the stresses placed on it. Areas of increased stress result in bone deposition. This theory has been extended to the remodeling of soft tissues. Collagen fibers organize themselves along lines of mechanical stress.[2] This is of particular importance when rehabilitating patients after ligamentous injuries. A gradual change in the mechanical stress through the injured tissue along biomechanically consistent lines can help strengthen the injured tissue and help it to resist reinjury.[2] It is important to place gradual mechanical stress on healing soft tissues by placing them in functional positions throughout the rehabilitation process. For example, when rehabilitating a patient with a medial deltoid ligament sprain to her ankle, the position of the foot during CKC exercises is important for controlling the amount of stress placed on the healing tissue. Allowing the subtalar joint to excessively pronate places an undesirable stress on the healing medial deltoid ligament.

Neurophysiologic Factors

Neurophysiologic support for using CKC activities in rehabilitation is provided by stimulation of the proprioceptive system. Proprioception is a specialized form of touch and is composed of the sensation of joint movement (ie, kinesthesia) and of joint position (ie, joint position sense).[28] The sensory receptors consist of mechanoreceptors and nociceptors found in muscles, joints, periarticular structures, and skin.[29] Four major types of joint receptors, the muscle spindle, the Golgi tendon organs, and cutaneous receptors have been identified as structures providing sensory input to the central nervous system (CNS).[29] Deformation and loading of the soft tissues surrounding a joint trigger the mechanoreceptors to convert this mechanical energy to electrical impulses.[28,30] The electrical impulses are transmitted to and integrated by the CNS to produce a motor response.[29,30]

Mechanoreceptors can be classified as rapidly or slowly adapting, depending on the type of stimulus. Rapidly adapting joint mechanoreceptors such as Pacini's corpuscles emit a rapid burst of impulses that declines quickly.[29,31] These rapidly adapting receptors are believed to detect a sudden change in joint motion (ie, acceleration or deceleration).[28,29] Slowly adapting mechanoreceptors emit a sustained level of impulse and are believed to detect the position of the limb in space and slow changes in position.[28,29]

The joint receptors include type I (Ruffini), type II (Golgi-Mazzoni or paciniform), type III (Golgi type), and type IV (free nerve endings) and are located in the joint capsules and ligaments.[31–33] Movement of a joint provides the CNS with continuous information about position and movement of that joint. Weight-bearing activities stimulate Type II and III joint receptors to generate a signal.[2,34]

Type I receptors are present in the fibrous layer of the joint capsule and are most widely distributed in the proximal joints.[34] These receptors monitor the rate and direction of joint movement and the angular position. Type I receptors respond when joint pressure is applied to the joint surfaces (ie, weight bearing).[31,32]

Type II receptors are small, encapsulated receptors found in tendon surfaces and the inner surface of the joint capsule. These receptors detect rapid joint movements and respond to deep pressure, perpendicular compression of the joint capsule as performed in a weight-bearing posture, and vibration.[32,34]

Type III receptors are present in intrinsic and extrinsic ligaments around joints.[31] Stimulation of type III receptors occurs according to the rate of joint movement and the force of gravity (ie, weight bearing).[31] CKC activities use the force of gravity to stimulate these receptors.

It has been hypothesized that a loss of mechanoreceptor feedback after joint injury results in the loss of protective muscular cocontraction, contributing to a cycle of repeated ligamentous injury and further joint instability.[35] The use of

CKC activities during rehabilitation can can stimulate these mechanoreceptors.[20,29] By encouraging muscular cocontractions through CKC exercises, the cycle of repeated ligamentous injury may be disrupted.[20]

Additional neurologic support for the use of CKC activities is provided by retraining balance and position sense after a joint injury. Balance (ie, postural control) is the ability of the body to maintain the center of mass over the base of support without falling.[36] This is an important motor skill. An individual senses her body position relative to gravity by combining visual, vestibular, and somatosensory (ie, proprioceptive) inputs.[36] Small adjustments in the ankle, hip, and knee are used to maintain the line of gravity over the base of support.[19,20,37] In a CKC movement, indirect forces from muscles of adjacent segments are transferred to and received from adjoining segments. The position of an adjoining segment of the kinetic chain can assist with proprioceptive input, helping to maintain equilibrium.[36] CKC activities focusing on balance and postural control should be an important part of any lower extremity program, particularly one with the goal of restoring normal kinesthesia.

Neural Adaptation

Neural adaptation involves changes in the ability of the nervous system to recruit the appropriate muscles to obtain a desired result.[38] When beginning a new exercise program, the strength gains that occur in the first few weeks can be attributed to improved coordination from neural adaptation as the person becomes more efficient in performing the activity.[38] In evaluating the aspects of neuromuscular re-education, understanding the three levels of CNS influence on motor control is helpful. The simplest level involves the spinal reflex and is responsible for reflex muscle splinting.[35] The second level of motor control involves interaction at the brain stem for control of posture and equilibrium. In the highest level of CNS involvement, the mechanoreceptors interact with cognitive awareness.

Continued practice of patterned motion requires less cognitive awareness, until it eventually becomes automatic or habitual and can be performed with ease.[21,35] Using functional CKC activities enhances the nervous system's ability to recruit groups of muscles to work together. Neural pathways are created that closely replicate functional demands. Proponents of motor learning describe the process of learning a new movement as beginning on a conscious cognitive level and, with repetition, moving to a more subconscious level. Rehabilitative programs should enhance functional outcomes by including functional CKC activities. For a quadriplegic patient who must use her upper body to perform transfers from the wheelchair to the bed, a new neural pathway of using the upper extremity in a closed fashion becomes necessary. Seated CKC triceps dips would be an appropriate activity to include in this patient's rehabilitation program to enhance development of this pathway.

Specificity of Training

CKC training relies on the principle of the specificity of training.[14,19,38] Studies involving strength training have shown movement pattern specificity; a greater increase in strength was measured when the test activity was similar to the actual training exercise.[38,39] This approach involves the use of the specific adaptations to imposed demands (SAID) principle.[40,41] Changes in the neuromuscular system can be accomplished by applying a specific type of mechanical stress (ie, imposed demands) to that system. In response to the stress, the body makes specific adaptations in muscle recruitment patterns. Using CKC training helps to replicate the imposed demands of activities of daily living and uses a more natural recruitment pattern of an eccentric muscle contraction to decelerate or control a movement, followed by a concentric muscle contraction. Using a 4-inch step to perform step-up exercises to gain the lower extremity hip and thigh strength needed to improve the functional performance of ascending stairs is an example of using the SAID principle with a CKC activity.

Stretch-Shortening Cycle

Plyometrics is a method of training the neuromuscular system to increase power (ie, work per time) by combining speed and strength of muscular contractions.[42–45] The increased power occurs from storing energy during the eccentric phase and using this stored energy during the concentric phase. Plyometrics involves rapid closing and opening of the kinetic chain[3] and is routinely prescribed as part of the rehabilitation of athletes after orthopedic injuries. Plyometric activities enhance the neuromuscular system's natural recruitment patterns through a decelerating motion followed by an accelerating motion.

A frequent goal of rehabilitation of athletes is to return their ability to change forward energy into vertical height, as in blocking a volleyball or dunking a basketball. The basic premise is that a muscle can perform more positive (concentric) work if it is stretched (eccentrically loaded) immediately before shortening.[42,45,46] Mechanically, the elastic components of the muscle and tendon (ie, myosin, actin, and other proteins) that are arranged in series are stretched during the eccentric portion, thereby storing energy. During the concentric portion, this energy is released as the elastic components return to their resting length.[2,42,45,46] This is similar to the way a spring stores energy as it is stretched and releases the energy as it returns to its resting length. It is believed that activation of the muscle spindle, inhibition of the Golgi tendon organs through the stretch reflex, and a marked increase in the chemical energy enhance muscular contraction.[42,45–47]

The result is improved neural efficiency and neuromuscular control with increased tolerance to stretched loads (ie, decreased injury) and an increase in the explosive ability of muscular contractions.[2,42,45] CKC activities that stimulate the use of the stretch-shortening cycle include running, jumping activities, box drills, and skipping.[3]

Influence of Motion on the Kinetic Chain

Understanding the influence of foot and ankle biomechanics on the entire kinetic chain is essential to ensure accurate prescription of CKC exercises. A brief description of how motion of the subtalar joint can influence the kinetic chain is provided to illustrate proper CKC training.

During closed chain pronation, motion of the subtalar joint involves calcaneal eversion and talar plantar flexion and adduction[48] (Fig. 15-1). Because of the association of the talus with the ankle mortise (ie, tibia and fibula), the lower leg follows the talus with internal rotation and a superior and anterior translation of the fibular head, talocrural joint dorsiflexion, and flexion with a valgus stress at the knee (Fig. 15-2). Motion occurring up the chain continues with femoral adduction and internal rotation as the hip moves into flexion.[49–51] The pelvis flexes and internally rotates in phase with the limb (the tibia, femur and pelvis all internally rotate, with the distal segment moving faster and through a greater range of motion [ROM]) as the lumbar spine extends and counterrotates.[49,50]

Jackson[50] describes the pelvis as the next triplane joint that has an intimate relationship with the subtalar joint. He feels that the axis of inclination of the subtalar joint dictates the amount of transverse and frontal plane rotation occurring at the pelvis and throughout the lower limb. Because the normal angle of inclination of the subtalar joint is 42 degrees, the amount of transverse and frontal plane motion should be equal. A high subtalar joint axis results in increased transverse plan motion of the pelvis and entire lower extremity. This configuration results in excessive subtalar joint supination coupled with external tibial rotation, knee extension, femoral external rotation, and abduction and external rotation of the ilium.[50] The clinical significance of a high subtalar joint axis is that the limb has difficulty with shock attenuation.[48] Low subtalar joint axis results in more frontal plane motion of the pelvis and lower extremity.[50] Excessive subtalar pronation (ie, calcaneal eversion) is coupled with the frontal plane motions of femoral adduction and an increased valgus stress on the knee. The clinical result is a limb that is inefficient during propulsion.[48]

Because motion of the foot and ankle is coupled with hip, knee, and pelvic motion, initiation of exercises in one segment of the lower extremity kinetic chain results in predictable movement of the other segments. The distal segment moves through a greater ROM and more rapidly than the proximal segment.[49]

The following example illustrates the influence of motion on the kinetic chain. A patient reports to physical therapy with the diagnosis of posterior tibialis tendinitis. During the evaluation, she displays prolonged subtalar joint pronation during the midstance phase of the gait cycle. Because prolonged pronation has resulted in an overuse injury to the posterior tibialis tendon, one of the goals of rehabilitation is to teach this patient to supinate the subtalar joint. Beginning in a seated position to control the amount of weight bearing, the patient should actively raise the arch in the foot. Dorsiflexing the hallux can be used to assist with raising the arch when plantar flexing the forefoot into the ground should be avoided. As the arch raises, external rotation of the lower leg can be seen and felt. Progress the exercise to standing; external rotation of the lower leg results in knee extension and external rotation of the hip. Dorsiflexing the hallux can be eliminated after the patient begins full weight bearing. The patient then reverses the exercise, beginning with tightening of the posterior gluteus medius, hip lateral rotators, and gluteus maximus. External rotation of the hip results in knee extension, external rotation of the lower leg, plantar flexion of the talocrural joint, and supination of the subtalar joint. The arch height raises. The patient should be encouraged to include contracting the hip musculature during the stance phase of gait to enhance supination of the subtalar joint. Research by Perry[52] supports this activity. Electromyographic (EMG) studies show that the gluteus medius and, to a lesser extent, the gluteus maximus and posterior tibialis are active in the stance leg during midstance of the gait cycle.

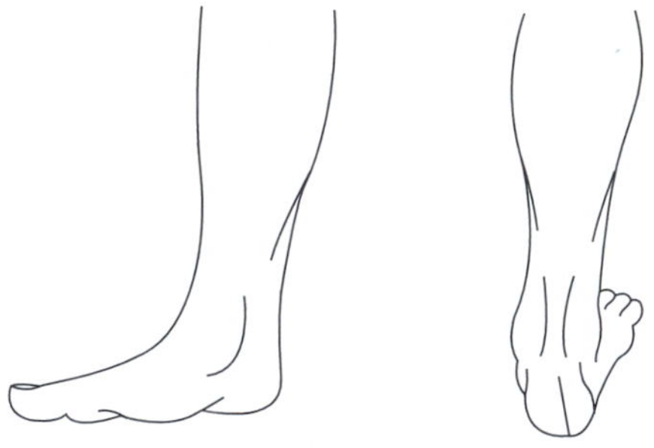

FIGURE 15-1 Closed chain pronation: calcaneal eversion, talar plantar flexion, and adduction.

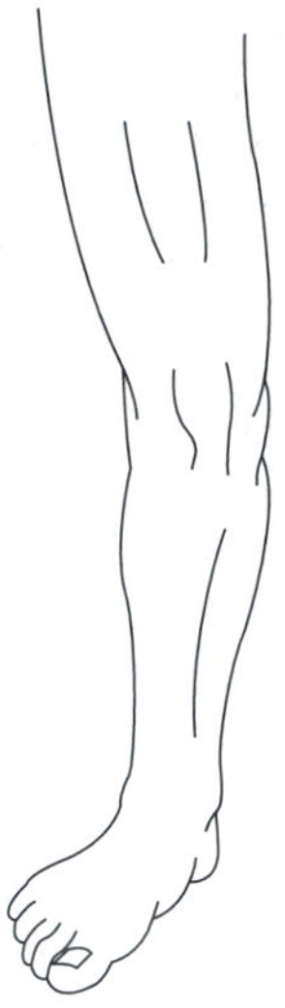

FIGURE 15-2 Closed chain pronation: internal rotation of the lower leg and flexion with valgus stress at the knee.

EXAMINATION AND EVALUATION

The evaluation of functional activities and documentation of improvements in function are critical issues facing the physical therapy profession. Many insurance companies base reimbursement of physical therapy services on documented improvements in function. CKC training has the unique advantage of "becoming the test"; the test becomes the exercise, and consequently, the exercise becomes the test. An example is testing of static balance. The patient presents with difficulty in single-limb stance during gait. The patient is asked to balance with shoes off, eyes open, and on one limb. Measurement is taken of the amount of time balance is achieved. The test ends when an alteration in position of the stance limb, the non–weight-bearing limb, touches or after 30 seconds. If less than optimal performance occurs, this activity becomes part of the patient's home exercise program. After the 30-second limit is reached, the difficulty of the test can be enhanced.[12]

Another example of an exercise is an excursion test in single-limb stance. Excursion tests are designed to measure the amount of motion that can be controlled at a joint.[12] For example, consider a patient who presents with decreased stride length on the left during gait. Beginning on the left leg, the patient is asked to extend the left hip with a successful return to the standing position while maintaining the single-limb stance. The degrees of hip extension in the sagittal plane is measured. If limited hip extension is measured, this activity becomes part of the patient's home exercise program.[12]

In *Lower Extremity Functional Profile,* Gray and Team Reaction[12] attempted to set standards for the measurement and documentation of functional testing in a CKC setting. The tests are designed with a set of rules using clear and consistent terminology and standards that can be easily documented. The tests evaluate the functional movements of static and dynamic balance, amount of motion (ie, excursion), and distance moved in a CKC environment.[12] Tests for the sport activities of step, hop, and jump also are presented.[12] Other researchers have devised functional tests to determine the readiness of an athlete to return to recreational activities.[53–55] Pylometric exercises are a form of CKC training. A few CKC submaximal tests can indicate the safety of performing plyometric exercises.[42,47] Before initiation of pylometric activities, Albert[42] and the National Strength and Conditioning Association[47] recommend that a person should be able to long jump her height in distance. This approach is useful when dealing with adolescents to ensure that their immature muscular and skeletal systems can handle the stress of increased loads. Comparative results of functional testing can be obtained from pretest and posttest values or by comparing right and left values.[12]

TREATMENT INTERVENTION

CKC training is a valuable form of exercise for enhancing patients' ability to function in their work, home, or recreational environments. Rehabilitation of muscular strength and neuromuscular coordination must take into account the position and function of the entire kinetic chain. The position of an adjacent segment directly affects the muscular contraction and applied force throughout the involved region. No longer is there rehabilitation of a "knee patient." A study by Bullock-Saxton[56] helps to justify this statement. The researcher compared two groups: an injured group who had sustained severe unilateral ankle sprains and a matched uninjured, control group. Changes in sensory perception (ie, vibration) and motor response (ie, hip extensor firing pattern) were found. The results showed significant delays in gluteus maximus recruitment on the ipsilateral and contralateral sides in the injured group.[56]

Rehabilitation of a patient with a knee injury focuses on functional limitations and rehabilitation of the entire limb. Resolving these functional limitations includes weight-bearing activities under task-specific conditions. The flexibility, simplicity, and creativity associated with CKC training affords countless possibilities for exercises to be included in a home exercise program.

Postural Considerations

To take full advantage of the benefits of CKC activities, some guidelines for implementation are helpful. Selecting CKC exercises includes special considerations:

- Placement of the center of mass
- Placement of the foot
- Relationship between the proximal and distal segments

Performing a knee flexion-extension exercise in a closed chain position can strengthen different muscle groups, depending on where the center of mass is placed relative to the knee. Figure 15-3 shows an example of a minisquat with the center of mass placed directly above the knee. The knee extensors must work to control the movement. In Figure 15-4, the center of mass is located behind the knee, resulting in more stress placed on the hip extensors to control the movement. Figure 15-5 shows a knee flexion-extension exercise in which the pelvis is forward relative to the knee. In this example, the gastrocnemius must work to control the knee movement. This is true in the daily activities of stair climbing, sit to stand movement, and forward progression of the body over the stance limb during the gait cycle. When prescribing these CKC activities, placement of the center of mass can directly influence muscle recruitment.

Placement of the foot can influence the efficiency of performing CKC exercises. When the subtalar joint is permitted to pronate excessively, internal rotation of the entire lower limb occurs with a resultant increased valgus stress at the knee.[34,48] This may contribute to patellofemoral pain or interrupt the healing of a medial collateral ligament strain. External devices can be used to position the foot and consequently the entire lower extremity in a better position. The use of an external device to support the subtalar joint

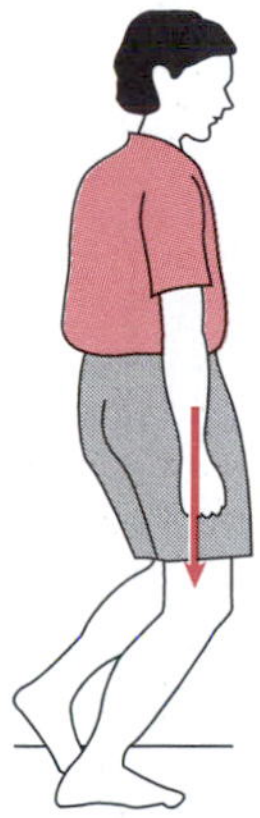

FIGURE 15-3 The center of mass is located directly over the knee.

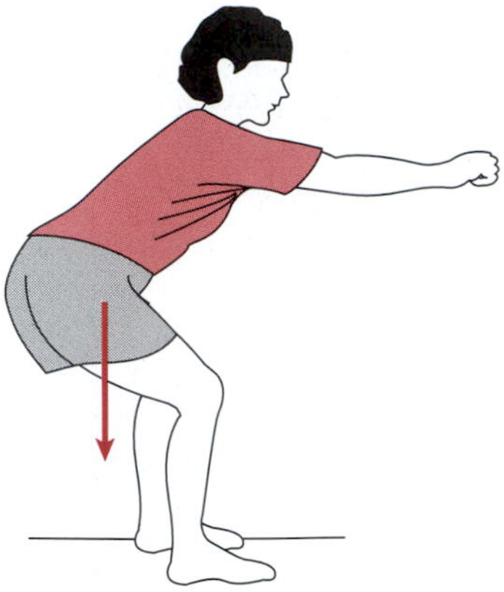

FIGURE 15-4 The center of mass is located behind the knees.

in a neutral or slightly supinated position when stretching the gastrocnemius in a CKC position can be used to limit subtalar pronation and enhance dorsiflexion of the talocrural joint (Fig. 15-6).

The relationship of the proximal and distal segments affects the movement as a whole. In a CKC functional activity, the proximal segment is moving on a more stationary distal segment. Closed chain knee extension is performed by the medial aspect of the femur moving posteriorly with an internal rotation component over a fixed tibia. Another example is the motion of ankle joint dorsiflexion. In a closed chain setting, ankle joint motion is accomplished by the tibia and fibula moving over a relatively stationary talus. With the knee extended, the eccentric muscular contraction of the gastrocnemius and soleus is responsible for controlling ankle joint dorsiflexion in a CKC activity.

In a CKC setting, motion occurs proximally and distally to the axis of rotation. It is important to understand the relation between the movement of the segments relative to each other and their speed of movement. Osteokinematically, the distal segment moves through a greater ROM more rapidly than the proximal segment.[49] For example, knee flexion is coupled with obligatory internal tibial rotation. To perform CKC knee flexion, the tibia must internally rotate more than the femur. If this rotation does not occur, the knee is unable to flex. Controlling knee flexion in a CKC

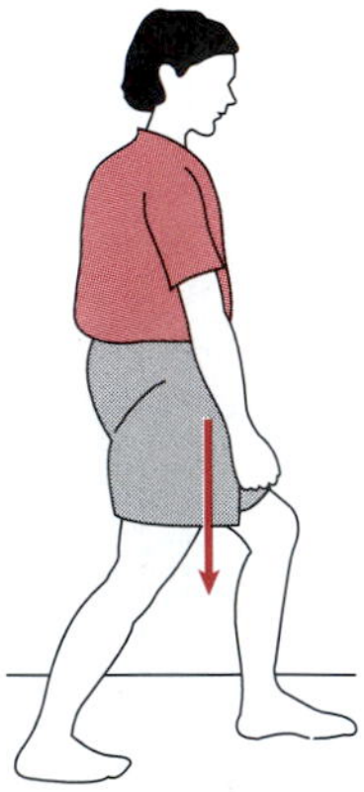

FIGURE 15-5 The center of the mass is located in front of the knee of the back leg.

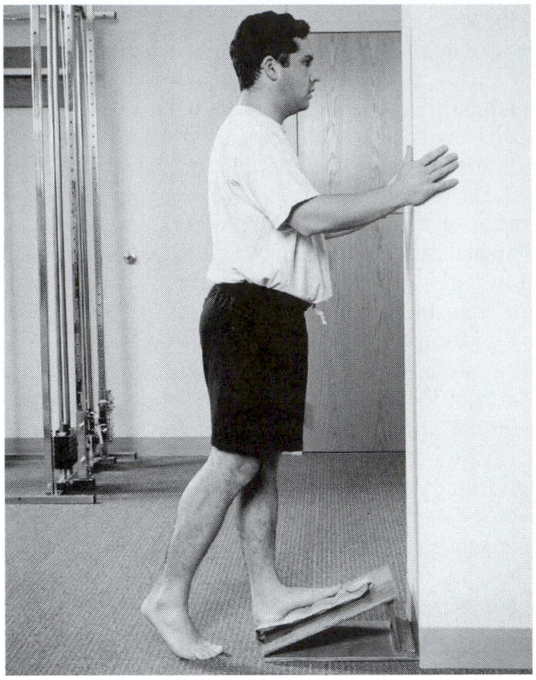

FIGURE 15-6 Supporting the subtalar joint in a neutral or slightly supinated position enhances ankle-talocrural joint dorsiflexion.

position requires muscular control of rotation of the tibia from below and of the femur from above. The tibia internally rotates through a larger excursion while the femur remains relatively laterally rotated as the knee flexes. If the femur and tibia rotated the same amount with the same speed, no relative motion would have occurred (Fig. 15-7). Controlling the rate and amount of subtalar joint pronation by eccentric contraction of the deep posterior calf muscle

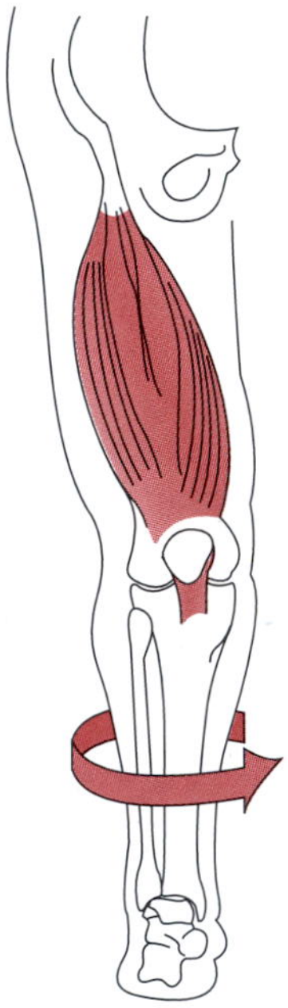

FIGURE 15-7 Relative rotation of the distal and proximal segments.

group and excessive hip internal rotation by eccentric contraction of the hip lateral rotators results in smooth, coordinated knee flexion.

The concept of the proximal segment moving over the distal segment becomes important when mobilizing joints after periods of immobilization. Standard mobilization techniques describe mobilization of the distal segment.[57] During function, the proximal segment is moving over the distal segment. Mobilizing joints, particularly those of the foot and ankle, in accordance with this principle can enhance function.[58] Incorporating CKC activity after joint mobilization should be considered to ensure proper CKC kinematics and recruitment patterns in a gained ROM (Fig. 15-8).

Dosage Guidelines

When using CKC exercises in a rehabilitation program, the variables of force, speed, complexity, and control of movement must be considered, alone and in combination.[19,34] Chapter 2 further details the gradation of exercise.

Earlier in the rehabilitative process, strength, neuromuscular control, and the healing tissue's tolerance to stress are less developed. Force should begin low in a gravity-eliminated or gavity-reduced posture. As the injured tissue heals and muscular strength and coordination develop, mechanical stress can be increased by increasing the weight-bearing forces.

CKC exercises should be performed slowly and in a controlled manner and then progressed as the healing tissue can tolerate stress and neuromuscular control improves. Currwin and Stanish[59] think that proper rehabilitation of patients with tendinitis injuries incorporates eccentric loading of the musculotendinous unit and increased velocity or the speed with which the eccentric loads occur. They believe that the inability of the musculotendinous unit to control the eccentric loads was one factor resulting in the injury.

Complex movements in multiple directions are a part of ADLs and athletic activities. Initiation of CKC exercises should begin in a single plane and then progress to include the frontal and transverse planes. An example of challenging the frontal plane during single-leg stance is lateral reach (Fig. 15-9). An example of challenging the transverse plane during single-leg stance is reaching with trunk rotation to the right (Fig. 15-10). Additional activities using an external object (eg, dribbling a basketball) should be incorporated to further challenge patients according to their functional needs.

Acquiring good postural control is important for efficient function and safety. Initially, the patient should be permitted to use an external support mechanism while performing balance and postural control. Gradation of the activity occurs by gradually removing the external support. For exam-

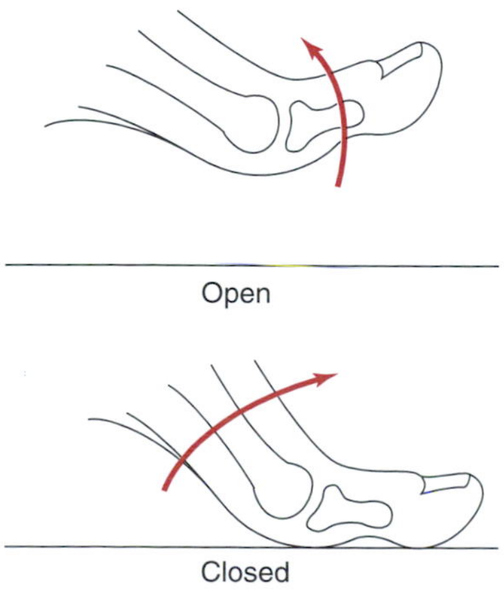

FIGURE 15-8 Incorporating closed kinetic chain activity to improve range of motion for the first metatarsal phalangeal joint.

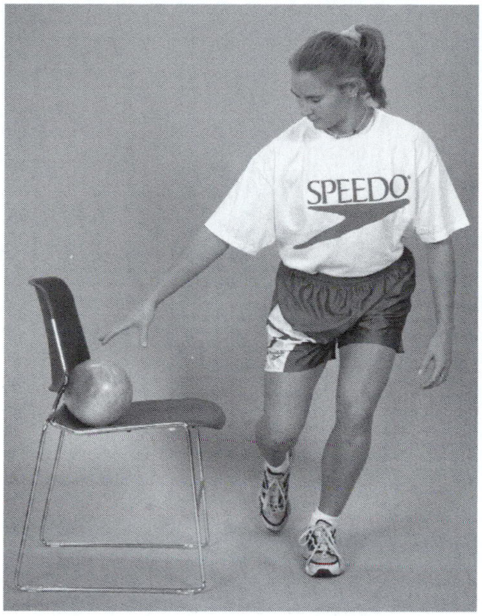

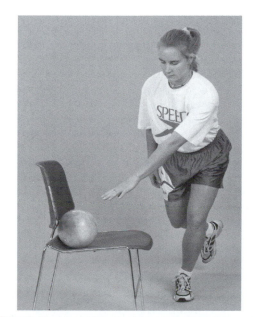

FIGURE 15-9 A lateral reach during a single-leg stance challenges the frontal plane.

FIGURE 15-10 Reaching with trunk rotation to the right during a single-leg stance challenges the transverse plane.

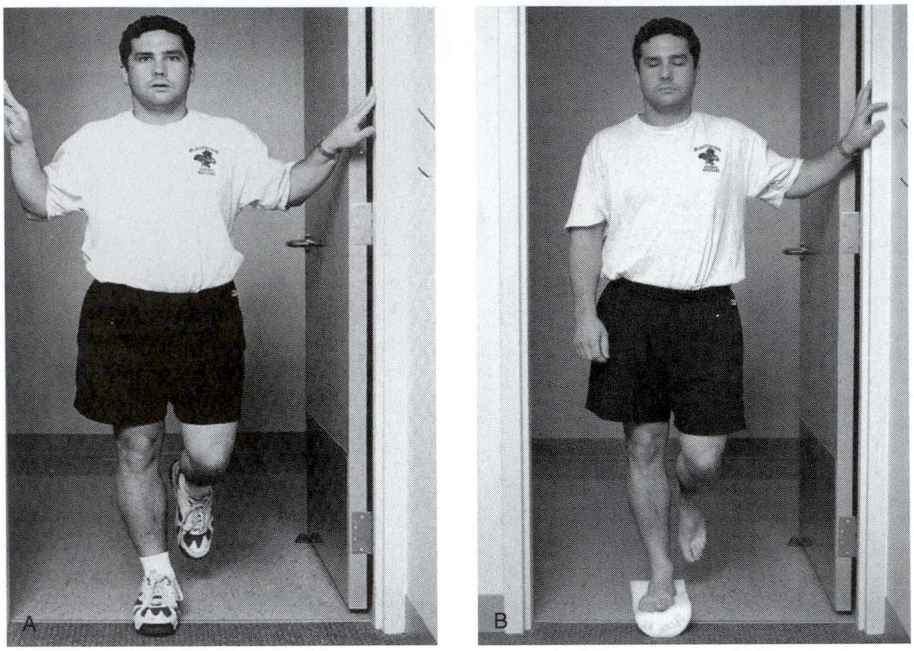

FIGURE 15-11 ***(A)*** Balance exercise using external support. ***(B)*** By altering the surface (use of a foam pad), the exercise becomes more challenging.

ple, improving static single-limb balance can be performed in a doorway with the shoe on and touching the doorway with both hands. As balance and the patient's confidence improves, the activity is progressed and the external support is removed. The shoe is removed, followed by touching the doorway with only one hand; this progresses to not touching the doorway during the exercise. Closing the eyes continues to remove external support, as does altering the supporting surface by placing a foam pad beneath the foot. The foam pad alters the mechanoreceptor input and the ground reaction force to the limb (Fig. 15-11).

Contraindications and Precautions

When choosing CKC training as a method of rehabilitation, the patient's safety is a primary concern. A rehabilitation program should begin submaximally and progress to functional goals the patient can tolerate. To safely progress a patient through the rehabilitative process, it is necessary to incorporate criteria for gradation of the exercise. When substitution of another component in the chain occurs and the intended link is unable to perform the activity, the exercise should be altered to an easier level.[28] For example, a patient could perform a lateral step down from a 6-inch step with the instruction to keep her knee over the second toe could continue until a substitution occurred. Inability to keep the knee over the second toe or an increase in symptoms should result in an alternation of the step down. The exercise could be performed on a 4-inch or 2-inch step. Proper performance of the exercise should be stressed over the number of repetitions.

Additional precautions when using CKC exercises include pain, joint effusion, and the inability of joints to handle the compressive forces. Environmental conditions must be evaluated so the activities are performed on a flat, hard surface with appropriate footwear.

Examples of Closed Kinetic Chain Exercises

Selected techniques of CKC exercises for common impairments are presented to demonstrate the treatment principles and stimulate creativity when using CKC activities as an integral part of a home exercise prescription. Sample exercises for mobility, balance, and muscle performance impairments are shown in Figures 15-6 and 15-11 and in all of the Self-Management displays in this chapter.

Upper Extremity Impairments

Research has been done to evaluate the necessity to perform CKC exercises for the upper extremity. Intramuscular EMG data have shown that a number of closed or partially closed activities should be incorporated into a shoulder rehabilitative program.[60,61] A classification system using nontraditional open and closed chain terminology is appropriate when discussing shoulder function,[15,62,63] because the conditions that apply to the lower extremity with weight-bearing forces do not routinely occur in the upper extremity.[63]

Numerous studies have evaluated the importance of having a "stable base" for performing these skill activities.[61,64] The study results confirm the findings of Sullivan and colleagues[21] about the stages of motor control. First, stability is necessary in the form of cocontraction around the glenohumeral joint, progressing to controlled mobility with proper scapulothoracic rhythm. Additional studies have demonstrated the necessity of an efficient kinetic chain to accomplish these complex skill movements by generating, transferring, and regulating forces created in the legs and trunk to the hand. Gray[34] observed the entire kinetic chain when rehabilitating patients with shoulder dysfunctions. He thinks shoulder position can be enhanced through different positioning of the lower extremity.

SELF-MANAGEMENT: Improving Hip Mobility—Backward Lunge

Purpose: To improve hip extension

Precautions and contraindications: Pain on exertion, acute injury, lumbar spine anteroposterior instability

Position: Standing with feet shoulder width apart, knees over second toes

Movement technique: Maintain arch height.

Lunge backward, and maintain a neutral spine position.

Extend the hip.

Hold for _______ seconds.

Slowly return to the start position.

Repeat ____ times

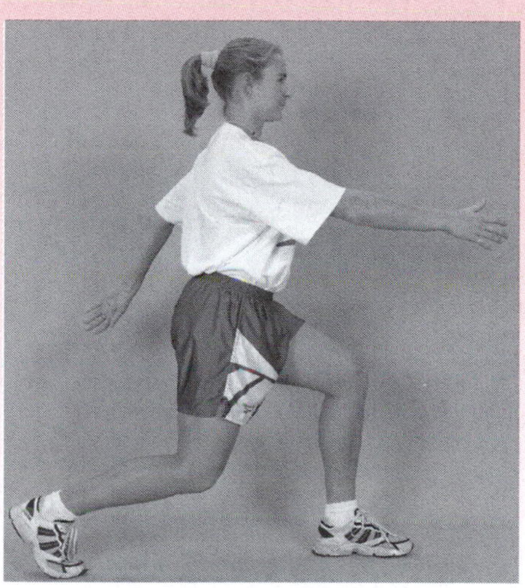

SELF-MANAGEMENT: Foot Intrinsic Muscle Strengthening

Purpose: To promote isometric intrinsic muscle strength

Precautions and contraindications: Pain on exertion, acute injury

Position: Begin seated; progress to single-leg stance

Movement technique: Maintain arch height.

Tighten the muscles in your arch.

Do not push the ball of your foot into the floor.

Hold for _______ seconds.

Repeat ____ times

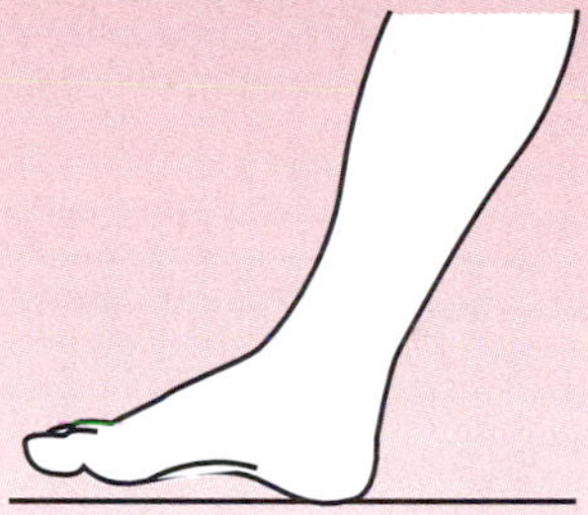

PATIENT EDUCATION

Education and training are provided to the patient in written and illustrated forms. Education focuses on the patient's independence with an effective home exercise program. Clear instructions on exercise dosage and precautions and safety considerations for each CKC activity are provided. Environmental safety is addressed as well.

Key Points

- CKC exercises use the forces of weight bearing and the effect of gravity to simulate functional activities.
- Common characteristics of CKC activities include interdependence of joint motion, motion occurring proximal and distal to the axis of rotation, greater joint compressive forces, stabilization afforded by joint congruency, recruitment of muscle contractions, and eccentric followed by concentric muscle contractions to provide a more normal functional pattern.
- Proximal segments move over more fixed distal segments.
- CKC training of the lower extremity involves movement of the foot, ankle, knee, hip, and pelvis in a predictable sequence.
- The success of using CKC activities in the rehabilitation of patients begins with understanding the kinetics and kinematics of the joints and subsequent kinesiology when the distal segment is attached to a supporting surface.

SELF-MANAGEMENT: Hip Strengthening—Sagittal Plane

Purpose: Strengthen hip and knee extensor muscles eccentrically; concentrically strengthen hip flexor muscles on open kinetic chain limb

Precautions and contraindications: Pain on exertion, acute injury

Position: Single-leg stance on ___-inch box

Movement technique:

Maintain arch height.

Step forward with the non–weight-bearing limb.

Control hip and knee flexion of the stance limb.

Take ___ seconds to complete the exercise.

Slowly return to the start position.

Repeat ____ times

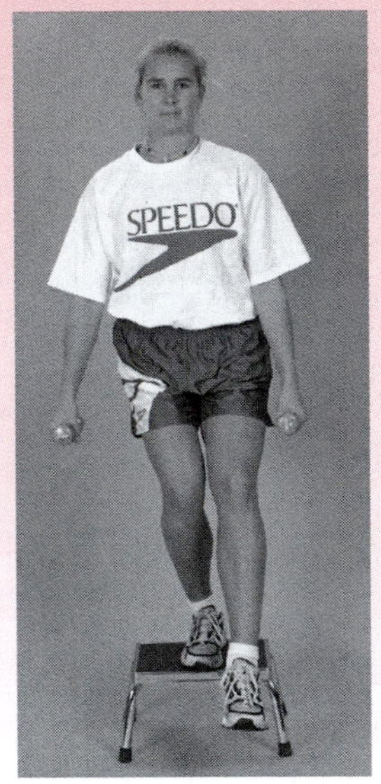

SELF-MANAGEMENT: Hip Strengthening—Transverse Plane

Purpose: Strengthen hip external rotator muscles eccentrically; concentrically strengthen hip external rotator muscles on open kinetic chain limb

Precautions and contraindications: Pain on exertion, acute injury, lumbar spine rotational instability

Position: Single-leg stance on ___-inch box

Movement technique:

Maintain arch height.

Externally rotate the non–weight-bearing limb.

Control internal rotation of the stance limb.

Take ___ seconds to complete the exercise.

Slowly return to the start position.

Repeat ____ times

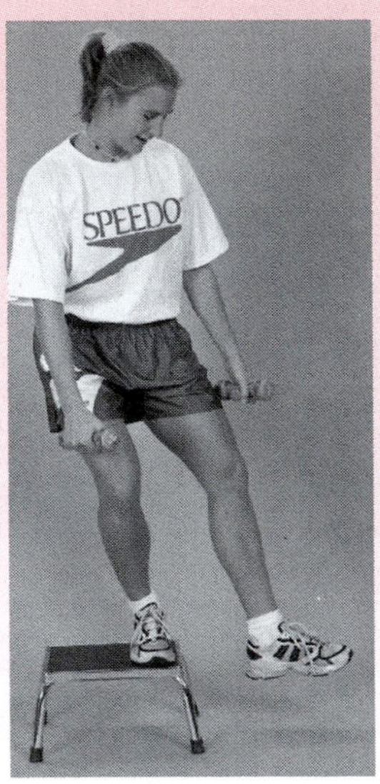

SELF-MANAGEMENT: Hip Strengthening—Frontal Plane

Purpose: Strengthen hip abductor muscles eccentrically; concentrically strengthen hip adductor muscles on open kinetic chain limb

Precautions and contraindications: Pain on exertion, acute injury

Position: Single-leg stance

Movement technique:
Maintain arch height.
Place Theraband around waist and anchor securely.
Laterally lunge on the non–weight-bearing limb.
Control adduction of the stance limb.
Take ___ seconds to complete the exercise.
Slowly return to the start position.

Repeat ____ times

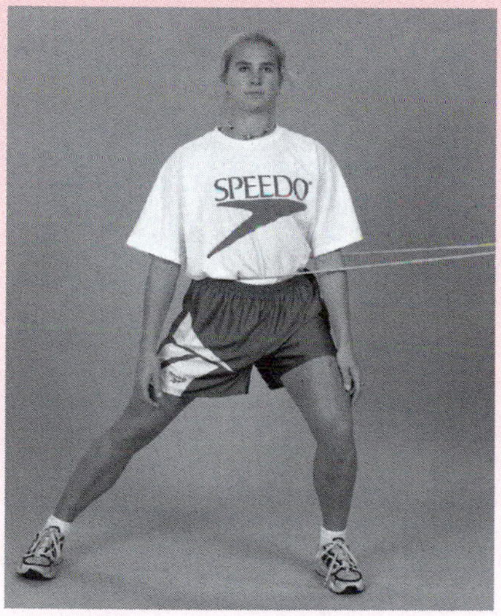

SELF-MANAGEMENT: Quadriceps Strengthening >30 Degrees (Wall Squats)

Purpose: To strengthen the quadriceps muscle eccentrically and isometrically

Precautions and contraindications: Pain on exertion, acute injury of posterior cruciate ligament (should consider supine leg press)

Position: Standing approximately 2 feet from the wall, feet shoulder width apart, knees over second toes

Movement technique:
Maintain arch height.
Stand with the back against the wall.
Slowly slide down the wall, bending the knees, stopping at ____ degrees.
Maintain knees over second toes.
Hold for 6 seconds.
Take 4 seconds to complete the exercise.
Slowly return to the start position.

Repeat ____ times

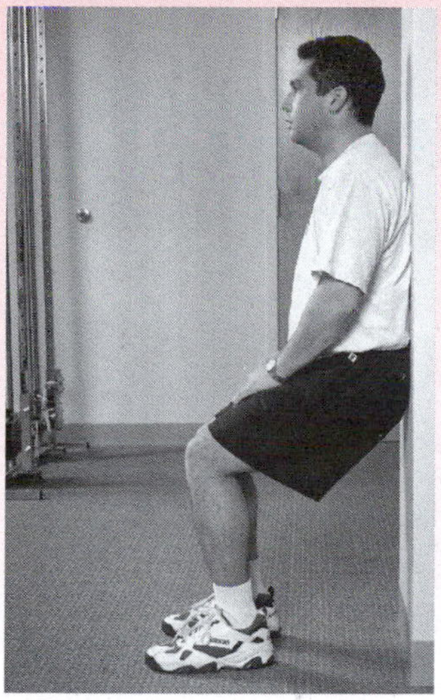

SELF-MANAGEMENT: Quadriceps Strengthening 0 to 30 Degrees (Retrowalking)

Purpose: To strengthen the quadriceps muscle concentrically, dynamic balance

Precautions and contraindications: Pain on exertion, acute injury, balance difficulties

Position: Standing on the treadmill with feet at the normal angle and base of gait, holding onto the side railing

Movement technique:

Walk backward, extending the right hip and landing on the ball of the right foot.

Extend the right knee, pressing the right heel into the bed of the treadmill.

Repeat the sequence by extending the left hip.

Repeat ____ times

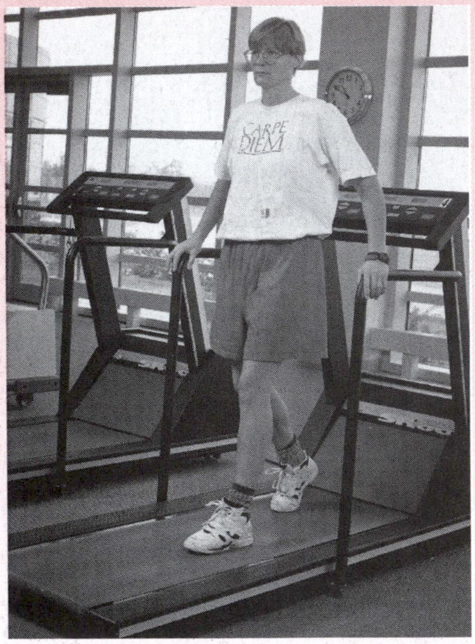

Positioning on treadmill

SELF-MANAGEMENT: Calf Strengthening—Single-Leg Heel Raise

Purpose: To strengthen the gastrocnemius muscle concentrically and eccentrically, enhance balance

Precautions and contraindications: Pain on exertion, acute injury, severe balance disorders

Position: Single-limb stance

Movement technique:

Maintain arch height.

Place a ball or rolled-up sock between the ankles.

Keeping your knee straight, squeeze the sock, and raise the heel off the floor.

Try to keep the weight evenly distributed over the first and fifth toes.

Take ___ seconds to raise heel off the ground.

Take ___ to slowly return to the start position.

Repeat ____ times

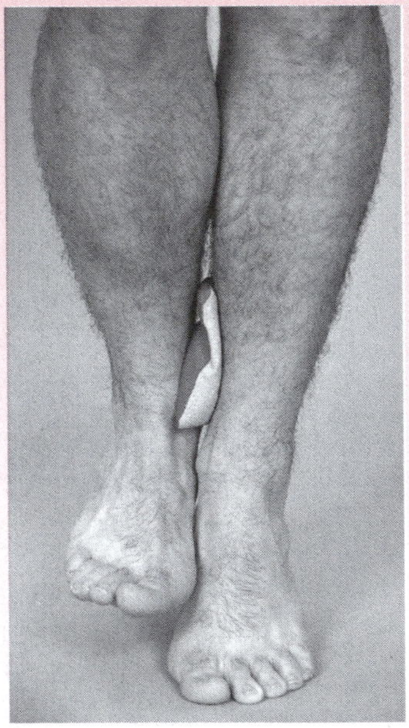

SELF-MANAGEMENT: Quadriceps Strengthening >30 Degrees (Forward Lunge)

Purpose: To strengthen the quadriceps muscle eccentrically and isometrically

Precautions and contraindications: Pain on exertion, acute injury

Position: Standing with feet shoulder width apart, knees over second toes

Movement technique:

Maintain arch height.

Lunge forward.

Keep the knee over the second toe, and behind the ankle.

Bend the knee forward until the thigh becomes parallel to the ground.

Hold for 6 seconds.

Take 4 seconds to perform the exercise.

Slowly return to the start position.

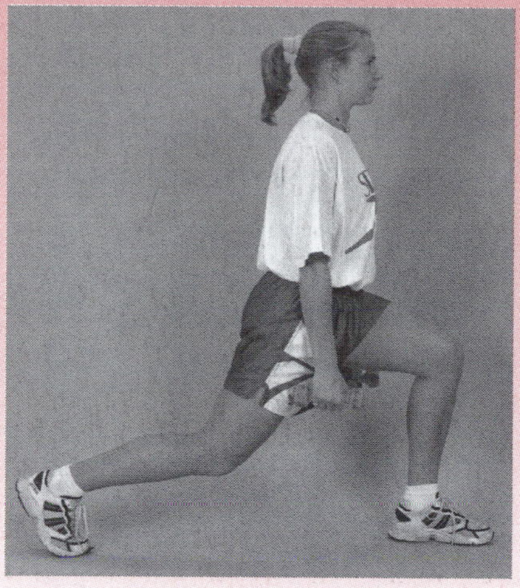

Repeat ____ times

SELF-MANAGEMENT: Quadriceps Strengthening 0 to 30 Degrees (Closed Kinetic Chain Short Arc Quads)

Purpose: To strengthen the quadriceps muscle concentrically, isometrically, and eccentrically

Precautions and contraindications: Pain on exertion, acute injury

Position: Standing with feet shoulder width apart and with the affected knee over the second toe, place the ball behind the knee and the heel against the wall.

Movement technique:

Maintain arch height.

Try to straighten your knee by pushing the back of your knee into the ball.

Hold this position for 6 seconds.

Slowly return to the start position.

Repeat ____ times

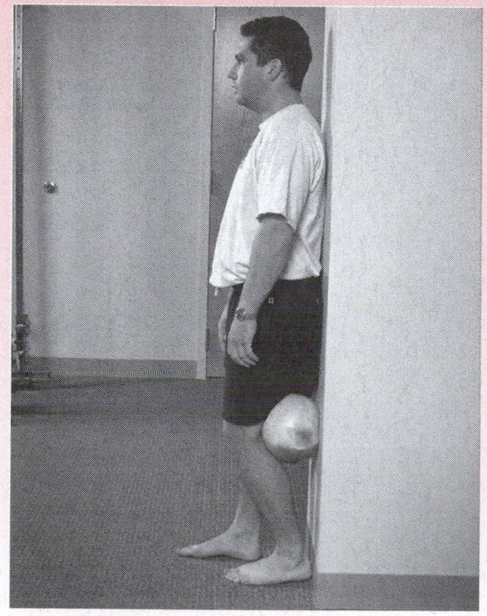

Starting position

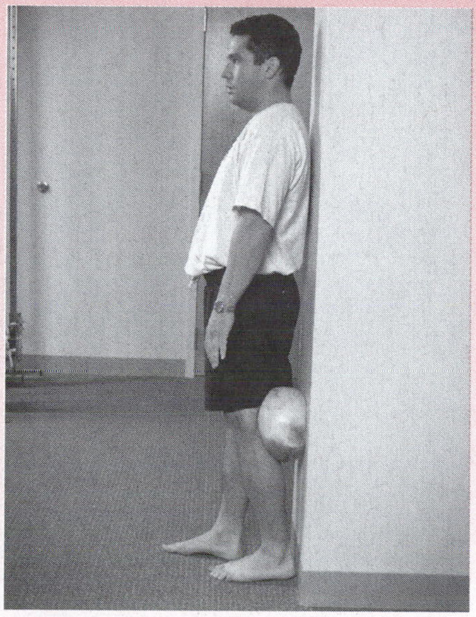

Ending position

SELF-MANAGEMENT: Lumbar Spine Strengthening

Purpose: To strengthen the lumbar paraspinals and gluteal musculature isometrically

Precautions and contraindications: Pain on exertion, acute injury

Position: Kneeling on hands and knees

Movement technique:

Maintain neutral spine.

Slowly extend your _______ arm and _______ leg.

Stabilize the pelvis on the weight-bearing limb.

Stabilize the shoulder girdle with the weight-bearing arm.

Hold ____ seconds.

Slowly return to the start position.

Repeat ____ times

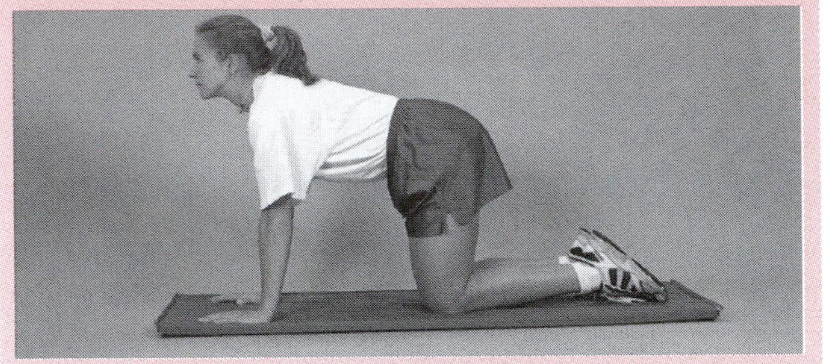

Starting position

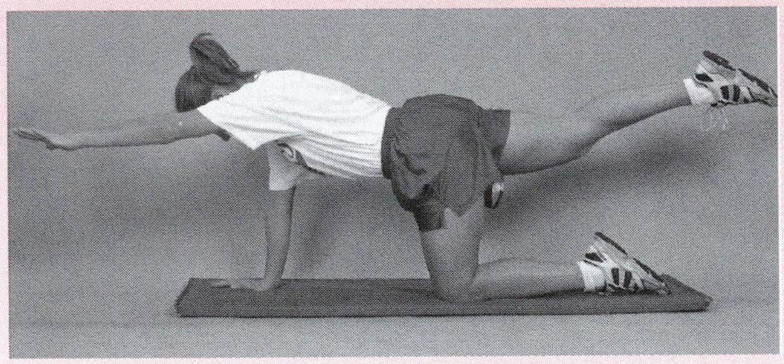

Ending position

SELF-MANAGEMENT: Hip Strengthening—Backward Lunge With Tubing

Purpose: To strengthen the hip extensor muscles concentrically

Precautions and contraindications: Pain on exertion, acute injury, lumbar spine anteroposterior instability

Position: Standing with feet shoulder width apart, knees over second toes

Movement technique:

Maintain arch height.

Place Theraband around the waist.

Lunge backward, and maintain a neutral spine position.

Extend the hip.

Hold for ____ seconds.

Slowly return to the start position.

Repeat ____ times

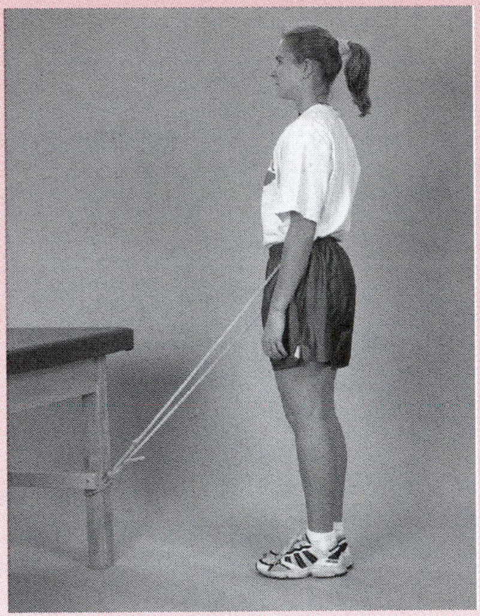

Starting position

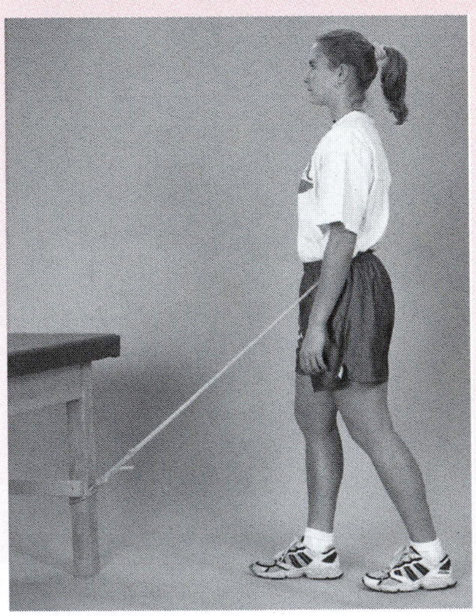

Ending position

SELF-MANAGEMENT: Hip Strengthening—Backward Squat

Purpose: To strengthen the hip extensor muscles eccentrically

Precautions and contraindications: Pain on exertion, acute injury

Position: Standing with feet shoulder width apart, knees over second toes

Movement technique: Maintain arch height.

Place a tall chair directly behind you.

Sit backward into the chair, pivoting around your knees.

As you sit back, move your arms forward to counterbalance the sitting motion.

Slowly return to the start position.

Repeat ____ times

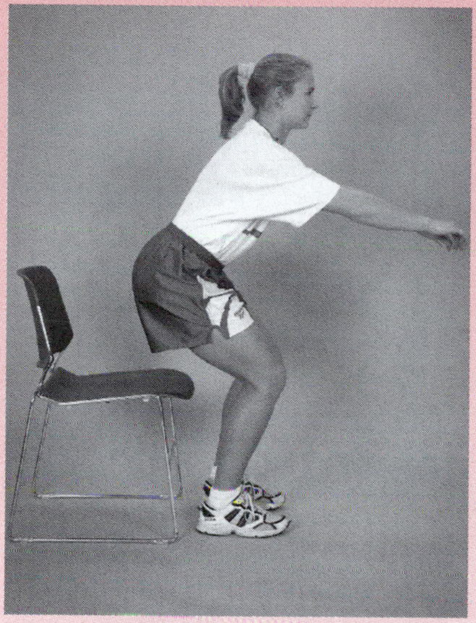

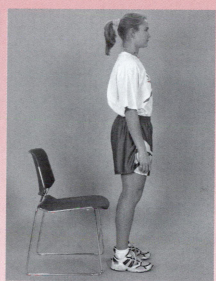

Starting position

Ending position

SELF-MANAGEMENT: Calf Strengthening—Forward Lean

Purpose: To strengthen the gastrocnemius muscle eccentrically

Precautions and contraindications: Pain on exertion, acute injury

Position: 8 to 10 inches from a wall, single-limb stance

Movement technique: Maintain arch height.

Place hands in front of your chest to catch yourself.

Keeping your knee straight, lean forward, leading with your waist.

Use your gastrocnemius muscle to control the forward motion.

Slowly return to the start position.

Repeat ____ times

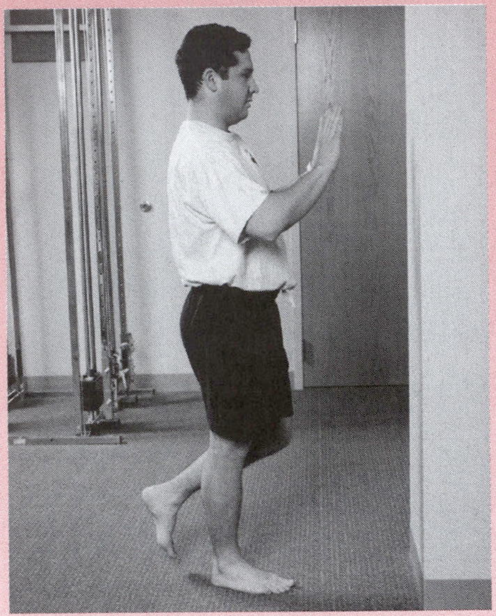

Starting position

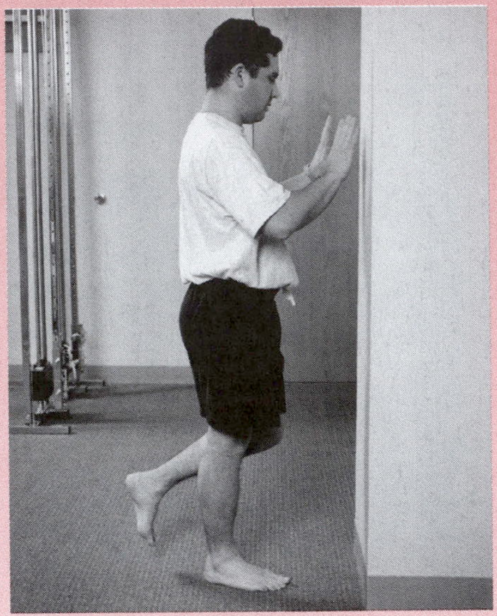

Ending position

SELF-MANAGEMENT: Calf and Hamstring Strengthening—Closed Kinetic Chain Knee Extension (Pelvis Forward)

Purpose: To strengthen the gastrocnemius and hamstring muscle eccentrically

Precautions and contraindications: Pain on exertion, acute injury, lumbar spine anteroposterior instability

Position: Normal walking stride

Movement technique: Maintain arch height.

Keep pelvis forward.

Place Theraband around the tibia, just below the knee, and anchor it to an immovable object.

Begin with your knee bent.

As the Theraband tries to extend your knee, slowly control knee extension.

Keep your pelvis forward.

Take ___ seconds to complete the exercise.

Repeat ___ times

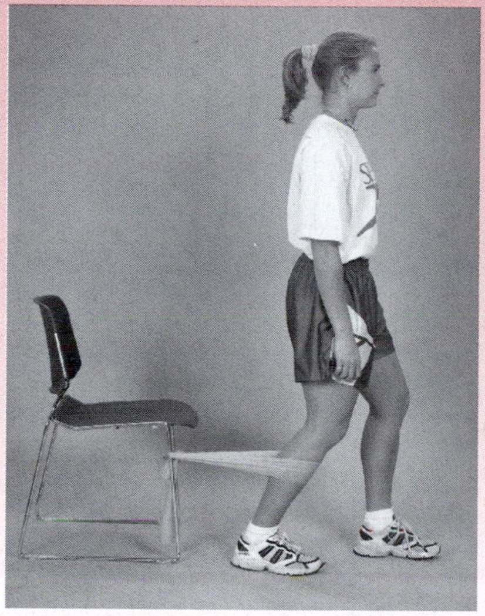

Starting position

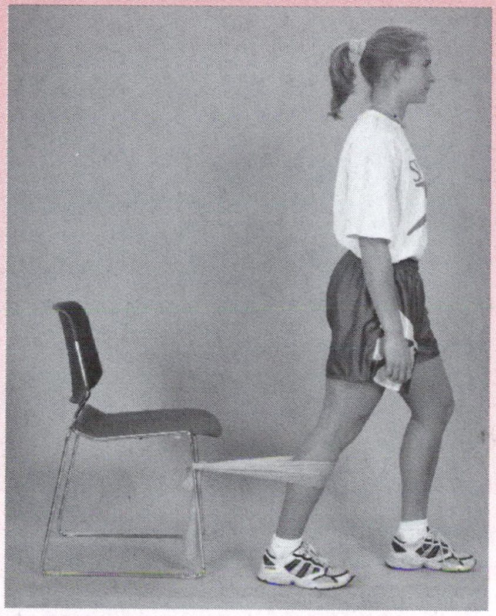

Ending position

SELF-MANAGEMENT: First Ray Stability—Windlass Mechanism

Purpose: To strengthen the peroneus longus in a functional position

Precautions and contraindications: Pain on exertion, acute injury

Position: Begin seated, progress to normal walking stride

Movement technique: Maintain arch height.

Extend *only* the hallux.

Gently push the knuckle of your big toe into the floor.

Hold ___ seconds.

Repeat ___ times

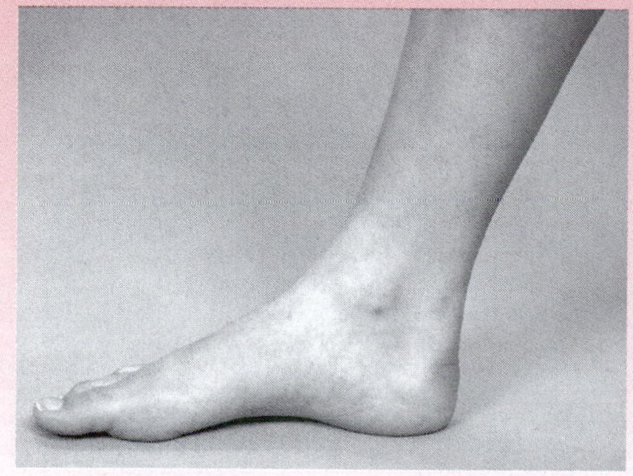

Starting position

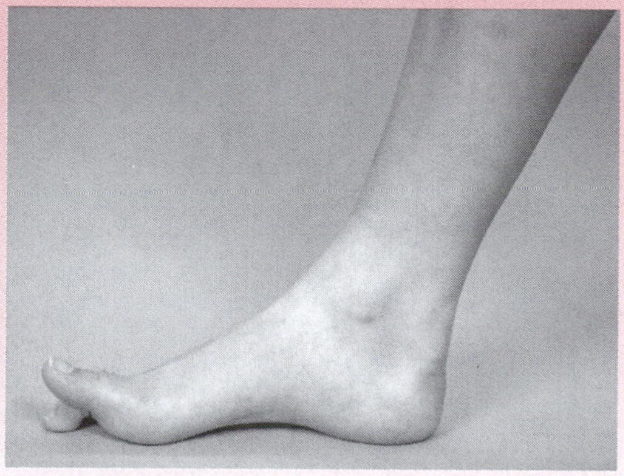

Ending position

SELF-MANAGEMENT: Subtalar Joint and Midtarsal Joint Pronation

Purpose: To promote controlled movement of the subtalar and midtarsal joints

Precautions and contraindications: Pain on exertion, acute injury

Position: Begin seated, progress to normal walking stride

Movement technique: Extend *only* the lateral four toes in a smooth and controlled manner.

Gently try to lift the lateral border of your foot off the floor.

Take ___ seconds to complete this exercise.

Repeat ____ times

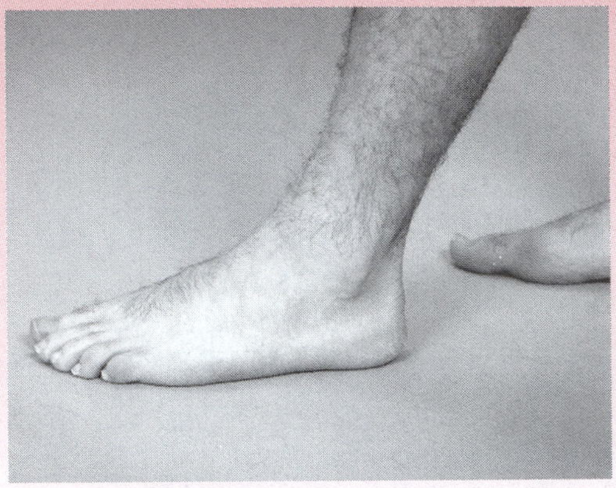

Starting position

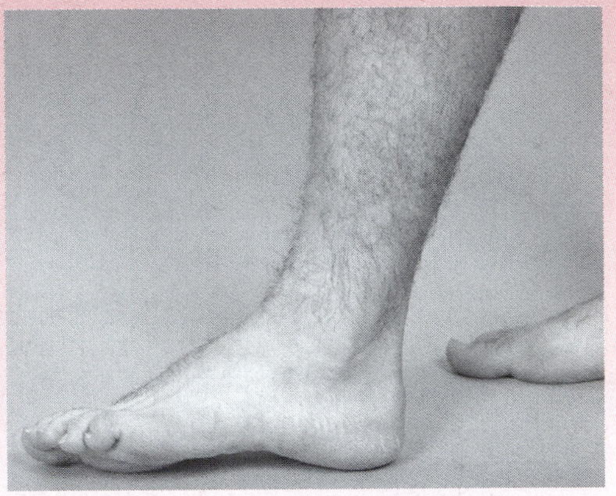

Ending position

SELF-MANAGEMENT: Subtalar Joint Pronation

Purpose: To promote controlled movement of the subtalar joint, enhance balance

Precautions and contraindications: Pain on exertion, acute injury, severe balance disorder

Position: Single-leg stance

Movement technique: Place Theraband around the outside of the foot, and attach it to an immovable object.

Raise the heel off the floor.

As you return the heel to the floor, control the motion of the Theraband pulling the subtalar joint into a pronated position.

Take ___ seconds to complete this exercise.

Repeat ____ times

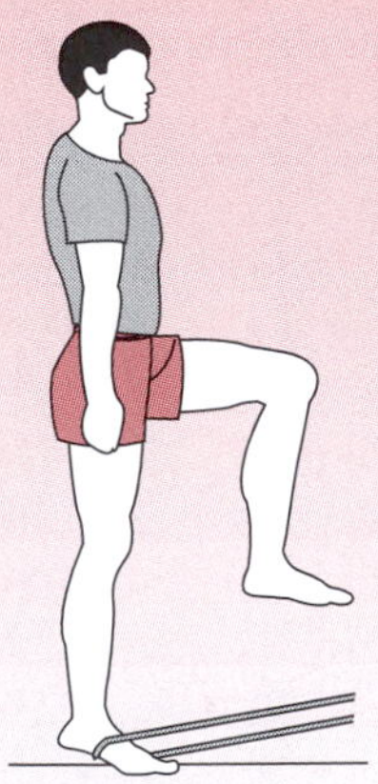

Starting position

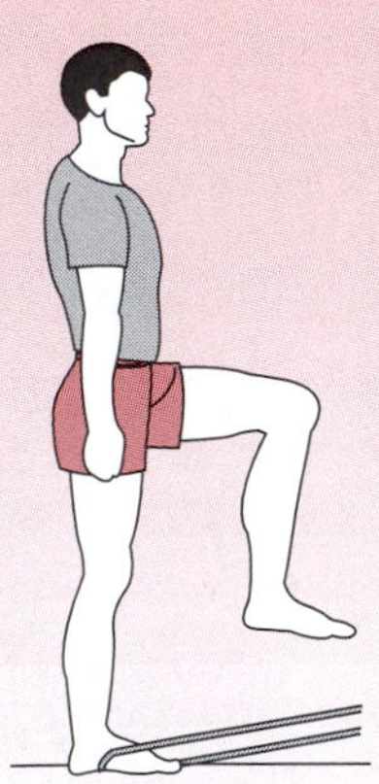

Ending position

SELF-MANAGEMENT: Hip Strengthening—Transverse Plane

Purpose: To strengthen hip external rotator muscles eccentrically, concentrically strengthen hip external rotator muscles on the open kinetic chain limb

Precautions and contraindications: Pain on exertion, acute injury, lumbar spine rotational instability

Position: Single-leg stance; place non–weight-bearing limb on a wheeled stool

Movement technique:

Maintain arch height.

Externally rotate the non–weight-bearing limb.

Control internal rotation of the stance limb.

Take ___ seconds to complete this exercise.

Slowly return to the start position.

Repeat ____ times

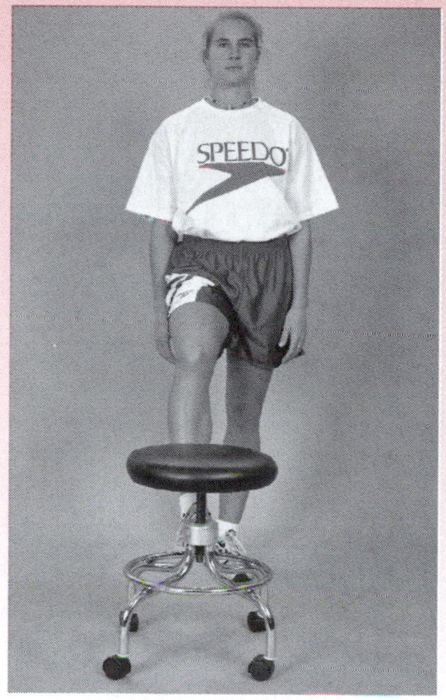

Starting position

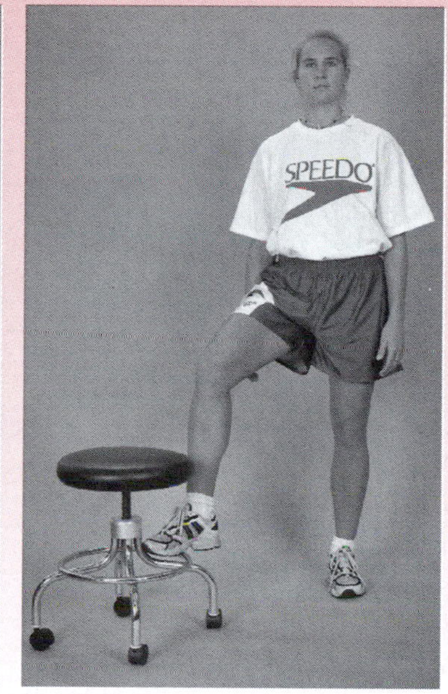

Ending position

SELF-MANAGEMENT: Quadriceps Strengthening 0 to 30 Degrees (Standing Stationary Cycling)

Purpose: To strengthen the quadriceps muscle concentrically

Precautions and contraindications: Pain on exertion, acute injury, balance difficulties

Position: Standing on the pedals of the bike

Movement technique:

Begin pedaling in an upright position.

Use the quadriceps muscle to control the knee as it moves into extension.

Repeat ____ times

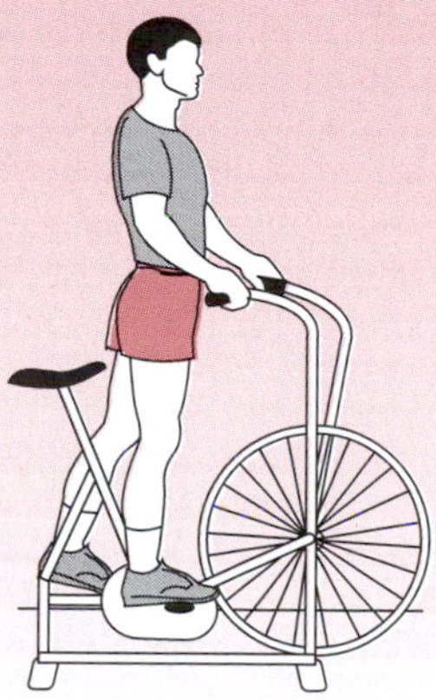

LAB ACTIVITIES

1. Choose three closed or pseudokinetic chain exercises (one for each segment of the lower extremity), and adapt each exercise to patients with the following injuries. Be prepared to demonstrate the exercises, give written home instructions (including dosage and precautions), and explain the scientific basis of your selection.
   a. Subacute extensor mechanism dysfunction in a college athlete
   b. Extensor mechanism dysfunction in a 70-year-old, sedentary woman
   c. Acute, excessive pronation of the subtalar joint in a 15-year-old recreational athlete
   d. Chronic, excessive pronation of the subtalar joint excessive pronation in a diabetic, hypertensive, slightly obese, 60-year-old man who is moderately active
   e. ACL-deficient knee in a 45-year-old firefighter who is preparing for return to work in 2 weeks
   f. ACL-reconstructed knee with medial collateral ligament strain 6 weeks after surgery
2. Choose three CKC exercises for the upper extremity. Incorporate at least two proprioceptive neuromuscular facilitation elements in your treatment for the following patients:
   a. A 3-year-old boy with a fracture of the clavicle 4 weeks after the injury.
   b. A 17-year-old high school senior softball player with an anterior instability of the glenohumeral joint, who has a good chance for a college scholarship if she performs well this season
   c. Chronic faulty movement pattern of the glenohumeral joint with dominance of the axiohumeral rotators (pectoralis major and latissimus dorsi) over the scapulohumeral rotators in a 48-year-old carpenter
3. Using the principle of the proximal segment moving over a fixed distal segment, mobilize the tibiofemoral joint to gain knee extension and talocrural joint to obtain dorsiflexion. Develop one CKC activity to be used as a home exercise to maintain mobility of each joint.
4. Develop an activity changing the center of mass over the base of support to alter muscle recruitment of the hamstrings, quadriceps and gluteals, and gastrocnemius and soleus in squat, sit to stand, and step-up activity.
5. Analyze the influence of forcing an excessively toed-in position of a patient with a naturally toed-out stance position on the ACL at the knee.
6. Develop five activities for each plane to enhance movement in the frontal, transverse, and sagittal planes during single-limb stance.
7. Describe the osteokinematics up the chain of the effect of subtalar joint supination.

REFERENCES

1. Steindler A. *Kinesiology of the Human Body Under Normal and Pathological Conditions.* Springfield, IL: Charles C Thomas; 1973.
2. Snyder-Mackler L. Scientific rationale and physiological basis for the use of closed kinetic chain exercise in the lower extremity. *J Sport Rehabil.* 1996;5:2–12.
3. Wilk KE, Naiquan Z, Glenn SF, Andrews JR, Clancy WG. Kinetic chain exercise: implications for the anterior cruciate ligament patient. *J Sport Rehabil.* 1997;6:125–140.
4. Lindal O, Movin A. The mechanics of the knee joint. *Acta Orthop Scand.* 1967;38:226–234.
5. Smidt GL. Biomechanical analysis of knee flexion and extension. *J Biomechanics.* 1973;6:79–92.
6. Paulos L, Noyes FR, Grood ES, et al. Knee rehabilitation after anterior cruciate ligament reconstruction and repair. *Am J Sports Med.* 1981;9:140–143.
7. Arms SW, Pope MH, Johnson RJ, et al. The biomechanics of the anterior cruciate ligament rehabilitation and reconstruction. *Am J Sports Med.* 1984;12:8–18.
8. Grood ES, Suntay WT, Noyes FR, et al. Biomechanics of the knee-extension exercise. Effect of cutting the anterior cruciate ligament. *J Bone Joint Surg.* 1984;66A:725–734.
9. Henning CE, Lynch MA, Glick KR. An in vivo strain gauge study of elongation of the anterior cruciate ligament. *Am J Sports Med.* 1985;13:22–26.
10. Renstrom P, Arms SW, Stanwyck TS, et al. Strain within the anterior cruciate ligament during hamstring and quadriceps activity. *Am J Sports Med.* 1986;14:83–87.
11. Hungerford DS, Barry M. Biomechanics of the patellofemoral joint. *Clin Orthop.* 1979;144:9–15.
12. Gray GW, Team Reaction. *Lower Extremity Functional Profile.* Adrian, MI: Wynn Marketing; 1995.
13. Panariello RA, Backus SI, Parker JW. The effect of squat exercise on anterior-posterior knee translation in professional football players. *Am J Sports Med.* 1994;22:768–773.
14. Palmitier RA, An KN, Scott SG, Chao EYS. Kinetic chain exercises in knee rehabilitation. *Sports Med.* 1991;11:402–413.
15. Dillman CJ, Murrary TA, Hintermeister RA. Biomechanical differences of open and closed chain exercises with respect to the shoulder. *J Sport Rehabil.* 1994;3:228–238.
16. Jorge M, Hall ML. Analysis of EMG measurements during bicycle pedalling. *J Biomech.* 1986;19:683–694.
17. Wozniak-Timmer CA. Cycling biomechanics: a literature review. *J Orthop Sports Phys Ther.* 1991;14:106–113.
18. Snyder-Mackler L, Delitto A, Bailey SL, Stralka SW. Strength of the quadriceps femoris muscle and functional recovery after reconstruction of the anterior cruciate ligament. *J Bone Joint Surg Am.* 1995;77:1166–1173.
19. Irrgang JJ. *Closed kinetic chain exercises for the lower extremity: Theory and application.* LaCrosse, WI: Sports Physical Therapy Home Study Course, Sports Physical Therapy Section of the American Physical Therapy Association; 1994.
20. Harter RA. Clinical rationale for closed kinetic chain activities in functional testing and rehabilitation of ankle pathologies. *J Sport Rehabil.* 1996;5:13–24.
21. Sullivan PE, Markos PD, Minor MAD. *An Integrated Approach to Therapeutic Exercise Theory and Clinical Application.* Reston, VA: Reston Publishing Company; 1982.

22. Knott M, Voss DE. *Proprioceptive Neuromuscular Facilitation*. 2nd ed. New York: Harper & Row; 1968.
23. Lutz GE, Palmitier RA, An KN, Chao EYS. Comparison of tibiofemoral joint forces during open-kinetic-chain and closed-kinetic-chain exercises. *J Bone Joint Surg Am.* 1993;75:732–739.
24. Yack HJ, Collins CE, Whieldon TJ. Comparison of closed and open kinetic chain exercise in the anterior cruciate ligament-deficient knee. *Am J Sports Med.* 1993;21:49–53.
25. Markolf KL, Bargar WL, Shoemaker SC, et al. The role of joint load in knee stability. *J Bone Joint Surg Am.* 1981;63:570–585.
26. Shoemaker SC, Markolf KL. Effects of joint load on the stiffness and laxity of ligament-deficient knees: an in vitro study of the anterior cruciate and medical collateral ligaments. *J Bone Joint Surg Am.* 1985;67:136–146.
27. Stormont DM, Morrey BF, An K, Cass JR. Stability of the loaded ankle. *Am J Sports Med.* 1985;13:295–300.
28. Lephart SM, Pinccivero DM, Jorge LG, Fu FH. The role of proprioception in the management and rehabilitation of athletic injuries. *Am J Sports Med.* 1997;25:130–137.
29. Grigg P. Peripheral neural mechanisms in proprioception. *J Sport Rehabil.* 1994;3:2–17.
30. Barrack RL, Lund PJ, Skinner HB. Knee joint proprioception revisited. *J Sport Rehabil.* 1994;3:18–42.
31. Umphred DA, McCormack GL. Classification of common facilitatory and inhibitory treatment techniques. In: Umphred DA, ed. *Neurological Rehabilitation*. 2nd ed. St. Louis: CV Mosby; 1990:111–161.
32. Werner J. *Neuroscience: A Clinical Perspective*. Philadelphia: WB Saunders; 1980.
33. Freeman MAR, Wyke B. The innervation of the knee joint: an anatomical and histological study in the cat. *J Anat*. 1964;101:505–532.
34. Gray G. *Chain Reaction: Successful Strategies for Closed Chain Testing and Rehabilitation*. Adrian, MI: Wynn Marketing; 1989.
35. Borsa PA, Lephart SM, Mininder SK, Lephart SP. Functional assessment and rehabilitation of shoulder proprioception for glenohumeral instability. *J Sport Rehabil.* 1994;3:84–104.
36. Nashner L. Practical biomechanics and physiology of balance. In: Jacobson G, Newman C, Kartush J, eds. *Handbook of Balance Function and Testing*. St. Louis: Mosby–Year Book; 1993:261–279.
37. Guskiewicz KM, Perrin DH. Research and clinical applications of assessing balance. *J Sport Rehabil*. 1996;5:45–63.
38. Sale DG. Neurological adaptation to strength training. In: Komi PV, ed. *Strength and Power in Sport*. Oxford: Blackwell Scientific Publications; 1992:249–265.
39. Sale DG, MacDougall D. Specificity in strength training: a review for the coach and athlete. *Can J Appl Sports Sci.* 1981;6:87–92.
40. Kegerreis S. The construction and implementation of functional progressions as a component of athletic rehabilitation. *J Orthop Sports Phys Ther.* 1983;5:14–19.
41. Roy S. Irvin R. *Sports Medicine: Prevention, Evaluation, Management and Rehabilitation*. New York: Prentice-Hall; 1983.
42. Albert M. *Eccentric Muscle Training in Sports and Orthopaedics.* New York: Churchill Livingstone; 1991:7.
43. Voight ML, Cook G. Clinical application of closed kinetic chain exercise. *J Sport Rehabil.* 1996;5:25–44.
44. Komi PV, Bosco C. Utilization of stored elastic energy in leg extensor muscles by men and women. *Med Sci Sports Exerc.* 1978;10:261–268.
45. Enoka R. *Neuromechanical Basis of Kinesiology*. Champaign, IL: Human Kinetic Books; 1988.
46. Bosco C, Komi P. Potentiation of the mechanical behavior of the human skeletal muscle through prestretching. *Acta Physiol Scand.* 1979;106:467–472.
47. National Strength and Conditioning Association (NSCA). *Plyometric Training: Understanding and Coaching Power Development for Sports* [video tape]. Lincoln, NE: National Strength and Conditioning Association; 1989.
48. Root ML, Orien WP, Weed JH. *Normal and Abnormal Function of the Foot*, vol II. Los Angeles: Clinical Biomechanics Corporation; 1971.
49. Inman VT, Ralston HJ, Todd F. *Human Walking*. Baltimore: Williams & Wilkins; 1981.
50. Jackson RJ. *Functional Relationships of the Lower Half*. Middleberg, VA: Richard Jackson Seminars; 1995.
51. Mann RA, Hagy J. Biomechanics of walking, running and sprinting. *Am J Sports Med*. 1980;8:345–350.
52. Perry J. *Gait Analysis: Normal and Pathological Function.* Thorofare, NJ: Slack; 1992:151–167.
53. Mangine RE, Kremchek TE. Evaluation-based protocol of the anterior cruciate ligament. *J Sport Rehabil.* 1997;6: 157–181.
54. Lephart SM, Perrin DH, Fu FH, Minger K. Functional performance tests for the anterior cruciate insufficient athlete. *J Athl Training.* 1991;26:44–49.
55. Risberg MA, Ekeland A. Assessment of functional tests after anterior cruciate ligament surgery. *J Orthop Sports Phys Ther.* 1994:19:212–217.
56. Bullock-Saxton JE. Local sensation changes and altered hip muscle function following severe ankle sprain. *Phys Ther.* 1994;74:17–31.
57. Kaltenborn FM. *Mobilization of the Extremity Joints, Examination and Basic Treatment Techniques.* Oslo: Olaf Norlis Bokhandel, Universitetsgaten Oslo; 1980.
58. Hoke BR, Lefever-Button S. *When the Feet Hit the Ground . . . Take the Next Step*. Toledo, OH: American Physical Rehabilitation Network; 1994.
59. Curwin S, Stanish W. *Tendinitis: Its Etiology and Treatment*. Lexington: Collamore Press; 1984.
60. Townsend H, Jobe FW, Pink M, Perry J. Electromyographic analysis of the glenohumeral muscles during a baseball rehabilitation program. *Am J Sports Med.* 1991;19:264–272.
61. Moseley JB, Jobe FW, Pink M, et al. EMG analysis of the scapular muscles. *Am J Sports Med.* 1992;20:128–134.
62. Lephart SM, Henry TJ. The physiological basis for open and closed kinetic chain rehabilitation for the upper extremity. *J Sport Rehabil.* 1996;5;71–87.
63. Wilk KE, Arrigo CA, Andrews JR. Closed and open kinetic chain exercise for the upper extremity. *J Sport Rehabil.* 1996;5:88–102.
64. Glousman R, Jobe FW, Tibone JE, Moynes D, Antonelli D, Perry J. Dynamic electromyographic analysis of the throwing shoulder with glenohumeral instability. *J Bone Joint Surg Am.* 1988;70:220–226.

RECOMMENDED READINGS

Beckett ME, Massie DL, Bowers KD, Stoll DA. Incidence of hyperpronation in the ACL injured knee: a clinical perspective. *J Athl Training*. 1992;27:58–60.

DeCarlo M, Shelbourne KD, McCarroll JR. Traditional versus accelerated rehabilitation following ACL reconstruction: a one year follow-up. *J Orthop Sports Phys Ther.* 1992;15:309–316.

Irrgang JL, Whitney SL, Cox ED. Balance and proprioceptive training for rehabilitation of the lower extremity. *J Sport Rehabil.* 1994;3:68–83.

CHAPTER 16

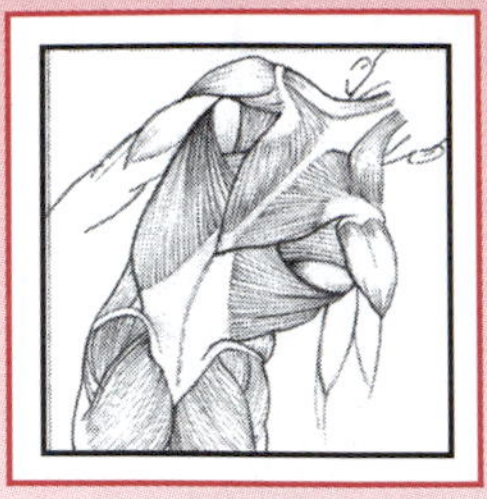

Alternative Movement-Related Therapies*

Donna Bajelis, Stuart Bell, Jeff Haller, Jack Blackburn, Judith Aston, and Daniel J. Foppes

In the field of rehabilitative therapies, alternative exercise paradigms are increasingly being included in an integrative approach to managing musculoskeletal and neurologic disorders. The recognition and use of these methods among medical professionals are based on a growing understanding of their efficacy in rehabilitation.

Only one of the approaches discussed in this chapter was created and developed by a trained medical professional, Dr. Milton Trager. The training and educational backgrounds of the developers of alternative exercise paradigms include biochemistry, physics, aerospace engineering, dance, and theater. Each creator contributed his unique perspective and understanding of the nature, structure, and expression of the human body and movement. All of these approaches strive to enhance the cognitive awareness of the individual's kinesthetic and proprioceptive function. Each approach requires proactive participation of the individual to learn and take responsibility for awareness of his body. These movement-oriented schools of thought provide an effective addendum to other forms of physical therapy treatment.

* Editor's note: This chapter was included because many physical therapists are beginning to incorporate alternative therapies into their treatment plans. The term alternative can be interpreted as meaning unfounded, nontraditional, or better than standard treatment. The definition used by the National Institutes of Health Office of Alternative Medicine emphasizes the lack of "sufficient documentation" of safety and effectiveness (Office of Alternative Medicine. Functional Description of the Office. Bethesda, MD: National Institutes of Health; 1993). *Physical Therapy* editor Jules M. Rothstein said, "The only reason some practices are called 'alternative' is that they haven't been researched. When the research is done, they won't be called 'alternative' any more; they'll be accepted into the mainstream, or they'll be rejected." This chapter describes movement-related alternative therapies to expand the awareness of students and clinicians about these approaches. Although some of these ideas are controversial, they remind us that no technique works for everyone. This text does not promote adoption of these alternatives without critical thought and study before, during, and after training in a given method.

HELLERWORK MOVEMENT

Hellerwork is an evolution of the Rolfing method. Joseph Heller, the founder, a mathematician and aerospace engineer, was trained by and worked closely with Dr. Ida Rolf and Judith Aston, the founder of Aston-Patterning. Hellerwork agrees with the principles of Rolfing in believing that structure determines function and that form follows function.[1] Like Rolfing, Hellerwork is a method of myofascial release that operates independent of a specific diagnosis. Hellerwork is unique in the field of myofascial release and movement therapies in that the practitioner consciously attempts to integrate the attitudinal and psychological aspects of posture and movement. As a Rolfer, Joseph Heller learned that the body, when organized about a vertical line, had improved efficiency and function of movement.[2,3] However, the structural changes that occurred in the body through Rolfing were not as long lasting as Heller thought they could be. While studying structural patterning with Judith Aston, Heller began to incorporate movement into his Rolfing sessions. The structural changes from the Rolfing sessions lasted longer when the client was taught how to use his body efficiently in movement.

Definitions and Goals

Hellerwork is a philosophy and way of being based on the inseparability of body, mind, and spirit. The process of Hellerwork integrates structural myofascial release, verbal dialogue, movement education, and energetics to create a human structure that supports healing and personal transformation. The theory of Hellerwork movement is based on personal awareness of body movement. The Hellerwork practitioner's intention is to educate and assist the patient in uncovering attitudes and unconscious beliefs that may contribute to and limit postural integrity and efficient movement dynamics.

Principles

Hellerwork movement has certain fundamental concepts and foundational principles:

- Structure determines function. Structural form limits what the body can or cannot do efficiently.
- Form follows function. The body forms itself according to how it is used.
- Body, mind, and spirit are inseparable.

Hellerwork recognizes the existence of a greater field in which we live, interact, and express ourselves: gravity. The purpose of Hellerwork is to enhance the individual's awareness of and relationship to that field. Within the context of a healing relationship, the Hellerwork practitioner works on body structure, psyche, and movement to improve function and well-being. The Hellerwork process follows an ordered sequence that organizes the body along the lines of gravity. This is accomplished through the guided touch of the practitioner, who educates the client to make changes toward a more functional movement pattern. The purpose of Hellerwork movement is to deepen a person's awareness about his movement patterns and how those movement patterns affect the development of his structure.

Examination and Evaluation

Hellerwork involves extensive evaluation about postural alignment and movement and the evaluation of myofascial length and tone across all the major joints of the body.[5] During the initial evaluation, the Hellerwork practitioner assesses whether the patient's major problems are physical or mechanical, an aberration of movement patterns, or psychophysiologic.

PHYSICAL OR MECHANICAL IMPAIRMENTS

Physical or mechanical impairments are those that are mechanically induced. The biomechanical alignment of myofascia can induce bones and joints into positions of abnormal stresses and create stress points. Stress points are load-bearing sites where major fascial planes cross joints in the body. For example, the thoracic lumbar fascia and trapezius muscle cross at approximately the 8th through 10th thoracic vertebrae, which corresponds to the bra line. Tension in either plane can create an increase in shear forces at T8 through L2, and these forces create an imbalance of load bearing from the upper to the lower torso. The result of excessive tension can be posterior displacement of the thorax in relation to the pelvis. An example of a complex, mechanically induced impairment is a patient presenting with a compound fracture of the right tibia and fibula. The results of a mechanical or physical injury are revealed in the specific site of injury and eventually throughout the whole body. The casting and immobilization of the leg may cause fascial and soft tissue displacement and restrictions of the leg.[6,7] Weight bearing is shifted to the uninjured left leg while the fracture heals. Favoring the left side of the body in movement establishes a pattern that affects vertical and horizontal alignment of the pelvis, torso, neck, and head, an effect that continues well after the injury to the right leg has healed.[8,9]

ABERRATION OF MOVEMENT PATTERNS

Aberration of movement patterns refers to impairments that result from habit or emulated behavior. Certain habits or attitudes cause postural changes. For example, a person who sits daily in a wheelchair may present with a forward head, extended chin, slumped shoulders, and sunken chest (Fig. 16-1). A self-conscious person may present with shrugged shoulders, retracted head and neck, and forward gaze and may have difficulty making eye contact with others. Attitude-induced postures may become true mechanical postures over time.[10]

PSYCHOPHYSIOLOGIC IMPAIRMENT

Psychophysiologic impairments are the result of somatoform responses to emotional trauma. For example, a woman who was told one evening by her husband that he wanted a divorce awoke the next morning with a painful, immobile shoulder, which continued to be a problem for 20 years. This chronic condition resolved when the woman was able to experience and release her grief and loss through Hellerwork.[10]

Treatment Intervention

Hellerwork movement teaches people to listen to their bodies as they move. The most important aspect of Hellerwork is to teach people to have a constant kinesthetic awareness of how they move throughout the day (eg, how they pick things up off the floor, orient their bodies to lift children, work at a computer). Rather than teaching one theoretically correct way of sitting, standing, bending, or lifting, Hellerwork

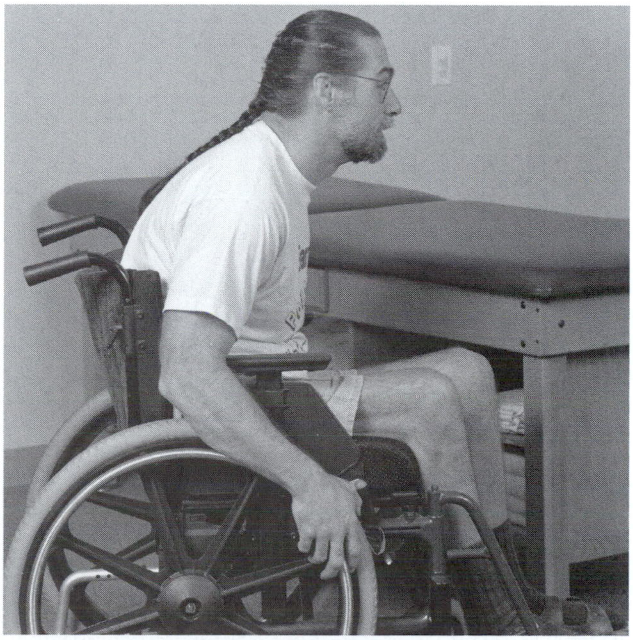

FIGURE 16-1 Poor posture from habitual sitting.

practitioners encourage their clients to explore, comprehend, and interpret their own kinesthetic perceptions of alignment and movement that are appropriate for their bodies. This is accomplished with the guided touch of the practitioner, which familiarizes the patient with his existing inefficient movement patterns (Fig. 16-2). The practitioner demonstrates, guides, and instructs the client about new, efficient patterns of movement.[11]

TRAGER MOVEMENT

For many years before his formal medical education, Milton Trager worked as a self-taught bodyworker and movement therapist. His early results with pain relief and movement re-education were dramatic. Trager successfully treated extremely disabling diseases such as cerebral palsy and postpolio paralysis.

Trager's treatments were different because the manipulations were gentle, rhythmic, repetitious, and painless. The client, though passive, was aware of pleasurable sensations in his body. Using his technique, Trager imparted the impulses of physical movement while the client lay passively on the table. He would then teach the patient to replicate these movements for himself.

Trager became a medical doctor in 1955. At the age of 42, he entered the University of Autonoma in Guadalajara, Mexico. He completed his internship in internal medicine and some residency in psychiatry at the Territorial Hospital in Kaneohe, Oahu, Hawaii. In 1957, he established a private practice in general medicine in Honolulu. Dr. Trager experimented with treating debilitating illnesses such as cerebral palsy and postpolio paralysis. Throughout medical school, he treated children affected by polio. He specialized in treating neuromuscular disorders. Originally, his method of bodywork and movement re-education was called psychophysical integration. He tried to get this approach accepted by the medical community. However, despite amazing success in treating difficult conditions such as muscular dystrophy, Parkinson's disease, and postpolio syndrome, he received a tepid response from his colleagues.[12] In 1977, at the age of 68, Trager retired from full-time medical practice but continued to see many "untreatable" patients and refine his techniques.

In 1975, Trager demonstrated his approach at the Esalen Institute in Big Sur, California. One of the staff members, Betty Fuller, a teacher and sponsor of Moshe Feldenkrais's work, was so impressed that she became Trager's first pupil. That same year, she started arranging training for bodyworkers and others to learn this technique from Trager. Betty and others founded the Trager Institute in 1980. Trager treated medical patients until 1989. He continued to teach and refine his approach until his death in 1997. He primarily worked with advanced practitioners after 1989.

Definitions and Goals

The intent of the Trager approach is to enable the client to release unconscious physical and mental limitations or holding patterns. The practitioner wants to create a new experience of feeling in the client through gentle guided movement. The work promotes deep relaxation and helps to increase physical mobility and mental clarity.

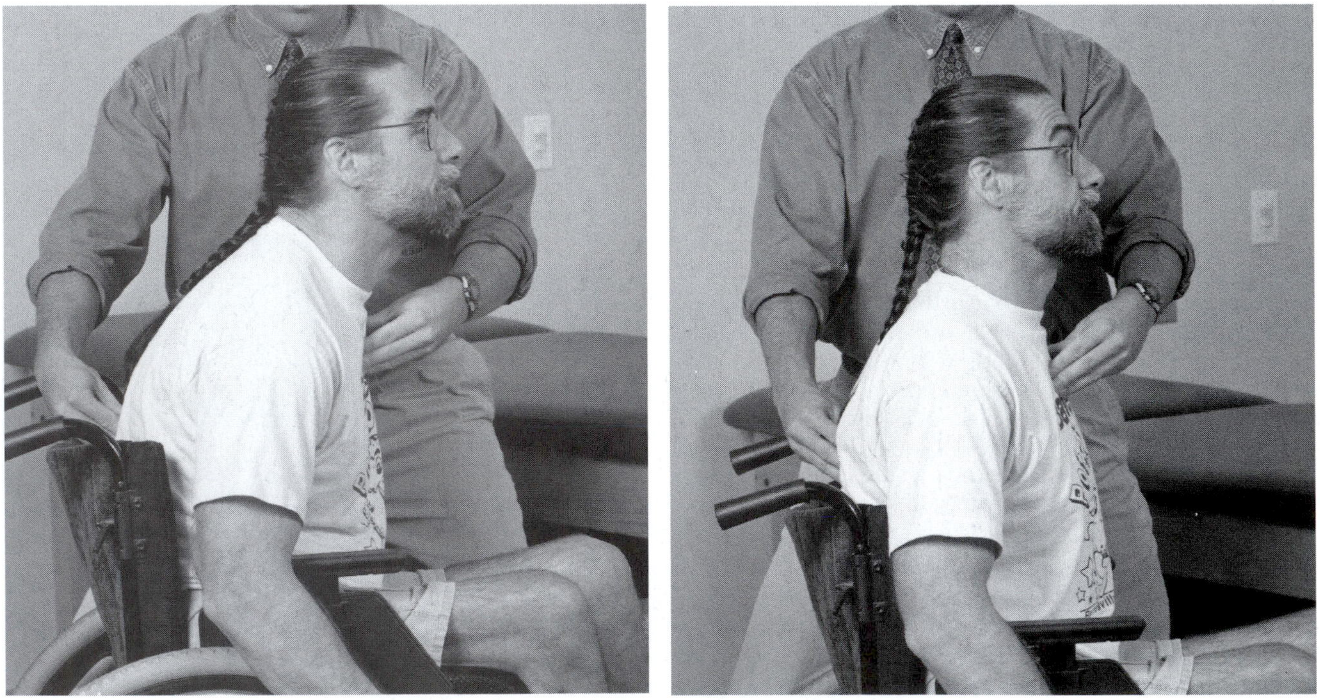

FIGURE 16-2 The practitioner uses guided touch to help the client explore his alignment and movement patterns.

Principles

Physiologic and psychological holding patterns are reactions to pain directed by the unconscious mind. Ordinarily, these holding patterns are released as the body heals itself. Pathology can be thought of as an interruption or delay in this healing process.[13] Bodily sensations provide a pathway into this unconscious holding pattern. The Trager practitioner imparts new, pleasurable sensations to reach and change the unconscious mind. Recall and reinforcement anchor these changes.

There is an underlying assumption that everything that takes place in the body is also reflected in the mind and vice versa. We can think of the mind as being distributed throughout the body to the cellular level through neural transmitters. Although we tend to regard the body and mind as separate entities, they are one soma or functional unit.

Our conscious mind is only selectively aware of this two-way communications link. When we experience fear, we are sometimes aware of changes that affect the sympathetic nervous system through sensations in our body. Through conscious monitoring, we can also become aware of sensations related to processes controlled by the autonomic nervous system, such as the breath and heart rates. We also can be consciously aware of the information involved in voluntary and involuntary muscle movement, although we mostly remain unaware of these information pathways.

Trager proposed that the body is replicated exactly in the unconscious mind, which also contains stored memories. He further postulated that most clients are unaware of their pain-induced patterns of resistance to available movement and bodily healing processes. For example, a person experiences trauma to the body with accompanying injury, pain, and other sensory data. To continue functioning without reinjury and avoid feeling more pain, the mind automatically and unconsciously splints the region through a neuromuscular response. The mind also stores the traumatic emotional information in the memory. Both of these responses are automatic and not consciously directed. We can think of these responses, respectively, as splinting or guarding and as numbing or avoiding the pain. The results often appear as deep-seated physical limitations and mental agitation.

Trager maintained that the unconscious mind holds a permanent record of all bodily transmitted experiences. Restimulation of this unconscious material can cause it to surface or become conscious again. The practitioner, by gently instilling pleasurable movement, introduces new information to that part of the unconscious mind. When the client feels these new sensations in an area that has a history of trauma, his mind has the option of selecting new data over the old. During the session, the practitioner reinforces this selection by calling attention to the experience so the client becomes consciously aware of the new sensations.

Evaluation and Examination

Before and after the tablework, a technique of the Trager approach, the practitioner performs an evaluation of the patient's awareness of sensation and quality of movement. Mentastics, another Trager technique, is used for assessing and improving the quality of movement and the awareness of sensation. The tablework and Mentastics are aimed at exploring what happens when restricted body parts are moved passively. Any positive changes are verbally and manually reinforced by the practitioner. It is important to evaluate how much the patient is aware of these changes.

Treatment Intervention

The Trager approach combines three main components in treating clients. These include tablework (ie, practitioner-initiated passive movement), Mentastics (ie, patient-initiated active movement), and mental presence or "hook-up." These techniques are used to alter the mind of the client through movement, feelings, and sensations.

TABLEWORK

During the tablework, the practitioner uses verbal cues to stimulate changes in the unconscious mind. The tablework involves a gentle rocking motion with traction, compression, torquing, and other forms of tissue stretch. The hands are used to isolate different joints, muscles, fascia, or other connective tissue. These portions of the client's body are supported and put into motion so that the momentum of the movement, while distributed throughout the client's body, can be anchored and vectored precisely (Fig. 16-3). The practitioner focuses the client's awareness on the sensations he is feeling. These sensations are unique, because most clients have not been supported and rocked in this way since they were infants. The movements are highly pleasurable and comforting and impose no painful stimuli.

The sensations in the body imparted by the movement become the medium for reaching or changing the mind of the client. This change of mind is the reason that the tablework in Trager is also called psychophysical integration. The client is intentionally guided to integrate the new information, such

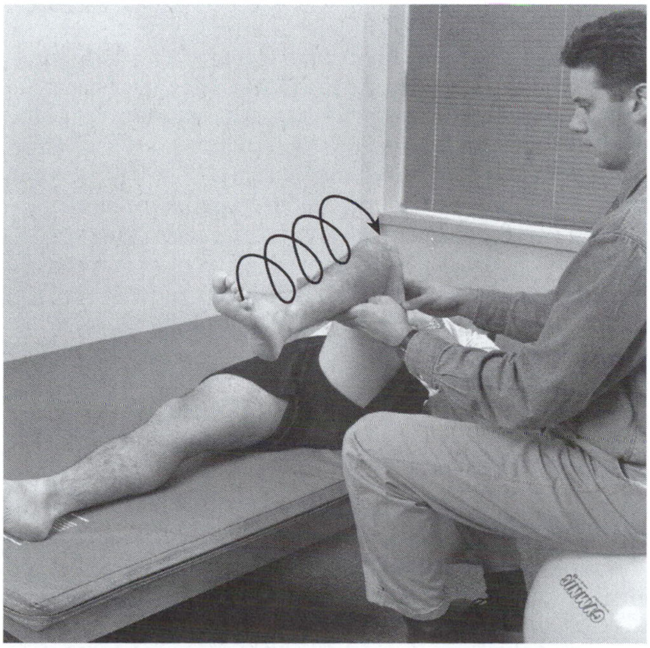

FIGURE 16-3 Trager tablework. The practitioner supports and gently moves the client's leg in a spiral motion.

as "I thought this shoulder could not move in this way without pain, but now that I feel it moving and bringing me pleasurable sensations, I have another option." At this point, the practitioner can reinforce this new awareness by teaching Mentastics to the client. These movements allow the client to reproduce the pleasurable sensations he experienced on the table.

MENTASTICS

The second component of the work is called Mentastics, a word Trager coined that combines "mental" and "gymnastics." Mentastics are movements developed by Trager to replicate what has happened in the tablework. Practitioners teach these movements to patients so that they can reproduce for themselves the feeling of the tablework. Mentastics are gentle and pleasurable movements. They use the gravitational field and momentum to stretch, open, and passively move the targeted joint or tissue. The movements are carefully designed so the muscles and joints being addressed are passively affected, just as they are in the tablework. During tablework, the client is encouraged to feel the sensations produced by the movement and to feel what it is like to use less and less effort. This awareness by the client can produce long-term changes in the client's holding patterns. Witt[14] said, "Instead of requiring the patient to control the movements, as in regular exercises, the patient is encouraged to 'let go'." In practice, this means the patient is instructed to initiate a movement and then let go of the muscle tension and allow the weight of the body part to carry the motion to completion.

HOOK-UP

The third component of the Trager approach is called hook-up. Trager coined this word to describe the mental state of the practitioner as she works. It means being connected to the client by sharing a common experience. Another way of describing this awareness is that the practitioner keeps her mind "present" by focusing on the sensations in her own body. This is a precise meditative technique for concentration. In a way, the client and the practitioner are sharing the same sensations or sensory information packets from the opposite ends. In this way they are hooked up. These information packets can include all the data of touch (ie, texture, tonus, and temperature) and all the components of the proprioception feedback loop. This shared information is the basis of the approach. An example of the hook-up experience is a dance couple who have such close bonding that each can anticipate the movements and thoughts of the other. While they are dancing, they seem to be of one mind. Trager places great emphasis on the hook-up portion of the work.

ASTON-PATTERNING†

Judith Aston, the founder and developer of Aston-Patterning, is a pioneer in the field of human movement, body mechanics, and the integration of body, mind, and environment. Realizing that current understanding of the human body was constrained by a linear viewpoint, she designed a new paradigm for body efficiency in static and dynamic postures. She has incorporated natural three-dimensional asymmetry and spiral patterns to create movement assisted by gravity and ground reaction force.

An innate gift for teaching has been at the core of Judith Aston's career. She was a college instructor of dance and movement for actors, dancers, and athletes from 1963 through 1972. She also trained therapists help their patients to identify and evolve individual patterns of expression. At Dr. Rolf's request, she developed and taught the movement program for the Rolf Institute from 1968 through 1977. She now maintains schedules of training and teaching throughout the United States, Europe, New Zealand, and Japan. She is a valued consultant in athletics, industry, and education.

Definitions and Goals

Aston-Patterning is a versatile and comprehensive system for therapeutic change, based on individuality as it manifests in the shapes, tensions, expressions, and motions of the body. The combined techniques enable each individual to pursue his ideal of his body in terms of posture and practical function. The primary focus is educational, promoting sophisticated choices in body use that reduce the element of chance in performance and personal healing.

Principles

The basic approach applied throughout this whole system emphasizes the quality of communication between the practitioner and patient. With the objective of providing positive reinforcement and building on success on subtle and obvious levels, practitioners use the concept of matching, which applies to patients' learning styles, belief systems, body shapes, tension patterns, and other pertinent aspects. Using Aston-Patterning techniques, practitioners facilitate change by matching what is presented, rather than imposing methods or ideas not appropriate to the client.

Aston-Patterning techniques are constructed around the principles of the Aston paradigm:

- Each individual is unique in all aspects of his body and person, and some degree of asymmetry of posture and movement is absolutely natural.
- Natural biomechanical efficiency involves negotiation of the body's asymmetries in three dimensions.[15]

Examination and Evaluation

The evaluation used in Aston-Patterning, along with the patient's history and mental, emotional, and physical status, combines visual observation of postural alignment and function with palpation of soft tissue to develop a whole picture of the body. During the evaluation of the patient, a body map is created that delineates alignment, dimensional relationships, and patterns of hypertension and hypotension[16,17] (Fig. 16-4). The body map is used to help develop cause-and-effect hypotheses, to formulate the appropriate

† Edited by Jenna Woods, BFA, CMT, with assistance from Judy Smith Huston, BMUS, both of whom are Aston-Patterning practitioners.

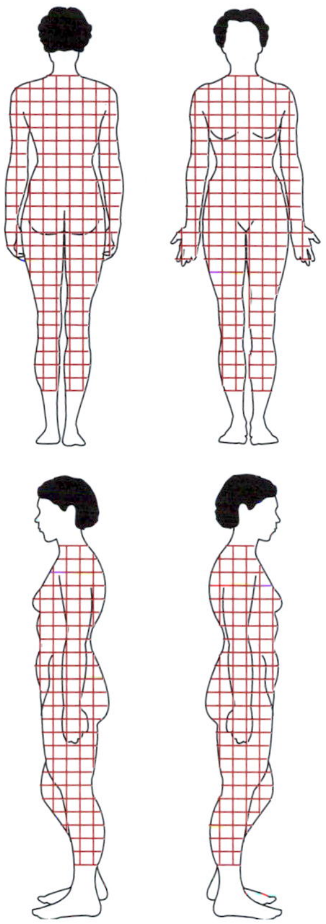

FIGURE 16-4 Example of body map used by Aston-Patterning practitioners.

work sequence, and to determine the appropriate combination of techniques. By referring to the whole picture, a practitioner is able to facilitate change in a balanced way throughout the body. After a session, the patient is reevaluated for changes in alignment, dimension, tension, and movement and for successful integration of the changes.

Treatment Intervention

The treatment intervention of Aston-Patterning includes bodywork, movement education, ergonomic consultation, and fitness training. These treatment methods are interwoven in individual sessions according to the sequence and combination the practitioner and patient find most appropriate to access the change needed at that time.

BODYWORK

Bodywork techniques in Aston-Patterning focus on working three dimensionally through the tissue and following the grain of the tissue. This is based on Aston's discovery that living tissue has directional grain and that it is spiral in nature.[15] The technique used specifically avoids compressing the tissue; the practitioner instead matches the shape by taking up slack and then releases holding patterns by following the grain and matching the tension in the tissue. Aston agrees with the idea that structural holding patterns, in which the fascia has tensed, impedes muscular flexibility. The Aston bodywork technique reduces stiffness of the fascia, allowing rehydration of tissue.[18] Bodywork is applied in three forms:

- Aston massage, which focuses on releasing functional holding patterns
- Myokinetics, which focuses on releasing structural holding patterns in soft tissue
- Arthrokinetics, which focuses on releasing structural holding patterns in joints and along bones

MOVEMENT EDUCATION

Attention to function is crucial to Aston-Patterning, because when the form of the body changes, reorientation is needed to avoid relapse and help the patient integrate the changes into everyday life. The movement work, called neurokinetics, is implemented through various basic movement units, each of which is used to explore aspects of movement in relation to body parts or specific tasks. Because of the simple-to-complex approach, the patient is able to learn an efficiency of movement that allows easier movement and that gives him the knowledge and control to change the patterns that were contributing to his discomfort. This work is extremely versatile and has been applied to everything from body awareness to rehabilitation to Olympic performance.

ERGONOMIC CONSULTATION

Aston ergonomic consultations developed as Judith Aston noticed how much and how easily the body is influenced by external factors. The purpose of this work is to enable a patient to understand how his body is affected by any object or arrangement of objects with which he physically interacts. Patients are shown different ways of modifying these objects or arrangements so they can feel the difference when their interactions are supportive and easy instead of awkward, difficult, or dangerous. Patients learn how to create individualized support in their environments.

FITNESS

Aston fitness training is an extension of neurokinetics that is applied to toning, stretching, and loosening or lubrication of tissues. Attention is focused on alignment, dimension, and cooperation of all appropriate muscle groups by customizing each exercise and program.

The first example is a patient with postpolio syndrome, which can be interpreted as the inability to further compensate for dysfunctions. An Aston-Patterning practitioner may include specialized exercise for increasing support, bodywork to release compensatory patterns of tension, ergonomics to accommodate the involved area, movement education to enhance the patient's ability to move comfortably and effectively work with the presented asymmetries, and certain toning exercises to stabilize the pattern.

The second example is an athlete in training for the Olympic gymnastics team who consistently is unable to execute a balanced landing after a series of three back handsprings. An Aston-Patterning practitioner may begin work with this client by researching the objectives, which may include watching successful performances of the series by other gymnasts before the first session with the client. The practitioner then may watch the athlete perform and have him experiment to discover whether there are any circumstances in which execution is successful, such as after only one back handspring. After watching and adding that visual information to the history and other initial assessment results, the practitioner may design an education program to elicit awareness of critical errors in timing, placement, speed, force, or movement design. Using bodywork and fitness exercises as needed to support the movement lessons, the practitioner can help the athlete learn to execute a more successful sequence of motions so that his objective is achieved.

The third example is a violinist whose complaint is severe pain in her right shoulder that occurs after only a few minutes of playing. After a visual assessment of the client standing and palpation of the area, the practitioner may ask the client to demonstrate playing. Using all available information, the practitioner would develop a working hypothesis about functional and structural causes of the difficulty. Knowing that there are immediate emotional issues, the practitioner may first use Aston massage or a brief movement lesson involving the breath to help release functional tensions and lessen the emotional distress. Over time, movement lessons, augmented with ergonomic changes in relation to the violin and bow and supported by appropriate Aston fitness exercises and bodywork, could be used to teach the client ways to prepare for playing, lessen tensions after playing, and learn a more efficient way to play. This allows her to circumvent the shoulder pain and, by reducing overall tension, to enrich the sound of her instrument.

ALEXANDER TECHNIQUE‡

At the turn of the last century, F. M. Alexander, who was employed as a Shakespearean reciter, was plagued by losing his voice during recitals. After many uneventful encounters with medical practitioners, who informed him that it was nothing organic, he began experiments to unearth the cause of the difficulty. After 9 years of careful and scientific experimentation, he determined that the trouble lay in the way he understood and used his body. He also determined that there were ways he could teach himself to overcome his misuse and misunderstanding. He was successful in permanently overcoming his own difficulties, and he developed a powerful technique for teaching others to overcome their difficulties.

Definitions and Goals

The Alexander technique is an educational process that promotes general re-education of the whole body and its uses. The goal is to achieve improved functioning by overcoming debilitating bodily reaction and habitual patterns. Because this technique addresses the whole body and all its uses, it has been successfully applied to many and varied functional, structural, and neurologic difficulties.[18]

‡Written by Stuart J. Bell.

Principles

Alexander discovered that we are all creatures of habit, and most of our habits are detrimental to our well-being. He found that our habits govern our sense of feeling, sense of ourselves, spatial awareness, and use patterns and that we cannot trust our feedback systems to help us overcome these habits. What feels to be correct alignment, posture, tone, or direction is probably not correct. He discovered there were ways that the habits could be undone and kept undone. These means were a new and different way of approaching the problem. His means involved "inhibiting" and unlearning habitual, unconscious control of the body and then learning a new, conscious thinking process for control of the body.[13]

Through consistent application of this conscious thinking and relearning process, Alexander was able to teach students to become more sensitive, more responsive, and more able to differentiate internal and external feedback. Overall use of the body, general functioning, and posture improve, and students look and feel better and move more comfortably than before learning this technique.

Examination and Evaluation

Alexander teachers rely primarily on visual and tactile evaluation within normal, functional ranges of motion and action. The teacher evaluates a student visually for overall posture and use from the moment they meet. The teacher looks for any diminution of stature, especially of length, but also of width and depth as the student is given a stimulus to action. Because the most generally used stimulus to action in an Alexander lesson is sitting down into and standing up from a chair, the student is evaluated visually as he sits and then stands. The Alexander teacher is especially interested in what occurs in the region of the head and neck and how these movements relate to the back, because how the person uses the head, neck, and back is considered to be the area of "primary control."

The Alexander teacher uses his hands to evaluate how the student reacts to various stimuli to action. For example, as the student sits and stands, the teacher senses the movements and internal responses and reactions with his or her hands placed gently on the student's neck and head. By using the hands, the teacher is able to evaluate shortening and narrowing that is not visually obvious.

Treatment Intervention

With the Alexander technique, the means for change are relatively simple:

- Pay attention to the current state of one's being and body use.
- Inhibit the usual habit and reaction patterns.
- Use thought processes to direct the body toward proper use.

Although a person can accomplish the technique alone, the invaluable sensory feedback and guidance of the Alexander teacher greatly accelerates the process and produces far superior, consistent, and reliable results. In an Alexander lesson, the teacher employs various activities or stimuli to action to guide the learning process. Chair work, squat, lunge, whispered "ahh," and tablework are commonly used activities. The idea is that an activity creates a stimulus for the student (eg, moving from a sitting to standing position). Then the teacher verbally guides and aids the student in negotiating the activity while reacting with awareness and with an objective process of thinking through the activity. The student learns the process of effectively directing himself (Fig. 16-5).

Lessons usually take about 30 to 45 minutes, depending on the teacher, and 30 to 40 lessons are needed to lay a solid neurologic foundation for change. Depending on the presenting condition or the interest of the student, more lessons may be valuable to refine awareness, improve use, correct newly made improper habits, and continue to chip away at older, more established patterns. It is very much like playing a musical instrument or learning an art, craft, sport, or skill. At first, many lessons from a teacher are useful for developing a strong, correct foundation. Then, from time to time, more lessons are useful for refining and improving the person's capabilities. Our bodies and their effective, graceful use can be seen as a wonderful, joyous, lifelong learning experience. Our bodies change, and our relationship with them changes over time. What is effective today may not be as effective in 10 years.[18]

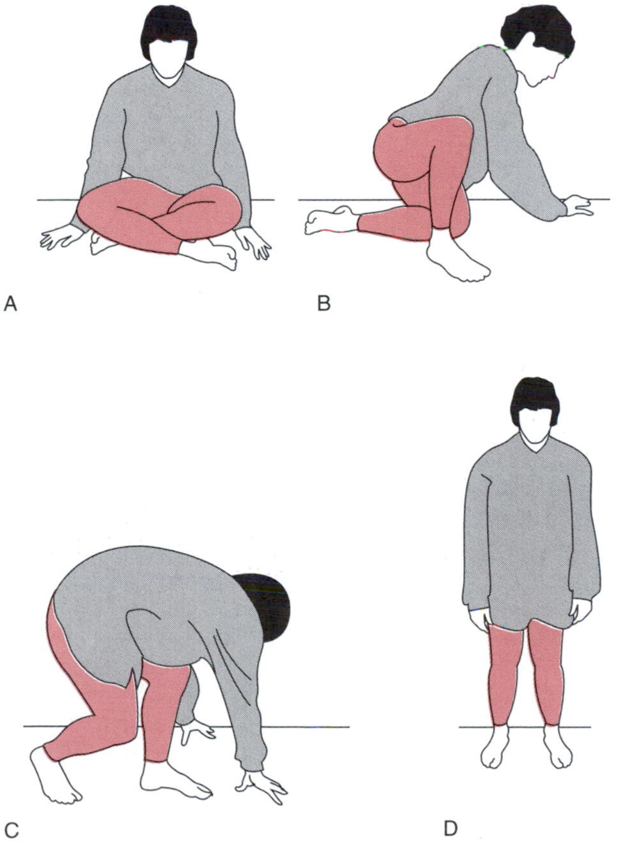

FIGURE 16-5 ***(A—D)*** During an Alexander lesson, the student negotiates a sit to stand activity learning to effectively direct herself.

FELDENKRAIS METHOD

The Feldenkrais method was founded by Moshe Feldenkrais (1914 to 1984). At the age of 14, he moved from Lithuania to Palestine, where he worked in construction and became interested in fighting techniques. As a young man, he developed a means of fighting that was based on using the fight or flight response elicited in an emergency rather than the responses based on years of training in fighting. He developed a manual for fighting. Years later, as a student of physics and electrical engineering at the Sorbonne in Paris, he had the opportunity to meet Jigoro Kano, the founder of judo (a martial art founded in Japan) who was traveling from Japan and giving demonstrations in Paris. He gave his manual to Kano, and he became one of the first Europeans to win a black belt in judo.

With his training, subsequent injuries, and insatiable curiosity about human functioning, he began to develop his method. His book, *Body and Mature Behavior*, was published in 1949.[19] He taught for more than 30 years and personally trained more than 250 practitioners in his style of teaching. His lessons in the use of self are classic and so well organized that no modern teacher has been able to improve on the method he invented.

Feldenkrais was an inventive and curious man whose thinking was extraordinarily global. His method was derived from abstract and theoretical ideas of the sciences and developed into concrete experiences for his students.[19] His work predates the modern cognitive sciences and systems approach to learning and human development. More than a decade after his death, much of his early thinking is gaining credibility in the cognitive sciences.

Definitions and Goals

Although the Feldenkrais method promotes relaxation, improves coordinated skillful movement, and promotes range of motion, none of these changes is the purpose of the lesson. The Feldenkrais method is an educational process through which the student learns how to learn. The Feldenkrais method uses movement as a means for persons to study and understand how they act so they can then refine their actions. The student learns to identify ineffective and efficient actions by observing minutely what they do. The Feldenkrais method explores functional movement from any position or orientation.

Principles

LEARNING PRINCIPLES

Learning in the context of the Feldenkrais method is not academic learning or skill learning that follows the example of the teacher; it is the kind of learning a child does. For example, think of a child standing in her crib. With one hand, she holds onto the upright bar for support. In the other hand, she holds a toy. As she stands, she looks around the room and at her toy. With the movements she experiences, she changes her balance and makes corrections to remain upright. At one point, she becomes so interested in the toy that she takes her hand from the bar to touch the toy and immediately falls down. After successive trials, the child eventually can let go of the bar, touch her toy, wobble about, and then put her hand back on the bar and remain standing. The child has not developed language yet. No one has demonstrated standing to her, but with many trials exploring many different ways, the child finds the path of least resistance,[20] refines her actions, and learns to stand.

Feldenkrais stated that learning means doing something that the person has not done previously. This could mean discovering how a person responds habitually to a situation and refining the habit so he can act in a more elegant, refined way, or it could mean learning and acquiring a completely new behavior. Feldenkrais did not consider a person to be skillful in his action unless he could complete an action in at least three different ways.

HUMAN ACTION

To Feldenkrais, the epitome of human action was the ability to move freely in all planes of action without preparation or hesitation. If a person has only one way of acting, it is compulsion. Two ways of acting are merely primitive choice. Until a person has three or more ways of accomplishing the same action, he is not free to act in the world with volition. Feldenkrais was interested in mature human action, which meant that the individual was able to stand on his own two feet in the world, maintain his individuality within a constantly changing environment, and respond with choice to each moment.

Feldenkrais used movement to improve human functioning because it is a unique way to study human action. It is difficult for a person to alter his thinking patterns. It is nearly impossible for a person to change how he senses information from the world or interprets that information. Those associations are deeply conditioned.[20] Persons can do little about how their emotional responses arise in different situations. It often takes many years to learn how to observe changes in our thinking and emotional states before we can have volitional control over these activities. However, movement can be readily refined and improved. When a person learns to act in an improved way, he may see how he maintained his conditioned or compulsive way of acting, even if it worked against his well-being. Any improved way of acting is reflected in a change of neuromuscular activity and in altered use of the skeletal, muscular, and soft tissue systems.

Examination and Evaluation

In the Feldenkrais method, the evaluation process is implicit within the intervention. As the practitioner works with the student so they can together discover the student's capabilities and the student's means of self-use, the student also begins to discover what is possible, and it becomes a part of his movement image. Through this process, the student learns how to change his action.

Treatment Intervention

Persons usually are not conscious of how they sit or move to a standing position. The Feldenkrais method strives to teach students three different ways of moving from sitting on the floor to standing.

A certified Feldenkrais practitioner develops an environment that stimulates students' learning. The environment offers minimal stimulation, and learning is done in a gentle manner, without effort or strain. If students are initially asked to make movements that are too intricate, too large, or made too powerfully, the complexity of the action overrides their ability to differentiate and feel what they do. The students are given plenty of time to explore and make mistakes. Competition, comparison, negative self-judgment, unnecessary effort, and trying are held to a minimum. Independence is encouraged. Students learn that they can refine their actions and make changes for themselves by paying attention to how they move. This gives them a sense of accomplishment.

For students to refine their behavior or learn new ways of acting, they must discover how they habitually act. During a lesson, students are verbally guided through movement explorations, but they are not shown how to do the movement. They experience it and all the alternatives to the movement provided by the teacher. Each person is guided into his own exploration. For example, if a student is asked to roll from his back to his side, he at first may not be able to distinguish how he initiates the movement. Does the movement begin by pushing a foot into the ground? Does he move his head first or his eyes? Does the movement originate in his pelvis? After a student knows how he habitually moves, he can begin to initiate the movement in alternative ways, discover possibilities for action he may not have known before, and adapt a better way of rolling (Fig. 16-6).

The student must be able to differentiate how he moves, and in time, the student learns to differentiate qualities of action. He begins to sense when he works with "parasitic effort" movements that are unnecessary for the efficient, elegant completion of the action.

The two techniques to implement the Feldenkrais method are called awareness through movement and functional integration. These techniques are different only in external appearance. Both processes use the same educational principles.

AWARENESS THROUGH MOVEMENT

Awareness through movement is a process taught in a group setting. In this process, the teacher provides a verbal map for the students to discover how they act. The student may be given the idea to study how he rolls from his back to his side. The teacher then provides the environment with the necessary verbal clues for the student to analyze his movement. Once he understands his unique movement patterns, the student is given information to help him find new ways of moving and discovering possibilities he probably did not know he could use or did not know were available to him. The simple act of rolling over can easily become an hour of exploration, which can lead to an elegant way of rolling and a quality of action previously not experienced by the student. Students can learn how they work with too much effort and learn to reduce the work put into the simplest actions. This understanding leads to feeling and acting with a muscular tone that is evenly distributed throughout the self; the movement not fixed by overuse in any particular area of the body. Feldenkrais recorded ap-

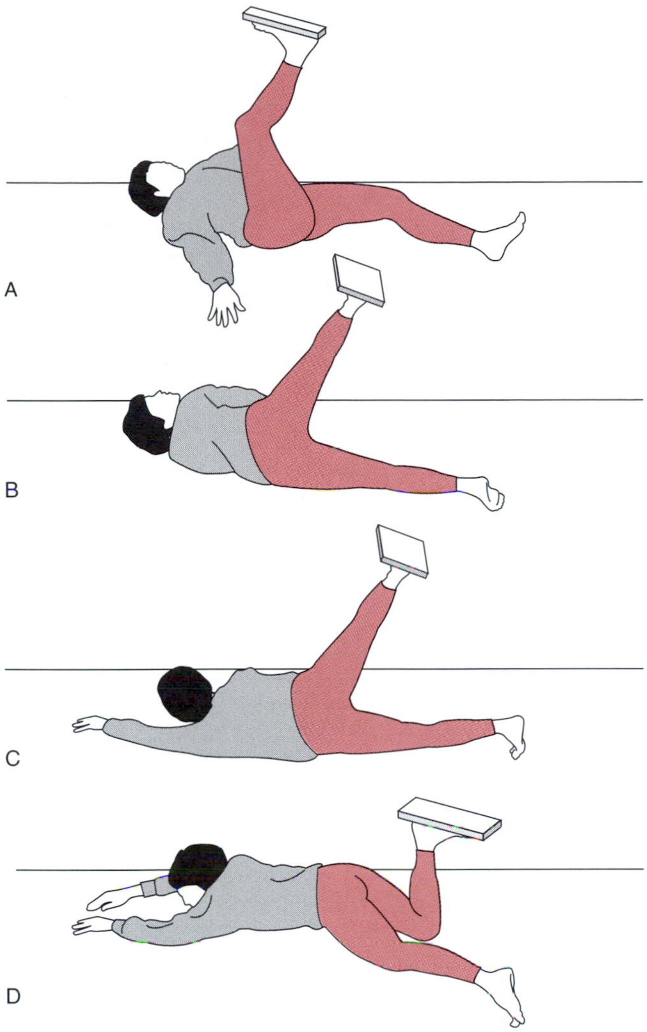

FIGURE 16-6 ***(A–D)*** During a Feldenkrais session the student explores how she rolls from her back to her stomach. In time, she will learn to differentiate the qualities of her movements.

proximately 1000 lessons about how we function in the world, including studies of flexion, extension, rotation, use of the eyes, movement of the head, relation of the breath to action, movements from rolling to sitting and sitting to standing, and use of the pelvis. All lessons are embodied within an educational philosophy instrumental to students developing their own mature behavior.

FUNCTIONAL INTEGRATION

Functional integration is the process Feldenkrais developed for working directly with a single student. Feldenkrais said functional integration is the relationship of the self to the environment, or "the relationship of the central nervous system to gravity." In most cases, it involves the student lying on a low table about the height of a chair. Through touch, the student is provided with an environment in which to explore his way of living in gravity. As he lies on the table, he is supported in such a way that unnecessary muscular activity can be discovered. The teacher provides the student with the opportunity to sense how he acts. For example, the teacher may roll the student's head or lift his arm. The teacher makes no effort to change the student's action. The student consciously or unconsciously feels whether it is easier to roll to the right or left, and each time his head is rolled, he finds the means to self-correct his action, provided that the rolling is done gently enough for the student to feel what is taking place. In the context of the lesson, the student is given the opportunity to explore this change in the use of movement of his head in relation to a function the teacher may help him find and explore.

In summary, functional integration is learning communicated through verbal and slow, gentle touch to provide new information directly to the neuromuscular system to improve problem-solving skills.[21] The Feldenkrais practitioner, because of his training, provides a rich environment of support, which is so comprehensive that the student is compelled to find movement improvement for himself.

Key Points

- Hellerwork is three-dimensional reconditioning of the body. Hellerwork involves deep connective tissue bodywork and myofascial release, movement education, and self-exploration of life issues through verbal dialogue.
- The Trager approach enables the client to release unconscious physical and mental limitations, also called holding patterns. The practitioner wants to create a new feeling experience in the client through gentle, guided movement, using tablework, Mentastics, and hook-up. The work promotes deep relaxation and helps to increase physical mobility and mental clarity.
- Aston-Patterning is a versatile and comprehensive system for therapeutic change, based on individuality as it manifests in the shapes, tensions, expressions, and motions of the body. The combined techniques, which include bodywork, movement education, ergonomic consultation, and fitness training, enable each individual to pursue his own ideal of his body in terms of posture and practical function. The primary focus is educational, promoting sophisticated choices in body use that reduce the element of chance in performance and personal healing.
- The Alexander technique is an educational process that promotes a general re-education of the whole body and its uses. The goal is to achieve improved functioning by overcoming debilitating bodily reactions and habitual patterns.
- The Feldenkrais method is an educational process through which the student learns how to learn. By implementing awareness through movement and functional integration, the Feldenkrais method uses movement as a means for persons to study and understand how they act so they can refine their actions.

REFERENCES

1. Rolf I. Rolfing: *Reestablishing the Natural Alignment and Structural Integration of the Human Body for Vitality and Well-Being.* Rochester, VT: Healing Arts Press; 1989:232.
2. Bajelis D. Hellerwork: the ultimate in myofascial release. *J Altern Complement Med.* 1994;12:26–30.

3. Barnes JF. *Myofascial Release: The Search for Excellence—A Comprehensive Evaluatory and Treatment Approach.* Paoli, PA: MRF Seminars; 1990:3.
4. Heller J, Henkin WA. *Bodywise.* Berkeley: Wingbow Press; 1991:29.
5. Kendall FP, Kendall McCreary E. *Muscle Testing and Function.* 4th ed. Baltimore: Williams & Wilkins; 1993.
6. Akeson WH, Amiel D, LaViolette D, Secrist D. The connective tissue response to immobility: an accelerated aging response? *Exp Gerontol.* 1968;3:289–301.
7. Woo SLY, Gomez MA, Woo YK, Akeson WH. The relationship of immobilization and exercise on tissue remodeling. *Biorheology.* 1982;19:397–408.
8. Akeson WH, Amiel D, Mechanic GL, Woo SLY, Harwook FL, Hamer ML. Collagen cross-linking alteration to joint contractures: changes in the reducible cross-linking in periarticular connective tissue collagen after nine weeks of immobilization. *Connect Tissue Res.* 1977;5:15–19.
9. Cantu RI, Grodin AJ. *Myofascial Manipulation: Theory and Clinical Application.* Gaithersburg, MD: Aspen Publications; 1992:25–62.
10. Kurtz R. *Body-Centered Psychotherapy.* Mendocino, CA: LifeRhythm; 1990:67–72.
11. Hanna T. Somatics. Reading, MA: Addison-Wesley Publishing; 1988:xi–xiv.
12. Liskin J. *Moving Medicine: The Life and Work of Milton Trager, MD.* xxx: Talman; 1996.
13. Miller B. Alternative somatic therapies. In: White AH, Anderson R, eds. *Conservative Care of Low Back Pain.* Baltimore: Williams & Wilkins; 1990.
14. Witt P. Trager psychophysical integration: a method to improve chest mobility of patients with chronic lung disease. *Phys Ther.* 1986;66:214–217.
15. Aston J. Overview: Seeing [course notes]. Mill Valley, CA: The Aston Training Center; 1987.
16. Hertling D, Kessler RM. *Management of Common Musculoskeletal Disorders: Physical Therapy Principles and Methods.* 2nd ed. Philadelphia: JB Lippincott; 1990.
17. Hoistad D, Greeley K. The Cervical Spine [course notes]. Seattle: xxx; 1994:51.
18. Alexander FM. *The Use of Self.* London: Chaterston; 1932:1–6.
19. Feldenkrais M. *Body and Mature Behavior: A Study of Anxiety, Sex, Gravitation and Learning.* New York: International Universities Press; 1949.
20. Feldenkrais M. *Awareness Through Movement: Health Exercises for Personal Growth.* New York: Harper and Row; 1972.
21. Reynolds JP. Profiles in alternatives. *Phys Ther.* 1994;2:52–59.

RECOMMENDED READINGS

ASTON-PATTERNING

Aston J, Miller B. A new approach to the dynamics of posture. *Phys Ther Today.* 1993;16:47–53.

Aston J, Molnar MA, Krier L. In your best shape with gravity's assistance. *Phys Ther Today.* 1992;15:50–59.

Aston J, Pollock J. Integrating Aston concepts into a massage therapy practice. *Massage.* 1996;March/April.

Burton Goldberg Group. *Alternative Medicine—The Definitive Guide.* Future Medicine Publishing; 1993:104–105.

Centeno K. An exclusive interview with Judith Aston. *Massage Bodywork.* 1996; spring.

Low J. The modern body therapies. *Massage.* 1988;16:48–50, 52, 54–55.

FELDENKRAIS METHOD

Feldenkrais M. *Awareness Through Movement.* New York: Harper & Row; 1977.

Feldenkrais M. *Body and Nature Behavior.* New York: International University Press, 1950.

Feldenkrais M. *Case of Nora.* New York: Harper & Row, 1997.

Feldenkrais M. *Elusive Obvious.* Capitula, CA: Meta Publications; 1981.

Feldenkrais M, Kimmey M, eds. *Potent Self: A Guide to Spontaneity.* San Francisco: HarperCollins; 1992.

Ruth S, Kergerreis S. Facilitating cervical flexion using a Feldenkrais method: awareness through movement. *J Orthop Sports Phys Ther.* 1992;16:25–29.

For further information: Feldenkrais Resources, Box 2067, Berkeley, CA 94702 [(800) 782-6716]; The Feldenkrais Guild, 524 Ellsworth Street S.W., P. O. Box 489, Albany, OR 97321-0143 [(800) 775-2118].

TRAGER MOVEMENT

Trager M, Guadagno C. *Trager Mentastics: Movement as a Way to Agelessness.* Barrytown, NY: Station Hill Press; 1987.

Liskin Jack. *Moving Medicine: The Life and Work of Milton Trager.* Barrytown, NY: Talman; 1996.

Juhan D. *An Introduction to Trager Psychophysical Integration and Mentastics Movement Education.* Mill Valley, CA: The Trager Institute; 1989.

Watrous I. The Trager approach: an effective tool for physical therapy. *Phys Ther Forum.* 1992;72:22–25.

Witt P. Experiencing chronic pain. *Whirlpool* 1987;spring:24–27.

HELLERWORK

Brugh J, Tarcher JP. *Joy's Way—A Map for the Transformational Journey.* New York: St. Martin's Press.

Dychtwald K, Tarcher JP. *Bodymind.* New York: St. Martin's Press.

Elson, Kapid. *Anatomy Coloring Book.* 2nd ed. New York: Harper & Row.

Fadiman, Frager. *Personality and Personal Growth.* 3rd ed. San Francisco: HarperCollins.

Heller J, Henkin WA. *Bodywise.* Berkeley, CA: Wingbow Press, 1991.

Juhan D. *Job's Body: A Handbook for Bodywork.* Barrytown, NY: Station Hill Press; 1987.

Kendall FP, Kendall McCreary E. *Muscle Testing and Function.* 4th ed. Baltimore: Williams & Wilkins; 1993.

Kurtz R. *Body-Centered Psychotherapy.* Mendocino, CA: LifeRhythm; 1990.

Platzer W. *Color Atlas and Textbook of Human Anatomy.* New York: Thieme Stratton.

Rolf I. *Rolfing: Reestablishing the Natural Alignment and Structural Integration of the Human Body for Vitality and Well-Being.* Rochester, VT: Healing Arts Press; 1989.

Travell JG, Simons DG. *Myofascial Pain and Dysfunction: The Trigger Point Manual: The Upper Extremities,* vol 1. Baltimore: Williams & Wilkins; 1983.

Travell JG, Simons DG. *Myofascial Pain and Dysfunction: The Trigger Point Manual: The Lower Extremities,* vol 2. Baltimore: Williams & Wilkins; 1992.

Warwick R, Williams PL, eds. *Gray's Anatomy.* 37th Br ed. London: Churchill Livingstone.

ALEXANDER TECHNIQUE

Alexander FM. *The Use of the Self.* London: Chaterston; 1984.

Barlow W. *The Alexander Technique.* New York: Warner Books; 1980.

Caplan D. *Back Trouble: A New Approach to Prevention and Recovery Based on the Alexander Technique.* New York: Triad; 1987.

Jones FP. *Body Awareness in Action: A Study in the Alexander Technique.* New York: Schocken Books; 1976.

For further information: Thomas Lemens, Director, Institute for the Alexander Technique, 15 The Parkway, Katonah, NY 10536 [(914) 232–8950].

CHAPTER 17

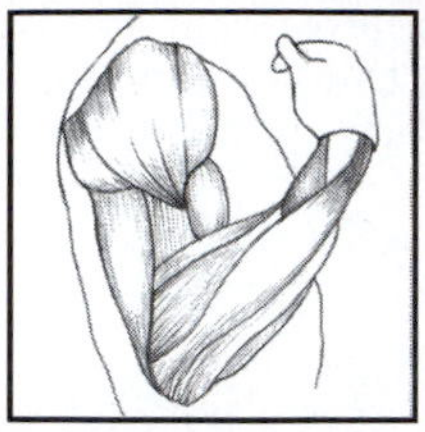

Aquatic Physical Therapy

Lori Thein Brody

Although water has been used therapeutically for centuries, only recently has its use become widespread in the rehabilitation community. Traditionally, water therapy has been limited to whirlpools used to debride wounds or to apply heat or cold treatments. However, the unique buoyant and resistive properties of water make it a useful tool for the rehabilitation specialist. The advantages of unloading and of immersion in a resistive medium are well recognized, and the use of water as a rehabilitative medium has developed. As a result, the body of knowledge surrounding aquatic rehabilitation has expanded exponentially.

As with other approaches to therapeutic exercise, it is important to realize that the water is a tool, with advantages and disadvantages. Not all patients are appropriate candidates for aquatic rehabilitation. The strengths and weaknesses of each treatment modality must be matched to the needs of the patient. Because water is such a unique environment, the clinician is advised to get in the pool and experience the effects of different exercises before prescribing them for patients. Often, exercises that appear to be simple can be quite difficult, and exercises that are difficult on land are easy to perform in the pool. The trunk stabilizing muscles are challenged with most arm and leg exercises and represent a very different task from the same activity performed on land.

Aquatic physical therapy can be defined as the use of an aquatic medium to achieve physical therapy goals. The purpose of this chapter is to acquaint the reader with the fundamental principles of aquatic exercise. It is intended to provide the framework for integration of water-based and land-based exercise to treat impairments, functional limitations, and disabilities.

PHYSICAL PROPERTIES OF WATER

The physical properties of water provide the clinician with innumerable options for rehabilitation program design. She should be familiar with these properties and the intended or unintended effects that may result from their interaction. For example, the effect of buoyancy on gait is that of unweighting, thereby reducing the amount of physical work of walking. However, this reduction may be offset by the frontal resistance encountered due to the water's resistance. As such, the clinician and patient should clearly define the goals of any given exercise in the pool to ensure progress toward overall functional goals.

Buoyancy

Archimedes' principle states that an immersed body at rest experiences an upward thrust equal to the weight of the same fluid volume it displaces.[1] As such, rather than a downward force resulting from gravity and body weight, individuals in the pool experience an upward force (ie, buoyancy) related to water depth and specific gravity. The specific gravity of an object (or an individual) is its density relative to that of water.[1] The specific gravity of water is almost exactly 1 g/cm^3; therefore, anything with a specific gravity greater than 1 g/cm^3 sinks, and anything less floats. This property forms the scientific basis for underwater weighing to determine body composition. The specific gravity of a person is determined by the relationship between lean body mass and body fat. Individuals with a higher relative lean body mass are more likely to sink, and those with a higher relative body fat have a tendency to float. These differences can be balanced by the appropriate use of water depth, flotation equipment, and waterproof weight equipment.

Buoyancy acts through the center of buoyancy, which is the center of gravity of the displaced liquid. If the body weight and the displaced fluid weights are unequal, a rotation about the center of buoyancy occurs until equilibrium is reached. The moment of buoyancy is the product of the force of buoyancy and the perpendicular distance from the center of buoyancy to the axis of rotation. As on land, the greater the distance, the greater is the force needed to move the limb.

> **DISPLAY 17-1**
> **Exercise Variables Used to Alter the Amount of Assistance Provided by Buoyancy**
>
> 1. Position or direction of movement
> 2. Water depth
> 3. Lever arm length
> 4. Flotation or weighted equipment

Buoyancy is one property of water that can be used to progress therapeutic exercise. The four main variables (Display 17-1) that can be manipulated to alter resistance or assistance are

1. Position or direction of movement in the water
2. Water depth
3. Lever arm length
4. Flotation or weighted equipment use

POSITION AND DIRECTION OF MOVEMENT

Like gravity, patient position and direction of movement can greatly alter the amount of assistance or resistance. Activities in the water can be buoyancy-assisted, supported, or resisted (Fig. 17-1). Movements toward the surface of the

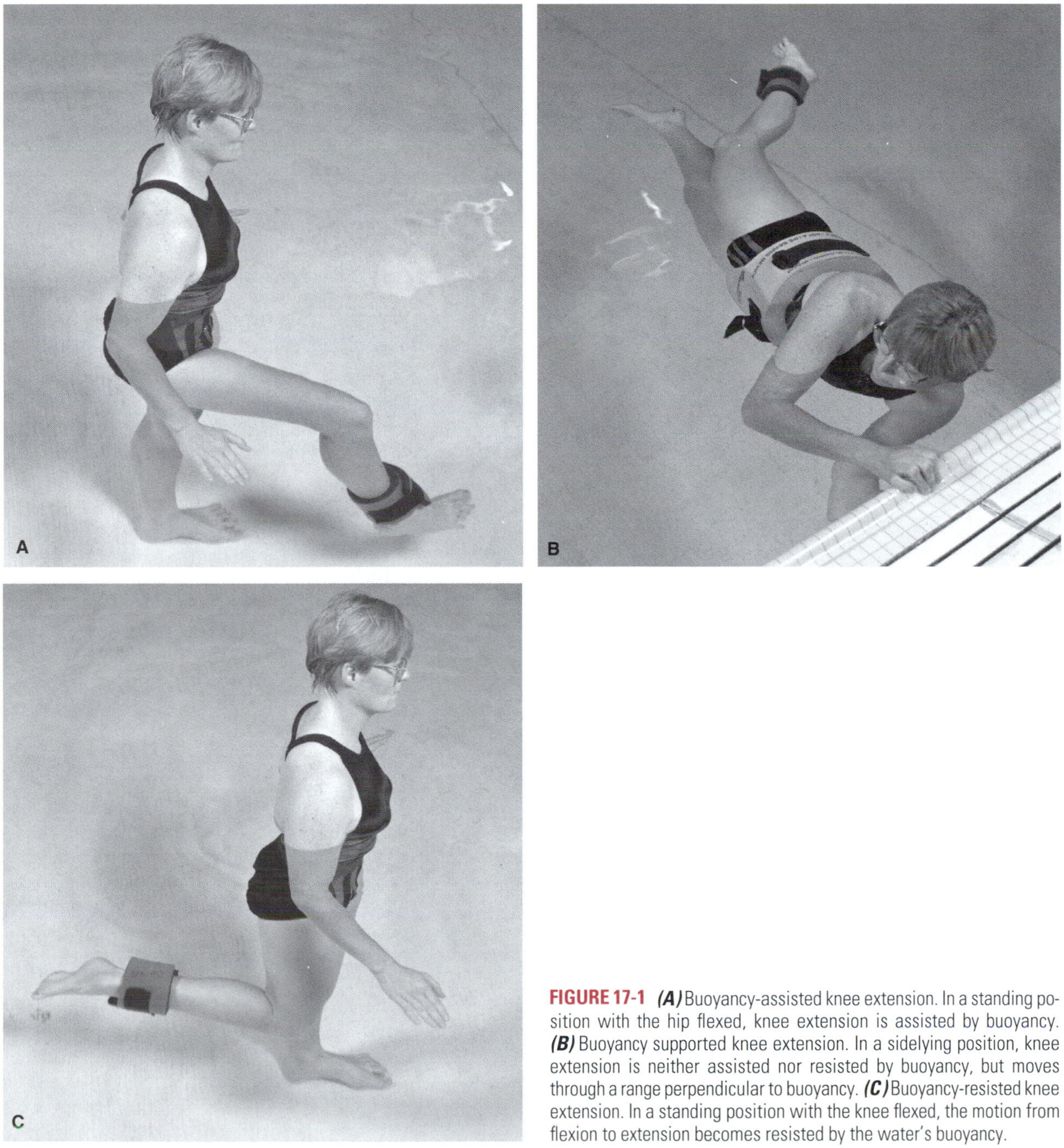

FIGURE 17-1 ***(A)*** Buoyancy-assisted knee extension. In a standing position with the hip flexed, knee extension is assisted by buoyancy. ***(B)*** Buoyancy supported knee extension. In a sidelying position, knee extension is neither assisted nor resisted by buoyancy, but moves through a range perpendicular to buoyancy. ***(C)*** Buoyancy-resisted knee extension. In a standing position with the knee flexed, the motion from flexion to extension becomes resisted by the water's buoyancy.

water are considered to be buoyancy-assisted exercises and are similar to gravity-assisted exercises on land. In this case, the movement is assisted by the water's buoyancy. In the standing position, shoulder abduction and flexion, as well as the ascent phase of a squat, are considered buoyancy-assisted exercises. In a prone position, hip extension can be buoyancy assisted. Movements parallel to the bottom of the pool are considered buoyancy supported and are similar to gravity-minimized positions on land. These movements are neither resisted nor assisted by buoyancy. In a standing position, horizontal shoulder abduction is an example of such an activity. Hip and shoulder abduction in a supine position are also examples of buoyancy-supported activities. Movements toward the bottom of the pool are buoyancy-resisted exercises. In a supine position, shoulder and hip extension are buoyancy-resisted activities, and the descent phase of a squat is resisted in a standing position. The ability of the clinician to position the patient a number of ways allows for a multitude of assisted, supported, and resisted activities.

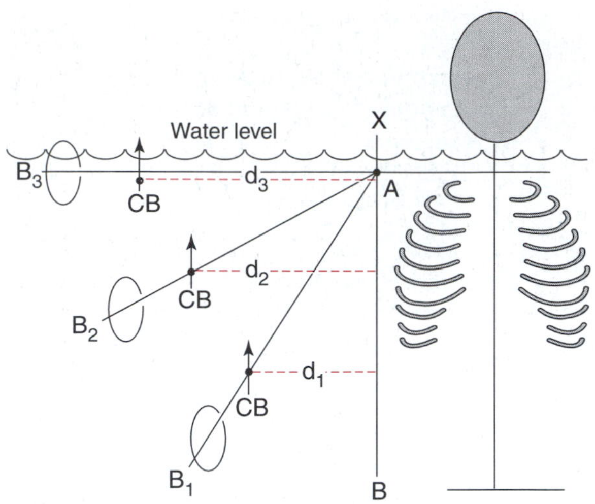

FIGURE 17-3 The effect of buoyancy with the edition of a float in the hand. (Adapted from Skinner AT, Thomson AM, eds. *Duffield's Exercise in Water.* 3rd ed. London: Bailliere Tindall; 1983.)

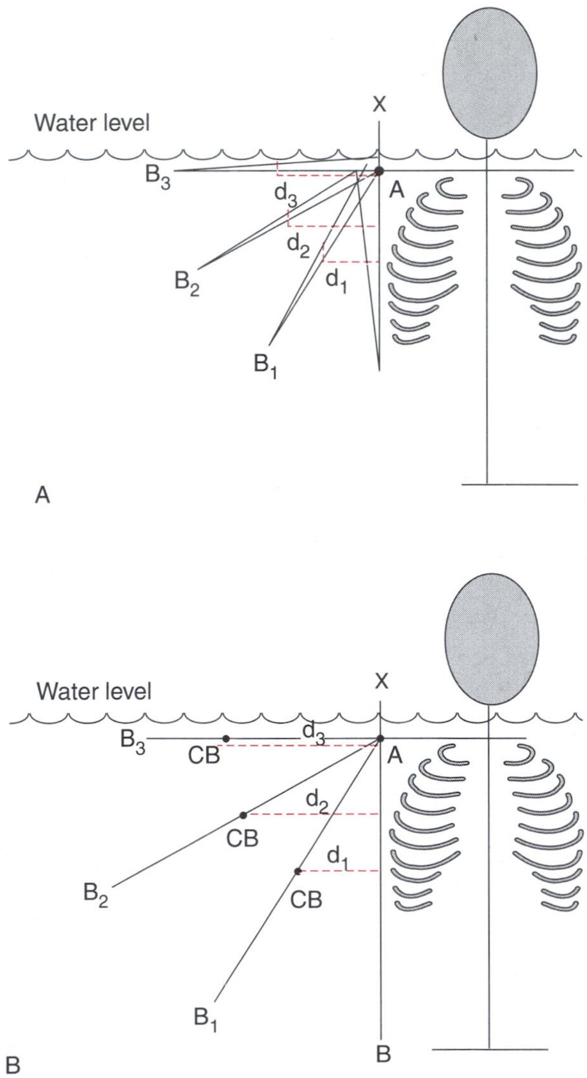

FIGURE 17-2 ***(A)*** The effect of buoyancy on shoulder abduction with a shortened lever arm (elbow bent). ***(B)*** The effect of buoyancy on shoulder abduction with a long lever arm (elbow extended). (Adapted from Skinner AT, Thomson AM, eds. *Duffield's Exercise in Water.* 3rd ed. London: Bailliere Tindall; 1983.)

WATER DEPTH

The water's depth is another variable that can alter the amount of assistance or resistance offered. For example, performing a squat in waist-deep water is easier than hip-deep water. Less support is provided by buoyancy in the shallower water. Walking can be easier or harder in deeper water, depending on the individual's impairment or disability. Someone with pain due to degenerative joint disease may find walking in deeper water easier because of the additional unloading of buoyancy, and someone with muscular or cardiovascular weakness may find the additional frontal resistance of deeper water more difficult. Estimates of percentage weight bearing at various depths have been obtained by Harrison et al.[2] The amount of weight bearing depends on the body composition of the patient, the water's depth, and the walking speed. Fast walking can increase the loading over the static condition by as much as 76%.[2] Occasionally, water depth options are limited by the available facilities. Modifications can be made by adding buoyant equipment to unload or by adding resistive equipment to increase frontal resistance.

LEVER ARM LENGTH

Just like exercise on land, the lever arm length can be adjusted to change the amount of assistance or resistance. Performing buoyancy-assisted shoulder abduction in a standing position is easier with the elbow straight (ie, long lever) than with the elbow flexed (ie, short lever). Conversely, buoyancy-resisted shoulder adduction is more difficult with the elbow extended because of the long lever arm (Fig. 17-2).

BUOYANT EQUIPMENT

To further increase the amount of assistance or resistance, buoyant equipment can be added to the lever arm (Fig. 17-3). A buoyant "bell" in the hand during shoulder abduction increases the assistance from buoyancy while in-

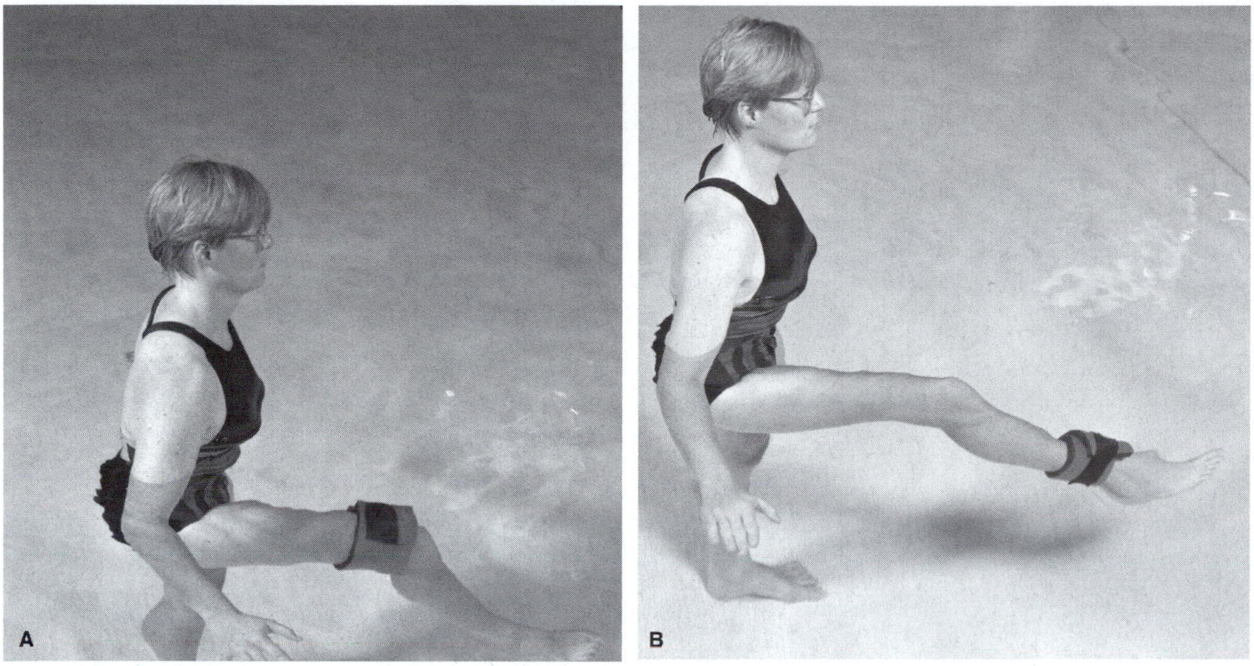

FIGURE 17-4 ***(A)*** Buoyant cuff added to the knee provides some assistance to hip flexion. ***(B)*** A buoyant cuff added at the ankle provides greater hip flexion assistance.

creasing resistance to the adduction return motion. Buoyant cuffs can be added anywhere along the lever arm to adjust the quantity and location of assistance or resistance (Fig. 17-4). Buoyant equipment is also used to support individuals in supine or prone positions as they perform exercises. Because buoyancy works in the direction opposite that of gravity, any land activity that would be resisted by gravity is assisted by buoyancy and vice versa.

Hydrostatic Pressure

The pressure exerted by the water at increasing depths (ie, hydrostatic pressure) accounts for the cardiovascular shifts seen with immersion and for the purported benefit of edema control. Pascal's law states that the pressure of a fluid is exerted on an object equally at a given depth.[1] The pressure increases with the density of the fluid and with its depth. Hydrostatic pressure is greatest at the bottom of the pool because of the weight of the water overhead. As such, the pool may be a good exercise option for individuals with lower extremity edema or joint effusion. The hydrostatic pressure also produces centralization of peripheral blood flow, which alters cardiac dynamics. This is discussed later in this chapter under Physiologic Responses to Immersion.

Viscosity

The viscosity of a fluid is its resistance to adjacent fluid layers sliding freely by one another.[1] This friction causes a resistance to flow when moving through a liquid. Viscosity is of little significance when stationary. The viscous quality of water allows it to be used effectively as a resistive medium, because turbulent flow is produced when the speed of movement reaches a critical velocity.[3] Eddies are formed in the wake behind the moving object, creating drag that is greater in the unstreamlined object than in streamlined objects (Fig. 17-5). In turbulent flow, resistance is proportional to the velocity squared, and increasing the speed of movement significantly increases the resistance. When moving through the water, the body experiences a frontal resistance proportional to the present-

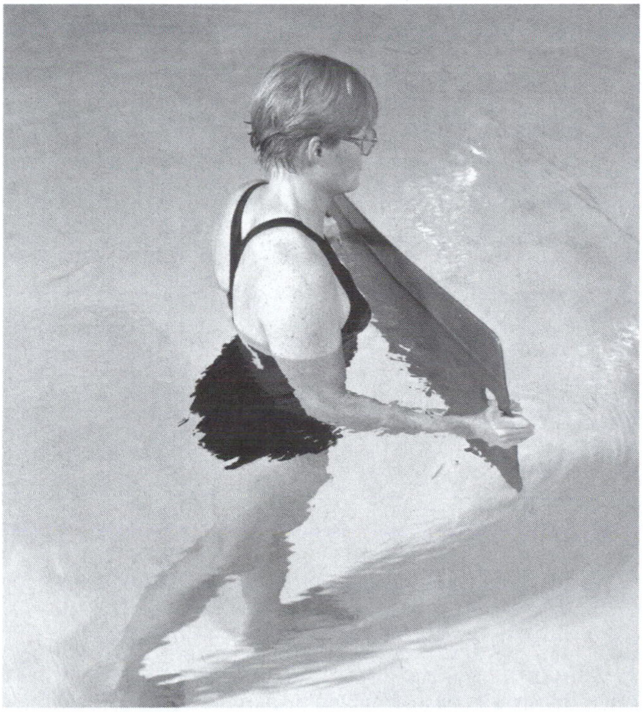

FIGURE 17-5 Using a plow while walking increases the surface area, creating eddies and drag.

ing surface area. Resistance can be increased by enlarging the surface area. The clinician has two variables to alter resistance produced by viscosity: the velocity of movement and the surface area or streamlined nature of the object.

VELOCITY OF MOVEMENT

Turbulence and resultant drag are created when movement reaches a critical velocity. Slow movement through the water produces little drag, and resistance is minimal. Buoyancy may be a more significant resistive or assistive property than viscosity during slow movement. However, when moving rapidly through the water, much resistance can be encountered that is proportional to the speed of movement. Individuals can progress resistance incrementally by gradually increasing the speed of exercise. This allows multiple gradations of an exercise rather than finite increases in weight, as is frequently necessary in land programs.

SURFACE AREA

In addition to altering the speed of movement, resistance can be modified by changing the object shape to provide more or less turbulence. The body can be positioned to alter turbulence, or equipment can be added. For example, less resistance is encountered in sidestepping than in forward or backward walking because of the more streamlined shape in frontal plane movement. Performing shoulder internal and external rotation with the elbows bent to 90 degrees with the forearms pronated produces much less resistance than performing this exercise with the forearms in neutral (Fig. 17-6*A* and *B*). Adding resistive gloves fur-

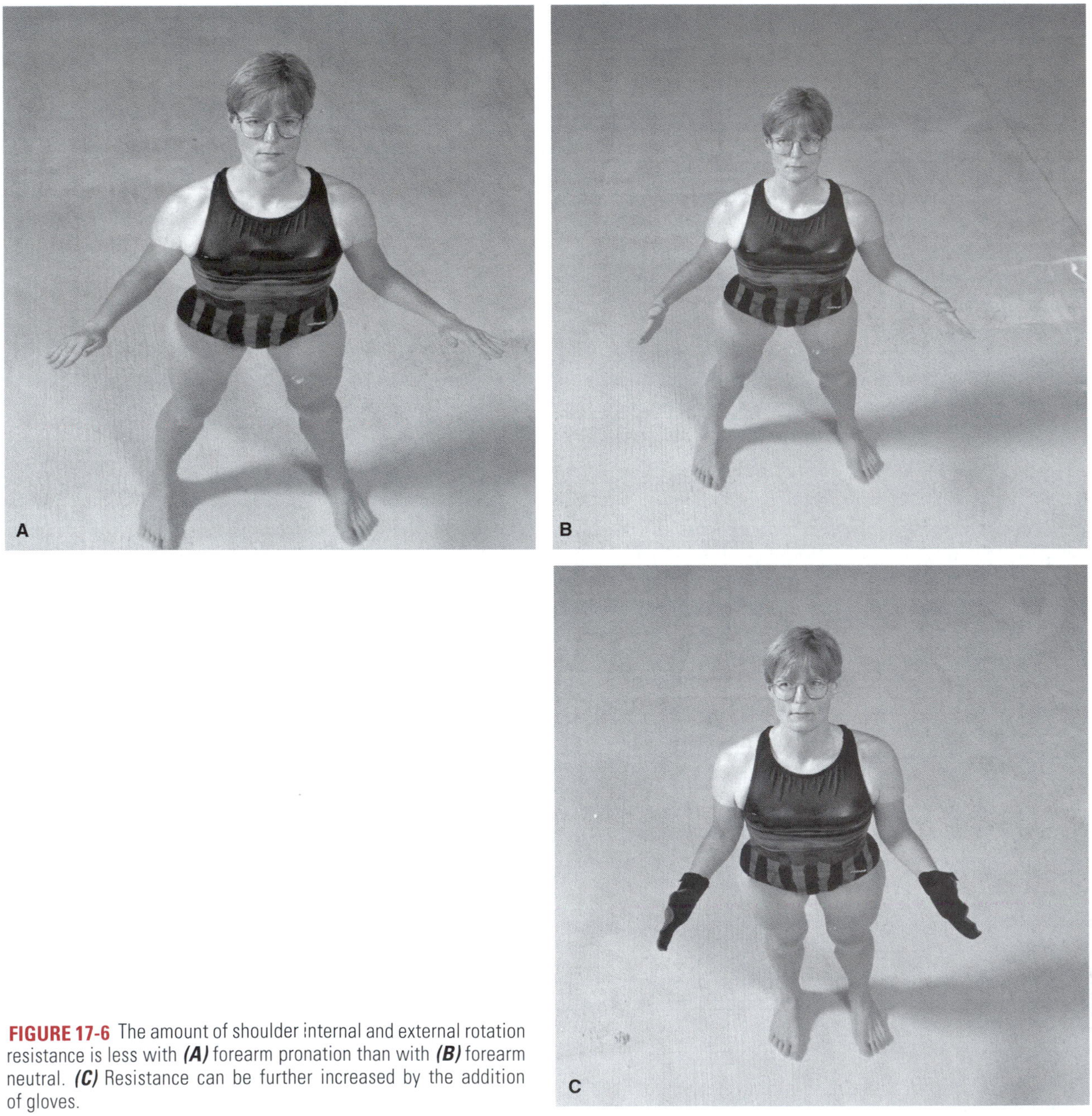

FIGURE 17-6 The amount of shoulder internal and external rotation resistance is less with ***(A)*** forearm pronation than with ***(B)*** forearm neutral. ***(C)*** Resistance can be further increased by the addition of gloves.

ther increases the resistance (Fig. 17-6*C*). Changing the pitch of the hand slightly between neutral and pronation alters the surface area and resultant resistance. This provides a multitude of resistive positions. Other equipment to increase the surface area and resultant turbulence are fins for the feet, a plow for resistive walking or other pushing and pulling activities, Hydrotone bells and boots, and paddles (Fig. 17-7).

PHYSIOLOGIC RESPONSES TO IMMERSION

Significant physiologic changes occur with immersion at various depths. Be aware of the changes that occur despite changes known to occur with exercise. These responses may produce desirable effects (eg, control of lower extremity edema) or undesirable effects (eg, limitation of lung expansion). Choose the appropriate water depth based on the specific health status of the patient and on the patient's physical therapy goals.

Effects of Hydrostatic Pressure

Immersion alone is not a benign action. The hydrostatic pressure encountered results in changes in cardiovascular dynamics even before exercise is initiated. Immersion to the neck results in centralization of peripheral blood flow.[4–8] Risch et al.[7] found that immersion to the diaphragm raised heart volume by approximately 130 mL, and further immersion to the neck increased heart volume by another 120 mL. Intrapulmonary blood volume increases 33% to 60%, and vital capacity has been shown to decrease 8%.[7] Immersion to the neck also increased central venous pressure at the height of the right atrium from 2.5 to 12.8 mm Hg.[7] The blood volume shift results in increased right atrial pressure of 12 to 18 mm Hg and increased left ventricular end-diastolic volume (ie, cardiac preload).[5,6,8] The cardiac preload produces a stroke volume (SV) increase through the Frank-Starling reflex. Studies have shown a SV increase of 35% and a cardiac output (CO) increase of 32% while immersed to the neck.[4,8] The heart rate (HR) remains unchanged or decreases because of the relationship of HR, SV, and CO such that HR × SV = CO. Risch et al.[7] demonstrated that raising the water depth from the symphysis pubis to the xiphoid decreased the HR 15%. These HR changes depend on the depth of immersion, the individual's comfort level in the water, water temperature, and type and intensity of exercise.

The cardiovascular changes due to centralization of blood flow are graded, and they occur with simple immersion before the onset of exercise. This accounts for much of the variability in HR changes with water exercise reported in the literature. The hydrostatic indifference point (HIP) is located approximately at the diaphragm and represents the point where the increase in hydrostatic pressure in the lower extremities and abdomen is precisely countered by the hydrostatic pressure of the water.[7] The effect of hydrostatic pressure on cardiovascular changes depends on the depth of immersion and on body position. For example, when the water level drops below the symphysis pubis, the positive effects of prevention of lower extremity edema are negated. The clinician should match the needs of the patient (eg, prevention of edema, cardiac history) with the risks and benefits of the various treatment modalities.

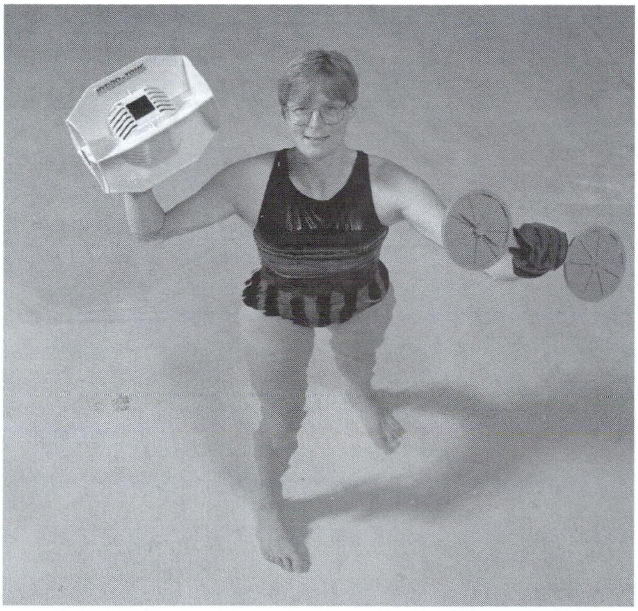

FIGURE 17-7 A variety of equipment is available to increase the surface area of moving limbs.

Effects of Water Temperature

Water temperature, like hydrostatic pressure, alters the cardiovascular challenge to the immersed subject in a depth-related fashion. Water that is too warm or too cold can add a significant thermal load to the cardiovascular system. Choukroun and Varene[9] found CO to be unchanged from 25°C to 34°C but significantly increased at 40°C; oxygen consumption was significantly increased at 25°C. Several studies have found a decreased HR in subjects exercising in cold water, and exercising in very warm water can increase HR.[10–14] Thermoneutral temperature is suggested to be approximately 34°C.[12–14] Most pool temperatures range from 27° to 35°C. Know the current pool temperature and potential effects on the patient.

PHYSIOLOGIC RESPONSES TO EXERCISE AND IMMERSION

In addition to the effects of immersion alone on cardiovascular dynamics, the clinician must consider the combination of changes due to immersion and changes due to exercise. Training in water produces physiologic adaptations similar to training on land, and aquatic training can be used to increase or maintain cardiovascular condition.[8,15–19] Deep-water running has been shown to maintain an individual's maximum oxygen consumption and 2-mile run time over a 6-week training period.[19] The pool can be used as a cardiovascular training tool alone or in combination with land-based training, providing the individual recovering from injury with alternative training mediums.

When training in the pool, the cardiac preload resulting from central volume increases persists despite the vascular shifts known to occur with exercise.[5] Despite the increase in blood flow to the working muscles (ie, peripheralization of blood flow), the increased cardiac load due to hydrostatic pressure (ie, centralization of blood flow) still occurs. Most studies have found the HR to be lower or unchanged compared with similar cardiovascular activity on land.[16,20–22] The depth of immersion affects the degree of cardiac changes, with increasing depth producing greater cardiovascular changes. Subjects studied while walking and jogging in ankle-, knee-, thigh-, and waist-deep water were found to work harder with increasing immersion up to the waist, at which point the increased resistance (due to surface area) was partially offset by buoyancy.[23] Water running and jogging in waist-deep water produces the same HR and oxygen consumption changes as exercise on land.[24,25] However, exercise while immersed to the neck will produce a HR of 8 to 11 beats per minute lower than similar land-based exercise.[26] A linear relationship between HR and cadence has been found during deep-water running.[27] Shallow-water running and deep-water running can be used for cardiovascular training. Mechanically, shallow-water running more closely resembles land-based running because of the foot contact on the bottom, but contact may also cause impact or friction problems.

When performing resistive exercise in the pool, it is important to realize that most muscle contractions are concentric because of the negation of gravity. Eccentric contractions can be generated if the water is shallow enough to minimize the effects of buoyancy or by resisting the force of buoyancy in an eccentric fashion. For example, performing a squat exercise in thigh-deep water requires eccentric contractions in the lower phase, but performing the same exercise in waist-deep water negates most of gravity's effects. If enough flotation equipment is used, an exercise can require eccentric resistance against buoyancy. With large flotation devices in the hand, the motion of shoulder abduction becomes an eccentric contraction of the shoulder adductors, resisting the force of buoyancy.

EXAMINATION OR EVALUATION FOR AQUATIC REHABILITATION

A full land-based examination should be performed by the clinician. This is the same evaluation the clinician performs when designing a land-based program, but the clinician must consider the physical properties of the water and the physiologic effects of immersion in determining the appropriateness of aquatic physical therapy for the patient. Some absolute and relative contraindications to exercise in the water exist. Individuals with excessive fear of the water, open wounds, rashes, active infections, incontinence, or tracheostomy should not be admitted to the pool. However, some physicians allow patients with open wounds to participate in aquatic rehabilitation with use of a Bioclusive dressing. This is commonly seen in patients with postoperative incisions.

Be aware of precautions to exercise in the water. The cardiovascular changes occurring with immersion should be of concern for the patient with a cardiac history. The hydrostatic pressure also limits chest expansion in those immersed in neck-deep water. This can create breathing difficulties for patients with pulmonary impairments or functional limitations. The hydrostatic pressure against the chest wall also can cause a sensation of an inability to breathe in persons who are uneasy in the water. The hydrostatic pressure produces diuresis, which can be avoided by emptying the bladder before entry to the pool.

Because of the sense of mobility experienced when exercising in the pool, many patients tend to overwork. Overexercise may occur because of the reduced gravity environment, the support of buoyancy, and the muscular relaxation associated with immersion, hydrostatic pressure, and water temperature. Frequently, the signs and symptoms of overwork do not manifest until later in the day or the next day. It therefore is better to err on the conservative side and underestimate the appropriate amount of exercise rather than overestimate.

AQUATIC REHABILITATION TO TREAT IMPAIRMENTS

After determination of the appropriateness of aquatic physical therapy with the patient, specific physical therapy goals must be developed. These goals should be written to address the specific impairments and functional limitations identified. The following sections describe principles of aquatic physical therapy to treat common impairments.

Mobility Impairment

Exercises to improve mobility and range of motion (ROM) can be easily performed in the water. The general muscular relaxation, support of buoyancy, and hydrodynamic forces occurring in water interact to provide an environment conducive to mobility activities. Be aware of the potential for overstretching while in the water. When designing a mobility program in the pool, the primary considerations are

1. The force of buoyancy and its effect on the desired motion
2. The position and available ROM at the joint
3. The direction of the desired motion
4. The need for any flotation or weighted equipment (Display 17-2).

DISPLAY 17-2
Considerations for Mobility Program Design

1. Force of buoyancy and its effect on the desired motion
2. Position and availage range of motion at the joint
3. Direction of the desired motion
4. Need for flotation or weighted equipment

Moreover, simple ROM exercises addressing impairments should progress to activities directed toward functional limitations and disabilities as quickly as possible. For example, exercises to increase hip and knee motion should progress to normal ambulation as soon as possible.

Buoyancy is the physical property used most often to facilitate ROM. Lever arm length and buoyant equipment are used to increase or decrease the amount of assistance from buoyancy. For example, hip flexion, shoulder flexion, and shoulder abduction are motions assisted by buoyancy in a vertical position. High marching steps can be performed with the knee flexed or extended, with or without flotation equipment. As soon as motion and weight bearing allow, this activity should be progressed to normal walking, running, or bicycling, depending on the patient's needs. Traditional stretching can also be performed using static structures in the pool such as steps, pool sides, and bars (Fig. 17-8).

Be alert to the use of proper technique when performing any exercise in the pool. Because of the water's refraction, it may be difficult to see the patient's posture and mechanics during exercise. The maintenance of proper spine position and osteokinematics during ROM activity is essential for the progression to functional limitation and disability-based exercises. It is often helpful to observe the patient's mechanics on land to ensure proper performance before pool exercise. Selected Intervention: Aquatic Therapy to Improve Upper Extremity Mobility and Selected Intervention: Aquatic Therapy to Improve Lower Extremity Mobility present examples of aquatic exercises that may be prescribed for clients with mobility impairment.

Muscle Performance and Endurance Impairment

Although buoyancy is the primary tool used to increase mobility, viscosity and hydrodynamic properties provide the greatest challenge to strength and endurance. The turbulence created during motion produces the greatest resistance and is influenced by the surface area, object shape, and speed of movement. The strength training principles and progressions used in water-based activities are the same as those used on land. Like techniques to increase mobility, traditional strength and endurance training exercises should be progressed to address functional limitations and disabilities as quickly as possible. For example, simple viscosity-resisted hip extension and knee extension exercises should be progressed to normal gait or rising from a chair as quickly as possible. Calisthenics, open kinematic chain, closed kinematic chain, diagonal patterns, and motor control exercises can be performed effectively in the pool.

Because the patient is immersed in a resistive medium, exercise in any direction can be resistive if given a critical velocity. A resistive motion in any direction requires a

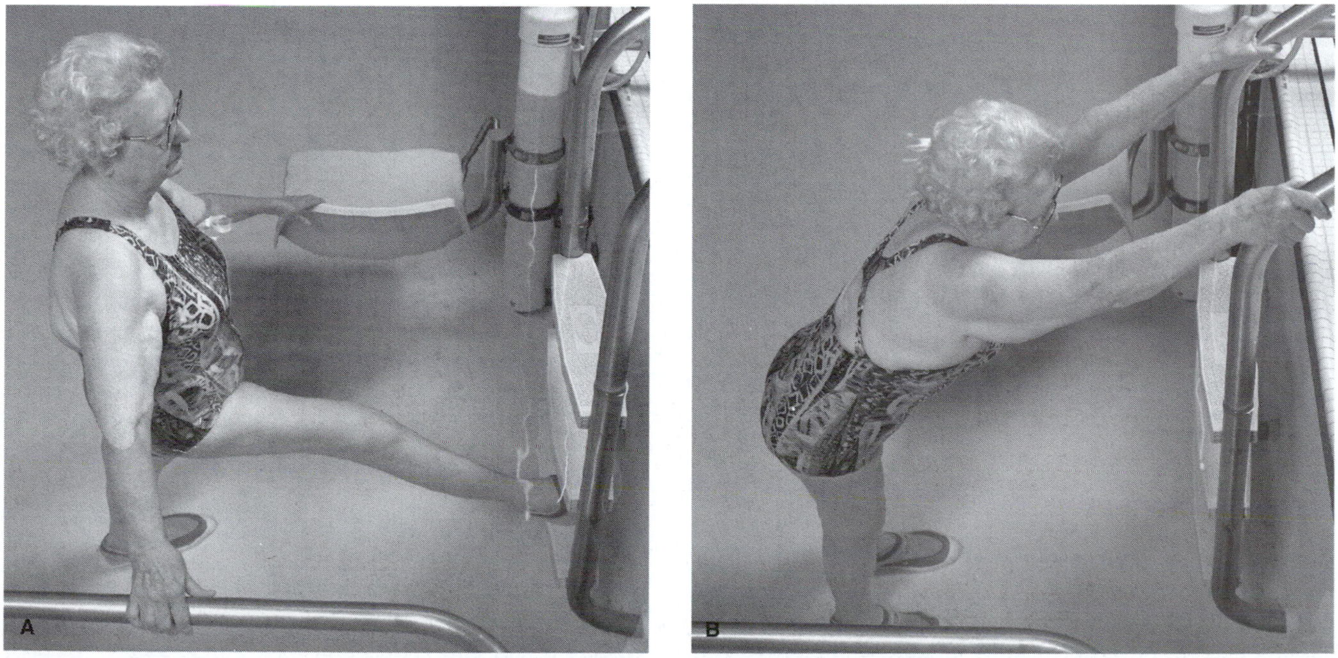

FIGURE 17-8 Stretching exercises for ***(A)*** hamstring muscles and ***(B)*** shoulder extensors can be performed using bars or the pool edge.

SELECTED INTERVENTION

Aquatic Therapy to Improve Upper Extremity Mobility

See Case Study #4

ACTIVITY: Shoulder internal rotation stretching

PURPOSE: To increase mobility in internal rotation and extension

ELEMENT OF THE MOVEMENT SYSTEM: Base

STAGE OF MOTOR CONTROL: Mobility

POSTURE: Standing in waist deep water holding a buoyant barbell behind the back

MOVEMENT: Squat slightly to increase the stretch

SPECIAL CONSIDERATIONS: Substitution such as forward trunk flexion or scapular protraction must be avoided. The patient should feel a medium to moderate stretching sensation.

DOSAGE: Patient should hold stretch for 30 seconds

EXPLANATION OF CHOICE OF EXERCISE: This exercise was chosen to increase shoulder mobility as one component of a comprehensive mobility, strength, and endurance program performed in the pool. This program is balanced with a home exercise program.

FUNCTIONAL MOVEMENT PATTERNS TO REINFORCE GOAL OF SPECIFIC EXERCISES: Reaching behind the back for hygiene, tucking in shirt, and hooking brassiere

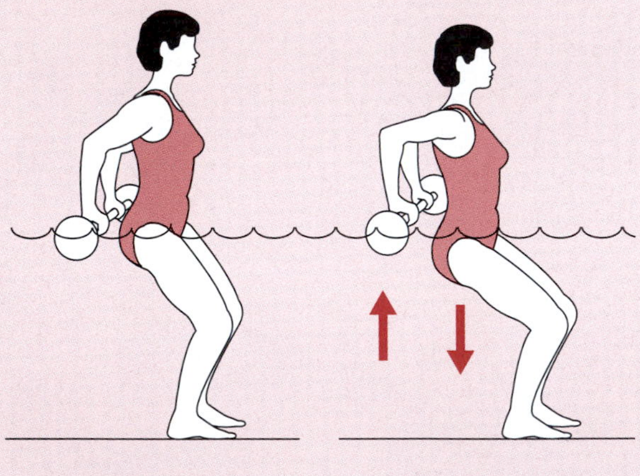

counterforce to stabilize against the turning effects of the center of buoyancy. For example, an individual standing in shoulder-deep water performing bilateral shoulder flexion from neutral to 90-degree flexion is pushed backward by the force generated with the arms (see Self-Management: Bilateral Shoulder Flexion). The leg and trunk stabilizers must fire to counteract and keep the individual from falling over. This can be an effective technique to train trunk stabilization. However, it is easy to overlook the additional muscular work necessary to provide stabilization against any kind of resistive movement in the pool, and this demand probably contributes to the overwork experienced by many patients. Be aware of which muscle groups are providing stability, the quantity of stabilization necessary, and the position or posture of the joints being stabilized. In the absence of external support (eg, hand hold, wall support), nearly any upper or lower extremity exercise places significant demands on the hip and trunk stabilizers.

As with exercises to increase mobility, equipment can be used to enhance resistive exercise. Buoyant cuffs or bells can be used to increase the resistance against buoyancy, and paddles, gloves, and other surface area–enhancing equipment can increase the resistance due to turbulence. It is important that the quality of the exercise not be sacrificed for an increase in resistance (see Self-Management: Bell Pushdowns).

Cardiovascular endurance can be increased in several ways, relying on the same principles of overload and progression used in land-based programs. The activity must be of sufficient intensity and duration, use primarily large muscle groups, and should be performed three to five times per week. Deep-water activities are especially useful for individuals with weight-bearing limitations. Deep-water running, bicycling, cross-country skiing, and vertical kicking are only a few of the activities that can be performed continuously or as intervals. Traditional swimming strokes complement these lower extremity dominant exercises. Shallow-water running makes an excellent cardiovascular conditioning exercise if impact is tolerated. Appropriate aquatic footwear must be worn when shallow-water running for any length of time. This minimizes the likelihood of impact injuries and friction injuries to the bottom of the foot.

Balance Impairment

The supportive medium of the water and its destabilizing forces provide an ideal environment for balance training. Other individuals in the pool create turbulence and create destabilizing forces. These forces can also be created by an individual's own movements. For example, kicking one leg forward produces a force pushing the individual backward (see Self-Management: Single-Leg Kicks). This must be countered with balance responses. Movements also occur slower in the pool due to the water's viscosity. As such, when balance is lost, the fall is slowed dramatically, giving the individual time to react and respond.

A variety of balance activities performed on land can be adapted to the pool. Any single-leg stance exercise with concurrent movement of the arms, opposite leg, or both can provide a wealth of balance exercise. Single-toe raises, stepups, and simple single-leg balance exercises can be performed with and without equipment (see Self-Management: Knee Flexion and Extension on a Single Leg). Selected Intervention: Aquatic Therapy to Improve Balance presents a sample of an aquatic exercise that may be prescribed for the client with balance impairment.

SELECTED INTERVENTION

Aquatic Therapy to Improve Lower Extremity Mobility

See Case Study #6

Although this patient requires comprehensive intervention as described in previous chapters, one specific exercise related to aquatic therapy will be described.

ACTIVITY: Lunge walking

PURPOSE: To increase mobility in the hip, knee and ankle, and force or torque generation and endurance in the lower extremities

RISK FACTORS: No appreciable risk factors

ELEMENTS OF THE MOVEMENT SYSTEM: Base

STAGE OF MOTOR CONTROL: Controlled mobility

MODE: Mobility and resisted activity in a gravity lessened environment

POSTURE: Maintain an upright trunk throughout the exercise

MOVEMENT: Walking in a normal heel-toe gait pattern, exaggerating the knee flexion of the loading response to 60 to 80 degrees of flexion, followed by full extension at midstance.

SPECIAL CONSIDERATIONS: Ensure an upright trunk avoiding forward lean. Avoid knee flexion beyond 80 degrees of flexion, and maintain a vertical tibia during the knee flexion component.

DOSAGE: Repetitions to form fatigue; performed 2–3 times week

EXPLANATION OF CHOICE OF EXERCISE: This exercise was chosen to improve mobility at the hip, knee and ankle, as well as dynamic muscular control at these joints. This movement was chosen to emphasize the knee flexion component in the loading response phase of gait.

FUNCTIONAL MOVEMENT PATTERN TO REINFORCE GOAL OF EXERCISE: Normal gait, ascending and descending stairs, and getting in and out of chair

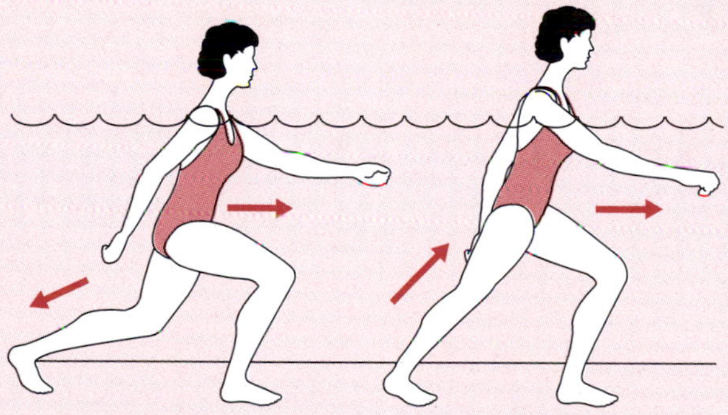

AQUATIC REHABILITATION TO TREAT FUNCTIONAL LIMITATIONS

Functional limitations represent restrictions in performance at the level of the whole person. Impairments involve losses at the tissue, organ, or system level but may or may not contribute to functional limitations. As the patient makes improvements in impairments, activities in the pool should be modified to emphasize the functional limitations. Functional limitations related to posture or position can be addressed in the pool. If prolonged sitting is a functional limitation, a variety of sitting activities can be performed in the pool. Many pools contain steps where the patient can sit with various levels of depth (ie, unloading). Chairs can be submerged in the pool, and buoyant equipment for sitting is available (Fig. 17-9). As sitting tolerance increases, the depth of water should be decreased, thereby more closely representing land situations. This same principle may be applied to deficiencies in prolonged standing or other positional limitations.

Functional limitations related to specific movement patterns (eg, gait, forward reaching) respond well to aquatic rehabilitation. Unloading the lower extremity or spine alone is frequently adequate to normalize gait mechanics. Verbal or tactile cuing may be necessary if gait changes have existed for some time. Any impairments such as limitations in motion, endurance, or strength must be addressed concurrently. As normal pain-free gait mechanics are achieved, the water depth should begin decreasing to replicate the land-based environment. Similarly, other functional limitations in movement can be

SELF-MANAGEMENT: Bilateral Shoulder Flexion

Purpose: Increased muscular strength and endurance in shoulder flexors and extensors

Increased trunk stability

Position: Standing with the feet in stride, arms at the side, and palms facing forward

Movement Technique: Level 1: Bring arms forward together; then turn palms facing backward and push arms backward. Turn palms forward and repeat.

Level 2: As above, but with feet in stance

Level 3: As above, with addition of resistive equipment

Level 4: As above, but standing on one leg

Level 5: As above, with eyes closed

Repetitions: ____ times

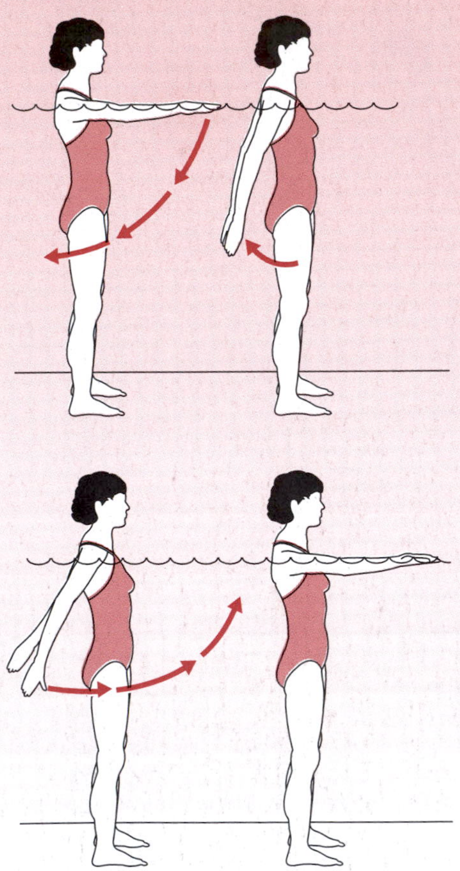

SELF-MANAGEMENT: Bell Push Downs

Purpose: Increased abdominal strength

Increased trunk stability

Increased shoulder and arm strength

Position: Standing in chest deep water, arms straight out in front with hands on a styrofoam bell

Movement technique: Level 1: Tighten abdominal muscles and pull bell straight down toward legs. Control the bell on the way back up.

Level 2: Move to deeper water.

Level 3: Increase size of buoyant bell.

Repetitions: ____ times ____

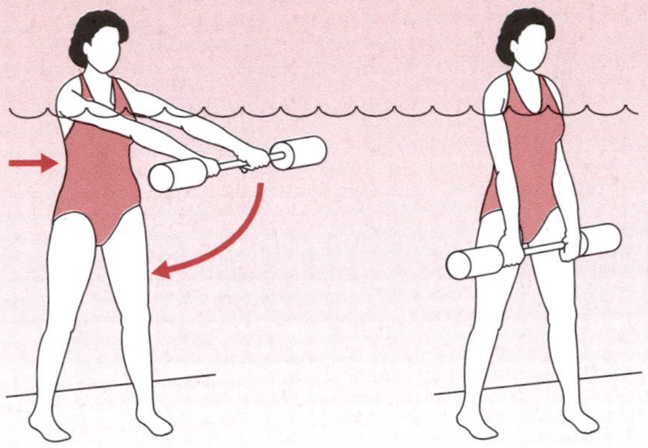

addressed in the same manner. For the individual with difficulty performing forward reaching, this activity can be assisted by buoyancy, which is progressed to buoyancy-supported and to bouyancy-resisted activity. Repetitive trunk flexion and extension, lifting, pushing, pulling, and squatting can be progressed in the same fashion (Fig. 17-10). Components of basic activities of daily living and instrumental activities of daily living can also be reproduced in the pool.

COORDINATING LAND AND WATER ACTIVITIES

One of the questions frequently asked by clinicians concerns the integration of water- and land-based activities. How much activity should be performed in the water, and when should land-based activity be incorporated? The advantages and disadvantages of aquatic rehabilitation and land rehabilitation should be matched to the needs of the individual patient, keeping in mind that humans function in a gravity environment. Because it is difficult to reproduce eccentric muscle contractions in the pool, the patient

SELF-MANAGEMENT: Single-Leg Kicks

Purpose: Increased hip mobility

Increased hip and knee muscle strength and endurance

Increased single-leg balance

Position: Standing on one leg in a neutral spine posture with abdominal muscles tightened. The non-weightbearing leg should be straight at the knee and flexed at the ankle. If working primarily on balance, stand near the edge, but do not hold on to steady yourself. Otherwise, hold on to the side for support.

Movement technique: Level 1: Kick leg forward and back, ensuring proper spine position. Avoid arching your back as your leg comes back, and avoid letting your trunk sway.

Level 2: Add resistive equipment to foot or ankle.

Repetitions: ____ **times** ____

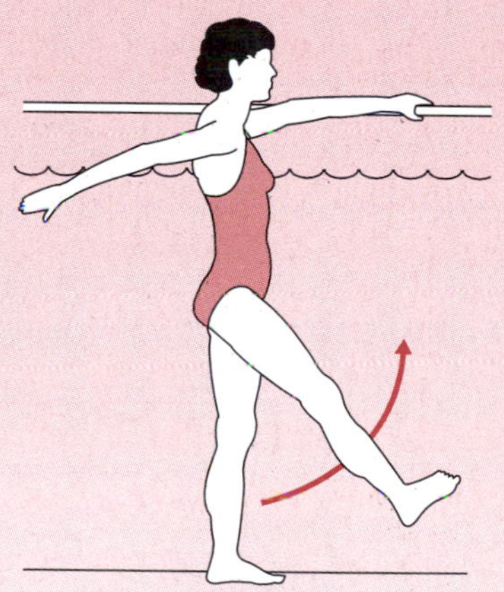

Starting position

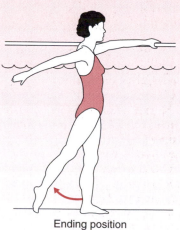

Ending position

SELF-MANAGEMENT: Knee Flexion and Extension on a Single Leg

Purpose: Increased knee mobility

Increased knee muscle strength and endurance

Increased trunk stability

Increased single leg balance

Position: Standing on one leg in a neutral spine posture, abdominal muscles tightened. The non-weight-bearing leg should be flexed to a comfortable position between 45 and 90 degrees at the hip and the knee bent. If working primarily on balance, stand near the edge, but do not hold on to steady yourself. Otherwise, hold on to the side for support.

Movement technique: Level 1: Flex and extend the knee through a comfortable range of motion.

Level 2: Add resistive equipment.

Repetitions: ____ **times** ____

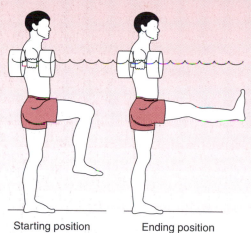

Starting position Ending position

should be progressed to land-based activities as quickly as tolerated. Early on, the patient may tolerate little land-based activity because of pain. Aquatic rehabilitation occupies most of the program at this time. As the patient is able to tolerate land-based activity, these exercises should be incorporated into the program. The quantity of water-based activity may remain unchanged, increase if tolerated, or decrease as the quantity of land-based exercise increases. The exact proportion and quantity of both land and water activity is determined by the needs and response of the patient. Occasionally, individuals respond better to alternate days in the pool, but others can progress to daily land-based exercises and discontinue pool exercise. The exercise program should be matched to the needs of the patient, with the goal of progressing to land-based exercise.

SELECTED INTERVENTION
Aquatic Therapy to Improve Balance

See Case Study #1

ACTIVITY: Single leg balance in chest deep water

PURPOSE: Train single leg balance through entire lower extremity and trunk without full weight on the limb.

RISK FACTORS: No appreciable risk factors

ELEMENT OF THE MOVEMENT SYSTEM: Modulator

STAGE OF MOTOR CONTROL: Stability

POSTURE: Single leg stance with arms in a comfortable position; lumboplevic region in neutral and knee in slight flexion

MOVEMENT: None; simply maintain balance

DOSAGE: Repetitions to form fatigue or pain; attempt to hold as long as possible

FUNCTIONAL MOVEMENT PATTERN TO REINFORCE GOAL OF SPECIFIC EXERCISE: Single leg stance of gait cycle

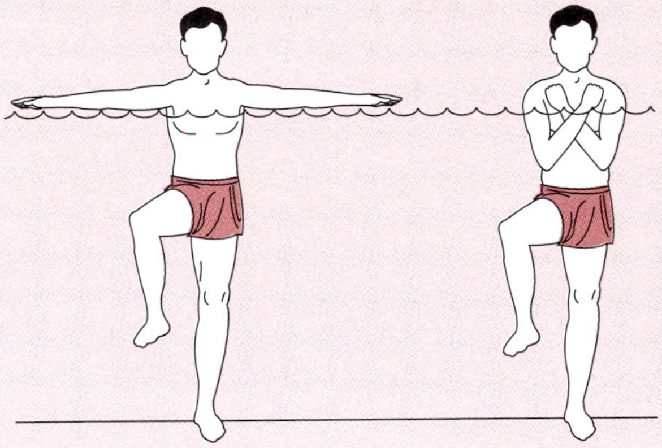

PATIENT EDUCATION

As with land-based exercise, patient education is a key component of the aquatic physical therapy program. The education program begins before entry into the water with a discussion of the fundamental properties of the water and the patient's expectations. Ensure patient comfort in the water; this is enhanced by educating the patient about the anticipated experience in the water. Identify the areas of entry and exit from the pool, the water's depth, and any other important safety features (eg, drop-offs, gutters, bars). Also familiarize the patient with the exercise program on land before entering the water to ensure proper exercise performance.

As the patient enters the water and the rehabilitation program proceeds, use this time as an opportunity to teach the patient about the expected benefits of the exercise. For example, when performing activities in single-leg stance, the patient frequently complains of an inability to maintain balance. Emphasize that developing balance is the purpose of the exercise and that any modification of the exercise to further destabilize the person is a progression of the exercise. When surface area-enhancing equipment is added, explain to the patient that it will increase the difficulty of the exercise. This also educates the patient on appropriate exercise program progression, and when the program is continued independently, the patient is able to self-manage and progress her own exercise program.

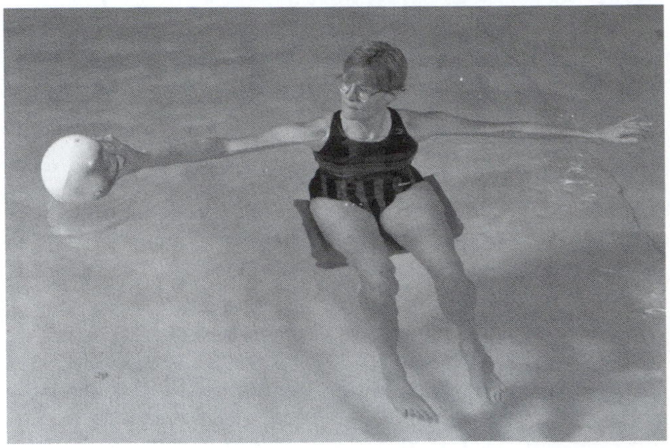

FIGURE 17-9 Posture exercises and reaching activities can be performed while sitting on flotation equipment.

Key Points

- The pool provides a unique environment for the rehabilitation of individuals with a variety of functional limitations and disabilities.
- The properties of buoyancy and viscosity can be used in a number of ways to achieve physical therapy goals.
- The effects of hydrostatic pressure and water temperature on the physiologic responses to activity must be considered to ensure patient safety.
- The water's viscosity provides much resistance and can be fatiguing for deconditioned individuals.
- Because a range of activities, from mobility and stretching to resistive and cardiovascular exercise can be performed in the pool, aquatic therapy can progress from the early stages through functional progression.
- Balance is challenged with nearly every arm and leg movement in the pool, and the effects of exercises on the trunk and leg stabilizers must be considered when designing the exercise program.
- The pool program must be balanced by a well-designed land-based program to ensure proper transition back to the land environment.

LAB ACTIVITIES

Pool Activities

1. Upper extremity
   a. Using a variety of positions (eg, supine, prone, standing) and equipment (eg, buoyant, resistive, wall, railings), develop an exercise program to increase a patient's shoulder, elbow, forearm, and wrist range of motion in all available ranges. Do this for a variety of motion limitations (ie, minimal loss to significant motion loss).
   b. Using a variety of positions and equipment, develop an exercise program to increase a patient's shoulder, elbow, forearm, and wrist strength and function. Progress from isometric exercise through a functional progression to activities of daily living, work, or sports. Perform open and closed chain exercises.
2. Lower extremity
   a. Using a variety of positions (eg, supine, prone, standing) and equipment (eg, buoyant, resistive, wall, railings) develop an exercise program to increase a patient's hip, knee, and ankle range of motion in all available ranges. Do this for a variety of motion limitations (ie, minimal loss to significant motion loss).
   b. Using a variety of positions and equipment, develop an exercise program to increase a patient's lower extremity strength and function. Progress from isometric exercise through a functional progression to activities of daily living, work, or sports. Perform open and closed chain exercises.
3. Trunk
   a. In an upright position, establish a neutral spine position and ambulate forward, backward, sidestepping, and braiding patterns. Vary step length, and observe resultant changes in range of motion.
   b. In an upright position, perform a variety of upper extremity exercises, and observe the challenges to the trunk stabilizers. Perform exercises with a wide stance, narrow stance, and standing on one leg.
   c. In an upright position, perform a variety of lower extremity exercises, and observe the challenges to the trunk stabilizers. Notice the differences between sagittal plane and frontal plane motions.

Land Activities

Develop land-based and aquatic rehabilitation programs for the following patient problems. Progress the program from the acute phase through to a functional progression.

PATIENT #1

A 54-year-old man has L4-L5 discogenic back pain. The patient has had recurrent episodes of pain over several years but has always been able to self-treat with a home exercise program designed by a physical therapist. Two weeks ago, the patient took a vacation requiring a long plane flight, followed by sleeping in a bed with a poor mattress. This patient has been unable to relieve the symptoms with self-treatment. His primary complaint is low back pain with occasional radicular pain to the left knee. Symptoms do not extend beyond the knee. The patient desires to return to walking as exercise and recreational golf. He works at a desk job.

Examination reveals an easily correctable lateral shift to the right, with decreased active and ROM in extension, left sidebending, and left rotation. Active motion is limited in flexion. Dural signs are positive for radicular symptoms, but deep tendon reflexes and sensation are intact throughout. The low back is diffusely tender, with a protective muscle spasm in the left erector spinae. Lower extremity strength is 5/5 to single repetition testing throughout.

PATIENT #2

A 60-year-old woman presents after a right proximal humeral fracture, which was cared for with sling immobilization for 6 weeks. She has a history of mild degenerative joint disease at the acromioclavicular joint. She is right handed and complains primarily of an inability to perform her daily activities because of motion loss and shoulder pain. Her goals are to return to activities of daily living, golf, and gardening.

Examination reveals loss of motion in all shoulder motions in a capsular pattern. Elbow, wrist, and hand motions are normal. Strength tests are limited by shoulder pain. Accessory motion is slightly decreased compared with the left in anterior, posterior, and inferior directions. Strength and sensation are normal throughout the rest of the right upper extremity.

PATIENT #3

A 17-year-old girl is seen 6 weeks after abrasion chondroplasty for an acute osteochondral lesion on the weight-bearing surface of her right knee medial femoral condyle. Her goals are to return to basketball, softball, and volleyball. She is partial weight bearing (50%) and can be progressed by 25% every 2 to 3 weeks until full weight bearing is achieved.

Active motion of the knee is S:0-10-90 and passive motion is S:0-5-100 with an empty endfeel. She maintains a 1+ effusion and has 4+/5 strength to manual muscle test, with visible atrophy of the quadriceps. Hamstring muscle testing is 4+/5, gluteus maximus is 4+/5, and gluteus medius 4/5. She ambulates with an antalgic gait pattern with bilateral axillary crutches. Overall, she has a varus knee alignment.

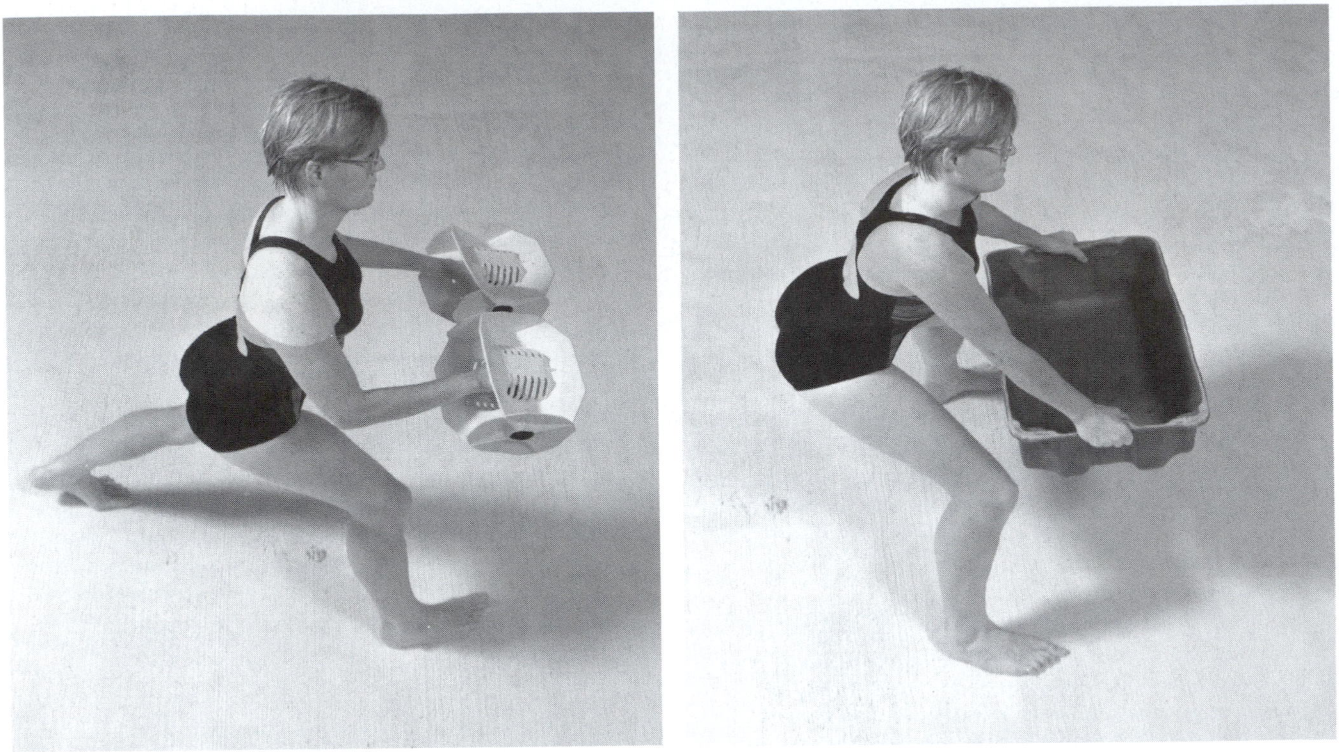

FIGURE 17-10 Work conditioning exercises such as ***(A)*** pushing and ***(B)*** lifting can be reproduced in the pool.

Critical Thinking Questions

1. How can the difficulty of the first selected intervention exercise (single-leg balance) be increased using the following?
   a. Arms
   b. Legs
   c. Equipment
   d. Other sensory systems
2. What factors might limit her ability to perform this exercise?
3. How is this exercise changed in different water depths?
   a. Waist deep
   b. Neck deep
4. How is the exercise in Self-Management: Bell Push Downs changed in different water depths?
   a. Chest deep
   b. Neck deep
5. How can mobility in internal rotation be improved while keeping the shoulders immersed?

REFERENCES

1. Beiser A. *Physics.* 2nd ed. Menlo Park, CA: The Benjamin/Cummings Publishing Co., Inc; 1978.
2. Harrison RA, Hillman M, Bulstrode S. Loading the lower limb when walking partially immersed: Implications for clinical practice. *Physiotherapy.* 1992;78:164–166.
3. Skinner AT, Thomson AM, eds. *Duffield's Exericise in Water.* 3rd ed. London: Bailliere Tindall; 1983.
4. Arborelius M, Balldin UI, Lilja B, Lundgren CEG. Hemodynamic changes in man during immersion with the head above water. *Aerospace Med.* 1972;43:592–598.
5. Christie JL, Sheldahl LM, Tristani FE, Wann LS, et al. Cardiovascular regulation during head-out water immersion exercise. *J Appl Physiol.* 1990;69:657–664.
6. Green GH, Cable NT, Elms N. Heart rate and oxygen consumption during walking on land and in deep water. *J Sports Med Phys Fitness.* 1990;30:49–52.
7. Risch WD, Koubenec HJ, Beckmann U, Lange S, et al. The effect of graded immersion on heart volume, central venous pressure, pulmonary blood distribution, and heart rate in man. *Pflugers Arch.* 1978;374:115–118.
8. Sheldahl LM, Tristani FE, Clifford PS, Kalbfleisch JH, et al. Effect of head-out water immersion on response to exercise training. *J Appl Physiol.* 1986;60:1878–1881.
9. Choukroun ML, Varene P. Adjustments in oxygen transport during head-out immersion in water at different temperatures. *J Appl Physiol.* 1991;68:1475–1480.
10. Craig AB, Dvorak M. Thermal regulation of man exercising during water immersion. *J Appl Physiol.* 1968;25:28–35.
11. Craig AB, Dvorak M. Comparison of exercise in air and in water at different temperatures. *Med Sci Sports Exerc.* 1969;1:124–130.
12. Golden C, Tipton MJ. Human thermal responses during leg-only exercise in cold water. *J Physiol.* 1987;391:399–405.
13. Golden C, Tipton MJ. Human adaptation to repeated cold immersions. *J Physiol.* 1988;396:349–363.
14. Sagawa S, Shiraki K, Yousef MK, Konda N. Water temperature and intensity of exercise in maintenance of thermal equilibrium. *J Appl Physiol.* 1988;2413–2419.
15. Avellini BA, Shapiro Y, Pandolf KB. Cardio-respiratory physical training in water and on land. *Eur J Appl Physiol.* 1983;50:255–263.

16. Hamer PW, Morton AR. Water running: Training effects and specificity of aerobic, anaerobic, and muscular parameters following an eight-week interval training programme. *Australian J Sci Med Sport*. 1990;21:13–22.
17. Vickery SR, Cureton KG, Langstaff JL. Heart rate and energy expenditures during aqua dynamics. *Physician Sports Med*. 1983;11:67–72.
18. Whitley JD, Schoene LL. Comparison of heart rate responses: Water walking versus treadmill walking. *Phys Ther*. 1987;67: 1501–1504.
19. Eyestone ED, Fellingham G, George J, Fisher AG. Effect of water running and cycling on maximum oxygen consumption and 2-mile run performance. *Am J Sports Med*. 1993;21:41–44.
20. Connelly TP, Sheldahl LM, Tristani FE, Levandoski SG, et al. Effect of increased central blood volume with water immersion on plasma catecholamines during exercise. *J Appl Physiol*. 1990;69:651–656.
21. McMurray RG, Berry MJ, Katz VL, Cefalo RC. Cardiovascular responses of pregnant women during aerobic exercise in the water: A longitudinal study. *Int J Sports Med*. 1988; 9:443–447.
22. Town GP, Bradley SS. Maximal metabolic responses of deep and shallow water running in trained runners. *Med Sci Sports Exerc*. 1991;23:238–241.
23. Gleim GW, Nicholas JA. Metabolic costs and heart rate responses to treadmill walking in water at different depths and temperatures. *Am J Sports Med*. 1989;17:248–252.
24. Evans BW, Cureton KJ, Purvis JW. Metabolic and circulatory responses to walking and jogging in water. *Res Q*. 1978;49: 442–449.
25. Yamaji K, Greenley M, Northey DR, Hughson RL. Oxygen uptake and heart rate responses to treadmill and water running. *Can J Sports Sci*. 1990;15:96–98.
26. Svedenhag J, Seger J. Running on land and in water: Comparative exercise physiology. *Med Sci Sports Exerc*. 1992;24: 1155–1160.
27. Wilder RP, Brennan D, Schotte DE. A standard measure for exercise prescription for aqua running. *Am J Sports Med*. 193;21:45–48.

UNIT 5

Functional Approach to Therapeutic Exercise of the Lower Extremities

CHAPTER 18

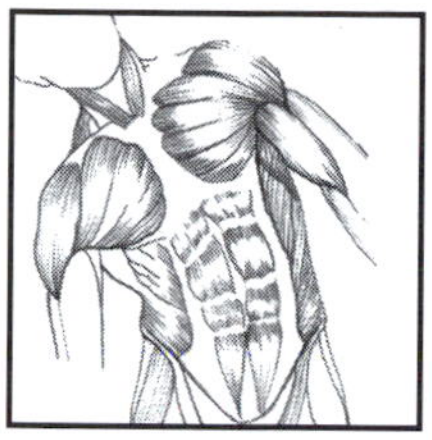

Therapeutic Exercise for the Lumbopelvic Region

Carrie Hall

A growing body of research has substantiated the use of exercise programs in the treatment and prevention of lumbopelvic syndromes.[1] Although improvement has been demonstrated with the use of exercise for lumbopelvic syndromes, the type of exercise prescribed remains controversial. Studies investigating different exercise programs report conflicting results. Many studies suffer from one or more design flaws, making it difficult to draw conclusions from their results. Underlying the difficulty in demonstrating the treatment effects of specific exercise protocols is the lack of consensus about classification of patients with lumbopelvic syndromes. Without a valid and reliable classification system, guidelines regarding exercise management for the patient with lumbopelvic syndrome-related signs and symptoms remain inexact.

Any classification system requires three criteria to guide conservative management of lumbopelvic syndromes:

1. Testing procedures and decision-making rules that are used for the classification of the patient must be operationally defined.
2. Clinicians must be well trained to carry out assessment and treatment procedures.
3. The classification system must result in successful outcomes in a cost-effective manner.

Various systems for guiding the conservative management of patients with lumbopelvic syndromes have been developed by McKenzie,[2] Delitto and Erhard,[3] Sahrmann,[4] and the Quebec Task Force,[5] but no consensus has been reached. The clinician therefore must base exercise management on a thoughtful and systematic examination and evaluation process and attempt to diagnose the origins of the presenting functional limitations and disability. Diagnosis requires taking a thorough history, performing a meticulous examination, evaluating physiologic impairments and functional limitations, and combining the data gathered from the physical therapy, medical, and psychological examinations. The impact of a psychological impairment on the presenting condition and prognosis must not be underestimated, but treatment of this impairment is beyond the scope of this text and is discussed only as part of the overall intervention.

Although it is tempting to develop an intervention based on a medical diagnosis or set list of physiologic impairments, this type of practice is not recommended. Effective intervention cannot be limited to treatment of disease or anatomic impairments; it must also address the physiologic and psychological impairments most closely associated with the cause of the patient's functional limitations and disability. Exercise prescription should be based on individual and ongoing assessment of the disability, functional limitations, and related impairments. There is no recipe approach for the prescription of exercises in the treatment of lumbopelvic syndromes. This chapter presents principles of exercise prescription with which to make decisions about appropriate therapeutic exercise interventions.

REVIEW OF ANATOMY AND KINESIOLOGY

The anatomy and kinesiology of the lumbopelvic region have received considerable attention in the literature,[6–10] which has enhanced clinical understanding of the function of the lumbopelvic region and emphasized the integrated nature of normal movement between the trunk and extremities. To properly examine, diagnose, and treat the lumbopelvic region, a thorough understanding of its anatomic and kinesiologic features is essential. Knowledge of lumbopelvic osteology and arthrology, osteokinematics and arthrokinematics, innervation, myology, and kinetics provides an important base for exercise prescription.

Lumbar Spine

The lumbar spine consists of five lumbar vertebrae. The first four lumbar vertebrae have a similar structure (Fig. 18-1), and the fifth lumbar vertebra has structural variations (Fig. 18-2).

ARTHROLOGY

The lumbar motion segment has distinct posterior and anterior elements. The primary features of the posterior element are the zygapophyseal joints and muscle attachments. The primary features of the anterior element are the vertebral bodies and intervertebral disks (IVDs).

The zygapophyseal joints have a distinctive shape and orientation in the lumbar spine. The angle that each joint makes with respect to the sagittal plane determines the amount of resistance offered to motion in the sagittal and transverse

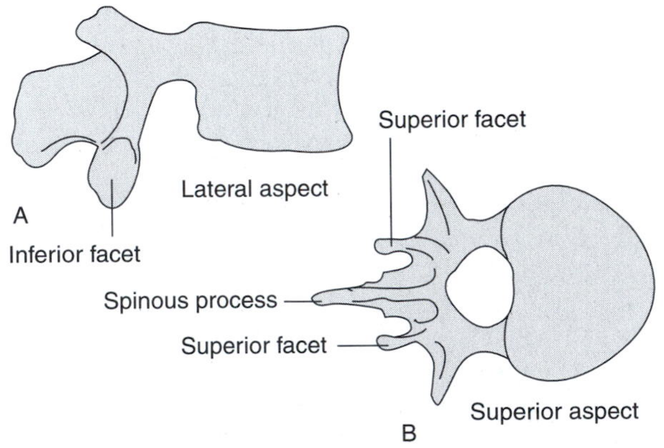

FIGURE 18-1 ***(A)*** Lateral view of a lumbar vertebrae. ***(B)*** Superior view of a typical lumbar vertebra shows the sagittal-plane orientation of the zygapophyseal joints. Sagittal-plane orientation resists rotation but not forward displacement.

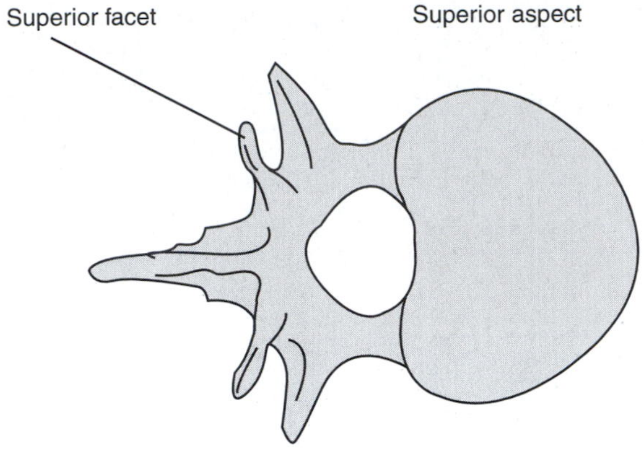

FIGURE 18-2 Superior view of a typical fifth lumbar vertebra. Note the more frontal plane orientation of the zygapophyseal joints. Frontal-plane orientation resists forward displacement but not rotation.

planes. The more the joint is oriented in the frontal plane, the more it resists sagittal plane motion, but the less it can resist transverse-plane motion; the converse is true for joints oriented in the sagittal plane (see Figs. 18-1 and 18-2).

From L1-L2 to L4-L5, the joint lies primarily in a sagittal plane, and the shape of the joint surface is in a variable J or C shape when viewed from above. The anteromedial part of the joint lies in or near the frontal plane and provides excellent resistance to anterior sagittal translation, a component of flexion. The posterolateral component is oriented more in the sagittal plane and provides excellent resistance to axial rotation, allowing only a few degrees of motion at each segment. In rotation, the posterior elements contribute approximately two thirds to the resistance of motion, and the anterior elements contribute the remaining one third.[11] Injury, disease, or developmental problems contributing to shape alterations (ie, anatomic impairments) of the zygapophyseal joints can lead to increased strain on the IVDs.[8,12] At L5-S1, the orientation of the joint is more frontal and therefore resists anterior shear more effectively than rotation. The frontal plane orientation resists the tendency of L5 to migrate forward on the anteriorly tilted sacral base. The fifth lumbar vertebra is additionally anchored by the strong and multibanded iliolumbar ligament.

The fibrous capsule of the zygapophyseal joint has posterior, superior, and inferior components, with fibers oriented more or less transversely from one articular process to the other. The anterior part of the capsule is formed entirely by the ligamentum flavum.[1] Some of the deep fibers of the posterior capsule attach directly into the outer edge of the articular cartilage. Posteriorly, a portion of the lumbar multifidus inserts directly into the capsule.[13] The pull of the multifidus may prevent entrapment of the capsule between the articular surfaces during movement.

The zygapophyseal joints typically demonstrate changes with aging. At birth, the joints are primarily oriented in the frontal plane, and they assume their more typical curved appearance during the first decade. The change may result from forces related to the development of bipedal gait in early childhood. Side-to-side joint asymmetry is common in adults and leads to articular tropism (ie, developmental alteration in the joint's shape) in a certain percentage of the population.[14] Some investigators feel that tropism may alter the biomechanics and increase the forces on some portions of the IVDs, thereby predisposing them to injury.[8,12,15]

Two other significant age-related changes occur in the zygapophyseal joints.[13] The cartilage of the anteromedial, frontal-plane-oriented portion of the zygapophyseal joint fibrillates, and the underlying subchondral bone scleroses in response to the forces of loading in flexion. In the posterior, sagittal-plane-oriented portion of the joint, a different type of cartilage damage occurs. The cartilage splits or shears vertically, probably because of the direct pull of the capsule (in part through the action of the multifidus) onto the cartilage.

The interbody of the lumbar spine involves portions of two vertebral bodies and an IVD. It is an adaptation that transmits vertical load, allowing movement and resisting torsion and shear. The IVD is made up of an annulus fibrosus (AF), a nucleus pulposus (NP), and an end plate. The fibers of each lamellae of the AF form concentric rings directed at an oblique angle of approximately 30 degrees from the horizontal. Each lamellae has an alternating orientation of collagen fibers such that the fibers in adjacent lamellae are at 90 degrees to each other. This orientation effectively resists compression, but horizontal translation and rotation are resisted by only a portion of the fibers.[8]

The NP is 70% to 90% water, depending on a person's age.[8,16] Because of its fluid nature and its complete containment within the AF and end plates, the NP exerts a force in all directions against the AF and end plate when pressure is increased through compression or weight bearing. This force braces the annulus from the inside, reducing its tendency to buckle under compressive loading. This structure also facilitates force transmission through the end plates. The end plate is associated more strongly with the IVD than with the vertebral body. It is situated on the superior and inferior part of the IVD. It is the weakest part of the IVD in compression.

Changes occur within the IVD with age. The most significant include loss of water (particularly in the NP), increasing collagen content, and an increasing similarity in the composition of the AF and NP. The result is a less efficient hydrodynamic bracing mechanism, which places increasing stress on the AF.

The IVD is the largest avascular structure of the body. However, it is metabolically active at a relatively slow rate.[8] The nutrition of the disk depends on diffusion. It receives its supply from the two closest vessel sources, which are those beneath the vertebral end plate and those at the periphery of the AF.[17] Although the primary mechanism of transport is thought to be diffusion,[7] a second mechanism may exist in which nutrients are exchanged along with the water that is routinely squeezed out of and drawn into the IVD during compression and decompression. Certain movements, possibly those in and out of flexion, may facilitate nutrition of the disk.[18,19] Although the metabolism is slow, it does result in turnover of some of the constituent structures of the IVD. When IVD injury occurs, healing transpires, but complete healing takes months to years. One of the direct benefits of exercise may be to facilitate the nutrition of the IVD.[6,20]

OSTEOKINEMATICS AND ARTHROKINEMATICS

The range of motion of the lumbar spine differs at various levels and depends on orientation of the facets of the intervertebral joints (see Figs. 18-1 and 18-2). Motion between two vertebrae is small and does not occur independently because all spinal movements involve the combined action of several motion segments. Skeletal structures that influence motions of the spine are the rib cage, which limits motion of the thoracic spine, and the pelvis and hip, which augment trunk motion by tilting the pelvis over the femoral head.

The lumbar facets from L1 to L4 lie primarily in the sagittal plane and favor flexion and extension over lateral flexion and rotation. The amount of flexion varies at each interspace of the lumbar spine, but most of the flexion takes place between the L4 and S1 levels. Lateral flexion is greatest in the upper lumbar levels and least at the lumbosacral level, whereas rotation is minimal from L1 to L4 and greatest at the lumbosacral level.

Flexion is a combination of anterior sagittal rotation (ie, osteokinematic motion) and a small amount of anterior sagittal translation (ie, arthrokinematic motion) (Fig. 18-3). It varies between 8 and 13 degrees per lumbar segment[21] and is limited primarily by the posterior ligamentous system and posterior IVDs, the zygapophyseal joint capsules, and compression of the anterior IVDs. Extension is a combination of posterior sagittal rotation (ie, osteokinematic motion) and a small amount of posterior sagittal translation (ie, arthrokinematic motion). It varies between 1 and 5 degrees per lumbar segment[21] and is limited by bony contact of the posterior elements. Rotation is limited to approximately 1 to 2 degrees per segment in each direction.[21] Initially, rotation occurs about a vertical axis, followed by a shift in the axis to the contralateral compressed zygapophyseal joint (Fig. 18-4). Rotation is limited primarily by bony engagement of the contralateral zygapophyseal joint, by tension of the capsule of the ipsilateral zygapophyeial

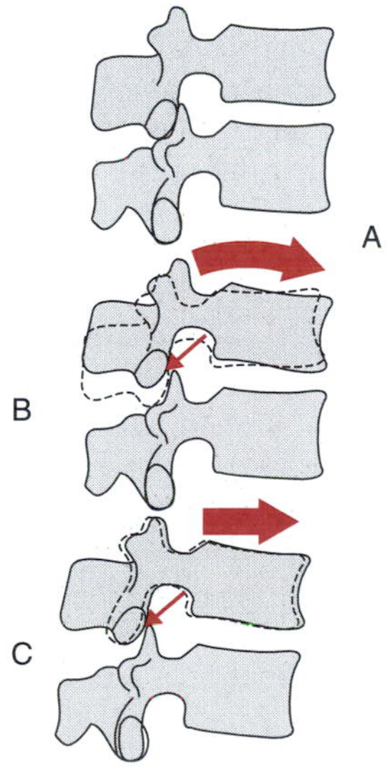

FIGURE 18-3 ***(A)*** Vertebral movement during flexion. Flexion of the lumbar spine involves a combination of anterior sagittal rotation and anterior translation. ***(B)*** As sagittal rotation occurs, the zygapophyseal joints separate, permitting the translation movement to occur ***(C)*** Translation is limited by compression of the inferior zygapophyseal joint of one vertebra on the superior zygapophyseal joint of the vertebra below.

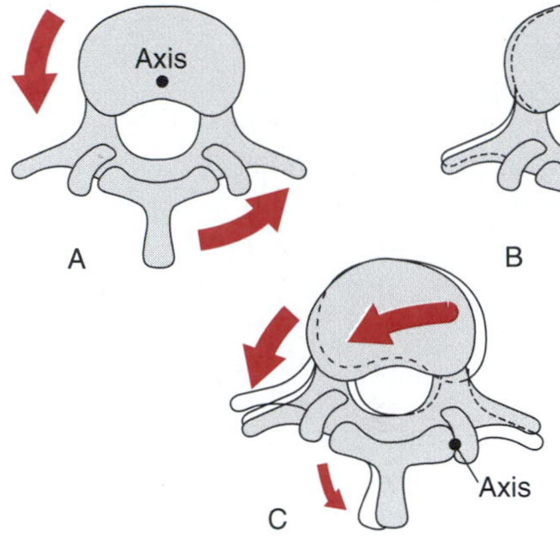

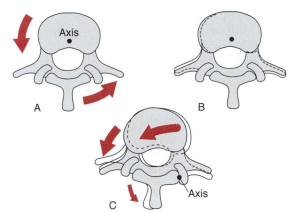

FIGURE 18-4 Vertebral movement during rotation: ***(A)*** Initially, rotation occurs around an axis within the vertebral body. ***(B)*** The zygapophyseal joints compress. ***(C)*** Further rotation causes the vertebra to pivot around a new axis at the point of compression.

joint capsule, and by approximately one half of the annular fibers as they are elongated. Rotation is usually coupled with side flexion in various patterns.[10] Likewise, lateral flexion does not occur in isolation in the lumbar spine but is coupled with rotation.

The coupling of motions in the lumbar spine, apart from L5-S1, where ipsilateral coupling of rotation and side flexion is known to occur,[22] is not consistent. Variation of coupled motions occurs between persons and at different segments within the same person. Individual patterning of motion coupling varies with sagittal position of the segment.[10] Because there appears to be a diversity of possible motion coupling, rules pertaining to coupled rotation and lateral flexion do not exist. Biomechanics must be assessed for each patient.

During flexion movements, the anterior AF and NP are compressed, the posterior AF is stretched, and the posterior NP is compressed on to the posterior wall. The posterior portion of the AF is the thinnest part, and the combination of stretch and increased pressure in this area may cause AF damage, causing the NP to bulge or herniate through the AF. Because of the alternating direction of the fibers of the AF, only one half of the fibers are stretched during rotation while one half relax. This stretch pattern may be one reason why the disk is more vulnerable to injury during combined flexion and rotation movements.

In a standing position, the lumbar spine moves in concert with the pelvic-hip complex to produce motion in the sagittal, frontal, and transverse planes. The best understood relationship of lumbar-pelvic-hip motion, the lumbar-pelvic rhythm (LPR), occurs in the sagittal plane during forward bending. LPR is a simultaneous movement in a rhythmic ratio of a lumbar movement to a pelvic rotation; the total movement consists of a person bending forward and returning to an erect position. At any phase of total-body flexion, the extent of lumbar spine flexion must be accompanied by a proportional degree of pelvic rotation.[23] Conversely, on return to an upright position, pelvic rotation should lead lumbar extension until full pelvic rotation to neutral has been achieved, with the remainder of the motion into upright occurring in the lumbar spine.[23]

INNERVATION

The outer one third to one half of the AF has a nerve supply[8] and is therefore capable of being a source of pain from the lumbar spine. The zygapophyseal joints and multifidus are supplied by the medial branch of the dorsal ramus of the spinal nerve. The capsule and synovial folds contain nociceptive fibers.[24] The ventral dura mater is innervated, but the dorsal is not.

Axons from segments L4 to S2 innervate the sacroiliac joint (SIJ). The superior gluteal nerves, the obturator nerves, the posterior rami of S1 and S2, and branches of the sacral plexus provide articular innervation.

KINETICS

The lumbar spine is a major load-bearing region of the body. Dynamic loads usually are higher than static loads because almost all body motion increases lumbar spine loads, from a slight increase during slow walking to significant increases during vigorous physical activity. Although it is beyond the scope of this text to review static and dynamic loads on the lumbar spine during all postures and activities, a few postures and movements are examined in the following sections.

Statics

In upright stance, the line of gravity of the trunk passes ventral to the center of the fourth lumbar vertebral body (Fig. 18-5).[25] It falls ventral to the transverse axis of motion of the spine, and the motion segments are subjected to a forward-bending moment, which must be counterbalanced by passive forces from the ligaments and erector spinae muscle and by active erector spinae muscle forces. Any displacement of the line of gravity alters the magnitude and direction of the moment on the spine, which must be counterbalanced by passive or active forces to maintain equilibrium. For the body to return to equilibrium, the moment can be counteracted by increased muscle activity, which causes postural sway. The erector spinae, abdominal muscles, and psoas are intermittently active in maintaining the upright position of the trunk.[26] However, small adjustments in the position of the head, shoulders, pelvis, knees, or ankles can decrease or abolish the need

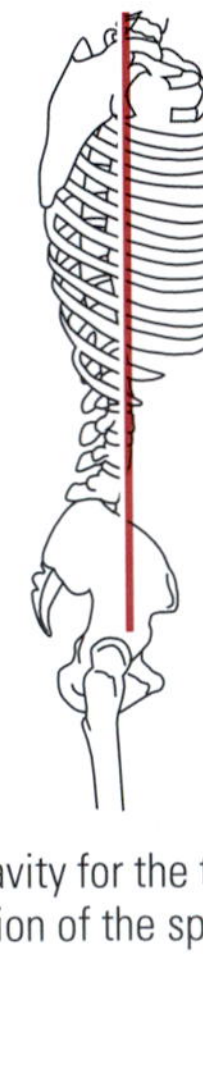

FIGURE 18-5 The line of gravity for the trunk (*solid line*) is usually ventral to the transverse axis of motion of the spine, and the spine is subjected to a constant flexion moment.

for muscle activity by restoring equilibrium. A person can rely solely on passive tension from ligaments or muscles being pulled taut to maintain equilibrium (eg, swayback posture).

Body position affects the magnitude of the loads on the spine. These loads are minimal during well-supported, reclined positions; remain low during relaxed, upright standing; and rise during sitting. During relaxed, unsupported sitting, the loads on the lumbar spine are greater than during relaxed, upright standing.[27] During erect sitting, forward tilting of the pelvis and an increase in the lumbar lordosis reduce the loads on the lumbar spine (Fig. 18-6), but these loads still exceed those produced during relaxed, upright standing. The loads on the lumbar spine are lower during supported sitting than during unsupported sitting. A backward inclination of the backrest and the use of a lumbar support further reduce the loads (Fig. 18-7).[28]

Loads on the spine are at their minimum when a person assumes a supine position with the hips and knees bent and supported. A further decrease in these loads is achieved by the application of traction.[29] Conversely, the highest loads on the spine usually are external loads that are produced by lifting.[27]

Dynamics

Almost all motion in the body increases the loads on the lumbar spine. This increase is modest during activities such as slow walking or easy twisting, but it can become substantial during various exercises.[27] In a study of normal walking at four speeds, the compressive loads at the L3-L4 motion segment ranged from 0.2 to 2.5 times body weight.[30] The

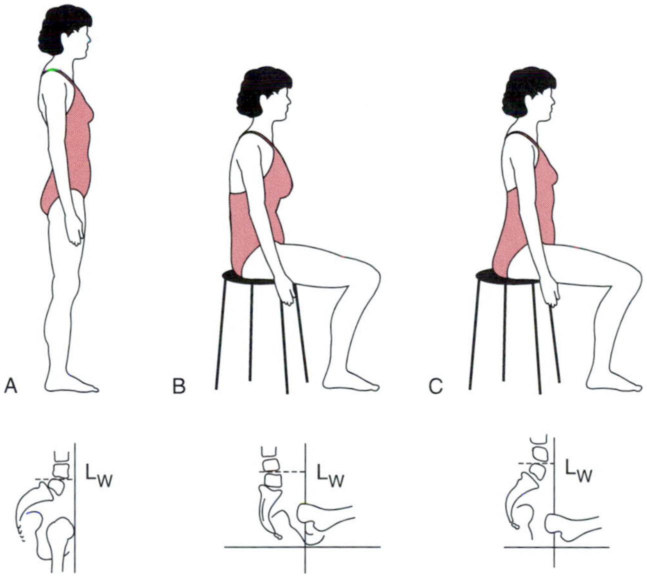

FIGURE 18-6 ***(A)*** Compared with relaxed upright standing, ***(B)*** the line of gravity for the trunk, already ventral to the lumbar spine, shifts further ventrally during relaxed, lumbar-flexed sitting. This shift creates a longer level arm (Lw) for the force exerted by the weight of the upper body. ***(C)*** During erect sitting with the pelvis in anterior pelvic tilt and the lumbar spine in extension, the line of gravity shifts dorsally, reducing the lever arm, but it is still slightly longer than during relaxed upright standing. (Adapted from Nordin M, Frankel H. *Basic Biomechanics of the Musculoskeletal System.* 2nd ed. Philadelphia: Lea & Febiger; 1989.)

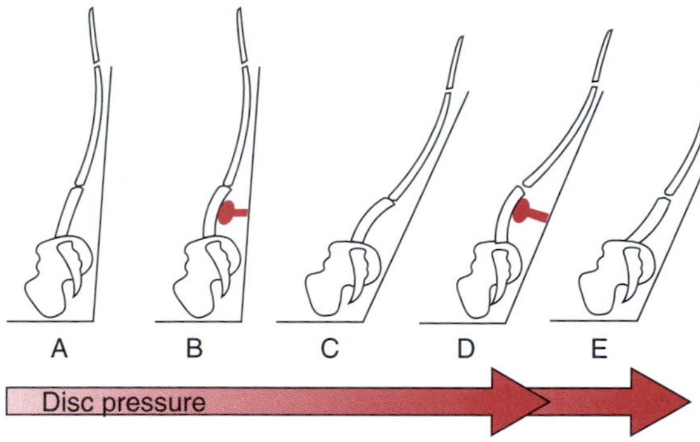

FIGURE 18-7 Influence of backrest inclination and back support on loads on the lumbar spine in terms of pressure on the third lumbar disk during supported sitting. ***(A)*** Backrest inclination is 90 degrees and disk pressure is at a maximum. ***(B)*** Addition of a lumbar support decreases disk pressure. ***(C)*** Backward inclination of the backrest to 110 degrees but with no lumbar support reduces disk pressure further. ***(D)*** Addition of lumbar support with same degree of backrest inclination further decreases pressure. ***(E)*** Shifting the support to the thoracic region pushes the upper body forward, moving the lumbar spine into flexion and increasing disk pressure. (Adapted from Andersson GBJ, Ortengren R, Nachemson A. Lumbar disc pressure and myoelectric back muscle activity during sitting. I. Studies on an experimental chair. *Scand J Rehabil Med.* 1974;6:104–114.)

loads were maximal at toe-off and increased linearly with walking speed.

Lifting and carrying an object over a distance is a common task required by any individual for work or as part of activities of daily living (ADLs), such as lifting groceries from the car and carrying them into the house, lifting a child from the floor or crib, or lifting the laundry basket from the floor to the washing machine. Several factors influence the loads on the spine during these activities:

- The position of the object relative to the center of motion of the spine
- The size, shape, weight, and density of the object
- The degree of flexion or rotation of the spine

However, following some general rules about body mechanics can lessen the load on the spine:

- Holding the object close to the body reduces the flexion moment on the spine.
- Reducing the size of the object can reduce the lever arm for the force produced by the weight of the object, lessening the load on the spine.
- Bending the hips and knees and keeping the back relatively straight reduces the load on the spine.

In considering transference of load through the pelvic girdle, passive and active mechanisms appear to contribute to pelvic girdle stability.[31] The passive mechanism contributes to stability because of the articular relationship of closely fitting joints, where no extra forces are needed to maintain the state of the system; this is called *form closure.*[7,32–35] Three factors contribute to form closure of any joint:

- The shape of the joint surface
- The friction coefficient of the articular cartilage
- The integrity of the ligaments that approximate the joint

The other mechanism is called *force closure*,[7,32–35] and it involves passive and active mechanisms to stabilize the joint. Force closure requires extra forces to keep the joint in place, such as that provided by ligaments and active muscle contraction. Form and force closure mechanisms prevent excessive motion of the innominates or sacrum. A 400- to 2600-pound force is necessary to disrupt the pelvic girdle.[36] An inherent disruption in form or force closure mechanisms must exist for instability to occur.

Pelvic Girdle

OSTEOLOGY AND ARTHROLOGY

Five sacral vertebrae are fused to form the triangular or wedge-shaped structure called the sacrum. The base of the triangle, which is formed by the first sacral vertebra, supports two articular facets that face posteriorly for articulation with the fifth lumbar vertebra. The two SIJs consist of the articulations between the left and right articular surfaces on the sacrum and the left and right iliac bones.

The shape of the SIJ is highly variable. In the skeletally mature individual, S1, S2, and S3 contribute to the formation of the sacral surface, and each part can be oriented in a different vertical plane. The sacrum is wedged anteroposteriorly. These factors provide resistance to vertical and horizontal translation. In the young, the wedging is incomplete, and the SIJ is planar at all three levels and is vulnerable to shear forces until ossification is complete in the third decade.[37]

The articular cartilage lining the SIJ is unusual. The sacral surface is lined with smooth hyaline cartilage, whereas the iliac surface is lined with a rough type of fibrocartilage. The conclusion of one study examining the friction coefficient of the SIJ suggested that the coarse cartilage texture contributes to the ability of the joint to resist translation.[34,35] The coarseness of the iliac cartilage increases with age.[38] The complementary ridges and grooves in the mature SIJ[34,35] also increase friction and thereby contribute to form closure.

The SIJ is surrounded by some of the strongest ligaments in the body (see Fig. 18-2). The dorsal sacroiliac ligament tightens when the sacrum counternutates (Table 18-1) relative to the innominate,[39] and the dorsal sacroiliac ligament is thought to control this motion. The sacrotuberous and interosseous ligaments tighten during sacral nutation (see Table 18-1) and control this motion.[40,41] The ventral sacroiliac ligament is the weakest of the group and is supported anteriorly by the pubic symphysis. These ligaments contribute to form and force closure.

Table 18-1. DEFINITIONS OF NUTATION AND COUNTERNUTATION

TERM	DEFINITION	SACRAL MOTION
Nutation	Sacral flexion	Base moves anteriorly and inferiorly Apex moves posteriorly and superiorly
Counternutation	Sacral extension	Base moves posteriorly and inferiorly Apex moves anteriorly and superiorly

ARTHROKINEMATICS

The amount of movement that is available at the articulation between the innominates and the sacrum is quite small and undoubtedly is the basis for much of the historical controversy regarding existence of movement of this joint. Movement has been studied in fresh and embalmed cadavers, in humans by a number of radiographic methods,[42–48] in humans by caliper measurement of the relationships of bony prominences, and at least once[36] by the insertion of Steinmann pins on the sacral and iliac side of the human joint. Motion does occur at the SIJ, but there are conflicting accounts of the precise model for SIJ motion and the axis through which motion occurs. These discrepancies may reflect the individual variability in joint anatomy and the variation that occurs in the early, middle, and extreme ranges of movement.

Movements of the innominates with respect to the sacrum occur primarily in the sagittal plane and are called anterior rotation and posterior iliosacral rotation.[45] Anterior iliosacral rotation occurs as the innominate rotates anteriorly in relation to the sacrum, with the ipsilateral anterior superior iliac spine (ASIS) moving anteriorly and caudally and the ipsilateral posterior superior iliac spine (PSIS) moving anteriorly and cranially. During posterior iliosacral rotation, the innominate rotates posteriorly in relation to the sacrum, with the ipsilateral ASIS moving posteriorly and cranially and the ipsilateral PSIS moving posteriorly and caudally. A small amount of posteroanterior translation of the innominate occurs with anterior rotation, and a small amount of anteroposterior translation occurs with posterior rotation. Anterior and posterior rotations of the innominate occur as normal osteokinematic motions during the gait cycle (see the Gait section).

Depending on the anatomic configuration of the innominate and sacral surfaces, a small amount of superoinferior translatory shear motion occurs.[49–51] The vertical movement occurs with limb loading and is most pronounced with static standing on one leg, especially if maintained for a prolonged period.[43]

Although SIJ mobility is normally limited, movement does occur throughout life.[7,32–34,53,54] The most widely accepted movement is that of nutation and counternutation (see Table 18-1).[55] Side bending and rotational movements have also been studied,[56,57] although the existence of these motions remains controversial. No definitive model exists to define the path of instant center of rotation of the joint, and the amount of motion present remains controversial.[58,59]

When the sacrum nutates relative to the innominates, a linear motion or translation between the two joint surfaces occurs. The SIJ is shaped like a boomerang with two arms at 90 degrees (Fig. 18-8). The short arm is oriented vertically, and the long arm is oriented horizontally. During sacral nutation, the sacrum glides inferiorly down the short arm and posteriorly along the long arm. During counternutation, the sacrum glides anteriorly along the long arm and superiorly up the short arm.

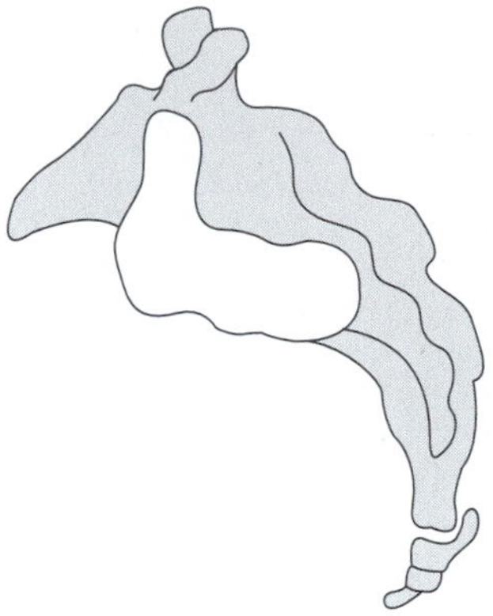

FIGURE 18-8 The sacral articular surface is shaped like an inverted "boomerang." It has also been described as a auricular "L" shape.

KINETICS

Stability of the pelvic girdle is important, because it must transmit forces from the weight of the head, trunk, and upper extremities and forces from the lower extremities upward. The pelvic girdle can be divided into posterior and anterior arches by a frontal plane passing through the acetabular fossa. Body weight is transferred from the L5 vertebra to the first sacral segment. The weight is then distributed equally along the sides of the sacrum across the arcuate line to the acetabulum. Ground reaction forces, which travel up the lower extremity, are transmitted superiorly through the same bony trabeculae and across the pubic rami to counterbalance the ascending forces from the contralateral limb.

Superincumbent body weight tends to force the sacral base anteroinferiorly. The components of the anterior arch act as a tie beam to prevent separation of the SIJ. If the pubic symphysis is unstable, there is a tendency for the two innominate bones to separate, allowing sacral tilting in an anteroinferior direction.

The angle of inclination of the articular surface of the sacrum is a significant factor in the stability of the SIJ.[48] The anatomic impairment of vertically oriented SIJs subject the ligaments to greater stress because less of the load is borne by the osseous structures of the posterior arch. Asymmetric loading may occur with asymmetry of the angle of inclination or postural asymmetry (eg, limb length discrepancy).

Myology

Optimal function of the lumbopelvic region requires an integration of the musculature of the posterior and anterior aspects of the spine, pelvis, and hips. In addition, the latissimus dorsi influences lumbopelvic mechanics. Because of the integration of musculature spanning the lumbopelvic region, myology is addressed in an integrated format for the entire region.

POSTERIOR LUMBOPELVIC MYOLOGY

The thoracolumbar fascia (TLF) and its powerful muscular attachments play an important role in stabilization of the lumbopelvic region.[60,61] Numerous muscular attachments into the TLF have been described, including attachments of transversus abdominis and some fibers of the internal obliques into the lateral raphe portion of the TLF and attachments of gluteus maximus, latissimus dorsi, erector spinae, and biceps femoris into the posterior layer of TLF (Fig. 18-9). This pattern suggests that the hip, pelvic, and leg muscles interact with arm and spinal muscles through the TLF.[60] The gluteus maximus and latissimus dorsi may conduct forces contralaterally through the posterior layer of the TLF, and the action of these two muscles may be linked to provide support to the SIJ and lumbar spine during gait and rotation of the trunk. This integrated system has also been proposed as a method of load transference between the spine and hips, in which the TLF is a centrally placed structure for the interaction of muscles from each region.

The spinal extensors may be broadly categorized as superficial muscles (ie, iliocostalis), which travel the length of the spine and attach to the sacrum and pelvis, and deep muscles (ie, longissimus and lumbar multifidus), which span the lumbar segments.

Even though the superficial spinal extensors do not attach directly to the lumbar spine, they have an optimal lever arm for lumbar extension by virtue of their attachments (Fig. 18-10). By pulling the thorax posteriorly, they create an extension moment at the lumbar spine. They function eccentrically to control decent of the trunk during forward bending and isometrically to control the position of the lower thorax with respect to the pelvis during functional movements.[62,63]

The attachment of the superficial spinal extensors also influences SIJ mechanics. Because of the attachment of the erector spinae aponeurosis to the sacrum, the pull of the erector spinae tendon on the dorsal aspect of the sacrum induces a flexion moment (ie, nutation) of the sacrum on the ilium (Fig. 18-11).

The deep erector spinae (ie, longissimus) have a poor lever arm for spine extension but are aligned to provide a dynamic counterforce to the anterior shear force imparted to the lumbar spine from gravitational force (Fig. 18-12).

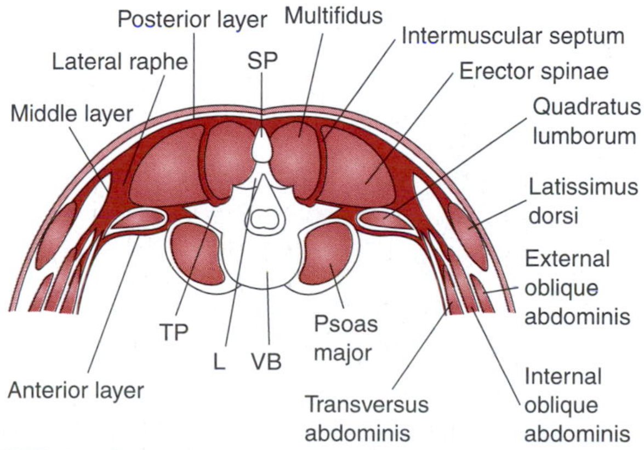

FIGURE 18-9 Cross section of the lumbar spine showing layers of the thoracolumbar fascia and the muscles that attach to it and are contained within it. The junction of the posterior and middle layers is the lateral raphe. (Adapted from Porterfield JA, DeRosa C, *Mechanical Low Back Pain: Perspectives in Functional Anatomy,* 2nd ed. Philadelphia: WB Saunders; 1998.)

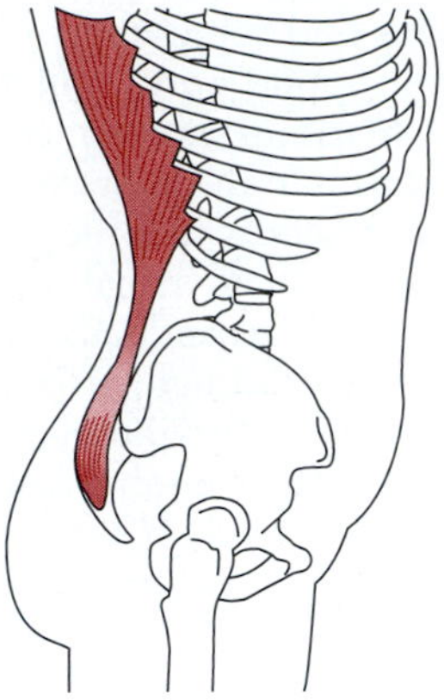

FIGURE 18-10 When viewed from the side, the superficial erector spinae can be seen to course superiorly from the pelvic attachment to the ribs. Movement of the right side of the pelvis forward or the rib cage backward (relative right spinal rotation) lengthens the superficial erector spinae on the right. The converse movements shorten the superficial erector spinae. (Adapted from Porterfield JA, DeRosa C, *Mechanical Low Back Pain: Perspectives in Functional Anatomy,* 2nd ed. Philadelphia: WB Saunders; 1998.)

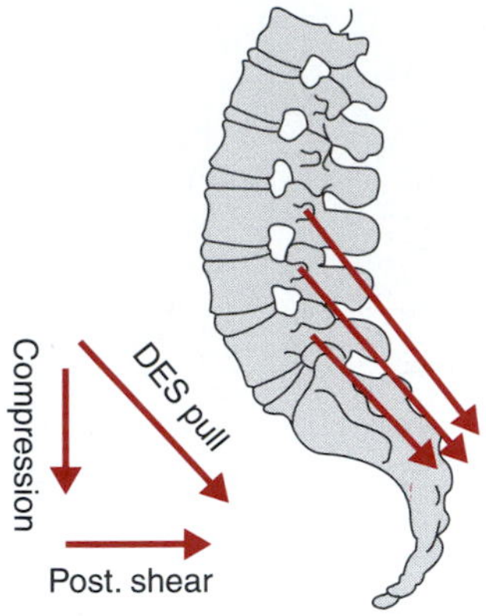

FIGURE 18-12 Because the deep erector spinae attach close to the axis of lumbar motion, the muscle group provides a dynamic posterior shear and compression force (*arrows*). This muscle can provide a force to prevent anterior translation. (Adapted from Porterfield JA, DeRosa C, *Mechanical Low Back Pain: Perspectives in Functional Anatomy.* 2nd ed. Philadelphia: WB Saunders; 1998.)

The attachment of the lumbar multifidus to the spinous process provides a strong lever arm for spinal extension (Fig. 18-13). During forward-bending motions, this muscle contributes to controlling the rate and magnitude of flexion and anterior shear.[64] Because of its deep location, short fiber span, and oblique orientation, the lumbar multifidus is thought to stabilize against flexion and rotation forces on the lumbar spine.[65,66] Several studies have illuminated its relationship with the vertebral segment.[67–69] The effect of dysfunction of this muscle, which is discussed in a later section, further emphasizes its important role in spine stabilization. The lumbar multifidus also contributes to dynamic stability of the SIJ. Because it is attached to the sacrotuberous ligament, tension on the ligament imparted as a result of multifidus muscle contraction potentially increases the ligamentous stabilizing mechanisms of the SIJ (Fig. 18-14).

ANTERIOR LUMBOPELVIC MYOLOGY

One of the most important muscle groups contributing to mobility and stability of the lumbopelvic region is the abdominal wall mechanism. The abdominal wall consists of, superficial to deep, the rectus abdominis, external oblique, internal oblique, and transversus abdominis. The rectus abdominis and obliques appear to serve a relatively more dynamic role than the transversus abdominis.

The transverse abdominis is circumferential, situated deeply, and has attachments to the TLF, the sheath of rectus abdominis, the diaphragm, iliac crest, and the lower six costal surfaces.[70] Because of its unique anatomic features, such as its deep location, its link to fascial support systems, its fiber type distribution, and its possible activity against gravitational load during standing and gait, the transverse abdominis is an important stabilizing muscle for the lumbar spine.[71–77] The transverse abdominis activates before the onset of limb movement in persons without low back pain,

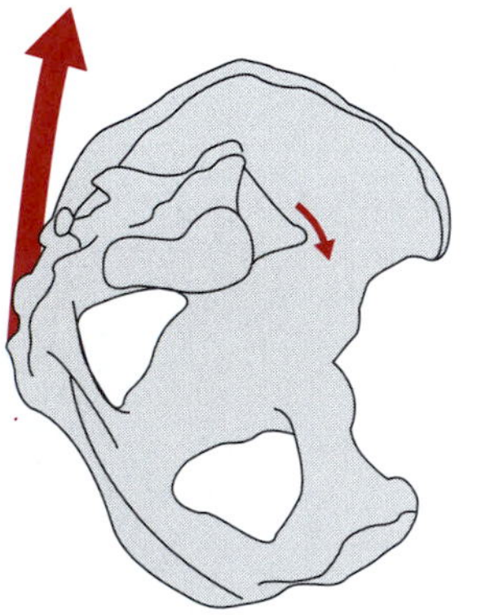

FIGURE 18-11 The attachment of the superficial erector spinae to the sacrum provides a potential force for sacral nutation (sacral flexion). Because nutation increases sacral stability, the superficial erector spinae may play a role in force closure of the sacroiliac joint. (Adapted from Porterfield JA, DeRosa C, *Mechanical Low Back Pain: Perspectives in Functional Anatomy.* 2nd ed. Philadelphia: WB Saunders; 1998.)

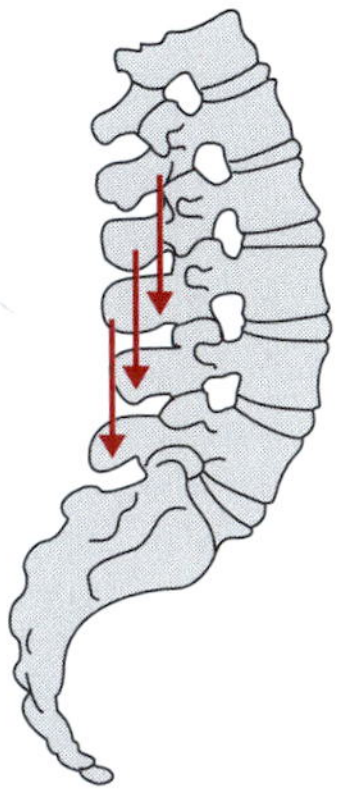

FIGURE 18-13 The lumbar multifidus provides a strong, dynamic force (*arrows*) for lumbar extension (Adapted from Bogduk N, Twomey LT. *Clinical Anatomy of the Lumbar Spine.* 1st ed. Edinburgh: Churchill Livingstone; 1987.)

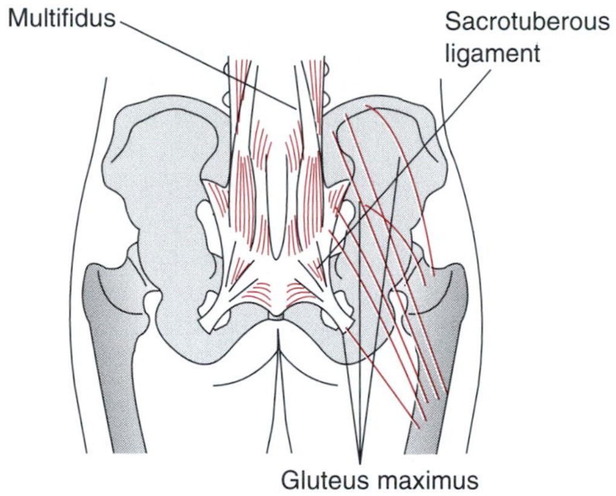

FIGURE 18-14 Anatomic relationship of lumbar multifidus to the sacroiliac joint, sacrotuberous ligament, and gluteus maximus. (Adapted from Porterfield JA, DeRosa C, *Mechanical Low Back Pain: Perspectives in Functional Anatomy.* 2nd ed. Philadelphia: WB Saunders; 1998.)

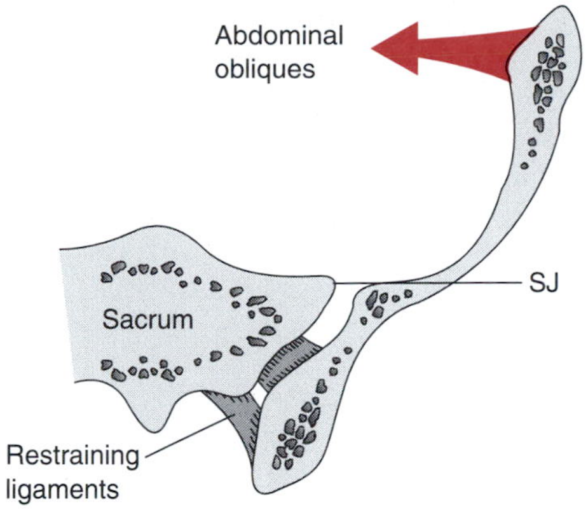

FIGURE 18-15 Contraction of the abdominal oblique muscles acting over the fulcrum of the interosseous ligament increases sacroiliac joint and pubic symphysis compression. (Adapted from Porterfield JA, DeRosa C, *Mechanical Low Back Pain: Perspectives in Functional Anatomy.* 2nd ed. Philadelphia: WB Saunders; 1998.)

but this function is lost in those with low back pain.[71] Current theory suggests that this muscle is a key background stabilizing muscle for the lumbar spine and that the emphasis of specific exercises for the abdominal wall should involve specific recruitment of the transverse abdominis instead of general strengthening or endurance.

The oblique abdominal muscles working synergistically provide an anterior oblique sling and, together with the posterior oblique sling (ie, TLF and associated structures), they assist in stabilization of the lumbar spine and pelvis in an integrated system of myofascial support.[32,33] The right external oblique works synergistically with the left internal oblique to produce rotation to the left and to prevent excessive rotation when necessary. The lumbar multifidus must synergically contract to prevent flexion imposed by the obliques so that pure rotation or transverse-plane stabilization can occur. The inferior and medial direction of the fibers of the external oblique are positioned to prevent anterior pelvic tilt and anterior pelvic shear. With respect to the SIJ, the oblique abdominals provide compressive forces between the two pubic bones and at the SIJ posteriorly (Fig. 18-15).

ASSOCIATED PELVIC, HIP, AND UPPER EXTREMITY MYOLOGY

Twenty-nine muscles originate or insert into the pelvis. Twenty of these link the pelvis with the femur, and nine link the pelvis with the spine. This implies that significant forces can be generated through the pelvis and subsequently through the lumbar spine by various combinations of knee and hip muscle activity.

The iliacus and psoas major have significant attachments to the spine and pelvis. If not counterstabilized by the abdominal muscles, the iliacus can exert an anterior rotation force on the pelvis, and the psoas major can exert an anterior translational force on lumbar segments.

The fibers of the gluteus maximus muscle run perpendicular to the plane of the SIJ and blend with the TLF and the contralateral latissimus dorsi.[7] Compression of the SIJ occurs when the gluteus maximus and the contralateral latissimus dorsi contract. This oblique system crosses the midline and is believed to be a significant contributor to load transference through the pelvic girdle during rotational activities and during gait.[7,32] The TLF is tensed by contraction of gluteus maximus, latissimus dorsi, and erector spinae muscles.

In addition to the attachment to the ischial tuberosity, the long head of the biceps femoris attaches to the sacrotuberous ligament. Contraction of the biceps femoris increases tension of the sacrotuberous ligament and pulls the sacrum against the ilium, effectively increasing the stability of the SIJ.[75]

In standing and walking, the pelvic girdle is stabilized on the femur by the coordinated action of the ipsilateral gluteus medius and minimus and by the contralateral adductor muscles. Indirectly, by maintaining a relationship between the hip, pelvis, and lumbar spine in the frontal plane, the gluteus medius, gluteus minimus, and adductors contribute to lumbar spine stability. Although these muscles are not directly involved in force closure of the SIJ, they play a significant role in pelvic girdle function.

The piriformis is considered to be part of the deep hip lateral rotator group and pelvic floor. It appears to play a vital role for stabilization of the SIJ. The piriformis attaches to the sacrum, the anterior surface of the sacrotuberous ligament, and the medial edge of the SIJ capsule. This muscle anchors the apex of the sacrum and controls sacral nutation. The link of pelvic floor function and lumbopelvic function should not be underestimated. One investigator found that some patients with chronic low back pain were unable to recruit the transversus abdominis without prior contraction of the pelvic floor.[76]

GAIT

Gait is an important functional activity. In the following sections, the biomechanics and muscle function of the gait cycle are described as they pertain to the lumbar spine and pelvic girdle.

Lumbar Spine

As the right lower extremity moves from initial contact and loading response to midstance, the right hip and iliac crest act as a post, and the left hip sinusoidally drops in preparation for swing through on that side. This relative elevation of the right hip creates bending to the right side and rotation to the left in the lumbar spine. This coupled motion is reversed on left heel strike.

Pelvic Girdle

Under normal physiologic circumstances, the pubic symphysis serves as the axis for anterior and posterior innominate rotation. A small amount of caudal-cranial vertical shear occurs on the weight-bearing side.

At initial contact on the right, the right innominate rotates posteriorly while the left innominate is in relative anterior rotation. At midstance on the right, the right innominate rotates relatively anteriorly toward neutral, and the left innominate rotates posteriorly toward neutral. At toe-off on the right, the right innominate begins to rotate anteriorly, past neutral, in preparation for swing, and the left innominate continues to rotate posteriorly in preparation for heel strike. The motion of the sacrum between the two innominates and adjacent fifth lumbar vertebra has been described as a complex, polyaxial, torsional movement that occurs about the oblique axes.[52,77]

Muscle Activity

LUMBAR SPINE MUSCLES DURING GAIT

The erector spinae muscles have two periods of activity that occur at initial contact and at terminal stance, just before preswing.[78] The bilateral activity of the erector spinae is presumed to prevent the body falling forward and to check rotation and lateral flexion of the trunk.

Little investigation of gait has been done with respect to the abdominal muscles. Two conflicting studies demonstrate activity of the rectus abdominis, obliqui externus, and internus[79] or absence of activity in the same muscle groups.[80] Perhaps the discrepancy in these studies is a result of various speeds of walking used in the testing conditions. The duration of electromyographic activity in the abdominal muscles increases with increased speed of gait.[79]

One study found evidence of abdominal and lumbar multifidus muscle activity in a feedforward manner in advance of the prime mover of the lower limb.[66] Although this study did not look specifically at gait, it did provide important information regarding the activity of the abdominal and multifidus muscles in response to a perturbation produced by movement of a limb similar to that occurring during gait. For the trunk muscles studied, only rectus abdominis and lumbar multifidus reaction time depended on the movement direction of the moving limb, suggesting that these muscles are involved in controlling the position of the center of mass within the base of support. Conversely, reaction time in the transversus abdominis and the internal and external obliques did not change with limb movement direction, indicating that these muscles are not influenced by the direction of the reactive forces. The transversus abdominis, a muscle largely ignored in the literature, was invariably the first muscle that was active. Contraction of these muscles appears to be linked with the control of stability of the spine against the perturbation produced by the movement of the limb. The conclusion drawn from this work is that clinicians should consider the function of these deep muscles, particularly the transversus abdominis, when attempting to train patients to control trunk stability during functional activities.

PELVIC GIRDLE MUSCLES DURING GAIT

Much of the muscle activity occurring across the pelvic girdle during gait is discussed in Chapter 20, but additional information regarding the link between the hip, the lumbopelvic region, and the upper extremity is provided in this section. The hamstrings become active just before initial contact,[81] which increases the tension in the sacrotuberous ligament and contributes to the force closure mechanism of the pelvic girdle with loading of the limb.[75,82,83]

At initial contact, the gluteus maximus muscle becomes active in conjunction with a counterrotation of the trunk and arm swing forward, resulting in lengthening of the contralateral latissimus dorsi muscle. Shortly thereafter, the arm swings backward, causing contraction of the contralateral latissimus dorsi. Lengthening and contraction of the latissimus dorsi contributes to increased tension in the TLF. The contralateral latissimus dorsi and ipsilateral gluteus maximus muscles together appear to tense the TLF, which continues to facilitate the force closure mechanism through the SIJ.[84] The superincumbant body weight is thereby transferred to the lower extremity through a system that is stabilized by ligamentous and myofascial tension. The gluteus maximus is considered key to force closure stabilizing mechanisms within the pelvis. Loss of function of the gluteus maximus as a result of disuse or neurologic impairment can hinder stability of the SIJ.

EXAMINATION AND EVALUATION

Symptoms originating in the lumbopelvic region often are experienced elsewhere in the lower quadrant. It is for this reason that a lumbopelvic scan is recommended before any lumbopelvic or lower quadrant examination. The purpose of the scan is to determine whether symptoms experienced in the lower quadrant are originating in the lumbopelvic region. If it is determined that symptoms are stemming from the lumbopelvic region, a more thorough lumbopelvic examination and evaluation is indicated. Display 18-1 lists the tests that should be included in any lumbopelvic scan examination.

If the examiner determines that the lumbopelvic region is at least one of source of the patient's signs and symptoms, a more thorough examination and evaluation of this region can be performed. The purpose of any assessment is to diagnose the cause of the presenting signs, symptoms, functional limitations, and disability. However, the spe-

> **DISPLAY 18-1**
> **Lumbopelvic Scan Evaluation**
>
> *Observation:* Posture scan in standing and sitting, local signs of skin color, texture scars, soft tissue contours
> *Active range of motion* (with overpressure if indicated): in standing, flexion, extension, lateral flexion; in sitting, rotation
> *Stress tests:* Supine lumbar compression and distraction, supine sacroiliac joint compression and distraction, sidelying sacroiliac joint compression, prone lumbar torsion stress
> *Provocative test:* Prone posteroanterior pressure to the lumbar spine
> *Palpation:* Palpate related lumbar-pelvic-hip musculature, assessing for tone changes, lesions, and pain provocation
> *Dural mobility tests:* Slump test, straight-leg raise, prone knee flexion
> *Neurologic testing:* Key muscles (see Table 18-2), reflexes, dermatomes

cific cause of symptoms originating in the lumbopelvic region is difficult to establish. A structural diagnosis is possible for approximately 70% of patients with chronic low back pain, if those patients with documented psychological aggravation of their symptoms are excluded.[85] Even when a structural diagnosis is provided, it cannot guide decisions regarding intervention in the management of lumbopelvic conditions. Structural changes do not necessarily correlate with or predict levels of pain or disability.[86] Removal or correction of structural abnormalities of the lumbar spine may fail to cure or even worsen painful conditions.[87] Without a diagnosis that can guide patient management, use of a traditional pathoanatomic model (ie, one that implies symptoms should be proportional to organ pathology) is limited.

Much effort has been devoted to developing diagnostic categories for low back pain to guide intervention and predict outcome. However, the basis for diagnostic classification has been highly variable. Pathoanatomic diagnostic systems operate by correlating the patient's symptoms and signs with the results of diagnostic imaging tests.[85] Because of the limitations of this approach, other diagnostic classifications have been developed to improve the classification of low back pain patients. The Quebec Task Force on Spinal Disorders developed a classification system based on a combination of time since onset and symptoms.[88] Some diagnostic systems have attempted to classify patients based on symptoms and response to treatment,[3] and another approach related physiologic impairments and symptoms to faulty postures and movement patterns.[4] The diversity of these approaches demonstrates the level of controversy and complexity surrounding the examination, diagnosis, and prognosis of lumbopelvic syndromes.

The emphasis of the evaluation discussed in this chapter is to determine the postures, movements, and related physiologic impairments that correlate with the patient's symptoms. The goal of the examination is to determine the pathomechanical rather than pathoanatomic cause(s) of symptoms. However, this examination can lead the examiner to a pathoanatomic diagnosis for the small percentage of patients in whom a precise structural fault can be ascribed. A pathoanatomic diagnosis can only be made by correlating the physical examination findings with the history and medical findings (ie, radiographic, neurologic, and laboratory study results). Such an approach is valuable for several reasons:

- It reveals to the examiner and the patient the type and direction of the mechanical stress that correlates with symptoms.
- It reveals physiologic impairments that correlate with the mechanical stress.
- It screens for pathology and anatomic and psychological impairments that affect the prognosis.
- It becomes the basis for a therapeutic exercise program and for posture and movement retraining.

The key to pathomechanical testing of the lumbopelvic region is determining the postures and movements that correlate with the patient's signs or symptoms. It can then be deduced what type and direction of forces exceed the tissue tolerance or adaptability and lead to mechanical or chemical stimulation of the nociceptive system. If the examiner is unable to correlate the history and physical examination findings with a mechanical cause, the source of the symptoms may be nonmechanical, and referral to a medical practitioner is indicated for further diagnostics (see Appendix 1).

The clinician examining a patient with a lumbopelvic syndrome has the responsibility of answering three critical questions by the end of the initial examination:

1. Is there a systemic or visceral disease underlying the pain (see Appendix 1)?
2. Is there evidence of neurologic compromise that represents a surgical emergency (eg, cauda equina symptoms)?
3. Are there mechanical findings that guide physical therapy intervention?

Data collected from the history and physical examination should provide an answer to all three questions.

Patient History

The patient's history is a critical component of the lumbopelvic examination. Information can be acquired through a patient questionnaire, through an interview, through review of medical charts, or all three forms. The history has several purposes:

- To establish an understanding of the mechanism of injury (if an injury precipitated the condition)
- To establish the pain location and pattern
- To assist in determining the nature, severity, and irritability of the condition
- To assess the effect of previous interventions
- To assist in determining whether the symptoms result from musculoskeletal or nonmusculoskeletal pathology
- To assist in determining whether signs of nonorganic pain behavior are present (see Special Tests section)
- To assess the patient's perceived functional limitations and disability and his understanding of the condition

The information gathered from the patient history should help guide the clinician toward specific tests to be included in the physical examination.

ALIGNMENT EXAMINATION

The therapist should perform a cursory evaluation of the patient's standing and sitting postures during the history portion of the examination. Posture also is examined formally as part of the evaluation process. The patient is aware of the scrutiny during the formal examination and may assume what he considers to be proper posture or posture that depicts the painful or emotional state he wishes to portray. The posture portrayed during this examination may be unconscious or intentional, and the motivation is not always easily discerned. Observation of posture without the patient's knowledge can be more revealing of the true contribution of posture to his signs and symptoms.

Several things should be observed while the patient is standing, including head position, shoulder girdle position, standing spine curves (ie, cervical, thoracic, and lumbar), and lumbopelvic, hip, knee, ankle-foot alignment should be examined about all three planes. The examiner is looking for asymmetry and possible relationships between segmental regions (eg, foot pronation and genu valgum on the side of a low iliac crest and apparent short limb).

Bony landmarks are assessed to visualize the position of the pelvis, including the iliac crest, PSISs, ASISs, and pubic symphysis. Ideal pelvic alignment is best visualized through the ASIS and pubic symphysis in the frontal plane.[89]

A hypothesis can be developed regarding the contribution of faulty lumbopelvic alignment to the pathomechanical cause of symptoms and the relationship of other body regions in perpetuating the faulty lumbopelvic alignment. Another hypothesis can be developed about muscle lengths. Assumptions can be made regarding muscle-fascial structures that are too long based on joint position, such as a long external oblique in an anterior pelvic tilt (Fig. 18-16). Muscle length testing is indicated to determine whether muscles are short because of joint position (eg, which hip flexors are short in anterior pelvic tilt). The results of positional strength tests performed later in the examination should correlate with the muscle length hypothesis.

Correction of standing alignment can reduce pathomechanical stress in the lumbopelvic region. The patient's symptoms may decrease with postural correction strategies. This is an early step toward the diagnosis of a pathomechanical cause of lumbopelvic functional limitations and disability.

The clinician should examine sitting posture in a supported and unsupported chair, paying particular attention to pelvic position and its relationship to hip alignment and spinal curves. If the patient is awakened from sleep by symptoms or experiences more pronounced symptoms on waking, the recumbent posture should be examined. Discomfort in the prone or supine position can correlate with extension stress (eg, short hip flexors can pull the pelvis into anterior pelvic tilt and lumbar spine into extension in the supine position), and discomfort in the sidelying position can correlate with stress in the transverse plane.

Correction of faulty alignment (eg, reduced anterior pelvic tilt in standing, reduced lumbar flexed posture in sitting, a pillow under the knees in supine or stomach in prone and between the legs in sidelying positions) reduces or relieves symptoms if the positional fault is correlated to the symptoms. This is another early step in determining a pathomechanical cause of lumbopelvic functional limitations and disability.

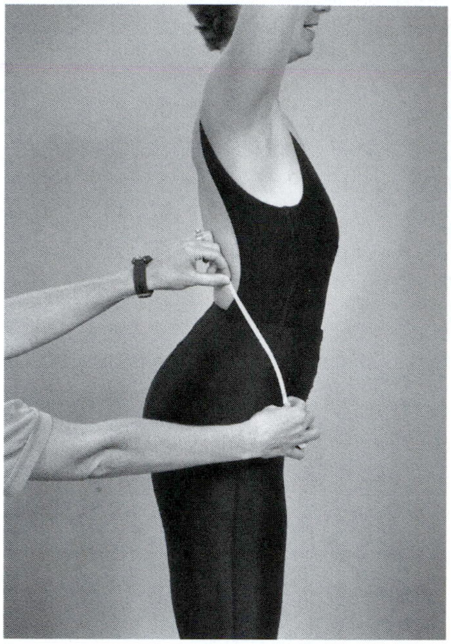

FIGURE 18-16 The lordotic posture and anterior pelvic tilt elongate the external oblique.

Gait Examination

Gait is a complex movement pattern that can demonstrate pathomechanical factors contributing to lumbopelvic signs or symptoms, particularly if the patient reports that walking increases or decreases symptoms. Analysis of gait should include observation of the foot-ankle complex, knee, hip, pelvis, spine, and upper quadrant movements about all three planes of motion during all phases of gait. Video analysis of gait is an efficient way to gain this information.

The relationship of other regions to the lumbopelvic region is important in ascertaining the mechanical stress imposed on the lumbar spine. For example, a rigid supinated foot that does not adequately pronate during the stance phase of gait may increase compressive stress on the lumbar spine. A hypermobile pronated foot may induce a transverse-plane stress on the lumbar spine by creating a short limb during the stance phase of gait. An asymmetric arm swing can promote transverse-plane stress in the lumbopelvic region. Short hip flexors limit hip extension mobility during terminal stance and may promote compensatory lumbar extension or rotation. Weak hip abductors can create a frontal-plane or transverse-plane stress on the lumbar spine by inducing a Trendelenburg or compensated Trendelenburg gait pattern (see Chapter 20). The natural lumbar extension that occurs during gait can reduce symptoms created by excessive flexion during prolonged sitting.

Mobility Examination

Tests examining for impairment in mobility in the lumbopelvic examination look at mobility along the continuum of hypermobility to hypomobility of the lumbar spine, pelvis, and adjacent regions (eg, shoulder girdle, other spine regions, hip, knee, ankle-foot complex). With this information, the therapist can better understand the physiologic impairments contributing to pathomechanical stress imposed on the lumbar spine. Mobility testing assists in diagnosing affected structures and staging the degree of irritability of the condition.

GROSS MOVEMENT TESTING

Gross movement testing is performed in standing for flexion and extension, lateral flexion, and quadrant movements; it is performed in sitting for rotation. All movement tests can be performed repeatedly to determine the effect of repeated movements on symptoms (eg, worsening of symptoms during repeated forward bending may indicate disk pathology). Overpressure can be used to reproduce symptoms. The intent of gross movement testing with respect to mobility assessment is fourfold:

1. To determine the patient's willingness to move
2. To reproduce symptoms
3. To determine the quantity of motion in the lumbar-pelvic-hip complex
4. To determine the quality of movement by assessing the LPR

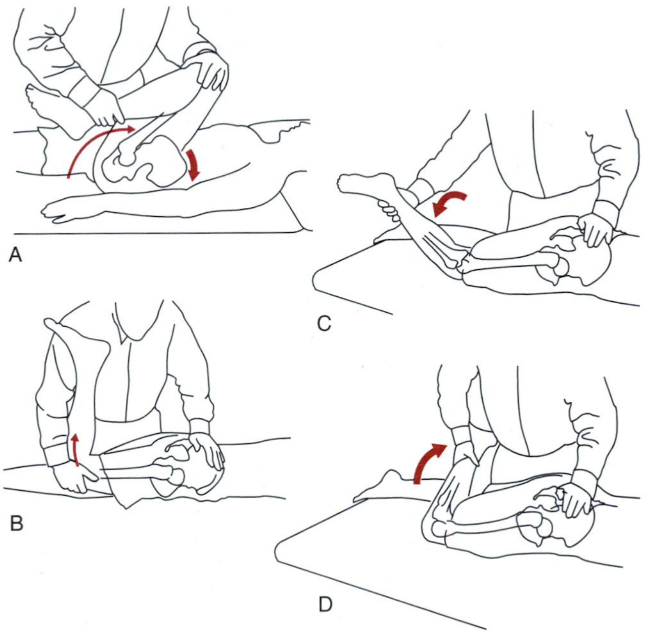

FIGURE 18-17 ***(A)*** Passive hip flexion can progressively stress the hip joint, followed by the posterior rotation of the ilium and spinal flexion. ***(B)*** Passive hip extension progressively stretches the anterior hip musculature and hip capsule, followed by anterior rotation of the ilium and extension of the lumbar spine. ***(C)*** Passive hip internal and ***(D)*** external rotation progressively stress the hip joint musculature, capsule, sacroiliac joint, and lumbar spine in a rotary direction.

NON–WEIGHT-BEARING PASSIVE AND ACTIVE OSTEOKINEMATIC HIP MOBILITY TESTING

Chapter 20 describes hip osteokinematic testing. The purpose of hip mobility testing is to determine hypomobility in the hip that may contribute to compensatory spine mobility, thereby imposing a pathomechanical stress on the lumbar spine. For example, a hip that is hypomobile in extension may cause compensatory spine extension, particularly during the terminal stance phase of gait or in the final phase of return from a forward bend. Passive hip joint mobility testing can be sequentially progressed to stress the iliosacral joint, lumbosacral region, and lumbar spine (Fig. 18-17) to provoke symptoms.

Active hip mobility testing can be used to assess movement patterns of the hip and stabilization patterns of the lumbopelvic region.[4] Faulty patterns can induce a pathomechanical stress on the lumbar spine and provoke symptoms. Correction of faulty patterns of lumbopelvic stabilization should reduce symptoms if the faulty pattern is contributing to pathomechanical stress on the affected structures. In this way, these tests can also be used to clear the hip joint of any possible involvement. If correction of lumbopelvic stabilization reduces symptoms, it is unlikely that the hip is the source of symptoms.

PASSIVE AND ACTIVE THORACIC OSTEOKINEMATIC MOBILITY

Thoracic mobility testing is described in Chapter 25. The purpose of thoracic mobility testing is to determine whether hypomobility of the thoracic spine is contributing to compensatory motion in the lumbopelvic region (eg, reduced or stiff thoracic spine rotation could contribute to excessive lumbar rotation).

PASSIVE ARTHROKINEMATIC LUMBOPELVIC TESTING

Passive arthrokinematic testing can be performed at each spinal level[90] and at the SIJ.[84] Arthrokinematic testing is used to determine the relative arthrokinematic mobility (eg, hypermobility versus hypomobility) and to stress the related spine and pelvic joints in an attempt to determine end feel, assess irritability, and provoke symptoms.

TESTS OF MUSCULAR EXTENSIBILITY

Tests of muscular extensibility across the pelvis and hip are described in Chapter 20. Data obtained from these tests provide the clinician with additional information about potential causes of pathomechanical stress on the lumbar spine. For example, during forward bending, short hamstrings can restrict pelvic forward rotation, resulting in flexion stress (Fig. 18-18*A*) on the lumbar spine. Short hip flexors can restrict pelvic backward rotation, resulting in extension stress on the lumbar spine during return to an upright position (Fig. 18-18*B*) or during backward-bending movements. Although not direct measures of trunk muscle extensibility, lumbopelvic forward bending, backward bending, and lateral flexion can test for posterior, anterior, and lateral trunk extensibility, respectively. Assessment of postural alignment can lead to a hypothesis about excessive trunk muscle length (see the Alignment Examination section).

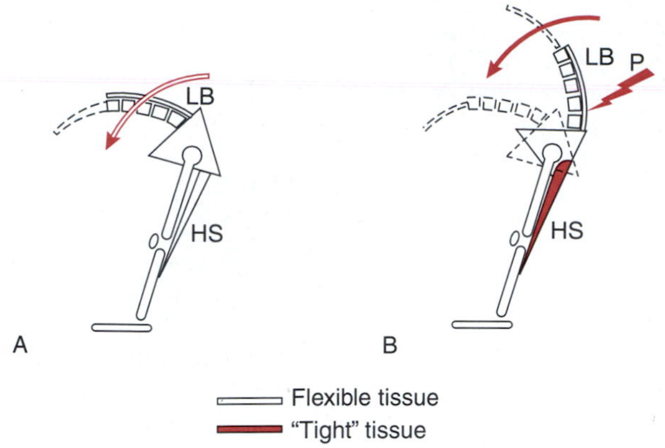

FIGURE 18-18 Reduced extensibility of the hamstrings (HS) can alter the lumbar-pelvic rhythm. Stiffness from the hamstrings slows (B) the rate and can potentially restrict the range of pelvic motion, causing excessive flexion stress of the lumbar spine. (From Calliet R. *Low Back Pain*. 3rd ed. Philadelphia: FA Davis; 1981:65).

All mobility tests should assess the effect that altered mobility of some structures has on lumbar and SIJ segmental movements. Reduced or excessive mobility in other regions affect mobility of the lumbar spine and pelvis. For example, excessive lumbar extension may be imposed on the L5 segmental level during active movement patterns because of relatively less extension mobility available in L1 through L4, thoracic segmental levels, or the hip or because of relatively less mobility in upper extremity flexion. By determining which segmental levels, what anatomic regions, and the sources of structural limitation (eg, muscle, capsule, bone), a specific intervention plan can be developed to address the related impairments.

Muscle Performance, Neuromuscular Control, and Endurance Examination

The ability for the abdominal, spinal extensor, and pelvic girdle muscles to carry out functions of mobility and stability must be carefully assessed to ascertain the pathomechanics of the lumbopelvic region. The sources of impaired mobility or stability of the spine include neurologic pathology, muscle strain, disuse or deconditioning, poor neuromuscular control, and lack of endurance. The impact of each of these causes of reduced muscle performance and endurance is discussed in more detail later in this chapter. Techniques for assessing these causes of impaired muscle performance and endurance are highlighted here.

MANUAL MUSCLE TESTING

Assessment of the force- or torque-generating capability of the spinal extensor and abdominal muscle groups can be performed with traditional manual muscle testing procedures as described by Kendall and colleagues.[89] Because of the numerous details regarding accurate assessment of the abdominal muscles, Kendall's work should be reviewed to ensure optimal manual muscle testing results.

ISOKINETIC TESTING

Although objective information about muscle force or torque production can be gathered from isokinetic testing, gross strength testing by this method may not be sensitive to the function of the deeper musculature surrounding the spine. Whereas many studies demonstrate an unequivocal relationship between impaired function of the deep abdominal and lumbar multifidus muscles and low back pain, studies comparing gross trunk strength in normal or low back pain patients have not consistently demonstrated such a relationship.[91–96] This difference may reflect the inherent limitations in conclusions that can be ascertained from studies examining maximal trunk strength in persons with low back pain. For example, pain can hinder maximal effort, and a test of a patient with low back pain may be more a test of the patient's tolerance to pain. This design problem may be responsible for the varied and seemingly contradictory results of trunk muscle strength reported in the literature.

Isokinetic testing of trunk muscle strength also focuses largely on the assessment of muscles primarily involved in and capable of producing large torques about the spine (eg, rectus abdominis, thoracolumbar erector spinae) rather than on muscles considered to provide stability and fine control (eg, deep abdominals, lumbar multifidus).[97,98] Most studies focus on maximal voluntary contractions, which are rarely carried out during the ADLs. In the chronic low back pain population, sudden, unexpected, and insignificant movement at low load can exacerbate symptoms just as commonly as tasks involving maximal exertion.[99,100]

NEUROMUSCULAR CONTROL

Isokinetic and traditional manual muscle testing may not be sensitive enough to assess the muscle performance of the deep trunk muscles (ie, transversus abdominis and lumbar multifidus). Testing of trunk muscle strength should also consider the function of the deeper musculature. Tests that examine the ability of the abdominal muscles to stabilize against various directional forces during active extremity movement can provide the clinician with an indication of the performance of the deep abdominal muscles. The lower abdominal functional strength test (see Self-Management: Lower Abdominal Progression) is one method of testing the neuromuscular control of the abdominal muscles to stabilize against sagittal (double-limb movements) and transverse-plane forces (single-leg movements) imposed by movements of the lower extremities.[4] Many repetitions can provide an indication of the endurance of the trunk muscles. When the spine is unable to remain stable against a specific force, it can indicate a lack of force or torque production or fatigue (depending on the focus of the test) of the associated trunk muscle. Similar tests assessing patterns of trunk stabilization have been developed by Sahrmann.[4]

RESISTED TESTING

In theory, resisted testing of the trunk muscles can also provide information about the integrity of the trunk muscles relative to imposed strain. However, resisted testing of the trunk muscles can also provoke other pain-sensitive structures and result in a weak and painful test, making it diffi-

SELF-MANAGEMENT: *Lower Abdominal Progression*

Purpose: To provide an alternative to sit-ups as an activity to strengthen and shorten weak and overstretched abdominal muscles, focus on an often ignored function of the abdominal muscles, and support the pelvis and lumbar spine in neutral during movements of the lower extremities

Starting position: Lie on your back on a firm surface, such as the floor, with knees bent and feet flat on the floor and shoes off. Place your fingertips on each side of your abdomen, just below your ribs (Fig. A). Take a deep diaphragmatic breath in (your physical therapist will teach you the correct technique for diaphragmatic breathing). As you exhale, make an "s" sound, and pull your abdomen in as if to pull your belly button closer to your spine. Do not concentrate on pushing your back flat but rather on lengthening your torso while pulling in your abdominals. To progress from one level to the next in this series:

The abdominal muscles must be pulled in, not *pooched* or distended. This occurs as increased strain is placed on the abdominal muscles from the progressively difficult leg movements.

The lumbar spine must remain in a neutral postion of a slight forward curve—just enough to fit your hand between your back and the floor—and not move into further forward curve or excessively flatten. You may use a small hand towel rolled under the small of your back to provide feedback as to the position of your spine.

Movement technique: Your physical therapist will check off the level(s) you are to perform with the appropriate dosage.

Level I: While keeping your abdomen pulled in, *slowly* lift one leg such that the hip is at a 90-degree angle. After you have completed the lift of the first leg, lift the other leg to the same postion. Return to the start position one limb at a time. Alternate the starting leg with each subsequent repetition. The abdomen must remain flat and not allowed to *pooch.* This ensures the abdominal muscles are contracting strongly enough to anchor the pelvis and lumbar spine against the weight of the legs.

A

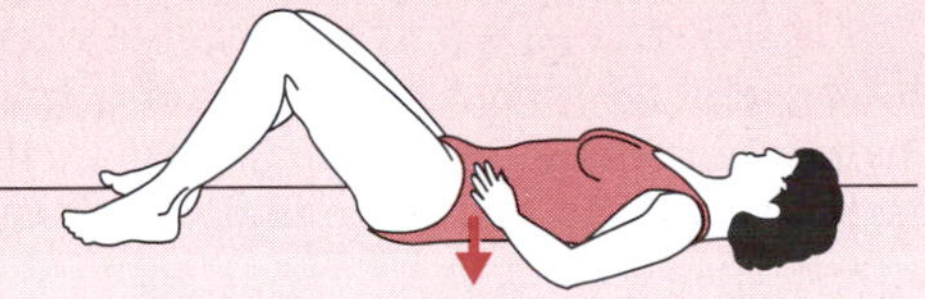

B

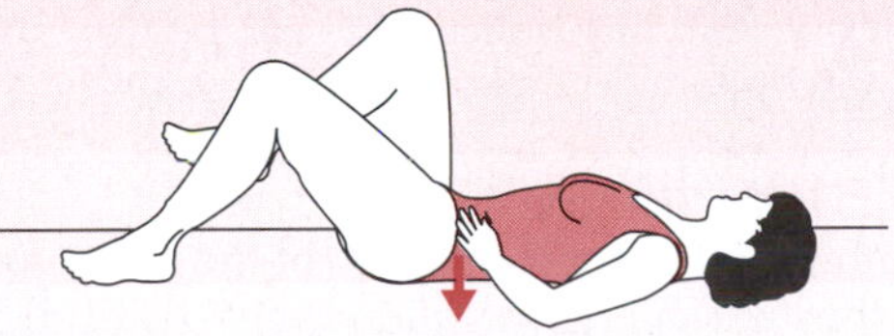

Dosage

Sets/repetitions ________________

Frequency ________________

Level II: Repeat level I, but instead of lowering the leg to the start position, **slide** one leg down to a fully extended position while keeping the opposite leg **elevated** off the floor. **Slide** the leg back to the same position as the nonmoving limb. Repeat with the other leg. As soon as you are unable to stabilize the pelvis and lumbar spine and the abdomen begins to *pooch,* stop and rest for a minute before continuing. If your hip flexors (front thigh muscles) are short, you will not be able to fully extend your leg without moving your spine out of neutral. In this case, stop sliding your leg when you notice your back moving from its neutral position. Eventually, your hip flexor muscles will lengthen as your abdominal muscles shorten and become stronger.

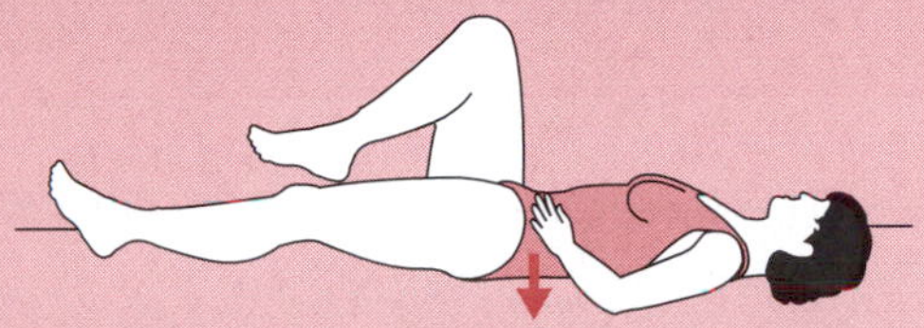

Dosage

Sets/repetitions ________________

Frequency ________________

Level III: Repeat level II, but instead of sliding your leg down and back, **glide** your leg down and back. The nonmoving leg should remain in a flexed position **off** the floor. It is easy to transition from a flat abdomen to a *pooched* abdomen at this level. Stop after completing two leg glides, and reset your muscles. Be sure to exhale with leg movements.

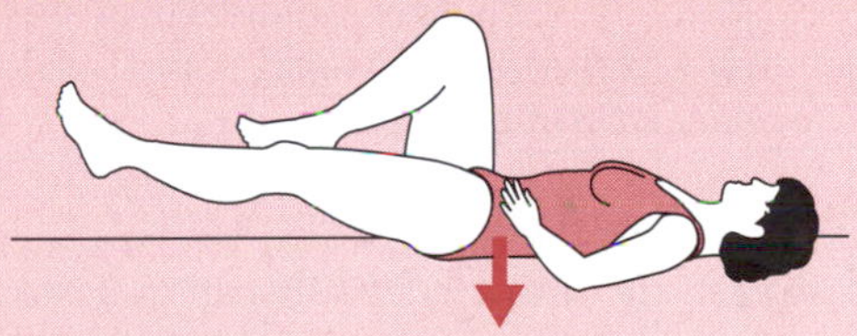

Dosage

Sets/repetitions ________________

Frequency ________________

Level IV: Begin from the start position, and lift **both** legs off the floor at the same time to the 90-degree position. Return to the start position by lowering both legs at the same time. **Slide** both legs simultaneously to the fully extended position, and **slide** both legs back to the start position.

A

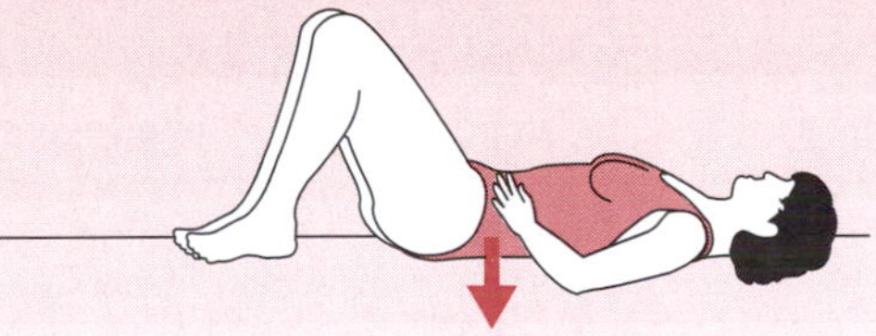

B

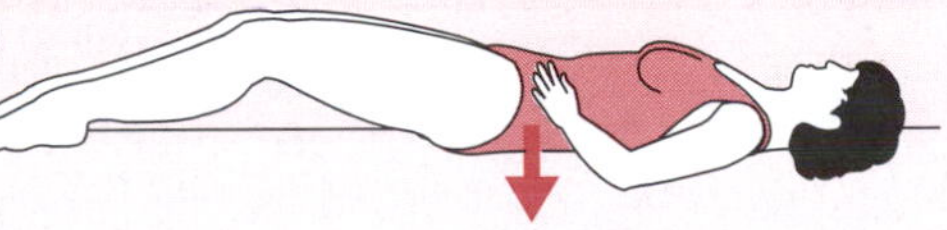

Dosage

Sets/repetitions ________________

Frequency ________________

(continued)

SELF-MANAGEMENT: *Lower Abdominal Progression* *(Continued)*

Level V: Repeat level IV, but **glide** both legs down and back to the start position.

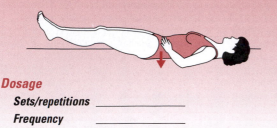

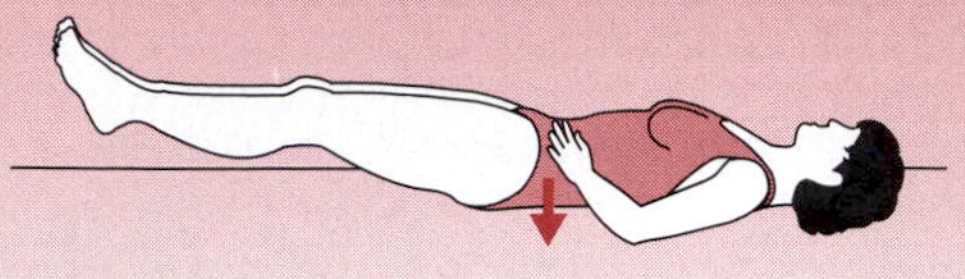

Dosage

Sets/repetitions ______________

Frequency ______________

cult to use resisted testing as a differential diagnostic test for trunk muscle strain.

MANUAL MUSCLE TESTING OF RELATED REGIONAL MUSCULATURE

Muscle strength testing of pelvic girdle and pelvic floor muscles can provide pertinent information about factors that may contribute to lumbopelvic dysfunction. For example, weakness in the gluteus medius results in excessive hip adduction and pelvic drop in the single-limb support phase of gait, which can impose frontal-plane stress on the lumbopelvic region and thereby contribute to lumbopelvic impairment or pathology. Chapters 19 and 20, respectively, provide recommendations for pelvic floor and pelvic girdle muscle performance testing.

RESISTED TESTS FOR NEUROLOGIC PATHOLOGY

Strength testing of the lower extremity can indicate potential nerve root or peripheral nerve involvement (Table 18-2). The specific pattern of weakness indicates whether the problem is nerve root or peripheral nerve in origin.

Table18-2. KEY MUSCLES AND CORRESPONDING NERVE ROOT AND PERIPHERAL NERVE IN THE LUMBOPELVIC REGION

KEY MUSCLE	NERVE ROOT	PERIPHERAL NERVE
Psoas	L2 (3)	Femoral
Quadriceps	L3 (4)	Femoral
Tibialis anterior	L4 (5)	Deep peroneal
Extensor hallucis	L5 (S1)	Deep peroneal
Gluteus medius	L5 (S1)	Superior gluteal
Peroneii	L5 (S1)	Superficial peroneal
Medial hamstrings	L5 (S1)	Sciatic
Gastrocnemius	S1	Tibial
Peroneii	S1	Superficial peroneal
Lateral hamstrings	S1	Sciatic
Gluteus maximus	S2	Inferior gluteal
Bladder and rectum	S4	

Pain and Inflammation Examination

The clinician examines pain in the lumbopelvic region with respect to many variables:

- Measurement of pain with respect to the level of disability it imposes on an individual with low back pain
- Examination techniques used to diagnose whether the pain is originating in the lumbopelvic region and, if possible, determine the potential sources of the pain
- Examination techniques to determine the potential causes of pain
- Examination techniques and clinical reasoning to determine the impact of pain on the physiologic function of the lumbopelvic region

Each of these components must be examined carefully to determine a plan of care and to provide sensitive measures of outcome.

MEASUREMENT OF DISABILITY

The measurement of disability resulting from low back pain may be accomplished with a variety of self-rated disability questionnaires or by clinical observation of tasks. A questionnaire usually is preferred to clinical observation because of its reliability, sensitivity, ease, and speed of application.[101] A sensitive measure of outcome can prove to be of great value to the patient, referring practitioner, and third-party payers by demonstrating a baseline level of disability and later showing that treatment has had an effect. Visual analog scales or other scales for rating pain that are used in isolation are not as discriminating an indicator of outcome as health status questionnaires.[101] The Disability Questionnaire (Fig. 18-19) and Pain Rating Scale (Fig. 18-20) are examples of disability indices that can be used as discriminating outcome measures of low back pain.[101]

DIFFERENTIAL DIAGNOSIS

Determining whether the source of the pain is originating within the lumbopelvic region requires careful and logical sequencing of examination techniques to exclude other possible sources of pain. It is often not possible to diagnose the specific source of pain within the low back, but determining that the lumbopelvic region is the source of

1. I stay at home most of the time because of my back.
2. I change position frequently to try and get my back comfortable.
3. I walk more slowly than usual because of my back.
4. Because of my back I am not doing any of the jobs that I usually do around the house.
5. Because of my back, I use a handrail to get upstairs.
6. Because of my back, I lie down to rest more often.
7. Because of my back, I have to hold on to something to get out of an easy chair.
8. Because of my back, I try to get other people to things for me.
9. I get dressed more slowly than usual because of my back.
10. I only stand up for short periods of time because of my back.
11. Because of my back, I try not to bend or kneel down.
12. I find it difficult to get out of a chair because of my back.
13. My back is painful almost all the time.
14. I find it difficult to turn over in bed because of my back.
15. My appetite is not very good because of my back.
16. I have trouble putting on my socks (or stockings) because of the pain in my back.
17. I can only walk short distances because of my back pain.
18. I sleep less because of my back.
19. Because of my back pain, I get dressed with help from someone else.
20. I sit down for most of the day because of my back.
21. I avoid heavy jobs around the house because of my back.
22. Because of my back pain, I am more irritable and bad tempered with people than usual.
23. Because of my back pain, I go upstairs more slowly than usual.
24. I stay in bed for most of the time because of my back.

When your back hurts, you may find it difficult to do some of the things you normally do.

This list contains some sentences that people have used to describe themselves when they have back pain. When you read them, you may find that some stand out because they describe you *today*. As you read the list, think of yourself *today*. When you read a sentence that describes you today, put a tick against it. If the sentence does not describe you, then leave the space blank and go on to the next one. Remember, only tick the sentence if you are sure that it describes you today.

FIGURE 18-19 Disability questionnaire. (Adapted from Roland M, Morris R. A study of the natural history of low back pain. Part II: Development of a reliable and sensitive measure of disability in low back pain. *Spine.* 1983;8:141–144.)

pain instead of the hip or nonmusculoskeletal areas (see Appendix 1) is critical to the plan of care. Although the lumbar spine clearing examination is designed to include or exclude spine involvement, it is often difficult to determine whether pain originates from the spine, SIJ, or hip joint. Additional tests performed during the lumbar examination (eg, hip clearing tests, see Chapter 20) can solidify the hypothesis.

DIAGNOSIS OF MECHANICAL CAUSES OF PAIN

After it has been determined that the lumbar spine or pelvis is the source of the pain (even if the exact source of the pain cannot be diagnosed), attempts must be made to determine the mechanical cause of the pain. The complexity of understanding the causes or mechanisms of pain is beyond the scope of this text. Much controversy exists about whether chemical or mechanical mechanisms initiate and perpetuate pain and about exactly what neurophysiologic and biochemical processes are responsible for pain.

The role of the physical therapist is to determine whether mechanical interventions can alter pain. During the examination process, the therapist can observe precise stabilization and movement patterns and correlate faulty patterns with the onset of or increase in pain. If altering the pattern of stabilization or movement reduces or eliminates the pain, the specific faulty movement patterns responsible for the pain can be diagnosed.[4]

Balance and Coordination Examination

There is evidence that low back pain patients present with alterations in righting and postural reflexes and changes in motor control patterns.[66,102–104] In light of this evidence, perhaps tests of balance and coordination should be incorporated into the examination of patients with low back pain. This approach may be particularly helpful if impairments in these elements of function are perceived to place the patient at risk for maintenance or recurrence of low back dysfunction. Chapter 7 provides information about balance tests.

Special Tests

NEURAL EXTENSIBILITY TESTS

Neural extensibility tests are commonly used for the lumbopelvic region. Because neural tissue (connective and conducting) can be a source of symptoms, tests of neurodynamics

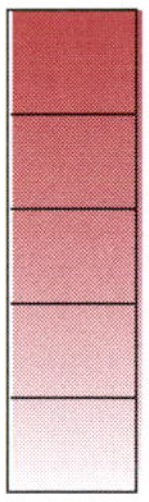

The pain is almost unbearable

Very bad pain

Quite bad pain

Moderate pain

Little pain

No pain at all

Now we want you to give us an idea of just how bad your back pain is at the moment.

Here is a thermometer with various grades of pain from "no pain at all" at the bottom to "the pain is almost unbearable" at the top. We want you to put a cross by the words that describe your pain best. Remember, we want to know how bad your pain is *at the moment.*

FIGURE 18-20 Pain rating scale. (Adapted from Roland M, Morris R. A study of the natural history of low back pain. Part II: Development of a reliable and sensitive measure of disability in low back pain, *Spine.* 1983; 8:141–144.)

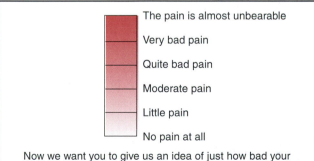

need to be included in most lumbopelvic examinations. Examples of tests of neurodynamics include the straight-leg raise, prone knee bend, and slump maneuver.

The clinician administering these tests should be skilled in the specialized features of handling and sequencing the components of the test and must understand what is considered to be a normal or acceptable response. Other sources[105] can provide more information on neurodynamic testing procedures.

WADDELL'S NONORGANIC SIGNS

As the cost of managing low back pain escalates, a reliable predictor of outcome is advantageous. Patients whose outcome is predicted to be poor at assessment require special management or redirection to more appropriate intervention. Waddell's signs can be used as a predictor of outcome for patients with lumbopelvic disabilities.[106] Waddell and coworkers[107] identified five nonorganic signs, and each can be detected by one or two tests. The tests assess a patient's pain behavior in response to certain maneuvers (Table 18-3). A patient presenting with a high Waddell score (ie, 3, 4, or 5 of 5 positive nonorganic signs) is believed to have a clinical pattern of nonmechanical, pain-focused behavior. The patient has significant enough psychological impairments that intervention focused on physiologic and anatomic impairments alone probably cannot produce a successful outcome. A high Waddell's score can be used as a predictor of functional outcome, as indicated by a low rate of return to work.[106] However, the practitioner must interpret this finding with caution. A high Waddell score only indicates a high degree of nonorganic or psychological impairments. It does not signify malingering, which is a judgment, not a medical or psychological diagnosis.[108] Patients with a high Waddell score should be referred to the appropriate practitioner for treatment before or in conjunction with further physical therapy intervention.

THERAPEUTIC EXERCISE INTERVENTION FOR COMMON PHYSIOLOGIC IMPAIRMENTS

It is not usually possible or desirable to set up a particular exercise regimen for the lumbar spine and pelvis based solely on the pathology or medical diagnosis. A pathoanatomic diagnosis usually cannot be reached. Even if a specific pathoanatomic diagnosis is reached, the presenting impairments, functional limitations, and disability of patients are often different, despite similar pathology or anatomic impairments. Classification schemes guiding conservative management of lumbopelvic syndromes have not been well developed. The choice of exercise intervention therefore must be based on the pathology and the physiologic, psychological, and anatomic impairments that are most closely related to the patient's functional limitations and disability.

Because this text is not presenting a treatment approach related to a specific classification system, the exercises are based on the physiologic impairments presented in Unit 2. Physiologic impairments have been separated for clarity of presentation. In reality, patients most often present with a complex interaction of pathology and anatomic, psychological, and physiologic impairments. Individual assessment determines which impairments are most closely related to the patient's functional limitations and disability and therefore warrant intervention. The exercise examples are not meant to demonstrate a comprehensive approach to the treatment of physiologic impairments; they were chosen to illustrate principles and a reasoned approach to the use of exercise for the lumbopelvic region. Principles related to work-conditioning programs, although often used in addressing lumbopelvic dysfunction, are not covered in this text.

Table 18-3. WADDELL'S SIGNS

TEST	SIGNS
Tenderness	Superficial—the patient's skin is tender to light pinch over a wide area of lumbar skin Nonanatomic—deep tenderness felt over a wide area, not localized to one structure
Simulation tests	Axial loading—light vertical loading over patient's skull in the standing position causes lumbar pain Acetabular rotation—back pain is reported when the pelvis and shoulders are passively rotated in the same plane as the patient stands; considered to be a positive test result if pain is reported within the first 30 degrees
Distraction tests	Straight-leg-raise discrepancy—marked improvement of straight-leg raising on distraction compared with formal testing Double-leg raise—when both legs are raised after straight-leg raising, the organic response is a greater degree of double-leg raising; patients with a nonorganic component demonstrate less double-leg raise compared with the single-leg raise
Regional disturbances	Weakness—cogwheeling or giving way of many muscle groups that cannot be explained on a neurologic basis Sensory disturbance—diminished sensation fitting a "stocking" rather than a dermatomal pattern
Overreaction	Disproportionate verbalization, facial expression, muscle tension and tremor, collapsing, or sweating

From Karas R, McIntosh G, Hall H, Wilson L, Melles T. The relationship between nonorgans signs and centralization of symptoms in the prediction of the return to work for patients with low back pain. *Phys Ther.* 1997;77:356. Reprinted with permission of the American Physical Therapy Association.

Pain and Inflammation

Pain is the most common reason persons with lumbopelvic syndromes seek health care. Pain is often perceived to be the cause of limitations in function and disability by individuals with lumbopelvic syndromes. The sources of pain within the lumbopelvic region are numerous and often difficult to diagnose because of the complex interaction of peripheral and central mechanisms responsible for the experience of pain. The physiologic and psychological impact that lumbopelvic pain has on the person can create profound disability. It is often difficult to determine the contribution of physiologic or psychological factors, necessitating treatment that deals with both categories of impairment. However, this section deals with the treatment of pain based solely on physiologic musculoskeletal factors.

Treatment of the physiologic musculoskeletal component of pain can include interventions along a vast spectrum of choices, ranging from pharmaceutical intervention in the form of oral medications or injections to physical therapy to surgery, applied individually or in any combination. The choice of intervention must be tailored to each case, ideally with input from all practitioners involved in the case. This section discusses therapeutic exercise as one type of intervention for the treatment of musculoskeletal lumbopelvic pain. Although the exercises suggested in this section were chosen to demonstrate activities or techniques to treat different causes of pain, many are used to treat other impairments, such as those of mobility, muscle performance, posture, and movement. Consequently, they may be referred to in later sections, illustrating the complex interaction of impairments and the diversity and versatility of the exercises.

To make informed decisions about the exercises chosen to treat pain, the clinician should understand the physiologic impact that pain has on the structures of the lumbopelvic region. There is evidence of segmental changes within the deep low back muscles in the presence of low back pain.[67,109–112] Atrophy has been found on the ipsilateral side and at the corresponding clinically determined level of symptoms in the lumbar multifidus, whose potential segmental stabilizing role in the lumbar spine is becoming increasingly well recognized.[113–114] Histologic changes have been found in the type I fibers of the lumbar multifidus in patients with herniated IVDs and chronic low back pain.[111,115–119] The changes identified in the type I fibers may result from pain-provoked, low-tension muscle contraction, which is not strong enough to stimulate type II fibers.[118] Others have hypothesized that the atrophy is consistent with pain-induced disuse.[112] Although the physiologic changes are not well understood, they do occur and contribute to impairments in muscle performance, neuromuscular control, and endurance, particularly in the lumbar multifidus.

A patient with chronic low back pain and poor segmental control over the stabilizing and movement functions of the motion segment is caught in a cycle of pain and dysfunction. Reducing the mechanical or chemical causes of pain is critical to breaking the cycle and allowing the structures affected by pain and inflammation to recover if provided with the appropriate stimulus.

Most structures in the lumbar spine can be a source of pain at some time under the right circumstances, making it difficult or impossible to diagnose a specific source of pain. The nerve root, disk annulus, facet joint, and muscle seem to be the most acceptable candidates for sources of pain.[120] The mechanisms of pain production are described as a combination of mechanical and chemical irritation of the nociceptive receptors within the tissues. It is not clear whether mechanical stresses lead to chemical irritation, which sensitizes the tissue, or chemical irritation makes tissue more sensitive to mechanical stress. The two mechanisms probably coexist.

In the spinal canal, the herniated nucleus pulposus (HNP) is a strong candidate for the cause of inflammation and irritation of nerve roots and nerve endings. Because of the juxtaposition of disk and nerve roots in the spinal canal, sciatica (ie, pain radiating from the low back into the buttock, posterior thigh, and leg) is likely to rise from compression of the dorsal root ganglion and inflamed nerve roots. When a painful condition is set in peripheral tissue, the consequent barrage of noxious signals into the spinal cord can sensitize somatosensory neurons in the dorsal horn. These sensitized neurons can contribute to a condition of chronic pain.[120]

The physical therapist is most interested in the mechanical cause of pain as it relates to movement. A systematic physical examination often reveals postures, stabilization, and movement strategies that contribute to the onset of pain, worsen existing pain, or conversely, abolish or reduce pain.

One philosophical approach[4] to treating mechanical causes of pain related to posture or movement is to teach the patient to avoid the posture or movement that is associated with the onset or worsening of pain. The therapist should instruct the patient in more desirable posture and movement patterns and treat the associated physiologic impairments contributing to the undesirable posture and movement strategies (eg, muscle extensibility, muscle performance, neuromuscular control). This approach probably intervenes mechanically by avoiding the postures and movements that are associated with pain and intervenes chemically by allowing the painful structures to "rest" and slow down or halt the inflammatory process. For example, in the patient who reports worsening of pain during forward bending, the LPR is faulty, with excessive motion in the low back relative to the hips. If the pain is reduced or abolished when the patient is instructed to bend with a greater contribution of movement from the hips and less movement from the low back, this information can be used to devise an exercise intervention. Examples of exercises to include in such a program are listed in Display 18-2.

In many cases, reducing the mechanical stress on the affected structures by improving mobility in adjacent regions, improving stability in the affected region, and making associated changes in posture and movement patterns are sufficient steps to resolve the episode of pain without need for other interventions. In other instances, complimentary interventions (eg, joint mobilization, physical agents, pharmaceutical intervention, psychological counseling) by the physical therapist or other practitioners involved in the case may be necessary to treat the mechanical, chemical, or psychological causes of pain.

DISPLAY 18-2

Exercises to *Improve* Hip Flexion Mobility and *Decrease* Lumbar Flexion Mobility

Exercises to improve hip flexion mobility

- Hand-knee rocking (see Self-Management: Hand-Knee Rocking in Chapter 20)
- Supine hip flexion without lumbar flexion (Fig. A)

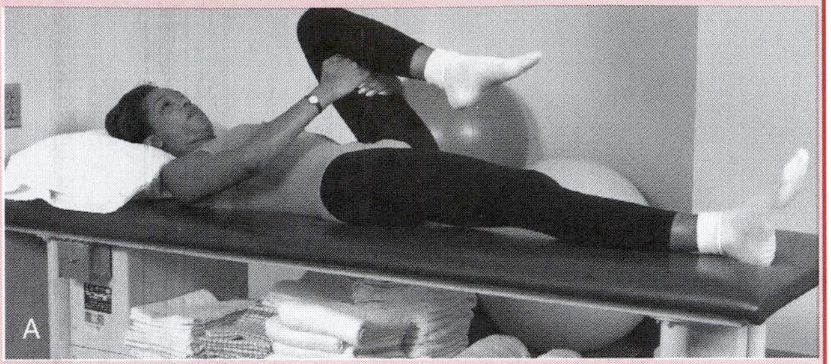

Exercises to reduce lumbar flexion mobility

- Seated knee extension (see Self-Management: Seated Knee Extension in Chapter 20)
- Waiter's bow (Fig. B)

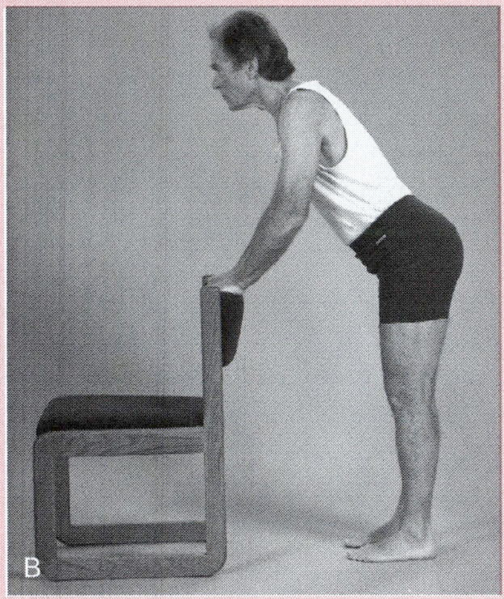

Instruction to alter posture and movement patterns

- Corrected Sitting Posture (see Patient-Related Instruction: Proper Sitting Posture in Chapter 19)
- Improved lumbarpelvic rhythm (see Patient-Related Instruction: Lumbar Pelvic Rhythm)

In another approach to the use of therapeutic exercise to treat pain, sagittal- and frontal-plane trunk movements are assessed with respect to symptoms.[121,122] A simplified example of this approach is the use of movements that reduce or abolish symptoms. Self-reports of postures related to pain, observation of posture, and single movements (eg, flexion, extension, lateral flexion) are used to assess the effect of posture and movement on symptoms. During the examination, each movement is rated according to terms used to describe a change in status (eg, improve, worsen, status quo). After the movement, the patient is asked to compare his symptoms with the baseline.

The concepts of peripheralization (ie, pain or paresthesia that moves distally away from the spine) and centralization (ie, pain or paresthesia that is abolished or moves from the periphery toward the lumbar spine) are used to determine which movements should be used in self-treatment. For example, if repeated forward bending peripheralizes symptoms and extension centralizes symptoms, extension-related exercises would be used in self-management to modulate symptoms (Self-Management: Prone Press-Up Progression). This approach to the treatment of acute low back pain has been effective in restoring function,[123] particularly if used in conjunction with a treatment-based classification approach to low back syndrome.[3]

Positional techniques can be used to modulate pain. For example, a patient can be taught to use positional traction if the goal is to separate joint surfaces to expedite relief of pain (Fig. 18-21). The theory behind positional traction is similar to that for other types of traction (see the Traction section) in that the technique is used to affect the mechanical causes of pain.[124]

Self-mobilization, or "prescriptive articular exercise," can be prescribed to correct articular dysfunction, particularly that which relates to the SIJ. For example, a patient who presents with recurrent sacroiliac articular dysfunction (eg, anterior innominate rotation) that is mechanically contributing to his pain should be able to self-treat the articular dysfunction rather than relying solely on the therapist to restore articular function.[125] An example of a prescriptive articular exercise is illustrated in Self-Management: Self-Mobilization for an Anterior Innominate Dysfunction. For this type of technique to be successful, the patient must learn to evaluate his dysfunction and to perform the appropriate technique with precision only until correction is achieved. It also must be emphasized to the patient that these techniques are not considered part of the regular exercise regimen; they should be used only for articular dysfunction that contributes to the patient's symptoms. Although pain is the most common symptom, paresthesias and weakness are also symptoms related to articular dysfunction and should be used as indications for this treatment technique.

For patients with chronic pain, posture and movement intervention may be prescribed to improve activity tolerance, which is the ability to tolerate a specific posture or movement deemed safe or necessary for function. The clinician should encourage patients to gain activity tolerance but not to completely ignore pain, because increased pain can serve as an impediment to progress.

A chemical process such as inflammation often dominates the clinical picture, and attempts at altering mechanical causes do not lessen the pain. The clinician must treat inflammation with the appropriate adjunctive modalities (eg, cryotherapy, electrotherapy), protective measures (eg, corset, SIJ belt), and controlled rest, but strict bed rest should be avoided (see Chapter 6). Moreover, the patient's physician should be alerted so that, if necessary, appropriate pharmacologic agents may be prescribed or modified.

Exercise is not contraindicated in the treatment of chemical causes of low back pain, but the primary goal is to reduce the inflammatory process, which is typically achieved by reducing mechanical stress on the region. Exercises encouraging controlled rest are prescribed to enable the pa-

SELF-MANAGEMENT: Prone Press-Up Progression

Purpose: To improve the mobility of your low back into extension, stretch the front trunk muscles, move your leg pain toward your back or abolish it completely, and progressively relieve the pressure on your lumbar disk

Your physical therapist may ask you to perform special exercises to reduce any shift you exhibit in your spine before the execution of this exercise.

Starting position: Face lying with legs straight.

Movement technique: Your physical therapist will inform you of the levels of this exercise you are to perform and the duration of time you should spend at each level.

You should *not* progress to the next level if your pain does not change in intensity or position (ie, does not move toward your spine) or moves further down your leg.

Level I: Remain on your stomach with your hands supporting your forehead.

Dosage

Duration ______________

Frequency ______________

Level II: Prop up onto your forearms. Be sure you relax your back.

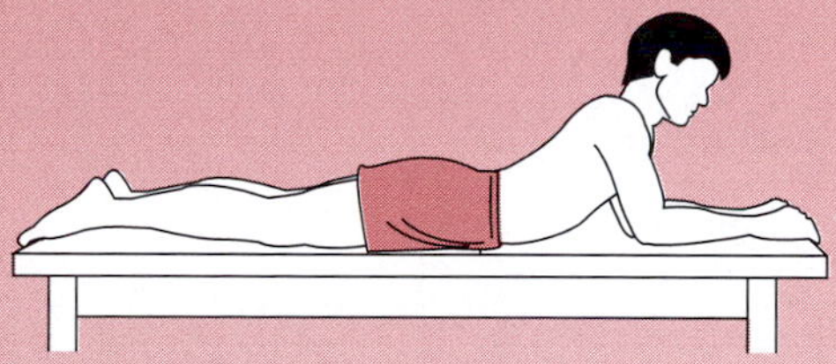

Dosage

Duration ______________

Sets/repetitions ______________

Frequency ______________

Level III: Place your hands next to your shoulders. Press your upper trunk upward with your arms through the prescribed range of motion. Be sure your back is fully relaxed.

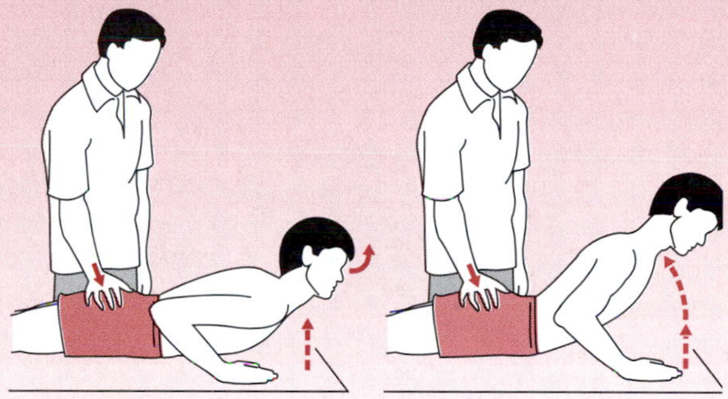

Dosage

Range of motion ______________

Sets/repetitions ______________

Frequency ______________

tient to perform basic movements without causing pain. To move without inducing a painful response, motion must be prevented at the affected lumbar spine segment or SIJ. Exercise may involve low-intensity isometric recruitment of the stabilizing muscles of the lumbar spine and SIJs with simultaneous small-range movements of the extremities.

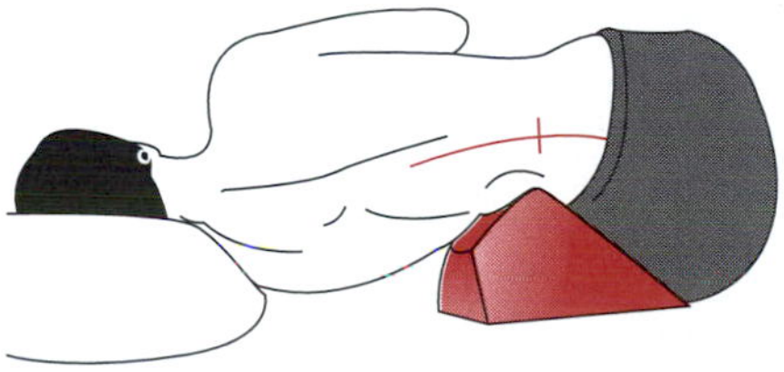

FIGURE 18-21 Positional traction. The use of a foam wedge allows maximal lateral flexion at a desired segmental level due to its sharp apex and ability to accommodate to the bony pelvis. The wedge easily can be made at a business that specializes in the manufacturing or design of foam products. The recommended density is CD-80. The preferred dimensions are $0 \times 8 \times 8 \times 18$ inches (small) and $0 \times 10 \times 10 \times 18$ inches (large).

Altering the length of lever arms, limiting the range of motion, and adjusting the position of the exercise to a gravity-lessened position are examples of altering the exercise to reduce the stress on the inflamed segments (Fig. 18-22) (see Self-Management: Gluteus Medius Strength Progression, in Chapter 20). Prophylactic range of motion exercises for associated regions and neuromeningeal mobility exercises[105] (see Self-Management: Neuromeningeal Mobilization) also may be used to maintain mobility and ensure forces through the inflamed region are kept to a minimum during movement.

As the acute pain reduces in intensity and irritability and as functional movement improves, a more advanced exercise program may be introduced, focusing on impairments in muscle performance, mobility, endurance, balance, and relatively more advanced postures and movement patterns. Transition to more advanced stages of care is rarely simple; it is often necessary to revert to more specific treatment of acute pain because of the difficulty in prescribing the optimal dosage for more advanced exercise. The dosage often stresses any given element of the movement system beyond its tolerance, resulting in increased pain and inflammation. Exercise

SELF-MANAGEMENT: Self-Mobilization for an Anterior Innominate Dysfunction

Purpose: To normalize the position and motion of your pelvis

Starting position: Supine on a firm surface

Movement technique: Keep your ____ hip and knee flexed. Pull your ____ knee toward your chest until you feel a mild barrier.

Gently squeeze your ____ gluteal muscles against an unyeilding force exerted by your hands keeping your knee to your chest. Hold your contraction for 8 to 10 seconds.

On relaxation, flex your hip and rotate your pelvis posteriorly until you feel a new barrier.

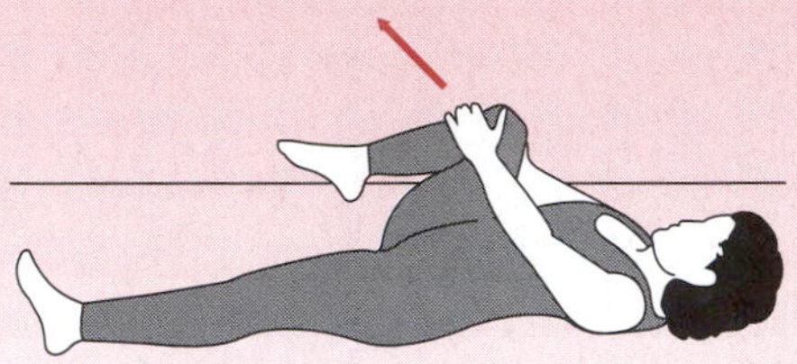

Dosage

Repetitions ____________

Frequency ____________

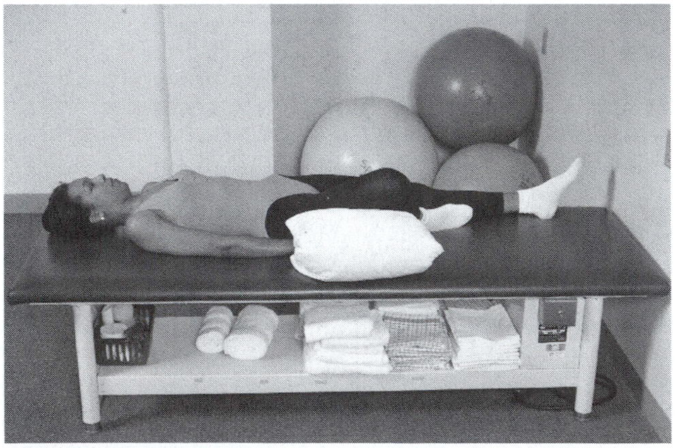

FIGURE 18-22 Supine with hip and knee flexion. Hip abduction and lateral rotation: This activity can be performed with several pillows under the thigh or next to a wall or couch that blocks movement of the hip into full abduction and lateral rotation. The use of props is indicated to decrease the excursion of the hip if the range of motion of the hip is limited, if there is lack of neuromuscular control, or if pain is felt early in the range. The patient is instructed to use the abdominal muscles to control pelvis and spine rotation as in Self-Management: Lower Abdominal Progression and to relax the adductors at end range before initiating the return to the starting position.

gradation should therefore err on the conservative side to avoid exacerbation of symptoms.

Patients should be educated about when to modify or stop exercise in light of increased symptoms (eg, numbness, paresthesia, pain) beyond acceptable time frames (eg, if symptoms are increased for more than 24 hours). Continuing to exercise when symptoms increase significantly or when increased symptoms exceed acceptable time frames can be counterproductive to progress. Educating the patient to heed the body's warning signs and to modify exercises appropriately (eg, decrease lever arms, work in gravity-lessened position, decrease repetitions, decrease frequency, longer rest periods) can prevent the complications of excessive stress on healing tissues.

The muscular changes that occurred as a result of lumbopelvic pain (eg, muscle performance capabilities, cross-sectional area, neuromuscular control) may not improve naturally after the pain has ceased and the patient resumes functional activities.[118,126] It probably will be necessary to teach specific, localized exercises that address impairments in muscle performance in the affected trunk muscles. This may require a lessening of load to allow the underused synergist to participate (Fig. 18-23) (see Self-Management: Lower Abdominal Progression, level I, and Self-Management: Prone Knee Bend) or a manually resisted exercise (Fig. 18-24) to provide the appropriate stimulus to improve muscle performance.

Muscle Performance Impairment

Examination and treatment of general muscle performance impairments in the lumbopelvic region have limitations. Evidence suggests that muscular dysfunction in the presence of lumbopelvic syndromes does not so much affect the strength of the trunk musculature as it influences the patterns of trunk muscle recruitment.[127–130] Subtle shifts in the patterns of muscle recruitment result in some muscles being relatively underused in the force couple, while other muscles relatively dominate the force couple.[4] The cause and effect relationships of these subtle shifts in muscle recruitment patterns cannot be determined and should be thought of as part of a continuous cycle of altered recruitment strategies and movement patterns.

Mechanisms such as muscle strain, pain, inflammation, neurologic pathology, or general deconditioning can contribute to underuse or disuse. The clinician must consider the possible mechanisms contributing to the subtle changes in muscle recruitment patterns to develop the appropriate exercise intervention. The following sections investigate the various causes of reduced muscle performance around the lumbar spine and recommend activities and techniques to alleviate muscle performance impairment.

NEUROLOGIC IMPAIRMENT AND PATHOLOGY

Mechanical (eg, compression, traction) and biochemical (eg, inflammatory response) factors arising from lumbopelvic dysfunction can result in nerve root pathology. For example, a HNP at the L5-S1 level can cause mechanical and biochemical irritation to the L5 nerve root and medial branch of the dorsal rami, resulting in weakness in the gluteus medius and same-level lumbar multifidus, respec-

SELF-MANAGEMENT: Neuromeningeal Mobilization

Purpose: To improve the mobility of your sciatic nerve and its branches into the calf and foot and to reduce the pain coming from a loss of mobility in the sciatic nerve

Assessment: Before beginning this exercise, you must first assess the status of your neural mobility.

Slump in your low back and pelvis as far as possible.

Bring your chin toward your chest.

Flex your foot as far as possible.

Slowly extend the knee on the side of symptoms as far as possible.

Notice the angle of your knee. You will recheck this angle after performing the exercise. You should be able to extend your knee further if you are successful with mobilizing your nerve.

If the angle is less, you have exacerbated your nerve and should repeat the series, reducing the range of motion of each movement in the series. Recheck the knee angle. It should be back to the original assessment position or may be improved.

Starting position: Slump in your low back, and roll your pelvis back as far as possible. *Slightly* flex your neck to take the stress off the forward head position the slumped posture placed your head in.

Movement technique

Knee mobilization: Keeping your ankle relaxed, extend your knee until you feel *mild* tension behind your knee. Relax back to the start position.

Dosage

Repetitions ______________

Ankle mobilization: Extend your knee about three fourths of the distance you found during the assessment. Flex and extend your ankle. (see Figure)

Dosage

Repetitions ______________

Neck mobilization: Extend your knee three fourths of the of the distance you found during the assessment. Flex your ankle toward your head about three fourths of the distance of its full range of motion. Actively flex your chin toward your chest and release to the start position. (see Figure)

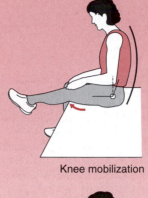

Knee mobilization

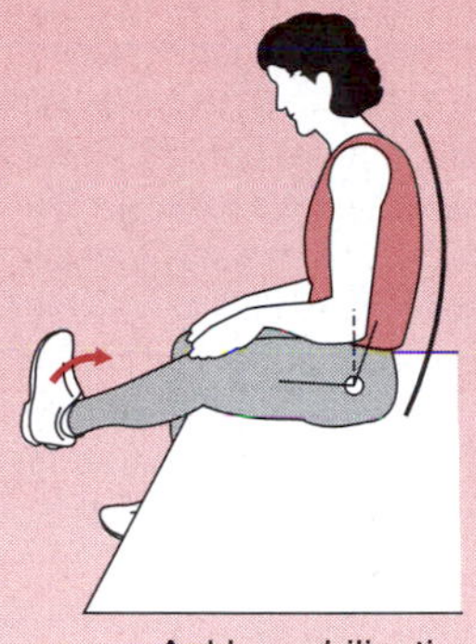

Ankle mobilization

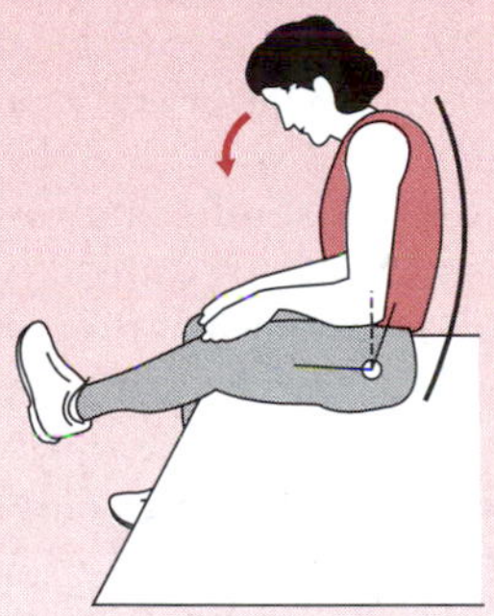

Neck mobilization

Dosage

Repetitions ______________

Reassess after the first cycle. If you have been successful as described under the assessment, repeat the cycle ___ times.

tively.[131] The underlying pathology or impairment causing the mechanical or biochemical irritation must be treated, if possible, to affect the efferent input into the corresponding musculature. Exercise to improve force or torque capability of the affected muscle without treating the underlying cause of the weakness is futile. Nonetheless, exercise may be a large part of the solution. For example, excessive mobility at a segmental level can lead to degenerative disk disease,[132] which can lead to nerve root compression and reduce efferent input into the associated musculature. Exercises to improve the stability of the offending segment coupled with exercises to improve the mobility of other segments or regions (eg, thoracic spine, hip joint) can reduce the mechanical stress on the nerve root, thereby contributing to restora-

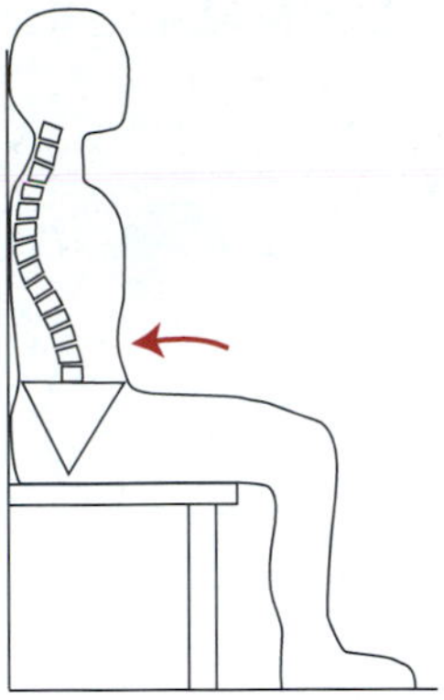

FIGURE 18-23 Sitting posterior pelvic tilt: This activity can be used by individuals with lordosis and anterior pelvic tilt, weak and overstretched abdominal muscles (particularly external oblique and transversus abdominus), and short hip flexors. The supine abdominal progression is often contraindicated for this type of patient due to the anterior translation and extension force exerted by the psoas and other hip flexors respectively. The patient sits with her back against a wall and is instructed to pull the umbilicus toward the spine to reduce the lordosis. Sitting takes the stretch off the hip flexors, and the pelvis should be able to move posteriorly with greater ease than in standing with the hip flexors on relative stretch. Use of a gluteal contraction over an abdominal contraction is discouraged. This exercise can be progressed to standing in slight hip and knee flexion (to release tension on the hip flexors) and then to standing upright. The advantage of this exercise is that it can be performed frequently throughout the day.

tion of neurologic input into the affected musculature. Appropriate strengthening exercises for the affected musculature (see Display 18-3) can be effective after the cause of the weakness is resolved.

Another neurologic cause of impaired muscle performance is nerve injury resulting in muscle paresis or paralysis, which can occur as a complication of surgery or from a traction injury to the nerve. Lumbar multifidus segmental atrophy at the surgical site has been reported in the chronic low back pain population after surgical intervention. It is thought to be the result of iatrogenic lesions of the dorsal rami and innervation failure of the low back muscles after surgery.[133] This finding is highlighted as a possible cause of "postoperative failed back syndrome" and is supported by histologic evidence.[134] Other investigators have reported denervation of segmental paraspinal musculature in patients with the radiologic diagnosis of segmental hypermobility.[137] These changes were thought to result from traction injury of the posterior primary rami segmentally supplying the muscle at the hypermobile segment. The ability for exercise to reverse the effects of denervation is related to the neurophysiologic recovery of the damaged nerve. Nonetheless, sustained mechanical stress from segmental instability delays or inhibits healing, and exercise targeted toward increasing segmental stability can reduce mechanical stress on the segment and augment healing.

If nerve regeneration occurs, specific exercises focused on improving force or torque generation are necessary to "re-educate" the previously denervated muscle.[110] Specific exercise recommendations are presented in Display 18-3.

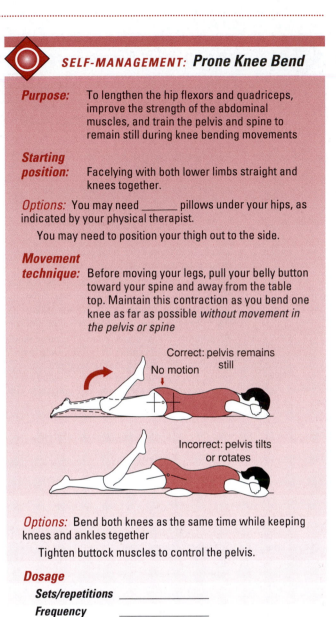

SELF-MANAGEMENT: Prone Knee Bend

Purpose: To lengthen the hip flexors and quadriceps, improve the strength of the abdominal muscles, and train the pelvis and spine to remain still during knee bending movements

Starting position: Facelying with both lower limbs straight and knees together.

Options: You may need _____ pillows under your hips, as indicated by your physical therapist.

You may need to position your thigh out to the side.

Movement technique: Before moving your legs, pull your belly button toward your spine and away from the table top. Maintain this contraction as you bend one knee as far as possible *without movement in the pelvis or spine*

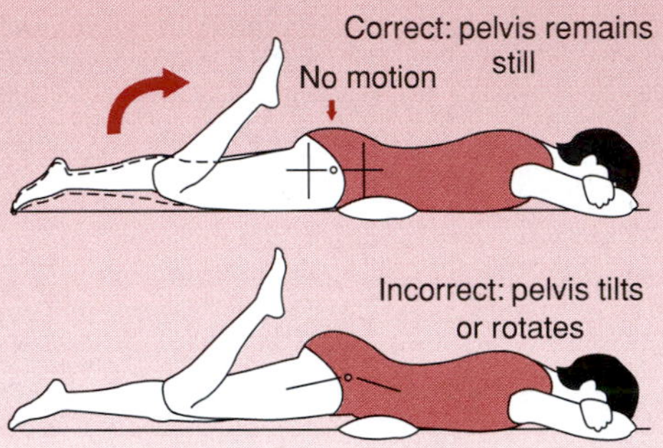

Options: Bend both knees as the same time while keeping knees and ankles together

Tighten buttock muscles to control the pelvis.

Dosage

Sets/repetitions _______________

Frequency _______________

MUSCLE STRAIN

Muscle strain can have many causes:

- Trauma (eg, spinal extensors and lumbar multifidus after a motor vehicle accident)
- Overuse (eg, oblique abdominal muscles in a competitive crew team member)
- Gradual continuous stretch (eg, external obliques in a swayback or lordotic posture)

Strain to lumbopelvic musculature, particularly if caused by trauma, is difficult to diagnose, because it often occurs with injury to other tissues in the motion segment. If a strain is suspected, the activity or technique, starting position, and dosage depend on the severity of the strain, the stage of healing, and the mechanism of injury. Severe strains in early stages of recovery and chronic strains with long-term disuse must start with low-intensity isometric exercises, as illustrated in Figure 18-22. Strains resulting from chronic stretch must

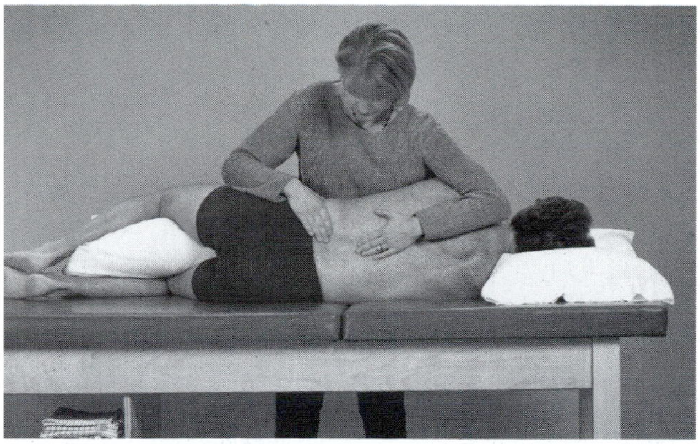

FIGURE 18-24 Sidelying manually resisted lumbar multifidus exercise. Restoration of lumbar multifidus activity may need to begin by facilitating the muscle at the level of spinal pathology with a manual tecnhique. Low-load rotary resistance is applied to the affected segment in a side lying position as if testing for passive physiologic intervertebral movement. The patient is encouraged to maintain the submaximal contraction against the therapist's resistance into rotation. The therapist palpates the segmental level to ensure multifidus activity. This can only be determined at the L5-S1 level, where the lumbar multifidus becomes superficial and can be palpated.

be supported and exercised with low initial loads and gradual progressions in the short range. For example, in the case of an external oblique strain due to marked lordosis and anterior pelvic tilt, use of an abdominal binder combined with low-load exercises (see Self-Management: Lower Abdominal Progression) is indicated in the early stages of recovery.

If the cause of the strain is overuse, ultimate recovery must involve improving the force or torque production and recruitment patterns of the underused synergist. For example, strain to the oblique abdominal muscles is a common injury among members on a crew team. It is caused by repetitive flexion and rotation. Changing the movement pattern to greater flexion and rotation occurring at the hips and improving the force and torque capability of the posterior spinal rotator muscle group and opposite oblique abdominal muscle group may be indicated.

Rarely does a patient progress from a trunk muscle strain in the expected time frame, primarily because of frequent reinjury of the muscle. Reinjury is most likely a result of poor protection of the injured area during postures and movement patterns the patient is unaware he is performing. It is the responsibility of the therapist to educate the patient to avoid postures and movement patterns most likely contributing to delayed healing and to use improved postures and movement patterns to promote the healing process.

GENERAL DISUSE AND DECONDITIONING

General disuse and deconditioning of the trunk and pelvic girdle muscles can result from the previously described causes. However, the trunk and pelvic girdle muscles also are susceptible to deconditioning as a result of decreased activity level. Trunk and pelvic girdle deconditioning may be a leading cause of lumbopelvic syndromes and therefore are critical areas to address in prevention. Individuals with general deconditioning require a careful examination so that a conditioning program is focused on the specific muscles in need of strengthening and that the program is initiated at the appropriate level of difficulty. The dilemma with most trunk-strengthening exercises performed to improve fitness (eg, bent-knee sit-ups, crunches, roman chair hyperextensions, abdominal or back strengthening machines) is that the exercise is often performed at a higher level than the muscles can safely execute the movement. When one synergist of a group is relatively weak, the other synergists often produce the necessary force or torque required to perform the desired movement, thereby reinforcing the muscle imbalance and increasing the risk of injury to the lumbopelvic region.

It is beyond the scope of this text to analyze all the common fitness exercises used to strengthen the trunk muscles. Because the ability to curl up to a sit-up should be considered a normal ADL and because the sit-up is still one of the most commonly performed abdominal exercises, a brief analysis of this exercise is provided.

The sit-up can be considered as two distinct phases of one movement: trunk flexion followed by hip flexion (Fig. 18-25). The rectus abdominis and internal oblique produce the trunk flexion phase, as indicated by rib cage depression (rectus abdominis) and rib angle widening (internal oblique), and the hip flexors produce the hip-flexion phase.[89] The role of the external oblique is to offset the anterior force on the pelvis and lumbar spine exerted by the hip flexor muscles as evidenced by a narrowing of the rib angle during the sit-up phase.[89] Although hip flexors may exhibit some weakness associated with postural problems (eg, weak hip flexors in the swayback posture), it rarely interferes with performing the hip-flexion phase of the sit-up. The problem in accurately performing a sit-up is usually weakness of the abdominal muscles, specifically the external oblique during the hip-flexion phase. As a result, the lumbar spine is vulnerable to the extension forces exerted by the hip flexor muscles.

Instruction in proper execution of the sit-up requires a complex level of analysis and decision making considering the performance of the abdominal muscles in relation to the hip flexor muscles and structural factors. Self-Management: Sit-Up offers a detailed description of the sit-up. It is important to teach the client to complete the trunk-curl phase before the sit-up phase for proper execution of this exercise.

The lower extremities constitute about one third of the body weight.[136] This means that the force exerted by the trunk in the supine position is greater than that of the lower extremities, and the feet need to be held down during the hip-flexion phase. However, if the spine flexes sufficiently as the trunk raises and the center of mass moves downward toward the hips, the trunk can be raised in flexion without having the feet held down. Most adolescents and women can perform the sit-up without having their feet held down because of a combination of body proportion (eg, upper body less mass relative to lower body) and segmental trunk flexion lowering the center of mass. In contrast, many men may need to have some added force applied (usually very little) at the point where the trunk curl is completed and the hip flexion begins because mass of the upper body is greater than that of the lower body. This may also be true for women with a stiff trunk because of the inability to segmentally flex the spine, which creates a longer lever arm and may require the feet to be held down during hip flexion. If it is necessary to stabilize the feet during the hip-flexion phase, the feet should be held down only during the hip flexion to ensure full trunk flexion before the hip-flexion phase begins. If the

DISPLAY 18-3

Resisted Exercises for the Lumbopelvic System

Stability Activities for the Anterior Aspect

- Leg slides (see Self-Management: Lower Abdominal Progression)
- Prone knee bend (see Self-Management: Prone Knee Bend)
- Hip and knee flexion, hip abduction and lateral rotation (see Self-Management: Bent-Knee Fall-out)

Stability Activities for the Posterior Aspect

- Manual lumbar multifidus facilitation (see Fig. 18-24)
- Sidelying small-range hip abduction
- Prone small-range hip extension (see Self-Management: Stomach Lying Hip Extension in Chapter 20)
- Prone neutral spine isometric

Stability Activities for Lumbopelvic Synergy

- Sitting upper extremity flexion, abduction, rotation (Figs. A and B)
- Quadruped arm lift (Fig. C)
- Standing resisted arm movements (see Fig. 18-29)

Controlled Mobility Activities for Lumbopelvic Synergy

- Trunk curl sit-up (see Self-Management: Sit-Up)
- Trunk sagittal and transverse plane motion in standing (see Fig. 18-30)

Skill Activity for Lumbopelvic Synergy

- Monitor performance of recreational or occupational skills

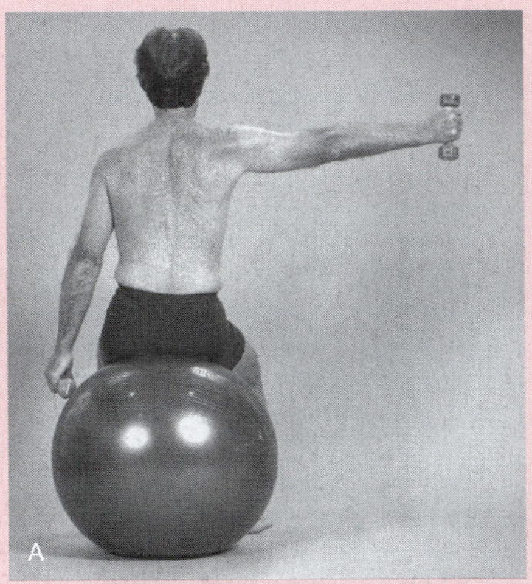
A

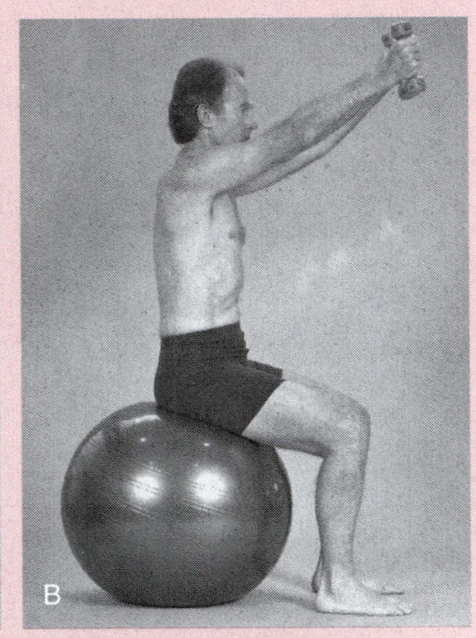
B

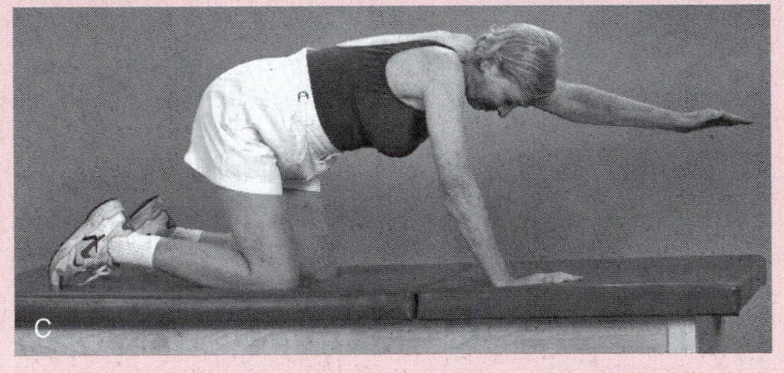
C

feet are held down prematurely or throughout the sit-up, the hip flexors are given fixation, and the trunk can be raised by hip flexion instead of trunk flexion.

Elevation of the feet during the sit-up can indicate abdominal muscle fatigue. For example, an individual may be able to curl the trunk through a specified arc of motion without the requiring the feet to be held down (or only during hip flexion) for the first few sit-ups. However, in subsequent sit-ups, the feet begin to rise before the specified arc of motion is completed. With the onset of abdominal fatigue, the feet elevate when previously elevation was not observed or rise earlier in the range if fixation is required during the hip-flexion phase, because the abdominal muscles are no longer producing enough force or torque to flex the trunk through the specified arc of motion and the hip flexors act earlier in the range to raise the trunk, with the feet rising as a result.

For many years, sit-ups were performed with the legs straight, but the emphasis has shifted to doing the exercise in the bent-knee position. For this reason, the bent-knee position is compared with the hip-extended position. The bent-knee sit-up has long been advocated as a means of minimizing or eliminating the action of the hip flexors, placing them "on slack" during the sit-up. This idea, which has persisted for many years among professionals and the public, is false and misleading. The abdominal muscles do not cross the hip joint and can therefore only flex the trunk. The sit-up, whether the hips are extended or flexed, is a strong hip flexor exercise; the difference is the arc of hip joint motion through which the hip flexors act (ie, hips extended 0 to 80 degrees, hips flexed 50 to 125 degrees). Because the hip joint moves to completion of hip flexion range of motion with the hips and knees flexed, high repetitions of this type

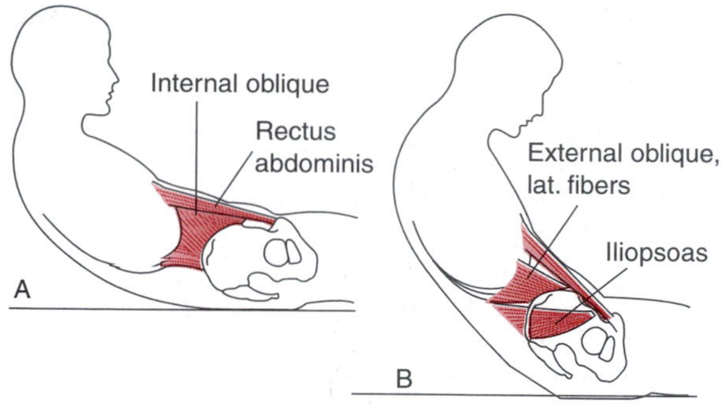

FIGURE 18-25 The sit-up can be considered a two-phase activity. ***(A)*** The first phase is the trunk curl. As trunk flexion is slowly initiated by raising the head and shoulders form a supine position, the rib cage depresses anteriorly (rectus abdominis) and the ribs flare outward, increasing the infrasternal angle (internal oblique). The pelvis tilts posteriorly simultaneously with the head and shoulders raising. ***(B)*** As the trunk is raised in flexion on the thighs, the sit-up enters the second or hip-flexion phase. As the hip flexors exert a strong force to tilt the pelvis anteriorly, the external oblique maintains the spine in flexion and the pelvis in posterior rotation. The infrasternal angle decreases, as evidence of the external oblique activity. (From Kendall FP, McCreary EK, Provance PG. *Muscles Testing and Function.* 4th ed. Baltimore: Williams & Wilkins; 1993:152).

of sit-up may be more conducive to the development of short hip flexors than the sit-up with the hips extended.

Although normal flexibility of the back is desired, excessive flexibility is not. A contraindication to performing a bent-knee sit-up is excessive flexibility of the lumbar spine. With the hips extended, the center of mass is slightly anterior to the first or second sacral segment. With the hips and knees bent, the center of mass moves cranially. The lower extremities exert less force in counterbalancing the trunk during the sit-up with the hips and knees flexed than with the hips extended. To sit up from the bent-knee position, the feet must be held down, or the trunk must flex excessively to move the center of mass downward. As the curl progresses, the center of mass moves distally toward the hip joint. In the hip-extended position, by the time the hip-flexion phase arrives, the center of mass has moved toward the hips, which encourages the hips (not the lumbar spine) to flex during the sit-up phase. With the hips flexed, the center of mass may not reach the hip joints by the hip-flexion phase, which encourages lumbar flexion. The persons most in danger of being adversely affected by repeated bent-knee sit-ups are children and youths because of their tendency toward excessive flexibility. Adults with low back pain associated with excessive flexion flexibility of the low back may also be adversely affected by this exercise.

A contraindication to performing a straight-leg sit-up is short hip flexors. In the supine position, a person with short hip flexors lies in anterior pelvic tilt and lumbar hyperextension. The danger with performing the sit-up from this position is that the hip flexors further extend the lumbar spine during the hip-flexion phase, causing lumbar hyperextension. The bent-knee position releases the downward pull of the short hip flexors, allowing the pelvis to tilt posteriorly and the lumbar spine to relatively flex. This relieves the extension stress on the low back. However, the hips and knees should be bent only as much as needed to allow the pelvis to reach neutral in the supine position. This position should be maintained passively by using a large enough roll or pillow under the knees. Prescribing bent-knee sit-ups (even in a partially bent-knee position) to individuals with short hip flexors is not the final solution, and this position should not be used indefinitely. Short hip flexors often accompany lengthened external oblique muscles because of the anterior pelvic tilt posture induced by the short hip flexors. The bent-knee sit-up neither addresses the short hip flexors nor the lengthened external obliques. Working toward a goal of being able to lie supine with the pelvis in neutral is accomplished by minimizing and gradually decreasing the amount of hip flexion permitted in the start position. Consequently, it is important to perform exercises to stretch the short hip flexors (see Self-Management: Prone Knee Bend), to strengthen and shorten the external oblique muscles (see Self-Management: Lower Abdominal Progression), and to attend to altered postural habits (eg, avoiding excessive anterior pelvic tilt and lumbar lordosis).

A trend in abdominal strengthening is a trunk curl or "crunch" performed without the hip-flexion phase. If the external oblique muscle is weak, making the lumbar spine vulnerable during the hip-flexion phase of the sit-up, performance of only the trunk-curl phase should be safe and effective for strengthening the abdominal muscles. There is less intradiskal pressure in performing the trunk curl than in a full sit-up.[27] However, the trunk curl focuses primarily on producing torque for movement rather than force or torque for stabilization of lumbar segments. Moreover, the trunk curl is contraindicated for any person with a thoracic kyphosis because of the stress thoracic flexion exerts on the kyphosis. Alternative exercises should be suggested for persons with poor lumbar stabilization and thoracic kyphosis (see Self-Management: Lower Abdominal Progression).

If the trunk curl is chosen, the therapist should determine the position in which the patient should start—a small towel roll under the knees, a wedge-shaped pillow under the head and shoulder, or a pillow under the knees. Before beginning the curl, the patient should activate the abdominal muscles with a resisted exhalation. It is important to take a deep diaphragmatic breath in and, on exhalation, make an "s" sound. While exhaling, the patient should pull the abdomen in so that the umbilicus moves toward the spine. With the arms extended forward, the patient should raise the chin toward the chest and continue to curl the upper trunk as far as the back can flex (see Self-Management: Sit-Up). The patient should not to come to a sitting position. If the subject cannot perform the curl to completion of his spine flexion because of abdominal weakness, a wedge-shaped pillow can be placed behind the head and shoulders to limit the range and the decrease the effect of gravity. As abdominal muscle strength improves, sequentially smaller pillows can be used. If the hip flexors are short, temporary use of a pillow under the knees can be used to decrease the pull of the hip flexors on the spine and allow the individual to lie in supine with the pelvis and spine in neutral.

Table 18-4 summarizes features related to the prescription of the sit-up and its variations. The sit-up, although used commonly, is not advocated as a sole means of improving performance of the abdominal muscles for the average person. Complex analysis is required when sit-ups are prescribed for high-level athletes (eg, divers, gymnasts) or industrial workers (eg, construction workers) requiring synergy among trunk and hip muscles for optimal sport or job performance. Display 18-3 presents alternative exercises to improve force or torque capability of the abdominal muscles.

SELF-MANAGEMENT: Sit-Up

Purpose: To strengthen the abdominal muscles and hip flexor muscles necessary to sit up from a supine position

Starting position: Backlying with hips and knees straight. Your physical therapist will determine if you are to begin this exercise in a supine position with hips and knees straight or with pillows under your knees. Your physical therapist will also determine if you will require fixation during the sit-up phase of this exercise.

Movement technique: To progress to higher levels of this exercise you must be able to

Curl your trunk to the same spine level with the selected arm position *and*

Maintain lumbar flexion and posterior pelvic tilt during the hip flexion phase.

In addition:

If you require fixation for your feet, do not use the fixation until the sit-up phase.

If you did not require fixation for level I, you should not require fixation at any level of the exercise. Ask your physical therapist if you have trouble keeping your feet down during the sit-up phase of level II or III. Premature lifting of your feet can be an indication of abdominal fatigue.

Level I: With your arms in front of your body, bring your chin to your chest, and slowly curl your trunk as you come to a full sitting position. Slowly reverse the curl and resume the start position.

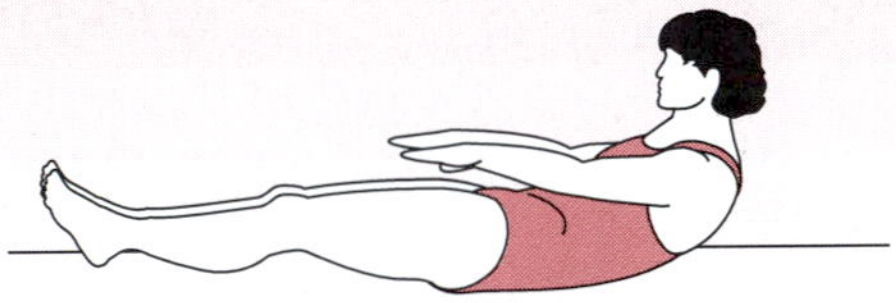

Dosage

Sets/repetitions ______________

Frequency ______________

Level II: Perform as in level I, but place your arms folded across your chest.

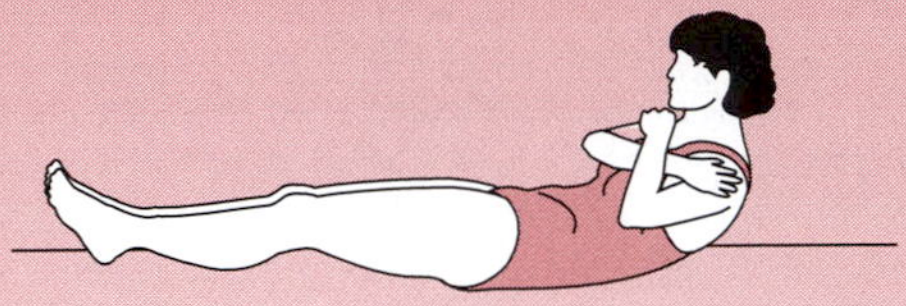

Dosage

Sets/repetitions ______________

Frequency ______________

Level III: Perform as in level I, but place your hands on top of your head.

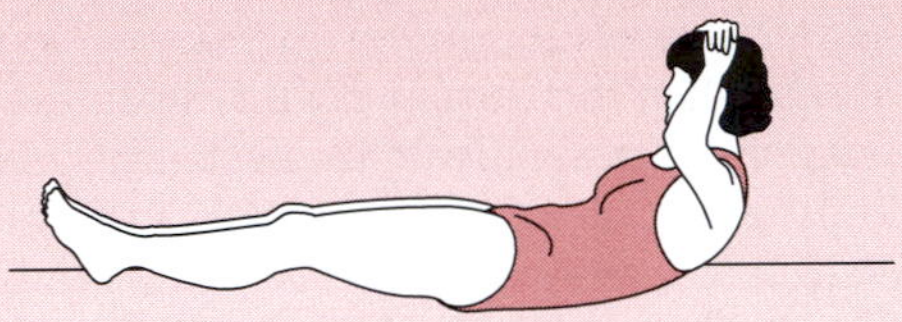

Dosage

Sets/repetitions ______________

Frequency ______________

EXERCISES TO IMPROVE NEUROMUSCULAR CONTROL, ENDURANCE, AND MUSCLE PERFORMANCE

Research has established a link between lumbar dysfunction and altered base (ie, muscle performance capability and endurance) and modulator (ie, neuromuscular control) function of the transversus abdominis, oblique abdominal muscles, and lumbar multifidus.[127–130,137,138]

General strengthening programs for the trunk muscles may not adequately recruit, strengthen, or improve the endurance of the deep and often underused trunk muscles. Localized and specific exercise aimed at training neuromuscular control of the lumbar multifidus, abdominal obliques, and transversus abdominis may be critical to improving subtle patterns of muscle recruitment necessary for optimal segmental stability in the lumbar spine. Similarly, specific exercises aimed at training neuromuscular control and force or torque production of the gluteus medius, gluteus maximus, hip rotators, lumbar multifidus, oblique abdominals, and transversus abdominis may be critical for optimal SIJ stability and load transference from the hip to the low back. Exercise recommendations geared toward improving neuromuscular control, endurance, and force or torque production for the trunk muscles are presented in Display 18-3. Exercise recommendations for the pelvic girdle muscles can be reviewed in Chapter 20.

Before presenting the exercise recommendations, three additional concepts must be addressed. First, exercises chosen should promote optimal length-tension properties of the trunk and pelvic girdle muscles. The affected muscles should be trained at the length desired for function. Too often, the abdominal muscles are strained during the trunk-

Table 18-4. SUMMARY OF INDICATIONS, CONTRAINDICATIONS, AND PRECAUTIONS IN PRESCRIBING THE SIT-UPS AND VARIATIONS

EXERCISE	INDICATIONS	CONTRAINDICATIONS AND PRECAUTIONS
Bent-knee sit-up	Lordosis	Short hip flexors, excessive trunk flexion flexibility, thoracic kyphosis
Temporary use of pillows under knees for sit-up	Short hip flexors	
Straight-leg sit-up	Good balance within abdominal muscles and between hip flexors	Short hip flexors, weak external oblique, disk pathology
Trunk curl (only)	Weak external oblique, disk pathology	Thoracic kyphosis
Temporary use of wedge	Weak internal oblique and rectus abdominis	

curl sit-up, particularly the external oblique and transversus abdominis. The mechanism by which a strain occurs is overstretch of the muscles while performing the trunk-curl sit-up (ie, abdominal distention or "pooching," that accompanies these exercises). Another disadvantage to strengthening the muscles in a lengthened range is the contribution this may have toward altered length-tension properties. The trunk muscles need to be of the right length to support the spine and pelvis in good static alignment and have the correct length-tension properties to continue to support the spine and pelvis during dynamic activities.

A second important principle is specificity of training or the principle of specific adaptation to imposed demands (SAID principle). For example, although a sit-up is a functional activity, it is not the primary function of all the abdominal muscles for ADLs and instrumental ADLs. It has been proposed that the lumbar multifidus, transversus abdominis, internal oblique, and external oblique are linked with the control of stability of the spine against the perturbation produced by movement of the limbs.[66] The primary role for the deep trunk muscles is to provide stability to the trunk during movements of the extremities. This is accomplished by performing exercises designed to improve the neuromuscular control and force or torque capability of the lumbar multifidus, oblique abdominal muscles, and transversus abdominis, such as those presented in Display 18-3.

A third principle governs exercise progression. The stages of motor control (ie, mobility, stability, controlled mobility, and skill) can be used to progress lumbopelvic exercise. Mobility and stability usually occur together in the lumbopelvic region. Stability is often a problem at the dysfunctional segmental level, and mobility is more likely to be a problem at an adjacent lumbar level or in some associated region (eg, hip, thoracic spine, shoulder girdle). To be most effective, mobility and stability impairments must be reconciled simultaneously. When developing a program focusing on stability, the chosen direction of force must be based on the directions in which the spine is most susceptible to motion and the directions most correlated with symptom reproduction.[4] After adequate mobility and stability are achieved, the patient is progressed to controlled mobility and then to skill-level activities.

According to a study by Richardson and Jull,[139] when patients followed a graded program of exercise to improve the force or torque capability and neuromuscular control of the lumbar multifidus and transversus abdominis, pain resolved within 4 weeks, with only a 29% recurrence rate at 9 months. These results were compared with a control group of low back pain patients who exercised aerobically by jogging and swimming. They too were pain free at 4 weeks, but they had a low back pain recurrence rate of 79% at 9 months. Specificity seems to be the key to the proper prescription of the exercises that correspond with improved neuromuscular control and force or torque production of the deep trunk muscles. This treatment approach demands a high level of skill by the instructor in teaching the exercise and a high level of patient compliance and attention to detail. Continual reassessment of muscle recruitment capabilities and force or torque production is necessary to progress or modify the exercise for optimal results.

One example of a specific, localized exercise is deep abdominal strengthening progression (see Self-Management: Lower Abdominal Progression). This exercise promotes specificity of muscle recruitment, with emphasis on the internal oblique, external oblique, and transversus abdominis. The patient can use resisted exhalation in the early stages of learning to facilitate localized transversus abdominis and oblique abdominal contractions. He is asked to inhale with a deep diaphragmatic breath. On exhalation, he is asked to contract the abdominal muscles so that the umbilicus moves toward the spine. The contraction must be isolated to the abdominal region from the umbilicus toward the pubic symphysis to localize participation of the transversus abdominis, not from the umbilicus upward toward the ribs (as evidenced by rib cage depression), which indicates dominance of the rectus abdominis and is a common mistake. If the patient is successful in localizing the transversus abdominis, the practitioner can observe the following:

- The umbilicus moves posteriorly toward the spine.
- The waistline becomes more narrow, as if a girdle were pulling the waist inward.
- The rib cage position remains unchanged (ie, the rib cage does not get pulled into depression by the rectus abdominis).

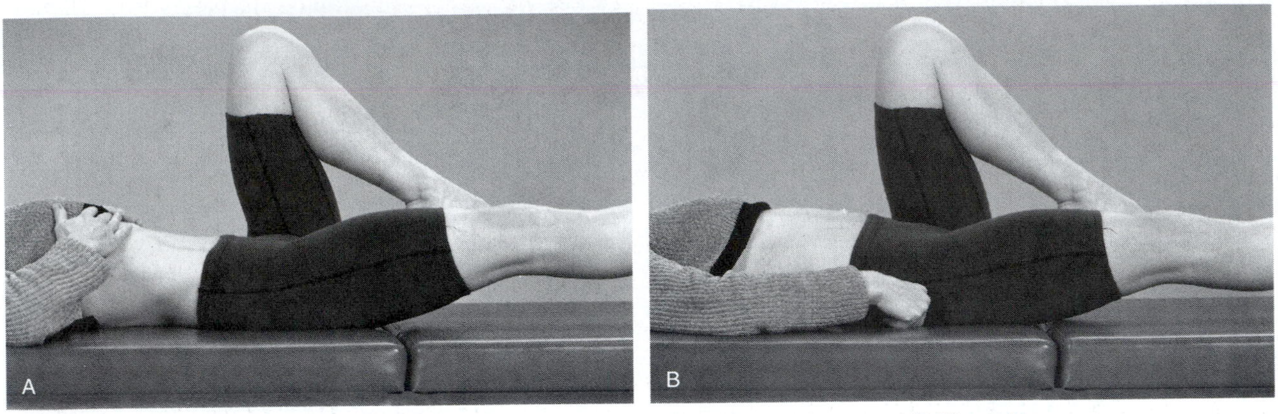

FIGURE 18-26 ***(A)*** Use of the oblique abdominal muscles and transversus abdominis in the short range. ***(B)*** Use of the abdominal muscles in a lengthened range. Note protrusion of the umbilicus.

These cues attempt to improve the synergy of abdominal participation and emphasize exercising at optimal length-tension relationships of the abdominal muscles. The patient is asked to use breathing to augment localized oblique abdominal and transversus abdominis recruitment during the leg-moving stages of each exercise. It is important to avoid performing leg movements with the abdominal muscles in a lengthened position (Fig. 18-26), particularly as the individual advances to higher loads imposed on the abdominal musculature by longer and heavier lever arms delivered by the lower extremities.

A pelvic floor contraction (see Chapter 19) can be incorporated to facilitate recruitment of the transversus abdominis. However, this should be used only as a temporary strategy to facilitate recruitment of the deep abdominal muscles, unless it is determined to be advantageous for the individual to use this synergy (see Chapter 19). For example, a pelvic floor contraction may be indicated for the chronic, unstable SIJ because of the shared muscle of the piriformis and the important supportive function of the pelvic floor to the pelvic girdle.

The individual should not progress to the next level unless the prescribed number of repetitions of the previous level can be achieved and the following criteria have been met:

- The lumbar spine should not deviate from the initial starting position, which should be in a neutral spine position (Table 18-5).
- The abdominal muscles, particularly the external oblique and transversus abdominis, should be functioning at optimal lengths (ie, not lengthened).
- The rectus abdominis should not be dominating the synergy, and a Valsalva maneuver is discouraged.

The exercise is progressed from level I to level V through a combination of progressively longer lever arms in the form of hip and knee extensions and increased loads in the form of moving one limb advanced to moving both limbs simultaneously. The direction of forces imposed on the spine also must be considered in advancing the exercise, particularly from level III to level IV. Level III and level IV may be interchanged with respect to difficulty, depending on which

Table 18-5. NEUTRAL AND FUNCTIONAL SPINE POSITIONS

SPINE POSITION	DEFINITION	CLINICAL JUDGMENT OF POSITION
Neutral spine position	Lumbar spine in slight extension. ASIS and pubic symphysis in the same vertical plane[90]	In supine, enough lumbar extension curve that the clinicians can reach the lumbar spinous processes, but not so much extension that the hand passes through to the other side.
Functional spine position	Position of greatest stability, least stress, fewest symptoms for an individual for any given activity	Varies with pathology, activity, and symptoms

ASIS, anterior superior iliac spine.

direction of force the patient has most difficulty controlling. Level III combines sagittal- and transverse-plane forces because of the unilateral limb movement, and level IV induces a strong sagittal-plane force because of the bilateral limb movement. If an individual has difficulty controlling rotational forces, progression from level II to level IV may be easier than to level III. These factors, combined with patient skill at accomplishing the criteria described previously, can guide the clinician in progressing the exercise.

Another abdominal exercise focusing on the ability of the abdominal muscles to stabilize the spine and pelvis is illustrated in Self-Management: Bent-Knee Fall-Out. Similar to level II and III illustrated in Self-Management: Lower Abdominal Progression, this exercise challenges the abdominal muscle's ability to stabilize against extension and rotation forces. An increased measure of difficulty can be introduced to both of these exercises by placing a half or full foam roll longitudinally along the spine. Foam rolls and gym balls are believed to facilitate recruitment of the deep trunk muscles and stimulate the proprioceptors and balance reactions that are necessary for function.[140] Care must be taken to introduce this variation when the patient is capable of using subtle recruitment patterns and does not fall into muscle dominance strategies to balance on the roll. Progression to a higher stage of motor control often suffices, unless the specific goal is to challenge balance and proprioception.

Another exercise is the early-stage lumbar multifidus strengthening exercise. This exercise challenges the lumbar multifidus and the deep abdominal muscles to stabilize the spine and pelvis. The key to this exercise is to facilitate a minor contraction to prevent the erector spinae from dominating the synergy. Patients often have initial difficulty in facilitating a lumbar multifidus contraction in a home exercise program. This is particularly true for patients with a chronic condition and for postoperative patients. Manual techniques can be used to help facilitate recruitment in the early stages of neuromuscular training. Figure 18-24 illustrates a manual technique for facilitating recruitment of deep abdominal and lumbar multifidus musculature. After a consistent contraction can be elicited with manual techniques, the patient can be instructed in progressive home exercises (see Display 18-3).

Exercises emphasizing stability through increased neuromuscular control and force or torque production can be progressed to sitting or standing. In sitting, extremity movements can be used in much the same way as in supine positions to challenge the spine to stabilize against various directional forces, with the emphasis on using the entire lumbopelvic stabilizing system in a synergistic manner. For example, sitting while raising the arm in the sagittal plane can challenge the spine to stabilize against flexion and extension forces, and changing the movement to a diagonal direction challenges the spine to stabilize against a transverse plane force. Sitting on a gym ball (Fig. 18-27), making the base of support unstable, can further challenge sitting. The patient is encouraged to use the appropriate trunk muscle activation strategy learned in previous localized exercises by presetting the contraction before arm or leg movements. Stabilization progressions can also be developed in standing. Standing on a half or full foam roll can further challenge a standing progression (Fig. 18-28).

SELF-MANAGEMENT: Bent-Knee Fall-out

Purpose: To train you to move your thigh independently of your pelvis, lengthen your inner thigh muscles, strengthen and shorten weak and overstretched abdominals, and train your abdominal muscles to stabilize against rotational forces

Starting position: Backlying with one leg straight and the other hip and knee bent with the foot flat on the floor. Place your hands on your pelvis as indicated by your physical therapist to monitor pelvic motion. Your physical therapist may ask you to place ____ pillows under the outside of the bent knee to let the knee fall into something.

Movement technique: Before moving your leg, take a deep diaphragmatic breath in. Your physical therapist will teach you how to breath with your diaphragm. On exhaling, make an "s" sound, and pull your abdominals in so that your belly button moves tward your spine. Let the bent knee fall out to the side. Do not allow motion to occur in the pelvis.

Relax the inner thigh muscles completely before returing to the start position.

You may need to use breathing to help with an abdominal contraction on the return from the fall-out position to the starting position.

Repeat ____ times

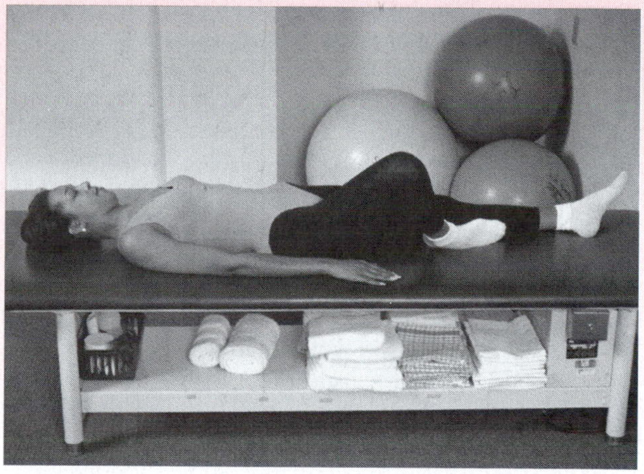

After neuromuscular control and adequate force or torque production are established to stabilize the spine against movements of the extremities and further strength is required from an occupation or recreational activity to achieve a functional outcome, higher forces are required than can be supplied by the extremities alone. Dumbbells, weighted balls, or ankle weights can be used to progress

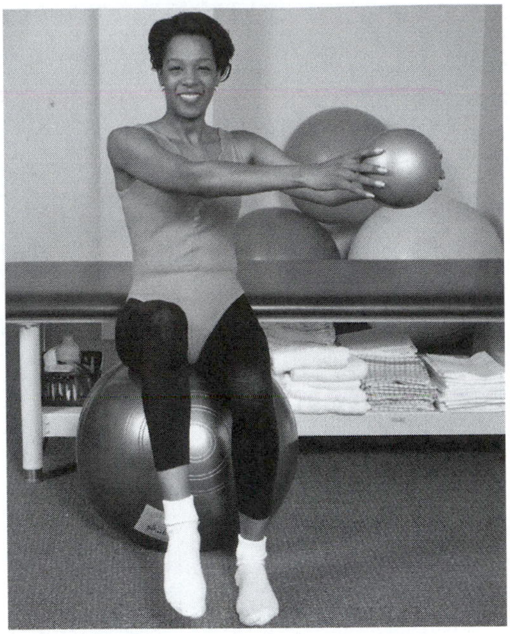

FIGURE 18-27 Sitting on a gym ball can add an element of difficulty to the stability phase of lumbo-pelvic exercise. Care must be taken to ensure quality of recruitment strategy as dominant strategies may emerge on the unstable surface.

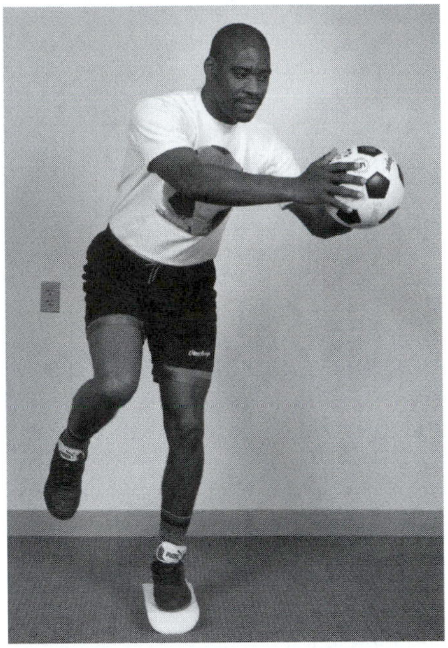

FIGURE 18-28 Standing on two foam rolls is easier than standing on one foam roll. For the stability phase, the goal is to reach to the side through movements at the hip with the spine in neutral. For controlled mobility, the goal is to move the hips and spine in a combined rotational movement pattern. However, movement should be emphasized at the hips and thoracic spine, with very little rotation occurring in the lumbar spine.

the previously described exercises. Pulleys or elastic tubing can also be used to increase the force requirements of the trunk musculature to stabilize the spine. For example, the patient can be challenged to maintain trunk stability with an isometric contraction while pulling the weight up or down, (Fig. 18-29*A*) side to side (Fig. 18-29*B*), or in a rotary motion. The emphasis initially is on dynamic motion at the hips, while avoiding motion through the trunk (ie, stability level of stages of motor control). This exercise requires effective stabilization of the trunk through the deep trunk muscles and active recruitment of latissimus dorsi, gluteus maximus, gluteus medius, adductors, and hip rotators. All of these muscles are important in stabilization of the lumbar spine and pelvic girdle through the posterior, anterior, and oblique muscular systems. The load is increased as tolerated, and the speed is maintained at a low level.

Preparation for high-level functional return requires more advanced strength training that incorporates spine motion as part of the total movement patterns (ie, controlled mobility and skill levels of stages of motor control). Programs of this nature may include spine motions involving concentric and eccentric work with variable resistance in all planes, such as controlled mobility in the sagittal plane (Fig. 18-30) and in combined planes. At this stage, the various isokinetic machines (eg, Medex, Medical exercise rotation trainer) and any pulley apparatus or resistive exercise tubing can be useful. The chosen movement pattern should be tailored to those required for the patient's occupational or recreational activities.

Rotation is often not well tolerated by those with a true articular instability of the lumbar spine or SIJ, particularly when the pelvis is fixed in an apparatus or in sitting. Patients with true articular instability should avoid motion in the affected region and should train strictly in isometric modes. Vocational counseling or recreational modification may be necessary for those with true articular instability. Counseling focuses on choosing activities that avoid rotational movement patterns.

As with all resistive exercise, after the force or torque capability has reached a functional level, functional activities must be added to the program. However, it is unnecessary to wait until the end of the rehabilitation program to train

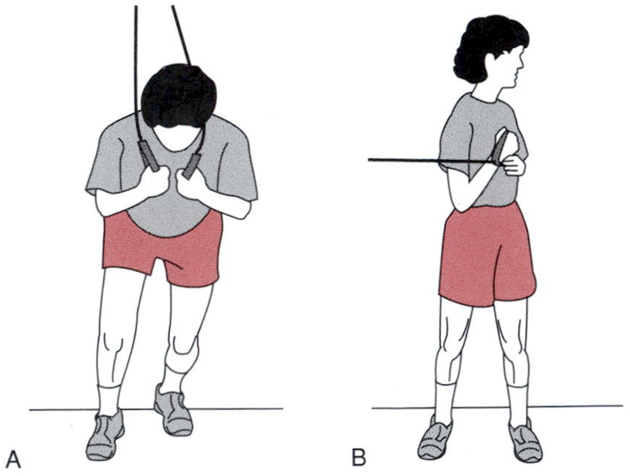

FIGURE 18-29 Tubing can be used to add resistance to a thorough stabilization exercise. The goal is to maintain the spine in neutral through isometric contractions of the trunk musculature while the arm (or leg) is moving in ***(A)*** sagittal- or ***(B)*** transverse plane, for example. As a result, most of the motion occurs in the hips.

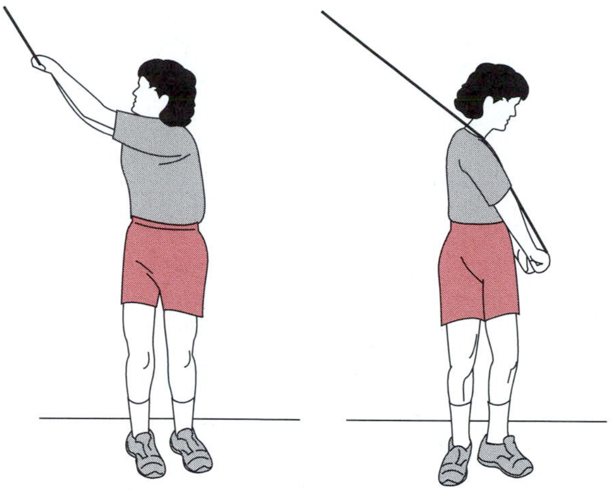

FIGURE 18-30 A progression from Figure 18-29 is controlled mobility. Instead of holding the trunk stable, the lumbar spine is incorporated into combined movement patterns with the remainder of the spine, hips, knees, ankles, and feet. Controlled mobility activities can be performed about separate planes of movement (eg, transverse plane). Resistance can be applied through pulleys, elastic tubing, or weighted balls. The patient can perform these activities on an unstable surface such as foam rolls or high-density foam squares. With controlled mobility drills, the motion can occur in the lumbar spine, but most of the motion should occur in the thoracic spine and hips, with the least occurring in the lumbar spine.

functional activities. These should be considered from day 1 in designing the plan of care. For example, a minimal expectation for a patient in acute pain is to perform hip and knee flexion (see Display 18-2) and bent-knee fall-outs (see Self-Management: Bent-Knee Fall-Out) in a supine position without pain. These duplicate movements necessary to get in and out of bed.

The definition of a successful functional outcome varies. Success for one person may be to perform light housework without pain or discomfort, and for another, success may mean resuming heavy lifting, playing a racket sport, or running long distance without pain or discomfort. The ability to return to desired functional activities, regardless of the level, requires neuromuscular skill to control motion of the trunk and pelvic girdle in relation to the other extremities. This requires interactive stabilization and movement strategies during total-body movement patterns. Exercises addressing force or torque generation of the trunk muscles should be part of a comprehensive rehabilitation program addressing other physiologic impairments. To achieve the neuromuscular skill level necessary to return to function at any level, functional exercises must be practiced with precise movement and recruitment patterns and for many repetitions frequently throughout the day. This requires a high level of commitment on the part of the patient. The exercises used to progress to a functional outcome are based on the postures and movement patterns used during ADLs and occupational and recreational activities. No two functional retraining programs should be the same, because each program is tailored to the individual's functional goals. Examples of functional activities are provided in the Posture and Movement Impairment section.

Mobility Impairment

Impairments in mobility in the lumbopelvic region must be considered in relation to the mobility continuum and the mobility of one segment or region relative to another. Mobility impairments include hypomobility, hypermobility, and instability (see Chapter 6).

Degenerative joint changes and factors increasing stiffness in myofascial tissues (see Chapter 6) contribute to relatively stiff or hypomobile segments. Hypermobility or instability can be caused by trauma (eg, motor vehicle accident resulting in an acceleration injury), pathology (eg, rheumatoid arthritis, degenerative joint changes), anatomic impairment (eg, spondylolisthesis, HNP, asymmetric tropic changes in the zygapophyseal joint), or repetitive movement patterns.

HYPERMOBILITY

Diagnosis of hypermobility and instability can be made from careful examination. The examiner should seek to discover the impairments contributing to the hypermobility.

Four factors can be responsible for the development of a hypermobile segment: trauma, pathology, anatomic impairment, or repetitive movement patterns. With repetitive movement, hypermobility can develop within the lumbopelvic region in response to a relatively less mobile segment or region. In a multijoint system with common movement directions, any given movement follows the segments providing the least resistance. Abnormal or excessive movement is imposed on segments with the least amount of stiffness. With repeated movements over time, the least stiff segments increase in mobility, and the more stiff segments decrease in mobility.

The site of abnormal or excessive motion is considered to be the site of relative stiffness or flexibility.[4] The term *relative* is key to this concept. For example, the fifth lumbar vertebra, because of its biomechanical and anatomic properties, is more adapted to produce rotation than any other lumbar segment. It is therefore relatively more flexible in the direction of rotation. This becomes a clinical problem or impairment only if the motion becomes excessive. A contributing factor is the relative stiffness at other spinal segments or hips in the direction of rotation. For example, playing golf involves a significant amount of total-body rotation to achieve a proper golf swing. If the hips, knees, or feet are relatively more stiff in rotation, this pattern may impose excessive rotation on the spine. If the thoracic spine or upper lumbar segments are stiff in rotation, this pattern may impose excessive rotation on the L5 segment. Excessive motion of rotation is imposed on the L5 segment to produce the desired total-body rotation. L5 is the site of relative flexibility in the direction of rotation.

The cause-and-effect relationship of relative flexibility can be addressed through a comprehensive program of improving mobility at the relatively more stiff segments or regions and improving stiffness at the relatively more mobile segment. It is important to improve the stiffness at the relatively more mobile segment because motion always follows the path of least resistance. Mobility only occurs naturally at the relatively more stiff segment if it is of equal mobility or more mobile than other segments. Stiffness should be increased at the site of relative flexibility by improving neuromuscular control, muscle performance, and length-tension relationships of the stabilizing muscles (see the Muscle Performance Impairment section) around the site of relative flexibility coupled with educating the patient and training postures and movement patterns (see the Posture and Movement Impairment section) that improve the distribution of mobility between associated regions and the lumbopelvic region.

A clinical example may provide insight into the complex relationships between the development of hypermobility and other physiologic impairments in the lumbopelvic region. A patient presents with low back pain. During the examination, the physical therapist notices that the pelvis and lumbar spine rotate during the initiation of active hip flexion and that this movement provokes low back pain. When the patient is properly cued to recruit the deep abdominal muscles, pelvic and spine rotation is reduced, and symptoms are eliminated. Other tests throughout the examination confirm that the L5-S1 segmental level is hypermobile in rotation.

All contributing impairments in mobility, muscle performance, neuromuscular control, endurance, posture, and movement should be determined by the end of the examination. In this scenario, it is possible that the patient presents with asymmetric weakness, poor neuromuscular control, and easy fatigability in the deep trunk muscles. The patient may present with short adductors unilaterally, positional weakness in gluteus medius unilaterally, excessive foot pronation unilaterally, and a functional limb length discrepancy and may provide a history of using a repetitive rotation movement pattern at work. To develop a program to improve the stiffness at the site of relative flexibility, each of the correlating impairments must be addressed. The program emphasizes achieving quality of total-body movement and training kinesthetic awareness to control spinal postures and movements in the direction associated with symptoms.

Exercises to reduce hypermobility at a segmental level or within the pelvis can be progressed according to traditional stages of motor control: mobility, stability, controlled mobility, and skill. The stage of mobility can be thought of as improving mobility at relatively stiff or hypomobile segments or regions. Activities and techniques to improve mobility are presented in the Hypomobility section.

The stage of stability can be thought of as improving neuromuscular control, muscle performance, and length-tension properties of the affected muscles to increase stiffness at the site of relative flexibility. Specific activities and techniques chosen to promote stiffness and stability at a site of relative flexibility should be based on the direction the segment is susceptible to excessive or abnormal flexion, extension, or rotation. To stimulate adaptive shortening in a lengthened muscle, exercises must be performed with the spine in neutral or functional positions with the muscles in the corresponding length. The patient must be educated to avoid habitual postures that place a lengthening stress on the muscle (eg, avoid standing in a swayback in the presence of lengthened external oblique). In some cases, immobilization in the short range (eg, use of an abdominal binder) may be necessary to facilitate adaptive shortening.

Controlled mobility focuses on the ability of the lumbopelvic region to move dynamically in all three planes with appropriate distribution of movement and forces within the lumbar region and between associated regions of the upper extremities, thoracic spine, SIJ, hip, knee, ankle, and foot. Skill is reached when the patterns of muscle activation become automatic and internalized by the patient during functional activities. Display 18-3 provides recommendations for exercises to develop stability through the stages of motor control.

To be most effective in reducing hypermobility with exercise, the clinician should educate each patient to use appropriate spine positions during all exercises and functional activities. There is no particular lumbopelvic functional position that is best for all patients and for all activities. Although the standard is the neutral position (see Table 18-5), it may not be achieved by all patients and for all activities, in which case the functional position of the spine should be used. The functional position (see Table 18-5) varies with physiologic status and stresses from ADLs and instrumental ADLs. It varies among individuals and circumstances. For example, to avoid symptoms, patients with spinal canal spondylolisthesis must avoid extension. The functional position may vary with the patient's activity. For example, flexion should be avoided during heavy lifting from the floor to the waist. Some authorities argue that the spine should be held in end-range extension for maximal protection and efficiency of motion.[141] However, end-range extension should be avoided during lifting from waist level to overhead, and the functional position may be biased toward flexion to avoid injury to the spine with this activity. Functional spinal posture may vary with the patient's behavior or symptoms. The more severe, irritable, and acute the condition, the more limited the functional position of the spine becomes to avoid symptoms.

HYPOMOBILITY

To be most effective, activities or techniques to reduce hypermobility must occur simultaneously with activities or techniques to increase mobility. Many activities or techniques can be used to increase mobility, such as manual techniques (eg, articular joint mobilization, muscle energy techniques, soft tissue mobilization); passive self-stretch or self-mobilization; or active assisted, active, and resisted exercise.

Passive intervention in the form of manual therapy or manual exercise without some form of active exercise should be avoided. One hazard in providing purely passive intervention is that the patient does not participate actively in the rehabilitation process. This may prevent the patient from achieving full recovery or contribute to recurrence, because the patient is unable to manage the condition independently. Whenever possible, active participation in the form of patient-related education and therapeutic exercise is encouraged in the place of passive intervention.

Active assisted range of motion, active range of motion, proprioceptive neuromuscular facilitation techniques (see Chapter 14), and passive stretching can be used to increase mobility (see Chapter 6). This discussion focuses on self-management exercises, emphasizing passive and active stretching.

Passive stretching may be necessary, particularly for muscle groups with adaptive shortness. Careful muscle length testing determines which trunk and pelvic girdle muscles require stretching. Trunk muscles, such as the rectus abdominis, quadratus lumborum, and lumbar erector spinae, and hip muscles, such as TFL or iliotibial band, semitendinosus or semimembranosus (medial hamstrings), biceps femoris (lateral hamstrings), hip adductors, hip rotators, iliopsoas, and rectus femoris, are susceptible to adaptive shortening.

Care must be taken when stretching muscles crossing the hip joint in individuals with lumbopelvic dysfunction, because the SIJ or lumbar spine often becomes the site of relative flexibility when the hip becomes hypomobile. Stabilization of the pelvic attachment while the distal attachment moves requires special attention in lumbopelvic patients because the spine or SIJ becomes the path of least resistance and therefore easily moves before the feeling of a stretch.

An example of proper stabilization for a diarthrodial muscle with attachments on the pelvis is the supine passive hamstring stretch. The hamstrings may be passively stretched in supine with one hip flexed and the ipsilateral knee extended (to the point of mild hamstring tension) and the foot against a wall while the contralateral hip and knee are extended. The lumbopelvic region is stabilized in part by the appropriate recruitment of the deep abdominal muscles and lumbar multifidus and by the underlying surface. The length of the hamstrings determines the distance from the wall and angle of straight-leg raise. Certain criteria are used for proper stabilization to facilitate the optimal stretch:

- The ipsilateral knee must be extended.
- The spine must be in neutral with respect to flexion, lateral flexion, and rotation.
- The opposite hip and knee must be in full extension.

The ipsilateral hip is flexed beyond the length of the hamstrings if the following movements are observed:

- Spine flexion or rotation, or both (Fig. 18-31*A*)
- Opposite hip flexion (Fig. 18-31*B*)

Medial or lateral hamstrings can be isolated by rotation of the hip (ie, lateral rotation isolates stretch to the medial hamstrings and vice versa for the lateral hamstring). The position is held until the feeling of mild tension disappears (usually up to 30 seconds). The patient then moves slightly closer to the wall to increase hip flexion and again creates mild tension. This action may be repeated up to three times. The goal is to achieve a significant increase in hamstring extensibility within one session.

A passive stretch should always be followed by an active movement pattern using the new extensibility of the muscle-fascial tissue. Examples of active movements using hamstring extensibility are illustrated in Display 18-2 (Fig. B). Without use of a chair for support, the hamstrings lengthen eccentrically during the lowering phase. The hamstrings can only be passively stretched if the person fully unloads his weight onto a table top surface so that hamstring activity is silent.

Active movements used during exercises focused on improving force or torque production, neuromuscular control, and length-tension properties can be used to stretch opposing muscles. For example, an individual with lumbopelvic pain who was diagnosed with lumbar hypermobility in the direction of extension and rotation may have worse symptoms after prolonged walking. During the stance phase of gait, the lumbar spine moves excessively into extension and rotation instead of the stance hip moving into extension. The impairments contributing to the relative flexibility in the direction of extension and rotation during walking may include weak, overstretched, and uncoordinated deep abdominal muscles and short hip flexors.

Self-Management: Lower Abdominal Progression demonstrates an exercise progression targeting the impairments in the deep abdominal muscles. Levels II through IV work on lengthening the hip flexors simultaneously. While the abdominal muscles contract in the short range, the hip flexor muscles elongate, and the site of relative flexibility becomes the hip joint rather than the lumbar spine. If the patient allows the hip flexors to pull the pelvis out of alignment,

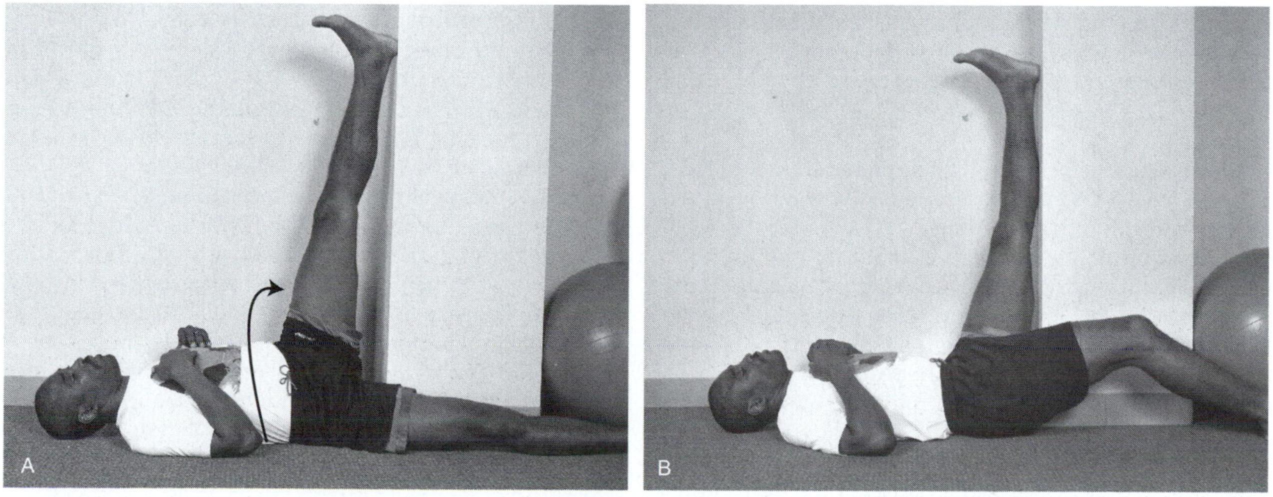

FIGURE 18-31 Supine passive hamstring stretch. Incorrect technique: ***(A)*** Spine flexion and rotation. ***(B)*** Opposite hip flexion.

the exercise becomes detrimental to altering the site of relative flexibility. In a patient with a hypermobile SIJ, the site of relative flexibility is the SIJ rather than the hip. The exercise must be monitored, focusing on movement of the innominate rather than the lumbar spine. For example, the patient monitors movement of the ASIS, stopping hip extension before movement of the ASIS in an anteroinferior direction.

In conjunction with this exercise, the patient can work on the same relationship in other positions, such as prone (see Self-Management: Prone Knee Bend). The lumbopelvic region is stabilized through appropriate abdominal recruitment, and the knee is flexed to the point of mild tension or just before the loss of lumbopelvic stabilization. Emphasis is placed on relaxation of the rectus femoris simultaneously with abdominal stabilization of the spine against the extension force imposed by the short diarthrodial hip flexor. The ultimate goal is for the patient to be able to stabilize the spine and elongate the hip flexor muscles during a functional activity, such as the stance phase of gait.

ADVERSE NEURAL TENSION

Adverse neural tension is a common sequela of many lumbopelvic conditions. It can affect motor performance and lumbopelvic mobility. Neuromeningeal mobility should be assessed and its influence determined. Specific exercises may be prescribed that are designed to improve mobility of the neural system (see Self-Management: Neuromeningeal Mobilization). The related anatomy, physiology, and application principles must be well understood for the effective and safe use of this type of treatment. This topic is worthy of more extensive coverage than is within the scope of this text. More information is provided by Butler.[142]

Balance and Coordination Impairment

The functional importance of proprioceptive training has been emphasized during rehabilitation of the spine.[143] Protection of the musculoskeletal system relies in part on adequate proprioception and reaction time of the neuromuscular system. This requires fine adjustments in neuromuscular activation patterns in response to a fluctuating load. True stability of the spine at the skill level requires precise and rapid responses to perturbations in the load imposed on the spine.

There is evidence that low back pain patients may be prone to excessive postural sway, poor balance reactions, and altered strategies for balance.[103] Low back pain patients have a tendency to fulcrum about the hips and low back to maintain upright postures during balance tasks; persons without low back pain tend to fulcrum about the ankle. Authorities[144] acknowledge the necessity of balance work in the rehabilitation of lumbopelvic patients, particularly when dealing with hypermobility and instability impairments.

Gym balls, wobble boards, slide boards, and foam rolls can be used to enhance proprioception and teach optimal balance strategies (eg, ankle versus back). Aspects of proprioceptive training can be incorporated at any stage of rehabilitation, as illustrated by examples focusing on balance and coordination discussed in other sections of this chapter. After an activity can be performed correctly on a stable surface, the patient can be positioned on a moving base of support, such as a gym ball (see Fig. 18-27) or foam roll (see Fig. 18-28). Any activity challenging balance and proprioception must be performed with precision, emphasizing correct body position and recruitment strategies. The rate of movement is progressed while accuracy is maintained.

An example of a high-level exercise challenging balance and coordination is standing on a half or full foam roller (the latter is the most difficult). The patient is instructed to shift his weight from side to side and forward to back from the ankles as trunk stability is maintained. Another variation is performance of squatting motions or upper extremity motions individually and then combined after proper trunk stabilization is accomplished. The ankles, knees, and hips are used as the fulcrum points for balance instead of the low back.

Endurance Impairment

In the treatment of lumbopelvic dysfunction, endurance can mean systemic aerobic endurance or local muscle endurance. Research supports the fact that aerobic exercise alone is not enough to prevent recurrence of low back pain,[139]although aerobic exercise is beneficial for patients with lumbopelvic syndromes. Aerobic exercise enhances healing, helps weight loss, and has favorable psychological effects, such as reduction of anxiety and depression.

Typically, the patient is limited by musculoskeletal pain in working at the optimal target heart rate necessary for producing aerobic gains. Aerobic exercise is initially prescribed "to tolerance" and is progressively increased as the patient's signs and symptoms improve. The mode of exercise (eg, biking, swimming, walking, jogging) should be based on the patient's desires and the postures and movements that relieve symptoms. For example, if walking relieves pain, but sitting increases pain, walking should be encouraged, and biking should be discouraged. If weight-bearing aerobic exercise is chosen, the physical therapist may need to counsel the patient in choosing proper footwear to ensure the best weight-bearing dynamics possible. Orthotic prescription may be necessary to optimize forces from the ground upward. If land exercise is unbearable, water is often a well-tolerated medium for aerobic exercise by a person with lumbopelvic dysfunction (see Chapter 17).

Many investigators have reported diminished trunk muscle endurance and increased rates of muscular fatigue in low back pain patients compared with individuals without low back pain, even when strength measures testing results are within normal limits.[95,96,128,145] Sophisticated electromyographic testing using a technique called power spectrum analysis has identified that the lumbar multifidus is the back extensor most susceptible to endurance changes.[128,137] These studies indicate the need to provide an endurance training component in the course of a total rehabilitation program. No special exercise recommendations are needed, because the dosage can be modified for exercises prescribed for force or torque production to satisfy endurance goals (ie, higher repetitions with lower loads).

Posture and Movement Impairment

Effective education in the area of posture and movement is essential to recovery from and prevention of recurrence of lumbopelvic syndromes. Posture and movement education covers a wide range of activities:

- Self-management in terms of correct positioning for relief of symptoms
- Advice on work station ergonomics and body mechanics
- Seating postures and ergonomic aids (eg, proper chair selection, lumbar supports)
- Advice on proper posture and movement patterns during ADLs and instrumental ADLs (eg, avoid excessive extension during the extension phase of forward bending in the presence of spinal stenosis)

Education regarding posture and movement should be initiated at the time of the first visit. By the end of the initial examination, the clinician should be aware of the postures and movements that exacerbate symptoms and therefore be able to instruct the patient in simple recommendations regarding sitting, standing, and recumbent postures. Basic movement patterns can be instructed, such as bed mobility (see Patient-Related Instruction: Bed Mobility), sit to stand, and bending (see Patient-Related Instruction: Lumbar-Pelvic Rhythm) and lifting maneuvers. The specific postures and movement patterns chosen to teach the patient should be based on the patient's pathology, impairments, functional limitations, and disability. For example, a person with a diagnosed HNP at L4 may have different sitting recommendations than a person with spinal stenosis. The former must avoid sustained, end-range flexion, and the latter must avoid sustained, end-range extension.

The clinician must consider specific posture and movement patterns for each prescribed exercise to be most effective. For example, allowing a patient to sit or move in lumbar flexion during sitting knee extension reduces the effectiveness of the hamstring stretch. The initial and ending posture and the spine position during the movement of knee extension must be emphasized. Similarly, allowing anterior pelvic tilt and lumbar extension during level II of the deep abdominal progression interferes with the goal of restoring muscle length-tension properties to the abdominal muscles relative to the hip flexor muscles. Attention to posture and movement during each exercise prescribed enhances its effectiveness.

The goal of any individual with a lumbopelvic syndrome is to achieve a desired functional outcome. This involves skill in total-body posture and movement patterns that use optimal stabilization and movement patterns. The entire therapeutic exercise intervention plan is geared toward this final goal. To achieve skill in posture and movement, the individual must pay close attention to precision of movement, regardless of the level of complexity (eg, bed mobility, playing golf) during specific functional exercises and during ADLs and instrumental ADLs. The clinician should teach or "coach" the patient in proper stabilization and movement strategies using the balanced foundation of neuromuscular control, muscle performance, endurance, mobility, and proprioception that the other impairment-based exercises have provided.

Aspects of posture and movement retraining can be incorporated into any stage of rehabilitation. Training begins by splitting complex movements into a number of simple component sequences. The choice of activity is determined by the functional requirements of the individual. At each progression of the program, more advanced posture and movement strategies are introduced. For example, an introductory postural strategy may be to teach the individual to sit properly in an ergonomic chair. Later, the patient may be progressed to improved sitting tolerance in a standard chair, while using the same educational concepts and improved physiologic capabilities. This progression requires improved muscle balance, joint alignment, and kinesthetic sense. The following list is an example of a movement pattern progression:

1. Simple bed mobility and sit to stand transfers
2. Gait (Fig. 18-32*A*) and stair stepping (Fig. 18-32*B*)
3. Occupational activities, such as lifting mechanics
4. Recreational activities, such as baseball (Fig. 18-33)

The more advanced the movement pattern, the more the task needs to be broken into simplified components to ensure that the proper amount of movement occurs in the segments where movement is desired and that stabilization occurs where no movement is desired. After skill is achieved at each component, simple movements are linked together to form the total activity sequence. Teaching skill in movement requires high levels of motivation and compliance from the patient and in-depth knowledge of concepts of motor learning and skill by the clinician. Chapters 8 and 16 further address exercise prescription for the treatment of posture and movement impairments.

Specific exercises may be linked together in a circuit-training format. Examples of functional circuits include lifting circuits to retrain occupational functional outcomes and sport or technique-specific circuits to retrain recreational activity functional outcomes. The lifting circuit may include a variety of manual handling procedures, such as single- and double-handed lifts with a variety of different shapes and weights, pushing and pulling activities, and reaching to high and low levels. A sport-specific circuit for soccer, for example, may include trapping, passing, dribbling, and shooting

Patient-Related Instruction

Bed Mobility

To reduce the stress on your low back, your physical therapist may ask you to get out of bed in a specific manner. The following instructions pertain to safe bed mobility.

- Pull your abdominal muscles in toward your spine, and slide one foot at a time up the bed until your knees are flexed and your feet are flat on the bed. Be sure to prevent your back from arching or rotating by using a strong abdominal contraction.
- If you are not close to the side of the bed, you must bridge and slide until you are close to the side of the bed. Be sure to use your gluteal muscles and keep your abdomen pulled in while bridging and sliding.
- Roll your body as one unit until you are lying on your side.
- Gently let your feet slide off the bed while simultaneously pushing yourself into the upright position with your hands.
- Note: Be sure to maintain an abdominal contraction during all components of this maneuver.

Patient-Related Instruction

Lumbar-Pelvic Rhythm

When you bend forward to pick up a light object, such as a shirt or a pencil, you can practice moving with the appropriate relationship between your low back and pelvis. The following are key points to keep in mind while bending forward:

Bending Forward (A to C)

- Leading with your head, slowly curl your spine as you bend forward.
- Think about relaxing at each vertebral segment.
- Try to keep your knees straight and minimize the backward shift of your hips.
- After you have reached the level of your low back in your forward bend, try to rotate your pelvis.
- Do not flex your low back further after your pelvis has stopped rotating.
- If you need to bend more to reach the desired distance, bend your hips and knees instead of flexing your low back beyond the rotation of your pelvis.
- At the end of the forward bend, relax your low back.

Return From Forward Bend (D to G)

- Lead with your hips and pelvis by contracting your gluteal muscles.
- Your low back should only extend after your pelvis has achieved its neutral position.
- At the end of the range, you may need to pull in with your abdominal muscles to achieve your neutral pelvic position.

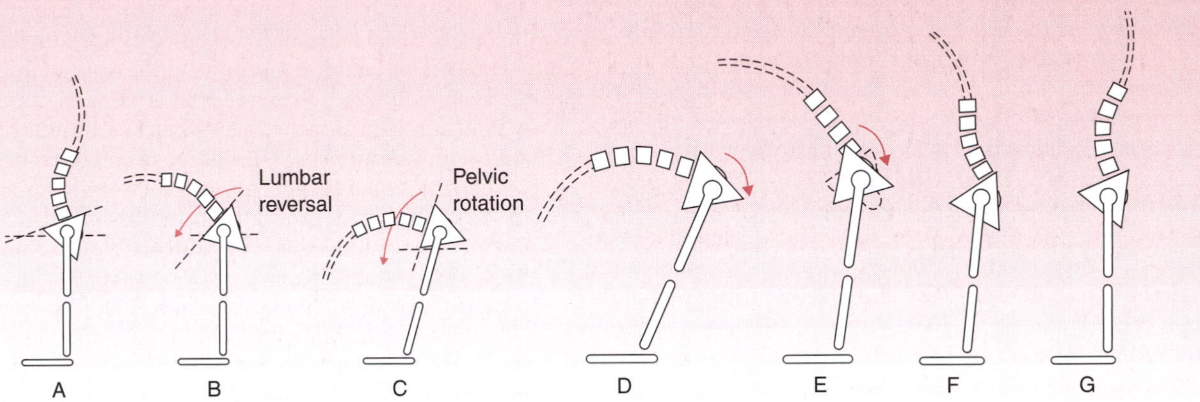

(From Calliet R. *Low Back Pain.* 3rd ed. Philadelphia: FA Davis; 1981.)

skills. With each movement, the aim is to maintain spinal stability during extremity motions so that the movement patterns become automatic or reach skill level.

Almost any piece of equipment, whether designed for a specific exercise, sport, or work activity, can be adapted to fit the principles of lumbopelvic functional movement retraining. Only imagination limits the exercise program after the principles are understood. Exercises can be adapted to meet the demands of the patient's work and recreation. The clinician must be careful not to progress the patient faster than he can learn to control motion with the optimal strategies. Diligence displayed by the patient and clinician is rewarded with fewer setbacks and higher gains in functional return.

THERAPEUTIC EXERCISE INTERVENTION FOR COMMON DIAGNOSES

Lumbar Disk Herniation

The peak incidence of herniated lumbar disks is in adults between the ages of 30 and 55 years.[146] Disk herniation without trauma can be thought of as one factor in a continuum of the spinal degenerative process. The degenerative process can progress from minor muscular or soft tissue injuries to abnormal spinal biomechanics, which ultimately can break down the underlying joint structure and create facet arthritis, disk degeneration, herniated disk, spinal stenosis, neurologic entrapment, and severe permanent disability.[147] A patient who suffers a spinal annular tear could develop spinal stenosis 10 years later. The job of clinicians involved in the treatment of lumbopelvic syndromes is to assist in the diagnostic process early, treat the sources (if known) and causes of dysfunction appropriately, and prevent severe pathologic conditions from developing. Unfortunately, the initial low back injury is often thought of as a benign muscular or ligamentous injury and is not heralded as the first sign of a process that can lead to severe pathoanatomy and disability.

The beginning of the degenerative process is an annular tear resulting in a disk protrusion or annular bulge. With a disk protrusion, the NP does not herniate from the disk; it is confined by the annular fibers. This may be the typical "back sprain" that results from bending, lifting, and frequent twisting. It often gives a person low back pain with little or no pain radiation into the legs. The pain is usually relieved quite rapidly with rest or curtailment of most bending or lifting activities for several days. Patients are usually fairly comfortable when on their feet, but when they change from a lying to a

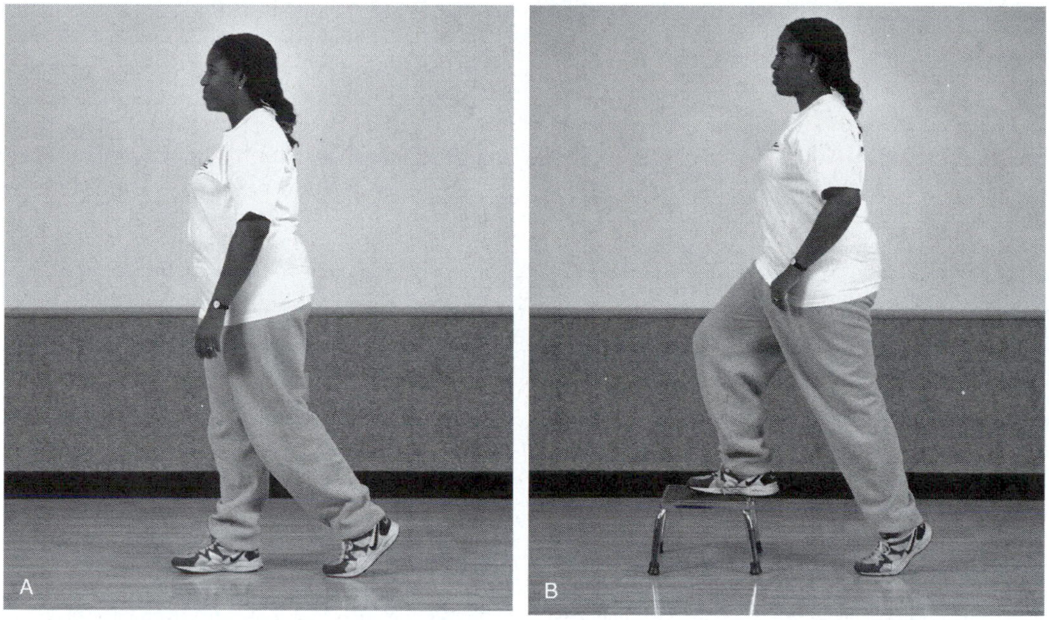

FIGURE 18-32 Controlled mobility and skill must be reinforced at the lumbar spine about all planes of motion and during all phases of gait. ***(A)*** A few of the critical aspects necessary to reduce stress or compensatory lumbar movements include: hip extension during terminal stance, thoracic rotation during swing, hip abductor stabilization during initial contact and loading. Stability is necessary in the lumbar spine for proper execution of a step-up. ***(B)*** During swing phase, the hip flexors must contract to form a stable base to prevent lumbar extension and lateral pelvic tilt. During stance phase, hip extensor and abductor muscles must contract strongly to prevent lateral pelvic tilt. The trunk muscles must work to prevent compensatory spinal sagittal, transverse, or frontal plane movements.

sitting position or from sitting to standing, the pain can be acute and disable them from fully standing. Pain probably is caused by the flexion forces imposed on the disk during these movements. These episodes, if not treated appropriately, can recur and become more frequent as time progresses. Eventually, they can lead to the more disabling disk herniation.

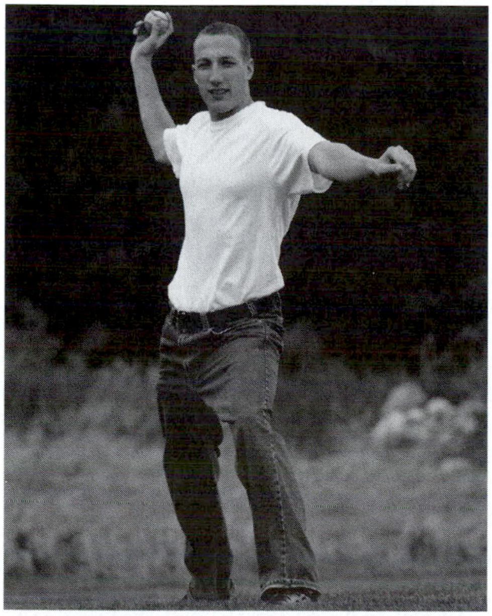

FIGURE 18-33 Skill is required for performing a baseball throw. During rotational movements, the emphasis should be on motion at the hips and thoracic spine. During sagittal-plane movements, emphasis should be on hip and knee motion.

If the annular tear progresses to full annular disruption, an HNP results. Penetration of the nuclear material into peripheral areas that are highly sensitive to mechanical and chemical stimulation may be the source of the disabling pain felt in disk herniation. HNP can be further classified into the following subsets:

- Disk prolapse: The annular fibers are disrupted, but the NP is still confined by a thin layer of AF.
- Disk extrusion: The outer AF is torn, and the NP is free of the annulus but is restrained by the posterior longitudinal ligament.
- Sequestrated disk: The NP moves beyond the posterior longitudinal ligament, and a fragment lies in the spinal canal.

Clinically, disk herniation can be divided into the following subsets:

- HNP without neurologic deficit
- HNP with nerve root irritation
- HNP with nerve root compression

HNP without neurologic deficit has signs and symptoms similar to those of an annular tear but is slower to recover and imparts slightly more disability. This condition may correlate with disk prolapse in which the pain may be severe but no encroachment has occurred on the nerve root. HNP with nerve root irritation has signs and symptoms, including sciatica, paresthesias, and positive straight-leg raise, but no neurologic deficit is diagnosed. HNP with nerve root compression has signs of nerve root irritation and reflex, sensory, and motor changes. A massive midline disk herniation may cause spinal cord or cauda equina compression, requiring immediate surgical referral. Fortunately, the cauda equina syndrome occurs in only 1% to 2% of all lumbar disk herniations that result in surgery.[146]

EXAMINATION AND EVALUATION FINDINGS

Sciatica is a symptom of nerve root irritation that could be caused by a lumbar herniated disk. Sciatica is defined as a sharp or burning pain radiating down the posterior or lateral aspect of the leg, usually to the foot or ankle, often associated with numbness or paresthesia. Sciatica caused by disk herniation is worsened by prolonged sitting and improved by walking, lying supine, lying prone, or sitting in a reclined position.[27] The pain is sometimes aggravated by coughing, sneezing, or the Valsalva maneuver. The absence of sciatica makes a clinically important lumbar disk herniation unlikely.[146,148] The estimated incidence of disk herniation in a patient without sciatica is 1 in 1000.[149]

Pain that is reproduced by flexion and that increases with repetitive flexion is consistent with disk pathology. The straight-leg raise test can be used as a factor in diagnosing a herniated lumbar disk. A symptomatic disk herniation tethers the affected nerve root. Pain results from stretching the nerve by straight-leg raising from the supine or sitting position. In the supine straight-leg raise test, tension is transmitted to the nerve roots after the leg is raised beyond 30 degrees, but after 70 degrees, further movement of the nerve is negligible.[150] A typical straight-leg raise sign is one that reproduces the patient's sciatica between 30 and 60 degrees of elevation.[146,151,152] The lower the angle producing a positive result, the more specific the test becomes, and the larger is the disk protrusion found at surgery.[153,154] Care must be taken to differentiate hamstring tension from sciatica. Sensitizing techniques (eg, neck flexion, ankle dorsiflexion) can be used to determine whether the pain experienced is originating from hamstring tension or nerve irritation.

Straight-leg raising is most appropriate for testing the lower lumbar nerve roots (L5 and S1), where most herniated disks occur.[146] Irritation of higher lumbar roots is tested with femoral nerve stretch (ie, flexion of the knee with the patient prone).

About 98% of clinically important lumbar disk herniations occur at the L4-L5 or L5-S1 intervertebral level,[146,154,155] causing neurologic impairments in the motor and sensory regions of the L5 and S1 nerve roots. The most common neurologic impairments are weakness of the ankle and great toe dorsiflexors (L5) or ankle and foot plantar flexors (S1), diminished ankle reflexes (S1), and sensory loss in the feet (L5 and S1).[146,154,155] In a patient with sciatica and suspected disk herniation, the neurologic examination can be concentrated on these functions. Among patients with low back pain alone (no sciatica or neurologic symptoms), the prevalence of neurologic impairments is so low that extensive neurologic evaluation is usually unnecessary.[149]

Higher lumbar nerve roots account for only about 2% of lumbar disk herniations.[146,154,155] They are suspected when numbness or pain involves the anterior thigh more prominently than the calf. Testing includes patellar tendon reflexes, quadriceps strength, and psoas strength.[146,156,157] Quadriceps weakness is virtually always associated with impairment in the patellar tendon reflex.[156]

The most consistent finding with a massive midline disk herniation is urinary retention.[158–160] Unilateral or bilateral sciatica, sensory and motor deficits, and abnormal straight-leg raising also are common examination findings.[158–160] The most common sensory deficit occurs over the buttocks, posterosuperior thighs, and perineal regions (ie, saddle paresthesia or amnesia).[158–160] Anal sphincter tone is diminished in 60% to 80% of cases.

There is a growing consensus that plain roentgenograms are unnecessary for every patient with low back pain because of a low yield of useful findings, potentially misleading results, substantial gonadal irradiation, and common interpretive disagreements.[149] The Quebec Task Force on Spinal Disorders suggests that early roentgenography is necessary only under the following conditions:

- Neurologic deficits
- Patient older than 50 or younger than 20 years of age
- Fever
- Trauma
- Signs of neoplasm[161]

Magnetic resonance imaging and computed tomography can be used even more selectively, usually for surgical planning.[149] The finding of herniated disks and spinal stenosis in many asymptomatic individuals[162,163] indicates that imaging results alone can be misleading. Valid decision making requires correlation with a comprehensive history and physical examination.

TREATMENT

There is no recipe approach toward the exercise management of low back pain, even if a specific structural diagnosis, such as HNP with nerve root irritation, is offered. Determining which interventions to use depends on diagnostic information regarding the pathoanatomic process and the physiologic impairments contributing to the pathomechanical process and on the psychological impairments, patient disability profile, and desired functional outcomes. The following concepts of care for specific stages of disk herniation can guide management of the degenerative disk process.

Acute Stage

In the acute stages of any injury, the immediate goals are often to relieve pain and to prevent or reduce inflammation so that the healing process can occur unimpeded. Early intervention and patient adherence to the recommendations addressing pain and inflammation in the case of HNP are essential for achieving a rapid recovery and for preventing chronic pain and disability.

Along with physical therapy intervention, the patient's physician usually prescribes steroidal or nonsteroidal anti-inflammatory medications and may suggest epidural steroid injection. The use of epidural steroid injection, performed by experienced physicians who have shown competence in the technical aspects of this procedure, has produced favorable outcomes, particularly if used in conjunction with physical therapy.[164]

Controlled rest is often recommended and may take the form of posture and activity modification (ie, avoidance of flexed postures, sitting, and bending or lifting activities) or local support (eg, corset, abdominal binder, tape). It is important to teach the patient to avoid flexed and asymmetric postures, flexion and rotation movements, and sitting (which elevates disk pressures) to enhance healing and prevent reinjury to the healing disk. The clinician also can teach the patient how to use cryotherapy at home to control inflammation. Traction also may be beneficial to relieve nerve root compression and radiculopathy or paresthesias in the acute phase (see the Adjunctive Interventions section).

Exercise can play a vital role in the treatment of pain and inflammation. For example, careful prescription of extension exercises (see Self-Management: Prone Press-Up Progression) may be useful in the early treatment of disk-related signs and symptoms. As with any mechanically induced injury, the causes of muscle or soft tissue injury must be avoided. In the acute phase of disk herniation, it is often difficult to determine the postures and movements associated with segmental dysfunction. However, it is useful to teach the patient basic movements (see Display 18-2 and Self-Management: Bent-Knee Fall-Out) and bed mobility (see Patient-Related Instruction: Bed Mobility) to avoid aggravating symptoms.

In the acute phase of disk herniation, the patient is often susceptible to the effects of immobilization as a result of the protective nature of this phase of care. Treatment to maintain or improve mobility of segments within the lumbar spine and thoracic spine and the extensibility of lower extremity muscles is vital for reducing stress on the injured segment and reducing the effects of immobilization that may play a role in recurrence of the condition. For example, joint mobilization of the thoracic spine and segments above and below the affected segmental level, along with soft tissue mobilization of the erector spinae group, can maintain joint mobility during the acute phase. Piriformis spasm is a common secondary effect of lower lumbar disk herniation. Soft tissue mobilization and passive stretching to this muscle can decrease pain associated with the spasm.

Treatment to maintain or improve mobility in the neural tissues also is critical in the acute stages. Tolerance is usually very low, and neuromeningeal mobility exercises must be performed with caution, usually in recumbent positions to prevent exacerbating symptoms. Neuromeningeal mobility exercises performed during the acute stage may prevent chronic complications from increased neural tension. Further guidance in prescribing these exercises has been provided by Butler.[105]

The clinician should encourage the patient to maintain some activity level, such as swimming or walking, during the acute stage. Swimming can be employed with the use of a kick board to prevent unwanted spinal motion while promoting aerobic fitness and lower extremity motion. Walking with a corset, wearing good shock-absorbing shoes, and walking on a soft surface (eg, gravel) may reduce disk pressure enough to tolerate the stress of walking. In addition to the benefits of movement, the benefits of low-level aerobic exercise are gained.

Subacute and Chronic Stages

After the acute pain has subsided and the patient has more freedom of movement, the treatment should focus on altering postures and movements and the associated impairments that produce symptoms. The ultimate goal is the return to the highest possible level of function with the safest and most desirable postures and movement patterns possible.

Review the sections on treatment of impairments to understand the concept of exercise intervention for mobility, muscle performance, balance, coordination, endurance, posture, and movement impairments and the progression through traditional stages of motor control. This information provides the basis for developing a progressive program of intervention for a patient with disk pathology beyond the acute stages of care.

Education is probably the most important intervention because of the chronic disability experienced by many persons with disk disease. The clinician must teach the patient to temporarily manage acute exacerbations with cryotherapy, positional techniques, or repeated shift correction and extension movements.[122] Instruction in body mechanics, ergonomics, and ongoing fitness activities are equally important in preventing recurrences. Evaluation of the work environment, work station design, preemployment musculoskeletal evaluation, and the development of industrial fitness programs are preventive strategies the clinician may implement. Perhaps the most important outcome of patient education is the sense of confidence gained by the realization that he can manage his back problem while continuing to function and lead a productive life.

Spinal Stenosis

Spinal stenosis is defined as an abnormal narrowing of the spinal canal (central) or the intervertebral foramen (lateral).[165] Central stenosis can result from osteophytic enlargement of the inferior articular process or vertebral bodies, congenitally decreased anteroposterior or mediolateral diameters of the spinal canal, hypertrophy of the ligamentum flavum, spondylolisthesis, or neoplasm that impinges on the cauda equina. Lateral stenosis is typically caused by subluxation of the facets as a result of disk narrowing. Extension and rotation positional faults of the segment produce further narrowing. Symptoms are usually segmental because of entrapment of the nerve root.

EXAMINATION AND EVALUATION FINDINGS

The characteristic history of persons with spinal stenosis is that of neurogenic claudication—pain in the legs and, occasionally, neurologic deficits that occur after walking. In contrast to arterial ischemic claudication, neurogenic claudication can occur on standing (without ambulation), may increase with cough or sneeze, is associated with normal arterial pulses,[166] and is relieved by flexion of the lumbar spine.

Increased pain on spine extension is typical of stenosis. Whereas flexion is usually painful with herniated disks, it can be a position of relief for patients with spinal stenosis. Patients feel more comfortable walking in a stooped position, cycling, walking behind a shopping cart or lawn mower, or walking up an incline or stairs, rather than walking on a flat surface, down an incline, or downstairs.[167,168]

TREATMENT

Treatment of spinal stenosis is based on symptoms related to postures and movements. If the patient has mild symptoms that fluctuate with mechanical, postural, and movement changes, he can be accommodated with appropriate patient-related education, exercise, external lumbar support, (i.e. corset), and nonsteroidal antiinflammatory medication. Although nonoperative measures cannot reverse a true anatomic impairment, they can accommodate it by increasing the foraminal or spinal canal diameter.

Exercise should focus on physiologic impairments that may contribute to foraminal or spinal canal narrowing:

- Weak oblique abdominals and transversus muscles
- Short hip flexors
- Thoracic kyphosis with overstretched and weak thoracic erector spinae
- Asymmetry of pelvic girdle and lower extremity muscle length and strength

Narrowing is typically associated with spine extension, extension and rotation, or shearing. Postures associated with relative extension (ie, kyphosis and lordosis), extension and rotation (ie, kyphosis and lordosis and limb length discrepancy), or shearing (ie, swayback) should be modified, and the patient should be told to avoid these postural habits.

The clinician should teach the patient to avoid movement patterns that require repeated extension, rotation, or shearing and instead to perform movement patterns that include flexion. For example, the patient should be taught to lead with hip extension and recruit hip extensors to return from a forward-bending position and, at the end of the extension cycle, to recruit abdominal muscles to avoid late lumbar extension (Fig. 18-34*B*) or anterior pelvic shift (Fig. 18-34*C*).

Limited ambulation is a frequent functional limitation among patients with spinal stenosis. Harness-supported treadmill ambulation for patients with leg pain brought on by walking can be used as a progressive return to walking without symptoms. The amount of unloaded force can be progressed until unloading force is no longer required to relieve pain during ambulation.[169]

Patients should be instructed in recreational activities that do not produce symptoms. Exercise biased toward flexion should be encouraged, such as walking on a treadmill with a slight incline, cycling or walking while pushing a stroller (eg, taking children for walks). Exercise biased toward extension should be discouraged, such as walking on a flat surface, walking downhill, or swimming.

Spondylolysis and Spondylolisthesis

Spondylolysis, a bilateral defect in the pars interarticularis, occurs in 58% of adults.[170] Approximately 50% of those never progress to any degree of spondylolisthesis, a condition of forward subluxation of the body of one vertebrae on the vertebrae below it.[170] Spondylolisthesis is not limited to any specific segment of the spine. How-

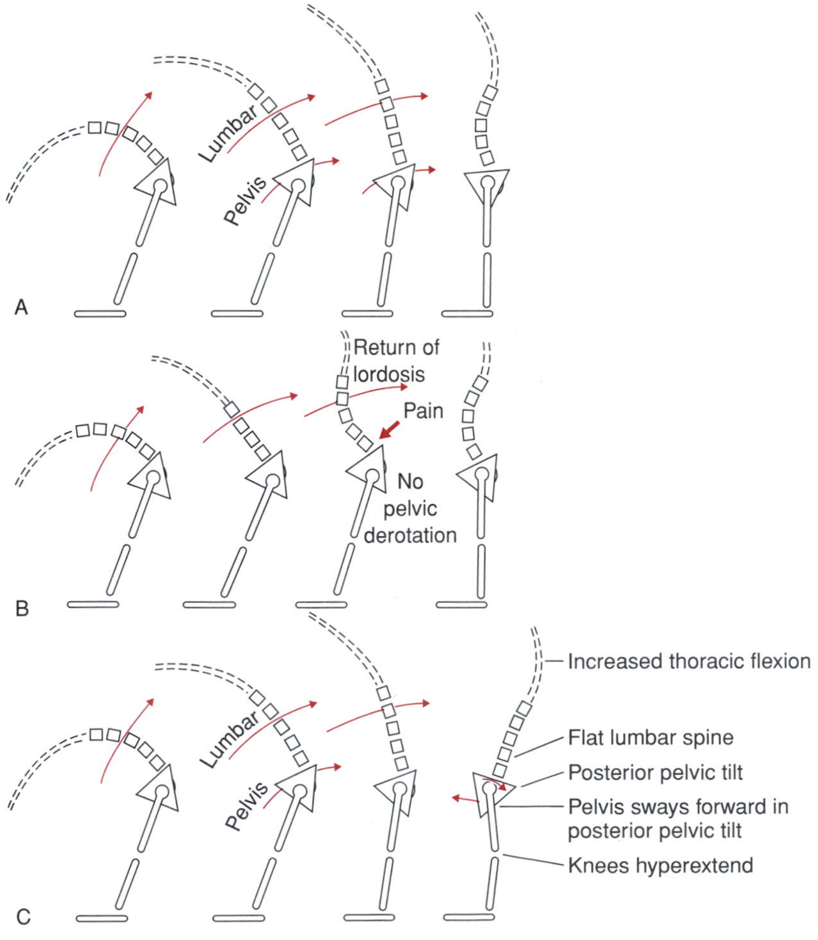

FIGURE 18-34 Proper versus improper flexion and re-extension. ***(A)*** Depicts proper simultaneous resumption of the lumbar lordosis with pelvic rotation. The pelvic rotation leads the re-extension phase, followed by lumbar extension after full pelvic rotation to neutral has been achieved. The result is neutral pelvic position and a normal lumbar extension curve. ***(B)*** Early lumbar extension without pelvic rotation causes an extension moment on the spine. The pelvis does not achieve neutral on standing, resulting in lumbar lordosis. This pattern should be avoided in an individual with stenosis or spondylolisthesis. ***(C)*** Another faulty re-extension strategy, often used by the individual with a swayback posture. At the end of the range, the pelvis sways forward causing an anterior shear to the lumbar spine, which should be avoided in an individual with stenosis or spondylolisthesis. (From Calliet R. *Low Back Pain.* 3rd ed. Philadelphia: FA Davis; 1981:132).

ever, it occurs most commonly at the L5-S1 segmental level, primarily because of the angulation of the L5 segment with respect to the vertical plane. Defects or impairment of any of the supporting structures can lead to subluxation of the superior segment on the inferior segment. Spondylolisthesis has been classified[23] by cause into five types:

1. Type I, isthmic: A defect in the pars interarticularis may be caused by a fracture or by an elongation of the pars without separation.
2. Type II, congenital: The posterior elements are anatomically inadequate because of developmental deficiency. This occurs rarely.
3. Type III, degenerative: The facets or the supporting ligaments undergo degenerative changes, allowing listhesis. There is no pars defect, and the condition worsens with age.
4. Type IV, elongated pedicle: The length of the neural arch elongates to allow listhesis. This is essentially an isthmic type. Traction forces are apparently contributory.
5. Type V, destructive disease: Metastatic disease, tuberculosis, or other bone disease may change the structure of the supporting tissues.

EXAMINATION AND EVALUATION FINDINGS

The patient may complain of back ache, gluteal pain, lower limb pain or paresthesias, hypesthesia, muscle weakness, intermittent claudication, or bladder and rectal disturbances. The physical examination may reveal that symptoms worsen on return from forward bending that is accompanied by lumbar extension at some point in the extension cycle. If the patient is cued to lead with the gluteals and to pull in with the deep abdominals, symptoms are reduced. The clinical diagnosis is suspected if this finding is accompanied by inspection and palpation of the spine in which a depression at the listhesis level is noticed. Percussion over the segment may elicit pain. Radiologic confirmation can be made by a lateral view of the lumbosacral region. A roentgenogram can diagnose spondylolysis or spondylolisthesis and the degree of subluxation, which can be graded.

TREATMENT

In general, treatment of spondylolysis or spondylolisthesis is nonsurgical.[174] Treatments include bracing, exercise, and nonsteroidal antiinflammatory medications. In children and adolescents, immobilization in a thoracolumbosacral brace, activity modification, and exercise expedite healing of the defect.[175,176]

Exercise, posture and movement retraining, and activity modification are the cornerstones of the rehabilitation program. As for the patient with spinal stenosis, lumbar extension and shearing forces should be avoided. Exercises focused on resolving the impairments associated with extension or shearing forces should be prescribed, and strong emphasis should be placed on abdominal strengthening and posture and movement retraining. If a brace is used in conjunction with physical therapy, the physical therapist should communicate with the physician regarding the prescribed immobilization period and weaning program. Most often, the patient can continue to participate in sports during the immobilization period and is encouraged to do so. However, activity modification also may be advised. Activities such as volleyball and gymnastics are associated with significant extension movements and shearing forces imposed on the lumbar spine. If movement patterns cannot be modified enough to reduce symptoms during these activities, the patient may need to be counseled to seek another form of recreation or athletic endeavor.

Sacroiliac Joint Dysfunction

The SIJ has the characteristics of synovial and fibrous joints; it contains synovium, articular cartilage, and a joint capsule, but it also has considerable fibrocartilage.[50] The joint surfaces of the ilium and sacrum assume an elongated boomerang shape with an irregular configuration. During load bearing, these surfaces approximate each other and form a tight interlock in what has been described as form closure.[174] The relatively large surface areas of these joints distribute loads over a considerable area. Although variable across populations, the available mobility of the SIJ is small. Considering the presence of fibrocartilage, the tight fit of the joint, the large surface area for force distribution, and the small available range of motion, it is not surprising that SIJ degeneration is less common than hip joint degeneration.

Conditions affecting the SIJ are nonetheless significant, not only because of the impact of an SIJ dysfunction on the function of the spine, pelvis, and lower extremity but also because an apparent musculoskeletal dysfunction may be signs and symptoms of a more serious disease process (Display 18-4). Before the clinician proceeds with treatment of a musculoskeletal dysfunction of the SIJ,

DISPLAY 18-4
Sacroiliac Joint Pathology

- Inflammatory conditions
  - Ankylosing spondylitis
  - Reiter's syndrome
  - Inflammatory bowel disease
  - Psoriatic sacroilitis
  - Rheumatoid arthritis
  - Juvenile chronic polyarthritis
  - Familial mediterranean fever
  - Behçet disease
  - Whipple disease
- Osteoarthritis
- Pyogenic infection
- *Brucella* sacroiliitis
- Tuberculosis
- Hyperparathyroidism
- Metastatic tumor
- Paget's disease

serious disease must be excluded. An SIJ dysfunction is a movement abnormality in the form of hypomobility, hypermobility, or instability.

EXAMINATION AND EVALUATION FINDINGS

Evaluation of the SIJ requires examination of the entire lumbopelvic girdle and hip complex to determine the interaction of impairments of each region and how the trunk, hip, and lower extremity affect SIJ function. Primary complaints include unilateral pain over the hypermobile (most often) or hypomobile SIJ and ipsilateral posterolateral buttock pain on the side of the dysfunctional SIJ.

It is often difficult to differentiate SIJ pain from lumbar and hip joint pain. Hip joint pain is more commonly perceived in the groin or lateral side of the thigh. With SIJ and hip joint dysfunction, patients rarely present with correlative neurologic findings unless some additional pathology is present. The physical examination can demonstrate joint dysfunction within the SIJ through a variety of specialized tests of iliosacral and sacroiliac osteokinematics and arthrokinematic motions. It is the clinicians's responsibility to determine the impairments contributing to force or form closure dysfunction. The clinician must determine the relationship between imbalances in muscle length, muscle performance impairments, neuromuscular control patterns, alignment, and movement patterns involving the lumbar-pelvic-hip complex.

TREATMENT

Treatment of SIJ dysfunction may require an array of joint mobilization and soft tissue techniques consistent with the presenting dysfunction. These manual therapy techniques require specialized skills in diagnosis and treatment that are beyond the scope of this text. Consistent with manual therapy techniques, patients can be taught self-mobilization techniques, as shown in Self-Management: Self-Mobilization for an Anterior Innominate Dysfunction. These techniques can assist the patient in maintaining joint alignment and function during the healing and restabilization process.

Although manual therapy is an important intervention for patients SIJ dysfunction, no manual therapy technique can improve stability across a hypermobile or unstable joint. To improve stability across a hypermobile SIJ, the clinician must focus on restoring muscle length balance, force or torque production, and neuromuscular control to the musculature involved in force closure (ie, latissimus dorsi, gluteus maximus, oblique abdominal group, hip adductors, and hip abductors). Hypomobility in the contralateral SIJ, hip joints, and trunk may be imposing excessive motion on the affected SIJ. Foot dynamics may also affect the SIJ by imposing a repetitive, asymmetric force up the kinetic chain.

With respect to therapeutic exercise, normalizing mobility within the pelvis and between the trunk, hip, and lower extremities is key to resolving dysfunction in the SIJ. The patient suffering from SIJ dysfunction can be thought of as a spine, SIJ, hip, knee, ankle, and foot patient. Impairments in any of these regions may affect the function of the SIJ and therefore require intervention. For example, a patient with dynamic foot pronation, excessive hip medial rotation, positive Trendelenburg sign, and weak deep abdominal muscles, gluteus medius, and gluteus maximus with an SIJ dysfunction may require intervention for each impairment to achieve permanent resolution of the SIJ dysfunction.

ADJUNCTIVE INTERVENTIONS

Bracing

Some form of motion restriction for excessive motion at a segmental level may be necessary in patients with hypermobility or instability in the lumbopelvic region.[175,176] Bracing is indicated when exercise alone, used to improve segmental stability and relative flexibility, has failed to produce a desirable functional outcome.

Support provided to the segmental levels with proper bracing can improve stiffness locally and encourage movement at segments requiring more relative mobility. For example, use of a lumbosacral corset can stabilize the lumbosacral region while promoting movement in the hips. Bracing theoretically should be able to improve length-tension relationships in affected trunk and pelvic girdle musculature. For example, overstretched abdominal musculature that often accompanies lumbar lordosis and anterior pelvic tilt is supported in the short range in a properly fitting lumbar support. With consistent use of a properly fitting support over time, the overstretched musculature may adaptively shorten. If accompanied by exercise, improved force- or torque-generating capability by the overstretched musculature may occur at a faster rate than with exercise or bracing alone. If the lumbar support stabilizes the spine during functional movement, it also can encourage movement across the hip joints in the desired directions, which can affect the extensibility of tissues surrounding the pelvic girdle.

Bracing is intended as an adjunctive measure to a comprehensive approach to the treatment of lumbopelvic syndromes. The choice of brace depends on the region requiring motion restriction (ie, upper lumbar, lumbosacral, or sacroiliac region) and the amount of immobilization required (ie, abdominal binder for minimal support to the abdomen versus a thoracolumbosacral corset with rigid stays for maximal support). The clinician must encourage the patient to continue with appropriate levels of functional activity and prescribed exercise while using the brace to improve strength, endurance, and mobility impairments and to prevent the undesirable effects of immobilization.

Traction

Lumbar traction is the application of forces to stretch the periarticular tissues and musculature,[36,177,178] separate joint surfaces, reduce intradiskal pressure,[179,180] and retract herniated disk material.[177,181] When lumbar traction is applied, the movement that occurs at the spinal segments is thought to be a combination of distraction of the vertebral bodies and gliding of facet joint surfaces. Results of research on traction use and effectiveness is mixed, but numerous authorities claim traction is an effective and beneficial method of treatment when used appropriately.[124,177,181,182–184] Others have shown poor results with treatment or found that the

Table 18-6. TRACTION TREATMENT PARAMETERS

DIAGNOSIS	PATIENT/STRAP POSITION	TYPE OF TRACTION	DURATION
HNP	Prone/anterior pull	Sustained	8–10 min
DDD/DJD	Supine/posterior pull; prone/anterior pull	Intermittent	10–15 min
Hypomobility			
Limited flexion	Supine/posterior pull	Intermittent	10–15 min
Limited extension	Prone/anterior pull	Intermittent	10–15 min
Facet impingement	Pt comfort/unilateral pull	Sustained or intermittent	10–15 min

positive effects of traction were of limited or marginal value.[185,188] Results of these studies must be considered judiciously, because most have studied traction as an isolated treatment. This puts unrealistic demands on a single treatment modality. Traction is intended as an adjunctive intervention to a total plan of care, including patient-related education and exercise instruction. Research that examines the use of traction in conjunction with a well-planned treatment regimen would help in defining the effectiveness of this form of treatment.

The type of lumbar traction used and the parameters of use can contribute to a rapid functional outcome. The types of lumbar traction include continuous, manual, positional, mechanical, and gravity assisted. Autotraction is another type that has been useful in the treatment of acute low back pain.[189] With this technique, the patient lies on an adjustable table and grasps bars at the head of the table. A traction belt is applied to the pelvis. Traction is performed by the patient pulling with his arms or pushing with his legs, allowing constant control of the force applied. The table can be manipulated three dimensionally and moved from horizontal to vertical.

The choice of which type of traction device to use is based on a thorough understanding of the physiologic effects of each type of traction coupled with the specific impairments related to the patient's condition. Several parameters that can be controlled with traction. The degree to which these can be modulated depends on the type of traction being used. Generally, a benefit of mechanical traction is that it has the most variables that can be manipulated. However, it must be performed in a clinical setting. Home traction (a form of mechanical traction) and positional traction do not have the benefit of manipulating several variables for the best patient prescription, but they can be performed independently at home.

Ideally, research should guide the type of treatment selected for given patient conditions. Unfortunately, few data are available to help clinicians select treatment parameters, and it is necessary to rely on theoretical arguments for parameter selection, tempered by common sense and clinical experience. Theoretical arguments regarding type of traction, intensity, patient position, direction of pull, treatment duration, and unilateral versus bilateral traction have been provided by Saunders.[190] Table 18-6 provides guidelines for selecting treatment parameters for four clinical conditions.

! Key Points

- A thorough understanding of the anatomy and biomechanics of the lumbopelvic region is a prerequisite to appropriate therapeutic exercise prescription for this region.
- Exercise must be based on a thoughtful and systematic examination process identifying the physiologic and psychological impairments most closely related to the individual's functional limitations and disability.
- Therapeutic exercise intervention for common physiologic impairments must be coordinated to address associated impairments and prioritized to address those most closely related to functional limitations and disability.
- Exercise management of common structural diagnoses must not follow a recipe approach, but rather relate to the patient's impairments, functional limitations, and disability.

? Critical Thinking Questions

1. Prioritize postures from the most to the least stressful on the lumbar spine.
2. Describe the principles for the use of optimal body mechanics during lifting.
3. Describe the biomechanical differences between the bent-knee and straight-leg sit-up.
4. How can exercise impact chemical causes of pain?
5. What postures place the external oblique in a lengthened position, making it susceptible to overstretch mechanism of strain.
6. Provide an example of relative flexibility or stiffness between the hip joint and lumbar spine in sagittal, frontal, and transverse plane movements.
7. What is the treatment for a relative flexibility or stiffness problem?
8. Define the anatomic injury that occurs with disk prolapse and the three subsets of disk herniation.
9. Define the three clinical categories of signs and symptoms associated with HNP.
10. Define spinal stenosis.
11. Discuss the difference between spondylolysis and spondylolisthesis.
12. Discuss the musculature involved in force closure of the SIJ.
13. Refer to Case Study #5 in Unit 7.

LAB ACTIVITIES

1. Pick up two loads of equal weight but different sizes. Which is easier to pick up, the larger or smaller size?
2. Analyze your partner's osteokinematic motions and muscle activity across the lumbar-pelvic-hip complex during each phase of gait about all three planes of motion. How does your partner deviate from the standard?
3. Analyze your partner's LPR. How would you retrain the pattern if the lumbar spine was relatively more flexible in the flexion phase? How would you retrain the pattern if the lumbar spine was relatively more flexible in the extension phase?
4. Teach your partner level II of the deep abdominal progression described in Self-Management: Lower Abdominal Progression. Be sure to incorporate resisted breathing into the exercise. What effect does a pelvic floor contraction have on performance of the exercise? Can your partner perform higher levels of the exercise? What is the main difference between level III and level IV? Can your partner perform level II on a half or full foam roll? Is it more or less difficult on a foam roll?
5. On your partner, perform manual resistance to the lumbar multifidus in sidelying. Can you palpate activity of the lumbar multifidus at the L5 level?
6. Analyze your partner performing bent-knee and straight-leg sit-ups. Does your partner require fixation of his or her feet during the hip-flexion phase of the bent-knee or straight-leg sit-up? During a straight-leg sit-up, how many sit-ups can your partner perform with arms straight before his or her feet lift up (or lift earlier in the range)? Arms crossed across the chest? Arms behind the head? What does lifting of the feet or lifting prematurely indicate?
7. Teach your partner how to passively stretch the hamstrings and hip flexors without lumbopelvic motion. Teach your partner an active movement that uses hip mobility without trunk mobility. What muscles must your partner use to stabilize the spine while actively stretching the hip flexors or hamstrings?
8. Teach your partner to stabilize against extension, flexion, and rotation forces (separately) while sitting on a flat surface and on a gym ball. Which one is easier? What would be the effect of sitting on a gym ball with your feet on a slippery surface (eg, slide board) performing upper extremity movements?
9. Teach your partner to stabilize against extension forces in standing on a flat surface and on a half and full foam roll. What type of balance strategy does your partner use (ankles, knees, or hips)?
10. Teach your partner controlled mobility activities in standing that challenge the spine to stabilize against flexion forces, extension forces, and rotation forces. Even though you are encouraging movement in the lumbar spine, where should most of the movement occur during total-body movements?
11. Teach your partner to perform a golf swing with appropriate motion occurring at the ankle-foot complex, knee, hip, pelvis, and spine. Where in the spine should most of the rotation occur?
12. Develop and teach your partner an exercise to improve the coordinated function of the latissimus and gluteus maximus to improve force closure of the pelvic girdle. (Hint: a step and elastic tubing are useful props). What other muscles are involved in force closure of the SIJ? Are you engaging all muscles at the appropriate length with the activity you devised?

a. Based on her history and physical examination findings, what is the likely medical diagnosis for this patient?
b. What are the faulty posture and movement patterns associated with onset of her symptoms?
c. What are the correlating physiologic impairments? List them under the headings used in this chapter (eg, mobility, muscle performance).
d. Develop an exercise program addressing all pertinent impairments related to her functional limitations and disability.
e. Be sure to include patient-related instruction tips.

REFERENCES

1. Yong Hing K, Reilly J, Kirkaldy-Willis WH. The ligamentum flavum. *Spine*. 1976;1:226–234.
2. McKenzie RA. *The Lumbar Spine: Mechanical Diagnosis and Therapy*. Lower Hutt, New Zealand: Spinal Publications; 1981.
3. Delitto A, Erhard RE, Bowling RW. A treatment-based classification approach to low back syndrome: identifying and staging patients for conservative treatment. *Phys Ther*. 1995;75:470–498.
4. Sahrmann SA. *Diagnosis and Management of Musculoskeletal Pain Syndromes*. St. Louis: Mosby; 1999.
5. Spitzer WO, Nachemson A. A scientific approach to the assessment and management of activity-related spinal disorders: a monograph for clinicians. Report of the Quebec Task Force on Spinal Disorders. *Spine*. 1987;12:51
6. Twomey L, Taylor J. Spine update: exercise and spinal manipulation in the treatment of low back pain. *Spine*. 1995;20: 615–619.
7. Vleeming A, Snijders C, Stoeckart J, Mens JMA. A new light on low back pain. Proceedings from the Second Interdisciplinary World Congress on Low Back Pain and Its Relation to the Sacroiliac Joint; November 9–11, 1995; La Jolla, CA.
8. Bodguk N, Twomey L. *Clinical Anatomy of the Lumbar Spine*. Melbourne: Churchill Livingstone; 1991.
9. Pearcy MJ, Tibrewal SB. Three dimensional x-ray analysis of normal movement in the lumbar spine. *Spine*. 1984;9: 582–587.

10. Vicenzino G, Twomey L. Side flexion induced lumbar spine conjunctrotation and its influencing factors. *Aust Physiother.* 1993;39:4.
11. Farfan HF, Cossette JW, Robertson GH, Wells R, Kraus H. The effects of torsion of the lumbar intervertebral joints: the role of torsion in the production of disc degeneration. *J Bone Joint Surg Am.* 1970;52:468–497.
12. Farfan HF, Sullivan JD. The relation of facet orientation to intervertebral disc failure. *Can J Surg.* 1967;10:170–183.
13. Taylor JR, Twomey LT. Age changes in lumbar zygapophyseal joints. Observations on structure and function. *Spine.* 1986;11:739–745.
14. Horwitz T, Smith R. An anatomical, pathological and roentgenological study of the intervertebral joints of the lumbar spine and of the sacroiliac joints. *AJR Am J Rontgenol.* 1940; 43:173–186.
15. Farfan HF, Huverdeau RM, Dubow HI. Lumbar intervertebral disc degeneration: the influence of geometrical features on the pattern of disc degeneration, a postmortem study. *J Bone Joint Surg Am.* 1972;54:492–510.
16. Beard H, Stevens R. Biochemical changes in the intervertebral disc. In: Jayson M, ed. *The Lumbar Spine and Backache.* 2nd ed. London: Pitman; 1980:407.
17. Maroudas A. Nutrition and metabolism of the intervertebral disc. In: Ghosh P, ed. *The Biology of the Intervertebral Disc.* Boca Raton, FL: CRC Press, 1988:137.
18. Twomey L, Taylor J. Sustained flexion loading, rapid extension loading of the lumbar spine, and the physical therapy of related injuries. *Physiother Pract.* 1988;4:129–137.
19. Adams MA, Hutton WC. The effect of posture on diffusion into lumbar intervertebral discs. *J Anat.* 1986;147:121–134.
20. Twomey L. A rationale for the treatment of back pain and joint pain by manual therapy. *Phys Ther.* 1992;72:885–892.
21. Pearcy M, Tibrewal M. Axial rotation and lateral bending in the normal lumbar spine measured by three dimensional radiography. *Spine.* 1984;9:582–587.
22. Bogduk N, Twomey LT. *Clinical Anatomy of the Lumbar Spine.* 1st ed. Edinburgh: Churchill Livingstone; 1987.
23. Caillet R. *Low Back Pain Syndrome.* Philadelphia: FA Davis; 1981.
24. Giles L, Taylor J. Human zygapophyseal joint capsule and synovial fold innervation. *Br J Rheumatol.* 1987;26:93–98.
25. Asmussen E, Klausen K. Form and function of the erect human spine. *Clin Orthop.* 1962;25:55.
26. Basmajian JV, DeLuca CJ. *Muscles Alive.* 5th ed. Baltimore: Williams & Wilkins; 1985.
27. Nachemson A, Elfstrom G. *Intravital Dynamic Pressure Measurements in Lumbar Discs: A Study of Common Movements, Maneuvers, and Exercises.* Stockholm: Almqvist & Wiksell; 1970.
28. Andersson GBJ, Ortengren R, Nachemson A. Lumbar disc pressure and myoelectric back muscle activity during sitting. I. Studies on an experimental chair. *Scand J Rehabil Med.* 1974;6:122–127.
29. Nordin M, Frankel H. *Basic Biomechanics of the Musculoskeletal System.* 2nd ed. Philadelphia: Lea & Febiger; 1989.
30. Cappozzo A. Compressive loads in the lumbar vertebral column during normal level walking. *J Orthop Res.* 1984;1: 292–301.
31. Panjabi MM. The stabilizing system of the spine. Part I. Function, dysfunction, adaptation, and enhancement. *J Spinal Disord.* 1992;5:383–389.
32. Snijders CJ, Vleeming A, Stoeckart R. Transfer of lumbosacral load to iliac bones and legs. Part 1: Biomechanics of self-bracing of the sacroiliac joints and its significance for treatment and exercise. *Clin Biomech.* 1993;8:285–300.
33. Snijders CJ, Vleeming A, Stoeckart R. Kleinrensink GH, Mens JMA. Biomechanics of sacroiliac joint stability: validation experiments on the concept of self-locking. Proceedings from the Second World Congress on Low Back Pain; 1995;San Diego, CA.
34. Vleeming A, Stoeckart R, Volkers ACW, Snijders CJ. Relation between form and function in the sacroiliac joint. Part 1: Clinical anatomical aspects. *Spine.* 1990;15:130.
35. Vleeming A, Volkers ACW, Snijders CJ, Stoeckart R. Relation between form and function in the sacroiliac joint. Part 2: Biomechanical aspects. *Spine.* 1990;15:133.
36. Colachis SC, Worden RE, Bechtol CO, Strohm BR. Movement of the sacroiliac joint in the adult male: a preliminary report. *Arch Phys Med Rehabil.* 1963;44:490.
37. Bowen V, Cassidy JD. Macroscopic and microscopic anatomy of the sacroiliac joint from embryonic life until the eighth decade. *Spine.* 1981;6:620–627.
38. Bowen V, Cassidy JD. Macroscopic and microscopic anatomy of the sacroiliac joint from embryonic life until the eighth decade. *Spine* 1981;6:620–628.
39. Vleeming A, Pool Goudzwaard AL, Hammudoghlu D, Stoeckart R, Snijders CJ, Mens J. The function of the long dorsal sacroiliac ligament: its implication for understanding low back pain. Proceedings of the Second World Congress on the Sacroiliac Joint and Its Relation to Low Back Pain; November 9–11, 1995; La Jolla, CA.
40. Vleeming A, Wingerden JP, Snijders CJ, Stoeckart R, Stijnen T. Loan application to the sacrotuberous ligament: influences on sacroiliac joint mechanics. *J Clin Biomech.* 1989;4: 205–209.
41. Vleeming A, Stoeckart R, Snijders CJ. The sacrotuberous ligament: a conceptual approach to its dynamic role in stabilizing the sacroiliac joint. *J Clin Biomech.* 1989;4:201–203.
42. Chamberlain WE. The symphysis pubis in the roentgen examination of the sacroiliac joint. *AJR Am J Roentgenol.* 1930; 24:621.
43. Dihlmann W. *Diagnostic Radiology of the Sacroiliac Joint.* Chicago: Year Book Medical Publishers; 1980.
44. Egund N, Alsson TH, Schmid H, Selnik G. Movements in the sacroiliac joints demonstrated with roentgen stereophotogrammetry. *Acta Radiol Diagn.* 1978;19:833–846.
45. Frigerio NA, Stowe RR, Howe JW. Movement of the sacroiliac joint. *Clin Orthop Rel Res.* 1974;100:370–377.
46. Mitchell FL Jr, Pruzzo NA. Investigation of voluntary and primary respiratory mechanisms. *J Am Osteopath Assoc.* 1971;70:149–153.
47. Reynolds HM. Three dimensional kinematics in the pelvic girdle. *J Am Osteopath Assoc.* 1980;80:277–280.
48. Solonen KA. The sacroiliac joint in the light of anatomical, roentgenological, and clinical studies. *Acta Orthop Scand Suppl.* 1957;27:11–15.
49. Snijders CJ, Vleeming A, Stoeckart R. Transfer of lumbosacral load to iliac bones and legs. Part 2: Loading of the sacroiliac joints when lifting in a stooped posture. *J Clin Biomech.* 1993;8:295–301.
50. Alderink GJ. The sacroiliac joint: review of anatomy, mechanics, and function. *J Orthop Sports Phys Ther.* 1991;13: 71–84.
51. Walheim GG, Olerud S, Ribbe T. Mobility of the pubic symphysis. *Acta Orthop Scand.* 1984;55:203–208.
52. Greenman PE. *Principles of Manual Medicine.* Baltimore: Williams & Wilkins;1989.
53. Walheim GG, Selvik G. Mobility of the pubic symphysis. *Clin Orthop Rel Res.* 1984;191:129–135.
54. Vleeming A, Wingerden JP, van Dijkstra PF, Stoeckart R, Snijders CJ, Stijnen T. Mobility in the SI joints in old people: a kinematic and radiologic study. *J Clin Biomech.* 1992;7: 170–176.
55. Kapandji IA. *The Physiology of the Joints,* vol 3. *The Trunk and Vertebral Column.* 2nd ed. New York: Churchill Livingstone; 1974.

56. Strachan WF. Applied anatomy of the pelvis and perineum. *J Am Osteopath Assoc*. 1939;38:359.
57. Strachan WF, Beckwith CG, Larson NJ, Grant JH. A study of the mechanics of the sacroiliac joint. *J Am Osteopath Assoc*. 1938;37:576.
58. Sturesson B, Selvic G, Uden A. Movements of the sacroiliac joints: a roentgen stereophotogrammetric analysis. *Spine*. 1989;14:162–165.
59. Mitchell FL, Moran PS, Pruzzo NA. *An Evaluation and Treatment Manual of Osteopathic Muscle Energy Procedures*. Valley Park, MD: Mitchell, Moran, Pruzzo Associates; 1979.
60. Vleeming A, Pool Goudzard A, Stoeckart R, et al. The posterior layer of the thoracolumbar fascia: its function in load transfer from spine to legs. *Spine*. 1995;20:753–758.
61. MacIntosh J, Bogduk N, Gracovetsky S. The biomechanics of the thoracolumbar fascia. *Clin Biomech*. 1987;2:78–83.
62. Morris JM, Benner G, Lucas DB. An electromyographic study of the intrinsic muscles of the back in man. *J Anat.* 1962;96:509.
63. Andersson GBJ, Ortengren R, Herberts P. Quantization electromyographics studies of back muscle activity related to posture and loading. *Orthop Clin North Am.* 1977;8:85–96.
64. Porterfield JA, DeRosa C, *Mechanical Low Back Pain: Perspectives in Functional Anatomy*. 2nd ed. Philadelphia: WB Saunders; 1998.
65. Aspden RM. Review of the functional anatomy of the spinal ligaments and the lumbar erector spinae muscles. *Clin Anat.* 1992;5:372–387.
66. Hodges PW, Richardson CA. Contraction of the abdominal muscles associated with movement of the lower limb. *Phys Ther*. 1997;77:132–144.
67. Hides JA, Stokes MJ, Saide M, Jull GA, Cooper DH. Evidence of lumbar multifidus muscle wasting ipsilateral to symptoms in patients with acute/subacute low back pain. *Spine*. 1994;19:165–172.
68. Rantanen J, Hurme M, Falck B, Alaranta H. The lumbar multifidus muscle five years after surgery for a lumbar intervertebral disc herniation. *Spine*. 1993;18:568–574.
69. Valencia F, Munro R. An electromyographic study of the lumbar multifidus in man. *Electromyogr Clin Neurophysiol*. 1085;15:205–221.
70. Williams P, Warwick R, Dyson M, Bannister L, eds. *Gray's Anatomy.* Edinburgh: Churchill Livingstone; 1987.
71. Hodges PW, Richardson CA. Neuromotor dysfunction of the trunk musculature in low back pain patients. Proceedings of the World Confederation of Physical Therapists Congress; Washington, DC; 1995.
72. Richardson CA, Jull GA. Muscle control, pain control. What exercises would you prescribe? *Manual Ther.* 1995;1:1–2.
73. Jull G, Richardson C. Rehabilitation of active stabilization of the lumbar spine. In: Twomey L, Taylor J, eds. *Physical Therapy of the Lumbar Spine.* 2nd ed. New York: Churchill Livingstone; 1994.
74. Richardson CA, Jull GA. Concepts of assessment and rehabilitation for active lumbar stability. In: Boyling JD, Palastanga N, eds. *Grieve's Modern Manual Therapy of the Vertebral Column.* 2nd ed. Edinburgh: Churchill Livingstone; 1994.
75. Wingarden JP, Vleeming A, Snidjers CJ, Stoeckart R. A functional-anatomical approach to the spine-pelvis mechanism: interaction between the biceps femoris muscle and the sacrotuberous ligament. *Eur Spine J*. 1993;2:140.
76. Hodges PW, Richardson CA. *Dysfunction of transversus abdominis associated with chronic low back pain*. Proceedings of the 9th Biennial Conference of the Manipulative Physiotherapists Association of Australia; 1995; Gold Coast, Queensland.
77. Beal MC. The sacroiliac problem: review of anatomy, mechanics and diagnosis. *J Am Osteopath Assoc.* 1982;81:667–679.
78. Battye CK, Joseph J. An investigation by telemetering of the activity of some muscles in walking. *Med Biol.* 1966;4:125–135.
79. Waters RL, Morris JM. Electrical activity of muscles of the trunk during walking. *J Anat*. 1972;111:191–199.
80. Sheffield FJ. Electromyographic study of the abdominal muscles in walking and other movements. *Am J Phys Med.* 1962;41:142–147.
81. Inman VT, Ralston HJ, Todd F. *Human Walking*. Baltimore: Williams & Wilkins; 1981.
82. Snijders CJ, Vleeming A, Stoeckart R. Transfer of lumbosacral load to iliac bones and legs. Part 1: Biomechanics of self-bracing of the sacroiliac joints and its significance for treatment and exercise. *J Clin Biomech*. 1993;8:285–294.
83. Vleeming A, Stoeckart R, Snijders CJ. The sacrotuberous ligament: a conceptual approach to its dynamic role in stabilizing the sacroiliac joint. *J Clin Biomech.* 1989;4:201–203.
84. Lee D. Instability of the sacroiliac joint and the consequences to gait. *J Manual Manipulative Ther.* 1996;4:22–29.
85. Frymoyer JW. Back pain and sciatica. *N Engl J Med.* 1988;318:291–298.
86. Saal J. The role of inflammation in lumbar pain. *Spine*. 1995;20:1821–1827.
87. National Center for Health Statistics, Vital and Health Statistics. Detailed Diagnosis and Procedures, National Hospital Discharge Survey 1986, 1987. Washington, DC: U.S. Department of Health and Human Services; 1988–1989.
88. Quebec Task Force on Spinal Disorders. Scientific approach to the assessment and management of activity-related spinal disorders a monograph for clinicians: report of the Quebec Task Force on Spinal Disorders. *Spine.* 1987;12(suppl 17):S1–S59.
89. Kendall FP, McCreary EK, Provance PG. *Muscles Testing and Function.* 4th ed. Baltimore: Williams & Wilkins; 1993.
90. Maitland GD. *Vertebral Manipulation.* 4th ed. London: Butterworths; 1977.
91. Addison R, Schultz A. Trunk strength in patients seeking hospitalization for chronic low back pain. *Spine*. 1980;5:539–544.
92. Mayer TG, Smith SS, Keeley J, Mooney V. Quantification of lumbar function. Part 2: Sagittal plane trunk strength in chronic low-back pain patients. *Spine*. 1985;10:765–772.
93. McNeil T, Warwick D, Andersson G, Schultz A. Trunk strengths in attempted flexion, extension, and lateral bending in healthy subjects and patients with low back disorders. *Spine*. 1980;5:529–537.
94. Pope MH, Bevins T, Wilder DG, Frymoyer JW. The relationship between anthropometric, postural, muscular, and mobility characteristics of males ages 18–55. *Spine*. 1985;10:644–648.
95. Holmstrom E, Moritz U, Andersson M. Trunk muscle strength and back muscle endurance in construction workers with and without back pain disorders. *Scand J Rehabil Med*. 1992;24:3–10.
96. Nicolaison T, Jorgensen K. Trunk strength, back muscle endurance and low back trouble. *Scand J Rehabil Med.* 1985;17:121–127.
97. Cresswell A, Grundstrom H, Thorstensson A. Observations on intraabdominal pressure and patterns of intramuscular activity in man. *Acta Physiol Scand.* 1992;144:409–418.
98. Wilke H, Wolf S, Claes L, Arand M, Wiesend A. Stability increase of the lumbar spine with different muscle groups. *Spine*. 1995;20:192–198.
99. Kirkaldy-Willis W, Farfan H. Instability of the lumbar spine. *Clin Orthop*. 1982;165:110–123.

100. Paris S. Physical signs of instability. *Spine*. 1985;10:277–279.
101. Roland M, Morris R. A study of the natural history of back pain. Part I: Development of a reliable and sensitive measure of disability in low back pain. *Spine*. 1983;8:141–144.
102. Dolce J, Raczynski J. Neuromuscular activity and electromyography in painful backs: psychological and biomechanical models in assessment and treatment. *Psychol Bull.* 1985;97:502–520.
103. Nies-Byl N, Sinnott PL. Variations in balance and body sway in middle-aged adults: subjects with healthy backs compared with subjects with low-back dysfunction. *Spine* 1991; 16:325–330.
104. Taimela S, Osterman K, Alaranta H, Kujula AS. Long psychomotor reaction time in patients with chronic low back pain. *Arch Phys Med Rehabil.* 1993;74:1161–1164.
105. Butler DS. *Mobilisation of the Nervous System.* Melbourne: Churchill Livingstone; 1991.
106. Karas R, McIntosh G, Hall H, Wilson L, Melles T. The relationship between nonorganic signs and centralization of symptoms in the prediction of return to work for patients with low back pain. *Phys Ther*. 1997;77:354–360.
107. Waddell G, McCulloch JA, Kummel E, Venner RM. Nonorganic physical signs in low back pain. *Spine*. 1980;5:117–125.
108. Hayes B, Solyom CAE, Wing PC, Berkowitz J. Use of psychometric measures and nonorganic signs testing in detecting nomogenic disorders in low back pain patients. *Spine*. 1993;18:1254–1262.
109. Fisher M, Kaur D, Houchins J. Electrodiagnostic examination, back pain and entrapment of posterior rami. *Electromyogr Clin Neurophysiol.* 1985;25:183–189.
110. Lindgren K, Sihvonen T, Leino E, Pitkanen M. Exercise therapy effects on functional radiographic findings and segmental electromyographic activity in lumbar spine and instability. *Arch Phys Med Rehabil.* 1993;74:933–939.
111. Mattila M, Hurme M, Alaranta H, et al. The multifidus muscle in patients with lumbar disc herniation: a histochemical and morphometric analysis of intraoperative biopsies. *Spine*. 1986;11:733–738.
112. Stokes M, Cooper R, Jayson M. Selective changes in multifidus dimensions in patients with chronic low back pain. *Eur Spine J.* 1992;1:38–42.
113. Wilke H, Wolf S, Claes L, Arand M, Wiesend A. Stability increases of the lumbar spine with different muscle groups. *Spine*. 1995.
114. Panjabi M, Abumi K, Duranceau J, Oxland T. Spinal stability and intersegmental muscle forces: a biomechanical model. *Spine*. 1989;14:194–199.
115. Fitzmaurice R, Cooper R, Freemont A. A histomorphometric comparison of muscle biopsies from normal subjects and patients with ankylosing spondylitis and severe mechanical low back pain. *J Pathol.* 1991;163:182A.
116. Ford D, Bagall K, McFadden K, Greenhill B, Raso J. Analysis of vertebral muscle obtained during surgery for correction of a lumbar disc disorder. *Acta Anat.* 1983;116:152–157.
117. Lehto M, Hurme M, Alaranta H, et al. Connective tissue changes of the multifidus muscle in patients with lumbar disc herniation. *Spine.* 1989;14:302–308.
118. Rantanen J, Hurme M, Falk B, et al. The lumbar multifidus muscle five years after surgery for a lumbar intervertebral disc herniation. *Spine*. 1993;18:568–574.
119. Zhu XZ, Parnianpour M, Nordin M, Kahanovitz N. Histochemistry and morphology of erector spinae muscle in lumbar disc herniation. *Spine*. 1989;14:391–397.
120. Cavanaugh JM. Neural mechanisms of lumbar pain. *Spine*. 1995;20:1804–1809.
121. McKenzie R. *The Lumbar Spine.* 1st ed. Upper Hutt, New Zealand: Wright & Carmen; 1981.
122. McKenzie R. Prophylaxis in recurrent low back pain. *N Z Med J.* 1979;89:22–23.
123. Erhard RE, Delitto A, Cibulka MT. Relative effectiveness of an extension program and a combined program of manipulation with flexion and extension exercises in patients with acute low back syndrome. *Phys Ther*. 1994;74: 1093–1100.
124. Saunders H. The use of spinal traction in the treatment of neck and back conditions. *Clin Orthop Rel Res.* 1983;179:31–38.
125. Ellis JJ, Spagnoli R. The hip and sacroiliac joint: prescriptive home exercise program for dysfunction of the pelvic girdle and hip. In: *Orthopedic Physical Therapy Home Study Course 971.* LaCrosse, WI: Orthopedic Section of the American Physical Therapy Association; 1997.
126. Hides J, Richardson C, Jull G. Multifidus recovery is not automatic following resolution of acute first episode of low back pain. *Spine*. 1996;21:2763–2769.
127. Grabiner M, Kohn T, Ghazawi AE. Decoupling of bilateral paraspinal excitation in subjects with low back pain. *Spine.* 1992;17:1219–1223.
128. Roy S, Deluca C, Casavant D. Lumbar muscle fatigue and chronic low back pain. *Spine*. 1989;14:992–1001.
129. Roy S, DeLuca C, Snyder-Mackler L, Emley M, Crenshaw R, Lyons J. Fatigue, recovery, and low back pain in varsity rowers. *Med Sci Sports Exerc.* 1990;22:463–469.
130. Haig A, Weismann G, Haugh L, Pope M, Grobler L. Prospective evidence for changes in paraspinal muscle activity after herniated nucleus pulposus. *Spine*. 1993;17:926–929.
131. Kelly JP. Reactions of neurons to injury. In: Kandel E, Schwartz J, eds. *Principles of Neural Science.* New York: Elsevier; 1985:187.
132. Risk factors for back trouble [editorial]. Lancet. 1989;8650: 1305–1306.
133. Sihvonen T, Herno A, Paljarvi L, Airaksinen O, Partanen J, Tapaninahos A. Local denervation of paraspinal muscles in postoperative failed back syndrome. *Spine.* 1993;18:575–581.
134. Kawaguchi Y, Matsui H, Tsui H. Back muscle injury after posterior lumbar surgery. *Spine*. 1994;19:2598–2602.
135. Sihvonen T, Partanen J. Segmental hypermobility in lumbar spine and entrapment of dorsal rami. *Electromyogr Clin Neurophysiol.* 1990;30:175–180.
136. Boileau JC, Basmajian JV. *Grant's Method of Anatomy.* 7th ed. Baltimore: Williams & Wilkins; 1965.
137. Biederman HJ, Shanks GL, Forrest WJ, Inglis J. Power spectrum analysis of electromyographic activity. *Spine*. 1991;16: 1179–1184.
138. Hodges P, Richardson C, Jull G. Evaluation of the relationship between laboratory and clinical tests of transversus abdominis function. *Physiother Res Int.* 1996;1:30–40.
139. Richardson CA, Jull GA. Muscle control pain control. What exercises would you prescribe? *Manual Ther.* 1995;1:2–10.
140. Bullock-Saxton JE, Janda V, Bullock MI. Reflex activation of gluteal muscles in walking. *Spine*. 1993;18:704–708.
141. Schipplein OD, Trafimow JH, Andersson GB, Andriacchi TP. Relationship between moments at the L5/S1 level, hip and knee joint when lifting. *J Biomech.* 1990;23:907–912.
142. Butler D. *Mobilization of the Nervous System*. Melbourne: Churchill Livingstone; 1991.
143. Lewit K. *Manipulative Therapy in Rehabilitation of the Locomotor System.* 2nd ed. Oxford: Butterworth Heinemann; 1991.
144. Panjabi MM. The stabilizing system of the spine. Part I. Function, dysfunction, adaptation, and enhancement. *J Spinal Disord.* 1992;5:383–389.
145. Suzuki N, Endo S. A quantitative study of trunk muscle strength and fatigability in the low back pain syndrome. *Spine*. 1984;8:69–74.

146. Spangfort EV. Lumbar disc herniation: a computer aided analysis of 2504 operations. *Acta Orthop Scand.* 1972; 5132:1–93.
147. Yong Hing KHB, Kirkaldy-Willis WH. The pathophysiology of degenerative disease of the lumbar spine. *Orthop Clin North Am.* 1983;14:491–504.
148. Alpers BJ. The neurological aspects of sciatica. *Med Clin North Am.* 1953;37:503–510.
149. Deyo RA, Rainville J, Kent DL. What can the history and physical examination tell us about low back pain? *JAMA.* 1992;268:760–765.
150. Brieg A, Troup JDG. Biomechanical consideration in the straight-leg-raising test: cadaveric and clinical studies of medial hip rotation. *Spine.* 1979;4:242–250.
151. Charnley J. Orthopedic signs in the diagnosis of disc protrusion with special reference to the straight leg raising test. *Lancet.* 1951;1:186–192.
152. Kosteljanetz M, Bang F, Schmidt-Olsen S. The clinical significance of straight-leg-raising (Lasegue's sign) in the diagnosis of prolapsed lumbar disc. *Spine.* 1988;13:393–395.
153. Shoqing X, Quanzhi Z, Dehao F. Significance of straight-leg-raising test in the diagnosis and clinical evaluation of lower lumbar intervertebral disc protrusion. *J Bone Joint Surg Am.* 1987;69:517–522.
154. Kortelainen P, Pruanen J, Koivisto E, Lahde S. Symptoms and signs of sciatica and their relation to the localization of the lumbar disc herniation. *Spine.* 1985;10:88–92.
155. Hakelius A, Hindmarsh J. The comparative reliability of preoperative diagnostic methods in lumbar disc surgery. *Acta Orthop Scand.* 1972;43:234–238.
156. Blower PW. Neurologic patterns in unilateral sciatica. *Spine.* 1981;6:175–179.
157. Aronson HA, Dunsmore RH. Herniated upper lumbar discs. *J Bone Joint Surg Am.* 1963;45:311–317.
158. Kostuik JP, Harrington I, Alexander D, Rand W, Evans D. Cauda equina syndrome and lumbar disc herniation. *J Bone Joint Surg Am.* 1986;68:386–391.
159. O'Laoire SA, Crockard HA, Thomas DG. Prognosis for sphincter recovery after operation for cauda equina compression owing to lumbar disc prolapse. *BMJ.* 1981;282: 1852–1854.
160. Tay ECK, Chacha PB. Midline prolapse of a lumbar intervertebral disc with compression of the cauda equina. *J Bone Joint Surg Br.* 1979;61:43–46.
161. Spitzer WO, LeBlanc FE, Dupuis M, et al. Scientific approach to the assessment and management of activity related spinal disorders: a monograph for clinicians: report of the Quebec Task Force on Spinal Disorders. *Spine.* 1987;12 (suppl 7):S16–S21.
162. Weisel SE, Tsourmas N, Feffer H, Citrin CM, Patronas N. A study of computer-assisted tomography. I: The incidence of positive CAT scans in an asymptomatic group of patients. *Spine.* 1984;9:549–551.
163. Boden SD, Davis DO, Dina TS, Patronas NJ, Weisel SW. Abnormal magnetic resonance scans of the lumbar spine in asymptomatic subjects. *J Bone Joint Surg Am.* 1990;72: 403–408.
164. Weinstein SM, Herring SA, Derby R. Contemporary concepts in spine care. Epidural steroid injections. *Spine.* 1995; 20:1842–1846.
165. Dirckx JH, ed. *Stedman's Concise Medical Dictionary for the Health Professional.* 3rd ed. Baltimore: Williams & Wilkins; 1997.
166. Turner JA, Ersek M, Herron L, Deyo R. Surgery for lumbar spinal stenosis: attempted metanalysis of the literature. *Spine.* 1986;11:436–439.
167. Dong GX, Porter RW. Walking and cycling tests in neurogenic and intermittent claudication. *Spine.* 1989;14: 965–969.
168. Porter RW. Spinal stenosis. *Semin Orthop.* 1989;1:97–111.
169. Fritz JM, Erhard RE, Vignovic M. A nonsurgical treatment approach for patients with lumbar spinal stenosis. *Phys Ther.* 1997;77:962–973.
170. Admundson GM, Wenger DR. Spondylolisthesis: natural history and treatment. *Spine.* 1987;1:323–328.
171. Zdeblick TA. The treatment of degenerative lumbar disorders: a critical review of the literature. *Spine.* 1995;20:126S–137S.
172. Steiner ME, Micheli LJ. Treatment of symptomatic spondylolysis and spondylolisthesis with the modified Boston brace. *Spine.* 1985;10:937–943.
173. Turner JA, Bianco AJ. Spondylolysis and spondylolisthesis in children. *J Bone Joint Surg Am.* 1971;53:1298–1306.
174. Vleeming A. Relation between for and function in the sacroiliac joint. Part I: Clinical and anatomical aspects. *Spine.* 1990;15:130–132.
175. Frymoyer JW, Krag MH. Spinal stability and instability: definitions, classification, and general principles of management. In: Dunsker SB, Schmidek HH, Frymoyer JW, et al, eds. *The Unstable Spine (Thoracic, Lumbar, and Sacral Regions).* Orlando, FL: Grune & Stratton; 1986:116.
176. Frymoyer JW, Akeson W, Brandt K, et al. Clinical perspectives. In: Frymoyer JW, Gordon SL, eds. *New Perspectives on Low Back Pain.* Park Ridge, IL: American Academy of Orthopedic Surgeons; 1989:222–230.
177. Onel D, Tuzlaci M, Saria H, Demir K. Computed tomographic investigation of the effect of traction on lumbar disc herniations. *Spine.* 1989;14:82–90.
178. Kane M, Karl RD, Swain JH. Effects of gravity facilitated traction on the intervertebral dimensions of the lumbar spine. *J Orthop Sports Phys Ther.* 1985;6:281–288.
179. Nachemson A, Elfstrom G. Intradiscal dynamic pressure measurements in the lumbar discs. *Scand J Rehabil Med.* 1970;51:10–40.
180. Bridger RS, Ossey S, Fourie G. Effect of lumbar traction on stature. *Spine.* 1990;15:522–524.
181. Gupta R, Romarao S. Epidurography in reduction of lumbar disc prolapse by traction. *Arch Phys Med Rehabil.* 1978; 59:322–327.
182. Crisp E. Discussion on the treatment of backache by traction. *Proc R Soc Med.* 1955;48:805–808.
183. Frazer E. The use of traction in backache. *Med J Aust.* 1954; 2:694–697.
184. Hood L, Chrisman D. Intermittent pelvic traction in the treatment of the ruptured intervertebral disc. *Phys Ther.* 1968;48:21–30.
185. Christie BGB. Discussion on the treatment of backache by traction. *Proc R Soc Med.* 1955;48:811–814.
186. Lindstron A, Zachrisson M. Physical therapy on low back pain and sciatica: an attempt at evaluation. *Scand J Rehabil Med.* 1970;2:37–42.
187. Pal B, Mangion P, Hossain MA, Diffey BL. A controlled trial of continuous lumbar traction in back pain and sciatica. *Br J Rheumatol.* 1986;2:181–183.
188. Weber H, Ljunggren AE, Walker L. Traction therapy in patients with herniated lumbar intervertebral discs. *J Oslo City Hosp.* 1984;34:62–70.
189. Larsson U, Choler U, Lidstrom A, et al. Autotraction for treatment of lumbago-sciatica: a multicentre controlled investigation. *Acta Orthop Scand.* 1980;51:791–798.
190. Saunders HD, Beissner KL. *Lumbar Traction.* LaCrosse, WI: Orthopedic Section of the American Physical Therapy Association; 1994.

CHAPTER 19

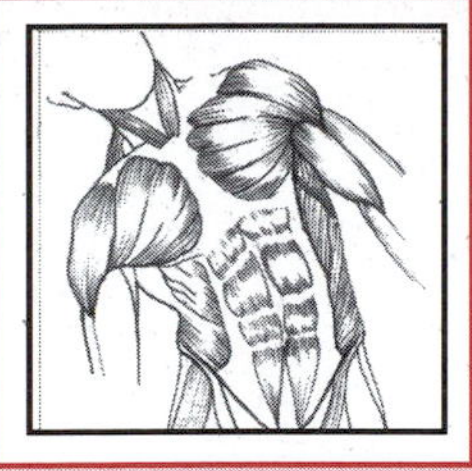

The Pelvic Floor

Beth Shelly

Impairments of the gynecologic, urinary, and gastrointestinal systems are often treated with medications or surgery. However, therapists have become increasingly involved in the rehabilitation of these patients, probably because of the positive outcomes seen with this type of treatment. Pelvic floor muscle (PFM) rehabilitation involves the skeletal muscles located at the base of the abdominal cavity. The *pelvic floor* refers collectively to tissues that span from the pubic bone to the coccyx. The area includes skeletal muscles under voluntary control, which respond to the same training techniques as other skeletal muscles in the body.

This chapter introduces students to the anatomy and kinesiology of the pelvic floor, physiology of micturition, and anatomic and psychological impairments of the pelvic floor. Management of common physiologic impairments of the pelvic floor, pelvic floor dysfunctions, and their impact on other areas of the body are described, and clinical applications are provided.

All physical therapists should screen patients for pelvic floor dysfunction and provide basic instruction in strengthening these skeletal muscles. This chapter provides screening and evaluation tools that do not require internal vaginal evaluation or surface electromyography (EMG) of the pelvic floor and explains how to teach pelvic floor exercises (PFEs), which strengthen the PFMs and specifically address impaired muscle performance. PFE is the proper term for PFM contractions without a device or object in the vagina. Arnold Kegel was an obstetrician who pioneered PFM strengthening in the 1940s. The Kegel exercise, as it is commonly known, is a contraction of the PFMs around an object, preferably a pressure biofeedback device. Patients often use Kegel exercises and PFE synonymously, and it may be less confusing for some patients to call all PFEs "Kegels." This chapter discusses pelvic pain associated with PFM dysfunction, but information about normal function of the lumbopelvic and hip structures should also be reviewed (see Chapters 18 and 20).

The therapist must know how to evaluate all of the structures of the pelvic floor to understand the medical diagnoses and treatment interventions for PFM dysfunction. A complete evaluation of this area requires intravaginal palpation and often includes surface EMG evaluation. This type of evaluation is usually not an entry-level skill, and postgraduate study is recommended for therapists interested in directly treating the PFMs.

REVIEW OF ANATOMY AND KINESIOLOGY

The many inconsistencies in labeling the structures of the pelvic floor found in the medical literature can make the study of these muscles confusing. This section outlines the current terminology used by most physical therapists. Kegel described the pelvic floor as five layers of fascia and muscles attached to the bony ring of the pelvis. Layers 1, 2, and 3 are skeletal muscles. Layer 4 is the smooth muscle sphincter of the bladder neck, and layer 5 is the endopelvic fascia. Because most patients with pelvic floor dysfunction are female,

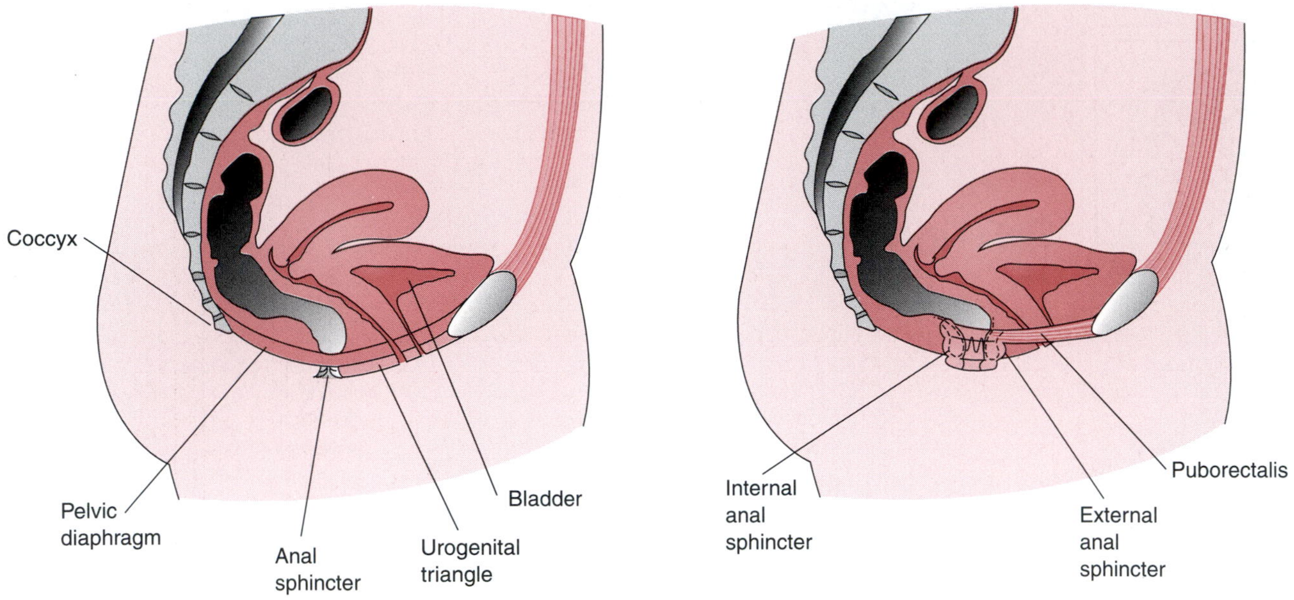

FIGURE 19-1 Pelvic floor muscle layers.

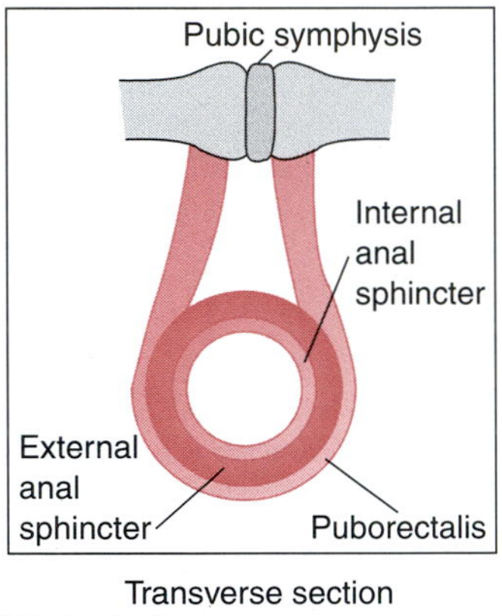

FIGURE 19-2 Anal sphincter.

female anatomy is discussed in this chapter, but the pelvic diaphragm layers and associated muscles are essentially the same in both sexes.

Skeletal Muscles

The skeletal muscles of the pelvic floor (Fig. 19-1) can be divided into four layers, from superficial to deep: (1) the anal sphincter; the urogenital triangle, which includes the (2) superficial perineal muscles and the (3) urogenital diaphragm; and the (4) pelvic diaphragm.

The *anal sphincter* (Fig. 19-2) is the most superficial skeletal muscle. The anal sphincter is made up of the internal anal sphincter (ie, smooth muscle) and the external anal sphincter (ie, skeletal muscle). These sphincters fuse superiorly with the puborectalis sling of the pelvic diaphragm muscle. These three muscles function together to provide fecal continence. Neurologic innervation is provided from the fourth sacral nerve and inferior branch of the pudendal nerve.

The *urogenital triangle* consists of the *superficial perineal muscles* (Fig. 19-3), which aid in the sexual function of the pelvic floor, and the *urogenital diaphragm* (Fig. 19-4), which is part of the continence mechanism of the pelvic floor. The three superficial perineal muscles are

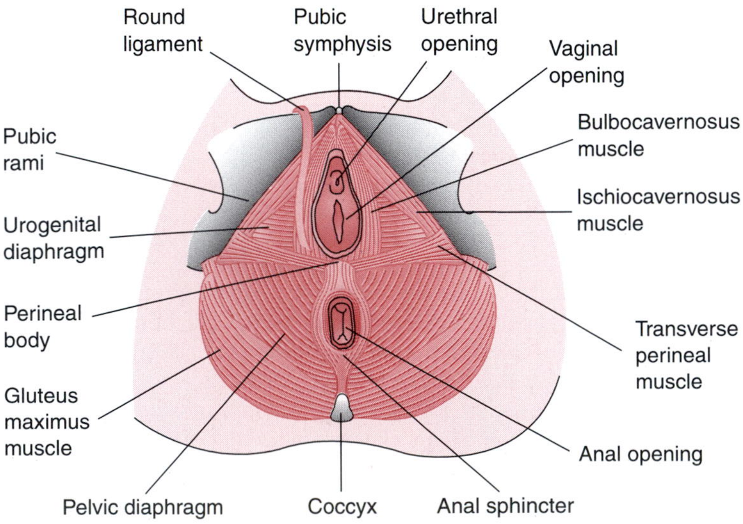

FIGURE 19-3 Female pelvic flow muscles—inferior view.

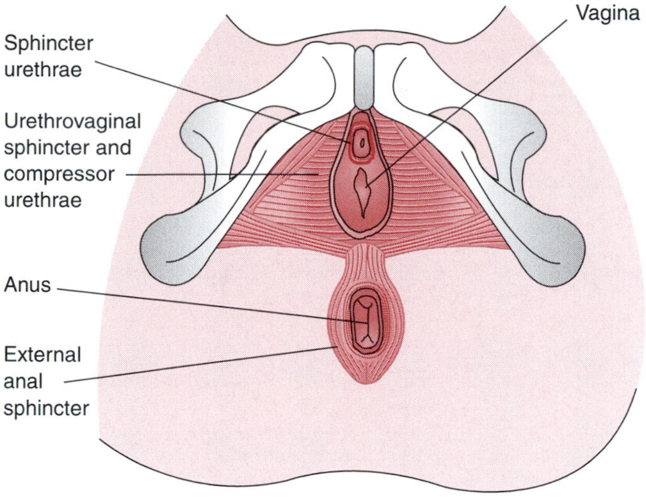

A

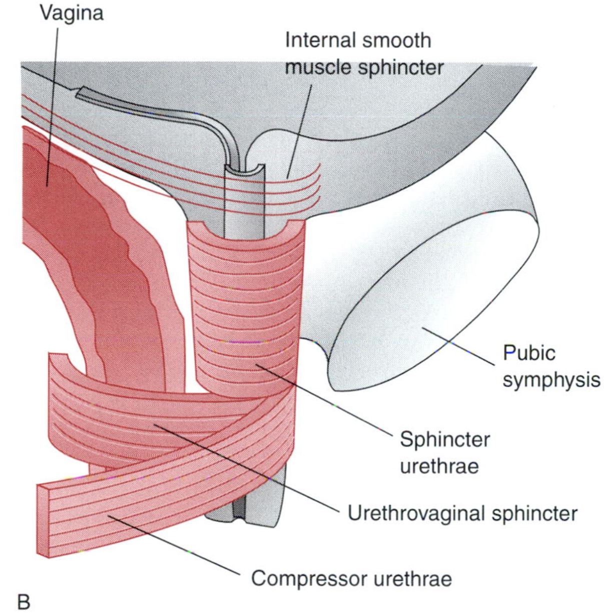

B

FIGURE 19-4 Female urogenital triangle: ***(A)*** Inferior view. ***(B)*** Side view. (Schussler B, Laycock J, Norton P, Stanton S, eds. *Pelvic Floor Re-education Principles and Practice.* New York: Springer-Verlag; 1994).

the bulbocavernosus, the ischiocavernosus, and the superficial transverse perineal. The three muscles of the urogenital diaphragm are the urethrovaginal sphincter, the compressor urethrae (formerly known together as the deep transverse perineal), and the sphincter urethrae[2–4] (Table 19-1).

Pelvic Diaphragm Muscles

The pelvic diaphragm (Fig. 19-5) is the largest muscle group in the pelvic floor and is responsible for most of the function or dysfunction of this area. This layer is divided into the coccygeus muscle and the levator ani muscles.

The coccygeus muscle originates on the spine of the ischium, inserts on the anterior portion of the coccyx and S4, and is innervated by the ventral rami of sacral nerves 4 and 5. In other mammals, this muscle controls tail movement. In humans, the coccygeus flexes the coccyx and may help stabilize the sacrum through its sacrococcygeal attachments.[4]

The levator ani muscle is further divided into the pubococcygeus and the iliococcygeus muscles. The iliococcygeus originates from the pubic ramus and arcus tendentious ligament (an extension of the obturator internus fascia) and inserts onto the coccyx. The pubococcygeus muscle is divided into the pubovaginalis and puborectalis muscles. The pubovaginalis originates at the posterior aspect of the os pubis and inserts on the perineal body and vaginal walls, forming a sling around the vagina. The puborectalis, originating from the pubic bone and obturator internus fascia and inserting onto the coccyx and lateral walls of the rectum, similarly forms a sling around the rectum. The innervation of the levator ani muscles is from the inferior rectal brace of the pudendal nerve of S2 through S4 and ventral rami of S2 through S4 (Table 19-2). The function of the levator ani muscles is to support the pelvic viscera and compress the vagina, urethra, and rectum for continence.

The pelvic diaphragm muscles are approximately 70% slow-twitch muscle fibers (type 1) and 30% fast-twitch muscle fibers (type 2).[2] Both types of muscle fibers have specific functions in the pelvic floor, and a complete exercise program must train both types of muscle fibers. The physiology of these muscles is similar to that of other skeletal muscles. The PFMs have the sensation of proprioception and deep pressure through the pudendal nerve. They respond to quick stretch and have extensive fascia throughout the muscle layers (see Table 19-2).

The PFMs contract as a unit to achieve various functions. Impairments can occur in a single layer or throughout the entire pelvic diaphragm. The remainder of the discussion of PFMs focuses on the pelvic diaphragm muscles because they are the largest in the pelvic floor and are responsible for most of its functions.

Related Muscles

The piriformis and the obturator internus are located with in the pelvis and can affect the function of the PFMs. The piriformis originates on the anterior surface of S1 to S4[5,6] (Fig. 19-6). Its inferior border is close to the superior border of the coccygeus muscle, and it inserts at the greater trochanter of the femur (Fig. 19-7).

The obturator internus originates at the inner rim of the obturator foramen and inserts onto the greater trochanter. The levator ani muscles attach to an extension of the obturator internus fascia (ie, the arcus tendinous, also called the white line). This muscle is best envisioned three dimensionally. It may help to look at a pelvic model with muscles to gain an understanding of the relationship of these two muscles. Impairments in length, strength, endurance, and patterns of recruitment of the piriformis and obturator internus muscles often contribute to PFM impairments and vice versa. Hip function may need to be considered with pelvic floor dysfunction and pelvic floor dysfunction with hip dysfunction.

The adductor muscle group also may participate in the PFM pain syndrome. Each muscle originates at the pubic

Table 19-1. MUSCLES OF THE UROGENITAL TRIANGLE

MUSCLE	ORIGIN	INSERTION	INNERVATION	FUNCTION
Superficial perineal				
Bulbocavernosus	Corpus cavernosum of the clitoris	Perineal body	Perineal branch of pudendal S2-S4	Clitoral erection
Ischiocavernosus	Ischial tuberosity and pubic rami	Crus of the clitoris	Perineal branch of pudendal S2-S4	Clitoral erection
Superficial Transverse perineal	Ischial tuberosity	Central perineal tendon	Perineal branch of pudendal S2-S4	Stabilizes perineal body
Urogenital diaphragm				
Urethrovaginal sphincter	Vaginal wall	Urethra	Perineal branch of pudendal S2-S4	Compression of urethra
Sphincter urethrea	Upper two thirds of urethra	Trigone ring	Perineal branch of pudendal S2-S4	Compression of urethra
Compressor urethrea	Ischiopubic rami	Urethra	Perineal branch of pudendal S2-S4	Compression of urethra

ramus and ischial tuberosity and inserts on the posterior femur and medial femoral condyle. The muscle is innervated by the obturator and sciatic nerves. Adductor fascia at the pubic rami is close to the superficial perineal muscle fascia.

The psoas minor and major muscles originate from vertebral bodies and disks of T12 through L5. The iliacus muscle originates at the medial iliac fossa. Both muscles fuse and travel in an anteroinferior direction under the inguinal ligament to insert onto the lesser trochanter of the femur. The iliopsoas muscle is innervated by the L2 through L4 spinal nerves. It is a key muscle to treat in lumbopelvic dysfunctions. Travell and Simons[5] call it the *hidden prankster* and stress its importance in pelvic dysfunctions.

Pelvic Floor Function

Kegel[7] defined the pelvic floor functions as supportive, sphincteric, and sexual.

SUPPORTIVE FUNCTION

The pelvic floor provides support to the pelvic organs. DeLancey and Richardson[3] stated that normal pelvic organ support is achieved by ligamentous support from above and PFM function from below. They also observed that recovery of organ support requires attention to restoring ligament support (ie, surgery) and restoring pelvic floor function (ie, pelvic floor rehabilitation). At rest, the PFMs maintain a minimal resting tone. The muscle activity increases with increased intra-abdominal pressure. The forces of gravity and increased intra-abdominal pressure (eg, laugh, cough, sneeze, vomit, lift, strain) encourage prolapse or protrusion of the pelvic organs. Strong PFMs help to support the organs against increased intra-abdominal pressure and enhance normal functioning. The supportive function is primarily performed by the tonic, slow-twitch muscle fibers.

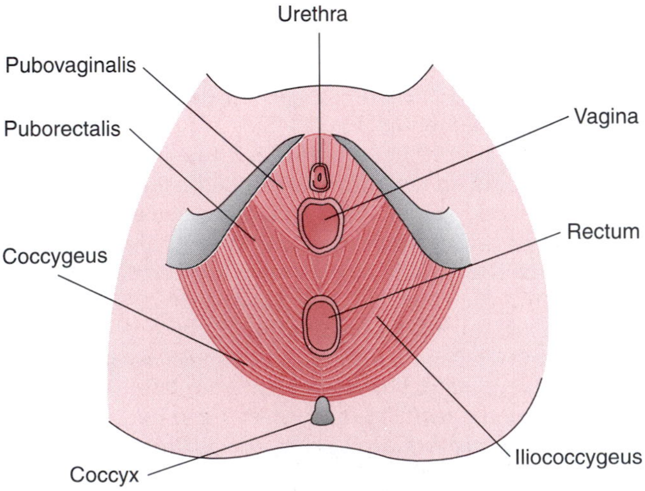

FIGURE 19-5 Female pelvic diaphragm—superior view.

SPHINCTERIC FUNCTION

The PFMs provide closure of the urethra and rectum for continence. During normal function, quick closure of the orifices is provided by the phasic, fast-twitch fibers of the pelvic floor. Closure during rest (ie, static resting tone) is provided by the slow-twitch muscle fibers. Continence is preserved when the pressure in the urethra (provided by several structures including the PFMs) is higher than the pressure in the bladder. Loss of sphincteric function may lead to incontinence. The medical literature commonly points out that incontinence is a symptom and not a disease; based on the terminology used in this book, incontinence results from impairments, not a pathologic condition. Intervention should be aimed at the impairments that contribute to the syndrome of incontinence.

SEXUAL FUNCTION

The vagina has very few sensory nerve fibers.[8] The PFMs provide proprioceptive sensation that contributes to sexual appreciation. Hypertrophied PFMs provide a smaller vagina and more friction against the penis during intercourse. This results in stimulation of more nerve endings and provides pleasurable sensation during intercourse. Strong pelvic floor contractions occur during orgasm. Patients with weak PFMs often cannot achieve orgasms.[8] In men, the PFMs assist in achieving and maintaining an erection.

Table 19-2. COCCYGEUS MUSCLE AND LEVATOR ANI MUSCLES

MUSCLE	ORIGIN	INSERTION	INNERVATION	FUNCTION
Coccygeus muscle	Spine of the ischium	Anterior portion of the coccyx and S4	Ventral rami, S4 and S5	Flex the coccyx
Levator ani muscles			Inferior rectal branch of the pudendal nerve, S2-S4, ventral rami, S2-S4	Support of the pelvic viscera, continence mechanism
Pubococcygeus				
Pubovaginalis	Posterior os pubis	Perineal body, vaginal walls		Compression of the vagina and urethra
Puborectalis	Pubic bone, arcus tendinous	Anterior coccyx, lateral rectum		Compression of the rectum
Iliococcygeus	Pubic rami, arcus tendinous	Coccyx		

Physiology of Micturition

Micturition refers to the physiologic process of urination and involves a complex set of somatic and autonomic reflexes. An explanation of micturition is provided in Display 19-1. This information is included so the therapist can explain the basics of normal bladder function to the patient and assist with basic bladder retraining.

Urine is produced steadily at about 15 drops per minute. Bladder filling is constant, except in the presence of bladder irritants, which increase urine production. There is always urine in the bladder. Urine continues to collect, and the bladder passively expands until approximately 150 mL of fluid is collected. Stretch receptors in the bladder then signal the brain that it may be necessary to get to the bathroom soon. This is called the first sensation to void. The detrusor muscle (ie, muscle of the bladder) remains quiet, and the PFMs maintain normal resting tone. Filling continues until 200 to 300 mL, when a stronger sensation of urgency is felt from increased activation of stretch receptors. The detrusor and PFMs remain unchanged. A severe urge to void usually occurs at 400 to 550 mL.[4] The brain eventually directs the person to a toilet, clothes are removed, and the person either sits on or stands over the toilet. The PFMs relax, the detrusor contracts, and urine flows out.[2] The PFMs return to resting tone when urine flow stops. Postvoid residual studies show how much urine is left in the bladder after urination. Normative values vary, but most practitioners think it is normal to have 5 to 50 mL of urine left in the bladder after a normal urination. It is neither necessary nor desirable to increase intra-abdominal pressure (ie, bear down) at any time during urination.

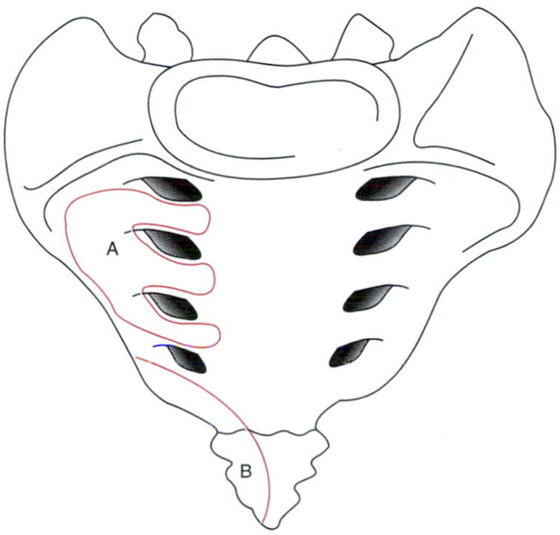

FIGURE 19-6 The anterior sacrum. Origin of the piriformis ***(A)*** and coccygeus ***(B)***.

Dysfunctions of micturition are complex. The screening questionnaires on page 360 can help identify patients with dysfunctions of micturition that may need further medical intervention and who should be referred to the physician.

ANATOMIC IMPAIRMENTS

Many factors contribute to normal function of the PFMs. Some of these factors cannot be changed by physical therapy interventions. The two major causes of anatomic impairments are birth injury and neurologic dysfunction.

Birth Injury

Vaginal delivery may result in tears, overstretching, or crush injury of the PFMs (ie, between baby's head and pubic rami) or may cause complete or partial denervation of unilateral or bilateral pudendal nerves (ie, stretch injury or avulsion of the nerve).

Birth injuries account for a significant percentage of PFM dysfunction. Mild and moderate injuries can be effectively treated with behavioral interventions (see the Impaired Muscle Performance section). However, severe trauma may result in severe muscle damage (usually unilateral) and decreased sensory or motor innervation sufficient to render the muscle ineffective. This type of trauma occurs in a very small percentage of births. Very fast deliveries do not allow time for tissue stretch and may result in a "burst" effect, extensively tearing the tissue. Deliveries with a pushing phase

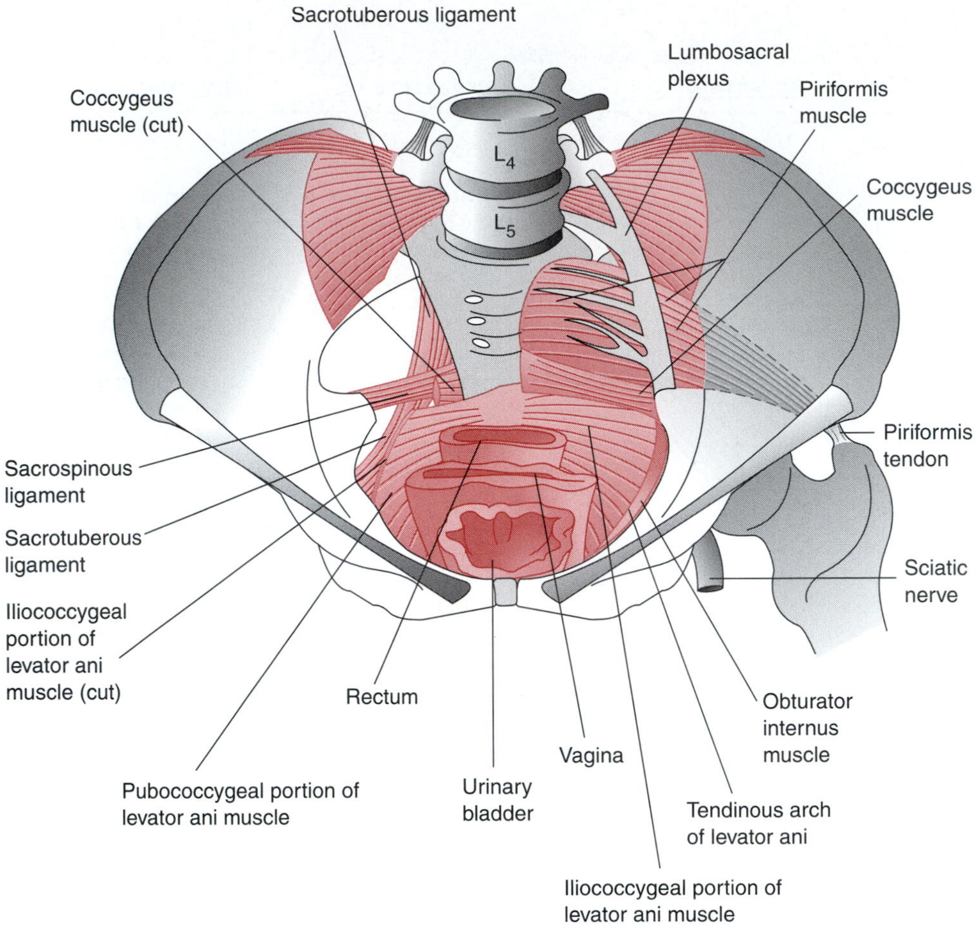

FIGURE 19-7 Piriformis and pelvic area—superior view.

longer than 2 hours may result in stretch injury to nerves and muscles. Use of forceps to assist delivery may result in increased trauma to the muscles. Many other factors during delivery may influence PFM outcomes, including the woman's position, leg position, size of the baby, medical interventions, and medications given. However, most women with vaginal deliveries sustain only minor, temporary dysfunctions and recover fully. To maximize birth recovery, all women of childbearing age should receive accurate preventative education on PFM health.

Neurologic Dysfunction

Many central and peripheral nervous system dysfunctions affect PFM function. Peripheral nervous system conditions, such as disk herniation and spinal cord injury, may result in sensory or motor denervation of the PFMs. Diabetes may result in sensory or motor denervation of the PFMs and autonomic neuropathy with disruption of bladder function. The pelvic plexus includes many small nerves that are often not visible during surgery. These nerves are not located in a consistent pattern in all patients. Radical pelvic operations, such as total hysterectomy and radical prostatectomy, may result in inadvertent disruption of the sensory and motor nerves to the bladder and PFMs. Patients may be able to strengthen the remaining innervated muscle to achieve full supportive and sphincteric function. Central nervous system diseases such as cerebrovascular accidents, multiple sclerosis, and Parkinson's disease may affect cognitive control of bladder and PFMs. These conditions may also affect the patient's ability to get to the toilet or to recognize the toilet and may affect the patient's social awareness of continence.

PSYCHOLOGICAL IMPAIRMENTS

Motivation

PFM strengthening requires motivation and persistence. Improvement in muscle function with PFM therapy can be quick and dramatic, but it is more often slow and gradual. Some patients do not have enough motivation to complete therapy and find it easier to wear incontinence pads. Incontinence affects patients' lives differently. Some patients are devastated and severely limited by a small amount of urine leaking two or three times per week. Other patients view large leaks two or three times per day as a mild inconvenience. The perceived severity of the condition helps determine motivation. Ask the patient, "On a scale of 0 to 10, how severely does your condition affect your life (0 = no effect; 10 = severely limiting)." Therapists must strongly encourage patients throughout therapy to maintain motivation. Depression and poor motivation may limit a patient's progress with PFE.

DISPLAY 19-1
Micturition Facts

- The bladder's job is to store urine and empty fully at the appropriate time and place.
- It is necessary to allow normal filling of the bladder for normal bladder function. A person should not go to the bathroom "just in case."
- It is important to drink six to eight 8-ounce glasses of fluid per day. Decreasing fluids does not decrease incontinence and may make urgency worse because concentrated urine is a bladder irritant.[9]
- It is normal to urinate six to eight times in a 24-hour period with normal fluid intake. More than eight times per day is called *urinary frequency.* In rare cases, the physician instructs patients to empty more frequently.
- The normal voiding interval is 2 to 5 hours.
- Normal nocturnal voiding frequency (after the patient has gone to bed for the evening) is zero to one time per night for children and adults younger than 65 years of age and one to two times per night for adults older than 65 years of age.
- Each urination stream should last 8 to 10 seconds. If urination is completed in 2 to 3 seconds, the voiding interval could have been longer.
- Squatting over the toilet may result in incomplete emptying of the bladder. Overflow from the adductors and gluteals to the PFM results in increased tone in the PFM and decreased urine flowing out.
- Many fluids can irritate the bladder, causing urgency and increasing urine production. The most common *bladder irritants* are caffeine (eg, coffee, tea, cola, medications, chocolate), alcohol, carbonated beverages, and nicotine. Many other substances can be irritants, including artificial sweeteners, citrus, and some over-the-counter and prescription medications. Eliminating or limiting bladder irritants decreases symptoms of urgency and urge incontinence.
- Women should always clean well after using the toilet by reaching around behind and wiping from front to back. This ensures that fecal matter is not introduced into the urethra and decreases the incidence of infection.

Sexual Abuse

An estimated one of three girls has been abused before the age of 14. Only one of five cases is reported. Some studies show that there is a higher incidence of incontinence, pelvic pain, and fibromyalgia among sexual abuse survivors. All therapists should be aware of symptoms of sexual abuse (Display 19-2) and should have some exposure to techniques to facilitate rehabilitation of these patients (Display 19-3). It is especially important to be sensitive to these issues when treating PFM dysfunction and pelvic pain. Therapists are encouraged to seek additional information on sexual abuse survivors (see the Recommended Reading section).

EVALUATION OR EXAMINATION

Every patient should be screened for PFM dysfunction. Understanding the risk factors for PFM dysfunction helps the therapist identify patients who may need more in-depth questioning about PFM function. Screening tools are provided to identify PFM impairments and dysfunctions. This section also outlines the information that is gathered by specialized therapists from internal vaginal examinations and from patient self-evaluations.

DISPLAY 19-2
Symptoms of Sexual Abuse

- Low self-esteem, feelings of loss of control
- Poor body awareness, often not trusting their own physical or emotional feelings
- Difficulty with anger and violence
- Difficulty with sexuality and intimacy; may avoid sex completely or compulsively seek sex
- Denies and forgets instructions or appointments
- Self-mutilating or addictive behaviors
- Controlling of environment, treatment, or your time
- Multiple personalities
- Dissociation (ie, avoidance of eye contact, distant look), an unconscious defense mechanism to separate the mind from the body and protect the mind from impending trauma; may occur during the treatment sessions

Risk Factors

The brief screening questionnaire should be given to all patients. Patients with medical histories that include many of these risk factors may be screened using the long form. Risk factors are related to the causes of various dysfunctions (Display 19-4).

Screening Questionnaires

Two types of screening questionnaires can be used to determine whether patients have dysfunctions of the pelvic floor. Questions should be clear and direct. A broad question such as "Are you incontinent?" usually results in a false-negative response.

BRIEF SCREENING QUESTIONNAIRE

Evaluation of all patients, especially those with the risk factors listed in Display 19-4, should include three questions:

DISPLAY 19-3
Guidelines for Therapy With Known or Suspected Sexual Abuse Survivors

- Give the patient control over as much as you can in the environment and in therapy.
- Offer names of community support services and psychologists skilled in the treatment of sexual abuse survivors.
- Do not touch the patient without her permission, and avoid hugging or other nonessential physical contact.
- Never allow the patient to disassociate.
- Be honest with the patient about your ability and knowledge (or lack of) in this area.

DISPLAY 19-4

Risk Factors for Supportive Dysfunction and Hypertonia Dysfunction

Supportive Dysfunction

- Vaginal childbirth
- Pregnancy
- Obesity
- Chronic or prolonged coughing, as with pulmonary diseases
- Severe bulimia with chronic vomiting
- Long-term incorrect lifting or straining with a Valsalva maneuver (ie, increased intraabdominal pressure with bearing down), including incorrect straining with exercise
- Chronic constipation
- Pelvic congestion or swelling
- Neurologic dysfunctions that may affect peripheral nerves of the pelvis and many central nervous system diseases
- Decreased awareness of pelvic floor muscles (PFM) with disuse atrophy
- Pelvic surgery

Hypertonia Dysfunction

- Back and pelvic pain with joint dysfunction, especially if related to a direct fall on the buttock or pubic bone
- Muscle imbalance of the hip muscles, abdomen or pelvis, or lumbar spine, including shortened muscles or connective tissue in the trunk and pelvis
- Habitual PFM holding (eg, excessive emotional stress)
- Abdominal adhesions and adhered scars in the pelvic region
- Deep episiotomy or perineal tearing with childbirth
- Pelvic surgery
- Pelvic inflammatory conditions, such as endometriosis or irritable bowel
- History of or current fissures or fistulas
- Connective tissue disease such as fibromyalgia
- History of sexual abuse
- History of or current sexually transmitted disease or recurrent perineal infections, including yeast infections
- Dermatologic conditions such as lichen sclerosis and lichen planus

- Do you ever leak urine or feces?
- Do you ever wear a pad because of leaking urine?
- Do you have pain during intercourse?

FULL SCREENING QUESTIONNAIRE

Therapists must understand the dysfunctions of the pelvic floor and their diagnostic classifications and the types of incontinence to fully understand interpretation of the results of this screening tool. The full screening questionnaire should be given if the patient responds affirmatively to the questions of the brief screening questionnaire. The longer version should be administered to a patient with pelvic, trunk, or back pain who is recovering slower than expected. The patient should respond with *never, sometimes,* or *often* to the questions:

1. Do you leak urine when you cough, laugh, or sneeze?
2. Do you lose urine when you lift heavy objects such as a basket of wet clothes or furniture?
3. Do you lose urine when you run, jump, or exercise?
4. Do you ever have such an uncomfortable, strong need to urinate that you leak if you do not reach the toilet? Do you sometimes leak with this strong urge?
5. Do you develop an urgent need to urinate when you hear running water?
6. Do you develop an urgent need to urinate when you are nervous, under stress, or in a hurry?
7. When you are coming home, can you usually make it to the door but then lose urine just as you put the key in the lock?
8. Do you have an urge to urinate when your hands are in cold water?
9. Do you find it necessary to wear a pad at any time because of leakage?
10. Does your bladder awaken you from sleep? How many times each night?
11. How often do you leak urine or feces?
12. How often do you inadvertently leak gas?
13. Do ever feel like you are "sitting on a ball" or that there is something "in the way" when you are sitting?
14. Do you ever feel like something is "falling out" of your perineal area?
15. Do you find it hard to begin urination?
16. Do you have a slow urinary stream?
17. Do you strain to pass urine?
18. Do you have pain during vaginal penetration, including intercourse, insertion of a tampon, or vaginal examination?
19. Do you have pelvic pain with sitting, wearing jeans, or bike riding?

Questions 1 through 14 may indicate a PFM supportive dysfunction or urgency that may be treated using PFEs. A positive response to questions 1 through 3 indicates symptoms of stress incontinence. A positive response to questions 4 through 8 indicates symptoms of urge incontinence. A positive response to questions 18 and 19 may indicate organ prolapse. Questions 13 through 19 may indicate hypertonia, incoordination, or obstruction. Patients with incoordination may benefit from PFEs. However, if the patient has symptoms of obstruction (ie, positive responses only to questions 15 through 17), she should be referred to the physician. If patient has symptoms of hypertonia (ie, positive response to questions 13 through 19), proceed with full evaluation of the sacroiliac, hip girdle, and pelvic fascia.

Results of the Internal Examination

A complete PFM evaluation is necessary to prescribe an appropriate exercise program for the PFMs. It includes an extensive history, symptom documentation, identification of associated factors, internal vaginal and rectal examinations, and surface EMG or pressure biofeedback evaluation. The specialized therapist obtains the following information from the internal examination of the PFMs:

Power is the ability to contract (manual muscle grade of 0 through 5). This grade provides information on how much lift (ie, supportive function) and closure (ie, sphincteric function) the PFMs have. The muscle bulk of the PFMs can be palpated to help determine possible duration of rehabilitation and rehabilitation potential. Patients with a small, thin PFMs require a longer rehabilitation time and generally have less rehabilitation potential than those with good PFM bulk.

Endurance is the ability to hold a slow-twitch muscle contraction and repeat the contraction. Therapists also determine how many fast-twitch muscle contractions can be done. The quality of the contractions is evaluated.

Resting tone between contractions is assessed, looking specifically for altered tone impairments.

Coordination of the muscles and contraction of other muscles, especially the gluteals, adductors, and abdominals, are assessed.

Other impairments, such as pelvic floor trigger points, decreased sensation, and scars or myofascial adhesions, may limit strengthening.

Internal examination of the PFMs is the gold standard evaluation. However, internal examinations cannot or should not be performed in some cases (Display 19-5).

Patient Self-Assessment Tests

When an internal evaluation cannot be performed, self-assessment tests can help patients and the therapist identify some of the impairments of the PFMs. Therapists can use the results of self-assessment tests to prescribe PFEs with some accuracy.

Two possible evaluation tools used when an internal evaluation cannot be performed include the stop test and digital vaginal self-examination (ie, finger in the vagina test). Begin with patient education, as outlined later in the Teaching Pelvic Floor Exercises section. This section also includes information about verbal cues for the proper contraction of PFMs. After a brief introduction to the PFMs and the exercise, the patient should be instructed in the stop test and digital vaginal self-examination test (see Patient-Related Instruction: Testing Your Pelvic Floor Muscle Ability by Performing the Stop Test and Digital Vaginal Self-Examination [Finger in the Vagina Test]). Digital vaginal self-examination is often accepted by female patients and can be taught to male patients (ie, finger in the rectum test) in the same manner if they are having trouble learning the correct contraction with other methods. Many factors influence continence and PFM function.

These tests cannot evaluate all aspects of muscle function, but they can give some indication of the muscles' abilities and provide guidance in prescribing exercises. Patient progress is judged by decreasing symptoms. Studies of stop test results have shown a positive correlation between PFM strength and the patient's ability to stop urine quickly.[10] Patients can perform the exercises at home and report to the therapist, or the exercises can be done in the clinic if sufficient privacy is available (ie, closed-door treatment room with a plinth or recliner is suggested). In the clinic, the therapist can briefly step out of the room while the patient performs the test or can remain in the treatment room with the patient adequately draped. The patient should provide the following information:

- Duration (in seconds) of slow-twitch muscle contraction hold
- Number of repetitions of slow-twitch muscle contractions
- Number of repetitions of fast-twitch muscle contractions
- Stop test grade

A third self-assessment test, the jumping jack test, is a test of advanced strength (see Patient-Related Instruction: Jumping Jack Test). It is usually not given to sedentary, incontinent patients. It is helpful for athletes and other active individuals who know how to do the PFE well. It is often used by patients to judge continued progress after active therapy has ended.

> **DISPLAY 19-5**
> **Contraindications to Internal Evaluation of the Pelvic Floor Muscle**
>
> - Pregnancy
> - Within 6 weeks of vaginal or cesarean delivery
> - Within 6 weeks after pelvic surgery
> - Atrophic vaginitis, a condition of fragile skin seen in cases of estrogen deficiency
> - Active pelvic infection
> - Severe pelvic or vaginal pain, especially pain during penetration or intercourse
> - Children and presexual adolescents
> - Lack of informed consent
> - Lack of therapist's training (The therapist should obtain specialized training in performing internal evaluations of the pelvic floor muscle. Training can be obtained in postgraduate courses or through individual instruction from a midwife, physician, nurse, or trained physical therapist.)

THERAPEUTIC EXERCISE INTERVENTIONS FOR COMMON PHYSIOLOGIC IMPAIRMENTS

This section outlines the physiologic impairments and possible treatments of the PFMs and related structures. Several types of impaired PFM function are possible:

- Impaired performance of the PFMs, abdominal muscles, and hip muscles
- Endurance impairments of the PFMs
- Pain and altered tone of the PFMs, hip muscles, and trunk muscles
- Mobility impairments causing PFM dysfunction as a result of adhesions, scar tissue, and connective tissue disorders
- Posture impairments
- Coordination impairments of the PFMs, PFMs during activities of daily living (ADLs), PFMs with the abdominals, and abdominal muscles alone

Impaired Muscle Performance

PELVIC FLOOR MUSCLES

Impaired muscle performance is the most commonly treated impairment of the PFMs. Impairments may include

Patient-Related Instruction

Testing Your Pelvic Floor Muscle by Performing the Stop Test and Digital Vaginal Self-Examination (Finger in the Vagina Test)

The following two tests can help you monitor your recovery. Perform these tests before beginning your pelvic floor exercise program and then periodically throughout the training period (finger in the vagina test approximately every 2 weeks and the stop test about every 4 weeks). Fluctuations in muscle ability occur in response to fatigue, medications, hormones, and other factors. The pelvic floor muscles are more likely to be weak at the end of the day, when you are sick, and just before menstruation.[8] For an accurate comparison, repeat these tests at the same time of the day and the same time of the monthly menstrual cycle as the original test. Any exercise program takes time and dedication. Like other muscles, the pelvic floor muscles may take 4 to 6 months to strengthen. After you have performed these two tests, report the following information to your therapist: stop test results, how many seconds you can hold the contraction, how many of these long-hold contractions you can do, how many quick contractions you can do.

The Stop Test

This test is used to determine the exercise position. Studies have shown that the ability to stop urine quickly correlates with good muscle function (ie, no leaking urine in most cases). This is not a direct measure of muscle strength, but it gives you some indication of the function of the muscle. Do not perform this test at your first morning urination. Sit down on the toilet and begin urinating. Try to stop the flow of urine abruptly and completely by squeezing the pelvic floor muscles. Men must hold the penis down into the toilet, because contraction of the pelvic floor causes the penis to move upward. If urine can be stopped abruptly and repeatedly, the muscle function is judged to be good (5/5). If you can stop the flow of urine once but cannot repeat this at the same sitting, your muscle function is fair (3/5). In this case, you should do the pelvic floor exercises in the upright sitting position against gravity. If your muscle function is poor (2/5), you can only slow the stream of urine. Very poor muscle tone (1/5) may not be able to slow the urine stream at all. If you are not able to stop the stream of urine, you should do the pelvic floor exercises lying down, eliminating the effects of gravity.

This technique is only a test. It should not be used as a regular exercise. The stop test should not be done more than once each month and is used only to determine in which position you should exercise. Repeated pelvic floor contraction during urination may disrupt the complex voiding reflexes and result in further bladder dysfunction.

TEST GRADE	DESCRIPTION OF FUNCTION	RESULTS OF STOP TEST	EXERCISE POSITION
5/5	Good	Urine stops abruptly and stopping can be repeated	All positions: stand, sit, lying down
4/5	Fairly good	Urine stops abruptly but can not be repeated	All positions: stand, sit, lying down
3/5	Fair	Can stop the flow of urine slowly and with difficulty	Sitting, lying down on back or side
2/5	Poor	Can slow the stream of urine but cannot stop it	Lying down on back or side
1/5	Very poor	Unable to slow the stream of urine	Lying down on back or side, hips in an elevated position

Digital Vaginal Self-Examination (Finger in Vagina or Rectum)

Place your finger into the vagina or rectum up to the level of the second knuckle. Palpate the muscle on either side of the vagina or rectum while you contract the pelvic floor muscle, pulling the muscles up and in. You should feel the muscles contract around your finger and pull your finger up and in. If you feel tissues pushing out of your body or bulging, ask your health care professional to evaluate the area. Determine how long you can hold the pelvic floor contraction and how many times you can repeat that contraction. Then perform quick maximal contractions (1-second hold). Count the number of quick contractions you can perform before the muscle tires.

weakness, increased length of PFMs or PFM tendons, or PFM atrophy.

PFM performance may be impaired by trauma during vaginal delivery, central nervous system (CNS) or peripheral nervous system (PNS) neurologic dysfunction, surgical procedures, decreased awareness of PFMs, disuse, prolonged increased intra-abdominal pressure, pelvic congestion or swelling, and back or pelvic pain. Impaired muscle performance is usually the primary impairment in the supportive dysfunction diagnostic classification, because loss of strength and increased length of muscle cannot fulfill the supportive function of the muscle. Weak, saggy muscles do not support the pelvic organs and result in supportive dysfunction of the PFMs. Lengthened muscles may result in pain and pressure in the perineum because structures "hang" on the ligamentous supports and stretch the nerves.

The treatment for impaired muscle performance is active PFEs. These strengthening exercises are explained later in in the Active Pelvic Floor Exercises section.

ABDOMINAL MUSCLES

Impaired abdominal muscle performance often results in a pendulous abdomen and can contribute to PFM dysfunction, especially incontinence. Restoring abdominal wall length and strength and avoiding Valsalva maneuvers are the goals of PFM dysfunction treatment.

Treatment of impaired abdominal muscle performance is described in Chapter 18. Patients with PFM dysfunction

> ***Patient-Related Instruction***
>
> ***Jumping Jack Test***
>
> This test is used only to evaluate pelvic floor muscle strength under physical stress. Do not perform this test until you can stop the urine flow at least once during urination. To begin, empty your bladder, and then perform five jumping jacks. If no urine leaks out, wait one-half hour, and do five more jumping jacks. If no leakage occurs, wait one-half hour, and repeat the five jumping jacks. The test proceeds until leakage occurs. Make a note of how long after urination and how many jumping jacks you could do before urine leakage occurs. There are no normative values for this test, but some therapists feel a patient should be able to do five to 10 jumping jacks 2 to 3 hours after urination without leaking.
>
> Circle the number jumping jack at which urine leakage occurs:
>
> Immediately—1 2 3 4 5
> ½ hr—1 2 3 4 5
> 1 hr—1 2 3 4 5
> 1 ½ hr—1 2 3 4 5
> 2 hr—1 2 3 4 5
> 2 ½ hr—1 2 3 4 5
> 3 hr—1 2 3 4 5
> 3 ½ hr—1 2 3 4 5
> 4 hr—1 2 3 4 5

should be taught not to bear down (ie, Valsalva maneuver) during exercises and ADLs. Valsalva maneuvers can contribute to incontinence and may increase the chance of pelvic organ prolapse.

HIP MUSCLES

Hip muscle impairment is often a primary impairment in hypertonia dysfunctions of the PFMs. Impairment and treatment of muscle imbalance around the hip is discussed at length in Chapter 20. The piriformis, obturator internus, and adductors are the most likely muscles involved because of their proximity to the PFMs. Any muscle impairment affecting the sacroiliac joint may also contribute to hypertonia dysfunction of the PFMs.

Active Pelvic Floor Exercises

PFEs strengthen the PFMs and specifically address impaired muscle performance. Proper contraction and relaxation of the PFMs are necessary for normal function and are the focus of treatment for most PFM impairments. Correct technique is essential.

TREATMENT AND DOSAGE INTERVENTION FOR ACTIVE PELVIC FLOOR EXERCISES

The therapist uses the results from the patient's self-evaluation (ie, stop test and digital vaginal self-examination test) to prescribe an individualized exercise program for PFM strengthening. The therapist also should consider the following parameters, even when prescribing PFE without the benefit of an internal examination. The therapist should remember the basic principles of overload (ie, the muscle must be challenged to its fullest capacity to improve strength) and specificity (ie, patients should exercise the muscle correctly in isolation). Patients can be taught these ideas and can learn to progress their own programs.[11] PFEs must be individualized for the patient to reach her full rehabilitation potential. Many well-intentioned publications give "cookbook" exercise programs that are too hard for the average incontinent patient (eg, hold for 10 seconds and repeat 10 to 15 times). Patients try to follow these instructions, realize that their symptoms are not changing, and ultimately abandon the exercises. These same patients have achieved good results with careful instructions and individualized programs.

Duration

How many seconds should the patient hold the slow-twitch muscle contraction? If the evaluation reveals that the patient can hold the contraction for 3 seconds (not uncommon for weak muscles), the therapist asks the patient to hold the pelvic floor contraction (ie, Kegel contraction) for 3 to 4 seconds before resting and repeating the exercise. Sustained PFM contractions are progressed to a maximum of 10 seconds.[12] This parameter shows the endurance of the muscles. Endurance impairments of PFMs are common.

Rest

How long should the patient rest between slow-twitch muscle contractions? Increased resting tone (ie, hypertonia) and weak muscles require longer rest times. Twice as much rest time as hold time is advised for a weak muscle (eg, 3-second hold, 6-second rest, and repeat). Rest time is decreased as strength increases (eg, 10-second hold, 10-second rest, and repeat). A quality PFM contraction requires complete relaxation at the end of each exercise. Incomplete relaxation does not train a muscle in its full range of motion and may result in hypertonia and pain. Complete relaxation between contractions produces a more functional muscle.

Slow-Twitch Repetitions

How many slow-twitch contractions should the patient do in one set before fatigue? For the patient previously described, the therapist would determine how many 3-second contractions the patient can complete. The average patient with an endurance impairment is able to perform only four to five repetitions before fatiguing. The exercise program must be individualized for maximum benefit.

Fast-Twitch Repetitions

How many fast-twitch contractions should the patient do in one set? A complete PFE program includes fast-twitch and slow-twitch muscle contractions. The therapist prescribes the number of fast-twitch muscle contractions based on how many can be done at the initial evaluation. Fast-twitch muscle contractions involve quick, maximal recruitment of the PFMs, followed by quick relaxation. These contractions are usually held for less than 2 seconds.

Sets

How many sets should the patient do in 1 day? Patients with weak PFMs should do a few contractions (as determined previously) several times during the day. The sets should be spaced throughout the day and performed up to five or six times per day, with a total of 30 to 80 pelvic floor contractions per day.[12]

Position

Gravity pulls down on the pelvic floor in upright positions. Patients with very weak PFMs should therefore do their exercises in the horizontal position (ie, gravity neutral). Patients with moderately strong PFMs can perform exercises in the sitting position (ie, against gravity) and advance to the standing position as they feel stronger. Results of the manual muscle test (MMT) using an internal examination of the PFMs provide the basis for prescribing exercise positions accurately. However, the stop test can give some guidelines for exercise positions when an internal examination is not possible. The stop test is an attempt to gain some information about the patient's PFM function in relation to gravity. The possible stop test results are listed in the Patient-Related Instruction: Testing Your Pelvic Floor Muscle Ability by Performing the Stop Test and Digital Vaginal Self-Examination (Finger in the Vagina Test). All patients should eventually progress to doing PFEs while standing, because it is necessary for the muscles to function well in this position (ie, most incontinence occurs while standing). Some publications recommend that women practice PFEs while driving or waiting in line. However, patients should learn these exercises in a quiet place so they can concentrate and perform the exercises correctly. After the exercises are learned well, patients can do them while waiting in line, driving, and watching TV.

Accessory Muscle Use

Contraction of the abdominal, adductor, and gluteal muscles can result in overflow to the PFMs.[13] The principles of overflow are used to facilitate strengthening of weak PFMs. Simply stated, overflow is the intentional contraction of associated muscles to increase recruitment of very weak muscles. This technique is usually reserved for patients with an MMT result of $1/5$ or $0/5$. Some patients with $2/5$ results need facilitation, but most therapists begin treatment without facilitation and add it later if the patient is not progressing as expected. Conversely, if the patient has an MMT result of $3/5$ or higher, the therapist discourages the use of accessory muscles. Eventually, all patients should learn to contract the PFMs without accessory muscles. Patients who are completely unable to slow the urine stream may benefit from facilitation, but if symptoms do not improve within 2 to 3 weeks, the patients should be referred to the physician, a therapist with specialized training in PFM rehabilitation, or both.

TEACHING PELVIC FLOOR EXERCISES WITHOUT AN INTERNAL PELVIC FLOOR MUSCLE EVALUATION OR SURFACE ELECTROMYOGRAPHY

Teaching PFE without internal palpation or biofeedback is difficult for the therapist and the patient. However, this section gives the therapist a comprehensive plan for teaching effective PFE, including patient education, verbal cues for proper PFM contraction, home exercise programs, and methods for putting the exercise program together. Therapists use the treatment dosage information in conjunction with the patient self-assessment and awareness exercises to prescribe an individualized PFE program.

Patient Education

Before teaching patients how to do the PFEs, they should be educated about the location and function of the PFMs, and the importance of normal PFM function should be explained.

Location. There are many commercially available charts, posters, and handouts that give a two-dimensional view of the location of the pelvic floor. However, many patients find three-dimensional models more helpful. Pelvic models that have the PFMs and obturator internus muscles in place help in explaining the proximity of the PFMs to the muscles of the buttocks and hips. Alternatively, the therapist can use a standard pelvic bone model and place her hand from the coccyx to the pubic bone to signify the muscles. The patient should understand that the PFMs are internal (approximately 2 inches into the vagina) and are in close proximity to the hip muscles. However, it is neither necessary nor desirable to contract the hip muscles while exercising the pelvic floor, unless the therapist is using overflow principles.

Function. An explanation of Kegel's three functions of the PFMs (the three Ss) is usually sufficient for the patient:

- Supportive: They hold the pelvic organs in.
- Sphincteric: They stop urine, feces, and gas from escaping until the person reaches the toilet.
- Sexual: They help women grip the penis and increase sexual feelings. They help men form and maintain an erection.

The therapist should to teach the differences in function between fast- and slow-twitch muscles. The analogy of sprinters and marathoners helps to explain the fast- and slow-twitch properties of the muscle. Sprinters depend on the fast-twitch muscle fibers, which are mainly responsible for the sphincteric function. The fast-twitch fibers contract quickly before a sneeze or cough. The marathoners are the slow-twitch muscle fibers, which provide the supportive function and hold up the organs. A combination of fast- and slow-twitch fibers assists sexual function.

Importance of Normal Muscle Function. The following points are examples of the importance of normal muscle function. The information can be individualized for each patient:

A well-exercised muscle has a good blood supply and may recover better from trauma such as childbirth or surgery. PFEs started during pregnancy result in less incontinence and pain after delivery.[14,15]

It is easier to learn these exercises before changes occur from surgery, pregnancy, childbirth, or aging. All women should have a basic knowledge of the PFMs and how they should be exercised (especially if they have any of the risk factors revealed by the screening questionnaires). PFEs should be a part of a woman's basic self-care, like brushing her teeth and showering.

Incontinence is a symptom not a disease. It is not an inevitable sequel of pregnancy, surgery, or aging, and 87% of patients can significantly reduce or eliminate incontinence with pelvic muscle exercises.[12]

Exercising these muscles before and after bladder suspension surgery may enhance the operative results. Some patients still have symptoms after bladder surgery or become incontinent several years later. Strengthening the PFMs may reduce the likelihood of recurring symptoms.

Weakness or spasm in this muscle group may result in stress to adjacent hip muscles and perpetuate functional limitations. Hip, buttock, and leg pain may not resolve unless this muscle group is functioning normally.

Verbal Cues for Proper Muscle Contraction. About 49% of patients verbally instructed in PFEs are doing them incorrectly.[16] Approximately 25% are pushing down on the pelvic floor.[16] This makes the dysfunction worse. The therapist must describe the exercises correctly and encourage patients to use the home exercises described in the next section. The following examples are ways to describe to a patient how to perform a pelvic floor contraction:

Tighten and lift the muscles around your vagina, and pull them up and inward, as if to stop urine flow.

Tighten the muscles that you would use to stop gas from escaping at a embarrassing time.

Pull your muscles up and in, as if you had the urge to urinate and could not stop to use the toilet.

Gently push out, as if to pass gas, and then quickly pull the muscles back up and in.

Home Awareness Exercises for Pelvic Floor Muscle Strengthening. Home exercises are an essential aspect of PFM strengthening. Before patients begin to perform these exercises on their own at home, they must have a complete understanding of their muscles and how to exercise them. The therapist should be aware of a patient's comprehension of the following exercises. Many patients nod and agree just to end the discussion of an embarrassing subject. The therapist should address this form of exercise with the same professionalism and completeness as she does for any other exercise. This approach can place the patient at ease, and it emphasizes the importance of the exercises.

Follow-up of the home exercise program is important. At subsequent sessions, ask patients how many, how long, and in what position they are doing the exercises, if they feel the contraction, if the muscles are getting stronger, and if the symptoms are decreasing. To improve compliance, it may be helpful for patients to keep a diary of the exercise routine and list how many times per day incontinence occurs.

These home exercises are used in conjunction with the self-assessment tests described in the evaluation section of this chapter (see Self-Management: Home Awareness Exercises). After going over the self-assessment tests and home awareness exercises with the patient, this information may be copied and given to the patient to take home with her. The patient should perform the tests and awareness exercises at home and then report to the therapist for documentation of results and development of an individualized PFE program.

PUTTING IT ALL TOGETHER—THE EXERCISE PROGRAM

The exercises described in Self-Management: Home Awareness Exercises are designed to help the patient identify and effectively contract the PFMs. However, it is important to create an exercise program that challenges the PFMs of each patient.

For example, if a patient's self-assessment test (eg, digital self-examination) shows that the PFM contraction was held for 5 seconds and repeated five times, that 10 quick contractions were performed, and that during the stop test she was able to slow the stream of urine but could not stop it, her evaluation results would be as follows:

- Duration of slow-twitch muscle contraction hold: 5 seconds
- Repetitions of slow-twitch muscle contractions: 5 times
- Repetitions of fast-twitch muscle contractions: 10 times
- Stop test: 2/5 (ie, poor muscle function)

With this information, the therapist could prescribe the following exercise prescription (Display 19-6). Five PFM contractions are held for 5 seconds with a 10-second rest between (double rest is given to patients with poor PFM function). Remind the patient to relax completely in between contractions. Ten quick PFM contractions are done to train the fast-twitch function of the muscle. Repeat the set four to six times per day; weak muscles need to exercise short sessions many times during the day. Exercises should be performed lying down. Most patients with a 2/5 stop test result do not need to use accessory muscles to perform the PFEs. The patient should contract the PFMs before and during stressful activities, such as coughing, sneezing, lifting, and straining. All patients should be given functional training activities such as "squeeze before you sneeze."

Self-assessment and modification of the exercise program continues periodically throughout rehabilitation. Remember to ask the patient how often and how many PFM exercises she can do. Ask if her symptoms are improving (ie, decreasing incontinence).

Endurance Impairment

The PFMs are 70% slow-twitch muscle fibers and do support pelvic organs against gravity in all upright positions. PFMs are postural muscles and must be able to maintain some baseline tone for long periods. Endurance impairment is the second most common PFM impairment treated. It is usually a primary impairment in supportive dysfunctions. Poor endurance of the PFMs is a common finding in many women without symptoms of PFM dysfunction. Most women probably have endurance dysfunction of the PFMs long before functional impairments of leaking urine or prolapse occur. Teaching PFEs to all adults may help to prevent PFM dysfunctions in the future. This is especially true with prenatal and postpartum women and women after menopause or gynecologic surgery. Endurance impairments are treated with PFEs.

Pain and Altered Tone Impairment

PELVIC FLOOR MUSCLES

PFM spasm with or without muscle shortening occurs in response to many situations outlined in the Hypertonia Dysfunction section of this chapter. Pain and altered tone impairments may be caused by lumbopelvic joint mobility impairment, tonic holding patterns of the PFMs, hip muscle imbalance and spasm, abdominal adhesions and adhered scars in the trunk and perineum, fissures, and fistulas. Pain

SELF-MANAGEMENT: Home Awareness Exercises

These exercises are used to help you understand what you should be doing during the Kegel or pelvic muscle exercise. Try the exercises at home, and report the results to your physical therapist. Remember that this is an internal muscle, and you should try not to contract the leg or buttock muscles. During these exercises try to identify

If you are doing the exercises correctly

How long you can hold the contraction (in seconds) up to 10 seconds

How many repetitions you can perform holding the contraction for the previous length of time

How many quick contractions you can perform

Index Finger on Perineal Body: Place your index finger on the perineal body (ie, the skin between the vagina or penis and the rectum) or lightly over the anus. This can be done over your underpants in some cases. Contract the pelvic floor muscles, and feel the perineal tissue moving away from your finger, up and into the pelvic cavity. If the pelvic floor is very weak, you may not feel much movement. However, you should never feel the anus or perineal tissue moving toward your finger or bulging. If you feel tissues moving toward your finger, stop exercising, and ask your physician, midwife, physical therapist, or other health professional to instruct you in the proper pelvic floor muscle contraction.

Finger Into Vagina or Rectum: Place your index finger into the vagina or rectum up to the level of the second knuckle. Palpate the muscle on either side of the vagina or rectum while you contract the pelvic floor muscles, pulling them in and up. You should feel the muscles contract around your finger and pull your finger up and in. If you feel tissues pushing out of your body or bulging, ask your health care professional to examine the area.

Visual Exercise:

Women Lie on your back with your knees bent and your head resting on several pillows. Hold a mirror so that you can see your perineal body and rectum. Contract the pelvic floor muscles up and in, and watch the perineal tissues moving up into the body. It may be difficult to see the movement if the muscles are very weak. Seek further professional instruction if any tissue comes toward the mirror or bulges outward.

Men Stand in front of a long mirror, and watch the penis as you contract the pelvic floor muscle up and in. The penis should move slightly upward during the contraction.

Sexercise—(for Women): Contract the pelvic floor muscles around the penis during intercourse. Ask your partner how long the contraction lasts and how many repetitions can be felt.

Squeezing Around an Object—(for Women): Contract the pelvic floor muscles around a tampon or similarly shaped object inserted into the vaginal canal. Many women feel the contraction of the pelvic floor muscles better if there is something in the vagina to squeeze.

and altered tone impairments are usually the primary impairments of hypertonia dysfunctions. Coccyx pain is rarely a result of sacrococcygeal joint mobility impairment, but it usually is caused by referred pain from spasm and trigger points in the surrounding muscles. The PFMs, obturator internus, and piriformis can refer pain to the coccyx (Fig. 19-8).

Treatment of PFM spasm includes manual soft tissue manipulation of PFM vaginally, rectally, or externally around the ischial tuberosities and coccyx. Surface EMG biofeedback and PFEs may also help restore the normal tone of the PFMs. In some cases, the PFMs become "frozen" and cannot relax or contract effectively (see Patient-Related Instruction: Importance of Relaxing the Pelvic Floor Muscles). Modalities such as electrical stimulation, ultrasound, hot, cold, and microcurrent are being used on the perineum to treat spasm. The therapist should learn the logistics of applying the modality on to the perineum. Modality parameters and other treatment considerations are the same as those used for spasm in other areas of the body.

DISPLAY 19-6

Sample Exercise Prescription

- Duration of slow-twitch muscle contractions: *5 seconds*
- Rest between slow-twitch muscle contractions: *10 seconds, double rest*
- Repetitions of slow-twitch muscle contractions: *5 times*
- Repetitions of fast-twitch muscle contractions: *10 times*
- Sets per day: *4 to 6 sets per day*
- Position: *gravity eliminated—lying down on back or side*
- Accessory muscle use: *not at this time*

HIP MUSCLES

Any muscle imbalance at the hip and trunk may contribute to hypertonia dysfunctions of the PFMs through sacroiliac joint mobility impairments. It is often difficult to pinpoint

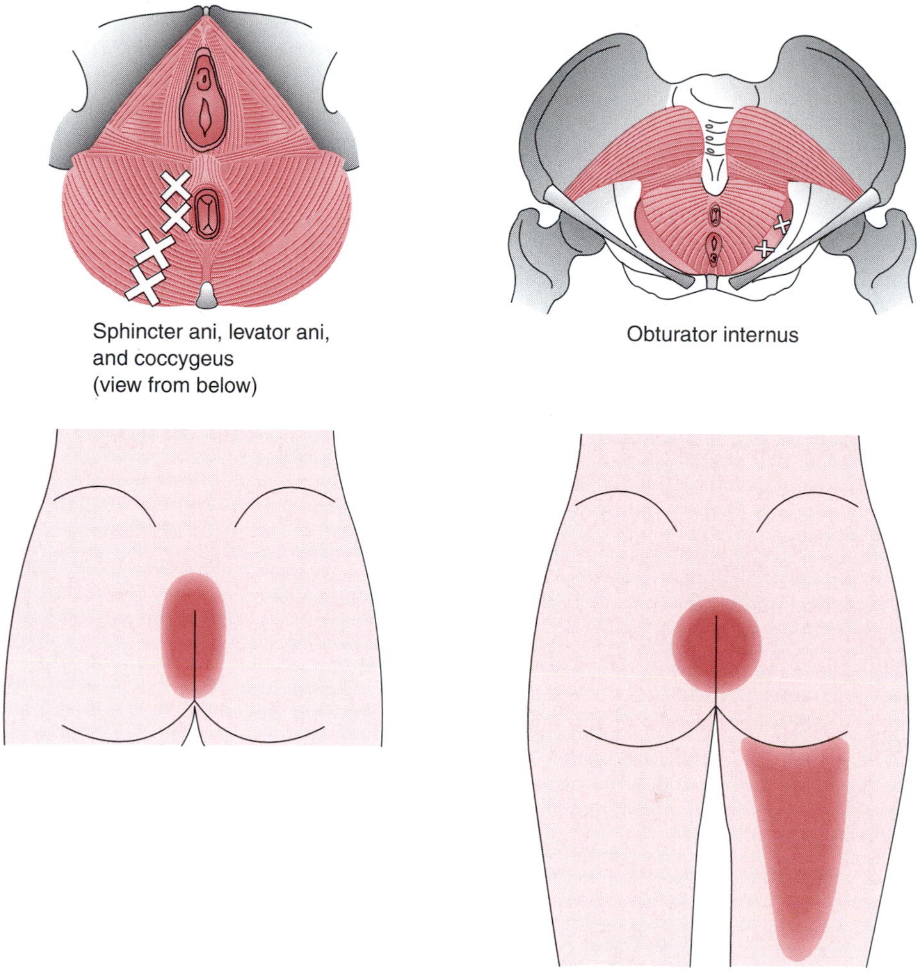

FIGURE 19-8 Trigger points (x) and their referral pain patterns *(shaded areas)*.

the origin of pain in the lower pelvic region. Muscle spasm and trigger points are a common cause of pain in the perineum, groin, and coccyx areas. Travell and Simons[5] describe referred pain patterns originating from trigger points in the adductors, PFMs, obturator internus, and piriformis (Figs. 19-8 and 19-9). Spasm and trigger points in these muscles may be primary or secondary impairments and should be treated in all patients with PFM dysfunction. Treatment for hip muscle spasms includes soft tissue manipulation, modalities (ie, ultrasound, electrical stimulation, hot or cold packs), therapeutic exercise for stretching and strengthening, and patient education about body mechanics and postures.

TRUNK MUSCLES

Iliopsoas and abdominal trigger points and spasm may be the primary muscular impairment in pelvic pain conditions. Iliopsoas spasm may irritate the pelvic organs that overlie

> ***Patient-Related Instruction***
>
> ### *Importance of Relaxing the Pelvic Floor Muscles*
>
> Pelvic floor muscles must be completely relaxed for normal function. For example, if you hold a brick in your hand all day and at the end of the day are asked to throw the brick 10 feet, you would probably not be able to throw it, because your arm muscles would be cramped and tired. Tonic holding of the pelvic floor muscles often results in a crampy pain in the groin or tail bone area. If you hold the pelvic floor muscles tense all day, you cannot contract the muscles more when you need them during coughing or sneezing. This may result in leaking urine. One goal of recovery is to be able to contract and relax the pelvic floor muscles well.

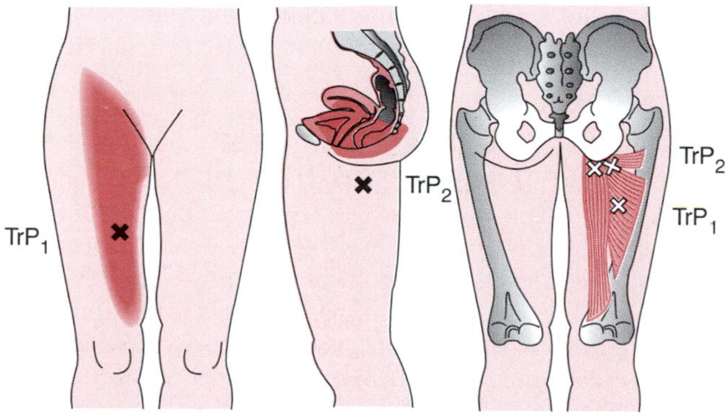

FIGURE 19-9 Trigger points (TrP) of the hip adductors (x) and their referral pain patterns *(shaded areas)*.

them and vice versa, making iliopsoas altered tone impairments an important condition to treat in cases of visceral dysfunction. Treatment of these muscles is essential to full recovery.

Mobility Impairment

Spasms of the PFMs are often related to sacroiliac, sacrococcygeal, pubic symphysis, and lumbar joint mobility impairments. These impairments may be primary or secondary and include hypomobility or hypermobility (see Chapter 6). Mobility restriction of scar tissue and connective tissue in the perineum and groin can also affect PFM function greatly.

MOBILITY IMPAIRMENTS CAUSING PELVIC FLOOR MUSCLE DYSFUNCTION

Hypomobility or hypermobility of the sacroiliac, pubic symphysis, or sacrococcygeal joint may cause the secondary impairment of PFM altered tone (ie, spasm). Pain from joint dysfunction may lead to a tonic holding pattern of the PFMs similar to that seen in the cervical muscles after an acceleration injury (ie, whiplash). Sacroiliac mobility impairments may also cause pain-induced PFM weakness. Any malalignment of the pelvis can alter the origin and insertion alignment of the PFMs and therefore affect function. A slight torque of the pelvis may impair muscle function by causing spasm or weakness. Significant joint impairments in all PFM dysfunctions should be treated to achieve full healing. These impairments are treated by joint mobilization, positioning, soft tissue mobilizations, therapeutic exercise, and other modalities.

Another example of mobility impairment causing PFM pain is vulvodynia. Vulvodynia is a complex and often idiopathic condition of pain in the external genitalia and vestibule. Some patients with symptoms of vulvodynia also have T12 through L2 joint mobility impairments, and these symptoms may decrease with treatment of lower thoracic and lumbar mobility impairments. The connection may be in the sympathetic innervation to the pelvic region. Vulvodynia may be a dysfunction of the sympathetic nervous system, similar to reflex sympathetic dystrophy. The hypogastric plexus (T10 through L2) provides sympathetic innervation to the pelvic and perineal area. Normal joint mobility in the T10 through L2 region may normalize sympathetic nerve output to the perineum and decrease symptoms. These hypotheses are based on clinical findings and have not been researched in experimental trials. Treatment of lumbar dysfunction usually is combined with many other treatment modalities for vulvodynia.

MOBILITY RESTRICTIONS RESULTING FROM PELVIC FLOOR MUSCLE DYSFUNCTION

Unilateral PFM spasms may contribute to and perpetuate pelvic joint mobility impairments. In some cases, untreated PFM spasm may be the reason for continued mobility impairments. This is seen commonly in the sacroiliac joint and less frequently in the sacrococcygeal joint. Because of PFM attachment onto the sacrum, unilateral PFM spasms can result in torque of the sacrum similar to the torque created by a unilateral piriformis spasm. Unilateral PFM spasms can occur as a result of trauma, such as groin strain with adductor insertion injury, birth injury, or a fall on the pubic rami. PFM spasm can be caused by sacroiliac joint mobility impairment and then become the reason for continued joint dysfunction. Whether it is the primary or secondary impairment, release of PFM spasm is needed to restore and maintain normal sacroiliac joint mobility in these cases.

MOBILITY IMPAIRMENTS RESULTING FROM ADHESIONS

Visceral adhesions may cause sacroiliac joint mobility impairments, especially if unilateral adhesions from organ to sacrum are severe. Specialized therapists use visceral mobilization techniques to manipulate organs and abdominal fascial tissue. These techniques are used to stretch adhesions and restore normal movement of lumbopelvic joints and pelvic organs. For example, in endometriosis, endometrial tissue implants in the abdominopelvic cavity outside the uterus. Like the tissue inside the uterus, the explanted tissue responds to hormones during the menstrual cycle with engorgement and then "sloughing off" (ie, bleeding during menses). Bleeding of this tissue inside the abdominal cavity leads to irritation, inflammation, and eventually scars and adhesions. Adhesions from endometriosis can be extensive throughout the abdomen and are often treated with laparoscopic laser surgery. Adhesions can pull on the ilium, coccyx, or sacrum and constrict bowels or fallopian tubes, altering joint and organ function. Soft tissue mobilizations of abdominal adhesions and organs can enhance organ function and may be the necessary link in maintaining normal mobility in the pelvic joints.

SCAR MOBILITY RESTRICTIONS

Episiotomy is a common obstetric procedure that involves making a cut in the perineal body immediately before vaginal delivery, usually to ease delivery (Fig. 19-10). Vaginal tissue may tear as an extension of an episiotomy or in lieu of an episiotomy at the time of delivery. Episiotomies and tears may result in adhesions and pain wherever the scar tissue occurs—at the perineal body, tissue inside the vagina, and even toward or into the rectum. Adhesion pain usually occurs in the immediate postpartum stage and abates in most women after 4 to 6 weeks. However, this

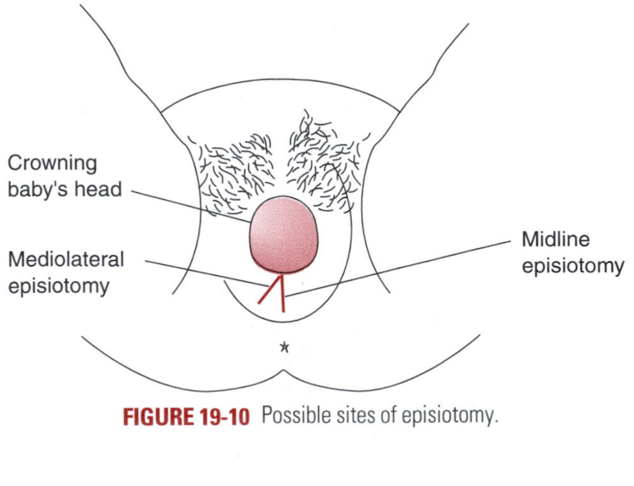

FIGURE 19-10 Possible sites of episiotomy.

pain persists in some women and can be so severe that intercourse is impossible and every bowel movement hurts. Sitting may be impossible, or sitting tolerance may be limited. Muscle spasm and adhesions are the most common impairments. Conversely, some patients demonstrate pain-inhibited PFM weakness. Treatment includes soft tissue manipulation and friction massage of scars externally and internally. Modalities, such as ultrasound, interferential electrical stimulation, hot packs, and cold packs also are used. PFEs and biofeedback are important in restoring the normal contraction and relaxation of muscles.

CONNECTIVE TISSUE MOBILITY RESTRICTIONS

Muscle strains often result in irritation to connective tissues and shortening of fascia and tendons. Groin injuries commonly traumatize the adductor muscle group. This is a very large muscle group that inserts onto the pubic ramus and ischial tuberosity. Physical therapists often treat the distal adductor muscle and fascia, whereas restrictions in connective tissue mobility and muscle spasms of the proximal adductor muscles are often left untreated. Tissue at the insertion of the adductor muscles to the pubic arch should be evaluated and treated in patients with persistent groin pain. A similar condition may occur in the hamstring muscles. The hamstring tendon sends a slip of connective tissue to the sacrotuberous ligament, which eventually fuses with the posterior sacroiliac ligaments. Impaired mobility of connective tissue at the proximal hamstring muscle may be related to persistent sacroiliac joint dysfunction. These conditions may occur with spasm of the PFMs. Treatment of connective tissue mobility impairment includes soft tissue mobilization, therapeutic exercise, and modalities (ie, ultrasound, electrical stimulation, hot packs).

Posture Impairment

Poor posture and body mechanics are commonly associated with joint mobility impairments. Education about proper posture and body mechanics is included in the treatment of all patients with joint dysfunction of the lumbopelvic area. Sitting posture demands special attention to PFM impairments (see Patient-Related Instruction: Proper Sitting Posture).

Patient-Related Instruction

Proper Sitting Posture

- Proper sitting posture is essential for relief of perineal and tail bone pain.
- Weight should be shifted forward on the two "sit bones" and thighs.
- There should be no pressure on the tail bone.
- Push your buttocks back in the chair so there is no space between your very low back and the chair.
- Use a small towel roll at your waist to maintain the inward curve if needed.
- A firmer chair can support your posture better and decrease pressure on the tail bone.

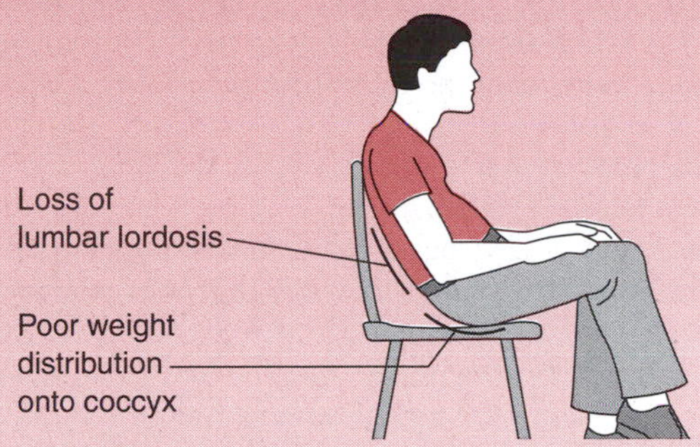

Poor sitting posture places weight on coccyx.

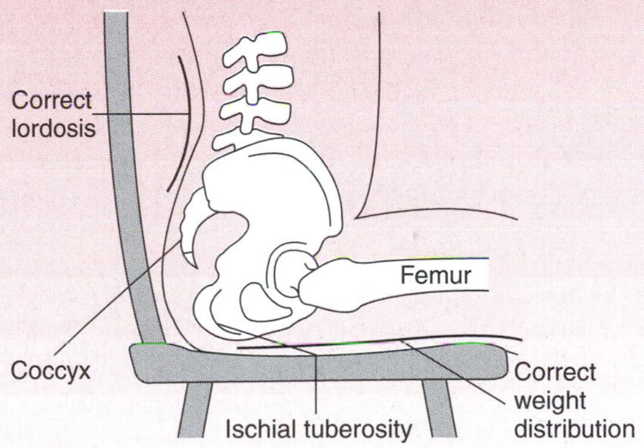

Proper sitting posture places weight on the ischial tuberosities and posterior thigh.

Coordination Impairment

Coordination impairment is related to inappropriate patterns of timing and recruitment of the PFMs and abdominal muscles. This impairment includes incoordination of the PFM contraction, incoordination of the abdominal contraction, incoordination of the PFMs during ADLs, and incoordination of the PFMs with the abdominals.

PELVIC FLOOR MUSCLES

Coordination impairment of the PFMs is the inability of all of PFMs to contract and relax at the appropriate times. Manual evaluation of the PFMs and biofeedback training may reveal the patient's inability to create and hold a synchronous contraction. This problem is usually related to decreased awareness of the PFMs. In non-neurologic conditions, the patient can usually learn the correct sequencing and timing of contraction through some form of biofeedback (eg, surface EMG; pressure; contracting around a finger, penis, or similar object).

PELVIC FLOOR MUSCLES DURING ACTIVITIES OF DAILY LIVING

Coordination impairment of the PFMs during ADLs is observed in stress incontinence, with urine leaking during lifting, coughing, and sneezing. In some cases, leaking results from impaired performance of the PFMs. However, some patients have fairly good PFM strength but do not contract the PFMs at the proper time during the activity. All patients must learn to contract the PFMs before and during

> **Patient-Related Instruction**
>
> ***Squeeze Before You Sneeze***
>
> Practice contracting the pelvic floor muscles immediately before sneezing, coughing, laughing, lifting, or straining. This is similar to training yourself to bring your hand to your mouth before you sneeze. By voluntarily contracting the pelvic floor muscles before increases in abdominal pressure, you will eventually create a habit, and the pelvic floor muscle will contract automatically.

increased intra-abdominal pressure (eg, cough, lift, sneeze) (see Patient-Related Instruction: Squeeze Before You Sneeze). One study showed that this type of training alone can decrease urine leakage up to 70%.[17]

PELVIC FLOOR MUSCLES WITH ABDOMINAL MUSCLES

The abdominal muscles participate in a synergy with the PFMs. The therapist should understand proper contraction of the PFMs with the abdominal muscles to correctly instruct the patient. For example, the therapist can instruct the patient to sit up tall in a chair and to pouch the abdominal muscles outward. As the patient keeps the abdomen pouched out and contracts the PFMs, she should notice the amount of effort needed and the force generated by the PFMs. Next, she should sit up in the chair and pull the abdominals inward, supporting the abdominal contents and the back. While she holds the abdominal contraction gently and contracts the PFMs, she notices the effort needed and the force generated by the PFMs. She then tries to contract the PFMs and bears downs, pouching out the abdominals. She next tries to contract the PFMs and then correctly pull the abdominal muscles inward.

Most persons feel a stronger PFM contraction when the abdominals are pulled inward properly. This is especially evident in the presence of PFM weakness. The PFMs cannot contract effectively when the abdominals pouch out, while bearing down, or during a Valsalva maneuver. In PFM training, it is especially important not to bear down and bulge the abdominals outward with the PFM contraction. All patients must learn to isolate the PFMs from the abdominal muscles at some point in the treatment.

Both sets of muscles respond to pressure changes in the abdominopelvic cavity. Forceful contraction of the abdominal muscles occurs with lifting, coughing, and sneezing. Urine leaks if a strong PFM contraction does not occur with the abdominal contraction during the increases in intra-abdominal pressure. A PFM contraction occurs with inward abdominal contraction. Conversely, bearing down is associated with PFM relaxation during bowel movement. PFM contraction during defecation is an example of PFM coordination impairment. This results in difficulty passing feces and often causes constipation and pain, which may be diagnosed as obstructed defecation. The patient must learn how to relax the PFMs at the proper time in association with the proper abdominal contraction for defecation (Table 19-3).

ABDOMINAL MUSCLES

Coordination impairment of the abdominal muscles result in an inability to pull the muscles inward. These impairments must be treated before considering PFM timing with the abdominals. See Chapter 18 for specific training techniques.

CLINICAL CLASSIFICATIONS OF PELVIC FLOOR MUSCLE DYSFUNCTIONS

Clinical classifications are groups of physiologic impairments that commonly occur together. The classification is the physical therapy diagnosis for the patient. Pelvic floor dysfunctions have four clinical classifications, which are used nationally by specialized physical therapists. Clinical classifications are intended to guide the therapist in treatment planning. However, the type and severity of physiologic impairments within the dysfunction vary, and treatments must be individualized. Each classification has a brief description of the syndrome and a discussion of the cause, common impairments, and functional limitations. There are many possible causes for these dysfunctions, which often result from a combination of pathologic conditions and comorbidities. In many cases, the primary cause is unknown. Therapists should have some understanding of the causes and comorbidities of the dysfunction they are treating, although it is not always necessary to pinpoint the cause for

Table 19-3. COORDINATION OF THE PELVIC FLOOR MUSCLE

ACTIVITY	NORMAL PFM ACTION	NORMAL ABDOMINAL ACTION	DYSFUNCTIONAL PFM ACTION	RESULT OF DYSFUNCTIONAL ACTION
Lifting	Contraction	Inward contraction by obliques	Relaxation or weak contraction	Leaking urine
Bowel movement	Relaxation	Bulging contraction by rectus abdominis with Valsalva maneuver	Contraction	Difficulty passing feces, constipation, pain

[a] In training of pelvic floor muscle (PFM) function, the patient must learn the coordinated functions of lifting and bowel movement and the isolated PFM contraction for training and strengthening.

effective treatment. It is necessary to identify the correct impairment for effective treatment.

Much of the information on PFM dysfunctions is based on the clinical observations of gynecologic physical therapists around the country. Unfortunately, few studies have been performed on the physical therapy treatment of these patients. All four clinical classifications are presented to provide a complete view of the dysfunctions treated by physical therapists. The medical diagnoses associated with supportive and hypertonia dysfunctions are discussed later in this chapter.

There are four diagnostic classifications:

1. Supportive dysfunction
2. Hypertonia dysfunction
3. Incoordination dysfunction
4. Visceral dysfunction

Supportive Dysfunction

Supportive dysfunction results from the loss of strength and integrity of contractile and noncontractile tissues; this dysfunction is weakness and sagging of the PFMs. Common medical diagnoses often associated with supportive dysfunction are stress incontinence, mixed incontinence, and pelvic organ prolapse (see Patient-Related Instruction: Boat at the Dock—Role of Pelvic Floor Muscles in Organ Prolapse). The supportive role of the PFMs in continence was discussed earlier in this chapter.

ETIOLOGY AND COMORBIDITIES

Severe birth injury may result in anatomic impairments of the PFMs and nerves in the area. More commonly, the trauma of vaginal delivery results in moderate or mild muscle impairments. Altered muscle length or tension may occur with stretch during delivery. Stretching of connective tissue or muscle beyond its elastic capacity renders the tissue permanently long. The increased length of connective tissue means that the muscle must generate more force to accomplish the same function. Functional weakness and impaired muscle performance result. Hypertrophy of the remaining muscles often produces the desired effect of improved support of the PFMs.

Muscle atrophy can result from central and peripheral nervous system dysfunction, including nerve damage from pelvic surgery. Temporary neurologic dysfunction, such as mild stretch to the pudendal nerve during delivery or Guillain-Barré syndrome, often responds well to PFE. In conditions of mild or incomplete nerve damage, the remaining PFMs often become hypertrophied and produce good functional outcomes. One study reported 15% to 20% of patients undergoing radical pelvic surgery had permanent voiding dysfunctions.[18] Pelvic surgery may result in complex anatomic changes that affect PFM function.

Many young children are taught not to touch or look at the perineum. In some cases, this early training results in adults with decreased awareness of the PFMs. Decreased awareness does not necessarily result in PFM weakness, but disuse atrophy may occur when decreased awareness is combined with other risk factors, such as menopause and bed rest. Decreased awareness of PFM contraction often exists concurrently with other impairments and makes rehabilitation more challenging. Many patients with severely decreased awareness can benefit from biofeedback instruction to identify the correct muscle contraction. The PFMs are used less when a Foley catheter is in place and while patients are on prolonged bed rest. These restrictions may result in disuse atrophy and impairment of PFM performance.

Prolonged increased intra-abdominal pressure may result in stretching of the PFMs or their tendons and may contribute to pelvic organ prolapse. Repeated, incorrect lifting or straining with Valsalva maneuvers and chronic or prolonged coughing or vomiting perpetuates incontinence and prolapse symptoms and slows recovery of PFM strength. These chronic increases in intra-abdominal pressure may initiate PFM impairment. Pregnancy and abdominal obesity increase intra-abdominal pressure. Obesity correlates with increased incontinence.

Patient-Related Instruction

Boat at the Dock—Role of Pelvic Floor Muscles in Organ Prolapse

- Imagine there is a boat tied to a dock (**A**). The pelvic organs (ie, bladder, uterus, and rectum) are the boat. The ropes holding the boat to the dock are the ligaments that support the organs from above. The water is the pelvic floor muscle.
- If the water level drops (**B**) (ie, loss of support or weakness of the pelvic floor muscles), the boat (organs) hangs on the ropes (ligaments). Eventually the ropes stretch out and break, resulting in the boat (organs) falling down (ie, prolapse).
- If you pull the boat back up by replacing the ropes (ie, organ suspension surgery) without raising the water level (ie, pelvic floor muscles strengthening) (**C**), the boat will continue to hang on the ropes and eventually falls down again (ie, prolapse). Falling happens quicker if you jump on the boat (ie, increase pressure in the abdomen from cough, sneeze, lift, or improper exercise).
- Long-lasting results are more likely if you raise the water level (ie, pelvic floor muscles strengthening) and stop jumping on the boat (ie, reduce unnecessary increases in abdominal pressure). In this case, the ropes (ligaments) may or may not need to be replaced (ie, ligament and pelvic organ surgery).

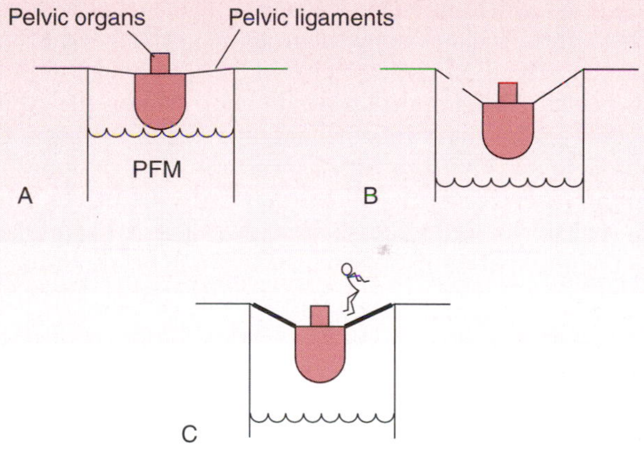

Pelvic congestion or swelling of the PFMs can occur during pregnancy and in some lymphedema conditions. Swelling in and around a muscle may inhibit its action sufficiently to cause impaired muscle performance. Hormones released during pregnancy loosen the connective tissue of PFM tendons, which causes the muscles to sag and results in supportive dysfunction. Because pregnancy is a temporary condition, most physicians and therapists are not concerned about symptoms of supportive dysfunction during pregnancy. However, 9 months of prolonged intra-abdominal pressure, especially with improper lifting at work, during exercise and ADLs, or in lifting another child, and prolonged, hormone-induced lengthening may result in significant postpartum supportive PFM dysfunction, even with a cesarean delivery.

COMMON IMPAIRMENTS

The most common physiologic impairments of supportive dysfunction are impaired PFM performance, including PFM weakness, increased PFM length, increased connective tissue length, and muscle atrophy; endurance impairment of the PFMs; and impaired abdominal muscle performance, including weakness and increased length of the abdominals.

The less common physiologic impairments associated with supportive dysfunction should also be treated for full recovery. Coordination impairment of the PFMs during ADLs often exists to some degree in supportive dysfunctions; coordination impairments of the abdominal muscles also occur with supportive dysfunction. When the PFMs are fairly strong and incoordination is significant, the patient is given the diagnosis of incoordination dysfunction. Pain impairments of the PFMs may be a concurrent problem that may lead to pain-induced weakness. In this case, the origin of pain must be treated to reach maximum muscle strength. Mobility impairment of the pelvic joints also may affect the PFMs (Display 19-7).

DISPLAY 19-7

Summary of Impairments and Possible Treatments for Supportive Dysfunctions

- Impaired performance and endurance of the PFM: weakness, increased length, atrophy
  - PFE: with facilitation, overflow, biofeedback or vaginal cones
  - Electrical stimulation (NMES)
- Coordination of the PFM: decreased awareness of how to contract correctly
  - PFE: with biofeedback and during ADLs
- Coordination and impaired performance of the abdominals
  - Therapeutic exercise for the abdominals
  - Proper contraction of abdominals with function
- Pain in PFM and mobility of pelvic joints
  - Soft tissue mobilization, scar mobilization
  - Joint mobilization, muscle energy techniques
  - Modalities such as heat, cold, ultrasound, and electrical stimulation

NMES, neuromuscular electrical stimulation; ADLs, activities of daily living.

FUNCTIONAL LIMITATIONS

Patients may exhibit symptoms of stress incontinence, mixed incontinence, and organ prolapse. Loss of urine with coughing, sneezing, laughing, lifting, or exercising often requires the use of absorbent products (ie, incontinence pads or diapers). Some patients limit or modify activities for fear of leaking urine. Patients may avoid shopping trips, overnight vacations, outdoor activities, and sports because of incontinence. Urinary frequency is urination more than seven times in a 24-hour period, and urination sometimes occurs as often as every 30 to 40 minutes. Frequency in conjunction with urinary urgency may require modification of ADLs, because patients usually do not venture far from the toilet. Lack of PFM support may be painful and result in decreased ability to ambulate or exercise.

Hypertonia Dysfunction

Hypertonia dysfunction is a complex category related to pain and spasm of the PFMs. Common medical diagnoses associated with hypertonia dysfunction include levator ani syndrome, pelvic floor tension myalgia, coccygodynia, vulvodynia, vestibulitis, vaginismus, animus, chronic pelvic pain, and dyspareunia. Hypertonia dysfunction may result from pelvic joint dysfunctions, hip muscle imbalance, and abdominopelvic adhesions and scars affecting the PFM function.

ETIOLOGY AND COMORBIDITIES

The cause of hypertonia dysfunctions is often more difficult to identify than the cause of other dysfunctions. Lumbopelvic joint mobility impairments or pathology is one of the most common impairments found in patients with hypertonia dysfunction. Injuries, such as a fall onto the coccyx or pubic ramus, are common for these patients. Pelvic joint dysfunction may result from PFM dysfunction or may directly or indirectly cause PFM spasm. Tonic holding patterns and spasm may result from the proximity of muscles to traumatized pelvic joints.

Hip muscle imbalance with coordination, pain, altered tone, and muscle performance impairments contributes to hypertonia dysfunction through its effect on the pelvic joints. Spasm of the associated muscles, particularly the obturator internus and piriformis, can directly irritate the PFMs, causing holding and spasm. Poor posture, disuse, and injury may contribute to hip muscle imbalance.

Abdominal or perineal adhesions and scars can cause hypertonia dysfunction. Pelvic organs must slide freely during physiologic functions such as peristalsis, bowel movement, or vaginal penetration during intercourse. Abdominal adhesions can restrict pelvic organ movement and cause pain and spasm of PFMs during bowel movement or intercourse. Severe adhesions of the uterosacral ligaments may restrict sacroiliac joint mobility. Adhesions may be a result of pelvic or abdominal surgery or an inflammatory condition of the abdomen, such as endometriosis. Perineal scars (often found in third- or fourth-degree episiotomies) can cause adhesions to the rectum and vaginal walls. These scars can be so painful that patients dread every bowel movement. Other painful conditions such as interstitial cystitis, endometriosis, fissures, and fistulas may also cause holding patterns in response to pain. Holding patterns of the PFMs may occur as a response to excessive generalized stress or reflect an emotional connection to the perineum. Excessive holding of the PFMs because of pain or stress often leads to trigger points, ischemic changes, and tissue shortening.

Connective tissue diseases such as fibromyalgia are associated with hypertonia dysfunctions, particularly vulvodynia. Pelvic pain, as discussed earlier, may be a problem for sexually abused individuals. The exact connection is unknown, but emotional holding of the PFMs and physical trauma to the perineum may play a part in the eventual development of hypertonia dysfunction.

COMMON IMPAIRMENTS

There are many possible primary physiologic impairments in hypertonus dysfunctions. Careful evaluation is necessary to determine the most significant impairments in each patient. The most common impairments of hypertonus dysfunction are altered tone of the PFMs, including spasm and trigger points; altered tone (eg, trigger points, spasm) of associated muscles of the hip, buttock, and trunk; impaired muscle performance and coordination impairments of the hip, leading to muscle imbalance around the hip; mobility impairments of pelvic joints, particularly the sacroiliac, pubic symphysis, and lower lumbar facet joints; mobility impairments of scar and connective tissue; and posture impairment, contributing to pelvic joint dysfunction. Pain impairment because of hypersensitivity of the perineal skin is common in vulvodynia, but it is not typical of other hypertonia dysfunctions (Display 19-8).

FUNCTIONAL LIMITATIONS

Hypertonia dysfunctions of the PFMs have functional limitations similar to other pelvic pain syndromes, such as low back and pelvic girdle pain. The ability to work (eg, lift, sit, push, drive, clean house), recreate, ambulate, sleep, and perform ADLs may be limited. Functional limitations unique to PFM hypertonia may result in a decreased ability or inability to sit because of severe perineal pain. Some patients cannot wear jeans or ride a bike. Routine pap smears can be painful or impossible. The affected woman often has a decreased ability or an inability to have sexual intercourse or sexual contact of any kind.

Many women and men are embarrassed to talk to their doctors, family, and friends about pelvic, perineal, or genital pain. It is difficult to explain the reasons for functional limitations if you are unable to tell someone the location or the nature of the pain. This creates emotional stress. Chronic pelvic pain patients often suffer in silence for many years before they find a medical professional who is able to treat them effectively.

DISPLAY 19-8
Summary of Impairments and Possible Treatments for Hypertonus Dysfunctions

- Altered tone of the PFM: muscle spasm and trigger points
  - Biofeedback for training the PFM to relax
  - Rhythmic contract and relax of the PFM (quick PFE)
  - Soft tissue mobilization, vaginally or rectally
  - Electrical stimulation on the perineum, vaginally or rectally
  - Relaxation training, autonomic nervous system balancing
  - Vaginal or rectal dilators
  - Ultrasound at the insertion of the PFM at the coccyx
  - Heat or cold over the perineum
- Altered tone of the associated muscles of the hip, buttock and trunk–muscle spasm
  - Soft tissue mobilization
  - Therapeutic exercises for stretching
  - Modalities such as ultrasound, electrical stimulation, heat, and cold
- Muscle impairments and coordination impairments of the associated muscles of the hip, buttocks, and trunk: muscle imbalances around the trunk and hip joint
  - Therapeutic exercises for strengthening and stretching
  - Coordination training of muscles around a joint (ie, around the hip) or between several areas (hip and abdominals)
- Mobility impairment of scar and connective tissue of the perineum, inner thighs, buttocks, and abdominals
  - Soft tissue mobilization, scar mobilization
  - Visceral mobilization
  - Modalities such as ultrasound, heat, and microcurrent
- Mobility impairments (eg, hypermobility, hypomobility) of pelvic joints: sacroiliac, pubic, lumbar, hip and sacrococcygeal
  - Joint mobilization, muscle energy techniques, strain and counterstrain, craniosacral therapy
  - Posture and body mechanics education
  - Therapeutic exercises for muscle imbalances
  - Modalities such as ultrasound, heat, cold, electrical stimulation, and TENS
- Faulty posture leading to undue stress on the pelvic structures
  - Instruction in proper sitting and standing posture and body mechanics
  - Use of cushions, lumbar rolls, and modified chairs
- Pain in the perineum with hypersensitivity of the skin and mucosa
  - Modalities such as cold, heat, ultrasound, and electrical stimulation
  - Education on avoiding perineal irritants

TENS, transcutaneous electrical nerve stimulation

Incoordination Dysfunction

Incoordination dysfunction can be divided into neurologic and non-neurologic syndromes. Detrusor sphincter dyssynergia is a type of incoordination resulting from a neurologic lesion in the spinal cord between the brain stem and T10. The PFMs and smooth muscle internal sphincter contract during a bladder contraction so that urine is unable to be expelled. This condition should be monitored by a physician. Symptoms of neurologic incoordination are similar to the obstructed voiding symptoms listed in the screening evaluation questionnaire. The therapist should refer the patient to the physician if neurologic incoordination or obstructed voiding is suspected.

Incoordination dysfunction may be a minor dysfunction with supportive or hypertonia dysfunctions, or it may occur as the primary dysfunction. Non-neurologic incoordination dysfunction is characterized by absent or inappropriate patterns of timing and recruitment of the PFMs. Common medical diagnoses associated with incoordination dysfunction include stress incontinence, constipation with obstructed defecation, and pelvic pain.

ETIOLOGY AND COMORBIDITIES OF NON-NEUROLOGIC INCOORDINATION DYSFUNCTIONS

The cause of pure non-neurologic incoordination dysfunction is often related to disuse and decreased awareness of the PFMs and abdominals. Muscle atrophy is not significant in this dysfunction. Decreased awareness may reflect an emotional condition or social conditioning. Pain in the pelvic or abdominal area may disrupt recruitment patterns. Surgical intervention may result in inhibition of the muscles—the muscles forget what to do, when to do it, and how it should be done. Some patients have never been aware of the PFMs and have developed poor recruitment patterns.

COMMON IMPAIRMENTS OF NON-NEUROLOGIC INCOORDINATION DYSFUNCTIONS

PFM weakness may be a minor impairment. Most of these patients are found to have good PFM strength on the MMT, and coordination impairment is the primary physiologic impairment. Coordination impairment of the PFMs, of the PFMs during ADLs, of the PFMs with the abdominals, and abdominal coordination impairment were discussed previously in the Coordination Impairment section.

FUNCTIONAL LIMITATIONS OF NON-NEUROLOGIC DYSFUNCTIONS

The most common functional limitation of incoordination dysfunction is stress incontinence with urine leaking during increased intra-abdominal pressure, such as during coughing, sneezing, or lifting. Patients also may have obstructed defecation with constipation and rectal pain.

Visceral Dysfunction

Visceral dysfunction is a pseudo-PFM dysfunction. It is an abnormality in mobility or motility of the abdominopelvic visceral tissues that leads to pain and musculoskeletal impairments. Detrusor instability, often found in patients with urge incontinence, is the most widely seen visceral dysfunction directly related to the PFMs. It is characterized by irritated detrusor contractions and is often related to PFM impairments. Urge incontinence responds well to supportive dysfunction treatments. The causes, impairments, and treatment of urge incontinence are discussed later in the Therapeutic Exercise Intervention for Common Diagnoses.

ETIOLOGY AND COMORBIDITIES

Visceral dysfunction encompasses several medical diagnosis: endometriosis, pelvic inflammatory disease, dysmenorrhea, surgical scars, irritable bowel syndrome, and interstitial cystitis. These conditions may result in impairments whose primary origin is abdominopelvic pain or adhesions caused by organ disease. Knowledge of the causes and medical management of these diseases is necessary to treat the resulting impairments. A multidisciplinary approach is optimal when dealing with visceral dysfunction. Treatment of comorbid musculoskeletal impairments often results in decreased pain and increased function.

COMMON IMPAIRMENTS

Weakness of the abdominal muscles, especially the oblique and transversus layers, may occur in response to pain in the abdomen, causing a pendulous abdomen with poor visceral and lumbar support. Secondary lumbopelvic joint mobility impairment and posture impairments may result. Altered tone (eg, spasm) or impaired muscle performance (eg, weakness) of the PFMs may also occur as a result of pain in the lower pelvic organs. Chronic pelvic pain postures often occur with long-standing abdominopelvic pain. These postures result in posture impairment; mobility impairments of pelvic and lumbar joints; altered tone, pain, and trigger points in trunk and lower extremity muscles; and impaired performance of the hip muscles with length and tension changes. Abdominal adhesions and scar mobility restrictions may result in decreased mobility or motility of abdominal and pelvic organs and pelvic joints. When organ mobility is restricted, cramping, pain, and altered organ function may result. For example, abdominal adhesions may form around parts of the bowel, constricting the bowel lumen and making passage of feces painful.

Mobility impairments play a major role in visceral dysfunctions. Visceral mobilization techniques are used by physical therapists to restore normal mobility of organs.

FUNCTIONAL LIMITATIONS

Functional limitations vary greatly in cases of visceral dysfunction. In the case of dysmenorrhea (ie, painful menstruation), patients may have 2 to 3 days each month of intense abdominal pain that confines them to bed. Other conditions result in constant abdominopelvic pain and cause functional limitations such as those of patients with trunk or back pain, who have a decreased ability to work, sit, walk, lift, have intercourse, play sports, exercise, or perform daily ADLs. Functional limitations may be directly related to organ dysfunction. For example, interstitial cystitis causes the person to urinate as often as every 15 minutes. Irritable bowel syndrome may result in alternating diarrhea and constipation, with many patients experiencing fecal incontinence with bouts of diarrhea. These functions are unpredictable and often force patients to remain near the toilet for fear of severe cramping or incontinence of feces.

THERAPEUTIC EXERCISE INTERVENTIONS FOR COMMON DIAGNOSES

This section describes the most common medical diagnoses for the pelvic floor region and suggests physical therapy interventions. The diagnostic classifications group physiologic impairments into common syndromes. The medical community uses a different classification system, and physical therapists should be aware of the medical classifications, testing, and medical treatment of these conditions to enhance their ability to provide effective physical therapy intervention.

The associated medical diagnoses discussed here are commonly associated with supportive and hypertonia dysfunctions. Medical diagnoses associated with supportive dysfunction usually fall into two categories—incontinence and organ prolapse. Both can be extremely complex conditions with many associated impairments and comorbidities. Some conditions associated with supportive dysfunctions are anatomic impairments and cannot be changed with physical therapy intervention.

The most common medical diagnoses associated with hypertonia dysfunction include chronic pelvic pain, levator ani syndrome, coccygodynia, vulvodynia, vaginismus, anismus, and dyspareunia. The most common physiologic impairments for each diagnosis is discussed with the diagnosis. Any impairment may be significant, and failure to address all significant impairments may limit the patient's progress. Any and all combinations of impairments listed for hypertonia dysfunction can be associated with these diagnoses. Each patient should be evaluated thoroughly, impairments identified, and treatment plans developed based on the severity and significance of each impairment.

Incontinence

Incontinence is defined as any loss of urine, feces, or gas at a time that is socially unacceptable. More than 13,000,000 persons in the United States have urinary incontinence. This figure includes approximately 50% of nursing home patients. Careful evaluation of these patients often reveals PFM weakness and treatable comorbidities. Approximately 80% of these incontinent patients can be significantly helped with noninvasive behavioral techniques used by physical therapists, occupational therapists, and registered nurses.[12]

Incontinence can be a limiting condition. It may occur during sports activities and cause embarrassment.[19] Nygaard[20] conducted a questionnaire study of women who exercised. She found that 47% had incontinence during exercise. Twenty percent of those women modified their exercise routines solely because of incontinence. Some women even stop exercising because of incontinence. This disruption in exercise ability may have a significant effect on physical therapy for other areas of the body. The therapist may encounter poor compliance with exercises that cause incontinence. The instructions included in this chapter may be enough to correct or minimize symptoms so that the patient can return to active exercises.

Incontinence also may limit elderly persons' activity levels. In some cases, incontinence causes embarrassment and may result in seclusion from social activities, family functions, and work. PFM strengthening can help these patients return to an active lifestyle without fear of embarrassing leakage. Incontinence also may result in secondary conditions such as skin breakdown, which can be a serious medical consequence for the elderly patient. All physical therapy patients should be questioned about leakage, and if appropriate, instructions should be given to help remedy the situation.

Understanding the most common types of incontinence assists therapists in developing treatment plans. Physicians broadly categorize bladder dysfunctions as the failure to store urine and the failure to empty urine. Stress, urge, and mixed incontinence are examples of a failure to store urine. Overflow incontinence is the failure to empty urine. The full screening questionnaire provided earlier helps to identify the type of incontinence. Stress and mixed incontinence are the two types directly related to supportive dysfunctions. Urge incontinence is a visceral dysfunction. Overflow and functional incontinence are usually not related to supportive dysfunction of the PFMs (Table 19-4).

Table 19-4. TYPES OF INCONTINENCE, SYMPTOMS, AND POSSIBLE TREATMENTS

TYPE OF INCONTINENCE	SYMPTOMS	DIAGNOSIS CLASSIFICATION	POSSIBLE TREATMENT
Stress incontinence	Small urine leak with cough, sneeze, exercise	Supportive dysfunction, PFM weakness	PFE, biofeedback, vaginal cones, electrical stimulation
Urge incontinence	Moderate or large urine leaks with strong urge to urinate	Visceral dysfunction, may have PFM weakness also	Bladder training, PFE if needed, biofeedback, electrical stimulation
Mixed incontinence	Symptoms of stress and urge incontinence	Supportive dysfunction, PFM weakness, visceral dysfunction	Bladder training, PFE, biofeedback, vaginal cones, electrical stimulation
Overflow incontinence	Small amounts of urine leaking constantly with cough and sneeze, straining to start urination, feeling of incomplete emptying	Possible incoordination dysfunction (PFM contraction during urination), visceral dysfunction (atonic bladder), hypertonia dysfunction (PFM spasm or pain)	Medical evaluation may be needed, advanced PFM rehabilitation with biofeedback, electrical stimulation, MFR, PFE, bladder training
Functional incontinence	Long or difficult trip to the toilet with leaking on the way	Mobility impairment of decreased ambulation ability, poor transfer ability, decreased finger coordination	Gait training, strengthening exercises for lower and upper extremities, environmental modifications

MFR, myofascial release

STRESS INCONTINENCE

Stress incontinence is defined as leaking of a small amount of urine during increased intra-abdominal pressure, such as during coughing, laughing, sneezing, and lifting. Continence is maintained when the pressure in the urethra is higher than the pressure in the bladder. Strong PFMs help to increase the pressure in the urethra. The urogenital diaphragm muscles play a large role in the closure of the urethra (see Fig. 19-4).

In stress incontinence, the patient coughs, and pressure in the abdominal cavity is increased, pressing down on the bladder. If urethral pressure is low (usually because the PFMs are not strong enough), the urethra is forced open slightly, and a small amount of urine leaks out (Fig. 19-11). The causes of stress incontinence are similar to the causes of supportive dysfunction. Physiologic impairments include impaired PFM performance, shortened endurance, and coordination impairments. Treatment for pure stress incontinence is PFM exercises, vaginal weights, and electrical stimulation.

URGE INCONTINENCE

Urge incontinence is defined as leaking urine associated with a strong urge to urinate. The normal urge to urinate is a result of activation of stretch receptors in the detrusor muscle. During this urge, the detrusor remains stable and does not contract. In some patients, a very strong urge to urinate is associated with inappropriate detrusor contractions. Unstable detrusor contractions are contractions of the bladder muscle at incorrect times (eg, when not positioned over the toilet). Strong, unstable detrusor contractions, as seen in detrusor instability, increase bladder pressure and may result in incontinence. The volume of urine leaked is usually larger than that with stress incontinence and may include the entire contents of the bladder. In some cases, urge incontinence may occur without unstable detrusor contractions (ie, sensory urgency).

The underlying cause of urge incontinence is often unclear and may include PNS or CNS nerve damage. It is suspected that poor bladder habits (especially going to the bathroom too frequently) and bladder irritants contribute to the condition. PFM weakness with impaired muscle performance and endurance impairment is often found in patients with urge incontinence. Coordination impairment of the PFMs during detrusor contraction may also be present. In this situation, the PFMs do not contract in response to the urge to urinate, and a small increase in bladder pressure may cause urine leakage. Primary treatment for urge incontinence can includes bladder retraining, avoiding bladder irritants, PFE, low-frequency electrical stimulation, and medications.

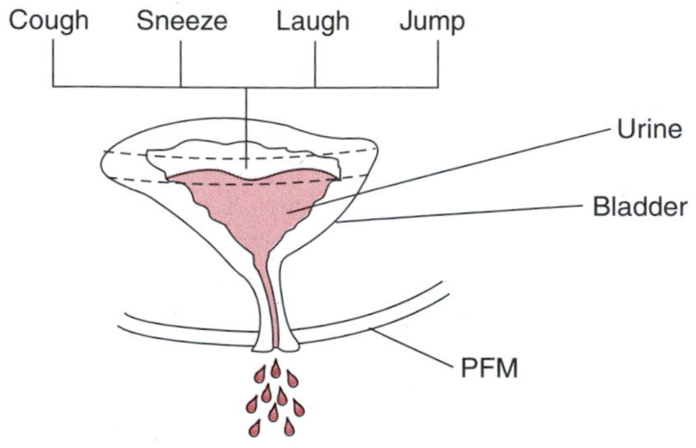

FIGURE 19-11 Stress incontinence.

MIXED INCONTINENCE

Mixed incontinence is a combination of stress and urge incontinence symptoms. These patients report leaking urine with increases in intra-abdominal pressure and with a strong urge to urinate. The causes of mixed incontinence are similar to the causes of supportive dysfunctions. The PFMs are usually weak. Treatment of this condition is similar to treatment for urge incontinence: bladder training, avoiding bladder irritants, PFM exercises, electrical stimulation, vaginal weights, and in some cases, medications.

OVERFLOW INCONTINENCE

Overflow incontinence results from a failure to empty the bladder fully. Obstruction of the urethra by tumor, scar tissue around the urethra, an enlarged prostate, or other mechanical blockage may prevent the bladder from emptying. Decreased contractility of the bladder from a neurologic deficit, such as peripheral nerve injury associated with radical pelvic surgery, cauda equina injury, or diabetes, also may contribute to overflow incontinence.

In overflow incontinence, the bladder does not empty fully, and high volumes of urine are maintained in the bladder. When the bladder pressure is higher than the urethral pressure, small amounts of urine "spill out." This small but constant leaking may or may not be related to increased intra-abdominal pressure and is characteristic of overflow incontinence. Physical therapy impairments may include pain and altered tone from spasm of the PFMs. Mobility impairment may be caused by adhered scars. Many cases involve neurologic incoordination of the PFMs or primary visceral dysfunction and require medical intervention. A full medical evaluation is essential. Therapists should refer the patient to the doctor if overflow incontinence is suspected. Physical therapy treatment by pelvic floor specialists may include biofeedback, electrical stimulation, myofascial release, PFEs, and bladder training.

FUNCTIONAL INCONTINENCE

Functional incontinence is defined as the loss of urine because of decreased mobility. Incontinence is a secondary condition in pure functional incontinence; the primary impairment is a mobility impairment—an inability to get to the toilet quickly enough. It is not unusual for an elderly or disabled patient to require 5 to 10 minutes to rise from a chair, ambulate with a walker to the toilet, maneuver in front of the toilet, lower her clothes, and sit down. Elderly patients often have less ability to store urine because of PFM weakness and less ability to defer the urge to urinate than younger persons. The mobility-impaired patient may leak urine on the long journey to the toilet. Patients may also have PFM dysfunction or anatomic impairments. However, treatment of mobility impairments and adjustments to the environment can improve function, and physical therapists are well suited to help these patients. Some ideas for helping these patients are detailed in Display 19-9.

DISPLAY 19-9
Helping Patients With Functional Incontinence

- Improve the speed of the sit-to-stand transfers by raising the height of the chair, providing a chair with arms, improving shoulder depression and elbow extension strength, and improving lower extremity strength in the quadriceps and gluteals.
- Improve the speed of ambulation to the bathroom by providing appropriate assistive devices, clearing obstacles from the pathway to the toilet, bringing the patient's chair closer to the toilet (eg, move the sitting room to the side of the house nearest the toilet) or bringing the toilet closer to the patient (eg, place a commode or urinal near the bed or sitting room), and improving balance and coordination, strength, and endurance of the lower extremities.
- Improve the speed of ambulation in the bathroom by clearing obstacles (especially rugs) and providing grab bars for ambulation without assistive devices if the bathroom is too small for the device to fit easily.
- Improve speed of lowering clothes by providing patient with Velcro-open pants, suggesting that women wear skirts and dresses, and improving finger coordination and dexterity to manage buttons and zipper more quickly.
- Improve stand-to-sit transfer onto the toilet by providing a raised toilet seat and handrails and by improving lower extremity function.
- Consider cognitive impairments in a patient's ability to recognize the bathroom. It may be helpful to place a picture of a toilet on or near the door or to leave the door open. In severe cases, even when patients are brought to the toilet, they may still not understand what to do.
- Absorbent garments (ie, diapers and pads) are available for men and women in a variety of sizes. Helping patients and caregivers to choose appropriate garments may allow increased participation in work, social, and recreational activities. Always make sure that the physician has been informed of the patient's incontinence and that conservative treatments have been tried.

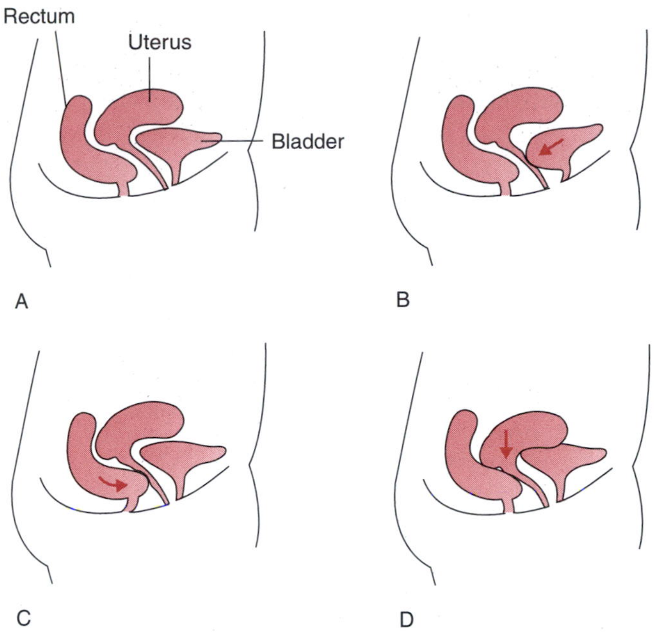

FIGURE 19-12 Common types of organ prolapse. ***(A)*** Normal organ positions. ***(B)*** Cystocele. ***(C)*** Rectocele. ***(D)*** Uterine prolapse.

Organ Prolapse

Organ prolapse is the second largest category of medical diagnoses associated with supportive dysfunctions. The cause of prolapse may be complex and is often associated with PFM supportive dysfunction and prolonged increases in intra-abdominal pressure. A simple explanation of prolapse and PFM function is presented in the Patient Related Instruction: Boat at the Dock. The most common types of organ prolapse (Fig. 19-12) are cystocele (ie, protrusion of the bladder into the anterior vaginal vault), uterine prolapse (ie, displacement of the uterus into the vaginal canal), and rectocele (ie, protrusion of the rectum into the posterior vaginal vault).

Common symptoms include a sensation of organs "falling out," feelings of pain or pressure in the perineum that may limit functional activities in standing, feeling that there is something bulging in the vagina, sensations of sitting on a ball, difficulty defecating (ie, rectocele), difficulty urinating (ie, cystocele), or painful intercourse (ie, uterine prolapse). All patients should learn how to protect the PFMs from undue stress. However, it is essential that patients with organ prolapse learn how to avoid increased intra-abdominal pressure. Physical therapy treatment involves educating patients on decreasing intra-abdominal pressure (see Patient-Related Instruction: Decreasing Intra-abdominal Pressure) and PFM exercises.

Chronic Pelvic Pain

Chronic pelvic pain is the most widely seen diagnosis associated with hypertonia dysfunction. It is analogous to the diagnosis of low back pain—it does not give specific information about what type of impairments may be present. The most common impairments are altered tone and performance impairments of the associated muscles of the trunk and hips, poor posture, and mobility impairments of the pelvic and lumbar joints. Therapists should remember the roll of the PFMs in sacroiliac dysfunctions. All patients with chronic pelvic pain should be screened for PFM dysfunction, evaluated, and treated if needed.

Levator Ani Syndrome

Levator ani syndrome is another diagnosis that may be used universally for patients with vaginal or rectal pain. Patients also report pain in the coccyx, sacrum, or thigh. Levator ani syndrome refers to spasm and trigger points in the pelvic diaphragm layer of the PFMs. Patients often report pain with defecation and increased pain with sitting. Some patients say they feel like they are "sitting on a ball" (this can also be a symptom of organ prolapse).

Pelvic floor tension myalgia is pain in the PFMs that is usually associated with spasm or chronic tension. This diagnosis is similar to levator ani syndrome, and many practitioners use the two names interchangeably.

Patient-Related Instruction

Decreasing Intra-abdominal Pressure

- Avoid constipation, and do not strain with defecation (ie, bowel movement). Drink lots of fluids to help avoid constipation and soften stools. Consult with a dietitian or physician about dietary changes and medications to avoid constipation.
- If you have difficulty getting out of the chair, scoot to the edge of the chair, lean forward, and push up with the arms. Avoid bearing down and breath holding. Instead, contract the abdominals inwardly, breathe out, and contract the pelvic floor muscles (PFM) while you stand up.
- Lift properly with inward contraction of abdominals and outward breath on effort. Avoid bulging the abdominals outward and bearing down.
- Exercise correctly using an inward abdominal contraction. Avoid bearing down and pouching the abdominal muscles outward. Unnecessary increases in intra-abdominal pressure may occur while lifting weights that are too heavy and with abdominal exercises that are too advanced. Curl-ups or sit-ups commonly cause the abdominals to bulge. Avoid curl-ups if you have organ prolapse. You should advance to weight lifting, advanced abdominal exercises, and jogging slowly and carefully if you have PFM weakness.
- If you are a postpartum woman, it is especially important to restore adequate PFM strength before returning to high-impact aerobics, jogging, and advanced weight lifting. The stop test and jumping jack test (see Patient-Related Instruction: Testing Your Pelvic Floor Muscles by Performing the Stop Test and Digital Vaginal Self-Examination) can be used to determine the ability of the PFM to withstand stress. You should score at least 3/5 on the stop test and should be able to do five jumping jacks one-half hour after urinating before returning to exercises that repeatedly increase pressure on the PFM. It is important to continue active rehabilitation of the PFM during your return to vigorous exercise. If incontinence persists or worsens, you may have to delay the return to vigorous exercises until more strength of the PFM is gained.
- It is important to seek medical treatment for chronic coughing or vomiting and to contract the PFM during coughing or vomiting. You can counterbrace the PFM by contracting during coughing and vomiting. Support the perineal tissue with gentle upward pressure of the hand over the perineum during coughing and vomiting spells.

Coccygodynia

Coccygodynia indicates pain at the coccyx bone. Pain at the coccyx is usually not related to the sacrococcygeal joint. More often, it is related to trigger points of the PFMs, obturator internus, or piriformis. Patients often have sacroiliac joint mobility impairments and less frequently have sacrococcygeal joint mobility impairments. Coccygodynia is a common sequel of falls directly on the buttocks. Patients report pain with sit-to-stand transfers, possibly because of gluteal muscle contraction or sacroiliac dysfunction. Coccygodynia patients have pain that limits sitting.

The most common impairments associated with levator ani, tension myalgia, and coccygodynia include altered tone of the PFMs and associated muscles; mobility impairments of scars, connective tissue, and pelvic joints; and faulty posture, especially in sitting. All patients with this diagnosis must learn to sit with their weight balanced on the ischial tuberosities and not on the tail bone (see Patient-Related Instruction: Proper Sitting Posture). Some patients need to use a special cushion to relieve pressure on the coccyx. The most effective cushion is a seat wedge approximately 2.5 inches tall with a small cut out in the posterior aspect (Fig. 19-13). A typical donut-shaped cushion places direct pressure on the coccyx and is therefore not recommended.

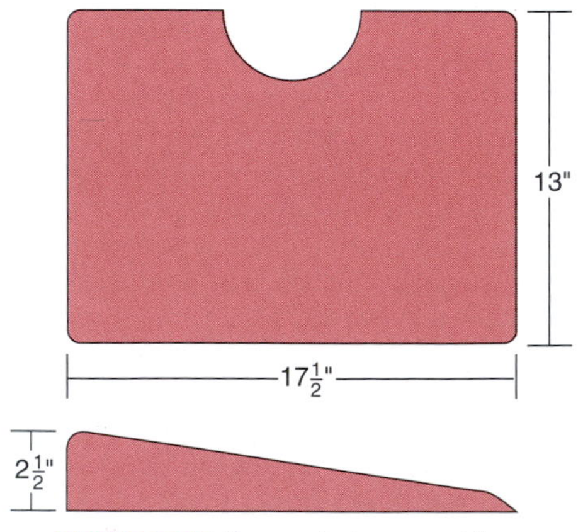

FIGURE 19-13 Coccygodynia seat cushion.

Vulvodynia

Vulvodynia is a broad diagnosis of pain in the external genitalia and vestibule. It can be a severe, often idiopathic condition that may or may not be associated with PFM dysfunctions. Patients report stabbing pain in the vagina and less commonly the rectum. Urination usually increases pain. Many patients are completely unable to have vaginal penetration of any kind (eg, intercourse, speculum evaluation, tampon insertion). Symptoms are increased with sitting and by wearing tight pants.

The causes of vulvodynia are complex and can include hypertonia dysfunction; metabolism of calcium, oxalate, and other substances; infection by bacterial and viral organisms (ie, yeast infections are common); pelvic surgery; environmental irritants or reactions; dermatologic conditions; and neoplastic conditions. Vulvodynia is a difficult condition to treat. A multidisciplinary approach is best. All impairments should be considered, especially mobility impairments of the pelvic and lumbar joints, mobility impairments of scars, and altered tone of the PFMs and associated muscles. These patients need special instructions in avoiding perineal irritants (see Patient-Related Instruction: Avoiding Perineal Irritants) and may benefit from pain-reducing modalities such as transcutaneous electrical nerve stimulation at the sacral nerve roots.

Vaginismus

Vaginismus is defined as a spasm of muscle around the vagina, usually the superficial muscle layer or urogenital diaphragm. It may be associated with vulvodynia. Patients report symptoms similar to those of vulvodynia, although to a lesser degree. Dyspareunia (ie, painful intercourse) is a

Patient-Related Instruction

Avoiding Perineal Irritants

Avoid unnecessary irritation to the vaginal tissue to encourage healing of the area. The vaginal tissue is like the tissue in your mouth. It needs to stay moist and should not be vigorously cleaned with harsh soaps. Here are some suggestions to decrease the irritation of the vaginal tissue:

Clothing

Avoid tight clothes, especially jeans and pantyhose. It is also helpful to avoid bike riding, because pressure and rubbing on the perineum can increase irritations.

Wear 100% cotton white underpants that are washed separately in hot water with a mild detergent; avoid bleach and fabric softeners.

Hygiene

Use white, unscented toilet tissue and pat dry after urination. Some women spray the vaginal area with a fine mist of plain water then pat dry.

Wash the vaginal area gently with mild soap (ie, natural glycerin-based soaps without deodorants or fragrances). Do not douche unless it is suggested by your doctor.

Avoid dripping shampoo or other soaps on the vaginal area while in the shower.

Soak in the tub with clear water—no bubble bath, bath beads, or other fragrance additives. Do not wash yourself in the tub; wash in the shower.

Menstruation

Avoid tampons if possible

Avoid pads with fragrances. Consider trying cotton washable menstrual pads.

Do not douche, unless suggested by your doctor

Medications

Speak to your doctor before using any prescription or over-the-counter cream on the perineum. Many creams can be irritating and make the situation worse.

Do not self-medicate for yeast infections.

Some contraceptive creams or jellies and lubricants can irritate. Speak to your doctor about an appropriate contraceptive method. Pure vegetable oil can be used as a vaginal lubricant without irritation by many women.

common symptom of vaginismus. Muscle spasms may be a secondary impairment in response to a medical condition, such as atrophic vaginismus or fistula (ie, a small opening in the skin similar to a small cut at the corner of the mouth).

Anismus

Anismus is a spasm of anal sphincter. It is similar to vaginismus in that it may be a secondary impairment caused by trauma, fissure, fistula, or hemorrhoids at the anal opening. Patients report severe pain with defecation, which often leads to constipation because patients delay defecation. The levator ani may or may not spasm.

Dyspareunia

Dyspareunia is the symptom of painful penetration and can be associated with all of the diagnoses previously described. It can be divided into two categories: pain at initial penetration or pain with deep penetration. Pain with initial penetration may be caused by superficial muscle spasm (ie, vaginismus), skin irritation (ie, vulvodynia), or adhered, painful episiotomy. Deep penetration dyspareunia may be related to spasm of the PFMs (eg, levator ani syndrome, tension myalgia) or organ prolapse with visceral adhesions. The most common impairments found in vaginismus, anismus and dyspareunia are altered tone of the PFMs and associated muscles and mobility impairment of scars and connective tissue.

OTHER MODALITIES AND TECHNIQUES

Many patient-related instructions have been included throughout this chapter. Education is essential for this patient population. When was the last time someone talked with you about how to urinate? Take time and make sure your patients understand anatomy and good bladder health, because they are often too embarrassed to admit that they do not know.

Physical therapy for the PFMs applies the same principles of treatment used for other weak and painful muscles. Therapeutic exercise principles are the same, and modalities are used for the same reasons. This section lists the modalities used in supportive and hypertonia dysfunctions. Several techniques are explored in more detail to enhance the therapist's ability to treat PFM impairments.

Various modalities and techniques may be added by the skilled practitioner to enhance the effect of active PFE for the treatment of supportive dysfunctions, including the diagnosis of incontinence. Modalities and techniques are chosen based on the patient's degree of muscle weakness. For a manual muscle grade of 0 to 2, the practitioner can include the following modalities or techniques:

- Facilitation with muscle tapping of the PFMs
- Overflow exercises of the buttocks, adductors, and lower abdominals
- Biofeedback with pressure or a surface EMG device
- Electrical stimulation
- Bladder training
- Coordination of PFMs during ADLs

For manual muscle grade of 3 to 5, the practitioner can include weighted cones inserted into the vagina and PFEs in more stressful activities, such as weight lifting. These patients continue to benefit from bladder training and biofeedback but should be weaned away from facilitation, overflow, and electrical stimulation.

Many other treatments are used in conjunction with exercise for the treatment of hypertonia dysfunctions (see Display 19-8). Treatments used for muscle spasms in other areas of the body can be used with PFM spasms as well. Later sections describe perineal scar mobilization and a method for externally palpating the PFMs.

Biofeedback

It is necessary to give all patients some form of feedback, whether it is with the finger in the vagina, a mirror, or with biofeedback machines during PFEs. Some practitioners use biofeedback machine evaluation and treatment with all PFM dysfunction patients. Surface EMG and pressure biofeedback are two methods of machine biofeedback. This type of biofeedback is especially helpful if the patient has decreased sensation or decreased motivation.

Pressure biofeedback involves an air chamber connected to a manometer, which records pressure changes. The air chamber is inserted into the vagina, and the patient contracts the PFMs around it. The PFM contraction creates increased in pressure in the vagina that is recorded and displayed for the patient and therapist. Some pressure devices collect specific data on pressure changes; others are used only for immediate feedback to the patient. Therapists must be careful to instruct PFE correctly, because bearing down increases pressure and may be misinterpreted as proper PFM contractions.

Surface EMG can provide even more information about the muscle contraction, patterns of recruitment, and resting tone. It is a powerful tool in treating PFM dysfunction. An internal vaginal or rectal probe or surface electrodes are used to pick up the electrical muscle activity of the PFMs so that it can be displayed. Stand-alone surface EMG units provide feedback in the form of a bar graph or line of lights. This gives information about one part of the contraction at a time. The units are helpful for home training. Computer-assisted surface EMG units can show the electrical muscle activity of the entire PFM contraction or several contractions in a row on one screen (Fig. 19-14). This allows the therapist to compare recruitment at different times in the contraction. Surface EMG is the ideal method of feedback in down training (ie, relaxation training) for patients with hypertonia dysfunction of the PFMs. Biofeedback therapy for patients with stress, urge, or mixed incontinence is given an A rating by the AHCPR guidelines on the management of urinary incontinence.[12] This means that properly designed research studies support the effectiveness of biofeedback for the treatment of these patients. These studies and guidelines have made it possible to get insurance reimbursement for biofeedback treatment in some patients.

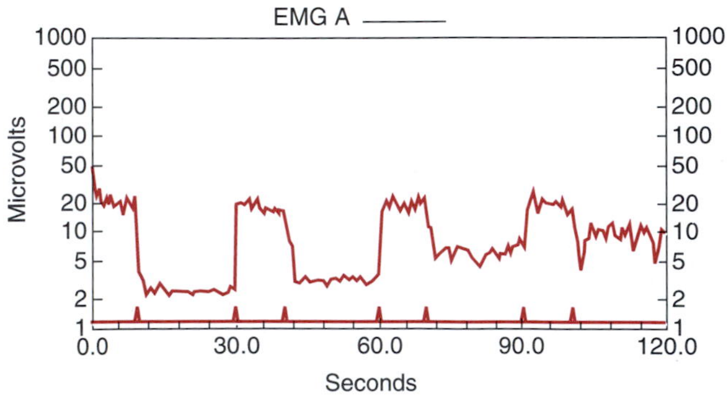

FIGURE 19-14 Print out of computer-assisted surface electromyographic treatment showing elevating baseline (From Shelly B., Herman, H., Jenkins, T. *Methodology for Evaluation and Treatment of Pelvic Floor Dysfunction.* The Prometheus Group; 1994).

Basic Bladder Training

Bladder training is scheduled voiding to regain normal voiding patterns. It is used in cases of urgency, frequency, urge incontinence, or mixed incontinence. Have the patient record the time she urinates in the toilet (ie, patients can count the number of seconds of the urine stream to give some indication of urine volume), the time of urine leakage (ie, incontinence), and why urine leaked (eg, cough, sneeze, lift). It is also helpful for the patient to record amount and type of fluid intake. Information should be collected for 3 to 6 days. This type of record is called a bladder diary (see Fig. 19-15). Bladder diaries can be simple or complex. The purpose of the simple bladder diary is to determine the following features:

MEASURE	PURPOSE
Average voiding interval	Determine average voiding interval
Frequency of voids in 24 h	Bladder habits and outcome data
Nocturnal voiding frequency	Bladder habits and outcome data
Number of incontinence episodes in 24 h	Outcome data
Cause of accidents	Stress or urge symptoms
Total fluid intake	Counsel on normal fluid intake
Number of bladder irritants per day	Counsel on decreasing bladder irritants

Some of the information gained from the bladder diary is to show improvement of the patient during treatment. The cause of the accidents helps identify the type of incontinence. Total fluid intake and the number of bladder irritants can be used to counsel patients on appropriate fluid intake. Bladder irritants must be limited for successful treatment of urge incontinence.

The average voiding interval (ie, average time between urinations) is the most important piece of information gained from the bladder diary for bladder retraining. Ask the patient to urinate in the toilet no sooner than the average voiding interval you determined from the bladder diary, whether they need to urinate or not. For example, if the average voiding interval was 1 hour, ask the patient to void in the toilet every 60 minutes—no sooner and no later. The bladder eventually becomes accustomed to the schedule, and urgency decreases. Most patients can increase the voiding interval by 0.5 hour every week. Do not increase the voiding interval if incontinence or urgency is worse or unchanged. Patients do not follow the bladder training schedule at night. Nocturnal voiding gradually improves as the daytime voiding interval increases. The goal is a voiding interval of 2 to 5 hours, with seven or fewer voids per day.

Urge deferment is taught to allow patients to maintain the voiding interval. If the urge arrives before the prescribed voiding interval, patients are encouraged to use the techniques in the Patient-Related Instruction: Urge Deferment. Patients need to practice several different techniques to find the most effective technique for them. After the urge has passed, patients should try to wait until the correct time to urinate.

Column # Directions

1 Urination in toilet: check, measure, or count # of seconds.
2 Make a check if a urine leak occurs, note small or large.
3 Note the reason for the accident (jump, sneeze, lift, water, urge).
4 Note type and amount of fluid intake.

Fill in the day and date at the top of each column.

Name________________________________ **Acct.#**________________________________

DAY												
	toilet	leak	reason	fluid	toilet	leak	reason	fluid	toilet	leak	reason	fluid
6 am												
7 am												
8 am												
9 am												
10am												
11am												
12am												
1pm												
2pm												
3pm												
4pm												
5pm												
6pm												
7pm												
8pm												
9pm												
10pm												
11pm												
12pm												
1am												
2am												
3am												
4am												
5am												
TOTAL												
# of pads												

Stop Test Results____________________________ **Patient's Signature**________________________________

Type of pad used____________________________

FIGURE 19-15 Bladder diary.

Patient-Related Instruction

Urge Deferment

- Sit down; pressure on the perineum helps calm the bladder.
- Relax and breathe; nervousness and anxiety contribute to urgency.
- Small pelvic floor muscle contractions help to reflexively relax the bladder.
- Keep the mind busy; attend to a task involving a lot of attention. Tell yourself you cannot stop to go to the bathroom, count backwards, or pretend you are in the car, and there is no bathroom available.
- Practice mind over matter; the mind has great influence over the bladder. For example, you are on a 2- or 3-hour car ride, and you feel the urge to urinate. If you say to your bladder, "Not now; calm down; I'll go later," the urge goes away. The bladder may become conditioned to produce the sensation of urgency and bladder contractions with certain activities (eg, before leaving home, before a speech, walking past the bathroom, arriving home, while unlocking the door). It is important to break these habits and establish control over the bladder. (Rather than the bladder controlling your actions.)

Patient-Related Instruction

Self-Mobilization of Scar Tissue

- Wash your hands thoroughly before beginning
- Choose one of the following positions:
  - Lying on the bed with pillows to prop the head up
  - Sidelying on the bed
  - In the tub
- Use your index finger to reach around from the back while sidelying, or use your thumb to reach the vagina from the front.
- Apply firm, downward pressure on the scar, usually located on the posterior vaginal wall. This probably feels uncomfortable but should not be extremely painful. Constantly holding pressure results in softening of tissue, similar to the feeling of your thumb sinking into a stick of butter.
- Maintain downward pressure for 1 to 3 minutes; then begin gentle oscillations in all directions. Do not allow your finger or thumb to slide over the skin; take the skin with you as your thumb oscillates. Continue these oscillations for several more minutes.
- Move on to another area of the scar, or finish the session.
- Use a hot towel on the perineum or soak in a hot tub to help dissipate any residual soreness.

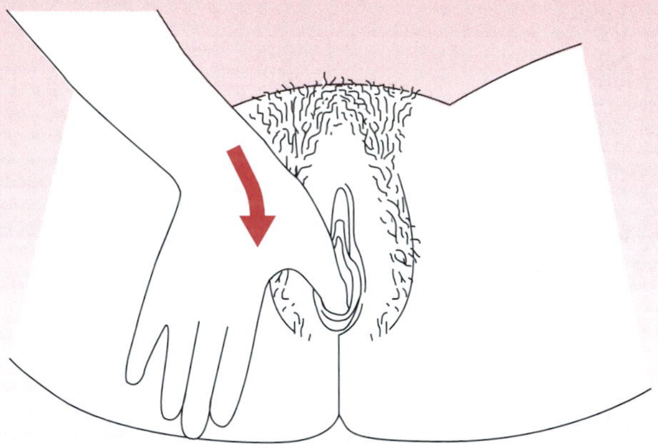

Episiotomy scar massage.

Scar Mobilization

Adhesion of perineal scars can cause pain with intercourse (ie, dyspareunia), pain with bowel movement, and weakness of PFMs. The goal of scar mobilization is to lengthen connective tissue and scar adhesions, allowing fascial layers to slide easily over one another. Complete scar management includes internal myofascial release of scars, mobilization of scars by patients or their partners, ultrasound, PFE, and heat if needed. One method for teaching mobilization of scar tissue is described in Patient-Related Instruction: Self-Mobilization of Scar Tissue.

The therapist can describe the technique using the patient's web space between the thumb and first finger as the posterior vagina (Fig. 19-16). This allows the therapist to give the patient the experience of the amount of pressure that is appropriate and to show how to perform the oscillations. Oscillations are similar to friction massage in that the goal is to slide the skin over the second layer of fascia, thereby breaking adhesions and restoring mobility.

Tolerance to scar mobilization varies with the severity of adhesions. Most women find that pain with deep myofascial release of scars decreases as the adhesions loosen. Dyspareunia usually decreases as scars loosen. Some women find it difficult to effectively massage their own vaginal

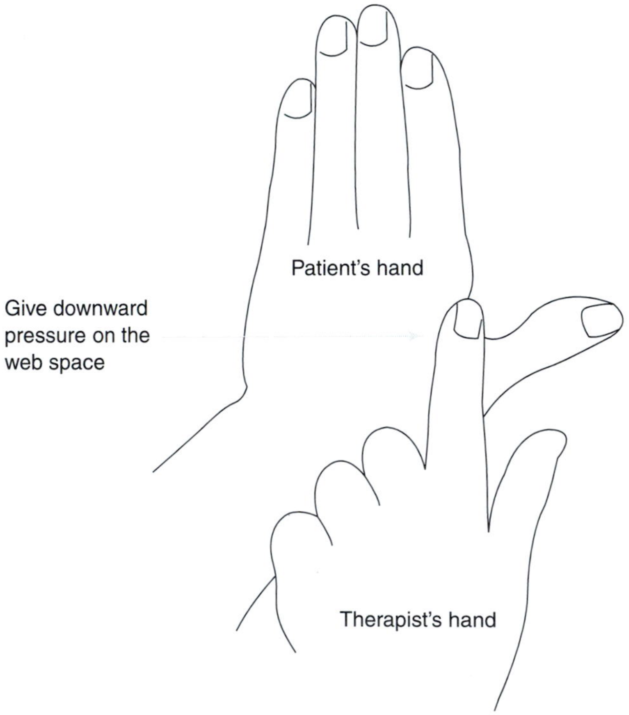

FIGURE 19-16 Describing self-mobilization of a vaginal scar using the patient web space.

scars. It may be difficult to reach the vagina, or it may be difficult to cause self-inflicted pain. In this case, partners can be trained in a similar manner to assist with treatment. Scar mobilization before intercourse can help decrease dyspareunia. Scar mobilization should not be performed in the presence of open wounds, rash, or infection. Postpartum women should wait at least 6 to 8 weeks after delivery and should check with the physician if questions arise.

Externally Palpating the Pelvic Floor Muscles

It is possible to palpate the PFMs externally at the insertion to the coccyx and along the length of the muscle at the medial ischial tuberosity. The benefits of this palpation are limited, but it is helpful in palpating and treating trigger points in some parts of the levator ani and obturator internus muscles. This method does not give access to all areas of the pelvic floor but helps in the treatment of myofascial pain syndromes. This palpation requires skilled instruction and practice to perfect. Patient position, therapist preparation, therapist position, hand positions, and technique are described in Display 19-10.

Key Points

- The pelvic floor tissues include the anal sphincter and three skeletal muscle layers: superficial perineal muscles (mostly related to sexual functioning), urogenital dia-

DISPLAY 19-10
Externally Palpating the Pelvic Floor Muscles

- **Patient position:** Place the patient in sidelying with the top leg in approximately 60 to 80 degrees of hip flexion and the knee comfortably bent. Put two or three pillows under the top leg to provide stability in neutral abduction or adduction, and allow the patient to relax the leg fully. Total patient relaxation is necessary for deep PFM palpation.
- **Therapist's position:** The therapist is positioned behind the patient and finds the tip of the ischial tuberosity on the uppermost ilium.
- **Therapist's preparation:** This palpation may be done through underpants but is more effective if the fingers are on bare skin. The therapist should wear a latex or vinyl glove on the palpating hand because it will be close to the anus and perineum.
- **Hand position:** The most effective hand position is supination, with the palm facing up and with all four fingers adducted in full finger extension. Keep the hand parallel to the table, and place the fingertips on the skin between the ischial tuberosity and the anus (just medial to the ischial tuberosity).
- **Technique:** Apply gentle inward pressure, directing your fingertips toward the anterior-superior iliac spine (ASIS) of the top ilium. Closeness to the ischial tuberosity results in the skin pulling taught and restricting deep palpation. In this case, reposition the fingers more medial to the ischial tuberosity, taking up some skin slack (see Figure). The levator ani muscles are rather deep, being the third layer in the pelvic floor. Depth from the skin varies greatly and can be more than 1.5 inches. When a firm resistance is felt, ask the patient to contract the PFMs. You should feel a firm PFM contraction pushing your fingers outward. This outward movement is not perineal bulging. A similar outward movement on correct contraction occurs with deep palpation into the abdominal cavity, followed by an abdominal contraction.

With the PFMs at rest, assess for pain, hypertonia, and connective tissue restriction in the usual manor. Angling the fingers anteriorly and posteriorly can give information about different areas of the levator ani muscle group. The obturator internus is a little more difficult to palpate. A review of anatomy is necessary to orient yourself to the location of the muscle in the sidelying position. Keep the palpating hand in the position described previously, and gently change the angle of the hand so that the wrist drops and the fingers move upward into the tissue above. The obturator internus is located in this area. The muscle should feel somewhat soft. Have the patient contract the muscle to ensure correct location. External rotation can be tested by asking the patient to lift the top knee upward toward the ceiling while keeping the foot on the supporting surface. The therapist resists this motion with a hand on top of the knee. A small isometric contraction should result in palpable muscle tension. The palpation depth is important. Shallow palpation results in palpation of the medial ischial tuberosity. In this case, continue straight, inward pressure until the tissue releases to a deeper level, and then angle the wrist down and the fingers upward. Myofascial release of muscle or connective tissue can be carried out in this position if impairments are identified.

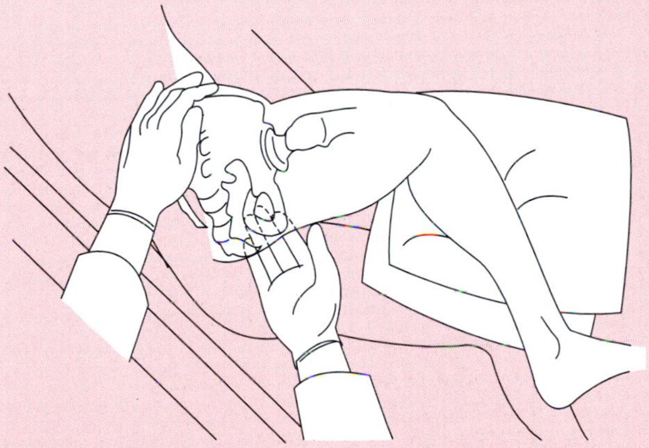

External palpation of pelvic floor muscles. (Adapted from Hoppenfeld, S. *Physical Examination of the Spine and Extremities.* New York: Appleton-Century-Crofts; 1976).

phragm (continence), and pelvic diaphragm (continence, pelvic support).

- The pelvic diaphragm includes the coccygeus and the levator ani muscles (pubococcygeus and iliococcygeus), the largest muscle group in the pelvic floor. These muscles are skeletal muscles under voluntary control and have 70% slow-twitch and 30% fast-twitch muscle fibers. They span from the pubic bone to the tail bone and between the ischial tuberosities. The pelvic floor is close to many hip muscles (ie, obturator internus and piriformis), but it is neither necessary nor desirable to move the legs while contracting the PFMs.
- The three functions of the pelvic floor are supportive (ie, prevents pelvic organs from prolapsing), sphincteric (ie, prevents involuntary loss of urine, feces, and gas from the urethra and rectum), and sexual (ie, increases sexual appreciation and maintains erection).
- All patients should be screened for PFM dysfunction with these simple questions. Do you ever leak urine or feces? Do you ever wear a pad because of leaking urine? Do you have pain during intercourse? If indicated, a more comprehensive questionnaire can be given to attempt to identify the type of incontinence and other limiting factors.
- Patients can be given self-assessment tests and taught self-awareness exercises: the stop test, jumping jack test, digital self-examination (finger into the vagina), index finger on the perineal body, visual exercise, sexercise, and squeezing around an object. These home exercises help to develop the exercise program and ensure patient is contracting the PFM correctly.
- Through home self-assessment, the patient reports the number of seconds a PFM contraction can be held, repetitions of holding contractions, repetitions of quick contractions, and results of the stop test.
- Impairments that affect PFM function include performance impairments of the PFMs, abdominals, and hip muscles; endurance impairments of the PFMs; pain and altered tone of the PFMs, hip muscles, and trunk muscles; mobility impairments causing PFM dysfunction as a result of PFM dysfunction, adhesions, scar tissue, or connective tissue; posture impairments; and coordination impairments of the PFMs, PFMs during ADLs, PFMs with the abdominals, and the abdominals themselves.
- PFM dysfunctions have four diagnostic classifications that are used by gynecologic physical therapists across the United States: supportive dysfunction (ie, loss of support usually as a result of impaired PFM performance); hypertonia dysfunction (ie, pain and altered tone impairment in the PFMs); incoordination dysfunction (ie, coordination impairment with poor timing and recruitment of PFMs); and visceral dysfunction (ie, dysfunctions of the pelvic viscera with possible PFM involvement). PFM dysfunctions can result in significant functional limitations and affect the quality of life.
- Incontinence is the most common result of supportive dysfunction. The most common types of incontinence are stress incontinence (ie, loss of urine and increased intra-abdominal pressure with a cough, sneeze, laugh, or lift); urge incontinence (ie, very strong urge to urinate, usually associated with a bladder contraction, which results in leaking urine); mixed incontinence (ie, combined stress and urge incontinence); overflow incontinence (ie, obstruction at the urethra or a flaccid bladder that allows high volumes of urine to collect in the bladder and spill over); and functional incontinence (ie, leaking of urine because of an inability to ambulate to toilet quickly).
- Organ prolapse is another common diagnosis resulting from PFM weakness. Forms include cystocele (ie, bladder prolapse into the vagina); uterine prolapse (ie, uterine displacement into the vagina); and rectocele (ie, rectal prolapse into the vagina).
- With the results of screening questionnaires, the physical therapist should be able to develop an exercise program, including the duration of slow-twitch contraction, rest between slow-twitch contractions, repetitions of slow-twitch contractions, repetitions of fast-twitch contractions, number of sets per day, exercise position, need for overflow facilitation from accessory muscle, and other treatments that may be helpful.
- All physical therapists should be aware of the PFMs and be prepared to give generalized strengthening instructions.
- Teaching PFEs involves educating the patient on the location and function of the PFMs and the importance of normal PFM function, providing accurate verbal clues, and teaching home assessment and awareness exercises. The most effective verbal cues seems to be "Pull your sphincter muscles up and in as if you do not want gas to come out." Many patients become discouraged and abandon PFEs. Therapists must continue to monitor the patient's progress and to actively encourage participation in the PFE program.

Critical Thinking Questions

1. Develop a PFE program for the following patients. Include the duration of slow-twitch muscle contractions, duration of rest between slow-twitch muscle contractions, and number of repetitions of slow-twitch muscle contractions, number of repetitions of quick contractions, number of sets per day, exercise position, whether to use accessory muscles or not, and any other treatment that may be helpful. Indicate which type of incontinence the patient may have and any risk factors that may limit her progress.
   a. A 64-year-old woman, a mother of three children, has a 10-year history of gradually worsening urinary leaking with coughing, sneezing, walking, lifting, and laughing. She wears three panty liners each day and leaks a small amount of urine an average of six times per day. The patient does not report a strong urge to urinate or difficulty urinating, and she has no complaints of pain. She does have a 5-year history of adult-onset diabetes. She expresses concern about the odor of her leaking and admits avoiding overnight trips, long car rides, and social activities that involve physical activity such as walk-a-thons or exercise classes.

      After the initial evaluation, the patient was taught the stop test and finger in the vagina test, with these results:

      Duration of hold: 3 to 4 seconds
      Repetitions of holding contractions: 3 times

LAB ACTIVITIES

1. Practice administering the screening questionnaire.
2. Develop a case study in which a patient needs to be instructed in PFEs. Practice explaining the location and function of the muscles and the importance of PFEs using words, posters, and models.
3. Explain the appropriate self-assessment test and home awareness exercises to the patient.
4. Perform the self-assessment test and self-awareness exercises at home, and develop an appropriate exercise program for yourself. Exercise programs should include the following:
   a. Results of the functional stop test and jumping jack test
   b. The number of repetitions and amount of hold time per contraction
   c. The amount of rest that should be taken between contractions
   d. The number of fast-twitch muscle contractions per set
   e. The number of sets per day
   f. Suggested position of exercises (ie, lying down or upright)
   g. Other methods of strengthening that should be considered
5. Practice palpating the PFMs externally at the ischial tuberosity (see Display 19-10). Evaluate for pain, trigger points, spasm, and connective tissue tension. Make sure you are on the correct muscle by having the patient contract that muscle.
6. Sit up tall in the chair, and pouch your abdominal muscles outward. Keep the abdomen pouched out, and contract the PFMs. Notice the amount of effort needed and the force generated by the PFMs. Next, sit up in the chair, and pull the abdominals inward, supporting the abdominal contents and the back. Hold the abdominal contraction gently and contract the PFMs. Notice the effort needed and the force generated by the PFMs. Next, try to contract the PFMs and bear down, pouching out the abdominals. Try to contract the PFMs and then pull the abdominal inward correctly.

Repetitions of quick contractions: 6 times
Stop test result: able to slow the stream of urine

Develop an exercise program.

b. A 25-year-old woman is the mother of a 12-month-old baby, who weighed 9 lb 2 oz at birth and was delivered vaginally after a long labor. Delivery required the use of forceps and a deep episiotomy. The woman presented with the primary complaints of having a strong urge to urinate and needing to urinate every 1 to 2 hours, and she occasionally leaks urine before reaching the toilet. She is an emergency room nurse in a major hospital and admits to very small amounts of leaking with lifting patients in and out of bed. Other significant medical history includes right sacroiliac pain since pregnancy and sacroiliac pain with intercourse. The patient reports voiding 10 to 14 times each day (two to three times each night), which significantly interferes with her work. She wears maxipads (two per shift) to work because she is unsure whether she will be able to leave a patient to urinate. The urologist has tried medication without success and feels the patient may have a permanent dysfunction.

After the initial evaluation, the patient was taught the stop test and finger in the vagina test, with these results:

Duration of hold: 7 seconds
Repetitions of holding contractions: 10 times
Repetitions of quick contractions: 15 times
Stop test result: can stop urine flow toward end of stream only once

Develop an exercise program.

2. Imagine you or someone you love is the patient in question 1b, and examine how you would feel about your situation. Describe the impact on your life (ie, work, family, social interactions, emotions). List some things you would be forced to change because of your condition.
3. You are treating a 30-year-old man who fell off a ladder onto his right buttock. After 3 weeks of quality treatment, he has experienced significant decrease in low back and sacroiliac pain, but he can only sit for one-half hour and experiences pain with sit to stand transfers and when going up stairs. He finally admits that his tail bone hurts and that it feels like he is "sitting on a ball." Your evaluation shows no dysfunction in the lumbar spine, and persistent hypomobility of right sacroiliac. Which muscles should you assess for dysfunction, and how would you treat them. Think about how you would explain to the patient that his pain may be related to the PFMs.

REFERENCES

1. Kegel A. Progressive resistance exercises in the functional restoration of the perineal muscles. *Am J Obstet Gynecol.* 1948;56:238.
2. Schussler B, Laycock J, Norton P, Stanton S, eds. *Pelvic Floor Re-education Principals and Practice.* New York: Springer-Verlag; 1994.
3. DeLancey J, Richardson A. Anatomy of genital support. In: Benson T, ed. *Female Pelvic Floor Disorders.* New York: Norton Medical Books; 1992.
4. Walters M, Karram M. *Clinical Urogynecology.* St. Louis: Mosby–Year Book; 1993.
5. Travell J, Simons D. *Myofascial Pain and Dysfunction: The Trigger Point Manual,* vol 2. Baltimore: Williams & Wilkins; 1992.
6. Mcminn R, Hutchings R. *Color Atlas of Human Anatomy.* Chicago: Year Book Medical Publishers; 1977:81.

7. Kegel A. Sexual function of the pubococcygeus muscle. *West J Surg Obstet Gynecol.* 1952;10:521.
8. Chiarelli P. *Women's Waterworks—Curing Incontinence.*, Snohomish, WA: Khera Publications; 1995.
9. Pearson B. Liquidate a myth: reducing liquid intake is not advisable for elderly with urine control problems. *Urol Nurs.* 1993;13:86–87.
10. Sampselle C, DeLancey J. The urine stream interruption test and pelvic muscle function. *Nurs Res.* 1992;41:73–77.
11. Woman's Hospital Physical Therapy Department. *The Bottom Line on Kegels.* Baton Rouge, LA: A Woman's Hospital Publication; 1997.
12. Urinary Incontinence Guidelines Panel. *Urinary Incontinence in Adults: Clinical Practice Guideline.* AHCPR Pub. No. 92-0038. Rockville, MD: Agency for Health Care Policy and Research, Public Health Service, U.S. Department of Health and Human Services; March 1996.
13. Bo K, Stien R. Needle EMG registration of striated urethral wall andpelvic floor muscle activity patterns during cough, Valsalva, abdominal, hip adductor and gluteal contractions in nulliparous healthy females. *Neurourol Urodyn.* 1994;13:35–41.
14. Nielsen C, et al. Trainability of the pelvic floor—a prospective study during pregnancy and after delivery. *Acta Obstet Gynecol Scand.* 1988;67:437–440.
15. Sampselle C. Changes in pelvic muscle strength and stress urinary incontinence associated with childbirth. *J Obstet Gynecol Neonatal Nurs.* 1990;19:5:371–377.
16. Bump R, Hurt G, Fantl A, Wyman J. Assessment of Kegel pelvic muscle exercises performed after brief verbal instruction. *Am J Obstet Gynecol.* 1991;165:322–329.
17. Miller J, Ashton-Miller J, DeLancey J. The knack: use of precisely timed pelvic muscle contraction can reduce leakage in SUI. *Neurourol Urodyn.* 1996;15:392.
18. Weih AJ, Barret DM. *Voiding Function and Dysfunction: A Logical and Practical Approach.* Chicago: Year Book Medical Publishers; 1988.
19. Bo K, et al. Prevalence of stress urinary incontinence among physically active and sedentary female students. *Scand J Sports Sci.* 1989;11:113–116.
20. Nygaard I, DeLancey J, Arnsdorf L, Murphy E. Exercises and incontinence. *Obstet Gynecol.* 1990;75:848–851.

RECOMMENDED READINGS

King P, Myers C, Ling F, Rosenthal R. Musculoskeletal factors in chronic pelvic pain. *J Psychosom Obstet Gynecol.* 1991;12 (suppl):87–98.

Sahrmann SA. Diagnosis by the physical therapist. *Phys Ther.* 1988;68:1703–1706.

PATIENT EDUCATION

Bass E, Davis L. *The Courage to Heal: A Guide for Women Survivors of Child Sexual Abuse.* 3rd ed. New York: Harper & Row; 1994.

Burgio K. *Staying Dry.* Baltimore: John Hopkins University Press; 1989.

PHYSICAL THERAPY BOOKS

Adams C, Frahm J. Genitourinary system. In: Myers R, ed. *Saunders Manual of Physical Therapy.* Philadelphia: WB Saunders; 1995.

American Physical Therapy Association. *Women's Health Gynecological Physical Therapy Manual, 1997.* 1-800-999-APTA, ext. 3237.

Polden, Mantle. *Physiotherapy in Obstetrics and Gynecology.* Stoneham, MA: Butterworth-Heinemann Publishers; 1990.

Schussler B, Laycock J, Norton P, Stanton S, eds. *Pelvic Floor Reeducation Principles and Practice*. New York: Springer-Verlag; 1994.

MEDICAL BOOKS

Benson T, ed. *Female Pelvic Floor Disorders.* New York: Norton Medical Books; 1992.

Wall L, Norton P, DeLancey J. *Practical Urogynecology.* Baltimore: Williams & Wilkins; 1993.

CHAPTER 20

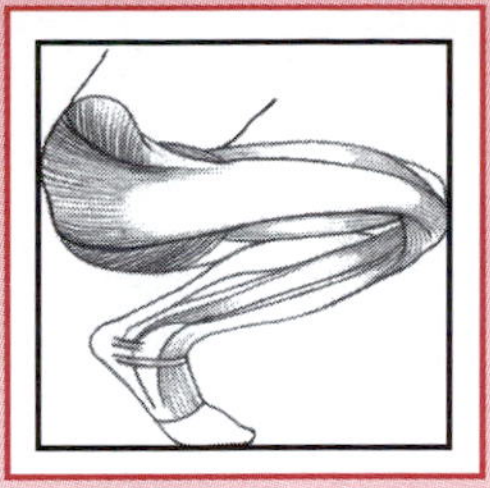

The Hip

Carrie Hall

The primary roles of the hip joint are (1) to support the weight of the head, arms, and trunk during standing erect postures and during dynamic weight-bearing activities such as walking, running, and stair climbing and (2) to provide a pathway for transmission of forces between the lower extremities and pelvis. The structure and function of the hip affect the function of the entire lower kinetic chain and the upper quadrants through its articulation with the pelvis proximally and the femur distally. The hip joint is a diarthrodial ball and socket articulation with a marked degree of inherent stability and relatively limited mobility. In this respect, it differs from the shoulder joint, which is an open ball and socket articulation with great freedom of movement at the expense of stability.

Neither structure nor function of the hip joint can be examined without considering the weight-bearing function of the joint and the interdependence with the other joints of the lower extremity and lumbopelvic region. These issues are examined in this chapter, which also provides a review of the anatomy and kinesiology of the joint. Common anatomic impairments and the components of examination and evaluation of the hip joint also are described. Therapeutic exercise interventions are suggested for the treatment of physiologic impairments and selected diagnoses of the hip joint.

ANATOMY AND KINESIOLOGY

The hip joint is composed of the head of the femur and the acetabulum of the pelvis (Fig. 20-1). The construction of this joint allows for the wide range of functions required for the activities of daily living (ADLs), such as sitting, squatting, walking, and stair climbing.

Osteology and Arthrology

The concave component of the hip joint is the acetabulum. The acetabulum is located on the lateral aspect of the pelvis, which is formed by the fusion of the ilium, ischium, and the pubis (see Fig. 20-1*A*). The acetabulum forms a true hemisphere, but only a horseshoe-shaped portion of the hemisphere is covered with articular cartilage.[1] A peripheral ring of fibrocartilage called the acetabulum labrum (see Fig. 20-1*B*) deepens the entire socket. The cavity of the acetabulum faces obliquely anteriorly, laterally, and caudally.

The femoral head is the convex component of the hip joint. The shape of the head of the femur varies among individuals, ranging from just slightly larger than a true hemisphere to almost two thirds of a sphere.[1] The femoral head is attached to the femoral neck, which is attached to the shaft of the femur between the greater and lesser trochanter (Fig. 20-2). The femoral neck angulates the head such that the head most commonly faces medially, superiorly, and anteriorly.

The angulation of the femoral head varies among persons and even from side to side in the same individual. The femoral neck has two angular relationships with the femoral shaft that are important to hip joint function: The *angle of inclination* is the angle formed between the neck and shaft of the femur in the frontal plane. The angle of inclination offsets the femoral shaft from the pelvis laterally and in most adults is about 125 degrees (Fig. 20-3).[2] The *angle of torsion* is formed as a projection of the long axis of the femoral head and the transverse axis of the femoral condyles

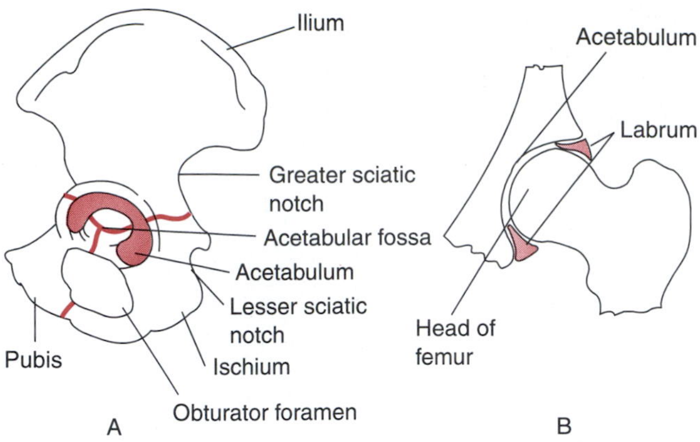

FIGURE 20-1 ***(A)*** Articulating surface of the acetabulum. ***(B)*** Lateral view of the hip joint shows the relationship of the acetabular labrum and femoral head.

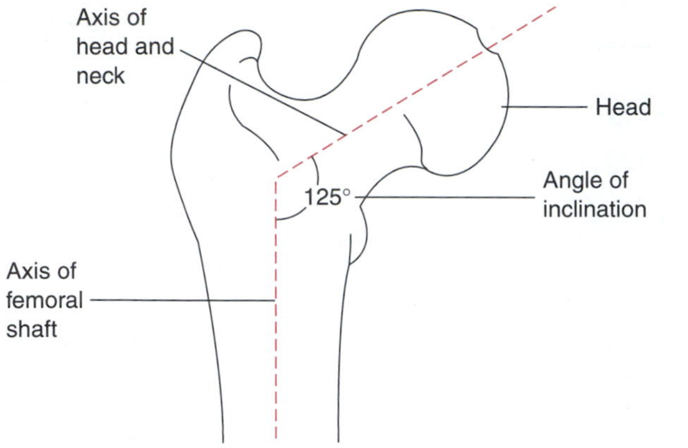

FIGURE 20-3 The axis of the femoral head and neck form an angle with the axis of the femoral shaft called the angle of inclination. The drawing illustrates the normal angle of inclination.

(Fig. 20-4). In adults this angle averages about 12 to 15 degrees but varies widely with age and sex.[2]

The head of the femur is covered with articular cartilage, except for a small central portion called the fovea. The cartilage covering is thickest in the medial central region and thinnest toward the periphery.[2] The variations in the cartilage thickness correlate with different strength and stiffness properties in various regions of the femoral head.[3] The articular capsule of the hip is very strong and dense, unlike the weak shoulder capsule. The hip joint capsule is attached to the entire periphery of the acetabulum by its attachment to the acetabulum labrum. The anterior portion of the capsule is stronger than the posterior portion, because it is reinforced by two strong ligaments, the iliofemoral ligament and pubofemoral ligament (Fig. 20-5*A*). The posterior capsule is reinforced by one, the ischiofemoral ligament (Fig. 20-5*B*).

The inverted-Y-shaped iliofemoral ligament is the strongest ligament at the hip, with its fibers taut in hip extension. The superior fibers of the iliofemoral ligament become taut during hip adduction, and its inferior fibers become taut during hip abduction. The pubofemoral ligament becomes taut in hip abduction and extension. The ischiofemoral ligament spirals anteriorly around the femoral neck and becomes taut in extension.

Because all the capsular ligaments are coiled around the femoral neck in a clockwise direction, combined extension and medial rotation of the hip tighten the ligaments, and combined flexion and lateral rotation uncoil the ligaments. Consequently, extension and medial rotation is the position of greatest stability for the hip, and flexion and lateral rotation is the position of least stability for the hip, particularly if combined with adduction, as in sitting cross-legged. A strong force up the femoral shaft toward the hip joint, with the hip in the latter position, may push the femoral head out of the acetabulum resulting in hip joint dislocation.[4]

The internal architecture of the femur reveals trabeculae systems that accommodate the mechanical stresses and strains created by the transmission of forces between the femur and pelvis. The medial trabeculae system (Fig. 20-6*A*) closely parallels the joint reaction force on the head of the femur during single-limb support.[1,2] The lateral trabeculae system (Fig. 20-6*B*) probably resists the compressive force on the femoral head produced by contraction of the abductor muscles (ie, gluteus medius, gluteus minimus, and tensor fascia lata).[2]

With aging, the femoral neck gradually undergoes degenerative changes. The cortical bone is thinned, and the trabeculae are gradually reabsorbed.[5] These changes may

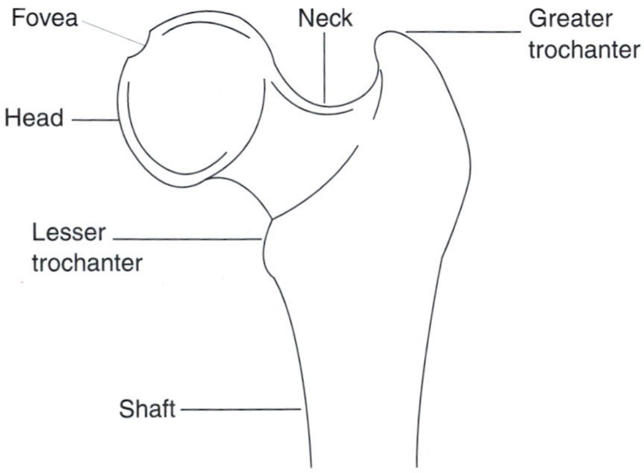

FIGURE 20-2 An anterior view of the proximal portion of the left femur shows the normal relationships of the head, neck and femoral shaft.

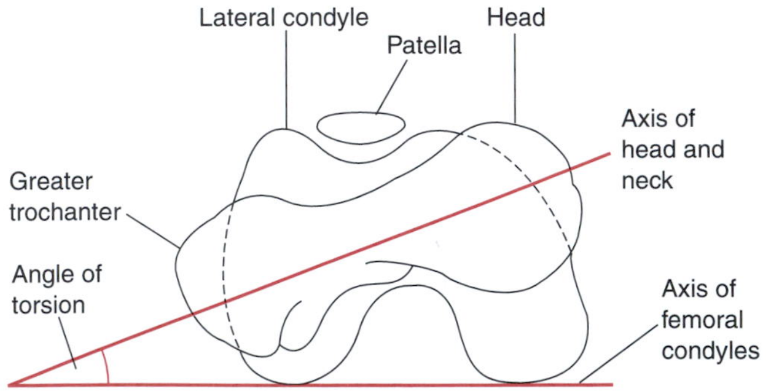

FIGURE 20-4 The normal angle of torsion of the right femur.

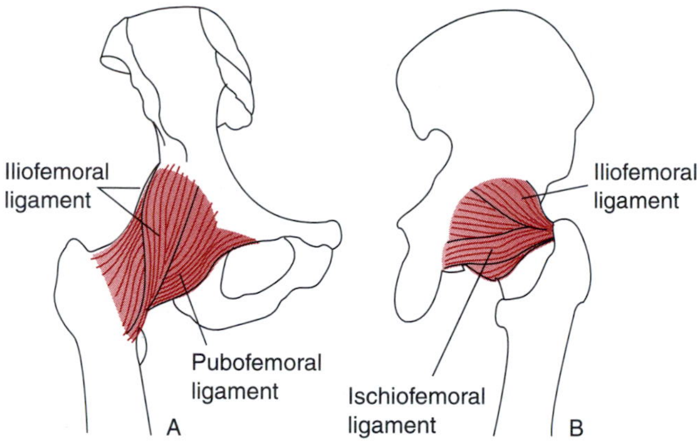

FIGURE 20-5 ***(A)*** Anterior view of the hip illustrating the iliofemoral and pubofemoral ligaments. ***(B)*** Posterior view of the hip illustrating the ischiofemoral ligament.

predispose the femoral neck to fracture, which is the most common fracture site in elderly persons.[2,5]

The greater trochanter is a large, bony prominence projecting posterosuperiorly from the junction of the neck and shaft of the femur (see Fig. 20-2). The gluteus medius and gluteus minimus attach along the lateral and anterior surfaces of the greater trochanter, respectively. The lesser trochanter (see Fig. 20-2) occupies the posteromedial junction of the neck and shaft of the femur and is the site of iliopsoas attachment.

Kinematics

In considering kinematics of the hip joint, it is useful to view the joint as a stable ball and socket configuration wherein the femoral head and acetabulum can move in all directions. Lack of mobility at the hip joint can result in compensatory increase in motion proximally or distally in the kinetic chain. However, the most common sites of compensation for lack of motion at the hip joint are the sacroiliac joints, lumbar spine, and knees.

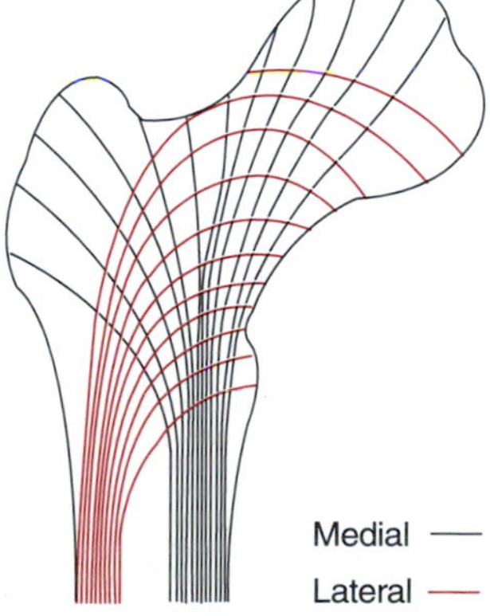

FIGURE 20-6 Femur showing the medial trabeculae and lateral trabeculae systems.

OSTEOKINEMATICS

Hip motion takes place in all three planes: sagittal (flexion and extension), frontal (abductionadduction), and transverse (medial and lateral rotation).

When not influenced by tension of the diarthrodial hip muscles (eg, hamstrings, rectus femoris), motion is greatest in the sagittal plane, where the range of flexion is 0 to approximately 120 to 135 degrees (or soft tissue approximation), and the range of extension is 0 to 15 degrees. With the knee in extension, placing passive tension on the hamstrings, the range of flexion is considerably less, approximately 90 degrees. The range of extension is notably less than that of flexion and is limited by the tension of the iliofemoral ligament. Ranges of flexion and extension can appear greater than actual if pelvic and lumbar motion is allowed to take place. For this reason, care must be taken in measuring the range of motion (ROM) at the hip. In measuring hip sagittal plane mobility, the examiner must stabilize carefully to prevent posterior pelvic tilt and lumbar flexion during hip flexion and prevent anterior pelvic tilt and lumbar extension during hip extension.

The range of abduction is 0 to 30 degrees, whereas adduction is somewhat less, 0 to 25 degrees. When measuring abduction at the hip, care must be taken to properly stabilize the pelvis from laterally tilting and the lumbar spine from side bending. Abduction is checked by impact of the femoral neck on the acetabular rim, but before this occurs, it is usually restrained by the adductor muscles and the iliofemoral and pubofemoral ligaments. Movement beyond physiologic adduction is also accompanied by tilting of the pelvis and side bending the lumbar spine. These associated movements must be controlled when measuring hip adduction ROM.

Discrepancies exist in the literature concerning rotation ROM, probably because of the method of measurement, age differences, and structural differences between men and women. The most acceptable method for measuring hip rotation ROM is with the patient in the prone position with the hips extended to tighten the anterior capsule.[6] If the ROM is tested in sitting, the hip is flexed and the anterior capsule relaxed, which allows a slightly greater range of lateral rotation. Stabilization of the lumbar, pelvis, and tibiofemoral joints is required to accurately measure hip joint ROM when tested in prone. With respect to the tibiofemoral joint, tibial lateral rotation can occur to allow greater hip joint lateral rotation because of the attachment of the tensor fascia lata (TFL)–iliotibial band (ITB) complex into the tibia, and tibiofemoral valgus can occur and give the appearance of increased hip medial rotation ROM. These joints must be carefully stabilized when measuring hip joint rotation ROM in addition to the lumbopelvic region.

Hip rotation ROM varies with the age and sex of the individual. Children younger than 2 years of age usually have a lateral rotation contracture of the hip resulting from an intrauterine position in which the hips are flexed and laterally rotated.[7] Standing provides the stimulus for the hips to rotate medially, reducing the lateral rotation contracture to the point where medial and lateral rotation ROM is roughly comparable throughout childhood. Later in life, lateral rotation becomes greater than medial rotation in men, but in women, they remain about equal, or in many instances, medial rotation is slightly greater.[8] In a study of 500 subjects, spanning 22 age groups from younger than 1 year old to 70 and older, medial rotation was greater in female subjects than in male subjects by a mean of 7 degrees.[9] For female subjects, from middle childhood on, the mean medial rotation ROM was about 50 degrees, and the normal range was 25 to 65 degrees. For male subjects, the mean ROM for medial rotation was about 40 degrees, and the normal range was 15 to 60 degrees. From middle childhood on, the mean lateral rotation ROM for both sexes was about 45 degrees, and the normal range was 25 to 65 degrees.[9]

The clinician should be aware of ROM requirements necessary to perform ADLs to assist the patient in developing appropriate functional goals. ROM values for gait are addressed in a subsequent section. The average ranges of motion required for basic ADLs are summarized in Table 20-1. Maximal motion in the sagittal plane is needed for tying the shoe and squatting to pick up an object from the floor. The greatest motion in frontal and transverse planes was recorded during squatting and shoe tying with the foot across the opposite thigh. The values obtained for these common activities indicate that hip flexion of at least 120 degrees and abduction and lateral rotation of at least 20 degrees are necessary for carrying out activities in a normal manner. If these values are not available at the hip, the body probably will find the path of least resistance and move excessively or abnormally in a compensatory joint to attain the desired movement. For example, during squatting, if 120 degrees of hip flexion is not available in one hip, the lumbopelvic region may compensate with excessive flexion or rotation motions. If this faulty movement pattern is used repeatedly, microtrauma may be imposed on the compensatory segments, potentially leading to pathology.

Table 20-1. MEAN VALUES FOR MAXIMUM HIP MOTION IN THREE PLANES DURING COMMON ACTIVITIES

ACTIVITY	PLANE OF MOTION	RECORDED VALUE (DEGREES)
Tying shoe with foot on floor	Sagittal	124
	Frontal	19
	Transverse	15
Tying shoe with foot across opposite thigh	Sagittal	110
	Frontal	23
	Transverse	33
Sitting down on chair and rising from sitting	Sagittal	104
	Frontal	20
	Transverse	17
Stooping to obtain object from floor	Sagittal	117
	Frontal	21
	Transverse	18
Squatting	Sagittal	122
	Frontal	28
	Transverse	26
Ascending stairs	Sagittal	67
	Frontal	16
	Transverse	18
Descending stairs	Sagittal	36

Data from Johnson, RC, Smidt, GL. Hip measurements for selected activities of daily living. *Clin Orthop*. 1970;72:205–215.

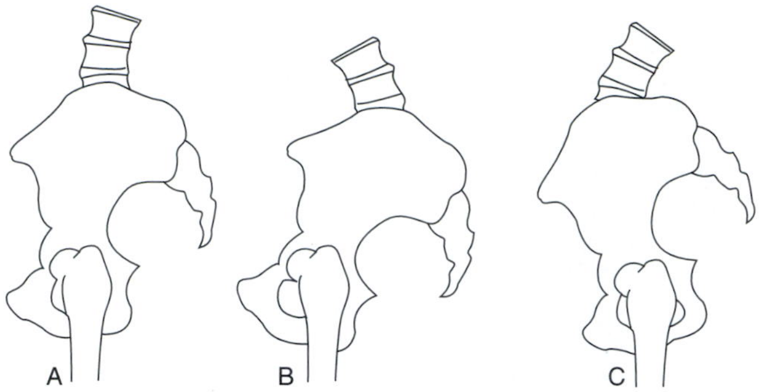

FIGURE 20-7 Relationship of movements in the sagittal plane of the pelvis and hip. ***(A)*** Normal position. ***(B)*** Posterior pelvic tilt and hip extension. ***(C)*** Anterior pelvic tilt and hip flexion.

In the closed kinetic chain, movement of the pelvis occurs over the head of the femur about all three axes of motion. The osteokinematic ROM and arthrokinematic relationships remain unchanged, regardless of the status of the kinetic chain (ie, open versus closed).

Anterior and posterior pelvic tilting occur in the sagittal plane about a frontal axis (Fig. 20-7). Motion of the pelvis in an anterior direction (ie, anterior pelvic tilt) produces hip flexion and lumbar extension, and motion of the pelvis in a posterior direction (ie, posterior pelvic tilt) produces hip extension and lumbar flexion. Lateral pelvic tilt occurs in the frontal plane about an anteroposterior axis (Fig. 20-8). In lateral pelvic tilt, one hip joint serves as the axis for motion, and the opposite iliac crest elevates or drops about that pivot point. The hip on the high iliac crest side is in relative adduction, and the hip on the low iliac crest side is in relative abduction.

Pelvic rotation occurs in the transverse plane about a vertical axis (Fig. 20-9). Rotation of the pelvis in a clockwise direction results in left hip lateral rotation and right hip medial rotation, and rotation of the pelvis in a counterclockwise direction results in right hip lateral rotation and left hip medial rotation.

ARTHROKINEMATICS

Because of the inherent structural stability of the hip joint, the arthrokinematic motion accompanying hip flexion and

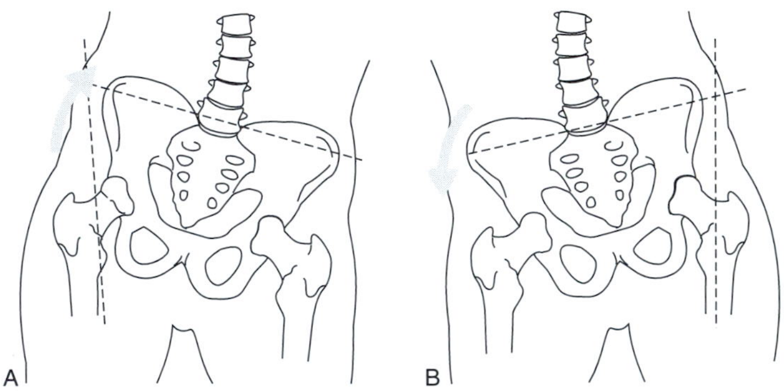

FIGURE 20-8 Relationship of movements in the frontal plane of the pelvis and hip. The hip on the high iliac crest side is in relative adduction, while the hip on the low iliac crest side is in relative abduction.

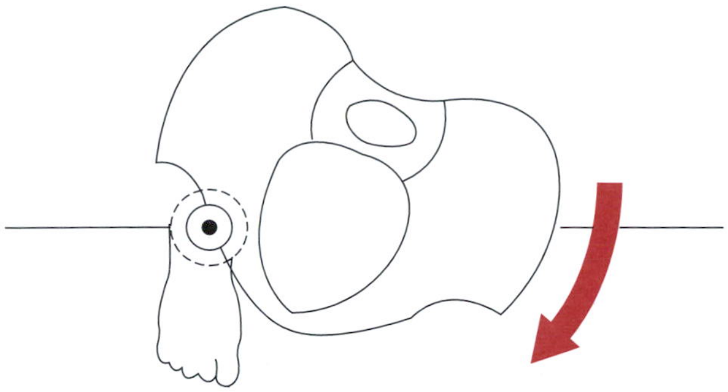

FIGURE 20-9 Relationship of movements in the transverse plane of the pelvis and hip. Rotation of the pelvis in a clockwise direction results in right hip medial rotation and left hip lateral rotation. (From Norkin CC, Levangie PK. *Joint Structure and Function: A Comprehensive Analysis.* 2d ed. Philadelphia: FA Davis; 1992:313.)

extension is nearly a pure rotation. The head rotates posteriorly in flexion, accompanied by a slight posterior glide, and the head rotates anteriorly in extension, accompanied by a slight anterior glide. The motions of hip abduction and adduction and of medial and lateral rotation also include combinations of rotation and gliding, which occur opposite to the motion of the distal end of the femur (when the femur is the moving segment).

Muscles

Numerous muscles cross the hip joint. Table 20-2 lists the muscles according to their function at the hip in an open kinetic chain. Review of Table 20-2 should be aided by an atlas of anatomy to help visualize the muscular relationships. Coordinated muscle function in the kinetic chain is discussed in the Gait section.

In considering the musculature that crosses the hip, the practitioner must consider the relationship of the hip muscles to the muscles of the trunk and the roles they play in moving or positioning the pelvis and spine. Dynamically, hip extensors and abdominal muscles posteriorly rotate the pelvis. Statically, postural hip flexion may result from a combination of short hip flexors, elongated anterior trunk musculature (ie, lower rectus and external obliques), and shortened posterior trunk musculature (ie, lumbar erector spinae and latissimus dorsi).

Musculature of the lower extremity acting at the knee, ankle, and foot affects the function of the hip and vice versa. For example, chronic hyperextension of the knee due to weak quadriceps and short ankle plantar flexors transmits an anterior force up to the head of the femur. This anterior force may contribute to anterior compression of the head of the femur in the acetabulum. Likewise, stretched and weak hip lateral rotators can lead to the hip functioning in chronic medial rotation, which may result in excessive pronatory forces at the foot.

Nerves and Blood Supply

Branches of nerves derived from the lumbosacral plexus innervate the hip joint and the rest of the lower extremity.

Table 20-2. MUSCLES OF THE HIP JOINT

FLEXORS	EXTENSORS
Iliopsoas	Gluteus maximus
Tensor fascia lata	Hamstrings
Rectus femoris	Posterior fibers of gluteus medius
Sartorius	Piriformis
Adductor magnus, longus, brevis	
Pectineus	
Gracilis	
Abductors	**Adductors**
Gluteus medius	Adductor magnus, longus, brevis
Tensor fascia lata	Quadratus femoris
Superior gluteus maximus	Pectineus
Gluteus minimus	Obturatur externus/internus
	Gracilis
	Medial hamstrings
Medial Rotators	**Lateral Rotators**
Tensor fascia lata	Piriformis
Gluteus minimus	Obturator internus/externus
Anterior fibers of gluteus medius	Gamellus superior/inferior
Adductor magnus/longus	Quadratus femoris
Semimembranosis/semitendinosis	Gluteus maximus
	Posterior fibers of gluteus medius
	Biceps femoris

From Norkin C, Levangie P. *Joint Structure and Function*. Philadelphia: FA Davis; 1983.

The hip joint receives branches from the obturator and femoral nerves (lumbar plexus [L1-L4]) and the superior gluteal nerve and the nerve to the quadratus femoris (sacral plexus [L4-S3]). Because of the innervation from the femoral nerve, pain experienced in the knee can be the result of pathology in the hip.

The blood supply to the head of the femur is of particular importance because of its significance in common pathologic conditions at the hip, including fractures, osteochondrosis (Legg-Calve-Perthes disease), and avascular necrosis of the femoral head. The head of the femur receives its vascularization from two sources: the artery of the ligament of the head of the femur (ligamentum teres) and branches of the medial and lateral circumflex arteries that ascend proximally along the neck of the femur.

Because of the relation of the medial and lateral circumflex arteries to the neck of the femur, they are subject to injury in the case of a femoral neck fracture. Because they are intracapsular, pressure caused by joint effusion may stop blood flow. This mechanism is thought to be a factor in osteochondrosis of the head of the femur and, in some cases, idiopathic avascular necrosis of the head.

Kinetics

Kinetic studies have demonstrated that substantial forces act on the hip joint during simple activities. The factors involved in producing these forces must be understood if rational rehabilitation programs are to be developed for patients with functional limitations and disability due to hip pathology and impairments.

STATICS

During double-limb support, the line of gravity of the body passes posterior to the hip joint, creating an extension moment. Because extension of the hip is a position of stability, erect stance can be achieved without muscle activity. When a person moves from double-limb support to single-limb support, the line of gravity shifts in all three planes, producing moments about the hip that must be counterbalanced by muscle forces. The magnitude of these forces depends on spinal alignment; the positions of the non–weight-bearing leg, trunk, upper extremities, and weight-bearing leg; and especially the inclination of the pelvis.[10] Fig. 20-10 demonstrates how the line of gravity in the frontal plane shifts with three different positions of the pelvis and upper body.

The shift of the gravity line and resulting change in the length of the lever arm of the gravitational force (GFLA, the perpendicular distance between the gravity line and the center of rotation in the femoral head), influences the magnitude of the moments about the hip joint (Fig. 20-11). The hip abductors must counterbalance the moment created by the GFLA. The GFLA and joint reaction force are minimized when the trunk is tilted over the hip joint (see Fig. 20-10*B*). Patients with hip pain may adopt this type of gait pattern, with maximal trunk tilt over the ipsilateral side, to reduce joint reaction forces and decrease pain. Patients with weak abductors may present with a Trendelenburg sign (see Fig. 20-10*C*) because of the inability of the hip abductors to generate enough force to counterbalance the GFLA.

DYNAMICS

Many investigators have studied loads imposed on the hip joint during dynamic activities.[11–16] The joint reaction force during gait in men and women without hip pathology varies. In men, two peak forces occur; one, just after initial contact, is approximately four times body weight, and a larger peak, just before preswing, is approximately seven times body weight.[17] In women, the force pattern is the same, but the magnitudes are somewhat lower, reaching a maximum of four times body weight during late stance phase.[17]

Kinetics and Kinematics of Gait

The pelvis, hip, knee, ankle, and foot work in synergy to produce the ideal gait pattern. Table 20-3 summarizes kinetics and kinematics of the gait cycle at the hip. This information is provided so that deviations from the norm are appreciated, and appropriate specific and functional exercises can be developed to treat impairments in movement patterns associated with gait.

Because motions at the ankle, knee, and hip in the sagittal plane are the most important in contributing to the critical events that occur in gait, they are the focus of the

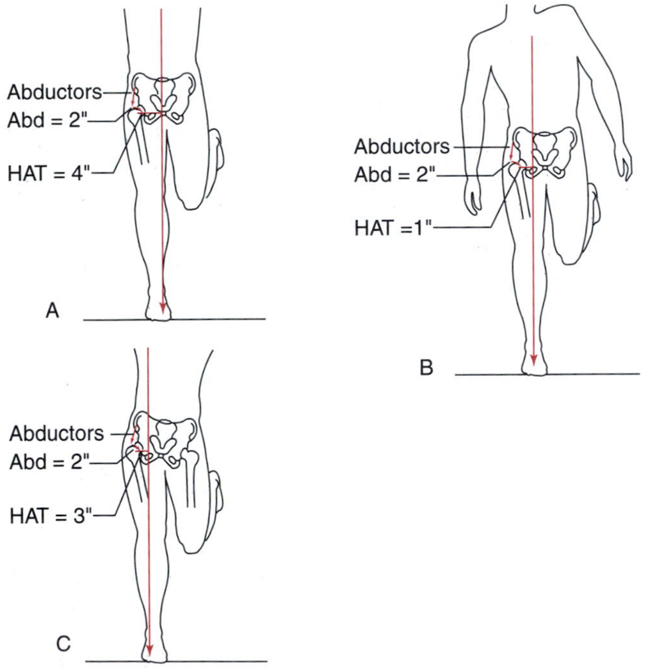

FIGURE 20-10 ***(A)*** In right unilateral stance, the weight of the head, arms, and trunk (HAT) act 4 inches from the right hip, producing an adduction torque around the right hip joint. The abductors, acting 2 inches from the right hip joint, generate a large force to produce an abduction torque sufficient to counterbalance the torque produced by HAT. ***(B)*** When the trunk is laterally flexed toward a stance limb, the moment arm of the HAT is substantially reduced, whereas that of the abductors remains unchanged. The result is a substantially diminished torque from the HAT and a corresponding decreased hip abductor force to counterbalance the HAT torque. ***(C)*** The pelvis drops on the opposite side of the stance limb when the abductor force cannot counterbalance the torque produced by HAT. This is called a positive Trendelenberg's sign.

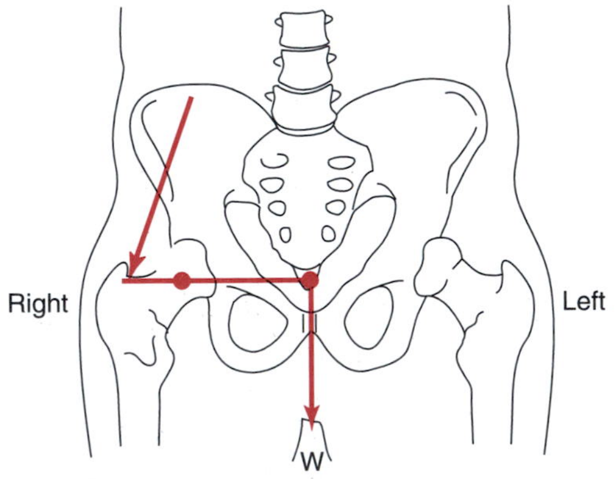

FIGURE 20-11 In right unilateral stance, a moment is created around the right hip joint that tends to produce a clockwise rotary force about the right hip. Activity of the right hip abductors is necessary to counteract the gravitational moment. The arrow indicates the action line of the right hip abductors in right unilateral stance. The distance from the action line to the right hip joint axis is about one-half the distance from the right hip joint axis to the body's center of gravity. The right hip abductors must be capable of exerting a force almost twice as great as the gravitational force to prevent lateral drop of the pelvis on the left.

Table 20-3. KINETICS AND KINEMATICS OF THE GAIT CYCLE AT THE HIP

PHASES OF THE GAIT CYCLE	RANGE OF MOTION	MOMENT	MUSCLE ACTIVITY	MUSCLE CONTRACTION TYPE
Initial contact	25 degrees of hip flexion	Rapid, high-intensity flexion moment	Hamstrings	Eccentric
			All hip extensors are active in preparation for loading response	Eccentric/isometric
Loading response	25 degrees of hip flexion	Flexion torque persists, second highest torque demand; adduction moment begins	All of the hip extensors to conteract the flexion moment	Eccentric
			Posterior TFL, gluteus medius, gluteus minimus, upper gluteus maximus to stabilize the pelvis in the frontal plane	Isometric/eccentric
Midstance	Extends to neutral	Decreased flexion moment; adduction moment continues	Hip abductor group is active as above	Isometric/eccentric
Terminal stance	Hip extends to 20 degrees (a portion of this apparent hip extension may come from pelvic rotation posteriorly 5 degrees	Adduction moment ends; hip extension moment keeps hip stable	Anterior TFL	Eccentric
Preswing	Moves toward neutral	Hip extension moment diminishes to 0 degrees	Adductor longus, rectus femoris	Concentric at the hip Eccentric to the knee
Initial swing	15 degrees of hip flexion	Not measured	Iliacus, gracilis, sartorius, adductor longus	Concentric
Midswing	25 degrees of hip flexion	Not measured	Iliacus, gracilis, sartorius cease	Concentric
			Hamstring begins	Eccentric
Terminal swing	Unchanged from midswing	Not measured	Hamstrings Lower fibers of gluteus maximus and adductors	Eccentric Isometric/eccentric

Adapted from Rancho Los Amigos Medical Center. *Observational Gait Analysis*. *Downey*, CA: Los Amigos Research and Education Institute; 1993.

summary information in Table 20-3. Other more subtle motions occur in all three planes at the foot, knee, hip, and pelvis. These motions should also be understood to analyze the gait cycle and appropriately treat pathologic gait. More detailed kinesiologic information about the gait cycle is provided by Perry.[18]

ANATOMIC IMPAIRMENTS

Four anatomic impairments of the hip joint are considered: angle of torsion, angle of inclination, center edge angle of the acetabulum, and limb length discrepancy (LLD). Each anatomic impairment independently or in combination with other impairments (anatomic or physiologic), warrants careful consideration about the impact on hip joint function and the function of joints proximal or distal to the hip. Anatomic impairments of the femur can contribute to dysfunction in the knee and hip regions.

Angles of Inclination and Torsion

The angles of inclination and torsion are normal anatomic relationships of the femur. However, the degree of inclination or torsion can become abnormal when the values are greater or less than normal. Abnormal angulations of the femur are considered anatomic impairments. These anatomic impairments of the femur can significantly alter hip joint mechanics, which can alter the mechanics of adjacent segments proximally and distally in the kinetic chain.

In the frontal plane, adduction and extension of the femoral shaft in relation to the femoral head causes the axis of the femoral neck and the femoral shaft to form an angle called the angle of inclination (see Fig. 20-3).[1] In early infancy, the angle is about 150 degrees because of the abducted position of the femur in utero. The angle decreases with age. The normal adult angle is about 125 degrees, and the normal older adult angle is about 120 degrees.[1] The angle is somewhat smaller in females and somewhat larger in males. A pathologic increase in the angle is called coxa valga (Fig. 20-12A), and a pathologic decrease is called coxa vara (Fig. 20-12B).

The medially rotated position of the femoral shaft in relation to the position of the head and neck creates an angulation in the transverse plane called the angle of torsion.[19] The angle is formed by a line parallel to the posterior femoral condyles and a line through the head neck of the femur (see Fig. 20-4). The newborn infant has a maximum angle of torsion of approximately 40 degrees. This decreases to an average of 32 degrees at the age of 1 year and further decreases to 16 degrees by the age of 16 years.[20] The angle is normally about 12 to 15 degrees in the adult, but it may range from 8 to 30 degrees and, like the angle of inclination, varies between sexes and among persons.[1,19] A pathologic increase in the angle of torsion is called anteversion (Fig. 20-13*A*), and a decrease is called retroversion (Fig. 20-13*B*). Anteversion and retroversion can be screened for during a clinical examination.

A pathologic increase in the angle of inclination (coxa vara) can be associated with hip anteversion and genu valgum, and a pathologic decrease in the angle of inclination (coxa valga) can be associated with genu varum. Although some conditions such as anteversion, coxa vara, and genu valgum may occur together, each may occur independently. Because the hip joint can only tolerate a limited amount of torsion (12 to 15 degrees) without jeopardizing the congruence of the hip joint, a pathologic increase (>15 degrees) or decrease (<12 degrees) in the angle of torsion is manifested distally at the femoral condyles. In the standing position, the femoral condyles of an individual with femoral anteversion are oriented medially, and in femoral retroversion, they are oriented laterally when the femoral head is in maximum congruence. The individual with femoral anteversion functioning with the femoral condyles facing laterally risks losing congruence of the femoral head in the acetabulum, similar to the the individual with femoral retroversion functioning with the femoral condyles facing medially. The practitioner must be aware of these anatomic impairments when guiding femoral alignment during exercise and function.

Center Edge Angle or Angle of Wiberg

A line connecting the lateral rim of the acetabulum and the center of the femoral head forms an angle with the vertical

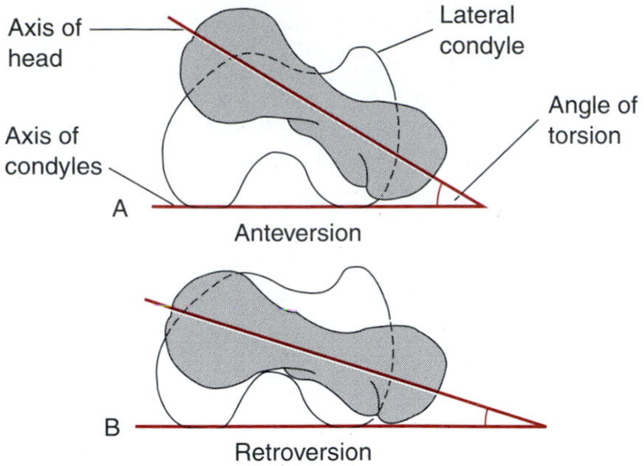

FIGURE 20-13 ***(A)*** A pathologic increase in the angle of torsion is called anteversion. ***(B)*** A pathologic decrease in the angle of torsion is called retroversion. (From Norkin CC, Levangie PK. *Joint Structure and Function: A Comprehensive Analysis.* 2d ed. Philadelphia: FA Davis; 1992:313).

known as the center edge angle, also called the angle of Wiberg (Fig. 20-14). The center edge angle for the average adult is 22 to 42 degrees.[21] Although this is a normal angle, variations in the angle can lead to altered stability of the femoral head, in which case it would be considered an anatomic impairment.

A smaller center edge angle (ie, more vertical orientation) of the acetabulum may result in decreased congruency of the head of the femur and the acetabulum, placing the head of the femur at increased risk of superior dislocation of the head of the femur. Children are at greater risk for this type of dislocation than adults, because the center edge angle normally increases with age.[22] It may be for this reason that congenital dislocation is more common at the hip joint than any other joint in the body.[23]

Limb Length Discrepancy

LLD, when measured from one common bilateral point of reference proximally to another common bilateral point of reference distally, is a unilateral difference in the total length of one leg compared with the other. LLD is commonly thought of as resulting from a structural fault in the anatomic length of the long bones or hemipelvis or asymmetric struc-

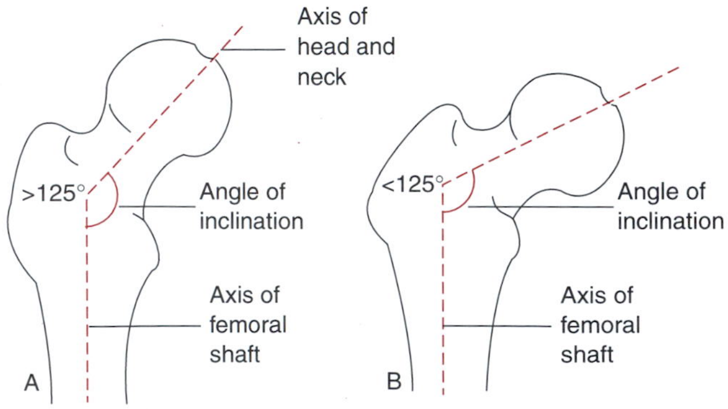

FIGURE 20-12 Abnormal angles of inclination. ***(A)*** A pathologic increase in the angle of inclination is called coxa valga. ***(B)*** A pathologic decrease in the angle of inclination is called coxa vara.

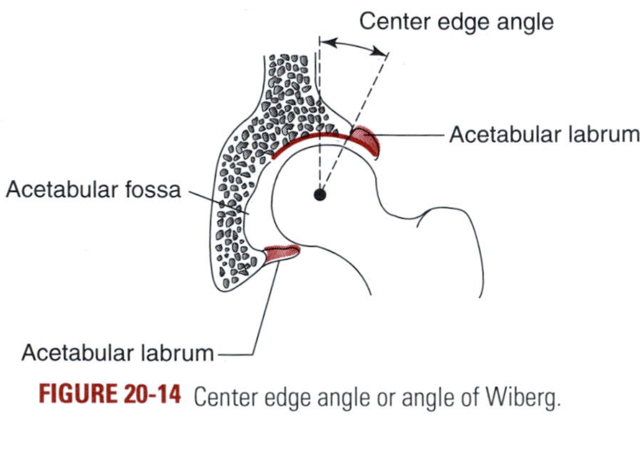

FIGURE 20-14 Center edge angle or angle of Wiberg.

tural development of the spine (ie, scoliosis), in which case it would be considered an anatomic impairment. However, LLD often is the result of the functional relationships of the spine, pelvis, long bones, and bones of the feet about all three axes of motion. For example, an individual standing in a neutral subtalar position, measured bilaterally from the tip of the medial malleolus to the horizontal plane (ie, flat surface), should have equal measurements of both limbs. If the individual is allowed to pronate one foot, the medial malleolus of the pronated foot moves closer to the ground. The difference in height may be as much as $^1/_4$ to $^3/_4$ of an inch. This would be considered a physiologic impairment, instead of an anatomic impairment, resulting in LLD.

Structural and functional LLDs are common clinical terms used to describe the two types of LLDs. Table 20-4 summarizes definitions of the clinical terms used to describe LLD.

LLD has been associated with hip pain, knee pain, and low back pain and with lower extremity stress fractures.[24–26] Studies have shown increased hip joint forces of up to 12% in the relatively short and long limbs with LLDs of 3.5 to 6.5 cm.[27] In general, an LLD of more than 2.0 cm results in asymmetry in contact time, first and second force peaks, and loading and unloading rates of the vertical ground reaction force in gait.[28] Because of the changes in forces incurred at the hip and gait asymmetries, it appears that more than 2 cm of LLD can affect kinetics and kinematics throughout the kinetic chain and therefore should be addressed. Treatment of LLD is addressed in a later section.

EXAMINATION AND EVALUATION

Examination and evaluation of the hip can be isolated to the hip in the case of specific hip pathology (eg, rheumatoid arthritis, osteoarthritis, avascular necrosis of the femoral head). However, even for a diagnosis isolated to the hip, evaluation of the knee, ankle-foot, and lumbopelvic regions may provide useful information. Similarly, the hip is commonly included in the examination and evaluation of other regions to assess anatomic or physiologic impairments of the hip that may be contributing to dysfunction in the affected region (eg, a stiff hip contributing to lumbar hypermobility).

The descriptive examination and evaluation information presented in this section is not intended to be comprehensive or reflect any specific philosophical approach; it simply serves as a general review of pertinent tests performed in most hip examinations. Several clearing examinations of related regions are described to provide a conceptual understanding of an integrated approach to examination of the lumbopelvic region.

History

The history, as in any regional examination, must attempt to establish several facts:

- Onset and progression of the current condition
- Location, nature, and behavior of symptoms
- Past and current health status
- Effect of intra-individual and extra-individual interventions
- Effect the condition has had on ADLs and social roles

Of particular importance is a history of congenital hip dysfunction (eg, congenital hip dysplasia), childhood hip conditions (eg, slipped capital epiphysis, severe anteversion treated with bracing), or a family history of osteoarthritis or rheumatoid arthritis. The hip rarely becomes injured as a result of trauma, but it is commonly affected by repetitive abnormal stress. In the latter case, it is important for the practitioner to gain an understanding of the ADLs, recreational, and occupational activities with which the patient is involved on a repetitive basis and which activities seem to provoke symptoms. Much of this information can be obtained through self-report forms (Display 20-1), and the formal interview can clarify subjective information.

Lumbar Spine Clearing Examination

The prevalence of lumbopelvic conditions in the general population, combined with the fact that pathology in the lumbopelvic region can manifest in referred pain patterns into the hip (eg, posterior buttock) and cause neurologically mediated weakness of hip joint musculature (particularly the gluteal musculature), supports routine lumbar screening during any hip examination. A typical lumbar scan examination is outlined in Chapter 18. Although this scan may seem extensive, excluding or diagnosing lumbar or sacroiliac joint involvement is critical to accurate diagnosis of lower quadrant pain. Positive test results for the lumbar scan examination can indicate a need for a more thorough lumbar or sacroiliac joint examination.

Other Clearing Tests

The practitioner should examine and evaluate associated regions. Although the hip may be the source of symptoms, it is common for multiple regions to be involved, particularly in

Table 20-4. DEFINITIONS OF STRUCTURAL AND FUNCTIONAL LEG LENGTH DISCREPANCIES

TERM	TYPE OF IMPAIRMENT	DEFINITION	MEASUREMENT TECHNIQUE
Structural	Anatomic	Actual osseous *length* difference between the hemipelvis, femur, and tibia	Standing anteroposterior x-ray film or ultrasound imaging[39]
Functional	Physiologic	*Position* of osseous structures as they relate to each other and to the environment during weight-bearing function	Actual difference between two pairs of identical reference points (eg, greater trochanter and medial malleolus)

DISPLAY 20-1

Self-Report Form

Functional Index

Walking

- ☐ Pain does not prevent me walking any distance.
- ☐ Pain prevents me walking more than 1 mile.
- ☐ Pain prevents me walking more than $^1/_2$ mile.
- ☐ Pain prevents me walking more than $^1/_4$ mile.
- ☐ I can only walk using a stick or crutches.
- ☐ I am in bed most of the time and have to crawl to the toilet.

Work

(*Applies to work in home and outside*)

- ☐ I can do as much work as I want to.
- ☐ I can only do my usual work, but no more.
- ☐ I can do most of my usual work, but no more.
- ☐ I cannot do my usual work.
- ☐ I can hardly do any work at all (only light duty).
- ☐ I cannot do any work at all.

Personal Care

(*Washing, dressing, etc.*)

- ☐ I can manage all personal care without symptoms.
- ☐ I can manage all personal care with some increased symptoms.
- ☐ Personal care requires slow, concise movements due to increased symptoms.
- ☐ I need help to manage some personal care.
- ☐ I need help to manage all personal care.
- ☐ I cannot manage any personal care.

Sleeping

- ☐ I have no trouble sleeping.
- ☐ My sleep is mildly disturbed (less than 1 h sleepless).
- ☐ My sleep is mildly disturbed (1–2 h sleepless).
- ☐ My sleep is moderately disturbed (2–3 h sleepless).
- ☐ My sleep is greatly disturbed 3–5 h sleepless).
- ☐ My sleep is completely disturbed (5–7 h sleepless).

Recreation/Sports

(*Indicate sport if appropriate* ____________________)

- ☐ I am able to engage in all my recreational/sports activities without increased symptoms.
- ☐ I am able to engage in all my recreational/sports activities with some increased symptoms.
- ☐ I am able to engage in most, but not all of my usual recreational/sports activities because of increased symptoms.
- ☐ I am able to engage in a few of my usual recreational/sports activities because of my increased symptoms.
- ☐ I can hardly do any recreational/sports activities because of increased symptoms.
- ☐ I cannot do any recreational/sports activities at all.

Acuity

(*Answer on initial visit.*)

- ☐ How many days ago did onset/injury occur? ____________ days

Stairs

- ☐ I can walk stairs comfortably without a rail.
- ☐ I can walk stairs comfortably, but with a crutch, cane, or rail.
- ☐ I can walk more than one flight of stairs, but with pain or weakness.
- ☐ I can walk less than one flight of stairs.
- ☐ I can manage only a single step or curb.
- ☐ I am unable to manage even a step or curb.

Uneven Ground

- ☐ I can walk normally on uneven ground without loss of balance or using a cane or crutches.
- ☐ I can walk on uneven ground, but with loss of balance or with the use of a cane or crutches.
- ☐ I have to walk very carefully on uneven ground without using a cane or crutches.
- ☐ I have to walk very carefully on uneven ground even when using a cane or crutches.
- ☐ I have to walk very carefully on uneven ground and require physical assistance to manage it.
- ☐ I am unable to walk on uneven ground.

Standing

- ☐ I can stand as long as I want without pain.
- ☐ I can stand as long as I want, but it gives me extra pain.
- ☐ Pain prevents me from standing for more than 1 hour.
- ☐ Pain prevents me from standing for more than 30 minutes.
- ☐ Pain prevents me from standing for more than 10 minutes.
- ☐ Pain prevents me from standing at all.

Squatting

- ☐ I can squat fully without the use of my arms for support.
- ☐ I can squat fully, but with pain or using my arms for support.
- ☐ I can squat $^3/_4$ of my normal depth, but less than fully.
- ☐ I can squat $^1/_2$ of my normal depth, but less than $^3/_4$.
- ☐ I can squat $^1/_4$ of my normal depth, but less than $^1/_2$.
- ☐ I am unable to squat any distance due to pain or weakness.

Sitting

- ☐ I can sit in any chair as long as I like.
- ☐ I can only sit in my favorite chair as long as I like.
- ☐ Pain prevents me sitting more than 1 hour.
- ☐ Pain prevents me sitting more than $^1/_2$ hour.
- ☐ Pain prevents me sitting more than 10 minutes.
- ☐ Pain prevents me from sitting at all.

Pain Index

Please indicate how much pain you feel at this time on the scale below

|____|

No Pain — Worst Pain Imaginable

PLEASE COMPLETE ON LAST VISIT ONLY

Improvement Index

Please indicate the amount of improvement you have made since the beginning of your physical therapy treatment on the scale below.

|____|

No Improvement — Complete Recovery

Work Status

1. No lost work time
2. Return to work without restriction
3. Return to work with modification
4. Have not returned to work
5. Not employed outside the home

Work days lost due to condition: ______________ days

Adapted from Therapeutic Associates Outcome System. Therapeutic Associates, Inc. 15060 Ventura Blvd., Suite 240, Sherman Oaks, CA 91403-2426 patients with long-standing impairments, functional limitations, and disability. A thorough examination of all involved regions permits the clinician to develop an integrated and comprehensive plan of care. For example, impairments of the pelvic floor may affect function of the hip. Screening for pelvic floor dysfunction can alert the practitioner to any associated pelvic floor conditions (see Chapter 19).

Visceral involvement or serious disease or disorders should be excluded. Pain in the hip and pelvic region can also result from visceral sources (see Appendix 1). A thorough history and physical examination and evaluation can alert the practitioner to visceral involvement or serious disease or pathology.

The hip must be excluded as the source of symptoms experienced in other regions. Because the hip is largely innervated at the L3-L4 level, hip pathology occasionally causes pain to be referred to the knee. A patient complaining of knee pain without apparent knee pathology or impairments should have the hip examined as a potential source of pain.

Standing Alignment

Specific lumbopelvic and lower quadrant alignment should be examined in all three planes. Hypotheses can be developed regarding the contribution of faulty alignments at the ankle, foot, knee, and lumbopelvic regions to the alignment of the hip, and hypotheses can be developed regarding faults in muscle lengths. The practitioner can make assumptions regarding muscles that are too long based on joint position, but muscle length testing is indicated to determine whether muscles are too short due to joint position. Initial screening for LLD should be performed by evaluating iliac crest heights and carefully observing spine, pelvic, femur, tibia, and foot alignments and the bony landmarks of the pelvis, knee, and ankle in all three planes of motion.

Gait

Gait evaluation is an important component of the examination of a person with a hip dysfunction. Analysis of gait should include observation of the foot, ankle, knee, hip, pelvis, lumbar spine, and upper quadrant in the frontal, transverse, and sagittal planes of motion during each critical event in gait (eg, initial contact, loading response, midstance). Of particular importance are the relationship of pelvic and hip motion (ie, amount of lateral pelvic tilt and hip adduction [Trendelenburg's sign]) and the relationship of hip and lower extremity motion (ie, hip medial rotation, tibial medial rotation, and foot pronation). Because the hip functions interdependently with other regions in the body, the relationship of distal and proximal segments to the hip must also be evaluated.

Video analysis can assist in this complex examination procedure, because the video can be taken from any angle and can be viewed in slow motion to allow precise observation of the components of gait. Hypotheses can be generated about the cause of any observed gait deviation that can be confirmed or negated as a result of the additional data collected.

Mobility

Mobility testing of the hip joint includes several assessments. *Quick tests* are functional movements that are used to ascertain the patient's willingness and ability to move and the requisite extent of the examination to follow. Such tests for the hip include flexing the hip and knee while putting the foot on a standard step height and during squatting. These actions are done first with feet flat and then up on the toes to determine ankle involvement.

Active and passive open chain osteokinematic ROMs are assessed. It is important to determine osteokinetic mobility of the hip joint along the continuum of hypermobility to hypomobility about all three axes of motion by carefully stabilizing the spine and pelvis during passive ROM examination techniques.

Passive arthrokinematic tests should examine mobility of the hip through caudal, anterior, posterior, medial, and lateral glides and by lateral distraction. The arthrokinematic examination should include mobility testing along the continuum of hypomobility to hypermobility.

Qualitative assessment of active and passive ROM combined with clinical reasoning can supply specific diagnostic information:

- Use of firm overpressure applied to a motion is used to exclude or diagnose joint pathology. Overpressure can also be used to determine the hip end-feel and therefore the structures providing the barrier to further motion.
- Assessment of the sequence of pain and limitation can grade the irritability of the condition and guide the intensity of treatment.[29]
- The pattern of restriction indicates the presence of a capsular pattern. This is an indication of joint inflammation.[29] Because the hip joint is deep in the pelvis, it is difficult to observe inflammation, and the presence of a capsular pattern can indicate signs of current or past joint inflammation. The capsular pattern of the hip is gross limitation of flexion, abduction, and medial rotation, slight limitation of extension, and little or no limitation of lateral rotation.[29]
- The combined results of passive and active movement testing can implicate a contractile or inert structure.[29] For example, the findings of passive movement painful in one direction and active movement painful in another implicate a contractile structure.

Tests of muscular extensibility are also important in assessing mobility of the hip. Common extensibility tests include determining the length of several muscles:

- Medial and lateral hamstrings (hamstring length should be examined as a group and individually as medial and lateral hamstrings)
- Iliopsoas (hip flexor length should be assessed individually for the iliopsoas, rectus femoris, and tensor fascia lata)
- Rectus femoris
- TFL/ITB
- Hip adductors
- Hip rotators

The examiner should assess for a lack of extensibility and for excessive extensibility. A hypothesis should be developed regarding what impact a lack of extensibility or excessive extensibility will have on the function of the hip and related regions.

Functional Movement Testing

Functional movement testing should also be observed to examine the integrated movement patterns of the lumbar spine, pelvis, hip, knee, ankle, and foot. Examples of functional movement testing for the hip include the following:

- Forward bending to observe lumbopelvic rhythm (see Chapter 18)
- Squatting (also used as a quick test)
- Ascending and descending steps
- Moving from sit to stand and back to sit
- Gait
- Running

Muscle Performance

Impairments in muscle performance can result from numerous sources, and tests of muscle performance combined with results of other tests should attempt to determine the presence and source of reduced muscle performance. The following discussion highlights specific types of muscle performance testing procedures used to diagnose the presence and source of impairment of muscle performance.

Specific *manual muscle testing* (MMT) of muscles surrounding the hip joint can provide information regarding muscle performance and the generating capability of each muscle or fiber direction of a single muscle (eg, anterior versus posterior gluteus medius).[30,31] Comprehensive MMT of the hip musculature also can determine the relationship of muscle performance capability of synergist and antagonist musculature around the hip (eg, posterior gluteus medius versus TFL as hip abductors).

Positional strength testing can determine the length-tension properties of the relevant muscle (see Chapter 4). If a muscle tests weak in the short range (ie, 3+/5 or less on a scale of 1/5 to 5/5 [30]) but strong in a middle range (4/5 or greater), it is most likely an elongated muscle (ie, adaptively lengthened beyond its normal length). Positional strength testing of the gluteus medius, gluteus maximus, iliopsoas, hip adductors, hip rotators, and TFL, combined with mobility tests and functional movement tests, can determine relationships of muscle length, strength, and function about the hip joint.

Selective tissue tension tests combine active and passive ROM with resisted tests of muscles around the hip joint complex. Results of these tests can assist the examiner in the differential diagnosis of a contractile or noncontractile lesion.[29] The major muscle groups (ie, hip flexion, extension, abduction, adduction, and rotation) should be tested one by one if a contractile lesion is suspected. Careful positioning of additional resisted tests can identify which synergist is at fault. For example, if the hip flexor group is implicated, it is possible through careful positioning to further differentiate the TFL from iliopsoas.

If a selective tissue tension test is positive, interpretation of the *resisted test* can indicate the severity of tissue lesion. Table 26-4 in Chapter 26 explains diagnostic findings with respect to resisted tests. Resisted tests can also screen for a neurologic cause of reduced force production, particularly in reference to the fatigability of the muscle being tested. Diagnosing the cause of the neurologic weakness can be challenging. Patterns of weakness coupled with the results of other clinical neurologic tests (eg, reflexes, sensory testing) can assist in the differential diagnosis of the neurologic weakness (eg, nerve root, peripheral nerve, neuromuscular disease). Electrodiagnostic, radiologic, and laboratory studies may be required to confirm a diagnosis.

Pain and Inflammation

Examination for pain and inflammation is done concurrently with other tests to determine the source. Inflammation is difficult to examine in the hip joint, because it is deep within the pelvis and cannot be readily palpated. Positive findings for a capsular pattern of hip mobility and end-feel assessment (ie, pain before limitation of motion is reached) indicate former or active inflammation.

Examination of the pain level should be incorporated into the subjective and objective portion of the examination. The patient should answer questions regarding pain level by using a visual, numeric, or verbal analog scale over a 24-hour cycle in relation to specific activities and in general.[32] During the physical examination, the patient should be questioned about the onset, location, and intensity of pain with respect to each test performed.

An attempt must be made to diagnosis the cause of the pain. The specific source of symptoms may not be diagnosed without additional tests that are beyond the scope of physical therapy practice (ie, radiologic, electrodiagnostic, and laboratory studies). However, in the event that symptoms were not induced by traumatic injury or disease, the cause of the symptoms can be diagnosed through careful examination and determination of the physiologic impairments that contribute to increased biomechanical stress to the hip joint.

Balance

Balance tests are often included in hip examinations because of the high incidence of falls resulting in hip injury and fracture. Balance testing should identify intrinsic (ie, related to the individual) and extrinsic (ie, associated with environmental factors) factors related to the risk of falling.

Low-tech balance assessments can identify risk factors for falls.[33] Strong correlations have been found among performance-based measures and fall risk, as well as between performance-based measures and self-report measures. Five variables are significantly related to fall risk[33]:

1. Berg Balance Scale (functional performance scale) score[34]
2. Dynamic Gait Index score[35]
3. Balance Self-Perceptions Test score[36]
4. History of imbalance
5. Type of assistive device used for ambulation

High-tech, computerized, force-platform balance devices commonly measure the ability to maintain the center of pressure within the base of support against progressive perturbations. This information is highly objective and is often used to track progress in developing postural balance.

Special Tests

Numerous special tests are used to confirm or negate symptoms or suspected diagnoses of the hip. For the commonly used special tests discussed in this section, specific information regarding the technique of application can be found in the related references.

The *Trendelenburg test* is used to evaluate the functional force or torque capability of the hip abductor muscle group. During gait, the patient may exhibit a positive Trendelenburg sign (see Fig. 20-10*C*) or compensated Trendelenburg sign (see Fig. 20-10*B*).[37] However, other gait deviations of the hip indicate hip abductor torque impairment, such as excessive hip medial rotation, pelvic counterrotation, or excessive lateral pelvic shift. These other gait deviations, although not traditionally called Trendelenburg signs, are also indicators of reduced hip abductor force or torque and are particularly related to positional weakness of the gluteus medius.

If the examiner suspects that one of a patient's legs may be shorter than the other, specific tests are indicated to determine whether a structural or functional LLD exists. Ultrasound techniques have been developed to measure LLD. This technique is superior to clinical measuring methods and radiologic examinations.[38] However, the most accepted method for accurate measurement of structural LLD is the standing anteroposterior roentgenogram.

Common clinical techniques for measurement of functional and structural LLDs are supine or prone measurements of limb length from paired anatomic sites.[37] In standing, the use of lifts under the apparent short side until visual symmetry is achieved can indicate the amount of LLD that exists with weight bearing. Without trauma to the long bones of the lower extremity or disorders of the joint surfaces, functional LLD should be suspected as the source of asymmetry.

The *clinical determination of the angle of torsion* is commonly called the *Craig test* and is used to diagnose anteversion or retroversion of the hip joints.[39] The patient should be lying in the prone position. To measure the right hip, the examiner stands on the contralateral side; the left hand is used to palpate the greater trochanter, and the right hand internally rotates the hip, with the patient's knee flexed to 90 degrees. At the point of maximal trochanteric prominence (representing the most lateral position of the greater trochanter), the angle subtended between the tibia and true vertical (representing the angle of torsion) is measured with a goniometer. This measurement correlates well with intraoperative measurements (Pearson correlation coefficient R value of 0.930 for the right hip and 0.877 for the left hip), and it is more accurate than radiographic techniques (Pearson correlation coefficient R value of 0.438 for the right hip and 0.399 for the left hip).[40]

In the *flexion and adduction test* or *Scour test*, movement is used to elicit joint signs when other movements are normal. The movement involves flexion and adduction through an arc from 90 to 140 degrees of flexion.[41]

The *FABER test*[42] is used to identify hip dysfunction. The examiner positions the hip in flexion, abduction, and external rotation. Caution must be used in interpreting a positive FABER test result as an indication of isolated hip dysfunction because the position and movement of the test probably place stress on the lumbopelvic region.

Functional Ability Assessment

Although measures of physiologic impairments are important for diagnosis, prognosis, and treatment planning, functional ability and quality of life are better indicators of outcome.[43] Functional ability can be measured directly through observation of functional tasks or by the use of self-report measures. Display 20-1 illustrates a general self-report measure with a specific section devoted to the hip. The Harris Hip Function Scale is another, but it is specific to degenerative conditions of the hip (Display 20-2). The Harris Hip Function Scale was originally designed to assess patient status after the onset of traumatic arthritis of the hip.[44] This scale combines a patient's report of pain and his capacity for ambulation and self-care. These tasks account for 91% of the score, and deformity and hip ROM account for 9% of the score. The advantages of this scale are that it is heavily weighted toward function, is easy to administer, and is familiar to most clinicians.

THERAPEUTIC EXERCISE INTERVENTIONS FOR COMMON PHYSIOLOGIC IMPAIRMENTS

After a thorough examination and evaluation of the hip and all related regions, the clinician should have a thorough understanding of the functional limitations affecting the patient and the related impairments. The diagnosis and prognosis are formulated, and an intervention is planned. One or more of the following specific impairments may be diagnosed:

- Hypermobility
- Hypomobility
- Decreased muscle performance
- Decreased endurance
- Altered balance
- Pain
- Inflammation
- Faulty postural habits
- Faulty movement patterns

The decision to treat any impairment lies in its relationship to the functional limitation and disability. Prioritization of impairments is critical to effective and efficient intervention. Exercise intervention should be kept as functional as possible. However, if the impairment is profound, specific exercise may be necessary to improve the level of performance until it can be incorporated into a functional activity. Specific exercise and functional activity examples are provided in the discussion of exercise intervention for each impairment.

Impaired Muscle Performance

The section on kinetics described the powerful forces required from the musculature surrounding the hip joint for accomplishing ADLs. The force-generating capability of any muscle around the hip joint may be compromised for one of the following reasons:

- Neurologic pathology (eg, peripheral nerve, nerve root, neuromuscular disease)

DISPLAY 20-2
Harris Hip Function Scale

(Circle one in each group)

Pain (44 points maximum)

None/ignores	44
Slight, occasional, no compromise in activity	40
Mild, no effect on ordinary activity, pain after unusual uses activity, aspirin	30
Moderate, tolerable, makes concessions, occasional codeine	20
Marked, serious limitations	10
Totally disabled	0

Function (47 points maximum)

Gait (walking maximum distance) (33 points maximum)

1. Limp:	
None	11
Slight	8
Moderate	5
Unable to walk	0
2. Support:	
None	11
Cane, long walks	7
Cane, full time	5
Crutch	4
Two canes	2
Two crutches	0
Unable to walk	0
3. Distance walked:	
Unlimited	11
Six blocks	8
Two to three blocks	5
Indoors only	2
Bed and chair	0

Functional Activities (14 points maximum)

1. Stairs:	
Normally	4
Normally with banister	2
Any method	1
Not able	0
2. Socks and tie shoes:	
With ease	4
With difficulty	2
Unable	0
3. Sitting:	
Any chair, 1 hour	5
High chair, 1/2 hour	3
Unable to sit 1/2 hour any chair	0
4. Enter public transport	
Able to use public transportation	1
Not able to use public transportation	0

Absence of Deformity (requires all four) (4 points maximum)

1. Fixed adduction <10	4
2. Fixed internal rotation in extension <10*	0
3. Leg length discrepancy less than 1 1/4 inch	
4. Pelvic flexion contracture <30*	

Range of Motion (5 points maximum)

Instructions

Record 10° of fixed adduction as "—10° abduction, adduction to 10°"

Similarly, 10° of fixed external rotation as "—10° internal rotation, external rotation to 10°"

Similarly, 10° of fixed external rotation with 10° further external rotation as "—10° internal rotation, external rotation to 20°"

	Range	Index Factor	Index Value*
Permanent flexion (1)______°	______°		
A. Flexion to			
(0–45°)		1.0	
(45–90°)		0.6	
(90–120°)		0.3	
(120–140°)		0.0	
	______°		
B. Abduction to			
(0–15°)		0.8	
(15–30°)		0.3	
(30–60°)		0.0	
C. Adduction to			
(0–15°)	______°	0.2	
(15–60°)		0.0	
D. External rotation in extension to	______°		
(0–30°)		0.4	
(30–60°)		0.0	
E. Internal rotation in extension to	______°		
(0–60°)		0.0	

*Index Value = Range × Index Factor

Total index value (A + B + C + D + E) ______

Total range of motion points (multiply total index value × 0.05) ______

Pain points: ______
Function points: ______
Absence of Deformity points: ______
Range of Motion points: ______
Total points (100 points maximum) ______
Comments:

Modified from Harris WH. Traumatic arthritis of the hip after dislocation and accetabular fracture; treatment by mold Arthroplasty. J Bone Joint Surg. *1969;51:737–755.*

- Muscle strain
- Altered length-tension relationships
- General weakness from disuse due to muscle imbalance, general deconditioning, or reduced muscle torque production for a specific performance level (eg, high-level athlete in training)
- Pain

NEUROLOGIC PATHOLOGY

Neurologic pathology can cause weakness of the hip. If neurologic pathology is suspected, a thorough examination and evaluation, combined with additional tests that are beyond the scope of physical therapy practice (ie, radiologic, electrodiagnostic, and laboratory studies), are used to diagnose the source of the pathology. To develop the appropriate plan of care, it must be determined whether the cause of the neurologically induced weakness is neuromusculoskeletal (eg, nerve root, peripheral nerve) or neuromuscular (eg, multiple sclerosis) in origin.

If the clinician has determined that the cause is neuromusculoskeletal in origin, it must then be determined whether the pathology is at the level of the nerve root or in a peripheral nerve. A dysfunction at the level of the lumbar spine can induce nerve root pathology that can manifest as weakness of the muscles innervated by the affected segmental levels.[45] The clinician must thoroughly screen the lumbopelvic region to confirm or negate the hypothesis of spinal influence on the reduced force-generating capability of muscles surrounding the pelvic girdle.

After a thorough examination and evaluation process, the neurologically induced hip joint weakness must be treated. Whether the source of the neurologic involvement is from the nerve root or peripheral nerve, the origin of the problem must be treated appropriately for the affected muscle torque production to improve.

Despite alleviation of neurologic factors, weakness contributing to functional limitation may still exist. The level of weakness depends on the duration of neurologic involvement. The residual weakness must be addressed at the appropriate level of intervention. For example, a 13-year-old gymnast has had a 5-month complaint of posterolateral hip pain. At the time of her initial evaluation, she was diagnosed with a gluteus medius strain. Appropriate treatment of her gluteus medius strain did not improve her condition after 3 months. At that time, her physician performed a thorough lumbar screen. Radiologic reports indicated a grade II L5-S1 spondylolisthesis with slight L5 nerve root compression occurring with end-range lumbar extension. As a result of the additional diagnosis of spondylolisthesis, she was treated with lumbosacral bracing and exercise to correct impairments related to the spine instability. During the next 3 months, her hip pain began to resolve, although only after a dual program was developed for treatment of the spondylolisthesis and gluteus medius strain.

The L5 nerve root innervates the gluteal musculature. Irritation of the nerve root at the unstable spinal level could interrupt the motor function of the L5 nerve root, resulting in neurologically induced weakness of the gluteus medius.[45,46] Without full afferent input into the gluteus medius, it may be vulnerable to strain, especially at the level of this patient's activity. Effective healing could not occur until afferent input into the gluteus medius was fully restored, which could not occur until the stability of L5-S1 segmental level was sufficient for her activity level. After the L5-S1 level became more stable and normal afferent input was restored to the affected musculature, a gradual conditioning program for the gluteus medius muscle was necessary.

An example of a progressive strengthening program for the gluteus medius is illustrated in Self-Management: Gluteus Medius Strength Progression. This progression begins in prone for the muscle with a 3/5 or lower MMT grade[30] and progresses to sidelying with increasing lever arms to increase the load on the muscle. As muscle torque and endurance capabilities improve, transition to functional positions and movements can be introduced. Self-Management: Walk Stance Progression can be progressed

(text continues on page 404)

SELF-MANAGEMENT: *Gluteus Medius Strength Progression*

Purpose: To strengthen the hip muscles that keep your hip and pelvis in good alignment when you walk (highest level of this exercise (level V). Helps to stretch the band on the outside of the thigh)

Level I

Start Position
- Lie on your stomach on a firm surface. Place ___ pillows under your torso as indicated in the illustration.
- Your legs should be in line with your hips and rotated *slightly* outward.

Movement technique
- Pull in your abdomen by bringing your belly button toward your spine.
- Squeeze your buttock muscle.
- *Slightly* lift your leg and move it sideways through as much range as your hip allows. The indication that your hip has moved through its full available range is that your pelvis begins to tilt sideways and your spine sidebends. Do not move your hip any further after you feel your pelvis or spine move. Hold this position for 10 seconds.
- Return your hip to a start position.

Dosage

Sets/repetitions ______

Frequency ______

Level II

Perform as in level I, but attach a ______ piece of elastic around your ankles.

Dosage

Sets/repetitions ________

Frequency ___________

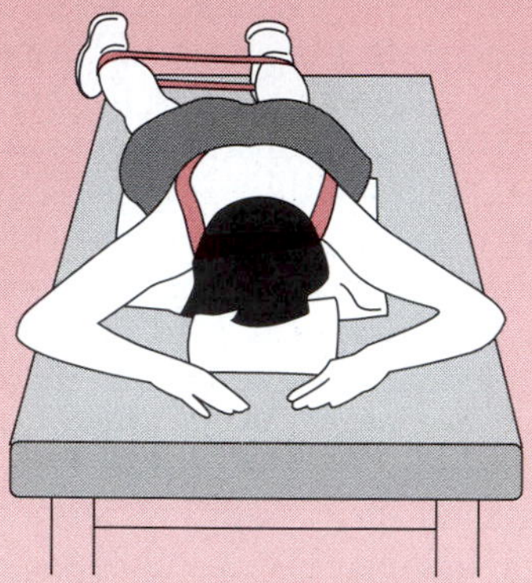

Level II: Prone hip abduction with elastic

Level III

Start position

- Lie on your uninvolved side, with your hips and knees bent and _____ pillows between your knees.
- Be sure you are on your side, with your head and neck in line with your spine and your spine in neutral, not rotated forward or backward.

Movement technique

- Keep your trunk still by pulling your belly button toward your spine to activate your abdominal muscles. Slowly turn your hip outward (like opening a clam shell). Hold this position for 10 seconds.
- Slowly return to the start position.

Dosage

Sets/repetitions ______

Frequency ___________

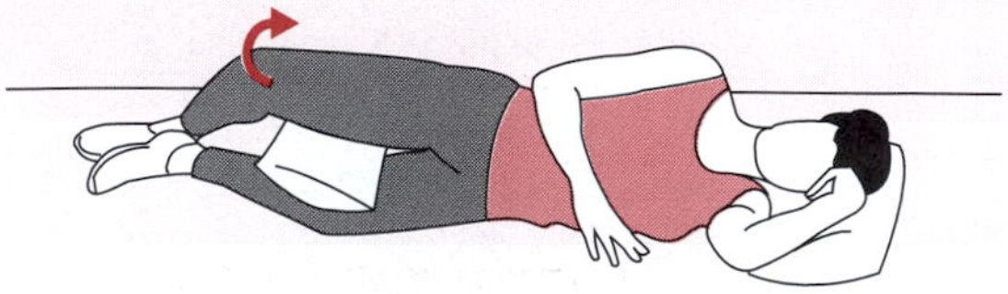

Level III: Sidelying hip lateral rotation

Level IV

Start position

- As in level III, but your knees should be only slightly bent.

Movement technique

- Turn out your hip without letting your pelvis or spine tilt backward or forward by activating your abdominal muscles as in level III.
- Lift your thigh upward and slightly backward through a full range of motion. Your pelvis will tilt and your spine will bend when you reach the end of your hip range. Do not move your pelvis or spine. Hold this position for 10 seconds.
- Keeping your hip turned outward, slowly lower your thigh to the start position.

Dosage

Sets/repetitions _______

Frequency ___________

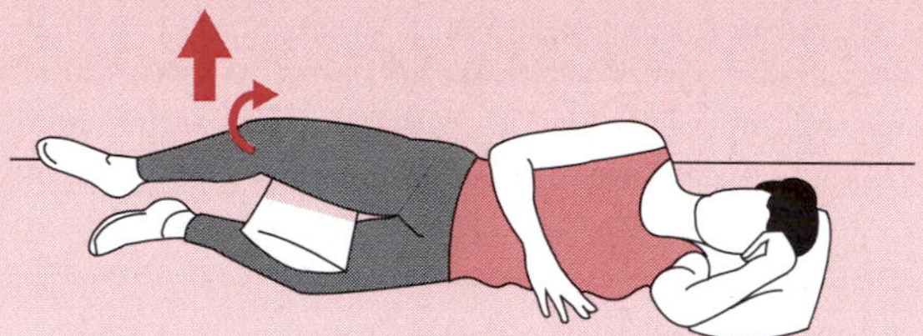

Level IV: Sidelying hip abduction—short lever arm

Level V

Start position

- As in Level IV, but with your hips and knees straight in line with your torso.
- It is helpful to lie against a wall, positioning your pelvis such that your pelvis is against the wall and both "cheeks" are touching the wall.

Movement technique

- As in level IV, but slide your heel up the wall through a full hip range of motion. Do not compensate by tilting your pelvis or sidebending your spine. Hold this position for 10 seconds.
- Keeping your hip turned outward, slowly lower your leg to the start position.

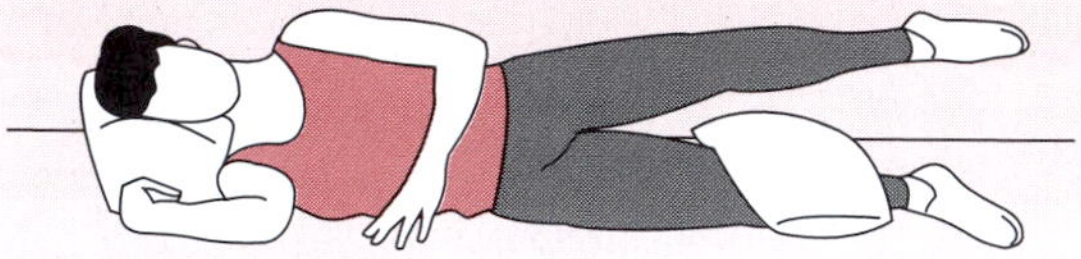

Level V: Sidelying hip abduction—long lever arm

Dosage

Sets/repetitions ______

Frequency ___________

SELF-MANAGEMENT: Walk Stance Progression

Purpose: To teach the correct pattern to move your body over your hip, teach a good strategy to balance on one leg, and strengthen your hip and other lower extremity muscles to support your lower extremities in good alignment for activities you perform in standing

Level I

Start position

- Stand in a staggered stance position with your involved leg in front of your uninvolved leg.
- Check the position of your feet, knees, hips, and pelvis.
- Feet should be facing straight ahead with arches in neutral.
- Knees should be facing straight ahead without turning in or out excessively (If you have anteverted or retroverted hips, the knee position may be modified).
- Hips and pelvis should be facing forward and level.

Movement technique

- Slowly bend your front hip and knee while leaning slightly toward your front leg.
- Do not bend your knee further than the length of your foot. Hold this position for 10 seconds.
- Squeeze your seat muscle
- Tighten your quadriceps
- Hold the arch of your foot up while you keep your big toe down

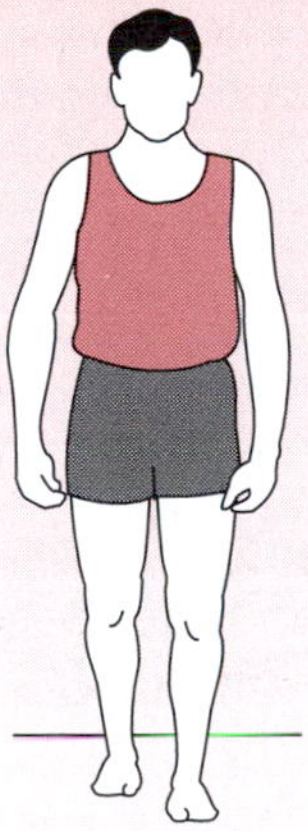

Level I

Dosage

Sets/repetitions ______

Frequency __________

Level II: Single limb stance

Start position

- The start position for this exercise is the end position of level I.

Movement technique

- Progress from the walk stance position by lifting your back heel upward as you straighten your front knee and hip (A).
- Be sure your feet, knees, hips, pelvis, and spine are in good alignment.
- Hold this position for 3 seconds.
- Slowly bring your back thigh forward by bending the hip and knee (as if to take a step forward) (B).
- Balance for up to 30 seconds.

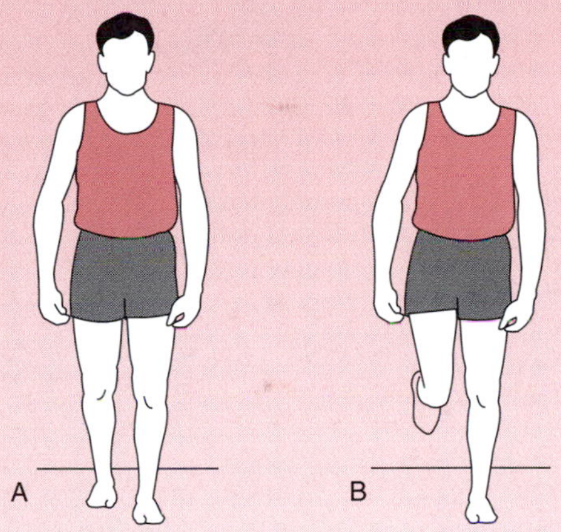

Level II

Dosage

Sets/repetitions ______

Duration__________

Frequency __________

Level III: Split squat

Start position

- Position yourself in a staggered stance with your involved leg forward.
- Lean toward your front limb as in Level I.
- Keeping your spine, pelvis, hips, knees, and ankles steady, slowly lower yourself until you see or feel your pelvis tilting or rotating out of the start position.
- The movement should be occurring at your hip and knee. Your front knee

should only bend as far as the length of your foot.
- Most of your weight should be over your front limb; if you feel your back limb straining, shift your weight onto your front limb.
- Slowly rise upward while keeping your weight shifted forward.
- Repeat up and down while remaining in a forward position over your front foot.

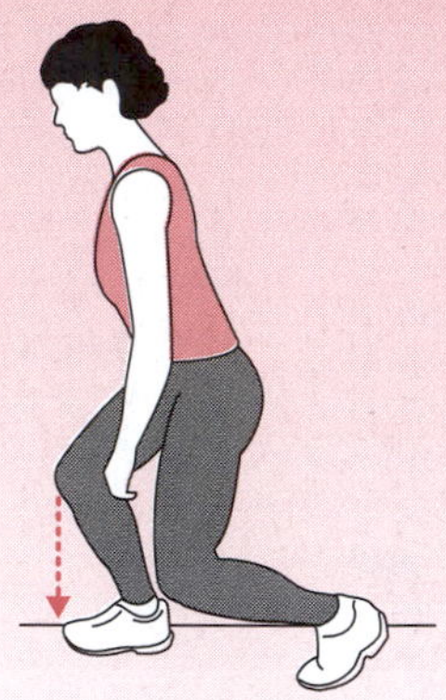

Level III

Dosage

Sets/repetitions ______

Frequency __________

Level IV: Lunge

Start position

- Stand with both feet on the floor and weight equally distributed between both limbs.
- Take a step forward and watch your pelvis, hip, knee, ankle, and foot position as in level I. Do not let your back arch.
- This is a ballistic exercise. Be extra careful about your position.

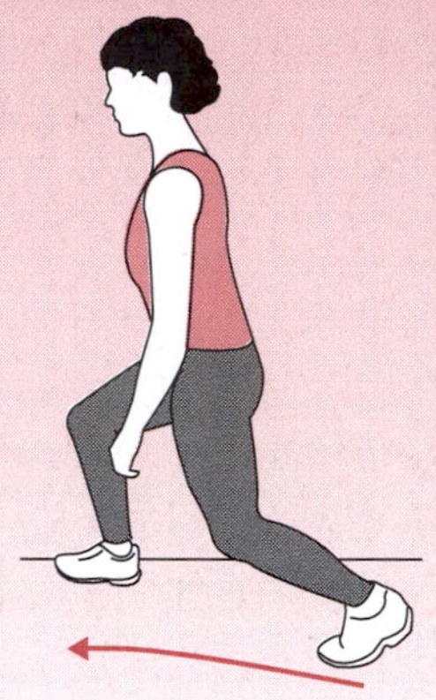

Level IV

Dosage

Sets/repetitions ______

Frequency __________

to a leap (Fig. 20-15), with the focus on controlling frontal and transverse plane forces at the hip with the gluteus medius on landing.

MUSCLE STRAIN

Force-generating capability may be compromised by an injury to the muscle in the form of muscle strain. Muscle strain may be the result of a sudden, injurious force, as in hamstring and rectus femoris strains, but it may also occur as a result of gradual, continuous stress to the muscle, as in overuse of one synergist or in a muscle functioning in a chronically stretched position.

The hamstring muscle commonly is strained as a result of overuse. It participates in force couples around the lumbopelvic hip complex, contributing to posterior pelvic rotation, hip extension, and indirectly, hip medial and lateral rotation. During gait, all portions of the hamstring are active from midswing to early loading response (see Table 20-3). From midswing to initial contact, the role of the hamstrings is to decelerate the hip. At initial contact and loading response, the biceps femoris is thought to decelerate tibial medial rotation that occurs with foot pronation.[47] Because of the multiple roles of the hamstrings, it is quite susceptible to overuse strain. Hamstring overuse may have several possible mechanisms:

- Subtle imbalances in force or torque production and endurance between the hamstrings and gluteus maximus may lead to excess demand on the hamstrings to decelerate hip flexion during late midswing and hip medial rotation at initial contact.
- Significant forefoot varus (see Chapter 22), combined with length-tension alterations and reduced force or torque production of the deep hip lateral rotators, may lead to overuse of the biceps femoris. Without optimal foot mechanics and hip lateral rotator function, the biceps femoris load is exaggerated because of the increased role it must play in decelerating femoral and tibial medial rotation at initial contact through the midstance phase of gait.
- Underuse of the oblique abdominal muscles may lead to overuse of the hamstrings because of the increased role they must play to exert a posterior rotational force on the lumbopelvic region.

Treatment of a hamstrings strain should follow the guidelines for tissue healing outlined in Chapter 10. However, for the hamstrings to fully recover, treatment must be focused on the *cause* of the strain. If the cause of the strain is overuse, the load must be reduced on the hamstrings during meaningful functional activities. Improving the force or torque production, endurance, and neuromuscular control

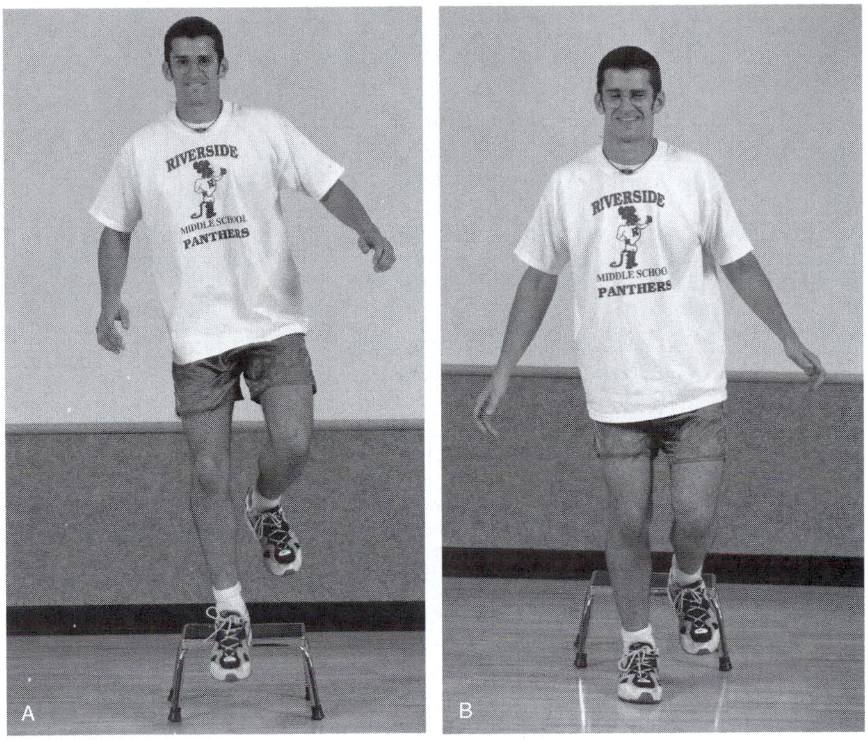

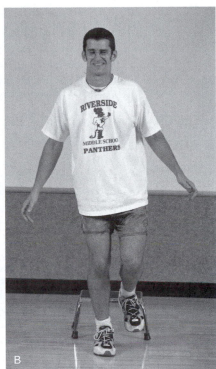

FIGURE 20-15 A step can be used to simulate a leap in a more controlled manner. ***(A)*** Jumping off the step with emphasis on height or distance. ***(B)*** Landing in an optimal spine, pelvis, knee, ankle, and foot alignment.

of the underused synergists and correcting for any biomechanical factors (eg, foot orthotic to correct for forefoot varus) constitute a recommended course of action.

Two commonly underused synergists involved in the cause of hamstring overuse strain are the gluteus maximus and deep hip lateral rotators. Examples of therapeutic intervention for progressive strengthening of the gluteus maximus and deep hip lateral rotators are shown in Self-Management: Stomach-Lying Hip Extension. The exercises illustrated are considered specific, nonfunctional exercises. There are two reasons to prescribe this type of exercise instead of more functionally relevant exercise. First, the force-generating capability of the muscle is inadequate to allow it to fully participate in a functional task. Second, the kinesthetic awareness of the muscle may be such that the patient's ability to selectively recruit it during a functional task may be insufficient.

After force-generating capability and kinesthetic awareness are improved sufficiently, graded functional activities can be initiated. Self-Management: Walk Stance Progression and Self-Management: Step-Up, Step-Down illustrate functional progressions of specific exercises that use the gluteus maximus, quadriceps, deep hip lateral rotators, and peroneus longus and posterior tibialis in sagittal-plane kinetic chain activities. Each of these muscles has a role during the exercises:

- The gluteus maximus muscle decelerates hip flexion in the lowering phase of the split squat, lunge, and step-down and accelerates hip extension during the rising phase of the split squat, lunge, and step-up.
- The quadriceps muscle decelerates knee flexion during the lowering phase of the split squat, lunge, and the step-down and accelerates knee extension during the rising phase.

SELF-MANAGEMENT: Stomach-Lying Hip Extension

Purpose: To strengthen the seat muscles, train you to move your hip independent of your pelvis and spine, and stretch the muscles on the front of your hip

Start position: Lie on your stomach on a firm surface, and place ______ pillows under your torso.

Movement technique

- Preset your spine and pelvic position by pulling your belly button toward your spine and squeezing your seat muscle.
- Use your seat muscles to lift your thigh *barely* off the floor.
- Return the thigh to the floor and repeat the lift with the other leg.

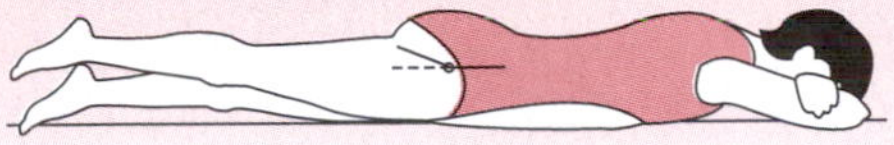

Dosage

Sets/repetitions ______

Frequency ______

SELF-MANAGEMENT: Step-Up, Step-Down

Purpose: To strengthen your spine, hip, knee, ankle, and foot muscles and to improve your balance in single limb stance

STEP-UP

Start position: Stand facing a step.

Movement technique

- Lift your leg onto the step, keeping your thigh in midline and your pelvis level.
- After your foot is on the step, check its position. The arch should be up with the big toe down.
- Lean toward the step, being sure that your knee is in line with your foot (NOTE: this may vary if you have anteverted or retroverted hips) and your pelvis is level.
- Step-up while keeping your pelvis level, knee over toes, and arch up. Be sure to lean into your hip, but do not let your pelvis tilt.

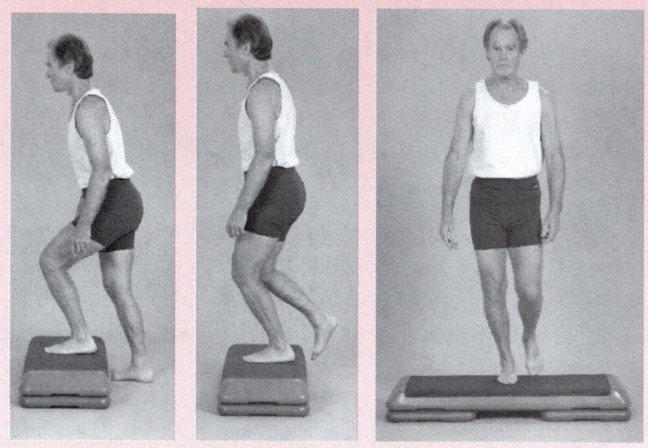

- ***Variation:*** You can stand to the side of a step and step-up sideways. This places even more stress on your outside hip-muscles. Be sure to keep your pelvis level.

Dosage

Sets/repetitions __________

Resistance (step height) __________

Frequency __________

STEP-DOWN

Start position: Stand on a step that is higher than you can control during a step-down movement.

Movement

- Flex the foot of the leg you are stepping down with.
- Bend the hip and knee of the foot remaining on the step as you lower your flexed foot toward the floor.
- Lean forward so as to bend at your hip.
- Do not completely step down, but stop just short of the floor and hold this position for up to 10 seconds.
- Be sure that your pelvis is level, your knee over your toes (NOTE: this may vary if you have anteverted or retroverted hips), and your arch up as you lower your leg. Do not deviate from this position.

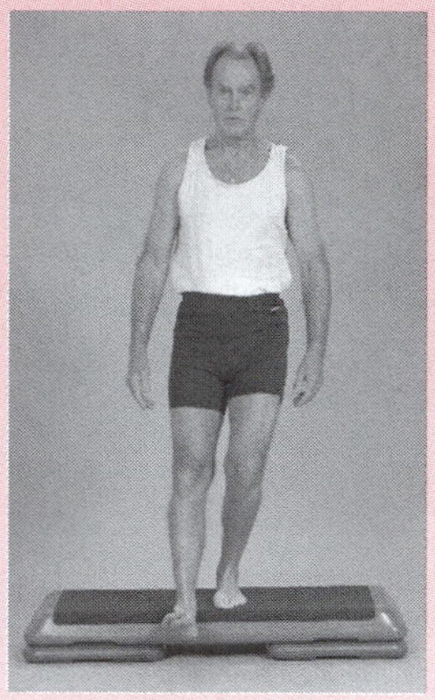

- **Variation:** You may need to use an external device to assist you in your balance
  - ____ Hold a ski pole, dowel rod, or upside down broom in each hand
  - ____ Hold a ski pole, dowel rod, or upside down broom in the opposite hand from which you are balancing
  - ____ Hold a weight in the hand of the hip on which you are balancing.
- **Variation:** After you can balance well during the lowering phase, you can further challenge your balance by using arm movements. When you have lowered yourself as far as you can control, raise the arm on the same side or opposite side of the leg on which you are balancing.
  - ____ Raise it up and down to the side
  - ____ Raise it up and down to the front
  - ____ Raise it toward and away from the midline of your body

Dosage

Sets/repetitions ________

Assistance (amount of weight in hand) ________

Resistance (step height) ______

Frequency ________

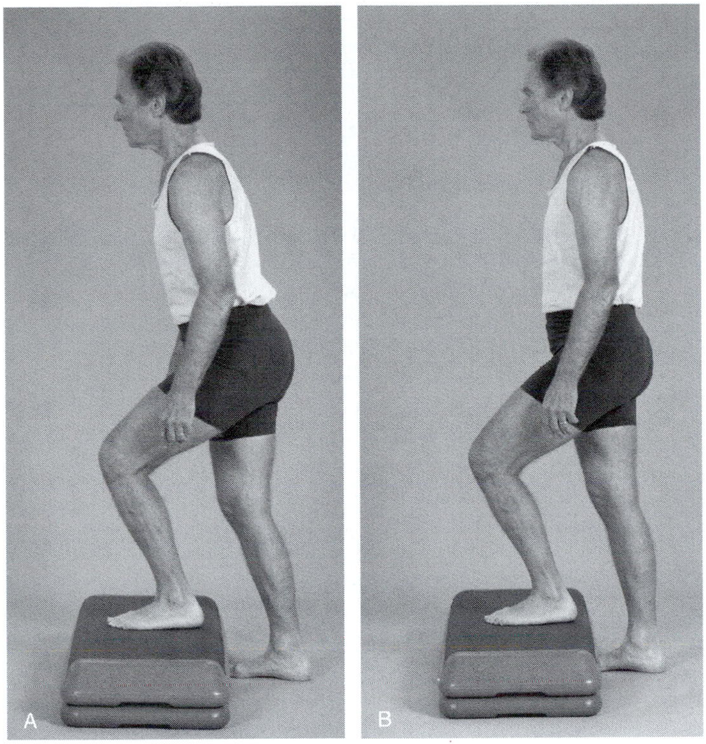

FIGURE 20-16 ***(A)*** Side view of step-up exercise with good spine, hip, knee and ankle/foot relationships. ***(B)*** Side view of step-up exercise with decreased hip flexion and center of mass posterior to the axis of rotation of the hip and knee. Step-up from this start position tends to use a hamstring and soleus strategy to pull the hip and knee into extension to raise the center of mass upward. This movement is opposite to the pattern shown in Figure 20-16*A*, which tends to use the gluteus maximus and quadriceps to raise the center of mass upward.

- The deep hip lateral rotators are recruited to prevent hip medial rotation during all phases of each exercise.
- The posterior tibialis and peroneus longus muscles control foot pronation during the stance phase of each exercise, which assists in controlling tibial and femur medial rotation up the kinetic chain.

Care must be taken to ensure recruitment of the underused synergists during each exercise. Subtle changes in the trunk, hip, knee, and ankle-foot angles during any phase of the split squat and step activity can diminish gluteus maximus, quadriceps, hip lateral rotator, or ankle-foot muscle activity and increase the load on the hamstrings (Fig. 20-16).

The gluteus medius muscle is commonly strained from gradual, continuous stretching, which can occur in an individual with a functional or structural LLD and with iliac crest height asymmetry. On the side of the high iliac crest, the hip is adducted, and the gluteus medius is in a stretched position. Eventually, the muscle may become strained because of functioning in a chronically stretched position. Treatment of this type of strain must involve exercises that resolve the contributing factors to the LLD in conjunction with treatment to improve the length-tension properties, force or torque production, endurance capacity, and neuromuscular control of the gluteus medius. In the early stages of recovery, taping (Fig. 20-17) can unload the muscle and support it at an appropriate length, providing an environment for healing. Severe strains may require use of a cane in the contralateral hand to unload the muscle enough to induce healing. Exercises to progressively strengthen the gluteus medius are depicted in Self-Management: Gluteus Medius Strength Progression and Self-Management: Walk Stance Progression.

DISUSE AND DECONDITIONING

Disuse and deconditioning of the hip joint musculature, particularly of gluteal and deep hip lateral rotator muscles, are common. Disuse or deconditioning can result from injury or pathology affecting the hip and surrounding structures or from acquired movement patterns that promote disuse. For example, weakness in the gluteal musculature in hip joint osteoarthritis is a common finding, but research has not determined whether it is the cause or the result of hip joint pathology.[48] Nonetheless, an exercise program that

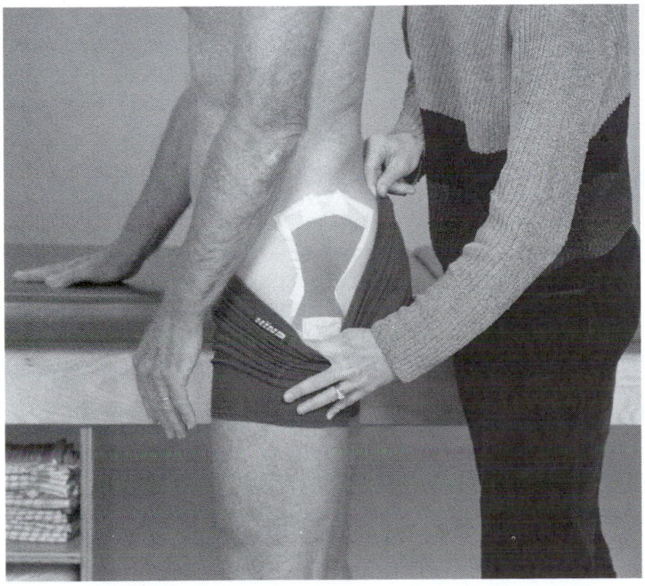

FIGURE 20-17 Taping to support a strained gluteus medius.

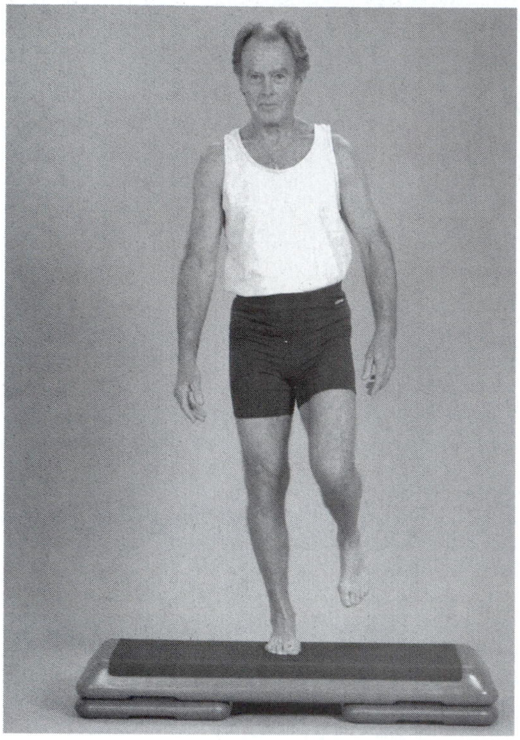

FIGURE 20-18 Use of a hip-hike strategy on the left to ascend the stairs.

addresses the force or torque capability of the atrophied gluteal muscles is indicated.

It is reasonable to consider that acquired posture and movement habits contribute to altered length-tension properties and disuse of the hip musculature. For example, a slightly high iliac crest, as commonly occurs in a handedness pattern on the dominant side, contributes to lengthening of the ipsilateral gluteus medius,[30] which affects its force-generating capability during function.[49] The muscle tends to function at its relatively lengthened state during gait (with the hip adducted).[49] Eventually, this movement pattern may become more exaggerated, contributing to excessive hip adduction during the stance phase of gait and further reliance on stability from passive tension of the ITB.[50] As the hip increases its use of the ITB for passive stability, gluteus medius participation may decrease. Subsequently, the gluteus medius is subject to further deconditioning. A deconditioned gluteus medius may lead to numerous hip, lumbopelvic, knee, and ankle-foot conditions.

Disuse weakness as a result of lack of participation in movement patterns can affect the iliopsoas, gluteus maximus, and hip lateral rotators. Because these muscles participate in gait and ascending stairs, reduced participation of these muscles can affect the performance of these ADLs.

The iliopsoas is active in the initial swing phase of gait and presumably in ascending stairs.[51] Its activity probably is related to the lateral rotation and hip flexion, which accompanies the initial swing phase of gait. Faulty patterns of hip flexion can indicate underuse of the iliopsoas and overuse of another synergist. The following examples describe faulty hip flexion patterns:

- Hip hike during the swing phase of gait or stair climbing suggests recruitment of lateral trunk musculature to hike the hip instead of using the iliopsoas to flex the hip (Fig. 20-18).
- Hip flexion with medial rotation (Fig. 20-19) suggests use of TFL as the predominant hip flexor instead of the iliopsoas.

Repetitive alteration in the optimal path of instant center of rotation of the hip during flexion and the resulting compensatory hip and lumbopelvic movement patterns predispose the hip and lumbopelvic region to further impairments and pathologic conditions. Specific exercises to improve the force-generating capability of the iliopsoas (see Self-Management: Iliopsoas Strengthening) and gradual movement re-education in hip flexion patterns are indicated to improve iliopsoas participation in the hip flexion force couple.

Reduced participation of the gluteus maximus profoundly affects gait and the ability to ascend stairs.[47] Gluteus maximus activity probably is related to deceleration of hip flexion at terminal swing and isometric extensor support of the flexed hip at initial contact and during the loading response phases of gait.[47] Lack of use of gluteus maximus during gait and stair ascension may impose greater stress on the hamstrings, which may predispose the muscle to strain. Bridging, squatting, step-ups, step-downs, and sit-to-stand exercises are functional methods for improving the gluteus maximus force-generating capability and its recruitment during functional movement patterns. These exercises can be graded to various performance levels (Fig. 20-20).

Hip lateral rotators are active from the initial contact to midstance of gait, presumably to decelerate the medial fem-

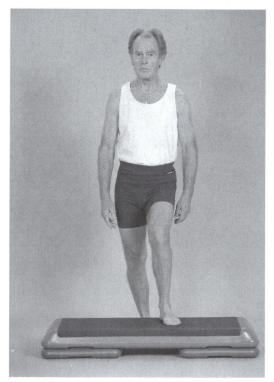

FIGURE 20-19 Medial femoral rotation of the left femur accompanying hip flexion during stair climbing.

SELF-MANAGEMENT: *Iliopsoas Strengthening*

Purpose: To strengthen the muscle deep in the front of your pelvis that lifts your leg and controls the forward rotation of your hip joint

Start position: Sit with your feet flat on a firm surface, back straight, pelvis erect, and arms resting at your sides.

Movement technique

Level I

- Use your hands to lift your knee toward your chest as far as possible without letting your lower back round or "slump" backward.
- Hold this position for the prescribed number of seconds.
- Lower your leg to the start position.

Level II

- Perform as in level I, but push against your knee with the opposite hand in a down and slightly outward direction for the prescribed number of seconds.
- Lower your leg to the start position.

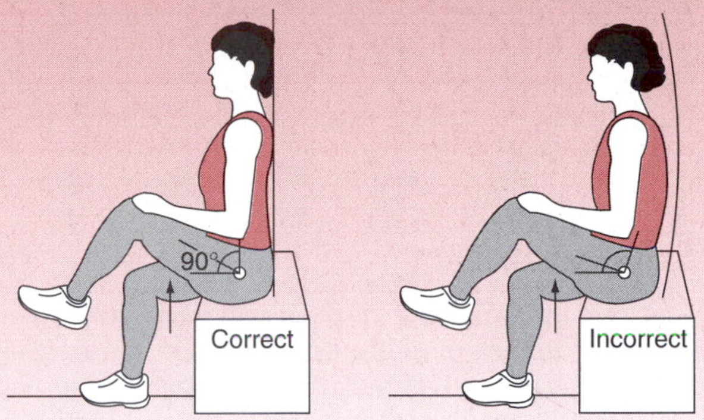

Dosage

Sets/repetitions ______

Duration _______

Frequency ______

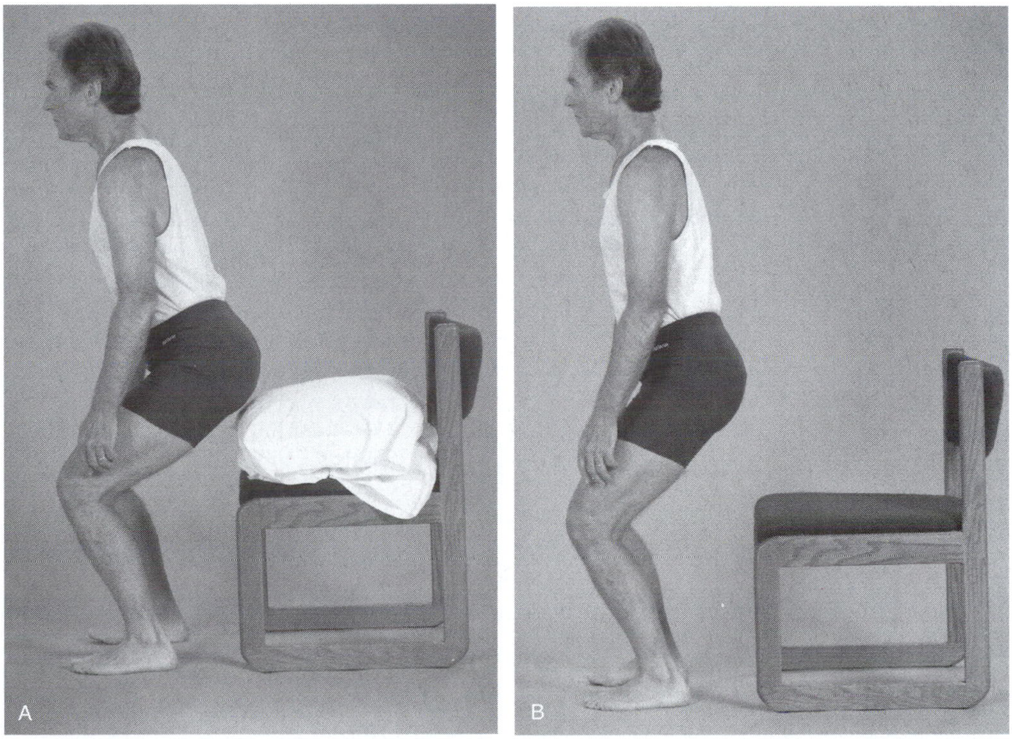

FIGURE 20-20 ***(A)*** Chair squats can be made easier with the use of pillows. ***(B)*** Gradually taking away the pillows can make the exercise more difficult.

oral rotation occurring as a result of foot pronation. Signs of excessive hip medial rotation during weight acceptance and the single-limb support phases of gait need to be examined to determine the cause (eg, excessive foot pronation, excessive hip medial rotation). If foot physiologic and anatomic impairments are excluded and hip lateral rotator force or torque production is inadequate, the excessive hip medial rotation probably is related to reduced hip lateral rotator eccentric control during the pronatory phase of gait. Use of orthotic support as a remedy for this problem should be avoided. Instead, specific exercise and functional retraining of the hip lateral rotator functional control should be emphasized (Fig. 20-21; see Self-Management: Walk Stance Progression).

Mobility Impairment

Mobility impairments of the hip can span the continuum of hypermobility to hypomobility. The extreme clinical manifestation of hypomobility is the arthritic hip with a capsular pattern of limitation. The extreme clinical manifestation of hypermobility is congenital dysplasia of the hip, creating chronic instability in the hip joint. Between these extreme conditions, more subtle mobility impairments can affect the function of the hip, lumbar spine, sacroiliac joint, knee, ankle, and foot.

HYPERMOBILITY

Because of the inherent stability of the hip, hypermobility is not commonly thought of as an impairment in the adult hip, but rather as an impairment in the developing hip. Treatment of the unstable developing hip usually consists of positioning, bracing, or surgery,[52,53] whereas treatment of the hypermobile (rarely unstable) adult hip usually consists of therapeutic exercise and movement retraining.

Hypermobility of the adult hip is defined as motion that exceeds the standard acceptable ROM for the hip in a given direction. Hypermobility generally occurs in the female hip, with a strong tendency toward excessive medial rotation ROM. Hypermobility into medial rotation during gait can predispose the person to several hip-related diagnoses:

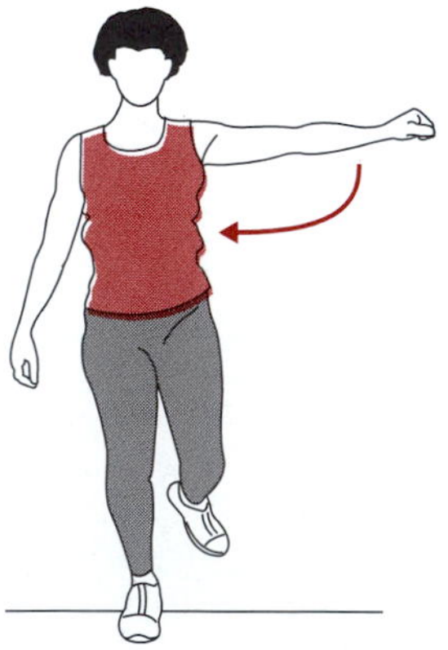

FIGURE 20-21 Single limb balance is accomplished with torsional destabilizing stress into medial and lateral rotation through movement of the upper extremities into horizontal abduction and adduction, respectively.

- Trochanteric bursitis
- ITB fascitis
- TFL strain
- Plantar fascitis
- Rotation-induced knee sprain
- Sacroiliac joint or lumbar dysfunction

Examination may reveal excessive medial rotation ROM relative to lateral rotation ROM bilaterally and excessive medial rotation ROM of the involved hip relative to the uninvolved hip. When excessive medial rotation ROM relative to lateral rotation ROM is diagnosed, care must be taken to screen for anteversion. If hip inflammation has occurred, early capsular changes may be reflected by a slight reduction in hip medial rotation and hip flexion mobility on the involved side compared with the uninvolved side. A common associated finding is weakness in the hip lateral rotators (ie, deep hip rotators, gluteus maximus, or posterior fibers of gluteus medius).

If the measured hip medial rotation is excessive, with mild to no anteversion, exercise to improve the force-generating capability of the lateral rotators is indicated. Lateral rotator–strengthening exercises, to be most effective, should be coupled with education about altering postural habits (eg, reduce the incidence of standing with the femur in excessive medial rotation) and movement training to improve recruitment of lateral rotators during closed chain function. See Patient-Related Instruction: Standing Knees Over Toes and Patient-Related Instruction: Walking With Knees Over Toes for examples of posture and gait education and training.

Individuals with hip anteversion can present with two unique hypermobility problems related to attempts to compensate for the anatomic impairment. Persons with hip anteversion may engage in activities that promote extreme hip lateral rotation, such as ballet or soccer. The anteverted hip is forced to function in extreme lateral rotation for accurate performance of the activity. The head of the femur can be forced to translate excessively anteriorly to achieve the laterally rotated femur position, often resulting in anterior groin pain. Hip joint hypermobility subsequently develops in the direction of anterior translation and lateral rotation. To prevent or alleviate the impairment, the patient should be educated about his unique lower extremity biomechanics and lateral rotation ROM limitations.

Another common movement impairment that develops in the individual with anteverted hips is to achieve lateral rotation ROM by laterally rotating the tibia on the femur, resulting in tibiofemoral problems. The person should also be educated about his unique lower extremity biomechanics and hip lateral rotation ROM limitations to prevent rotational hypermobility problems at the tibiofemoral joint.

HYPOMOBILITY

Hypomobility impairments, particularly in the direction of flexion and medial rotation, can be found in the young, middle-aged, and elderly adult hip joint. Subtle losses in mobility may indicate early arthritic changes[29] or hypomobility caused by chronic lack of use as a result of altered movement patterns. Marked hypomobility also is a hallmark finding for the arthritic hip.[29]

Pain need not be an essential component of early arthritic changes and hypomobility findings. For example, osteo-

Patient-Related Instruction

Standing Knees Over Toes

Your neutral hip position may vary depending upon the structure of your hips. Your physical therapist will instruct you as to your neutral position if you have a structural variation in your hips.

From the Front

- Your weight should be distributed equally between both feet.
- Your pelvis should be level from side to side
- The left side of your pelvis should be in line with the right side of your pelvis (ie, your one side of your pelvis should not be in front of the other side)
- Your knees should be in line with your feet; if you bent your knees, your knees would be directed over the midline of your feet.
- Your feet should be hip-width apart and *slightly* turned outward.
- The arch of your foot should be *slightly* elevated, with your big toe down.

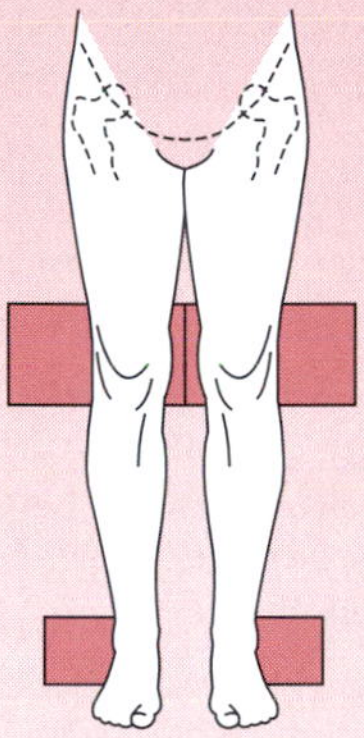

Ideal alignment

From the Side

- Your pelvis should be in neutral, with the front hip bones in the same plane as your pubic bone.
- Your knees should not be bent or locked.
- Your ankle should fall below your knee, with your lower leg at a 90-degree angle with respect to your foot.

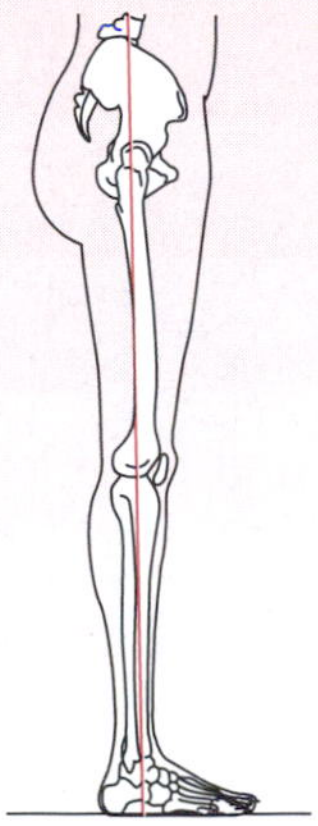

Patient-Related Instruction

Walking With Knees Over Toes

When you walk

- Do not let your knee lock back as you bring your weight over your foot. Your knee should be slightly bent when your heel contacts the floor and should slightly straighten as your body weight moves over your foot.
- At the time your heel hits the ground, think of squeezing your buttocks to prevent your knee from turning in as your body weight moves over your foot.
- Think of using your foot muscles to prevent your arch from dropping too low as your body weight moves over your foot.
- Keep your abdomen pulled in toward your spine to prevent your pelvis from tilting forward. This is particularly important as your body weight moves in front of your foot and your hip must extend. If you do not hold your abdominal muscles tight, your pelvis may tilt or rotate instead of your hip extending.

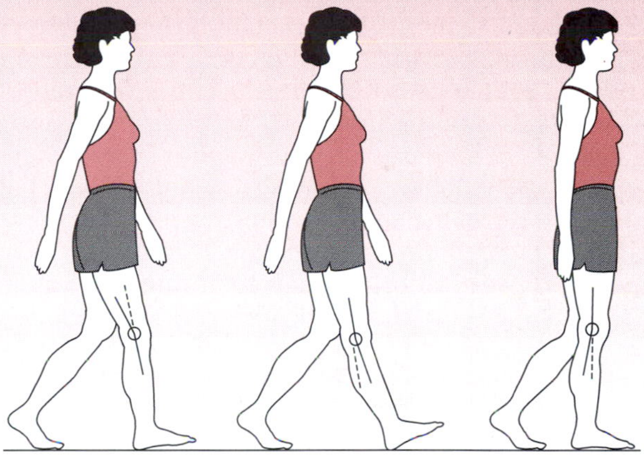

arthritis (confirmed radiologically) leading to considerable restriction of range in the capsular pattern may not cause pain, even when the capsule is stretched quite hard.[29] This is a typical finding in middle-aged men with a capsular pattern of restriction at the hip. Commonly, they have no complaints of hip pain or related functional limitation, but they may complain of low back pain because of the movement imposed on the back as a result of decreased hip mobility. Treatment of the hypomobile hip in the form of mobilization, stretching, strengthening antagonists, and retraining movement using the new hip mobility is indicated to reduce the stress on the low back.

Subtle capsular pattern findings are common in young and middle-aged women with a history of hip-related conditions (eg, groin pain, posterior buttock pain, trochanteric bursitis, ITB fascitis). This may be the result of hip joint hypermobility causing intraarticular inflammation, which leads to capsular changes. The examination findings may include the following findings:

- Slight reduction of hip medial rotation and flexion on the involved side relative to the uninvolved side

- Hip rotation asymmetry within and between limbs (ie, despite capsular changes on the involved side, medial rotation ROM may still be greater relative to lateral rotation ROM within the involved hip, although medial rotation may be less on the involved side when compared with the uninvolved side)
- Weakness in the hip lateral rotators

Treatment may include mobilization and stretching to restore hip medial rotation and flexion ROM to bilateral symmetry, but strength training and neuromuscular training also are required to gain control over excessive medial rotation movement patterns to prevent recurrent hip joint irritation (see exercise suggestions in the Hypermobility section).

Hip joint hypomobility may also develop as a result of altered lumbopelvic movement patterns because of a combination of anthropometric (eg, high center of mass), occupational, and environmental (eg, sports, recreation, hobbies) factors. It is hypothesized that ultimately, as hip mobility decreases, lumbar mobility increases. This finding has been demonstrated in measuring lumbopelvic rhythm during forward bending,[54–58] particularly in the early phase of forward bending.[58] The investigators of these studies found a significant relationship between a relative loss of hip flexion mobility and relative increased lumbar flexion mobility. Knowledge of this relationship is critical for the clinician prescribing exercise and retraining movement patterns. Functional activities such as bending forward to brush one's teeth, making the bed, and reaching into the refrigerator involve moderate amounts of hip and lumbar flexion. Hip stiffness resulting from reduced extensibility in capsule, ligament, or myofascial structures may impose excessive motion on the lumbar spine during forward-bending activities, which may ultimately lead to microtrauma and macrotrauma of the lumbar spine. Exercises to increase hip flexion mobility and lumbar stability, combined with retraining lumbopelvic rhythm during forward-bending activities, are important to mitigate impairments associated with the cause of low back pain in this particular patient subset. A useful exercise to retrain hip and lumbar movement is illustrated in Self-Management: Hand-Knee Rocking.

The hamstrings have been implicated as a potential source of hip stiffness.[58] A common stretch for the hamstrings is illustrated in Fig. 20-22. Care must be taken to ensure that the stretch occurs in the hamstrings without any associated lumbar flexion or rotation (see Fig. 20-22*B* and *C*). A selective medial or lateral hamstrings stretch can be induced by rotating the hip in the medial direction to stretch the lateral hamstrings and lateral direction to stretch the medial hamstrings. Because the hamstrings are a diarthrodial muscle, knee extension must be maintained while the hip flexes to ensure optimal stretch stimulus. After the hamstrings have been stretched passively, an active exercise should be performed to ensure the new length is used during function. One exercise that uses hamstring length during an active movement pattern is illustrated in Self-Management: Seated Knee Extension.

Another joint in the kinetic chain that may become stressed because of a relative to loss of mobility in the hip joint is the knee. During squatting movements, loss of motion at the hip may impose increased motion on the lumbar spine and the knee joint (Fig. 20-23). Loss of hip joint mobility is a common finding in persons complaining of overuse-related knee conditions such as patellofemoral dysfunction and patellar tendinitis. Improved hip joint mobility and force-generating capability of the gluteus maximus enable increased hip flexion and de-

SELF-MANAGEMENT: Hand-Knee Rocking

Purpose: To improve the flexibility of your hips, stretch the posterior hip muscles, and train independent movement between your hips, pelvis, and spine

Start position
- Position yourself on your hands and knees so that your hips are directly over your knees and hands are directly under your shoulders.
- Knees and ankles should be hip width apart with feet pointing straight back
- Your spine should be flat with a slight curve downward in your low back and your pelvis tilted so that your hip joint is at a 90-degree angle.

Movement technique: Rock backward at the hip joint only. Stop at any sensation of movement in your back.

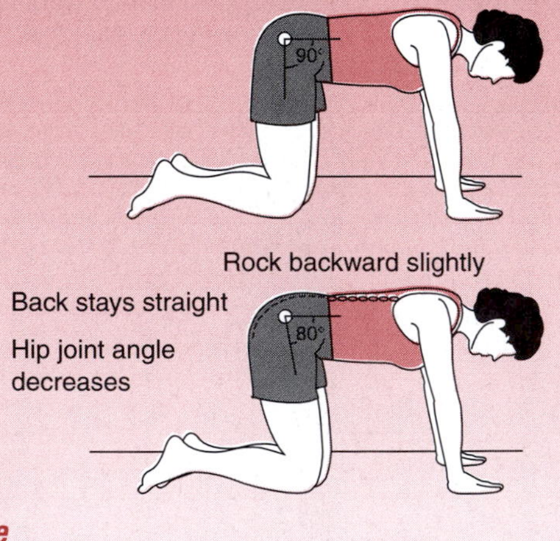

Dosage

Sets/repetitions ______

Frequency ________

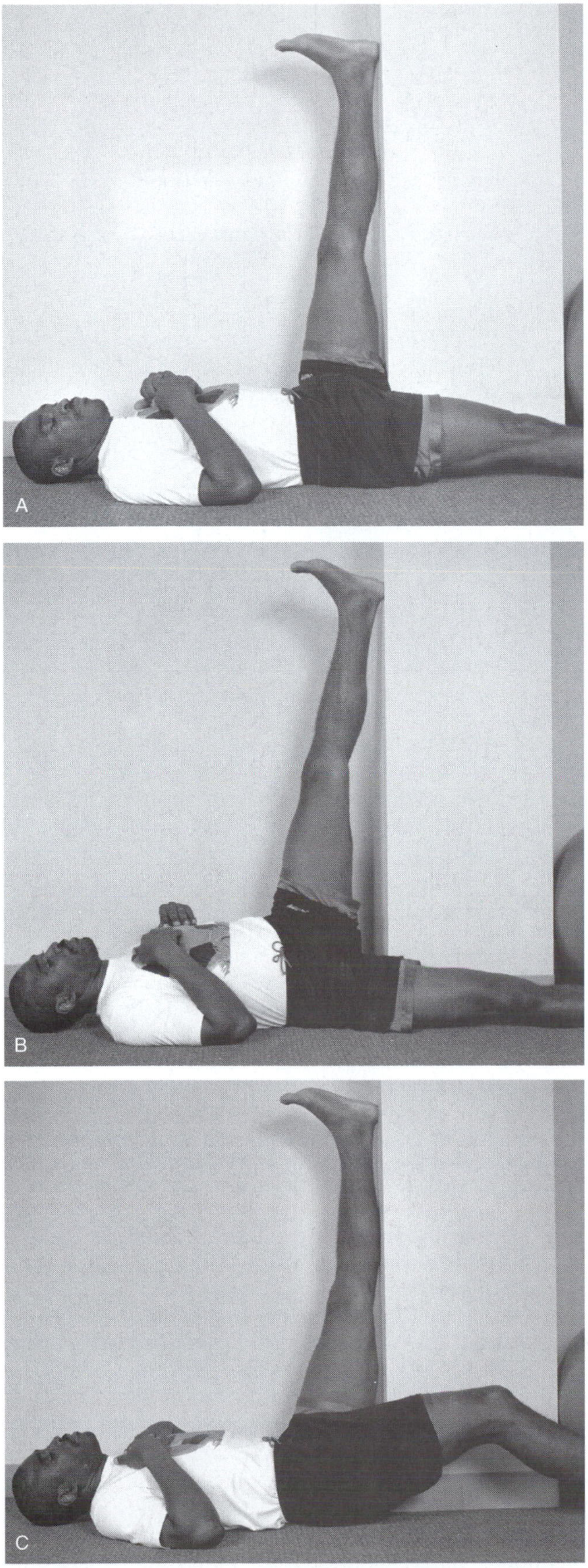

FIGURE 20-22 *(A)* Supine passive hamstring stretch. *(B and C)* Faulty technique associated with supine passive hamstring stretch.

SELF-MANAGEMENT: Seated Knee Extension

Purpose: To stretch the hamstring and calf muscles and train independent movement between your low back and pelvis and your hip and lower leg

Start position: Sit with your back straight, pelvis erect, and arms resting at your sides.

Movement technique:

- Slowly straighten your knee, being sure not to let your pelvis rock backward. Stop when you feel tension developing behind your knee. Hold this position for the prescribed number of seconds.

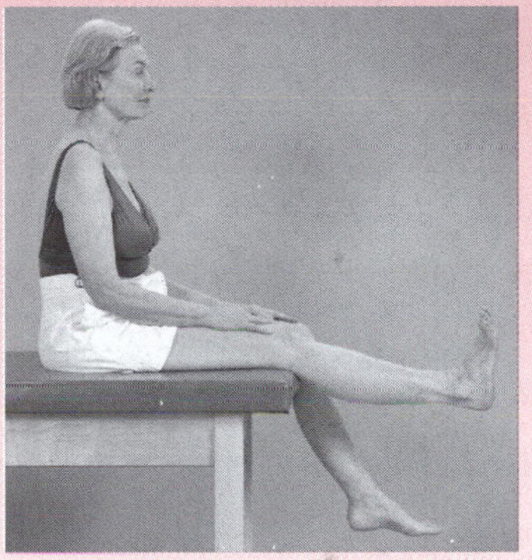

- **Variations**
  - ____ After your knee has moved as far as possible, move your ankle so that your foot points upward toward your knee.
  - ____ Rotate your hip and knee outward before you begin the stretch.
  - ____ Rotate your hip and knee inward before you begin the stretch.

Dosage

Sets/repetitions ______

Duration ______

creased knee flexion during squatting movements. Progressive squatting exercises with shared forces at the hip and knee are recommended to decrease excessive forces at the low back and knee (see Self-Management: Progressive Squat).

Emphasis has been placed on hip flexion and medial rotation hypomobility impairments, but loss of hip extension ROM is another common finding, particularly in patients with end-stage hip arthritis or low back pain. With capsular, ligamentous, or muscular stiffness or adaptive shortening

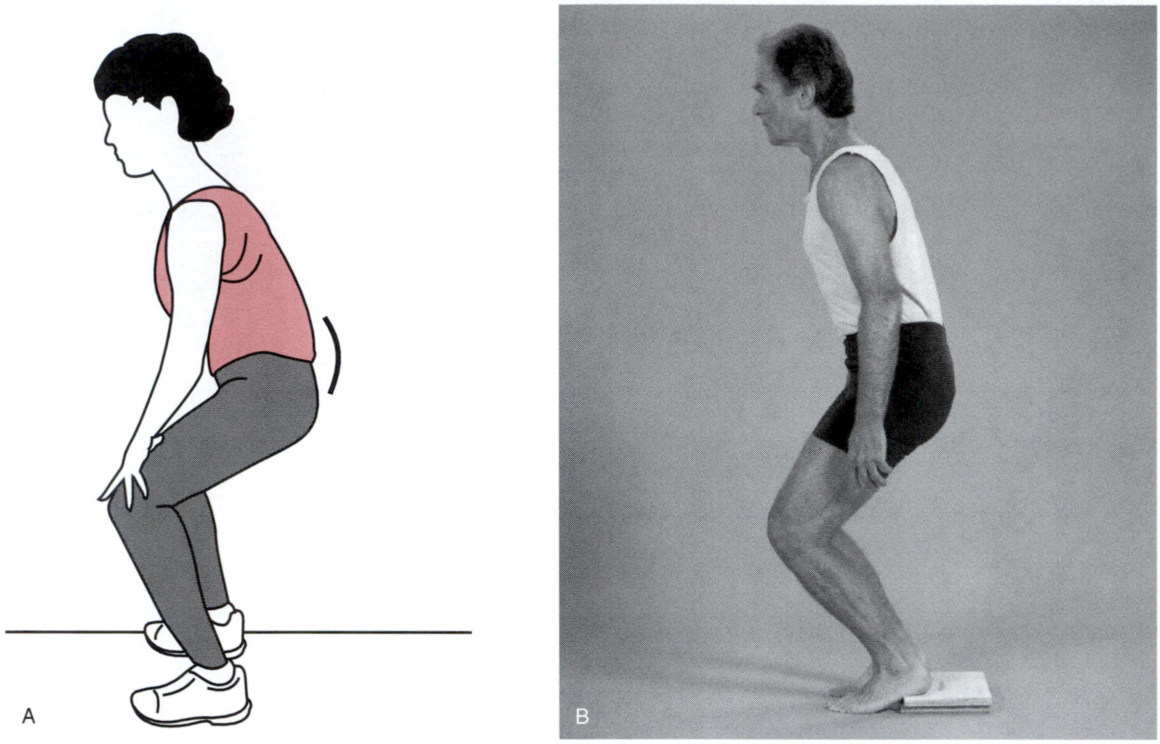

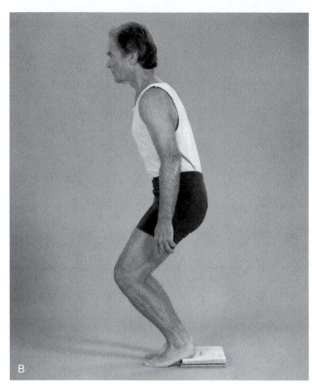

FIGURE 20-23 Squat. ***(A)*** Faulty squat technique performed with increased lumbar flexion as compensation for decreased hip flexion. ***(B)*** Faulty squat technique performed with increased knee flexion as compensation for decreased hip flexion.

across the anterior hip, the pelvis may rest in a relative anterior tilt in relaxed standing. This posture may contribute to a relative increase in lumbar extension to achieve an upright position (see Fig. 20-7*C*). During gait, hip extension is unable to be achieved, which may result in excessive lumbar extension or rotation. On return from the forward bend, the pelvis does not achieve a neutral position, and excessive lumbar extension is imposed on the lumbar spine (Fig. 20-24).

A common finding associated with loss of hip extension ROM is positional weakness in the external obliques, lower rectus abdominis, and transversus abdominis because of the chronically anterior tilted pelvis. Treatment of this impairment requires careful stretching of the affected hip flexor muscles and positional strengthening of the appropriate abdominal muscle groups (see Chapter 18).

Specific muscle length tests reveal which hip flexor muscles are contributing to the lack of hip extension ROM. Often, the diarthrodial hip flexors (ie, rectus femoris and TFL/ITB) are stiff or short. Traditional stretches for the diarthrodial hip flexors do not follow the basic guidelines for optimal stretching because proximal stability is often not maintained (Fig. 20-25). Alternative stretches are recommended for optimal results. Self-Management: Hip Flexor Stretch illustrates an isolated passive diarthrodial hip flexor stretch, and Self-Management: Prone Knee Bend in Chapter 18: illustrates an active diarthrodial hip flexor stretch. The latter stretch uses active movement of knee flexion in an extended hip position to place repeated stretch on the diarthrodial hip flexors while contracting the abdominal muscles to stabilize the pelvis. As the diarthrodial hip flexors elongate with this type of stretch, the abdominal muscles should become stronger in the short range (ie, neutral pelvic position).

For maximal results with passive and active stretches, it is critical to maintain the stability of the pelvis and spine while maintaining the femur and tibia in a neutral position during knee flexion. To isolate the stretch to the TFL, slight lateral rotation of the femur at end-range hip and knee flexion may place a transverse plane stress on this structure. The patient must be cautioned to maintain tibiofemoral alignment. Compensatory tibial lateral rotation may occur to avoid stretching the TFL.

To ensure that gains in hip extension mobility are used in a functional context, the clinician must confirm that proper movement patterns are being used during functional activities:

- During the late stance phase of gait (see Patient-Related Instruction: Walking With Knees Over Toes)
- During sit to stand
- During the return from forward bending (see Patient-Related Instruction: Return From Forward Bending With a Neutral Pelvis), precise performance of these movement patterns requires hip extension mobility and abdominal control to prevent anterior pelvic rotation.

Endurance Impairment

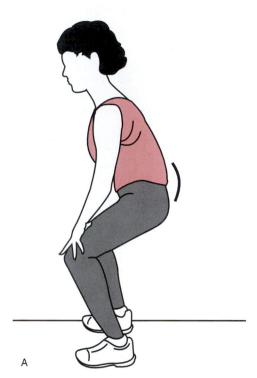

Endurance impairments at the hip must be thought of in light of the tremendous force-generating requirements of the gluteal musculature during functional activities. En-

SELF-MANAGEMENT: Progressive Squat

Purpose: To progressively strengthen your hip girdle muscles and train independent movement between your hips and spine

Start position: Stand with weight equally distributed between both feet and pelvis and spine in neutral. Your neutral hip position may vary depending on the structure of your hips. Ask your physical therapist for instructions on your neutral hip position.

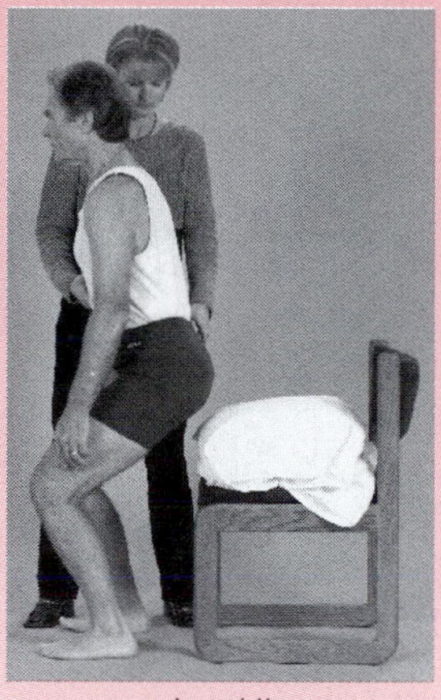

Level II

Movement technique:

Level I: Small knee bend

- Slowly bend your hips and knees.
- Do not bend your knees farther than the length of your feet. Think of sitting back slightly.
- Be sure that your feet are facing ahead, with knees over toes and pelvis level as you bend
- Return to the upright position by using your seat and front thigh muscles. Be sure to complete the rising phase by returning to the neutral spine and pelvic position.

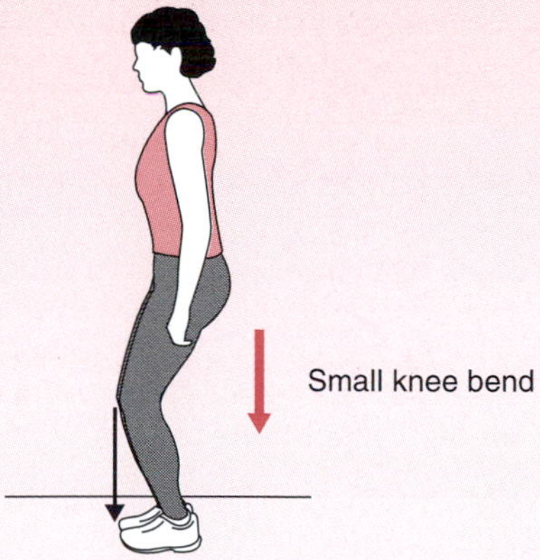

Level I

Level II: Chair squat

- Perform as in level I, but lower yourself to a chair with ___ pillows.
- Try not to collapse into the chair, but rather slowly lower yourself.
  - Return to the upright position by using your seat and front thigh muscles. Be sure to complete the rising phase by returning to the neutral spine and pelvic position.

Level III: Partial squat

- Perform as in level II, but do not use a chair as a stopping point; instead, lower yourself as far as is comfortable.
- As you move deeper into the squat, you will need to bend your hips more (remember that your knees should not bend further forward than the length of your feet) to keep your balance.

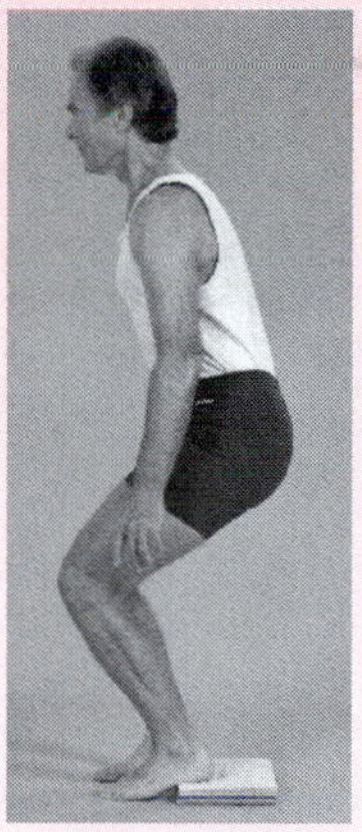

Level III

- ***Variation***

  Perform level III with a dumbbell in each hand

  Perform level III in a squat rack with a barbell

Dosage

Sets/repetitions ________

Frequency ________

Weight ________

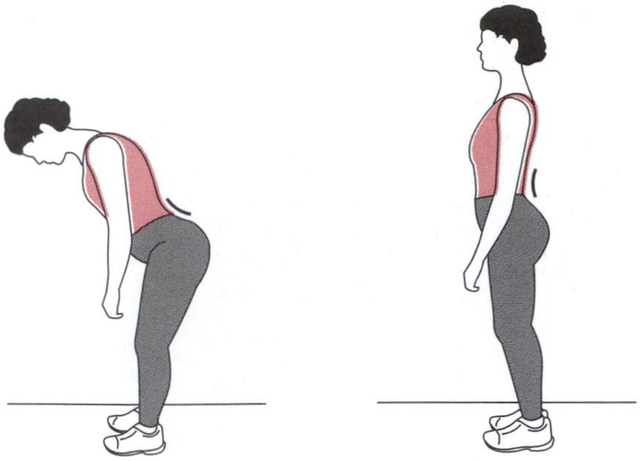

FIGURE 20-24 On the return from forward bend, if the pelvis stops rotating posterior before it reaches a neutral position, excessive lumbar extension is imposed on the spine to achieve an upright posture.

durance is required to meet the repetitious demands of walking. Proper synergy among all muscles involved in the gait cycle keeps the intensity of muscle action at an aerobic level. When one muscle in a synergy group reduces its function, it imposes greater demands on other muscles, potentially rendering them anaerobic and therefore far less energy efficient,[47] or causes compensatory strategies, such as reliance on the ITB for stability or a compensatory Trendelenburg pattern to reduce the need for muscle force to keep the center of mass (COM) within the base of support (BOS). Dosage parameters depend on the performance level desired by the individual (eg, walking 50 feet without pain, running a marathon in the best time possible), with an emphasis on high repetitions instead of maximal force production.

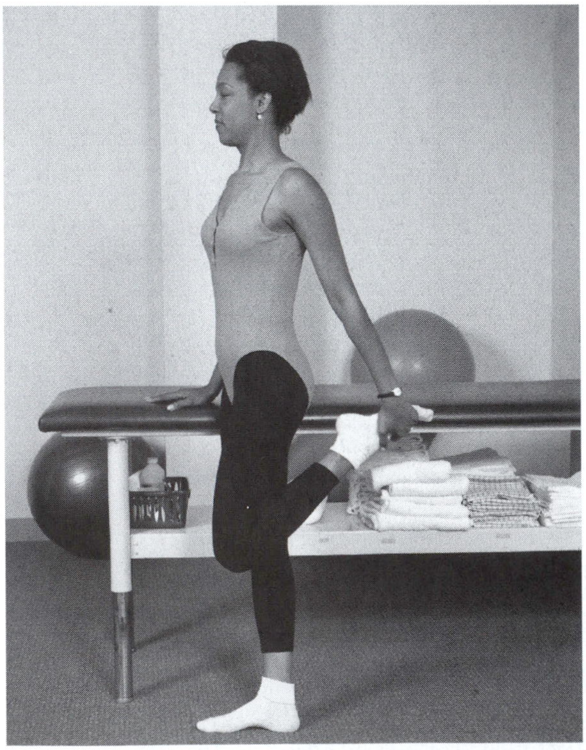

FIGURE 20-25 Traditional standing hip flexor stretches do not effectively stabilize the spine and pelvis.

SELF-MANAGEMENT: Hip Flexor Stretch

Purpose: To stretch the front thigh muscles

Start position
- Sit on the edge of a table so that your thigh is halfway off.
- Lie back while bringing both knees toward your chest.
- Pull your knees toward your chest until your low back just touches the tabletop surface.

Movement technique
- While grasping behind your knee, lower your other leg toward the floor, keeping your knee bent to 90 degrees.
- Keep your thigh in the midline; do not let it drift to the side.
- Do not let your thigh rotate inward
- Hold for ______ seconds.

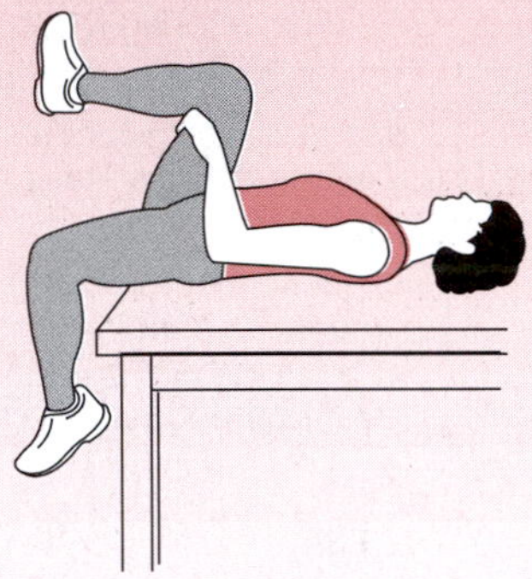

Dosage

Sets/repetitions ________

Frequency ________

Balance

Approximately 25% to 35% of persons older than 65 years experience one or more falls each year.[59–61] Falls are a leading cause of morbidity and mortality of persons older than 65 years,[62,63] and many of the falls result in hip fractures. Improved postural stability and balance (Display 20-3) can improve fear of falling and delay the onset of fall events for the well elderly.

Treatment of impaired balance must focus on the intrinsic and extrinsic factors related to the balance disorder. This requires extensive examination and evaluation of strength, mobility, vestibular function, balance reactions, and environmental factors.

Patient-Related Instruction

Return From Forward Bending With a Neutral Pelvis

When you come up from bending forward

- Lead with your hips by activating your seat muscles.
- Do not arch your back. Avoid this by pulling your abdomen in toward your belly button.
- Complete the motion by bringing your pelvis back to neutral before finishing the spine movement.

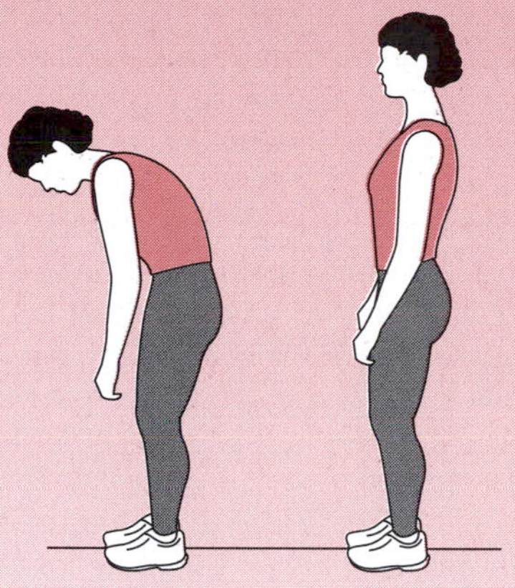

When You Rise Upward From a Squatting Motion

- Be sure to complete the motion by fully extending your hips until your pelvis reaches neutral.
- You may need to activate your abdominal muscles to rotate your pelvis to neutral.

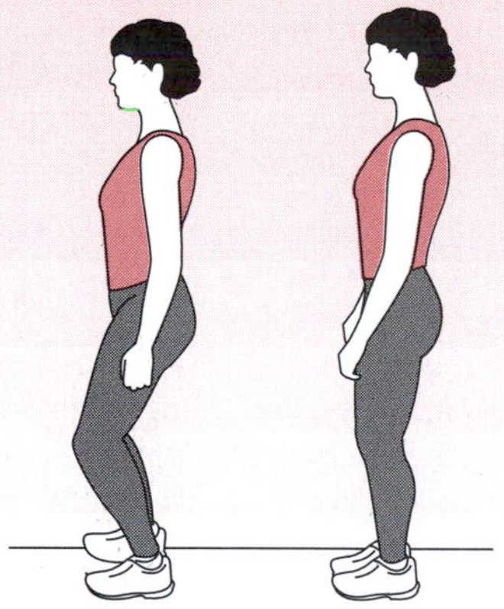

T'ai chi has been valuable in promoting posture stability and balance control in the well elderly.[64,65] The t'ai chi progression (ie, bipedal weight shifting to uniped positions) focuses less on centering the COM within the BOS and more on learning corrective strategies for instability. The advanced forms serve the purposes of destabilizing the individual in a controlled fashion, engaging new movement strategies and facilitating the confidence level of the participant.

Force-platform biofeedback systems can also be used to train posture stability and balance control. However, the focus of force-platform biofeedback systems is different than that of t'ai chi balance training. The former is typically concerned with learning to enhance COM or center-of-pressure movement within the limits of stability, and the latter is concerned with learning controlled motions as those limits are passed. Controlled clinical studies have not demonstrated a reduction in falls or delays in fall occurrences among older persons using force-platform biofeedback systems.[65] This may be because the ability to control the center of pressure during quiet standing or with the added provision of random but moderate perturbations, used during typical machine-based postural training, may not translate well into a functional situation, thereby not resulting in decreased fear of falling or delayed onset of fall events for older adults.

General guidelines can assist the practitioner in developing balance training activities for the hip:

- When training balance control, stepping and grasping reactions are not just strategies of last resort. These strategies can be initiated very early, well before the COM is near the stability limits of the BOS.[66] One goal of balance training may be to reduce the incidence of stepping and grasping strategies as posture stability and balance are increasingly challenged. Display 20-4 provides examples of progressive uniped balance tasks. The goal of the exercise would be to balance on one limb, with the progressive self-induced perturbations (eg, arm movements), without using a grasping or stepping strategy to prevent a fall.
- For anteroposterior perturbations, the fixed-support ankle strategy (ie, ankle muscular response to arrest the motion of the COM) may provide an early defense against destabilization, followed by a stepping or grasping strategy.[66] When using an anteroposterior destabilizing force (eg, uniped with sagittal arm movements), expect the ankles to provide the stabilizing force to maintain postural stability.
- A fixed-support hip strategy (ie, hip muscular response to arrest the motion of the COM) may be limited to a special task condition that precludes the option of stepping or grasping.[66] Use of a fixed-support hip strategy would be inappropriate under normal conditions.

DISPLAY 20-3

Definitions of Terms

- *Posture stability* is the development and execution of a controlled strategy that enables the individual to successfully maintain sitting, biped, and ultimately uniped positions while controlling the environment.
- *Balance* is the development and execution of a (successful) strategy that prevents a fall from occurring.

Wolf SL, Barnhart HX, Ellison GL, Coogler CE. The effect of t'ai chi quan and computerized balance training on postural stability in older subjects [author response]. Phys Ther. *1997;77:383–384.*

DISPLAY 20-4
Examples of Progressive Balance Tasks

- Balance on one leg on a firm surface is progressed to an unstable surface such as dense foam.
- Balance on one leg while rotating the head on a firm surface is progressed to dense foam.
- Balance on one leg with frontal, sagittal, or transverse plane arm movements on a firm surface is progressed to dense foam.
- Perform the previous balance task, but follow the arm movements with the eyes and head.
- Balance on one leg and move the trunk and upper body into contralateral flexion and rotation (ie, reach for inside of ipsilateral ankle and foot) and ipsilateral extension and rotation (ie, reach for object superior, lateral, and posterior to the head), and follow the arm movements with the eyes and head.
- Perform the previous three exercises while holding a weighted ball.

- Lateral destabilization complicates the control of compensatory stepping because of anatomic or physiologic restrictions on the lateral lower extremity movement and the associated prolonged uniped balance demand. Aging appears to be associated with increased difficulty in controlling lateral postural stability, which may be of specific relevance to the problem of lateral falls associated with hip fractures.[66] Exercises designed to provide frontal-plane destabilizing forces (eg, uniped with frontal-plane arm movements) would especially be indicated in the aging population. Side-stepping strategies for recovery to prevent a fall are important skills for this population to learn.

In treating balance impairments with training programs, including t'ai chi, progressive drills (see Display 20-4), and computerized balance devices, the specific demands of compensatory stepping or grasping reactions that are found to cause difficulty (eg, lateral weight transfer, rapid foot or arm movement, crossover steps) should be addressed. These skills can be addressed through unpredictable exercise conditions, such as the use of dense foam or having an outside perturbation such as a partner pushing or pulling the patient off balance). Cautious progression toward uniped motions is indicated, especially because this position is experienced by most older persons before falling.

Assistive devices can aid the individual in balance control before developing functional balance control through a comprehensive training program. Use of a cane in the nondominant hand has reduced the rate of falls by up to fourfold.[68] Cutaneous information from fingertip contact, through a cane, and from a stable surface is more powerful than vision in stabilizing sway in stance.[68]

The ability to effectively treat patients with balance disorders can be enhanced by a clearer understanding of the problems underlying balance. Clinicians trained in balance-related rehabilitation have shown that compliance with a multidimensional, individualized exercise program, addressing the impairments and functional limitations associated with balance deficits, can improve balance and mobility function and reduce the likelihood of falls.[36]

Pain and Inflammation

Pain from the hip joint can be referred anteriorly to the groin, referred laterally in the region of the greater trochanter, or radiate down the anterior and medial thigh to the knee. Occasionally, referred knee pain can occur with little or no pain in the hip. This pain pattern is so common in adolescents that a hip evaluation should always be done in conjunction with a knee examination for a complaint of knee pain.

Pain posterior to the hip or in the buttock is frequently associated with lumbar spine pathology, but it can also arise from the hip. Pain from the spine commonly radiates down the posterior thigh, occasionally to below the knee, but hip pain rarely radiates below the knee. Severe synovitis or acute arthritis can produce pain in the entire hemipelvis. Pain related to ITB fascitis is experienced in the lateral thigh and can be mistaken for lumbar radiculopathy. Because this condition occurs commonly in the elderly, spinal stenosis can be incorrectly implicated as the source of the lateral thigh pain.

Before prescribing exercise to abate pain and inflammation impairments, it is critical to determine the source and the cause of the pain and inflammation. Treatment must work toward alleviating impairments related to the source and cause of pain and inflammation for long-term resolution. Treatment of the cause of the pain and inflammation often relieves symptoms without specific treatment of the source. Several examples of treatment of the cause of pain and inflammation are presented throughout this chapter. Treatment of potential sources of hip pain and possible contributing factors can follow these general guidelines:

- *Activity modification:* Initially, the clinician should encourage patients to maintain force or torque, endurance, and mobility of the hip; while avoiding risk activities, such as running, carrying heavy loads (especially contralateral to the painful hip[69]), or prolonged standing.
- *Physical agents or electrotherapeutic modalities:* The use of cryotherapy, moist heat, or electrotherapeutic modalities may help modulate pain or decrease inflammation. Because of the anatomic position of the hip, these modalities may have limited effectiveness in treating intraarticular inflammation or sources of pain.
- *Manual therapy:* Appropriate use of joint and soft tissue mobilization can improve physiologic impairments related to pain and inflammation, such as joint mobility and tissue extensibility. Joint mobilization can also be used to modulate pain.[41]
- *Therapeutic exercise intervention:* Gentle active ROM exercises in the pain-free range can be used to modulate pain, similar to the grade III joint mobilizations described by Maitland.[41]
- *Assistive devices:* When a person has a limp caused by pain, use of an assistive device in the contralateral hand is necessary to reduce the load on the hip. A cane

in the contralateral hand of a patient can reduce the joint reaction force by as much as 30%.[69] Patients often are reluctant to use an assistive device for fear of "giving in to the condition." Patient-related instruction must include an explanation that temporary use of an assistive device will reduce the load at the hip and allow the pain and inflammation to resolve. Exercise to improve mobility and force- or torque-generating capability of the appropriate musculature is required to discontinue use of the assistive device without risk of recurrence of symptoms.

- *Weight loss:* Overweight persons must work diligently on weight loss through proper nutritional counseling and aerobic activity tolerated by a painful hip, including non–weight-bearing activity such as aquatic activities or cycling.
- *Biomechanical support:* Carefully prescribed foot orthotics can improve skeletal alignment and contact forces at the hip.

Posture and Movement Impairment

Posture impairments at the hip affect alignment of the hip and the alignment of other joints in the kinetic chain. Bilateral or unilateral alterations of hip joint alignment about any plane of motion affects alignment of the lumbar spine, sacroiliac joint, knee, ankle, and foot. For example, excessive femur medial rotation can contribute to altered alignment of the knee, ankle, and foot (Fig. 20-26*A*). Hip flexion can contribute to altered alignment of the pelvis and lumbar spine (see Fig. 20-7*C*). Hip extension can contribute to altered alignment of the knee (Fig. 20-26*B*).

Movement impairments at the hip, as with posture impairments, can be affected by impairments at other segments. The cause of any given hip movement impairment must be diagnosed from the data collected during the examination of the patient. For example, limited hip flexion during a step-up activity may result from a loss of hip flexion mobility, weakness in the hip flexors, or limited knee or ankle mobility. Only a thorough examination can reveal the cause of the movement impairments.

Although posture and movement retraining are ultimate goals in most physical therapy interventions, changes in posture and movement patterns require basic skills in mobility, force or torque production, and motor control. To effect a posture or movement change, mobility, length-tension properties, force or torque production, and endurance must be at functional levels, and kinesthetic awareness about joint position, joint motion, or a specific muscle recruitment pattern must be developed.

The initial focus of any intervention should be on developing physiologic impairments to a functional level. Use of electromyography for biofeedback while performing an exercise can improve kinesthetic awareness about specific muscle recruitment and movement patterns. After physiologic impairments have achieved a functional level of capacity, gradual transition from specific exercises addressing physiologic impairments to greater emphasis on posture and movement patterns used during functional exercise, and activities should occur until the primary emphasis is on functional retraining. Examples of exercises to improve posture and movement of the hip joint are presented throughout this chapter.

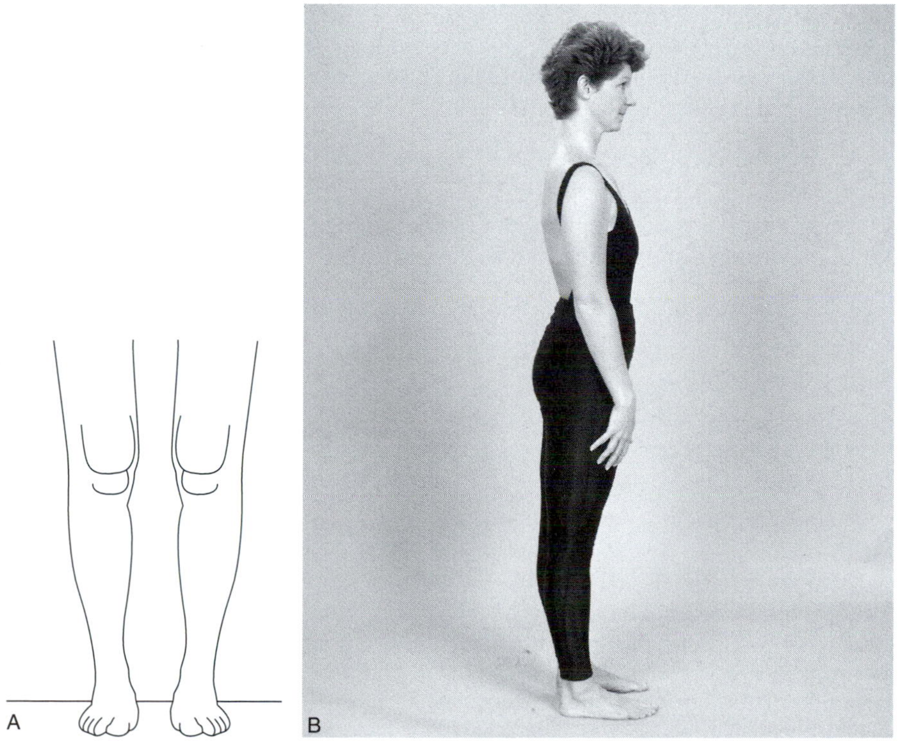

FIGURE 20-26 ***(A)*** Excessive femur medial rotation can contribute to tibial lateral rotation and foot pronation. ***(B)*** Excessive hip extension can contribute to genurecurvatum.

Limb Length Discrepancy

Although LLD is not considered a postural impairment isolated to the hip, it is discussed here because of its functional implication at the hip as the transmitter of forces from the ground and lower extremities to the trunk and upper extremities. Functional LLD is the most difficult form to diagnose and treat. Nearly any movement of an osseous segment out of its normal plane of reference in relation to other bones can create a shorter or longer distance between proximal and distal reference points. Altered osseous positions can occur about any axis of motion and in any segment. Minor alterations in position in any one segment, when added to minor alterations in position of other segments, can lead to a substantial LLD.

To further complicate matters, functional LLD can coexist with structural LLD–sometimes exaggerating the LLD and sometimes compensating for the LLD. For example, a structurally longer limb may compensate for its length with genu recurvatum or knee flexion, genu valgum or genu varum, or foot pronation. After the type of LLD and the segments involved are accurately diagnosed as functional, structural, or combined LLD, appropriate intervention must be determined.

STRUCTURAL LIMB LENGTH DISCREPANCY

Add the appropriate full-sole lift inside the shoe or outside the shoe. A general rule of thumb is that no more than $^1/_4$ inch of a full-sole lift is tolerated inside the shoe. If an equinus anatomic impairment exists, a heel lift is more appropriate than a full-sole lift. The amount of lift depends on the limb length difference and the patient's physiologic tolerance to change. Individuals with long-standing, significant structural discrepancies generally do not tolerate significant, rapid change because of the osseous and soft tissue adaptations that have developed over time. Minimal height adjustments at infrequent intervals should be made until the maximal necessary change has occurred.

FUNCTIONAL LIMB LENGTH DISCREPANCY

Treatment of functional LLD should consider the physiologic impairments at each involved segment and the interactions between levels. For example, a functionally short limb caused by femoral and tibial medial rotation and by foot pronation could have associated impairments of

- Lengthened or weak hip lateral rotators
- Lengthened or weak foot supinators
- Forefoot or rearfoot varus

Appropriate exercises, biomechanical support, and posture and movement training are necessary to alleviate the related impairments.

Patients with functional LLD related to lower extremity kinetic chain pronation (ie, femur medial rotation, genu valgum, and foot pronation) may benefit from temporary or permanent foot orthotics to assist in controlling pronation throughout the kinetic chain. However, caution must be used in prescribing orthotics to remedy physiologic impairments up the kinetic chain. Exercises to alleviate physiologic impairments contributing to pronation should be attempted first. If performance demands exceed the ability to control pronation, a temporary use of orthotics may be a necessary and useful adjunct.

Caution should be heeded in using sole or heel lifts to compensate for a functional LLD. The faulty strategy of displacing the COM over BOS used by a patient with a functional LLD does not necessarily alter with a lift. The more common scenario is for the individual to continue with the same faulty strategy, enhancing the functional LLD. For example, during initial contact phase of gait, the short limb may be functionally short as a result of positioning the hip in adduction with minimal displacement of the COM over the BOS (Fig. 20-27). After adding a lift, a similar gait strategy may continue to be used, causing further exaggeration of the LLD. Often, training the patient to properly position the hip and accurately displace the COM over the BOS alleviates the LLD (see Self-Management: Walk Stance Progression, levels I and II).

COMBINED FUNCTIONAL AND STRUCTURAL LIMB LENGTH DISCREPANCY

Combined functional and structural LLDs are treated with a combination of interventions. For example, if a tibial fracture through the growth plate contributed to some of the limb shortening, a combination of lift and exercise would be indicated.

THERAPEUTIC EXERCISE INTERVENTIONS FOR COMMON DIAGNOSES

Although it is beyond the scope of this text to present a comprehensive description and intervention plan for all diagnoses affecting the hip joint, a few selected diagnoses are presented. A brief overview of the cause, examination findings, and proposed treatment plan, with emphasis on therapeutic exercise intervention, is presented for each diagnosis.

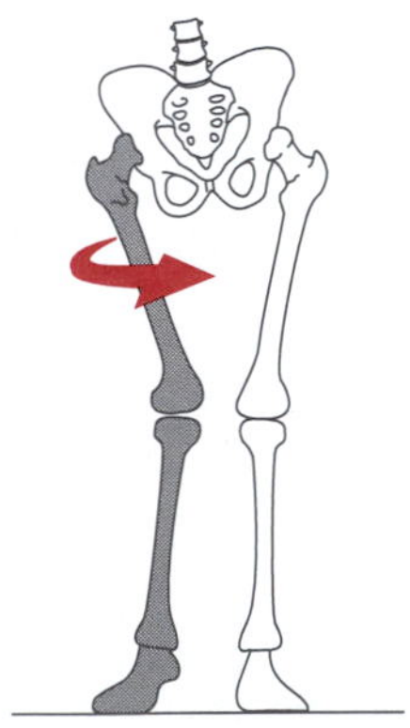

FIGURE 20-27 At initial contact phase of gait, an adducted and medially rotated femur and pronated foot may functionally shorten a limb.

Osteoarthritis

Arthritis is defined as any condition that results in cartilage damage, causing pain and limitation of the motion of a joint. Hip arthritis can be divided into several broad categories (Table 20-5). Because there is wide variation in the medical management of inflammatory arthritis, only the management of osteoarthritis is reviewed. Primary and secondary types of osteoarthritis are treated in a similar fashion. Chapter 11 provides information about the cause of osteoarthritis.

DIAGNOSIS

Proper diagnosis of a patient with hip osteoarthritis requires a careful history, physical examination, and review of appropriate radiographic and laboratory studies. The presence of radiographic changes (eg, joint space narrowing, moderate malalignment, osteophytes at the marginal aspects of the joint) should correlate with positive examination findings at the hip joint to arrive at a diagnosis of hip osteoarthritis. A positive radiographic finding alone does not indicate that the hip osteoarthritis is the source of symptoms, because many other musculoskeletal and nonmusculoskeletal sources can mimic hip joint pain. Hip osteoarthritis is a common sequelae of aging and is not always symptomatic.

Laboratory tests may not detect serum abnormalities unless their presence is related to another disease process. The rheumatoid factor test is generally negative. If the rheumatoid factor is found in the serum of older patients, its presence may be unrelated to the arthritis because false-positive results for rheumatoid factor increase with age in the normal population.[71]

Gradual, progressive, chronic pain can be associated with osteoarthritis. Intraarticular pain is usually described as deep, aching pain and can be experienced in the groin, around the greater trochanter, medial knee, and posterior buttock. The patient may induce or aggravate pain with moderate to vigorous activity and experience relief of pain with rest. Long periods of rest, however, may result in joint stiffness. The stiffness of osteoarthritis is not as severe as that of rheumatoid arthritis. Mild activity usually dissipates the stiffness.

Certain examination findings are typical of a patient with hip osteoarthritis:

- *Alignment:* anterior pelvic tilt, hip flexion, and hip lateral rotation.
- *Gait:* positive Trendelenburg sign, but more commonly a compensated Trendelenburg or antalgic gait (see Fig. 20-10*B*)
- *Mobility:* hypomobility in a capsular pattern with associated myofascial length changes
- *Decreased force or torque:* weakness most commonly in the gluteus medius and maximus.

Table 20-5. CATEGORIES OF ARTHRITIS

CATEGORY	TYPES	ETIOLOGY
Osteoarthritis	Osteoarthritis	Idiopathic Congenital Developmental Avascular necrosis Posttraumatic
Inflammatory arthritis	Rheumatoid arthritis Ankylosing spondylitis Psoriatic arthritis Systemic lupus erythematosus	Autoimmune
Infectious arthritis	Pyogenic	Bacteria
Other	Crystals Hemophilia	Gout, pseudogout Hemosiderin deposition

TREATMENT

The treatment for most patients with hip osteoarthritis is nonoperative.

- Nonsteroidal anti-inflammatory medications
- Physical therapy
- Intra-articular injection of corticosteroids
- Assistive devices
- Modification of activities

The focus of this chapter is physical therapy intervention for hip osteoarthritis, with primary emphasis on therapeutic exercise to treat the functional limitations and related physiologic impairments.

Pain and Inflammation

Management of pain and inflammation for hip osteoarthritis can follow the general guidelines discussed in a previous section. Activity modification may be one of the most significant aspects of treatment for pain and inflammation. The changes may include modification of basic and instrumental ADLs. The patient should be instructed in techniques to reduce joint stress during ADLs. The patient can be instructed in proper joint protection during prolonged postures (ie, standing with equal weight bearing on both feet) and common movement patterns (ie, carrying heavy loads in the hand on the involved side or in both hands equally).[69] The patient can covert vigorous weight-bearing activities (eg, running, tennis) to non–weight-bearing activities (eg, biking, swimming, water aerobics).

Specific to hip osteoarthritis, treatment addressing the cause of the pain should focus on altering the biomechanics of the hip. The degeneration in osteoarthritis is caused by a breakdown of chondrocytes, which are an essential element of articular cartilage. This breakdown is thought to be initiated by biomechanical stress. A primary goal of the intervention should be to alter biomechanical forces acting on the joint. Restoring joint mobility and tissue extensibility in flexion, extension, and medial rotation and restoring force or torque production and endurance of gluteus medius and maximus enable the joint to function in improved alignment and movement patterns.

Mobility

Specific exercises to improve joint mobility and tissue extensibility may include passive stretching in the affected directions (Fig. 20-28). However, active exercises should be employed whenever possible. Active exercises improve joint

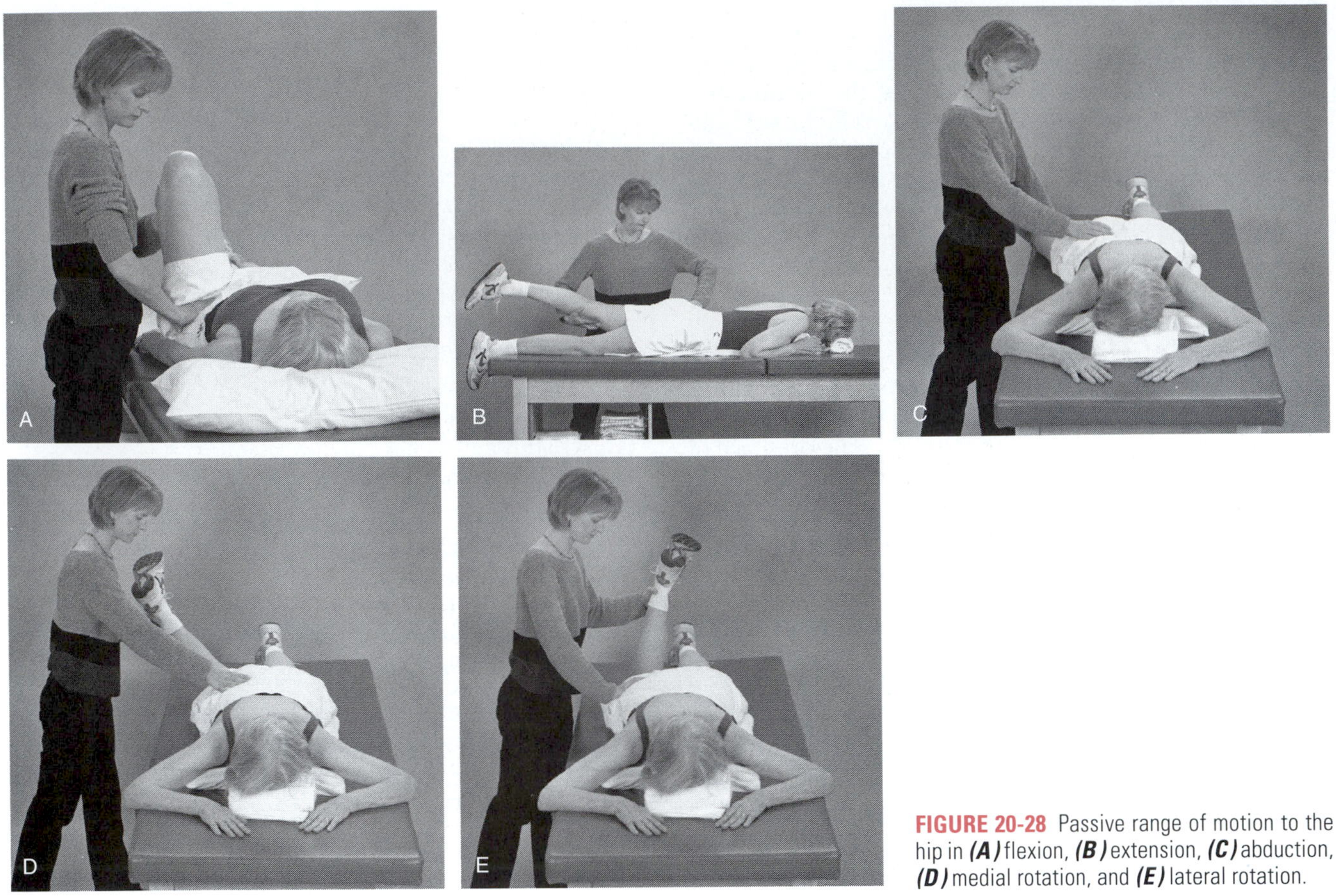

FIGURE 20-28 Passive range of motion to the hip in ***(A)*** flexion, ***(B)*** extension, ***(C)*** abduction, ***(D)*** medial rotation, and ***(E)*** lateral rotation.

mobility and recruit the muscles necessary to move the joint in the desired direction during function. Examples of active exercises to improve hip mobility in persons with hip osteoarthritis are shown in Self-Management: Gluteus Medius Strength Progression; Self-Management: Hand-Knee Rocking; Self-Management: Progressive Squat; and Figure 20-29. Another useful technique to teach the patient with osteoarthritis in the hip is self-traction (Fig. 20-30). This technique can assist in decompressing the joint to modulate pain and serves as a capsular stretch.

Muscle Performance and Endurance

The patient can be instructed in specific exercises to improve the force-generating capability and endurance of the hip extensors and abductors (see Self-Management: Gluteus Medius Strength Progression and Self-Management: Stomach-Lying Hip Extension). Whenever possible, functional exercises should be employed. For example, standing on the involved hip in neutral hip joint alignment and lifting the uninvolved hip onto a step can stimulate hip abductor recruitment on the weight-bearing side. However, weight-bearing exercises on a hip with osteoarthritis may exacerbate symptoms, particularly if the alignment is faulty. Adjunctive use of a cane, walking stick, ski pole, or dowel rod in the contralateral hand during weight-bearing exercise can reduce the amount of work necessary for the ipsilateral hip abductors. This approach reduces the joint reaction force and joint pain and increases tolerance to weight-bearing exercise.

Another method to reduce the joint reaction force enough to allow weight-bearing exercise is to hold a weight in the hand on the involved side.[69] The amount of weight can be graded to use the least amount necessary to reduce pain and allow optimal alignment during the step-up activity.

Regardless of the method used to unload the hip, the appropriate strategy for unilateral balance must reinforced. The gluteus medius and TFL are synergistic hip abductors. It is common for the TFL to dominate the stance recruit-

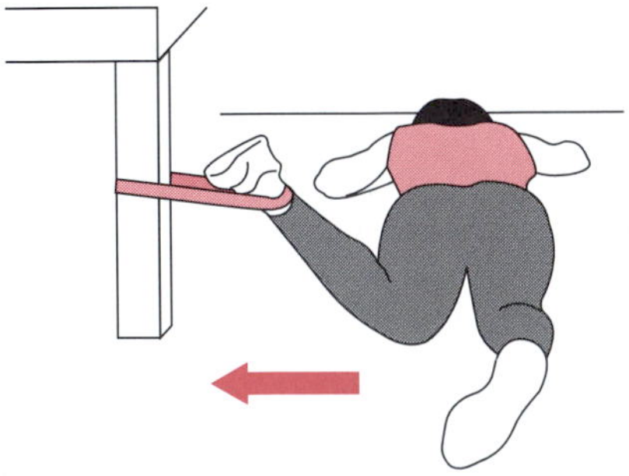

FIGURE 20-29 Prone hip medial rotation stretch with elastic. The patient is instructed to stabilize the pelvis in sagittal and transverse planes. It is important to keep the head of the femur in contact with the floor to ensure a precise rotational stretch. If the hip flexors are short, use of a pillow under the hips can allow the knee to flex 90 degrees without compensatory hip flexion.

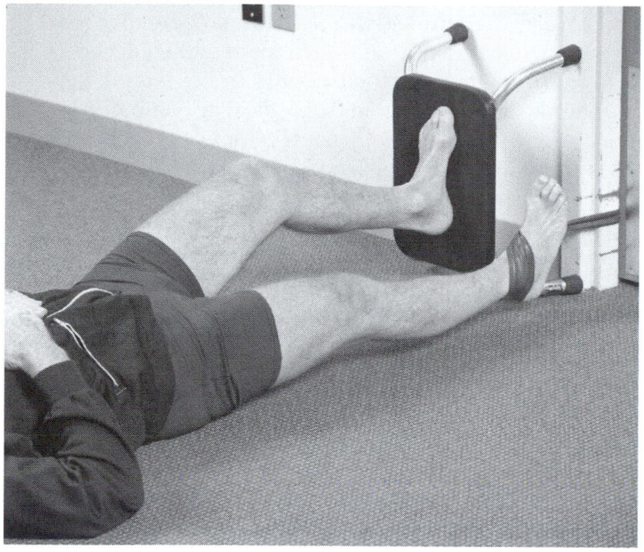

FIGURE 20-30 Self-traction of the hip.

ment pattern, particularly if the hip is in flexion or medial rotation. Education regarding the neutral position of the hip and gluteus medius recruitment is critical to the optimal outcome of this exercise. This may require additional activity from the lower abdominal muscles to control anterior pelvic tilt.

Step-up activities stimulate hip extensor recruitment[47] and facilitate hip flexion mobility, particularly if emphasis is placed on hip flexion during the step-up (Fig. 20-31), and step-down activities stimulate gluteus medius recruitment.[47] Care must be taken during stepping activities to prevent Trendelenburg patterns and to reinforce proper length-tension properties of the gluteus medius (ie, hip should not adduct more than 5–8 degrees, and femoral medial rotation should be kept to a minimum). All stepping activities can be graded by altering the step height or adding weight. A small step height (4 inches) and carrying a weight in the involved side hand reduces the force-generating requirements of the hip extensors and abductors. Conversely, larger step heights (8 to 12 inches) and carrying a weight in the contralateral hand increase the force-generating requirements.

Dosage parameters regarding repetition for these exercises depend on whether the goal is to improve force or endurance capabilities. Higher repetitions with a decreased load focus on endurance, and lower repetitions with a higher load focus on force production.

Balance

Injury to a joint and musculotendinous structures, as in hip osteoarthritis, probably results in altered somatosensory information that can adversely affect motor control.[73] Progressive balance training can have a positive effect on function of the arthritic hip. Self-Management: Walk Stance Progression levels I and II can be useful in training an individual to balance on one limb with correct form. After the patient is able to stand on one limb with appropriate muscle recruitment and joint loading strategies and without experiencing pain, balance activities can be added to the program. Progression should be taken slowly to prevent an inflammatory reaction in the hip, which would be counterproductive to improved function.

Posture and Movement

Patient-related instructions regarding improved weight-bearing habits are critical to the long-term effectiveness of therapeutic exercise. The person with hip osteoarthritis must be cautioned to avoid positioning the involved limb in the capsular pattern (ie, hip flexion and lateral rotation). During function, use of assistive devices such as canes, crutches, or walkers can be quite effective in reducing joint stress during ambulation. Problem solving to develop improved posture and movement patterns to allow continued participation in social and occupational activities is time well spent with a patient.

Adjunctive Interventions

Because the hip is a weight-bearing joint, it is important that the individual maintains optimal weight through proper nutrition and aerobic activity. Non–weight-bearing aerobic activities are recommended for persons with hip osteoarthritis. Use of a stationary bike with the seat relatively high can serve as means of maintaining aerobic activity with minimal weight-bearing stress on the joint. Pool activities are also recommended for persons with hip osteoarthritis. Swimming, non–weight-bearing exercise with inflatable supports, or weight-bearing exercises in a pool (see Chapter 17) minimize stress on the hip joint.

Total Hip Arthroplasty

If all nonoperative management fails to improve the function and quality of life of a patient with hip osteoarthritis,

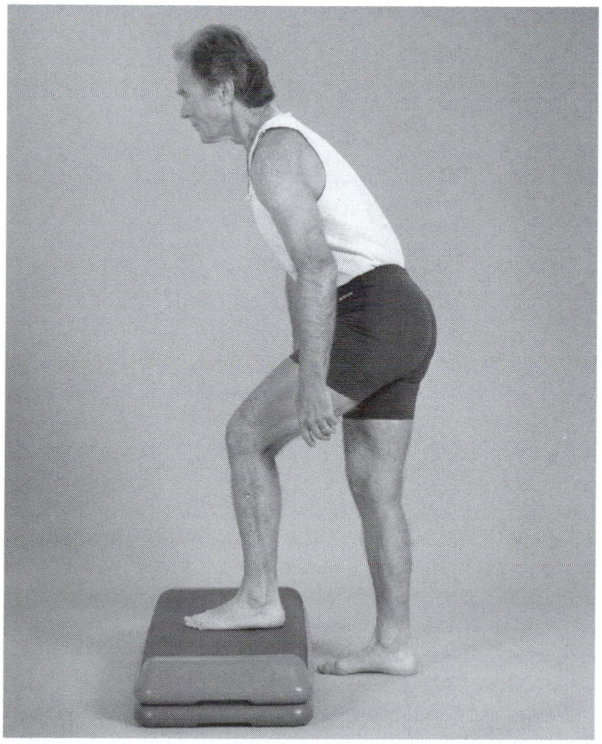

FIGURE 20-31 Side view of a step-up exercise with exaggerated hip flexion to focus on hip flexion mobility and gluteus maximus recruitment.

operative management is the next step. Total hip arthroplasty (THA) has been available for approximately 30 years. More than 120,000 artificial hip joints are being implanted annually in the United States.[73] The primary goal of THA is to relieve pain, although it is also used in cases of comminuted fractures of the femoral head when bony healing is unlikely. Pain relief can be accomplished in more than 95% of patients and lasts approximately 15 years or longer.[74]

There are two broad categories of hip prosthesis—cemented and uncemented—and three primary techniques to approach the hip surgically—posterior, anterolateral, and transtrochanteric. Each of these choices influences the postoperative management and rehabilitation of the patient. It is beyond the scope of this text to describe the details of each component selection and surgical approach, but the major differences are highlighted as they affect postoperative exercise management.

COMPONENT SELECTION: CEMENTED OR UNCEMENTED

A critical element with respect to postoperative care in terms of component selection is the weight-bearing restriction imposed on an uncemented femoral component. In the cemented THA, the femoral and acetabular components are cemented into position. Studies using the modern cement technique have reported a 0%–2% failure rate for the femoral component at 5 years.[75] Acetabular component fixation has not improved significantly and continues to demonstrate a combined radiographic loosening and revision rate of up to 40% at 11 years of follow-up.[76] However, the advantage of the cemented components is that weight bearing is permitted immediately postoperatively.

Concern about bone reabsorption and loosening, particularly in the acetabular component, led to the search for techniques to attach the implants to bone without the use of bone cement. Direct attachment of the implant to bone could allow long-term fixation. To minimize motion of the prosthesis within the bone, excellent initial stability must be obtained intraoperatively by precise preparation of the bone and firm impaction of the implant into the femur. When a femoral component is not properly inserted or it is inserted in poor-quality bone, weight bearing tends to piston the prosthesis into the canal. This motion can prevent bone growth into the surface. Consequently, many surgeons restrict weight bearing during the first 6 to 12 weeks. Significant variability has been reported regarding the revision rate for uncemented femoral components: 0%–13% at 2 to 7 years of follow-up.[77]

Uncemented femoral fixation can be complicated by thigh pain associated with loosening of the femoral stem. Thigh pain can occur in 5% to 20% of cases with uncemented femoral fixation.[78] The pain begins 4 to 6 months postoperatively and occasionally decreases after 18 to 24 months, perhaps as the femur remodels to accommodate to the femoral prosthesis.

Unlike the findings for uncemented femoral components, the clinical results for uncemented porous acetabular components have been excellent. In one 10-year follow-up study of uncemented acetabular components, 95% of the acetabular components were considered stable, and the Harris Hip rating scale had improved from a mean preoperative score of 52 points to a mean postoperative score of 90 points.[79]

Because of the excellent results of cemented femoral components and uncemented acetabular components, the concept of a hybrid THA was developed. It incorporated the best of both components, and it allows immediate weight bearing postoperatively, facilitating rehabilitation. In 1994, a consensus panel of orthopedic surgeons at the National Institutes of Health recommended that hybrid fixation be used in most patients receiving THAs.[73] Table 20-6 summarizes factors related to component selection.

SURGICAL APPROACHES

The three basic surgical approaches to THA are posterior, anterolateral, and transtrochanteric approaches. The surgical approach to the hip must provide adequate exposure to allow for careful preparation of the femur and acetabulum. The critical element for each approach is the treatment of the gluteus medius and greater trochanter, because this affects weight bearing and exercise restrictions postoperatively. Each surgical approach creates a different weakness in the hip capsule and renders it vulnerable to dislocation in that direction.

Posterior Approach

The posterior approach is the most commonly used approach for THA in the United States. The gluteus medius is left entirely intact, facilitating early rehabilitation. If the components selected permit full weight bearing immediately postoperatively, many patients progress rapidly from using a walker for 3 weeks to using a cane. By 6 weeks postoperatively, many have no need for a cane. The disadvantage of the posterior approach is that it is the most vulnerable to dislocation. Avoidance of hip flexion, adduction, and medial rotation should be strictly adhered to for a minimum of 6 weeks postoperatively.

Anterolateral Approach

For the anterolateral approach, the incision is made through the anterior capsule of the hip. Dissection of the gluteus medius is performed. To protect the muscle reattachment, some surgeons place the patient on restricted

Table 20-6. COMPONENT SELECTION FOR TOTAL HIP ARTHROPLASTY

COMPONENT	WEIGHT-BEARING RESTRICTIONS	REVISION RATE
Cemented femoral and acetabular components	Immediate postoperative weight bearing	Poor
Uncemented femoral and acetabular components	Restricted weight bearing for 6–12 weeks	Fair
Hybrid: cemented femoral component and uncemented acetabular component	Immediate postoperative weight bearing	Excellent

weight bearing and active or resisted gluteus medius exercise for up to 6 weeks postoperatively. The dissection of the gluteus medius can result in weakness for 4 to 6 months. Weakness persisting after 6 months may be caused by detachment or denervation of the gluteus medius. The advantage of the anterolateral approach is the low incidence of postoperative dislocation. The position of dislocation for this approach is extension, adduction, and lateral rotation.

Transtrochanteric Approach

This approach involves osteotomizing the greater trochanter from the proximal femur. As for the anterolateral approach, many surgeons restrict weight bearing for the first 6 to 8 weeks to allow healing of the osteotomy. The incidence of and position for dislocation is similar to those for the anterolateral approach. A significant advantage of this approach is that the trochanter can be reattached distal to its anatomic location to improve soft tissue tension and stability if the soft tissues are lax after the reconstruction. Table 20-7 summarizes weight-bearing restrictions and the positional and functional precautions for each THA surgical approach.

POSTOPERATIVE MANAGEMENT

Management of the patient should begin preoperatively with education about postoperative pulmonary exercises, dislocation precautions, use of vascular support, walking progression, and exercise progressions. This preoperative education is becoming increasingly important because cost-containment policies have reduced the inpatient stay after THA to 4 days or less.

Stability after THA is a primary precaution. The factors that affect stability can be divided into three major categories:

1. Patient factors, such as previous surgeries, patient height, and compliance with hip precautions postoperatively
2. Surgical factors, including component selection, component position, and soft tissue tension
3. Postoperative factors, such as trochanteric union, gluteus medius reattachment, and excessive ROM of the hip

Hip precautions are summarized in Table 20-7. Precautions appropriate to the surgical approach should be strictly adhered to for the first 6 weeks after surgery.

Postoperative management of THA can follow a general protocol with the understanding that individual cases may have slight variations during postoperative rehabilitation. The surgeon best understands the details of the surgical procedure for each case and therefore should guide the postoperative rehabilitation if there is a deviation from the traditional protocol.

Early Postoperative Management

Early postoperative management includes many exercises and activities. The patient should be transferred to a chair on the day of surgery, and he begins physical therapy, including early ROM with THA surgical approach precautions, on the first postoperative day (see Table 20-7).

Dynamic ankle pumping is performed, as is isometric exercise for the hip musculature. Caution should be used with isometric contractions of gluteus medius for anterolateral and transtrochanteric approaches. Submaximal contractions are recommended to protect the surgical site immediately after surgery. Physician approval is recommended for initiation of maximal isometric contractions and active exercise of the gluteus medius for patients with these surgical approaches.

Force or torque exercises are progressed to dynamic activities over 4 days after surgery if tolerated by the patient and the surgical approach is not a contraindication. Examples of dynamic exercises include:

- Prone hip abduction (to facilitate concentric and eccentric contractions of the gluteus medius versus TFL) can be progressed from active assisted, to active, and to light elastic resisted exercises (see Self-Management: Gluteus Medius Strength Progression). This exercise should be delayed for up to 6 weeks after anterolateral and transtrochanteric approaches.
- Prone hip extension, with emphasis on gluteus maximus recruitment and abdominal stabilization, can be progressed from active assisted, to active, to resisted (see Self-Management: Stomach-Lying Hip Extension).
- Prone hip rotation, to facilitate concentric and eccentric control of hip lateral rotators, can be progressed

Table 20-7. RESTRICTIONS AND PRECAUTIONS FOR TOTAL HIP ARTHROPLASTY SURGICAL APPROACHES

APPROACH	POST-OP WB STATUS	ROM RESTRICTIONS	FUNCTIONAL MOVEMENT PRECAUTIONS	ADDITIONAL CONSIDERATIONS
Posterolateral	Immediate full WB	Flexion >90 degrees, abduction, medial rotation	In/out chair, on/off toilet, don/doff shoes/socks	Extra precaution with tall patients
Anterolateral	Restricted WB for minimum 6 weeks	Extension, adduction, lateral rotation	Turning away from the surgical hip	
Transtrochanteric	Restricted WB for minimum 6 weeks	Extension, adduction, lateral rotation	Turning away from the surgical hip	

WB, weight bearing.

from active assisted, to active, and to resisted exercises with light elastics (see Fig. 20-38).

Assisted ambulation with a walker may begin as early as postoperative day 1 with appropriate weight-bearing restrictions (see Tables 20-6 and 20-7). Progression from a walker to crutches occurs within 4 days postoperatively. Progression to stairs must occur before discharge.

If a patient is not suitable to be discharged to a home environment, discharge plans are made for a short-term rehabilitation facility. Discharge to the home can be initiated when the following short-range goals are achieved:

- Independent ambulation with a suitable stable gait pattern
- Demonstrates the ability to function independently in a home environment

The patient must be supplied with patient-related instructions, including the following information:

- The safe performance of ADLs and instrumental ADLs required to be independent in the home. This may require a referral to an occupational therapist for demonstration of assisted ADL equipment such as a sock donner, slip-on shoes, a reacher-grabber, and sponge stick.
- Hip precautions with respect to ADLs, (eg, dressing, bathing, reaching low places, getting into and out of a car). These should be demonstrated by the clinician and practiced by the patient and caregivers.
- Exercise progressions

Intermediate Postoperative Management

Between 4 and 6 weeks after surgery, exercise is progressed as described. Exercises to improve mobility of the hip can include stretching, with education about the limits imposed by the surgical approach (see Table 20-7). After a posterior approach, stretching into hip flexion should not begin until 6 weeks or longer. The functional goals of stretching are to allow the patient to put on and take off his own socks and shoes. This should be done with a combination of hip flexion, abduction, and lateral rotation. Additional stretching is of limited benefit and may place the patient at risk for late instability.[81]

Exercises to improve force or torque production can be progressed. After weight bearing is permitted, with or without assistance, the following exercises can be initiated:

- Gluteus medius recruitment can be facilitated by using light elastics to resist abduction to the uninvolved extremity while standing on the involved extremity.[82]
- Step-ups, step-downs, and sit-to-stand activities can stimulate gluteus maximus and medius activity and can be graded by altering the step and chair height. Attention to posture and movement patterns is essential. Compromise in form must not take place; the exercise should be modified until the form is precise.
- Ambulation can be progressed to using a cane by 2 weeks postoperatively if the patient has no gait restrictions and demonstrates adequate strength and balance.

The quality of gait should be emphasized. Often, habits developed preoperatively, such as a Trendelenburg pattern, need to be modified postoperatively. Faulty gait patterns should be corrected to minimize abnormal stresses through the prosthesis. Extended use of an assistive device postoperatively may be necessary until the faulty gait patterns are minimized.

If the patient is discharged from the hospital to a short-term rehabilitation facility, discharge to home requires that the patient be fully independent in basic ADLs and instrumental ADLs in the home setting. This may require assessment of the home setting with intervention directed at overcoming or modifying recognized obstacles. The assistance of an occupational therapist and social service worker may be needed to return the patient safely to the home environment.

Advanced Management

The most critical long-term goal for most patients with a THA is to maintain a high quality of life with as little pain as possible. This may require some restriction of activity, such as those with high-impact loading—running, racquet sports, and basketball. These activities may reduce the functional life of the THA. Certain activities should be encouraged:

- Walking
- Swimming
- Cycling
- Moderate weight training
- Use of a ski trainer
- Use of a stair-climber

Sports such as golf, hiking, cycling, cross-country skiing, and occasional light doubles tennis also are acceptable.

Patients need to be educated regarding a lifetime of regular exercise for optimizing the life of the THA. Patients should be encouraged to attend scheduled follow-up appointments with the surgeon to provide a means of early detection of a mechanical problem.

POSTOPERATIVE COMPLICATIONS

The physical therapist should be aware of postoperative complications, which may include thromboembolic disease, prosthetic dislocation, heterotopic ossification, and deep sepsis.

Thromboembolic Disease

Thromboembolic disease includes deep vein thrombosis and pulmonary embolism. The clinical detection of deep vein thrombosis is extremely inaccurate. If the patient has painful calf swelling that does not respond to elevation, referral to the physician is mandatory, because this condition is considered a medical emergency.

Prosthetic Dislocation

Dislocation has been discussed in relation to postoperative precautions. The postoperative precautions should be emphasized, depending on the approach, for a minimum of 6 weeks. The patient should be cautioned that the reconstructed hip will always be more vulnerable to dislocation than the natural hip. If dislocation occurs, referral to the physician is necessary so that the decision to surgically or nonsurgically reduce the hip can be made and the patient can be given the proper brace for immobilization after the dislocation.

Heterotopic Ossification

The incidence of heterotopic ossification formation around a THA is 5% to 25%.[82] Frequently, the condition does not compromise the functional result. Loss of mobility is the indicator for this complication. Rapid loss of mobility postoperatively warrants a referral to the surgeon to exclude or confirm heterotopic ossification. Some persons are more at at risk for this complication:[82]

- Patients with hypertrophic arthritis
- Men older than 65 years
- Those with heterotopic ossification after prior surgery
- Persons with ankylosing spondylitis

Deep Sepsis

The most devastating complication after THA is deep sepsis.[83] Early detection is critical to an optimal outcome. If detected within the first 2 weeks postoperatively, open debridement and synovectomy combined with intravenous antibiotics may be successful. The worst-case scenario is the presence of a highly virulent and resistant pathologic organism. In this case, removal of all prosthetic components and cement is necessary. Reimplantation may be delayed for up to 12 months. During this time, the patient may be mobile by non–weight-bearing ambulation with a walker, if tolerated. Reimplantation may proceed when the wound is sterile if sufficient bone stock and tissue integrity remain. Pain and swelling concurrent with a fever are warnings of deep sepsis.

Iliotibial Band–Related Diagnoses

The extensive deep fascia that covers the gluteal region and the thigh like a sleeve is called the fascia lata. It is attached proximally to the external lip of the iliac crest, the sacrum and coccyx, the sacrotuberous ligament, the ischial tuberosity, the ischiopubic rami, and the inguinal ligament. Distally, it is attached to the patella, the tibial condyles, and the head of the fibula. The dense portion of the fascia lata situated laterally is designated the ITB. The TFL and three fourths of the gluteus maximus insert into the ITB so that its distal attachment serves as a conjoint tendon of these muscles. For the purposes of this discussion, dysfunction of the ITB is presented only as it relates to the TFL/ITB complex.

The TFL can be functionally differentiated into anteromedial and posterolateral fibers. The anteromedial fibers have a greater mechanical advantage for hip flexion, and the posterolateral fibers have a greater mechanical advantage for hip abduction and medial rotation (Fig. 20-32).[84]

During walking, the anteromedial fibers generally are quiet, whereas the posterolateral fibers are active near initial contact.[84] With sequentially increased locomotor velocity, anteromedial fiber activity increases near preswing and initial swing, presumably to decelerate the extending hip and accelerate flexion of the thigh, and posterolateral activity increases at initial contact.[84] The posterolateral fibers of the TFL/ITB complex have been implicated in providing stability against varus stress at the knee.[84] The anteromedial fibers are active during the hip flexion phase of the step-up, and the posterolateral fibers are active during the loading phase of the step-up.

Because of the vast functional roles of the TFL/ITB complex, it is prone to overuse and strain injuries. A few of the more common TFL/ITB–related diagnoses include

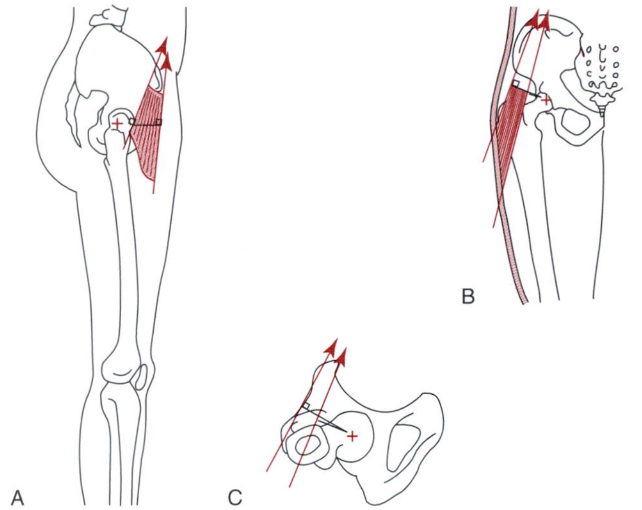

FIGURE 20-32 ***(A)*** The anteromedial fibers of the TFL have a greater mechanical advantage for hip flexion. ***(B)*** The posterolateral fibers of the TFL have a greater mechanical advantage for hip abduction and ***(C)*** medial rotation. (From Pare EB, Stern JT, Schwartz JM. Functional differentiation within the tensor fascia latae. *J Bone Joint Surg Am.* 1981;63A:1457).

- ITB fascitis
- ITB friction syndrome
- Greater trochanter bursitis
- Patellofemoral dysfunction
- TFL strain
- Faulty movement patterns at the hip and tibiofemoral joints

The cause of each of these diagnoses is reviewed separately. Treatment recommendations are provided for the related impairments and functional limitations shared by each of these diagnoses.

ILIOTIBIAL BAND FASCITIS

A condition, sometimes mistakenly diagnosed as sciatica, is that of pain associated with inflammation of the fascial band from overuse of the TFL, commonly called ITB fascitis. Pain may be limited to the area covered by the fascia along the lateral surface of the thigh or may extend upward over the buttocks and involve the gluteal fascia. Painful symptoms may extend below the knee, with associated symptoms of paresthesia in the region of the lateral calf.

A review of the anatomy of the lateral aspect of the knee demonstrates the relationship of the peroneal nerve to the muscles and fascia in this area. Peroneal nerve irritation can result from pressure from rigid bands of fascia in a short ITB or from the effect of traction from taut bands of fascia in an overstretched ITB. Peroneal nerve irritation can manifest as symptoms in the lateral calf.[30]

Symptoms are often worse in the morning and improve with minimal weight bearing, but they then worsen with continued weight bearing. Tests to differentiate ITB fascitis from sciatica are summarized in Display 20-5. Presumably, this condition results from overuse of the TFL/ITB. Concurrent with any overuse syndrome is underuse of the related synergists about any axis of motion in which the affected muscle

DISPLAY 20-5

Key Tests for Differential Diagnosis of Iliotibial Band Fascitis from Sciatica

Key Tests

- Palpation over the length of the fascia lata may elicit tenderness, especially over the greater trochanter or near the point of insertion lateral to the patella.
- Hip flexion, abduction, and medial rotation (TFL manual muscle test) may test painful.
- The Ober test (test for ITB length) reveals shortness of the TFL/ITB, and further stretch may elicit pain. Paresthesias along the peroneal nerve distribution may worsen with ankle inversion.[30]
- Lumbar spine clearing test results are negative for reproduction of the patient's symptoms.

Associated Findings

- Hip rotation ROM may reveal excessive medial rotation relative to lateral rotation ROM.
- Positional weakness of the synergistic muscles of the gluteus medius, gluteus maximus, iliopsoas, and quadriceps.
- Hip anteversion.
- Excessive medial rotation, positive Trendelenburg sign, or limited hip extension in gait.

functions. The more deconditioned the underused synergists become, the greater the force-producing requirements become for the TFL/ITB complex, until finally the force-producing requirements exceed the muscle and fascial capability, and inflammation results. Display 20-6 summarizes the synergist relationships that may become imbalanced, leading to TFL/ITB overuse.

OTHER ILIOTIBIAL BAND AND TENSOR FASCIA LATA OVERUSE SYNDROMES

Similar causes exist for the remaining TFL/ITB diagnoses, although with slightly different symptoms. Although some of these diagnoses manifest at the knee, treatment must focus on the cause of the condition, which is TFL/ITB overuse. The treatment focuses on the physiologic impairments associated with TFL/ITB overuse at the hip. Display 20-7 summarizes the signs and symptoms of other TFL/ITB overuse syndromes.

DISPLAY 20-6

Potential Synergist Relationships With TFL/ITB overuse

- The anteromedial TFL can dominate the hip flexion force couple, contributing to underuse of the iliopsoas.
- The posterolateral TFL can dominate the hip abduction and medial rotation force couples, contributing to underuse of the gluteus medius, upper fibers of the gluteus maximus, and gluteus minimus.
- Because the ITB can provide stability to the knee, overuse of the ITB may contribute to underuse of the quadriceps.
- The hip tends to function in medial rotation patterns, thereby contributing to underuse of the hip lateral rotator force couple, including the deep hip rotators, posterior fibers of the gluteus medius, and lower fibers of the gluteus maximus.

TREATMENT

Treatment of each of these diagnoses should be related to the presenting functional limitations, related impairments, and the stage of healing.

Pain and Inflammation

In the acute phase, treatment should be directed toward alleviating the pain and inflammation with medication (ie, nonsteroidal antiinflammatories), physical agents (ie, cryotherapy), electrotherapeutic modalities, and unloading (eg, use of a cane, taping, proper positioning at night with pillows between knees if sidelying). As acute symptoms subside, succeeding treatments should be directed toward resolving the impairments and functional limitations associated with the condition.

Mobility

Mobility impairments are most often associated with a stiff or short TFL/ITB complex. Stretching the TFL/ITB complex is indicated but can pose a challenge to the clinician and patient. The TFL/ITB has many actions at the

DISPLAY 20-7

Tensor Fascia Lata and Iliotibial Band Overuse Syndromes

- **ITB friction syndrome:** In **ITB friction syndrome,** pain and tenderness are localized to the lateral femoral condyle because of a short ITB exerting pressure over the lateral femoral condyle.
- **Trochanteric bursitis:** In **trochanter bursitis,** the bursa becomes inflamed due to the pressure exerted by a short ITB moving back and forth over the greater trochanter during movement.
- **Patellofemoral dysfunction:** Shortness of the ITB can contribute to **patellofemoral dysfunction** because of its insertion into the lateral retinaculum of the patellofemoral joint and its tendency to dominate over the quadriceps for knee stability **(see Chapter 21).**
- **TFL strain: TFL strain** can occur from overuse of a short TFL/ITB or a stretched TFL/ITB complex. The former is more common, but there are instances of strain of the stretched TFL/ITB. The TFL/ITB on the side of the adducted hip (usually the high iliac crest), if there are no associated hip medial rotation or hip flexion alignment or movement faults, is subject to continuous tension and therefore strain.
- **Faulty movement patterns at the hip and tibiofemoral joints:** Faulty movement patterns of the hip and tibiofemoral joints related to the TFL/ITB are critical to understanding the effect of muscle imbalance on the function of these joints. Sahrmann provides more information on this subject.*

*(*Sahrmann SA.* Diagnosis and Exercise Management of Musculoskeletal Pain Syndromes. *St. Louis: Mosby; 1999).*

hip. For an optimal stretch, the TFL/ITB must be elongated simultaneously in all directions opposite its actions. It is critical that the stretching be specifically directed to the area in need of stretch, and some commonly prescribed TFL/ITB stretches do not meet these criteria (Fig. 20-33).

An assisted stretch emphasizing the posterolateral fibers is shown in Fig. 20-34. This stretch ensures the most precise positioning for the best outcome. Rarely can the patient self-stretch in this position, but he may be able to master the control required after a series of hip abduction exercises with the emphasis on eccentric control of the gluteus medius (see Self-Management: Gluteus Medius Strength Progression). This exercise also emphasizes improving the force-generating capability and kinesthetic awareness of the gluteus medius—a critical, underused synergist. Another self-stretch exercise for the TFL/ITB is shown in Fig. 20-35. This stretch is directed more toward the anterolateral fibers and is considered an active stretch because of the activation of the abdominal muscle group and gluteus maximus to rotate the pelvis posteriorly.

TFL/ITB stretching should not be used in isolation with the hope that the stretch will permanently improve the length. The clinician must seek the related impairments and functional limitations that perpetuate the shortness. For example, short posterolateral fibers of the TFL/ITB do not remain stretched if the person stands and moves with the hip in excessive medial rotation. Education regarding postural habits and neuromuscular training of new movement patterns is essential to restoring length to the ITB on a more permanent basis.

Muscle Performance and Endurance

Improving the force-generating capability of the underused synergists is often a prerequisite to neuromuscular training. The TFL/ITB is not able to reduce its participation in movement patterns if the underused synergists cannot meet their physiologic and biomechanical requirements. Progressive iliopsoas, gluteus medius, gluteus maximus, and quadriceps strengthening may be required to reduce the load on the TFL/ITB.

The prescribed exercise depends on the positional strength of these muscles. For example, the iliopsoas may require active assist initially, progressing to active holding, resistive holding, and dynamic and more functional exercises (see Self-Management: Step-Up, Step-Down and Self-Management: Iliopsoas Strengthening). The emphasis is on end-range isometrics before dynamic movements to improve the positional strength of the iliopsoas at end range, thereby improving length-tension relationships of

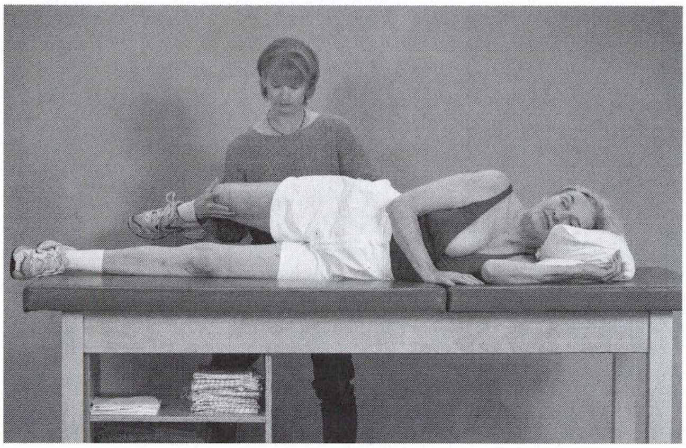

FIGURE 20-34 Assisted Ober stretch position.

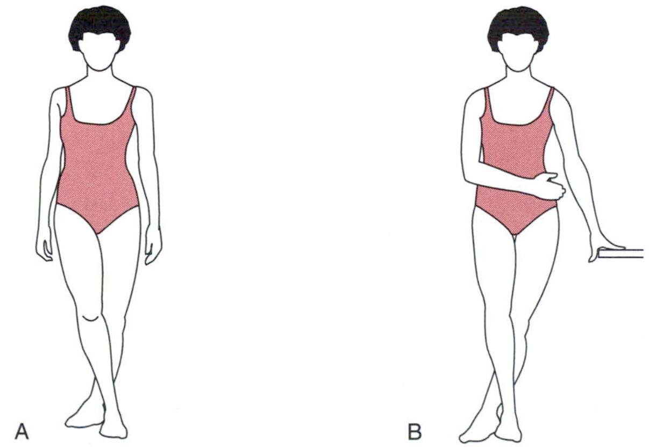

FIGURE 20-33 Commonly prescribed TFL/ITB stretch that does not stretch the TFL/ITB in all directions opposite its actions. ***(A)*** Crossing the legs places the hip joint in flexion and internal rotation. ***(B)*** Swaying laterally, with the hip flexed and internally rotated, stretches the gluteus medius more than the TFL/ITB.

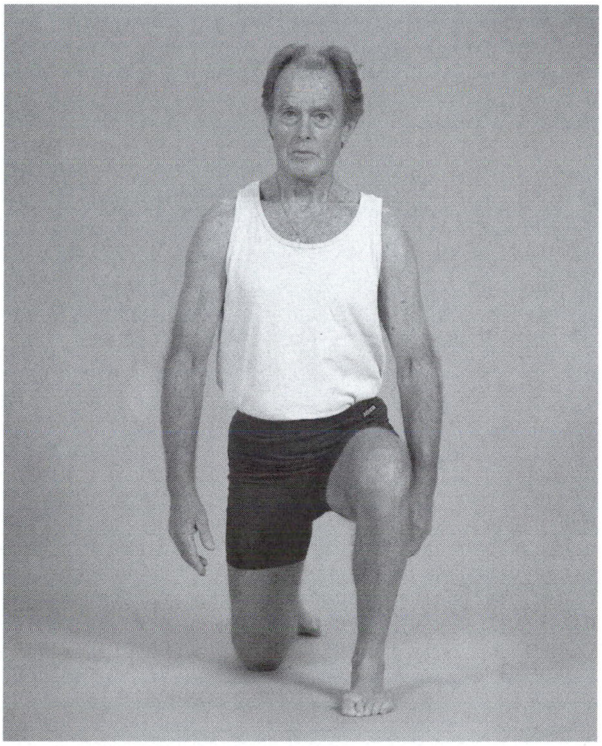

FIGURE 20-35 In the half-kneel stretch position, the patient is asked to maximally drop the contralateral pelvis to adduct the ipsilateral hip. The patient also is asked to extend the hip by means of posterior pelvic tilt (using the gluteus maximus and lower abdominal muscles). A slight hip lateral rotation can be added to stretch the PL fibers.

the relatively lengthened, weaker synergist to the TFL/ITB in hip flexion.

Adjunctive Intervention

For a strained TFL/ITB due to continuous tension, use of taping as illustrated by Kendall[30] (Fig. 20-36*A*) can unload the strained structure. Because the femur must not function in excessive medial rotation, taping the hip in a slight amount of lateral rotation may be indicated. An alternative taping technique is illustrated in Fig. 20-36*B*. Applying firm pressure over the TFL while applying tape over this area may unload the TFL and therefore encourage more gluteus medius participation during functional activities.

DISPLAY 20-8

Summary of Piriformis Function

- Decelerates hip medial rotation
- Accelerates hip lateral rotation
- Assists in decelerating hip adduction
- Assists in accelerating hip abduction
- Assists in the control of anterior pelvic tilt
- Assists in stabilization of the sacroiliac joint
- Functions as a portion of the pelvic floor

Stretched Piriformis Syndrome

The piriformis muscle has been implicated as a potential source of sciatica symptoms.[85] Although there may be numerous cases in which the sciatic pain is associated with a short piriformis, this discussion focuses on irritation of the sciatic nerve associated with a stretched piriformis. The piriformis arises with a broad origin from the anterior aspect of the sacrum and inserts into the superior border of the greater trochanter. Display 20-8 summarizes piriformis function.

In a faulty standing position with the femur in adduction and medial rotation and the pelvis in anterior pelvic tilt, the piriformis muscle is placed on stretch. The piriformis muscle is pulled taut, potentially entrapping the sciatic nerve. Pressure on the sciatic nerve may result from tension from the adjacent taut piriformis muscle. If the nerve pierces through the piriformis, an injurious tension may be imposed on the sciatic nerve along with the stretched muscle. Because the piriformis is actively used during gait, abnormal gait patterns can impose stress on the piriformis and related sciatic nerve. With a stretched piriformis, repetitive movements of the hip in medial rotation and adduction and movements of the pelvis in anterior pelvic tilt can impose friction on the nerve, resulting in inflammation of the neural tissue. Strain of the piriformis can ensue as a result of the muscle functioning in a chronically stretched position.

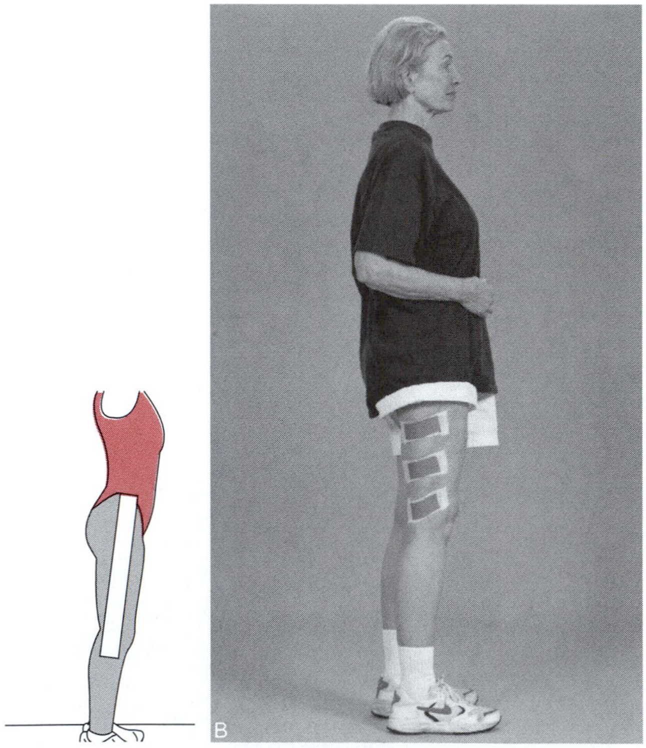

FIGURE 20-36 Taping techniques to unload the ITB. ***(A)*** Unloading the TFL/ITB with lateral longitudinal taping using a technique developed by Florence Kendall. ***(B)*** Unloading the TFL/ITB with anterior to posterior strips positioned proximally over the TFL and placed every 2 to 3 inches distally. The patellofemoral joint may need to be taped medially to prevent lateral displacement from the stretch placed on the ITB distally.

DIAGNOSIS

Pain caused by piriformis strain can be felt deep in the buttock. Resisted testing, particularly at end range, often elicits pain and weakness. Symptoms of sciatic nerve damage are often experienced below the level of involvement. Symptoms of sciatica related to a stretched piriformis can be experienced from the posterior buttock extending inferiorly to as far as the toes. Symptoms of pain or tingling may appear in the cutaneous areas supplied by the sciatic nerve before symptoms of numbness or signs of weakness become apparent.

Tests that are positive for cases of stretched piriformis syndrome are summarized in Table 20-8. These key tests aid in developing a differential diagnosis that includes a stretched piriformis, a shortened piriformis, lumbar radiculopathy, or referred pain.

TREATMENT

Treatment is based on the functional limitations, related impairments, and stage of the condition. The underlying problem of the stretched piriformis must be addressed for long-term resolution of the problem. Support of the muscle in the optimal length is critical to long-term changes. Whether this support is provided by taping, orthotic support, or posture and exercise is decided on a case by case basis, but it must be addressed in some fashion and for a period sufficient to allow recovery. Periodic ROM measures combined with positional strength testing and dynamic functional testing can indicate the status of recovery of muscle length and length-tension properties. The following sections provide guidelines for the treatment of stretched piriformis syndrome, with an emphasis on therapeutic exercise.

Table 20-8. DIFFERENTIAL DIAGNOSIS OF STRETCHED PIRIFORMIS SYNDROME

KEY TESTS	SIGNS
Standing alignment	Lordosis and anterior pelvic tilt Hip flexion and medial rotation High iliac crest on involved side
Selective tissue tension tests	<90 degrees of hip flexion, with adduction and medial rotation reproduces symptoms Passive or active lateral rotation and abduction reduces symptoms Resisted knee flexion is negative
Range of motion	Excessive hip medial rotation relative to lateral rotation within the involved side Excessive medial rotation of the involved side relative to the uninvolved side
Palpation	Tenderness elicited in region of the sciatic notch
Positional strength	Weakness in hip lateral rotators and posterior gluteus medius
Functional tests	Tendency to function in hip medial rotation, hip adduction, and anterior pelvic tilt during functional activities Repetitive movements in medial rotation and/or adduction, with the pelvis in anterior tilt, reproduce symptoms Lateral rotation, abduction, and neutral pelvic alignment relieves symptoms Symptoms diminish or disappear when not bearing weight
Lumbar clearing examination	Negative for reproduction of symptoms

Pain

Patients should be instructed in positions that relieve nerve pain. Relief may be achieved by placing the involved leg in lateral rotation and abduction in lying and standing positions. Sitting with the hips in lateral rotation (ie, legs crossed at the ankles) with periodic gluteal isometrics can alleviate symptoms while sitting.

Posture and Movement

Permanent changes with respect to postural habits are encouraged rather than extreme postural changes to relieve symptoms. For example, instruction should be offered regarding weight bearing equally on both feet with neutral femur (particularly with respect to medial rotation) and pelvic positions during relaxed standing, transitioning from sit to stand, and during stance phase of gait. Orthotic devices may be necessary to correct foot impairments contributing to the tendency to posture and function in excessive femoral medial rotation.

Muscle Performance

Exercises such as prone foot pushes (Fig. 20-37), prone hip extension with pelvic stabilization (Self-Management: Stomach-Lying Hip Extension), and sidelying hip abduction (Self-Management: Gluteus Medius Strength Progression), with emphasis on lateral rotation and prone hip lateral rotation in the short range (Fig. 20-38), can improve length-tension properties and positional strength of the lengthened lateral rotators. However, caution must be used with dosage parameters for the stretched piriformis. The force-producing capabilities may be significantly compromised because of the altered length-tension properties. The positional weakness may be compounded further by disuse weakness.

Strengthening the abdominal muscles (see Chapter 18) in the short range may be necessary to address an associated anterior pelvic tilt. Strengthening the ipsilateral gluteus medius may be necessary to improve the frontal plane alignment of the hip.

After the force capability of the piriformis has improved to maintain the femur in neutral while bearing weight, strength and endurance exercises can be progressed to standing to train the femur to function in less medial rotation (see Self-Management: Walk Stance Progression; Self-Management: Step-Up, Step-Down; Self-Management: Progressive Squat; and Fig. 20-21.)

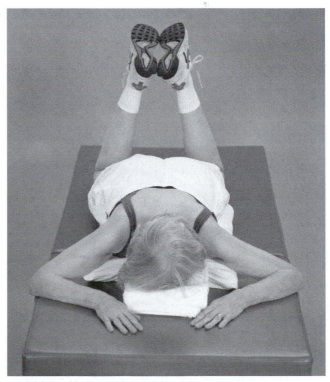

FIGURE 20-37 Prone foot pushes strengthen the piriformis isometrically in the short range.

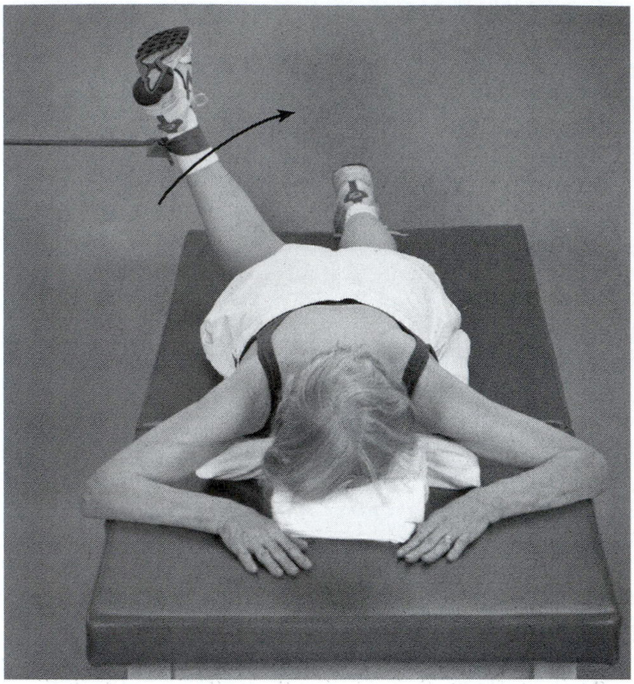

FIGURE 20-38 Prone hip lateral rotation with elastic. The patient is instructed to stabilize the pelvis in the sagittal and transverse planes while rotating the hip from medial rotation to midline or slight lateral rotation. The slow release back to medial rotation emphasizes eccentric control of the lateral rotators.

Mobility

Stretching the piriformis or movement through full medial rotation ROM is contraindicated during the recovery period. However, stretching the opposing medial rotators may be necessary if the opposing stiffness or shortness contributes to the hip functioning in medial rotation and imposes tension on the lengthened piriformis. Stretching the medial rotators (eg, posterolateral fibers of the TFL, gluteus minimus, anterior gluteus medius) can be difficult to perform alone. Assisted stretching with the patient in a prone position into lateral rotation, with careful stabilization of the pelvis and the tibia, ensures optimal stretch to the medial rotators (see Fig. 20-28E). The pelvis must be stabilized actively or passively to prevent anterior pelvic tilt and lumbar extension while stretching the TFL/ITB complex.

Stretching the low back muscles (see Self-Management: Hand-Knee Rocking) may be necessary to address the anterior pelvic tilt. Stretching the ipsilateral hip adductors (Fig. 20-39) may be necessary to improve frontal plane alignment of the hip.

Balance

Because the piriformis has important deceleration functions about all axes of motion, balance drills can train the muscle to control excessive forces against frontal (ie, prevent hip adduction), sagittal (ie, assist in preventing anterior pelvic tilt), and transverse (ie, prevent hip medial rotation) plane perturbations. Progression from level I to level II of Self-Management: Walk Stance Progression is

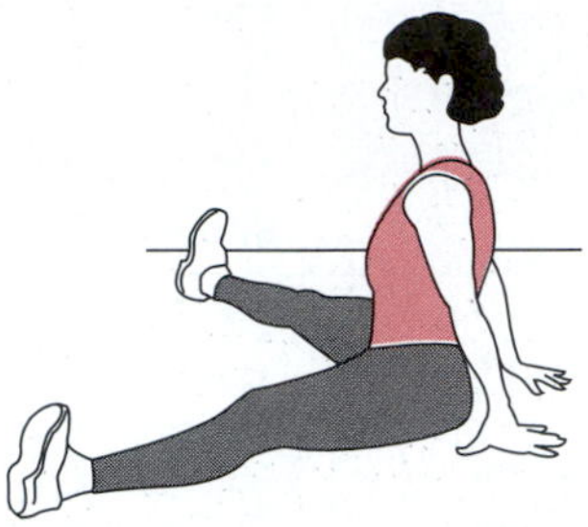

FIGURE 20-39 A method of stretching hip adductors. The patient is instructed in maintaining a neutral pelvis (sitting with the back against the wall can help prevent posterior pelvic tilt) and increasing the range of hip abduction versus trunk forward bend (as is commonly depicted in adductor stretches).

a prerequisite to any uniped balance drills. After uniped balance with good femur and pelvis alignment is achieved, progressive balance drills can be prescribed. Monitoring control over medial rotation is probably the most important function of this muscle, and the object of any balance drill should be to prevent excessive medial femoral rotation. Determination of what is considered excessive must be made on a case by case basis and consider factors such as irritability, stage of healing, the presence of anatomic impairments (ie, hip anteversion), and the type and level of activity to which the individual desires to resume.

Adjunctive Interventions

Taping behind the knee can serve as "biofeedback" to prevent excessive medial rotation tendencies during standing exercises and function (Fig. 20-40).

Key Points

- The structure of the hip joint is designed for stability and to withstand high kinetic forces.
- The angles of inclination and torsion are critical to ideal functioning of the hip joint.
- The ligaments of the hip provide significant stability to the hip, particularly in hip extension, adduction, and medial rotation.
- The tension of the ligaments correspond to positions of stability and instability of the hip.
- Hip osteokinematic ROM is closely linked to the lumbopelvic region. Limitation in hip mobility may manifest in compensatory lumbopelvic mobility and at the knee, ankle, and foot, although to a lesser degree.
- Hip arthrokinematic motions follow convex moving on concave rules with rolling and translation (minimal as it may be) moving opposite in direction to the distal end of the femur.
- It is important to understand the function of the muscles that cross the hip and the relationships they have with the lumbopelvic region and the knee joint.
- Kinetic forces at the hip can rise to four to seven times body weight in the gait cycle.
- A thorough hip examination is necessary to understand the anatomic and physiologic impairments in the hip and

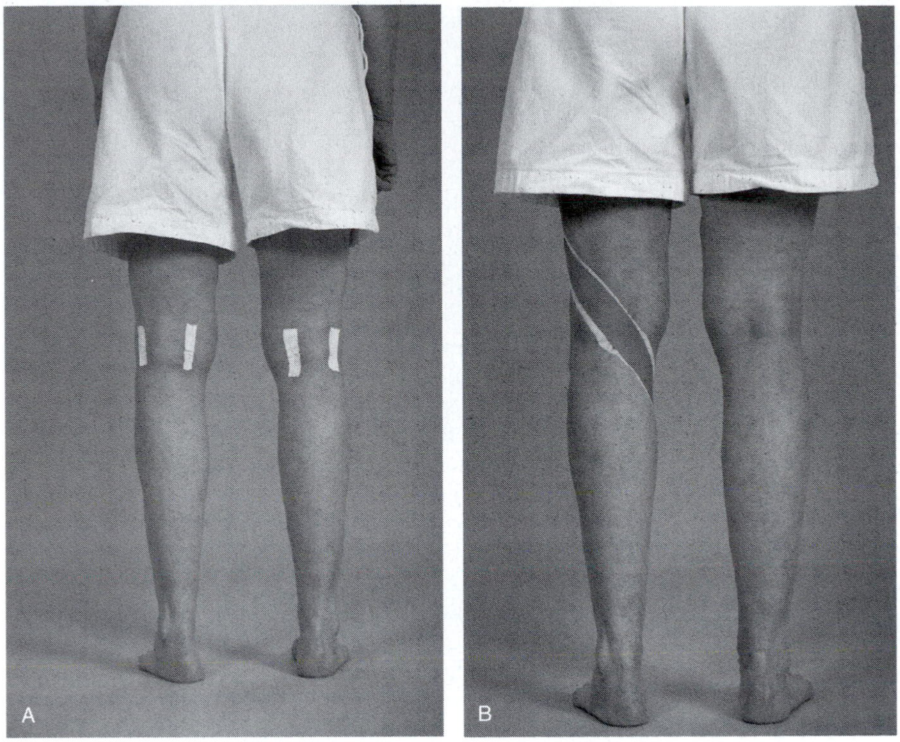

FIGURE 20-40 Excessive medial rotation of the femur in standing as shown by ***(A)*** tape on the hamstring tendons. ***(B)*** Corrective taping posterior to the knee. To encourage hip lateral rotation and tibia medial rotation, the tape is applied from the lateral femur distally to the medial tibia and from the medial tibia proximally toward the lateral femur. ***Note:*** Because this taping procedure does not anchor the tape to any bony prominence, its ability to prevent unwanted tibiofemoral movement is questionable. At best, it can provide temporary feedback to the patient until the tape has sufficiently stretched.

those in related regions that affect the patient's functional limitations and disability.

- Impairments in mobility, force or torque, endurance, balance, pain, and posture and movement commonly occur together in hip-related conditions. Treatment must focus on the impairments most related to the presenting functional limitations and disability. The initial focus should be on restoring functional capacity of each relevant impairment and gradual progression toward functional activity.
- The primary focus of treatment of hip osteoarthritis is to improve joint loading. Restoring proper joint mobility and force or torque are often prerequisites to restoring endurance and improving posture. Balance skills are the final element to restoring more optimal movement patterns and joint loading.
- Treatment after hip THA must follow strict guidelines to prevent the complication of hip dislocation. Postoperative protocols focus on restoring mobility, force or torque, and gait skills. The clinician must educate the patient regarding postoperative precautions and complications.
- Numerous ITB-related syndromes exist. The focus of treatment is to improve the force or torque and functional recruitment of the underused synergists in meaningful functional movement patterns.
- The stretched piriformis syndrome can mimic lumbar radiculopathy. Correct differential diagnosis from lumbar radiculopathy, short piriformis syndrome, and hamstrings strain is mandatory for a successful outcome. Treatment focuses on improving the movement patterns and associated physiologic impairments that contribute to femur medial rotation and adduction and on anterior pelvic tilt, all of which can contribute to stress on the piriformis and the sciatic nerve.

Critical Thinking Questions

1. To which type of knee alignment does coxa vara and coxa valga contribute?
2. What direction are the femoral condyles oriented in femoral anteversion and retroversion? If a patient with femoral anteversion participates in ballet, what type of mobility problem could he develop? If a patient with femoral anteversion participates in soccer, what type of mobility could he develop. What are your recommendations for the alignment of the femur during sport activities?
3. After posterior THA, what is the position for hip dislocation? Why? What would be a position for hip dislocation from a trauma?
4. What would be the compensatory lumbar motions and what phases of the gait cycle would be involved if right hip mobility were restricted in flexion, extension, or medial rotation?
5. If the hip were restricted in flexion, what movement patterns would you be concerned about contributing to this hip flexion restriction? What movement patterns would you retrain to improve hip flexion mobility? What muscle force or torque impairments would you be concerned about that could help perpetuate the hip flexion restriction? Answer these same questions with respect to restrictions in hip extension and medial rotation. What is

LAB ACTIVITIES

1. How would you progress a patient with osteoarthritis in standing exercises to improve weight acceptance and single-limb support phases of gait? Would you use any assistive devices?
2. Demonstrate to your partner how you should transfer in and out of a car, put on your shoes, get on and off a toilet, and in and out of the bathtub 4 weeks after THA performed with a posterior approach. Do the same for the transtrochanteric and anterolateral approaches.
3. With respect to Critical Thinking Question 5, develop a program of exercises that improve the mobility and associated force or torque impairment for each scenario. Teach this program to your partner. Assume that all manual muscle test grades are 3+/5. Progress specific nonfunctional exercises to functional exercises.
4. With respect to Critical Thinking Question 6, how would you begin to improve the force or torque production of a gluteus medius underused synergist with a positional strength grade of $^{3-}/_{5}$. How would you progress this exercise as the positional strength improved? Teach your partner these exercises. Can you feel the TFL trying to dominate the exercise movement pattern? What is the associated pattern of movement with TFL dominance? Can you progress this exercise to standing functional exercises. How does the foot alignment contribute to the hip position in closed chain positions and movements?
5. Practice the balance progression described in Display 20-4. What type of balance strategy are you using? Develop balance drills that stress the frontal plane and crossover stepping strategies.
6. With respect to Critical Thinking Question 7, progress hip lateral rotator exercises from specific, nonfunctional exercises to functional exercises. How would you stress the lateral rotators in a single-limb balance drill (be creative)?
7. Refer to Case Study #9 in Unit 7. Develop a complete therapeutic exercise intervention plan using the intervention model developed in Chapter 2.
8. Refer to Case Study #10 in Unit 7. Develop a complete therapeutic exercise intervention plan using the intervention model developed in Chapter 2.

this pattern of restriction (ie, restricted hip flexion, medial rotation, extension) called?

6. Describe the Trendelenburg pattern of gait. Can you describe other hip joint movement patterns that could indicate hip abductor weakness?
7. In TFL/ITB overuse diagnoses, why is the hip the focus of treatment? What are the common underused synergists that contribute to TFL/ITB overuse?
8. How would you differentially diagnose a stretched piriformis syndrome from a short piriformis syndrome, lumbar radiculopathy, or strained hamstrings?

REFERENCES

1. Singleton MC, LeVeau BF. The hip joint: stability and stress: a review. *Phys Ther.* 1975;55:957–973.
2. Frankel VH, Nordin M. *Basic Biomechanics of the Skeletal System.* Philadelphia: Lea & Febiger; 1980.
3. Kempson GE, Spivey CJ, Swanson SAV, Freeman MAR. Patterns of cartilage stiffness on normal and degenerate human femoral heads. *J Biomech.* 1971;4:597–609.
4. D'Ambrosia RD. *Musculoskeletal Disorders: Regional Examination and Differential Diagnosis.* 2nd ed. Philadelphia: JB Lippincott; 1986.
5. Cummings SR, Nevitt MC. A hypothesis: the causes of hip fracture. *J Gerontol Med Sci.* 1989;44:M107–M111.
6. Kling TF, Hensinger RN. Angular and torsional deformities of the lower limbs in children, *Clin Orthop Rel Res.* 1983;176: 136–147.
7. Engel GM, Staheli LT. The natural history of torsion and other factors influencing gait in childhood. *Clin Orthop.* 1974;99:12–17.
8. Steheli LT. Torsional deformity. *Pediatr Clin North Am.* 1977;24:799–811.
9. Staheli LT, Corbett M, Wyss C, King H. Lower extremity rotation problems in children: normal values to guide management. *J Bone JT Surg Am.* 1985;67:39–47.
10. McLeish RD, Charnley J. Abduction forces in one-legged stance. *J Biomech.* 1970;3:191–209.
11. Rydell N. Forces in the hip joint. Part II: Intravital measurements. In: Kenedi RM, ed. *Biomechanics and Related Bioengineering Topics.* Oxford, UK: Pergamon Press; 1965:351–357.
12. Rydell N. Forces acting on the femoral head prosthesis: a study on strain gauge supplied prostheses in living persons. *Acta Orthop Scand Suppl.* 1966;88:11–32.
13. Rydell N. Biomechanics of the hip joint. *Clin Orthop.* 1973;92:6.
14. Seireg A, Arvikar RJ. The prediction of muscular load sharing and joint forces in the lower extremities during walking. *J Biomech.* 1975;8:89–102.
15. English TA, Kilvington M. In vivo records of hip loads using a femoral implant with telemetric output (a preliminary report). *J Biomed Eng.* 1979;1:111–115.
16. Draganich LF, Andriacchi TP, Strongwater AM, Galante JO. Electronic measurement of instantaneous foot-floor contact patterns during gait. *J Biomech.* 1980;13:875–880.
17. Paul JP. *Forces at the human hip joint.* University of Chicago; 1967:Thesis.
18. Perry J. Gait Analysis: *Normal and Pathological Function.* New York: McGraw-Hill; 1992.
19. Steindler A. *Kinesiology of the Human Body.* Springfield, IL: Charles C. Thomas; 1973.
20. Fabray G, MacEwen GD, Shands AR. Torsion of the femur: a follow-up study in normal and abnormal conditions. *J Bone Joint Surg Am.* 1973;55:17–26.
21. Anda S, Svenningson S, Dale LG, Barnum P. The acetabular sector angle of the adult hip determined by computed tomography. *Acta Radiol Diagn.* 1986;27:443–447.

22. Svenningsen S, Apalset K, Terjesen T, Anda S. Regression of femoral anteversion. *Acta Orthop Scand.* 1989;60:170–173.
23. Williams PL, Warwick R, eds. *Gray's Anatomy.* 37th ed. Philadelphia: WB Saunders; 1985.
24. McCaw ST. Leg length inequality: implications for running injury prevention. *Sports Med.* 1992;14:422–429.
25. Rothenberg RJ. Rheumatic disease aspects of leg length inequality. *Semin Arthritis Rheum.* 1988;17:196–205.
26. Tjernstrom B, Olerud S, Karlstrom G. Direct leg lengthening. *J Orthop Trauma.* 1993;7:543–551.
27. Brand RA, Yack HJ. Effects of leg length discrepancies on the forces at the hip joint. *Clin Orthop.* 1996;333:172–180.
28. Kaufman KR, Miller LS, Sutherland DH. Gait asymmetry in patients with limb length inequality. *J Pediatr Orthop.* 1996;16: 144–150.
29. Cyriax J. *Textbook of Orthopedic Medicine*. 7th ed. vol 1. London: Bailliere Tindall; 1978:64–103.
30. Kendall FP, McCreary EK, Provance PG. *Muscles Testing and Function.* 4th ed. Baltimore: Williams & Wilkins; 1993.
31. Daniels L, Worthingham C. *Muscle Testing: Techniques of Manual Examination.* 4th ed. Philadelphia: WB Saunders; 1980.
32. Duncan GH, Bushnell MC, Lavigne GJ. Comparison of verbal and visual analogue scales for measuring the intensity and unpleasantness of experimental pain. *Pain.* 1989;37: 295–303.
33. Shumway-Cook A, Galdwin M, Polissar NL, Gruber W. Predicting the probability for falls in community-dwelling older adults. *Phys Ther.* 1997;77:812–819.
34. Berg KO, Wood Daphinee SL, Williams JT, et al. Measuring balance in the elderly: validation of an instrument. *Can J Public Health.* 1989;41:302–311.
35. Shumway-Cook A, Woollacott MH. *Motor Control: Theory and Practical Applications.* Baltimore: Williams & Wilkins; 1995.
36. Shumway-Cook A, Gruber W, Baldwin M, Liao S. The effect of multidimensional exercise on balance, mobility, and fall risk in community-dwelling older adults. *Phys Ther.* 1997;77:46–57.
37. Hoppenfeld S. *Physical Examination of the Spine and Extremities.* New York: Appleton-Century-Crofts; 1976.
38. Krettek C, Koch T, Henzler D, Blauth M, Hofmann R. A new procedure for determining leg length and LLD inequality using ultrasound. *Unfallchirug.* 1996;99:43–51.
39. McGee DJ. *Orthopedic Physical Assessment.* Philadelphia: WB Saunders; 1987.
40. Ruwe PA, Gage JR, Ozonoff MB, Deluca PA. Clinical determination of femoral anteversion. *J Bone Joint Surg Am.* 1992;74:820–830.
41. Maitland GD. *Peripheral Manipulation.* 2nd ed. London: Butterworths; 1977.
42. Magee DJ. *Orthopedic Physical Assessment.* 2nd ed. Philadelphia: WB Saunders; 1992.
43. Jette AM. Using health-related quality of life measures in physical therapy outcomes research. *Phys Ther.* 1993;73:528–537.
44. Harris WH. Traumatic arthritis of the hip after dislocation and acetabular fracture: treatment by mold arthroplasty. *J Bone Joint Surg Am.* 1969;51:737–755.
45. Kelly JP. Reactions of neurons to injury. In: Kandel E, Schwartz J, eds. *Principles of Neural Science.* New York: Elsevier; 1985:187.
46. Hause M, Kikuchi S, SakauyamaY, Ito T. Anatomic study of the interrelation between lumbosacral nerve roots and their surrounding tissues. *Spine.* 1983;8:50.
47. Lyons K, Perry J, Gronley JK, Barnes L, Antonelli D. Timing and relative intensity of hip extensor and abductor muscle action during level and stair ambulation. *Phys Ther.* 1983;63: 1597–1605.
48. Long WT, Dorr LD, Healy B, Perry J. Functional recovery of noncemented total hip arthroplasty. *Clin Orthop Rel Res.* 1993;288:73–77.
49. Neumann DA, Soderberg GL, Cook TM. Electromyographic analysis of hip abductor musculature in healthy right-handed persons. *Phys Ther.* 1989;69:431–440.
50. Inman VT. Functional aspects of the abductor muscles of the hip. *J Bone Joint Surg.* 1947;29:607–612.
51. LaBan MM, Raptou AD, Johnson EW. Electromyographic study of function of iliopsoas muscle. *Arch Phys Med Rehabil.* 1965:676–679.
52. Mubarak SJ, Leach JK, Wenger DR. Management of congenital dislocation of the hip in the infant. *Contemp Orthop.* 1987;15:29–44.
53. Pemberton PA. Osteotomy of the ilium with rotation of the acetabular roof for congenital dislocation of the hip. *J Bone Joint Surg Am.* 1958;40:724.
54. Mellin G. Correlations of hip mobility with degree of back pain and lumbar spinal mobility in chronic low back pain patients. *Spine.* 1988;13:668–670.
55. Thurston AJ. Spinal and pelvic kinematics in osteoarthrosis of the hip joint. *Spine.* 1985;10:467–471.
56. Offerski CM, Macnab I. Hip-spine syndrome. *Spine.* 1983;8:316–321.
57. Esola MA, McClure PW, Fitzgerald GK, Siegler S. Analysis of lumbar spine and hip motion during forward bending in subjects with and without a history of significant low back pain. *Spine.* 1996;21:71–78.
58. Li Y, McClure PW, Pratt N. The effect of hamstring muscle stretching on standing posture and on lumbar and hip motions during forward bending. *Phys Ther.* 1996;76:836–849.
59. Tinetti ME, Ginter SF. Identifying mobility dysfunctions in elderly patients; standard neuromuscular examination or direct assessment. *JAMA.* 1988;259:1190–1193.
60. Tinetti ME, Speechly M, Ginter SF. Risk factors for falls among elderly persons living in the community. *N Engl J Med.* 1988;319:1701–1707.
61. Nevitt MC, Cummings SR. Risk factors for recurrent nonsyncopal falls: a prospective study. *JAMA.* 1989;261: 2663–2668.
62. Kanten DN, Mulrow CD, Gerety MB, et al. Falls: an examination of three reporting methods in nursing homes. *J Am Geriatr Soc.* 1993;41:662–666.
63. National Safety Council. *Accident Facts and Figures.* Chicago: National Safety Council; 1987.
64. Tse S, Baily DM. T'ai chi and postural control in the well elderly. *Am J Occup Ther.* 1992;46:295–300.
65. Wolf SL, Barnhart HX, Ellison GL, Coogler CE, Horak FB. The effect of t'ai chi quan and computerized balance training on postural stability in older subjects. *Phys Ther.* 1997;77: 371–384.
66. Maki BE, McIlroy WE. The role of limb movements in maintaining upright stance: the "change in support" strategy. *Phys Ther.* 1997;77:488–507.
67. Ashton-Miller JA, Yeh MWL, Richardson JK, Galloway T. A cane reduces loss of balance in patients with peripheral neuropathy: results from a challenging unipedal balance test. *Arch Phys Med Rehabil.* 1996;77:446–452.
68. Jeka JJ, Lackner JR. Fingertip contact influences human postural control. *Exp Brain Res.* 1994;100:495–502.
69. Neumann DA, Cook TM, Sholty RL, Sobush DC. An electromyographic analysis of hip abductor muscle activity when subjects are carrying loads in one or both hands. *Phys Ther.* 1992;72:207–217.
70. Denham RA. Hip mechanics. *J Bone Joint Surg.* 1959;41: 550–557.
71. Price SA, Wilson LM. *Pathophysiology: Clinical Concepts of Disease Processes*. 2nd ed. New York: McGraw-Hill:1982.
72. Irrgang JJ, Whitney SL, Cox ED. Balance and proprioceptive training for rehabilitation of the lower extremity. *J Sports Rehabil.* 1994;3:68–83.

73. National Institutes of Health. *Total Hip Replacement: NIH Consensus Statement.* Bethesda, MD: US Dept. of Health and Human Services: 1994;12:1–31.
74. Schulte KR, Callaghan JJ, Kelly SS, Johnston RC. The outcome of Charnley total hip arthroplasty with cement after a minimum of twenty-year follow-up: the results of one surgeon. *J Bone Joint Surg Am.* 1993;75:961–971.
75. Russoti GM, Coventry MB, Stauffer RN. Cemented total hip arthroplasty with contemporary techniques: a minimum five year follow-up study. *Clin Orthop Rel Res.* 1988;235: 141–147.
76. Mulroy RD, Harris WH. The effect of improved cementing techniques on component loosening in total hip replacement: an 11 year radiographic review. *J Bone Joint Surg.* 1990;72: 757–760.
77. Engh CA, Bobyn JD, Glassman A II. Porous coated hip replacement: the factors governing bone ingrowth, stress shielding, and clinical results. *J Bone Joint Surg.* 1987;69: 45–55.
78. Engh CA, Culpepper WJ. Long term results of the use of the anatomic medullary locking prosthesis in total hip arthroplasty. *J Bone Joint Surg.* 1997;79:177–184.
79. Tomkins GS, Jacobs JJ, Kull LR, Rosenberg AR, Galante JO. Primary total hip arthroplasty with a porous-coated acetabular component: seven to ten year results. *J Bone Joint Surg* 1997;79:169–176.
80. Daly PJ, Morrey BF. Operative reconstruction of an unstable total hip arthroplasty. *J Bone Joint Surg Am.* 1992;74: 1334–1343.
81. Leiby KW, Neece PJ, Phipps SH, Hughs CJ. A comparison of two methods of resistance training on ipsilateral/contralateral hip abduction strength [abstract]. *J Sports Phys Ther.* 1995;21:52.
82. Maloney WJ, Krushell RJ, Jasty M, et al. Incidence of heterotopic ossification after total hip replacement: effect on the type of fixation of the femoral component. *J Bone Joint Surg Am.* 1991;73:191–193.
83. Fitzgerald RH. Infected total hip arthroplasty: diagnosis and treatment. *J Am Acad Orthop Surgeons.* 1995;3:249–262.
84. Pare EB, Stern JT, Schwartz JM. Functional differentiation within the tensor fascia latae. *J Bone Joint Surg Am.* 1981;63: 1457–1471.
85. Freiburg AH, Vinke TH. Sciatica and sacroiliac joint. *J Bone Joint Surg.* 1934;16:126–136.

RECOMMENDED READING

New perspectives on balance [special series]. *J Am Phys Ther Assoc.* 1997;77 and 77 [complete issues].

CHAPTER 21

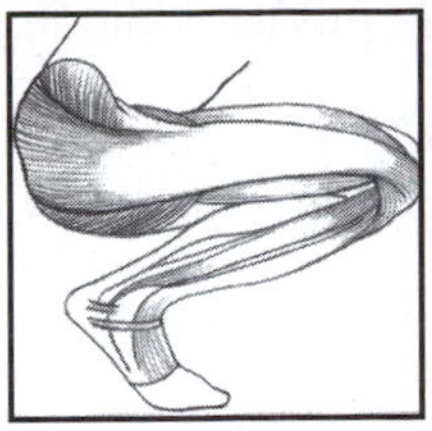

The Knee

Lori Thein Brody and Linda Tremain

The knee is one of the most frequently injured joints in the body. The quadriceps muscle spans the anterior thigh and crosses the tibiofemoral joint, producing knee extension when tensed. The patella enhances muscle performance across the longest lever arm of the body. Impairments at the knee joint can produce significant functional limitations and disability. The closed chain demands of daily activities such as walking, standing, and rising from a chair require smooth, coordinated action of the lower extremity neuromuscular system.[1–5] When considering knee impairments, the impact of these impairments on the related joints in the kinetic chain also must be addressed.

REVIEW OF ANATOMY AND KINESIOLOGY

A thorough understanding of the anatomy and kinesiology of the knee joint is necessary to comprehend the impact of impairments on function of the kinetic chain. The unique kinematic relationships of lower extremity joints depend on the local anatomic structures.

Anatomy

OSTEOLOGY

The femoral component of the tibiofemoral joint is composed of two large condyles separated by the intercondylar notch. The asymmetric medial condyle extends farther distally than the lateral, and the lateral condyle is slightly wider at the center of the intercondylar notch.[6–9] Viewed from the tibial surface, the medial condyle appears to be shorter, but is on average two thirds of an inch longer to accommodate the medial angulation of the femoral shaft.[8,9] This medial angulation varies from individual to individual and contributes to the quadriceps angle and degree of varus or valgus alignment. The lateral condyle is more directly in line with the femoral shaft.[10]

The condylar asymmetry contributes to the screw home mechanism, which occurs during terminal knee extension. The screw home mechanism is the femoral internal rotation coupled with tibial external rotation that occurs during the last few degrees of terminal extension (Fig. 21-1). A small prominence of bone, the adductor tubercle, can be palpated at the superior aspect of the medial femoral condyle, and it serves as the attachment for the adductor magnus muscle. This tubercle is an important landmark used when assessing the patellofemoral joint for malalignment or instability.

Two concave plateaus on the tibia correspond with the femoral condyles. The medial and lateral tibial plateaus are separated by the intercondylar tubercles, two bony spines that enter the intercondylar notch when the knee is in extension. The lateral tibial plateau is smaller, circular, and concave, whereas the medial plateau is more oval and flat.[10] The larger size of the medial plateau and its increased articular cartilage thickness support the larger medial femoral condyle.

The patella is the largest sesamoid bone in the body. Its triangular shape is divided into two major concave facets (medial and lateral) that glide on the two convex surfaces of the femur. Each of the medial and lateral facets are divided by two transverse ridges into superior, middle, and inferior facets. A seventh facet, also called the odd facet, lies on the most medial aspect of the patella, and articulates with the femur only in extreme flexion.

ARTHROLOGY

The bicondylar synovial tibiofemoral joint is supported by a fibrous joint capsule and lined with synovial membrane. Stability of the knee depends on the integrity of the capsule and its ligamentous and tendinous supporting structures. Posteriorly, the capsule is attached to the femoral and

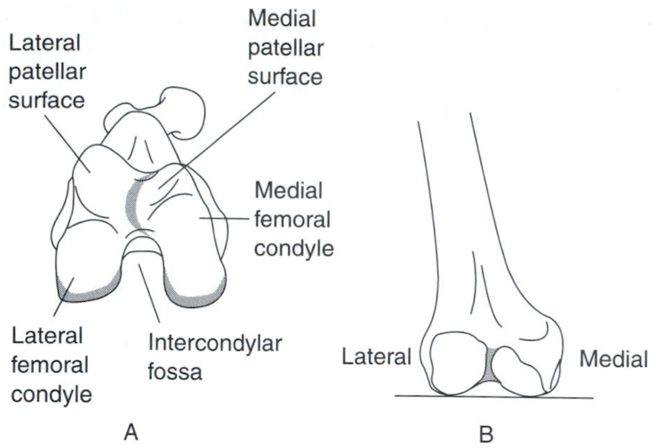

FIGURE 21-1 ***(A)*** View of the femoral surface from the inferior articulating surface. Note the more anterior prominence of the lateral femoral condyle. ***(B)*** The medial femoral condyle is longer than the lateral, and the lateral femoral condyle lies more directly in line with the shaft than the medial. However, the prominence of the medial femoral condyle results in a horizontal articulating surface. (Adapted from Norkin CC, Levangie PK. *Joint Structure and Function: A Comprehensive Analysis.* 2d ed. Philadelphia: FA Davis; 1992:340.)

tibial condyles just beyond their articular margins and is strengthened by the oblique popliteal ligament. Laterally, the capsule extends from the femur distally to the tibia and fibular head and is separated from the lateral collateral ligament (LCL) by fat and neurovascular tissues. Medially, the capsule extends from the femur to the tibia just beyond their respective articular margins and is reinforced by the medial collateral ligament (MCL). The medial structures have been divided into three layers. The most superficial is in the fascial plane, the middle layer consists of the superficial MCL, and the deep layer is composed of vertically oriented, thickened capsular tissue known as the deep medial ligament.[9]

Anteriorly, the capsule blends with the expansions of the vastus lateralis and vastus medialis to attach to the patellar margins and patellar tendon. The expansion continues medially and laterally to the respective collateral ligaments and inferiorly to the tibial condyles.[7,10] The medial and lateral expansions are called the *medial and lateral patellar retinacula,* sometimes known as the extensor retinaculum.[11] The retinacula provide the static balance for the patellofemoral joint, which is influenced by differences between the medial and lateral retinacula. The medial retinaculum is weak and thin compared with the lateral retinaculum, which is thick and strong. The medial retinaculum can be stretched or torn with a lateral patellar subluxation or dislocation, and the medial pain is often mistaken for a MCL sprain. Tightness in the lateral retinaculum contributes to lateral patellar tracking. The structure can be divided into superficial fibers affecting lateral glide and deep fibers contributing to lateral tilt (Fig. 21-2). Distally, the joint capsule attaches to the meniscal rim, and both are connected to the tibia through the coronary ligaments.

Some controversy exists about the classification of the anterior layers of the knee. Dye[12] describes five layers, discussed in order from deep to superficial:

1. The deep capsular layer is composed of capsular thickenings, which span from the patella to the medial and lateral menisci.[12]
2. The deep transverse layer provides a static guide system for the patella, with lateral fibers blending with the iliotibial band and medial fibers inserting near the medial femoral epicondyle.[12] This association of the iliotibial band, the transverse fibers, and the patella suggest a relationship between iliotibial band tightness and patellofemoral pain.
3. The middle layer (deep longitudinal) is composed primarily of fibers from the rectus femoris.
4. The oblique layer contains fibers from the rectus femoris, vastus medialis, and vastus lateralis.
5. The superficial arciform layer has mostly transverse fibers over the patella.[12]

The capsule is reinforced anteriorly by the patellar tendon, or ligamentum patella, which continues from the apex of the patella to the tibial tuberosity. The fibers originate from a broad area on the inferior pole and from the undersurface of the patella, and the most superficial fibers are continuous over the patella as the extension of the quadriceps. The deepest fibers are most affected in individuals with patellar tendinitis. Medially and laterally, the tendon is continuous with the medial and lateral patellar retinacula.[10]

The infrapatellar fat pad can be a source of anterior and inferior knee pain because of its innervation. When the infrapatellar fat pad becomes enlarged or inflamed, it can cause a significant amount of pain because of increased pressure from the inferior pole of the patella. Patella infera, caused by shortening of the patellar tendon in response to injury or surgery, can increase pressure and pain originating from the fat pad (Fig. 21-3).

The synovial membrane of the knee is the most extensive and complex in the body and generally adheres to the inner surface of the capsule. The synovium may invaginate between muscle and the femoral condyles on the medial and lateral aspects of the joint, creating medial and lateral gutters. Fibrosis after trauma or surgery to the knee can result

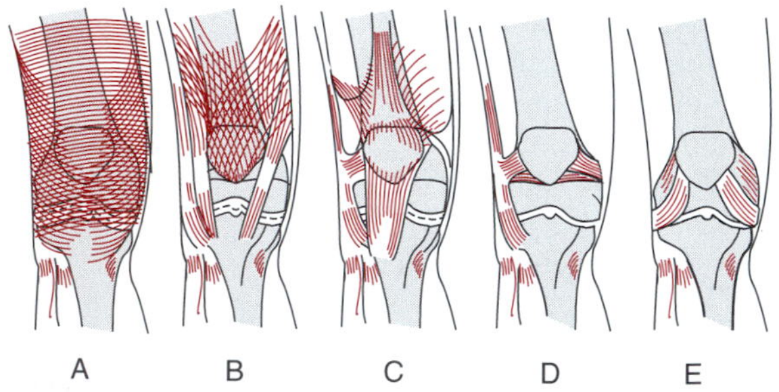

FIGURE 21-2 The multiple soft tissue layers affect the patellofemoral joint: ***(A)*** the superficial arciform layers with transverse fibers over patella and patellar tendon; ***(B)*** the intermediate oblique layer with chevron-oriented fibers from the rectus femoris, vastus lateralis, and vastus medialis; ***(C)*** the deep longitudinal layers, which are extremely adherent to the anterior surface of the patella; ***(D)*** the deep transverse layer blending with fibers of the iliotibial band; and ***(E)*** the deep capsular layer composed of the medial and lateral patellomeniscal ligaments. (Adapted from Dye SF. Patellofemoral anatomy. In: Fox JM, Del Pizzo W, eds. *The Patellofemoral Joint.* New York: McGraw-Hill, 1993:5.)

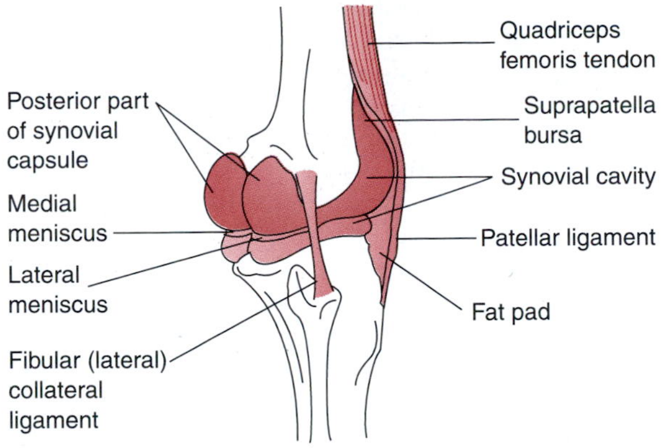

FIGURE 21-3 Posterolateral view of the knee indicating the extent and subdivisions of the synovial cavity. Note the size and relationship of the fat pad to the anterior structures. (Adapted from Pratt NE. *Clinical Musculoskeletal Anatomy.* Philadelphia, JB Lippincott; 1991:198.)

in scar tissue accumulating in these gutters and blocking extension motion. Embryonic remnants of the synovial septa may remain into adulthood, forming synovial plicae. The most common are the infrapatellar plica or fold (ie, ligamentum mucosum), suprapatellar plica, and mediopatellar plica.[8,10] These plicae may mimic or contribute to patellofemoral pain.

Several ligaments about the knee provide static stability. The MCL (tibial) is a broad, flat structure whose superficial portion is located in the second layer of the medial tissues. It contains vertical (anterior) and oblique (posterior) fibers originating slightly posteriorly from the medial epicondyle, and the ligament courses distally to the medial meniscus and tibia.[9,10] Because of its meniscal attachment, the medial meniscus is at risk when the MCL is torn. The LCL (fibular) is a more distinct, ropelike structure than the MCL and courses from the lateral epicondyle to the fibular head, blending with the insertion of the biceps femoris tendon. Unlike the MCL, the LCL does not attach to its respective meniscus, placing it at less risk with an LCL injury.

The cruciate ligaments can be found within the knee joint, just posterior to the articular center. They are named by their relative tibial positions and are intracapsular but extrasynovial. The anterior cruciate ligament (ACL) attaches on the anteromedial tibial plateau and courses posterolaterally, twisting on itself to attach at the posteromedial aspect of the lateral femoral condyle. It is composed of fascicles grouped into anteromedial and posterolateral bundles, named by their relative tibial attachments. The ACL passes through the intercondylar notch, pressing against its roof in full extension. Individuals with a small notch may be more susceptible to ACL injuries.[13,14] Moreover, scar in the notch after ACL reconstruction or poor graft placement can result in roof impingement, preventing full knee extension (Fig. 21-4). The posterior cruciate ligament (PCL) is more vertically oriented near the longitudinal axis of the knee. Its tibial origination is from a depression on the posterior tibia between the two plateaus, and it ascends anteromedially, attaching to the lateral surface of the medial femoral condyle. This origin is important in total knee arthroplasty, in which the PCL may be spared because of its attachment distal to the joint line. Like the ACL, the PCL is composed of two functional bands, the anterolateral and the posteromedial, which provide a continuum of stability throughout most of the range of motion (ROM).[15]

The menisci, or semilunar cartilages, are two crescent-shaped fibrocartilaginous structures with peripheral borders that are thick, convex, and triangular in cross section and taper to a thin, concave mobile edge centrally.[10,16] Each covers approximately two thirds of the tibial surface. The superior surface of each menisci is concave and articulates with the femoral condyles; the inferior surface is flat and rests on the tibial articular surface. The *medial meniscus* has a semilunar shape and is broader posteriorly and narrower anteriorly, where it attaches to the intercondylar area anterior to the ACL. Around its periphery, the medial meniscus is attached to the capsule and to the tibia through the coronary ligament. It is further stabilized by its attachment to the undersurface of the MCL. The semimembranosus muscle also attaches indirectly to the medial meniscus through its capsular arm.[16] The *lateral meniscus* is nearly circular, constituting approximately four fifths of a ring, and covers a larger portion of the tibial plateau than the medial meniscus.[10] Its peripheral attachments to a lax capsule and lack of attachment to the LCL partially account for the increased mobility of the lateral meniscus. This mobility contributes to the lower incidence of lateral meniscal tears.

MYOLOGY

The muscles crossing the knee joint consist of one-joint and two-joint muscles acting as agonists, antagonists, and stabilizers. Because the complex interactions of the hip, knee, ankle, and foot are beyond the scope of this chapter, the discussion of muscle function is limited to actions occurring at the knee joint (see Chapters 20, 21, and 22).

The primary *anterior muscles* are the quadriceps femoris, which act as the principle knee extensors. Of the four quadriceps muscles, only the rectus femoris is a two-joint muscle. It originates proximal to the hip joint at the anterior inferior iliac spine.[17] Dynamically, the length of the rectus femoris and the patellar tendon are critical to allow free patellar gliding during flexion and extension. Shortening

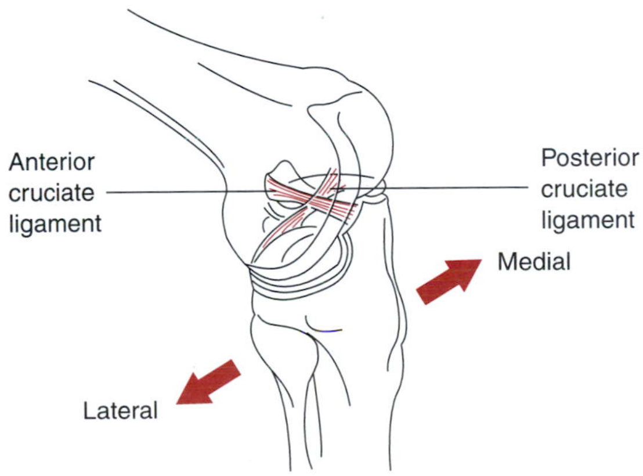

FIGURE 21-4 Anterolateral view of the knee illustrating the location of the cruciate ligaments relative to the intercondylar notch. (Adapted from Pratt NE. *Clinical Musculoskeletal Anatomy.* Philadelphia,: JB Lippincott; 1991:196.)

of the patellar tendon (ie, patella baja or patella infera) or shortening of the rectus femoris can contribute to increased compressive forces and inequitable force distribution over the patellar facets. The three vastus muscles—vastus lateralis, vastus intermedius, and vastus medialis—originate from the femur, crossing only the knee joint. These four muscles converge into a tendinous expansion proximal to the patella to insert on the proximal border of the patella and extend distally through the patellar tendon to insert on the tibial tuberosity. Compared with the vastus lateralis, the vastus medialis has greater bulk, inserts more distally, has a more oblique orientation (approximately 55 to 65 degrees), has a shorter tendon, and has a separate nerve supply.[12] Another anterior muscle, the sartorius, originates from the anterior superior iliac spine and the proximal half of the notch just distal to the spine and courses inferiorly and laterally to attach on the medial tibial surface anterior to the gracilis and semitendinosus insertions. The sartorius flexes, laterally rotates, and abducts the hip while it flexes and assists in knee flexion and medial rotation of the tibia.

The main *posterior muscles* are the hamstring muscles—biceps femoris, semitendinosus, and semimembranosus. The long head of the biceps originates from the ischial tuberosity by a tendon common to it and the semitendinosus, and the short head has a lengthy origination from the lateral linea aspera proximally almost to the gluteus maximus and distally nearly to the lateral femoral condyle.[10] As the fusiform long head descends, it joins the fibers of the short head and forms a common tendon that inserts into the fibular head, lateral tibial condyle, and deep fascia. Together, the biceps femoris flex and laterally rotate the tibia, whereas the long head assists in extension and lateral rotation of the hip. The semitendinosus muscle also originates from the ischial tuberosity by a common tendon with the long head of the biceps and is known for its exceptionally long tendon. The fusiform muscle descends along the posteromedial aspect of the thigh to insert on the medial tibial metaphysis in conjunction with the gracilis tendon.[10] The semitendinosus is a flexor and medial rotator of the tibia, and it assists in extension and medial rotation of the hip. The semimembranosus originates from the ischial tuberosity, descending posteromedially anterior to the biceps femoris and semitendinosus to divide into several distal insertions. Most notable of these insertions are the posteromedial aspect of the medial tibial condyle and the capsular arm attaching indirectly to the medial meniscus. Like the semitendinosus, the functions of the semimembranosus are to flex and medially rotate the tibia and to assist in extension and medial rotation of the hip.[17] After knee injury or surgery, patients frequently use the hamstrings as hip extensors to passively extend the knee rather than using the quadriceps. The therapist must closely observe muscle firing to ensure proper quadriceps activity.

Medially, the gracilis and adductors longus, magnus, and brevis function primarily at the hip but may provide dynamic stability to the knee joint. The *lateral musculature* acts primarily at the hip, with no direct action at the knee. The tensor fasciae latae arises from the anterior aspect of the iliac crest and the lateral aspect of the anterior superior iliac spine. It courses distally between and attached to the layers of the iliotibial tract at the mid-thigh, with the tract continuing to the lateral femoral condyle. At the knee, the tensor fasciae latae produces extension and lateral rotation through the iliotibial tract, and it assists in flexion, medial rotation, and abduction at the hip. The gluteus maximus also inserts into the iliotibial tract, with its origin from the posterior gluteal line of the ilium, the posterior surface of the distal sacrum and side of the coccyx, the aponeurosis of the erector spinae, the sacrotuberous ligament, and the fascia covering the gluteus medius.[10] Distally, the largest portion inserts into the iliotibial tract, with the deep fibers attaching into the gluteal tuberosity of the femur. The gluteus maximus extends, laterally rotates, and the lower fibers assist in adduction of the hip, and the upper fibers assist in hip abduction. Through the iliotibial tract, the gluteus maximus indirectly helps to stabilize the knee in extension. In addition to receiving fibers from the tensor fasciae latae and gluteus maximus, the iliotibial tract has superficial fibers that ascend laterally to the iliac crest and deeper fibers that blend with the hip joint capsule.[10] Distally, the tract is attached to the lateral tibial condyle, the lateral femoral condyle, and fibular head and to the patella through the horizontal fibers.

Kinematics

TIBIOFEMORAL JOINT

The knee is considered to be a tricompartmental joint, with medial, lateral, and anterior (patellofemoral) compartments. The arthrokinematic and osteokinematic motions at the tibiofemoral joint result in six degrees of freedom, including three rotations—flexion and extension, medial and lateral, valgus and varus—and three translations—anterior and posterior, medial and lateral, distraction and compression.[18] Normal ROM in the sagittal plane from extension to flexion is approximately 0 to 140 degrees, with extension limited by the ACL and PCL, the posterior capsule, and the anterior horns of the menisci. Flexion is limited by the cruciate ligaments and the posterior horns of the menisci. Motion may be limited by quadriceps, hamstrings, and gastrocnemius muscle lengths. Normal knee extension is accompanied by anterior glide of the tibia on the femur, and posterior tibial glide is associated with knee flexion. The motions of flexion and extension in the sagittal plane are accompanied by rotational motion in the transverse plane. The differential size of the femoral condyles and the static soft tissues contribute to the screw home mechanism of terminal knee extension.[8,18,19]

Motion in the frontal plane is minimal when the knee is held in full extension. For this reason, any varus or valgus stress is more likely to damage the collateral or cruciate ligaments as the knee approaches full extension. As the knee is flexed to 30 degrees, the LCL, posterolateral joint capsule, arcuate complex, and cruciate ligaments provide restraint against varus forces.[19] On the medial side, the MCL, the posteromedial capsule, and the cruciate ligaments stabilize against valgus forces. Normally, greater varus motion than valgus motion is found because of the greater laxity in the lateral structures and the breadth and orientation of the MCL.

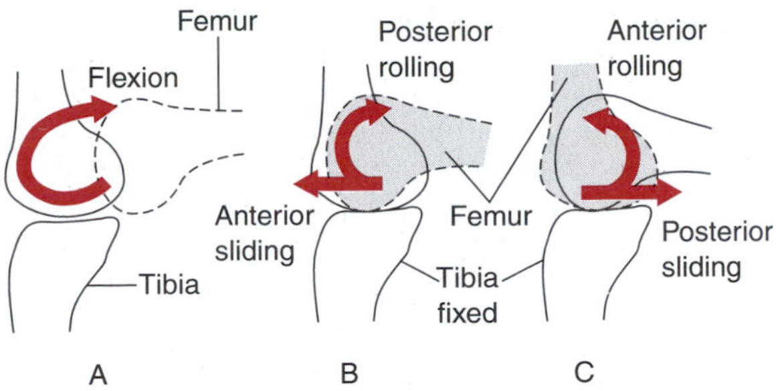

FIGURE 21-5 ***(A)*** Pure rolling of the femur on the tibia. The femur would roll off the tibia if no gliding occurred. ***(B)*** Posterior rolling and anterior gliding occur with flexion, while ***(C)*** anterior rolling and posterior gliding occur with extension. (Adapted from Norkin CC, Levangie PK. *Joint Structure and Function: A Comprehensive Analysis.* 2d ed. Philadelphia: FA Davis; 1992:355.)

In the transverse plane, medial rotation is limited by the ACL rotating on the PCL, the LCL, menisci, and the posterolateral capsule. Lateral rotation is restricted by the MCL, the posteromedial capsule, and menisci. The amount of medial and lateral rotation increases as the angle of knee flexion increases up to about 120 degrees. Minimal rotation can occur as the knee approaches full extension because of the articulation of the femoral condyles with the menisci and tightening of the ligaments. Any excessive rotation near full extension is likely to damage the menisci and ligaments.

The instant center of rotation is the axis about which the tibia rotates during flexion and extension at any instant in time.[18] Because of the arthrokinematic motion occurring during flexion and extension, the instant center of rotation changes throughout the ROM. As the knee moves from extension to flexion, the pathway moves posteriorly and superiorly in an elliptic fashion. At the initiation of flexion, the femur rolls on the tibia for approximately the first 15 degrees of flexion, after which gliding and spinning occur. If only rolling occurred throughout the range, the femur would roll off the back of the tibia before reaching full flexion (Fig. 21-5). Alterations in the instant center of rotation have occurred with internal derangements of the knee such as ligament and meniscal tears.[18,19] These alterations can produce focal areas of increased articular cartilage loading.

PATELLOFEMORAL JOINT

As the knee flexes from the fully extended position, the inferior pole first contacts the femur at approximately 20 degrees. As flexion proceeds to 90 degrees, the contact area includes more of the central portion of the patella, and it is not until 135 degrees that the medial odd facet contacts the medial femoral condyle.[20] This habitual noncontact and secondary cartilage underloading may contribute to the degeneration seen at the odd facet.

In ideal static alignment, the patella is situated slightly laterally because of the screw home mechanism that lateralizes the tibial tubercle. As the knee flexes and the tibia derotates, the patella is drawn into the trochlear groove. The patella remains in the trochlear groove until approximately 90 degrees of flexion. With continued flexion, the patella moves laterally and completes a lateral C-shaped curve. This motion occurs passively as the knee flexes through a ROM. However, this tracking changes during active knee extension, and the patella moves superiorly along the line of the femur if the vastus medialis obliquus (VMO) and the vastus lateralis (VL) are in balance.

KINEMATICS OF GAIT

A ROM of 0 to 60 degrees at the knee is necessary for normal gait. However, this presumes normal mobility at the pelvis, hip, ankle, and foot. Any limitations may require additional motion at the knee. When the foot makes initial contact with the ground, the knee is fully extended. The knee then flexes to 15 degrees during the loading response of gait. After this initial flexion, the knee begins to extend until it reaches full extension at midstance. As the body weight passes over the limb, the knee passively flexes to 40 degrees. As the knee moves into the initial swing phase, the knee further flexes to 60 degrees to assist the foot clearing the floor. The knee then continues to extend through the midswing and terminal swing phases, achieving full extension before initial contact (Table 21-1).

Table 21-1. KINETICS AND KINEMATICS OF THE GAIT CYCLE AT THE KNEE

PHASE OF THE GAIT CYCLE	RANGE OF MOTION (DEGREES)	MOMENT	MUSCLE ACTIVITY	MUSCLE CONTRACTION TYPE
Initial contact	0	Flexion	Quadriceps Hamstrings	Isometric At hip, isometric
Loading Response	Flexes 0 to 15	Flexion	Quadriceps	Eccentric
Midstance	Extends to 5 flexion	Flexion moving toward extension	Quadriceps	Concentric
Terminal stance	Extends to 0	Extension	Minimal	
Preswing	Flexes to 40	Flexion	Minimal	
Initial swing	Flexes from 40 to 60		Hamstrings	Concentric
Midswing	Extends from 60 to 30		Mostly passive with some hamstrings	Eccentric
Terminal swing	Extends from 30 to 0		Hamstrings Quadriceps	Eccentric Concentric

Kinetics

TIBIOFEMORAL JOINT

Ground reaction forces and muscle activation combine to create significant forces about the knee joint. Malalignment in any plane can result in considerable focal increases in force. Motions occurring in the sagittal plane result primarily in activation of the knee flexors and extensors. During the loading response phase of the gait cycle, a flexion moment requires quadriceps activation isometrically and eccentrically to counteract the moment. As the knee approaches midstance, the flexion moment is moving toward an extension moment, and the quadriceps muscles are active until the knee is fully extended. Subsequently, muscle activity about the knee is minimal because of the passive nature of the terminal stance and preswing phases despite the respective extension and flexion moments. As the leg enters the swing phase, the hamstrings are active to flex the knee in initial swing and to decelerate the leg in terminal swing, whereas the quadriceps are active only in terminal swing to extend the leg (see Table 21-1).

Ground reaction forces, muscular forces, and the normal lower extremity alignment combine to produce important loads in the frontal plane. During the stance phase, the varus moment produces a relative compression in the medial compartment and distraction in the lateral compartment of the knee. This puts greater loads on the medial articular structures (eg, articular cartilage, meniscus) and on the lateral stabilizing structures (eg, LCL, joint capsule). Force plate analysis demonstrates that ground reaction vertical force rarely exceeds 115% to 120% of body weight during normal ambulation. However, during jogging and running, ground reaction forces approach 275% of body weight.[18]

PATELLOFEMORAL JOINT

In addition to ground reaction forces, joint reaction forces are created at the patellofemoral joint by tension in the quadriceps and the patellar tendon. As the knee flexes in a weight-bearing position, greater quadriceps torque is required, and joint reaction force increases. For example, the quadriceps torque during level walking is one-half of the body weight, stair climbing is three to four times the body weight, and squatting is seven to eight times the body weight.[21] These compressive forces can be minimized by a properly aligned patella, which disperses the force over a large surface area. Patellar subchondral bone with a strong, well-organized trabecular arrangement also minimizes joint reaction forces. Pathology, such as degeneration of patellar or femoral chondral surfaces, further reduces the capability of responding to patellofemoral joint reaction forces.

The balance between the VMO and VL appears to be critical for maintaining normal patellar tracking. Results of surface electromyography (EMG) have suggested an approximately 1:1 ratio of VMO to VL input in normal individuals and less than 1:1 in those with patellofemoral pain.[22,23] Small amounts of swelling (as little as 20 mL of fluid) may inhibit the VMO.[24]

ANATOMIC IMPAIRMENTS

The primary anatomic impairments at the knee occur in the frontal plane. Alignments of the hip, knee, and ankle combine to form an integrated kinetic chain, which must be considered in its entirety. The position of the hip affects the position of the knee, and the position of the knee dictates foot position. The anatomic impairments at the knee must be evaluated in light of the posture of the lumbopelvic, hip, ankle, and foot joints.

Genu Valgum

The femur descends obliquely from the hip in a distal and medial direction. This medial angulation with a vertical tibia results in a valgus angle at the knee, or genu valgum (Fig. 21-6*A*). This medial angle is 5 to 10 degrees. Any angle greater than this is considered to be excessive genu valgum. This valgus position places greater load on the lateral compartment of the knee and relatively unloads the medial compartment. Over time, development of degenerative joint disease in the lateral compartment produces physiologic lengthening of the MCL as the lateral compartment compresses and the medial compartment is unloaded. Increases in the angulation increase the lateral pull of the quadriceps, placing excessive loads on the patellofemoral joint and increasing the risk of patellar dislocation. This angulation is measured at the quadriceps angle (Q angle), which is measured from the tibial tubercle to the anterior superior iliac spine, with the axis in the center of the patella. Genu valgus is associated with coxa varum at the hip and excessive pronation at the subtalar joint.

Genu Varum

When the angulation of the femur and tibia is vertical (0 degrees) or laterally oriented, the condition is referred to as genu varum (Fig. 21-6*B*). Genu varum increases the loads in the medial compartment of the knee and relatively unloads the lateral compartment. Genu varum is associated

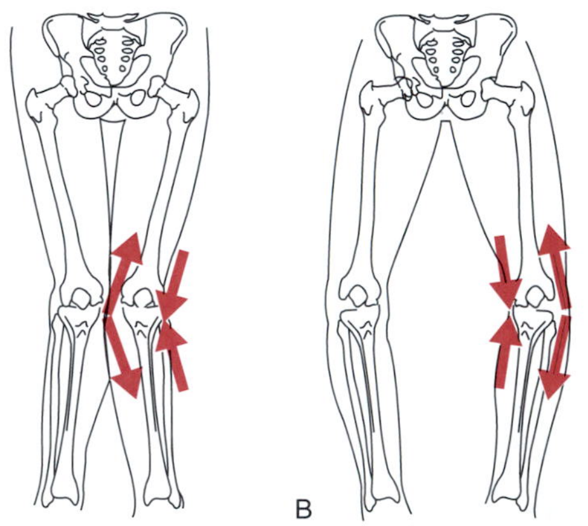

FIGURE 21-6 ***(A)*** Decreased tibiofemoral angle associated with coxa vara results in genu valgum. ***(B)*** Increased tibiofemoral angle associated with coxa valga results in genu varum. (Adapted from Norkin CC, Levangie PK. *Joint Structure and Function: A Comprehensive Analysis.* 2d ed. Philadelphia: FA Davis; 1992:344.)

with coxa valgum, and because the heel contact occurs in a calcaneal varus position, excessive pronation occurs to orient the calcaneus vertically.

EXAMINATION AND EVALUATION

As with all the joints of the lower extremity, a comprehensive knee examination includes the adjacent joints and the lumbopelvic region. The choice of specific tests and measures for the examination depend on the situation. The following sections discuss key aspects of knee joint examination (Display 21-1).

Subjective Data

The most important data to be gathered first is subjective information, which guides the objective examination and provides the clinician with important information about functional limitations and disability. Key questions focus on which symptoms are most disabling for the patient, who may experience pain, instability, mobility loss, weakness, catching, or other aggravating symptoms. From this information, the clinician chooses tests to match the patient's symptoms and designs a treatment program to address the functional limitations and disabilities described by the patient.

DISPLAY 21-1
Components of the Knee Assessment

- **I. Pelvis or hip**
  - A. Length of
    1. Hip rotators
    2. Hamstrings
    3. Iliotibial band
  - B. Hip alignment
  - C. Strength of
    1. Hip rotators
    2. Hip abductors
    3. Hip extensors
  - D. Hip capsule mobility
- **II. Knee**
  - A. Range of motion
  - B. Ligamentous stability tests
  - C. Meniscal tests
  - D. Extension overpressure response (infrapatellar fat pad testing)
  - E. Palpation for local tenderness
- **III. Patella**
  - A. Patellar orientation
  - B. Relationships of vastas medialis obliquus and vastas lateralis
  - C. Lateral retinacular tightness
- **IV. Tibia**
  - A. Tibial torsion
  - B. Tibial varum or valgum
  - C. Tibial rotation
- **V. Foot**
  - A. Pronation or supination
  - B. Rearfoot or forefoot alignment

Objective Data

The objective examination should begin with observation of posture and the position of the limb. Clearing tests for the lumbopelvic and hip regions should be performed. Any of these areas may refer pain to the thigh, knee, or calf. Several observations are important:

- Plumb line landmarks anteriorly, posteriorly, and laterally
- Genu recurvatum, flexion, valgum or varum
- Hip anteversion or retroversion
- Q angle
- Position of the patella, including glide, tilt, and rotation
- Muscle tone of the lower extremities
- Tibial internal or external torsion
- Foot posture, including pronation and supination
- Ecchymosis, swelling, or redness
- Ability to place weight on the limb

MOBILITY EXAMINATION

Mobility examination at the knee includes osteokinematic and arthrokinematic testing. Examination must include the tibiofemoral joint and the patellofemoral joint. These two joints work in unison to produce smooth, coordinated movement at the knee joint. The following tests of mobility should be performed:

Tibiofemoral joint
- Active and passive ROM overpressure for flexion and extension (ie, osteokinematic motion)
- Distraction, anterior and posterior glides (ie, arthrokinematic motion)

Patellofemoral joint
- Position during active ROM, including glide, tilt, and rotation
- Passive glide superiorly, inferiorly, medially, and laterally

Muscle extensibility
- Medial and lateral hamstrings
- Quadriceps
- Iliotibial band
- Iliopsoas
- Gastroc-soleus
- Hip rotators

IMPAIRED MUSCLE PERFORMANCE

Muscle function at the hip, knee, foot, and ankle should be tested in a logical order based on the subjective information and clinician's impressions after examination. The strength of most muscles acting at the knee exceeds the strength of most clinician's manual muscle test skills. The test results for many patients indicate normal strength although they have deficits. Other testing, such as isokinetics or the use of hand-held dynamometers, may be more suitable at the knee. However, the clinician should ensure that the limb is positioned so the muscle is tested at the correct length. These muscles are commonly tested in patients with knee complaints:

- Medial and lateral hamstrings
- Quadriceps

- Gluteal muscles
- Iliopsoas
- Gastroc-soleus
- Hip rotators
- Posterior tibialis

PAIN AND INFLAMMATION EXAMINATION

The pain and inflammation examination is performed as part of the subjective examination, and results are further clarified during the objective examination. Complaints of warmth, swelling, and local tenderness are symptoms of pain and inflammation. Palpable tenderness and warmth over specific anatomic structures are objective tests of pain. This information is correlated with subjective information to guide the remaining examination and treatment planning.

SPECIAL TESTS

Special tests are used to assess the integrity of structures about the knee. Specific tests for ligament laxity, apprehension in the case of patellar dislocation, and meniscal tests are a few of the many used. Magee's *Orthopedic Physical Assessment*[25] offers a complete description of special tests. Some of the most common special tests are listed in Display 21-2.

THERAPEUTIC EXERCISE INTERVENTION FOR PHYSIOLOGIC IMPAIRMENTS

After a thorough examination and determination of the diagnosis and prognosis, the treatment plan is implemented. Any impairments found must be correlated with a functional limitation or disability, with this aspect of the patient's care treated concurrently. However, some impairments must be improved before their associated functional limitation or disability can be addressed.

DISPLAY 21-2

Commonly Used Tests of the Knee

- Valgus stress at 0 and 30 degrees
- Varus stress at 0 and 30 degrees
- Lachman's test
- Anterior drawer
- Posterior drawer
- Pivot shift test
- Flexion rotation drawer test
- Posterior sag test
- External rotation recurvatum test
- Reverse pivot shift test
- Patellar apprehension test
- Fluctuation test
- McMurray's test
- Patellar tendon reflex

Mobility Impairment

HYPOMOBILITY

The first step in treating mobility impairment at the knee is determination of the cause. Mobility is decreased because of musculotendinous or capsular shortening. Mobility can be diminished by pathologic abnormalities such as an incorrectly placed ligament graft or a hypertrophic fat pad. Examination of the pattern of limitation and the patient's localization of pain can identify the cause of mobility impairment. Hypomobility at the knee joint results in compensation at associated joints. For example, squatting down with limited knee motion requires additional motion at the hip, ankle, and low back, and these joints are at risk for injury from the excessive demands placed on them.

Capsular restriction is common after immobilization, total knee arthroplasties, and multiple operations. Capsular limitations can occur at the tibiofemoral joint, patellofemoral joint, or both, and the source of the limitation must be ascertained. Full knee extension requires superior glide of the patella and anterior glide of the tibia on the femur. Knee flexion requires inferior glide of the patella along with posterior glide of the tibia on the femur. Capsular restrictions are treated with the respective glides and joint distraction techniques (Fig. 21-7). Quadriceps setting is an excellent exercise to increase and maintain superior patellar glide. (see Self-Management: Quadriceps Setting Exercise). However, if adhesions in the suprapatellar pouch limit the excursion of patellar glide, these exercises may increase patellar pain. Patellar mobilization in the direction of limitation can be performed by the therapist or by the patient in a home program (see Self-Management: Patellar Mobilization Per-

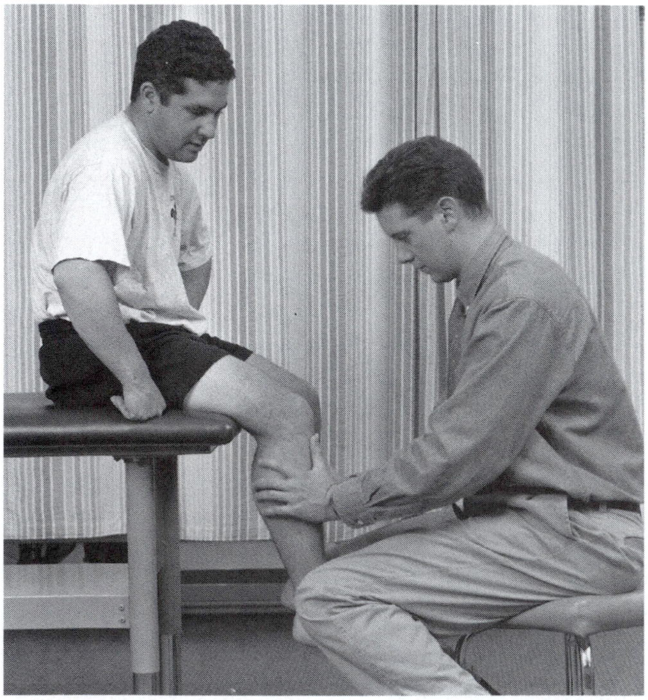

FIGURE 21-7 Joint distraction and posterior glide of the tibia on the femur can be performed simultaneously to increase knee joint flexion mobility.

formed by the Patient). This choice of exercise reinforces the necessity of a thorough examination.

Limitations caused by muscle shortening usually are treated with stretching exercises. The quadriceps and hamstring muscles may be lengthened in several positions, but care must be taken to ensure proper positioning of the spine, pelvis, and hip. Incorrect positioning can increase the stress in these areas and decrease the effectiveness of the stretch. The quadriceps may be stretched across the knee only or, with the addition of rectus femoris stretching, across the hip (Fig. 21-8). The pelvis must be prevented from tilting anteriorly, increasing lumbar extension during this stretch (see Self-Management: Quadriceps Stretching While Avoiding Lumbar Extension). Stretching the quadriceps at the knee may also be performed in prone with an abdominal support to prevent excessive lumbar extension (Fig. 21-9).

The hamstrings are easily stretched in a sitting position with the knee extended and the lumbar spine held in neutral. Posteriorly tilting the pelvis and flexing the lumbar spine must be avoided. This exercise can be performed throughout the day at a variety of workstations (Fig. 21-10). The medial hamstrings may be emphasized by laterally rotating the leg, and the lateral hamstrings may be emphasized by medially rotating the leg. Horizontally adducting the hip with internal rotation of the hip enhances stretching of the iliotibial band and its associated lateral structures (Fig. 21-11).

In addition to the major muscle groups acting at the knee, the closed chain nature of the lower extremity necessitates assessment at adjacent joints. For example, shortening of the medial rotators of the hip or the gastroc-soleus

SELF-MANAGEMENT: Quadriceps Setting Exercise

Purpose: To strengthen quadriceps muscle, mobilize patella superiorly, stretch tight tissues behind the knee, and re-educate the quadriceps how to work

Position: Sitting with the legs straight out, toes pointed up to the ceiling; a small towel may be placed behind the knee

Movement technique:

Level 1. Tighten the quadriceps muscle on top of your thigh. You should see your kneecap move up toward your hip. Your knee may push down toward the floor, and your foot may come up off the floor. You should be unable to manually move your kneecap when doing a quadriceps set correctly. If you are having difficulty, try doing a quadriceps set on the other leg at the same time. Be sure your hip muscles stay relaxed.

Level 2. Perform the same quadriceps set in a standing position.

Repetitions: _______ times

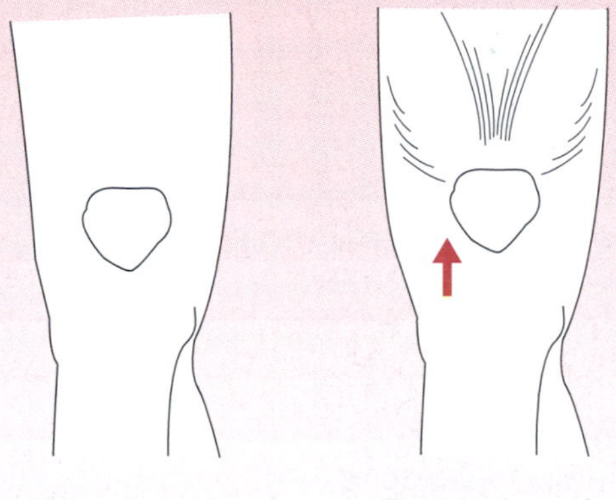

SELF-MANAGEMENT: Patellar Mobilization Performed by the Patient

Purpose: To increase the mobility of the kneecap in all directions

Position: Sitting with the legs straight out, toes pointed up to the ceiling

Movement technique: Using your fingers or the heel of your hand, push your kneecap ***(A)*** down toward your foot, ***(B)*** toward the outside, ***(C)*** toward the inside, and ***(D)*** up toward your hip. Hold each position for a count of five. These movements should not be painful.

Repetitions: _______ times

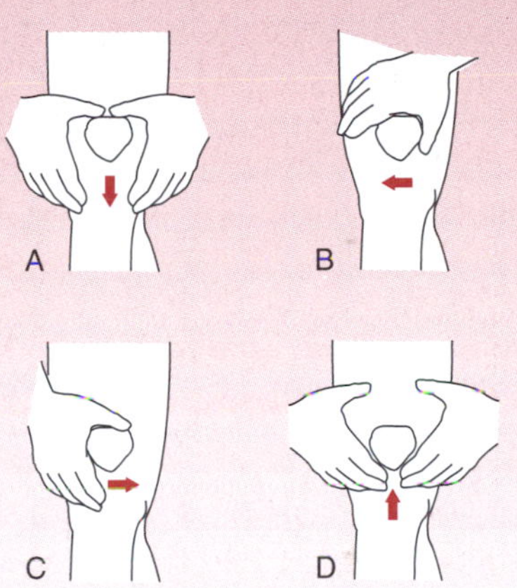

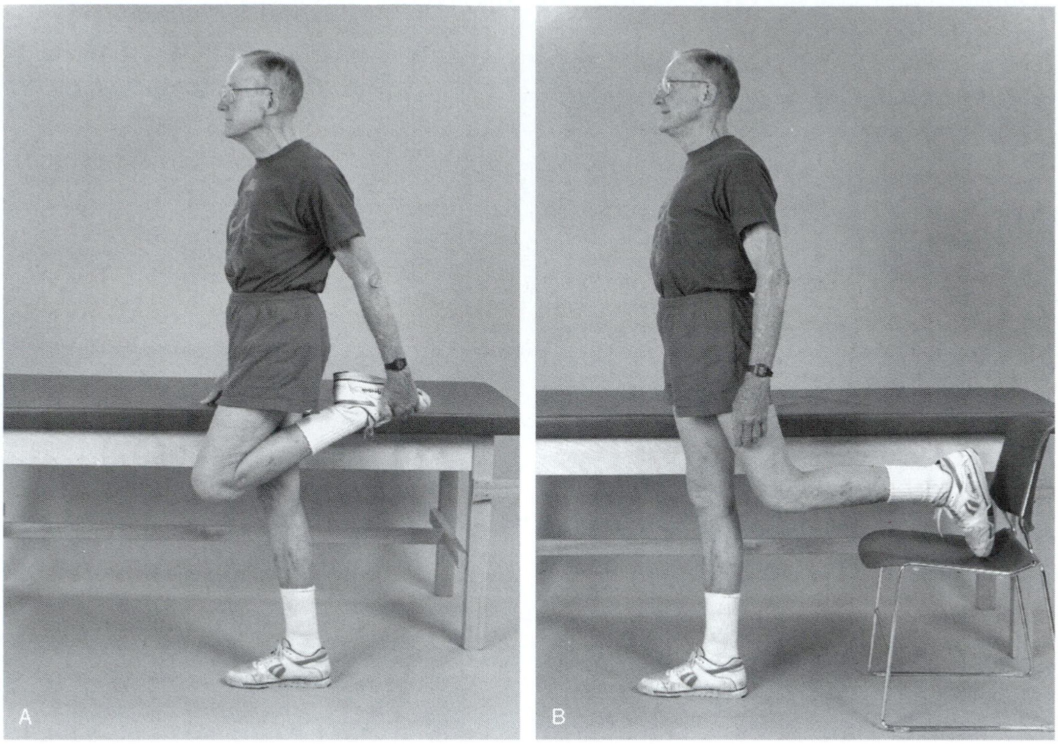

FIGURE 21-8 Quadriceps stretching while standing. ***(A)*** Across the knee only. ***(B)*** Across the hip and knee.

can contribute to patellofemoral pain at the knee. These tissues must be examined over all the appropriate joints.

HYPERMOBILITY

Hypermobility at the knee joint is associated with patellar instability and possible increased risk for ACL injuries.[13] Hypermobility is associated with clinical signs such as knee recurvatum and subtalar joint pronation. This combination may predispose individuals to patellofemoral pain at the knee.

Treatment of hypermobility at the knee joint requires postural education and retraining. This education is focused at all lower extremity joints and the lumbopelvic area. Good posture requires an integrated approach throughout the entire kinetic chain. Any further training must be superimposed on correct postural mechanics. After this posture is achieved, closed chain activities emphasizing cocontraction of lower extremity musculature enhance postural stability (Fig. 21-12). High-repetition, low-resistance activity is used to enhance stability.

Impaired Muscle Performance

NEUROLOGIC CAUSES

Muscle performance can be impaired at the knee by neurologic disorders. The most common cause is a lumbar spine injury or disease. In addition to directly affecting the quadriceps or hamstring musculature, lumbar spine pathology affecting proximal or distal musculature necessarily affects gait and other movement patterns. Altered movement patterns affects knee joint mechanics and ultimately the joint itself. Any complaints of knee joint impairments should prompt examinations of the spine and proximal and distal joints.

Other neurologic disorders, such as multiple sclerosis or Parkinson's disease, profoundly affect the ability to produce torque about the knee. Each of these situations must be evaluated within the context of the disease process. Because many muscles and movement patterns are affected, a more global examination is necessary to determine the treatment strategy.

Some authorities have suggested there is a neurologic component to patellofemoral pain. Studies of different quadriceps activation patterns in response to a patellar tendon tap have suggested timing differences in those with or without patellofemoral pain.[22,26,27]

The key consideration when designing interventions for those with neurologically mediated impaired muscle performance is ensuring use of the desired muscle. Neurologic weakness produces alterations in firing patterns to accomplish movement in the most efficient manner possible. Synergists may accommodate for weakness, or biomechanical modifications may enhance the activity of other muscles as compensation for the weakness. For example, a forward lean during stair ascent allows the hip extensors to compensate for weak quadriceps (Fig. 21-13). Close monitoring of exercise quality is necessary to ensure training of the desired muscle.

STRAIN AS A CAUSE

The ability to produce torque at the knee can be affected by muscular strain injuries. The quadriceps and hamstring muscle groups are the most commonly injured. The quadriceps and hamstring muscles can be injured by sudden

SELF-MANAGEMENT: Quadriceps Stretching While Avoiding Lumbar Extension

Purpose: To increase flexibility of the quadriceps muscles

Position: This exercise can be performed in several positions. Pick a position that is comfortable or convenient for you, but avoid arching your back when stretching; tighten your abdominal muscles to keep your back steady.

1. In a sidelying position, with abdominal muscles tightened ***(A)***
2. In a standing position, with some support, abdominal muscles tightened, and knees close together ***(B)***
3. On your stomach, with a small pillow or towel under your hips and abdominal muscles tightened ***(C)***

Movement technique: Grasp your ankle or a strap attached to your ankle, pulling it toward your buttocks until you feel a gentle stretch in the front of your thigh. Hold each stretch for 15 to 30 seconds.

Repetitions: ________ times

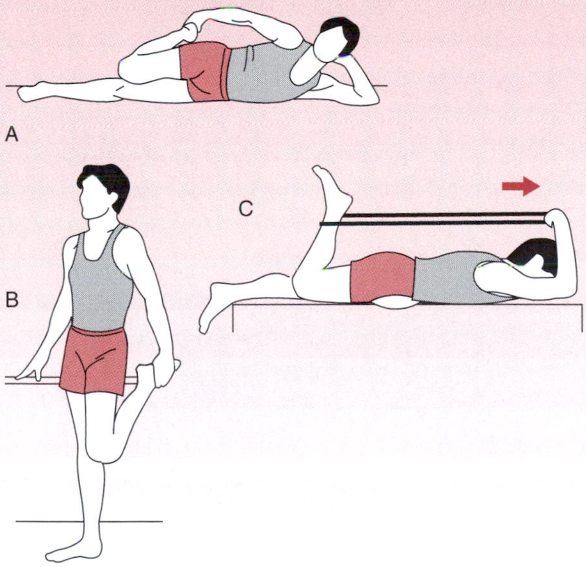

decelerative forces. The quadriceps decelerate the flexing knee during the loading response of the gait cycle, and the hamstrings decelerate the forward swinging shank during the terminal swing phase. These muscles may be injured as the result of a contusion. As with neurologic injuries, the first step in restoring the ability to produce torque is the development of kinesthetic awareness. Once this is developed, overload techniques as described in Chapter 4 can be applied. Rehabilitation techniques to improve force production in these muscles are described in Chapter 20. When returning the patient to function, the role of the affected muscle in should be retrained to fit the expected activity. For example, the runner with a hamstring strain injury as a result of the swing phase of gait should be trained in an open chain, decelerative function. Inertial exercise or other forms of repetitive decelerative exercise also can be used (Fig. 21-14).

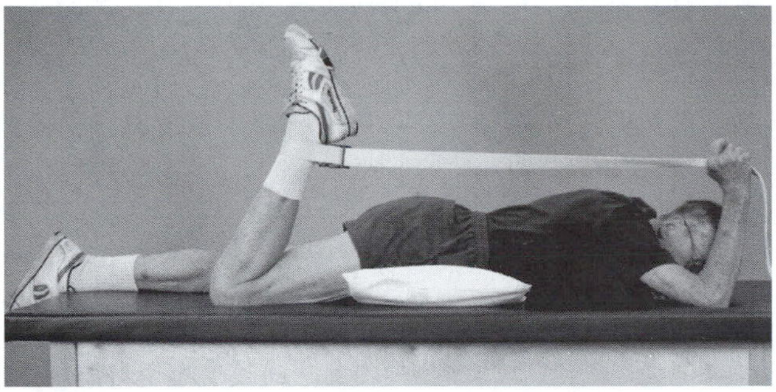

FIGURE 21-9 Prone quadriceps stretching with a pillow under the abdomen. These exercises can be performed with or without weights on the ankle for additional stretch.

DISUSE AND DECONDITIONING AS CAUSES

Disuse of the knee musculature occurs primarily in the quadriceps and may occur as a result of an injury at the knee or from any other joint in the kinetic chain, including

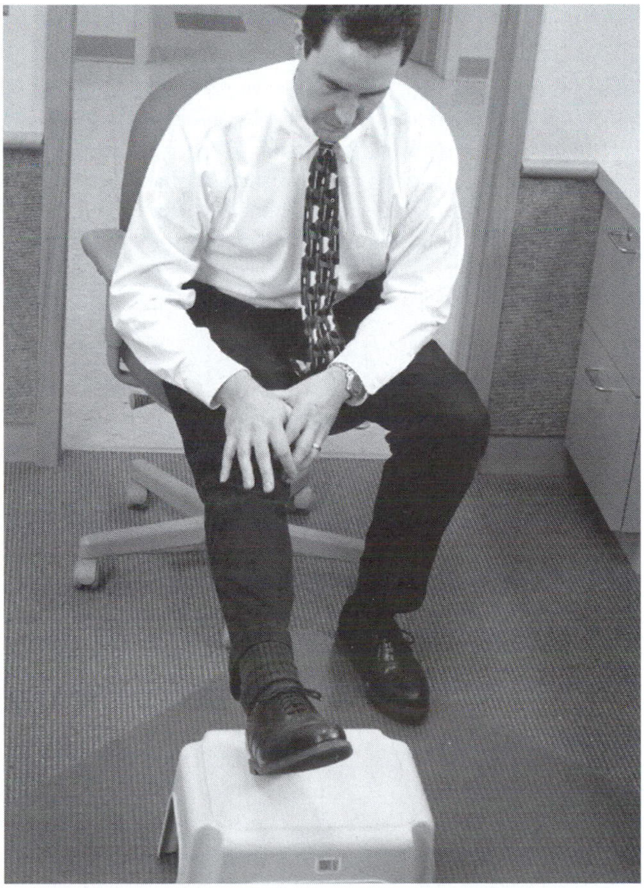

FIGURE 21-10 Hamstring stretch while seated at a workstation.

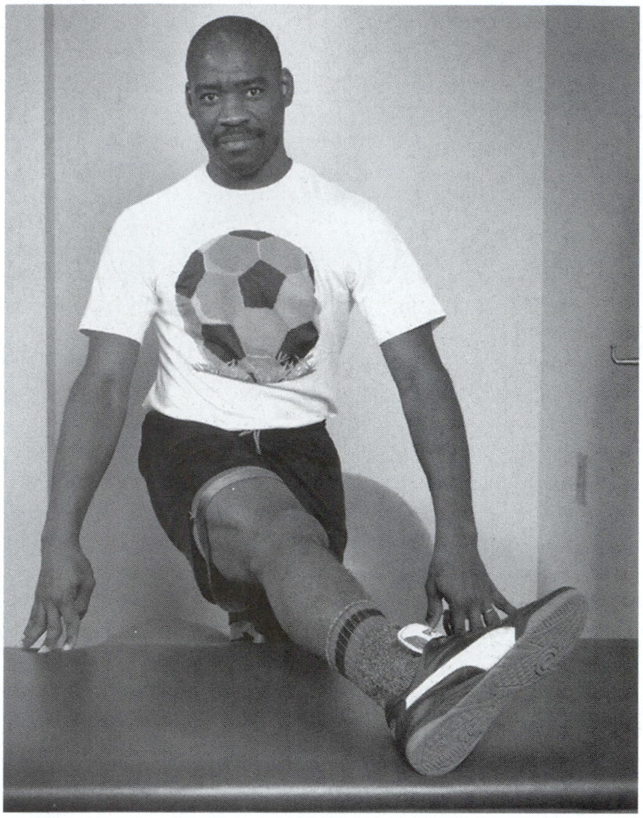

FIGURE 21-11 Lateral hip and leg stretch. Close observation prevents trunk rotation substitution for hip adduction.

the low back. An injury at an associated joint can prevent participation in usual activities, leading to disuse of musculature throughout the kinetic chain. Disuse of the quadriceps affects the loading and midstance phases of the gait cycle, during which the quadriceps decelerate the flexing knee, followed by a change of direction and acceleration into knee extension. This quadriceps action decreases loads on the joint surfaces and is critical in maintaining the health of the knee joint.

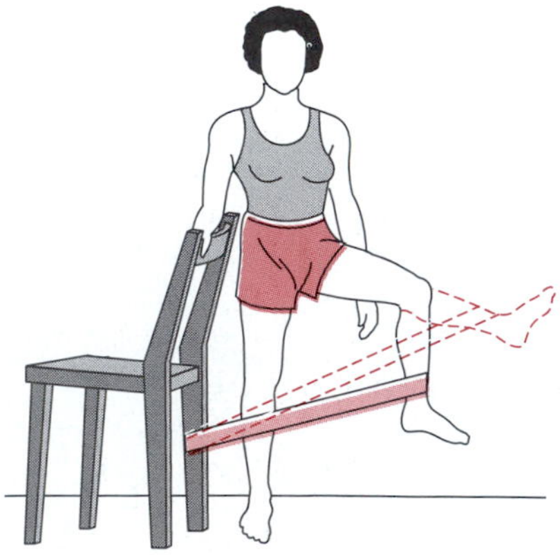

FIGURE 21-12 Knee extension exercise using tubing and with a focus on posture. This is a closed chain exercise on the weight-bearing side, and an open chain exercise on the non–weight-bearing side. It requires considerable balance and postural control.

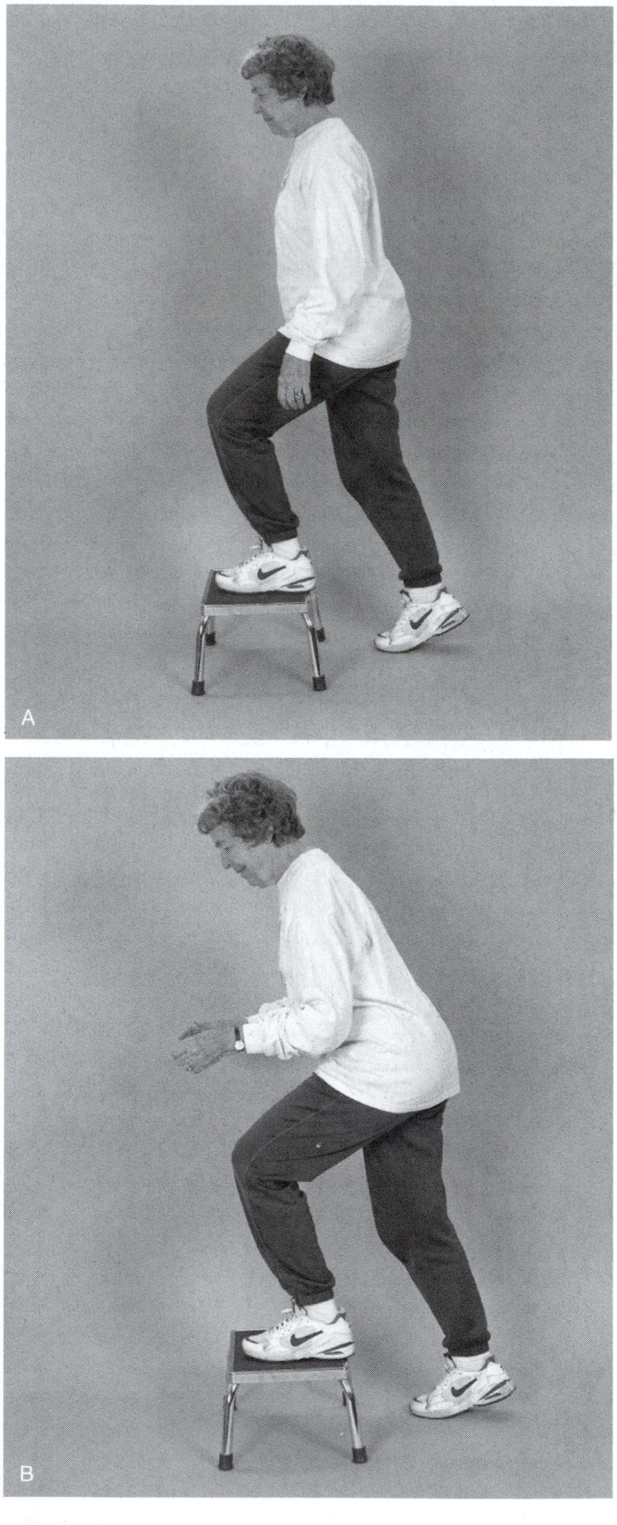

FIGURE 21-13 ***(A)*** Ascending stairs using proper mechanics. ***(B)*** Ascending stairs with the hip extensor muscle substituting for a weak quadriceps muscle.

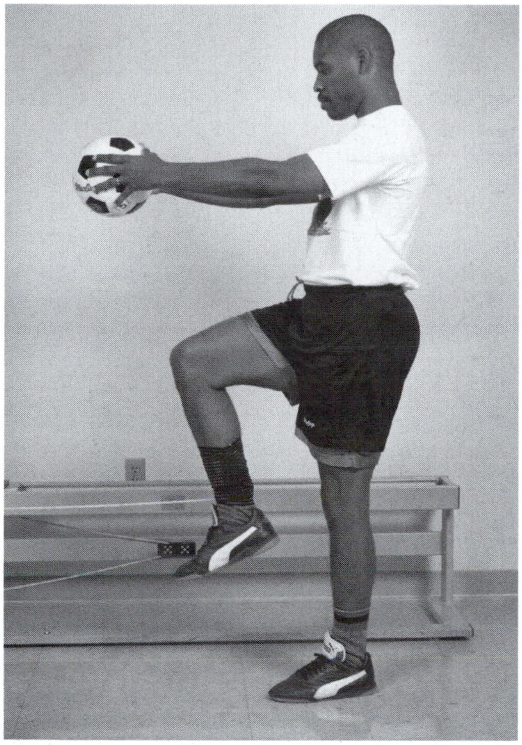

FIGURE 21-14 Hamstring muscle training with inertial exercise for high-repetition, low-resistance acceleration and deceleration training.

The quadriceps muscles work to decelerate the body when descending stairs and, along with the hip musculature, to ascend stairs and arise from a sitting position. Disuse can lead to profound changes in how activities of daily living (ADLs) are performed. Failure to perform these activities efficiently and continuously places additional loads on adjacent joints.

THERAPEUTIC EXERCISE INTERVENTION FOR COMMON DIAGNOSES

Ligament Injuries

ANTERIOR CRUCIATE LIGAMENT

The ACL is one of the most commonly injured ligaments in the knee and is the ligament injury resulting in the most controversy about treatment. In the past, an ACL tear could end the career of an athlete or result in the need for surgery and a year or more of rehabilitation. The long-term morbidity associated with an ACL injury with or without reconstructive surgery has made this injury the nemesis of many athletes. Fortunately, the ACL injury has become better understood and better managed, resulting in significant decreases in morbidity. The ACL tear usually occurs as the result of a quick deceleration, hyperextension, or rotational injury and does not involve contact with another individual. Injury to the ACL is frequently associated with injuries to the MCL, the medial meniscus, and the lateral meniscus. In the adolescent, the ACL may avulse from the tibial spine rather than tear in the midsubstance, and it should be surgically repaired with bone-to-bone fixation.

Although functioning independently, the ACL and PCL guide the instant center of rotation of the knee, thereby controlling the joint arthrokinematics. Any alteration in normal kinematics can produce focal areas of increased articular cartilage and other soft tissue loading. Sequelae such as degenerative joint disease and tendinitis must be considered when determining prognosis and treatment approach. Injury to the ACL can result in significant functional limitations and potential disability because of its role as the primary restraint against anterior tibial translation. Rupture of the ACL results in substantially increased anterior translation, with the maximum occurring between 15 and 45 degrees of flexion.[18] The posterior horn of the medial meniscus provides secondary restraint against anterior tibial translation and is at risk for injury after an ACL rupture. The ACL provides stability against tibial medial and lateral rotation and against varus and valgus stresses.

Because of its role in controlling the instant center of rotation, some individuals experience episodes of instability after ACL injury and subsequently fail conservative treatment. They may have surgery using static restraints to reconstruct the ACL. These tissues include the central one third of the patellar tendon, the hamstring tendon, and iliotibial tract. It is difficult to predict which persons may require reconstruction and which may be able to continue their normal activities without instability. Those involved in high-demand sports usually have more difficulty returning to activities without symptoms. Continued vigorous activity with an unstable knee can lead to meniscal tears, especially at the posterior horn of the medial meniscus.

Clinical examination procedures to detect an ACL tear start with an accurate history, including the mechanism of injury and time of onset of effusion. Acute injuries to the ACL are associated with an immediate, tense effusion. Lachman's test remains the gold standard for assessing excessive anterior tibial translation.[25] Instrumented laxity testing, as with the KT-2000, is routinely used to compare laxity with that of the contralateral knee and with population norms. Instability testing can be performed by several special tests, including the pivot shift, flexion rotation drawer, and the jerk test.[25]

Significant impairments, functional limitations, and disabilities occur after ACL tears. The acute ACL rupture is characterized by acute hemarthrosis, pain, and instability. Impairments such as effusion, loss of motion, inability to bear weight, loss of strength, poor balance and coordination, and pain are evident early in the course. Functional limitations include an inability to ambulate without an assistive device, limitations in basic and instrumental ADLs, and difficulty negotiating stairs. For individuals involved with sport and leisure activities or work that necessitates physical labor, an ACL injury can lead to significant disability. The inability to lift and carry heavy objects or to walk moderate distances can lead to the loss of functional and social interactions on many levels. Chronic impairments include instability, effusion, weakness, poor balance and coordination, and pain. These impairments can lead to functional limitations such as an inability to ambulate moderate distances without a brace or assistive device, difficulty ascending or descending stairs, or limitations in lifting and carrying objects. Persons may become disabled because these limitations prevent return to work, leisure activities, or basic or instrumental ADLs.

Rehabilitation issues of concern when treating the individual after ACL injury include the impairments, functional limitations, and disabilities identified during the evaluation and any concomitant injuries. Associated injury to the MCL or a small peripheral meniscal tear affects the rehabilitation program. The arthrokinematic changes and potential for secondary injury guide rehabilitation. Resistive open chain quadriceps exercises between 15 and 45 degrees are often avoided because of the increased anterior tibial translation found with this type of exercise. This translation is minimized in a closed chain exercise, which is frequently chosen after ACL injury. Because of the difficulty in returning to deceleration and cutting maneuvers, the rehabilitation program should include these types of movements along with resistive, balance, and coordination activities in multiple planes. Exercises may include resisted lateral movements, resisted rotational movements, and activities on unstable surfaces.

POSTERIOR CRUCIATE LIGAMENT

The PCL injuries represent an estimated 1% and 30% of all knee ligament injuries.[28] Most injuries occur as the result of a trauma such as a motor vehicle accident, with fewer PCL injuries occurring in sports.[28] The mechanism producing a PCL injury is most often a blow to the anterior aspect of the tibia, forcing it posteriorly. Less commonly, the PCL is injured as a result of hyperflexion, hyperextension, or a varus or valgus injury. In the case of hyperextension, the ACL is usually injured first. In the varus or valgus injury, the respective collateral ligament is injured, and in some cases, the ACL is injured before the PCL injury.

The clinician must examine the patient for concurrent injuries. The PCL injury is missed more often than the ACL injury because the PCL rupture does not usually result in significant instability. The individual may not present for examination or may be misdiagnosed because of an inaccurate examination. Some persons with multiple ligament or soft tissue injuries undergo reconstruction of the PCL using static restraints such as the central one third of the patellar tendon, Achilles tendon, or allograft.

The PCL is the primary restraint to posterior subluxation of the tibia on the femur, providing approximately 95% of the resistance against posterotibial translation.[29] A tear of the PCL results in significant increases in posterior tibial translation, with the greatest occurring between 70 and 90 degrees.[30] The PCL resists varus or valgus translation and is a secondary restraint to lateral tibial rotation.[28] Along with the ACL, the PCL helps control the instant center of rotation at the knee and joint arthrokinematics. The alteration in joint arthrokinematics after PCL rupture can result in significant disability. Articular cartilage contact pressures in the medial and anterior compartments are increased after PCL rupture, with peak medial pressures at 60 degrees and peak anterior compartment pressures at 90 degrees.[28] The individual with a PCL rupture generally complains of pain related to these changes, rather than frank instability. The natural history of the PCL-deficient knee is difficult to assess because of the heterogeneity of most populations studied. Many patients remain asymptomatic and are able to return to their preinjury activity levels, but others develop osteoarthritic changes in the medial and anterior compartments.[31] The clinician must consider the possibility of these changes and modify the rehabilitation program appropriately.

Clinical examination procedures to assess the PCL injured knee begin with a thorough history. The mechanism of injury and the symptoms are different from those of an ACL injury and should alert the clinician to a PCL injury. The posterior drawer test, performed at 90 degrees of flexion, is the gold standard for detection of PCL rupture.[25] However, the PCL injury is often misdiagnosed as an ACL rupture because of the clinician's inability to correctly determine the neutral position of the knee. In the 90-degree position, the tibia may sag posteriorly from the weight of gravity, and no further posterior translation is found, although excessive anterior translation may occur. This is translation from the posteriorly subluxed position to the neutral position, rather than from neutral to an anteriorly displaced position. The clinician should accurately determine the neutral position of the knee before laxity testing by assessing the relationship between the tibial and femoral condyles. The posterior sag and active quadriceps tests also can assess posterior translation, and the reverse pivot shift and external rotation recurvatum procedures test posterolateral instability. Instrumented laxity testing using the KT-2000 can provide objective comparisons of translation with the contralateral side or with population norms.

The extent of impairments, functional limitations, and disabilities after PCL rupture depends on associated injuries. Immediately after injury, the individual may present with effusion, loss of motion, weakness, poor balance and coordination, and an inability to ambulate without an assistive device. Functional limitations may include an inability to ambulate moderate distances, climb stairs, drive, or stand for extended periods. The resulting disability can affect the person's ability to participate in community, work, and leisure ADLs. When patients are seen for chronic functional limitations because of PCL deficiency, the subjective complaints usually are related to medial and anterior compartment pain and difficulty ambulating down a decline or stairs.

The issues affecting the rehabilitation approach are related to the potential medial and anterior compartment changes. Any additional ligament injuries that could further alter arthrokinematics or medial meniscal damage that could modify articular cartilage pressures have the potential to exacerbate compartmental changes. Comorbidities such as underlying osteoarthritic changes, a varus alignment, or history of patellofemoral pain negatively alter the prognosis. These issues should be the framework from which the rehabilitation program is designed. As in treating the ACL-deficient knee, open chain resistive exercise (knee flexion in this case) can increase posterior tibial translation, and closed chain activities are an important therapeutic exercise mode.

MEDIAL COLLATERAL LIGAMENT

The MCL consists of the tibial collateral ligament and the middle one third of the medial capsule (deep portion), which is subdivided into a thin anterior third, a strong middle third, and a moderately strong posterior third.[32] The incidence of MCL injuries is significantly higher than that of LCL injuries, and the MCL has been reported to be the most frequently injured ligament of the knee.[33] Damage to the MCL occurs less frequently at the femoral insertion compared with the tibial insertion because of differences in the insertion site structures. The MCL is usually torn as a result of a valgus stress by a lateral blow or by forced abduction of the tibia, as occurs when catching the inside edge of a ski. Associated injuries may include the ACL and medial meniscus. In the adolescent, injury to the femoral or tibial growth plate often precedes injury to the MCL and should be considered in the differential diagnosis.

The MCL is the primary restraint against valgus loads, and it resists tibial medial rotation. Unlike the cruciate ligaments, the MCL has the capacity for repair without surgical intervention. Most MCL injuries heal well without any long-term damage to the knee, despite some residual valgus laxity.[34,35] For this reason, most MCL injuries are treated conservatively. In the individual with a combined MCL and ACL injury, a short period of recovery usually is allowed, followed by reconstruction of the ACL. Injuries to the MCL in the presence of ACL ruptures do not heal as well as isolated MCL sprains.[36] Repairing the MCL or ACL risks the loss of extension ROM. The effects of lengthy immobilization on the ligament substance and insertion sites have been studied.[36] In dogs, surgical repair followed by 6 weeks of immobilization of MCLs resulted in inferior mechanical and structural properties, even at 48 weeks. Woo[36] reported that a remobilization period six times longer than the time of immobilization might be required for recovery. However, individuals with bony avulsions should have them surgically reattached.

Examination of the knee after MCL injury begins with a thorough history, including determining the mechanism of injury. The individual may present with localized swelling over the MCL or with an effusion if concomitant damage to the capsule has occurred. Because the MCL is taut in full extension, the knee may be held in a position of slight flexion. Overpressure to full extension reproduces medial knee pain. The midrange is the least painful, with pain increasing as the MCL begins to tighten again at approximately 70 degrees of flexion. Point tenderness may be found vertically along the length of the ligament, rather than transversely along the joint line (indicative of meniscal injury), and greater tenderness is generally found at the midsubstance and the tibial insertion than at the femoral insertion. Valgus stress testing at 30 degrees of flexion assesses the integrity of the MCL, and valgus loading in full extension tests the MCL, ACL, and PCL. Comparisons with the contralateral side must always be performed because of individual differences and physiologic laxity.

The impairments, functional limitations, and disabilities seen after acute MCL sprains are similar to those of cruciate ligament sprains. The prognosis after isolated MCL sprain is generally good because of the ligament's ability to heal well. Some individuals may experience difficulties with lateral and rotational movements or with activities on uneven surfaces. Persons returning to physical work or recreation are most at risk for limitations in these areas. Although the clinical examination may be benign after 6 to 8 weeks of rehabilitation, the lengthy ligament remodeling process may limit the MCL's tolerance for high-demand loading.

The most significant rehabilitation issues in the isolated MCL injury are the fact that the remodeling process lags behind the clinical examination findings and the need for frontal and transverse plane rehabilitation techniques. Traditional clinical examination procedures are not sensitive enough to determine readiness to return to high demand activities. Frequently, the individual has full ROM, symmetric strength, minimal or no valgus laxity, no effusion, and no tenderness to palpation after a few weeks of rehabilitation. However, the MCL is not stressed much in ordinary daily activities or even in sagittal plane activities such as straight-ahead running. The ligament must be loaded and trained just like muscle tissue to ensure adequate remodeling for high-demand activities. Loading in the frontal and transverse planes must occur to strengthen the ligament and its bony attachments and to ensure a safe return to physical activities (Figs. 21-15 and 21-16).

LATERAL COLLATERAL LIGAMENT

Injuries to the LCL are much less common than injuries to the MCL, and like MCL injuries, they heal well and without significant long-term disability. The LCL is the primary restraint to varus stress, and because of its location in the posterior one third, it also resists hyperextension, especially in the presence of a varus stress.[32] Lateral collateral ligament injuries usually result from hyperextension varus forces, with or without contact with another individual. Complete tears occur in the ligament midsubstance or

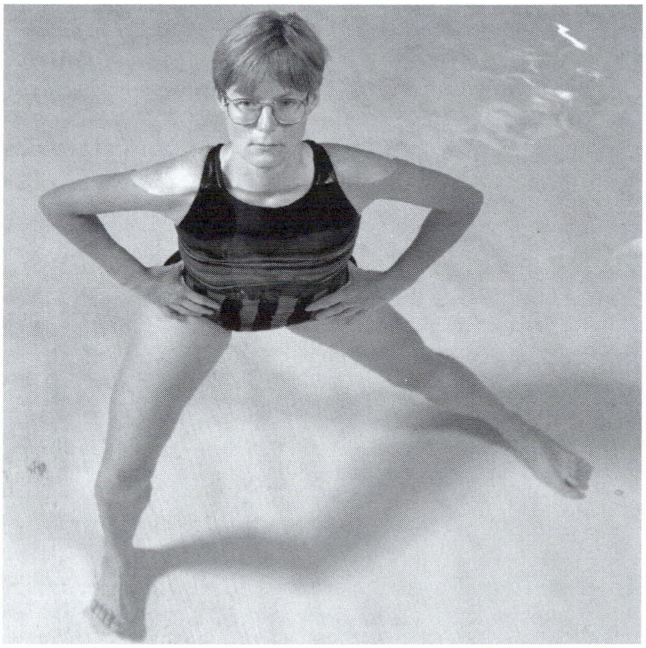

FIGURE 21-15 Side stepping in the pool is an early lateral movement activity.

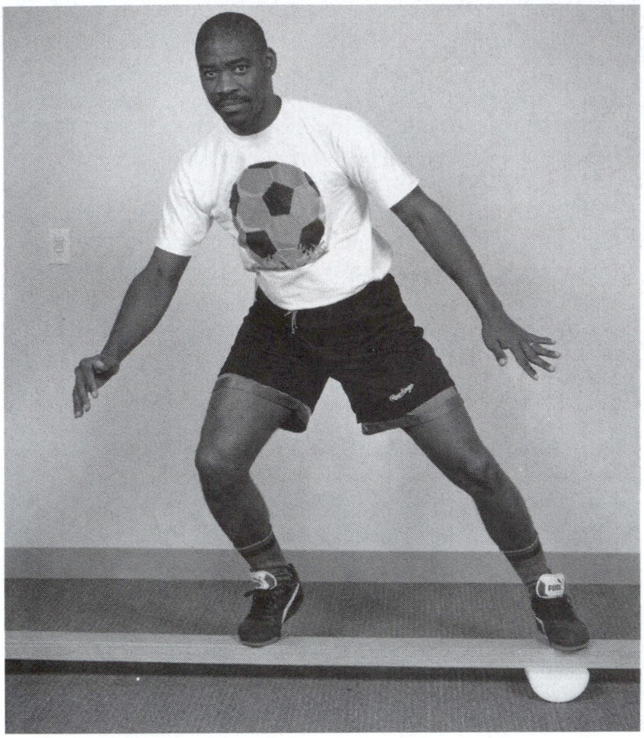

FIGURE 21-16 More challenging lateral movements include side stepping on a balance beam on foam rollers.

at the fibular insertion. Associated injuries may occur to the posterolateral structures, including the joint capsule, arcuate ligament, biceps femoris or popliteus tendons, or cruciate ligaments. In the adolescent, injury to the growth plate usually precedes ligament injury and should be considered in the differential diagnosis.

The natural history of the LCL injury rarely includes long-term disability because of its healing potential. Surgical repair of the isolated LCL is rarely performed. Individuals with significant varus deformities may experience instability after this injury and may require surgical stabilization. A bony avulsion should be surgically reattached. More extensive posterolateral corner injuries typically are reconstructed using static restraints or biceps femoris tenodesis.

The subjective history of an individual with isolated LCL injury includes varus, hyperextension, or both forces, with or without a "pop." Like the MCL, the extraarticular position of the LCL precludes a true joint effusion unless damage to the joint capsule coexists. Localized swelling may occur over the ligament. Because the LCL is most taut in full extension, the individual may experience lateral knee pain with overpressure into full extension. The ligament is tender to touch, but the joint line should not be tender. The varus stress test at 30 degrees of flexion best assesses the integrity of the LCL.

The functional limitations and disabilities seen after a LCL injury are fewer than those seen with an MCL injury. Most individuals are minimally limited after this injury, except in the case of a third-degree tear or concomitant ligament or capsular injury.

Rehabilitation issues are similar to those for MCL injuries. The prolonged course of ligament remodeling must be considered, along with the importance of retraining the individual and loading the ligament in the frontal and sagittal planes.

TREATMENT OF LIGAMENT INJURIES

Interventions should be aimed at achieving specific goals related to impairments, functional limitations, and disabilities. Impairments should be addressed if they are associated with a functional limitation or disability or if continued impairment could lead to disability in the future. Pain and effusion can be managed in the short term with physical agents, mechanical and electrotherapeutic modalities, and gentle therapeutic exercise. Cold packs, ice massage, compression therapies, and electrical stimulation are commonly used to minimize pain and effusion. Therapeutic exercise such as active and passive ROM activities within a comfortable range can provide lubrication to joint surfaces and can assist resorption of excessive joint fluid. The patient should receive instruction in the application of these procedures at home and guidance in modifying activities to minimize pain and effusion.

Traditional physiologic stretching and active and passive ROM activities facilitate restoration of preinjury joint motion. Occasionally, joint mobilization techniques may be necessary, although ligamentous injury generally results in too much mobility rather than too little. However, lengthy immobilization or an inability to fire the quadriceps may result in a loss of knee extension ROM. Neuromuscular reeducation exercises such as quadriceps setting, hamstring setting, and other muscle activation techniques can restore the ability to fire muscles, which is a prerequisite for normalization of movement patterns. The home program should include exercises to facilitate ROM increases and neuromuscular re-education exercises to advance gains made in the clinic (Fig. 21-17) (see Self-Management: Performing Flexion and Extension Mobility Exercises During the Day and Self-Management: Prone Hang for Knee Extension).

The pool is an excellent environment for performing mobility, normalizing gait, and initiating balance and gentle strengthening exercises. The water's buoyancy minimizes weight bearing while the hydrostatic pressure controls effusion. Walking, physiologic stretching, leg kicks, toe raises, single-leg balance, and minisquats can be easily accomplished in the pool (Fig. 21-18).

As the patient progresses out of the acute phase, more functional exercises may be initiated. Continuation of ambulation training and progression to ambulation without an assistive device are primary considerations for the return to normal activities. Land-based, closed chain exercises such as wall slides, minisquats, step-ups, stair stepping, and leg presses can facilitate functional activities such as stair climbing, rising from a chair, and getting in and out of a car (Fig. 21-19). Balance and coordination exercises such as step-ups, biomechanical ankle platform system (BAPS) board, single-leg pulleys, and toe raises without support can retrain balance reactions. Any impairments in motion, strength, pain, or effusion that are related to functional limitations should be addressed concurrently. Traditional progressive resistive

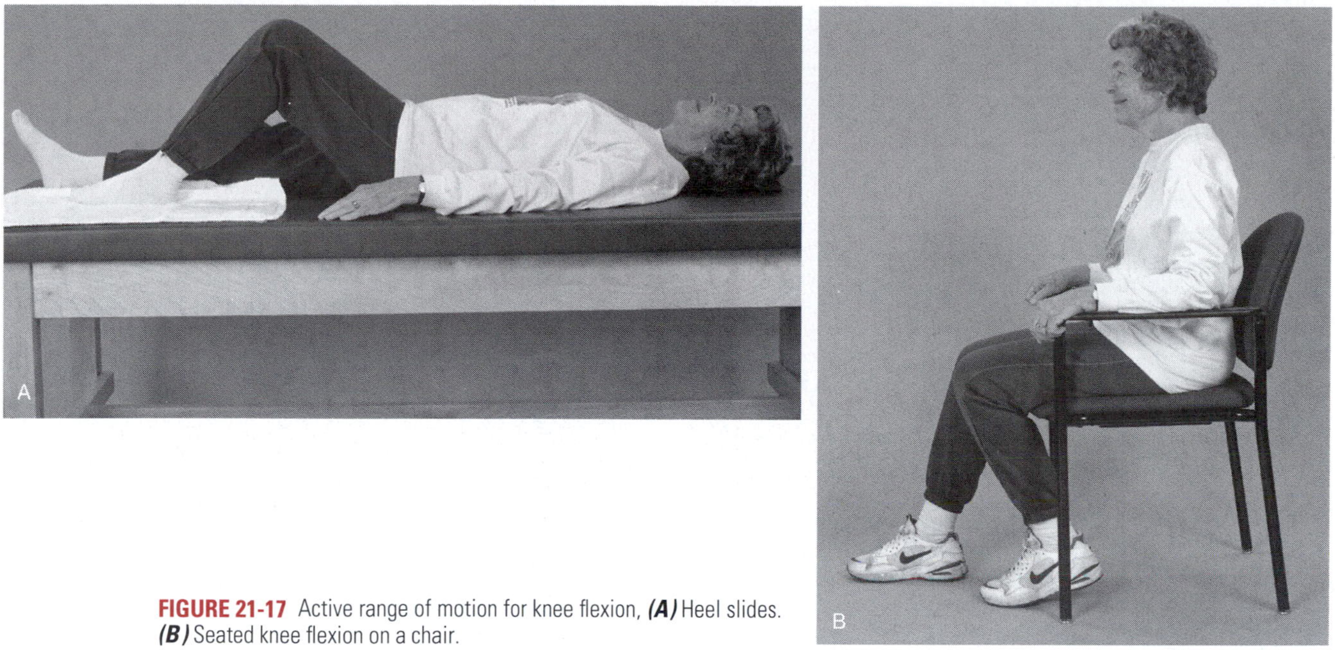

FIGURE 21-17 Active range of motion for knee flexion, ***(A)*** Heel slides. ***(B)*** Seated knee flexion on a chair.

SELF-MANAGEMENT: Performing Flexion and Extension Mobility Exercises During the Day

Purpose: To increase mobility in the knee

Position: Sitting or in another position of comfort

Movement technique: Actively extend the leg as far as possible and then bend it back as far as possible. You may use your other leg to help lift it the last little bit or to push it back a little farther.

Repetitions:_______ times

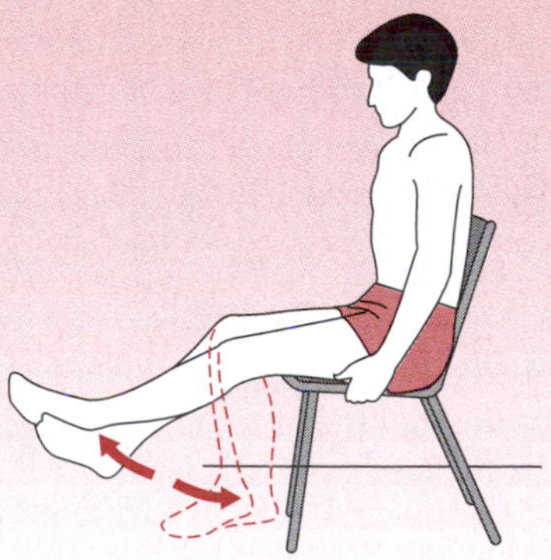

SELF-MANAGEMENT: Prone Hang for Knee Extension

Purpose: To increase mobility in knee extension and stretch tight tissues behind the knee

Position: On your stomach, with your knee just over the edge of the table; a towel under your thigh may be more comfortable.

Movement technique: Let your knee straighten by hanging over the table's edge. Your clinician may want you to put weight on your ankle or to use your other leg to increase the stretch. Hold for 1 to 2 minutes.

Repetitions:_______ times

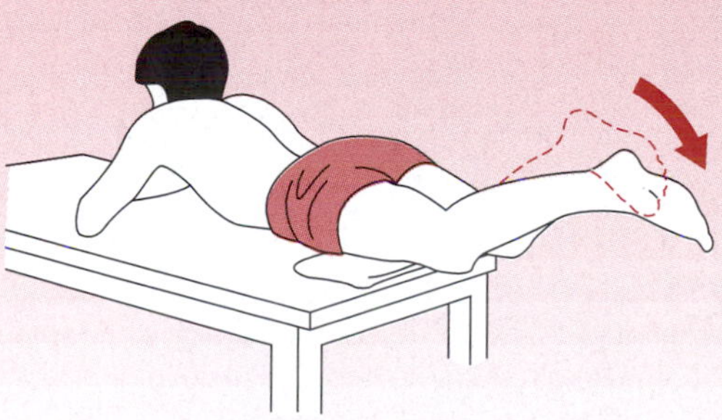

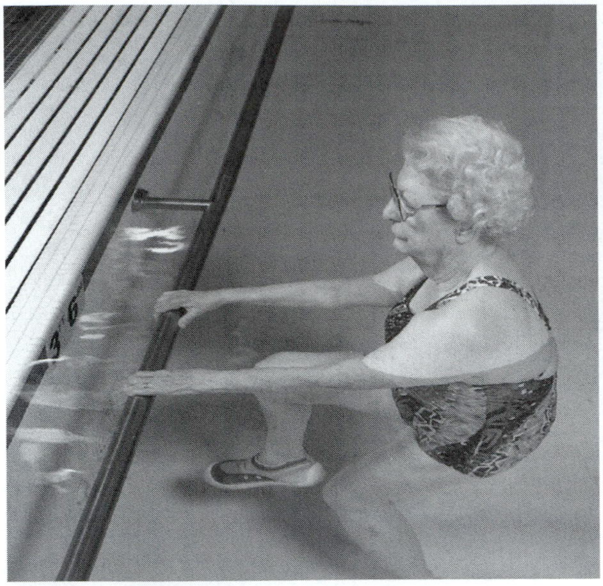

FIGURE 21-18 Single-leg minisquats in the pool are performed to increase mobility and strength.

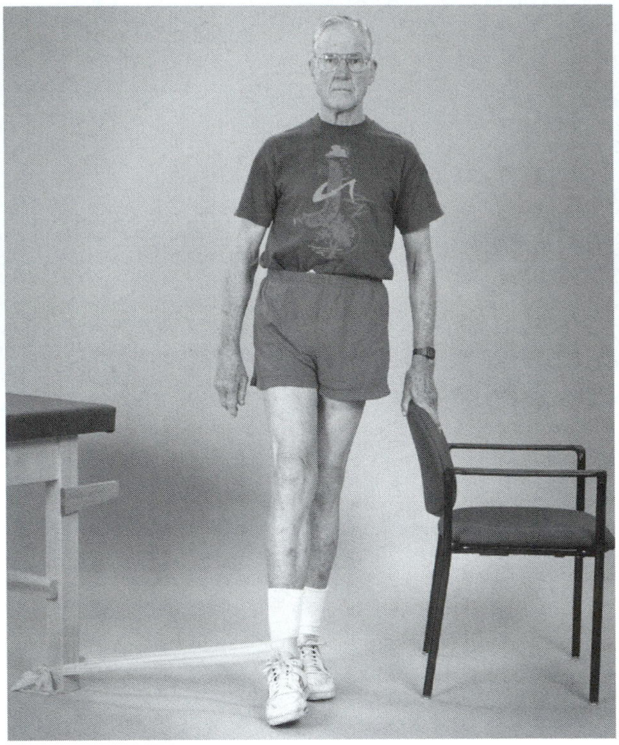

FIGURE 21-20 Resisted hip adduction using a resistive band.

exercises can be incorporated, keeping in mind the arthrokinematic issues. Weight machines, free weights, isokinetic devices, pulleys, and body weight are means to accomplish increases in the ability to produce torque. The clinician must be aware of the loads placed on the knee ligaments with various exercises and use caution to avoid overstressing a healing ligament. For example, resistive hip adduction using a resistive band around the ankle places a significant load on the MCL, which may be fine in the late stages but too much in the early stages (Fig. 21-20). At home, the use of body weight as resistance in the form of wall slides, squats, lunges, and step-ups is convenient and cost effective (see Patient-Related Instruction: Performing Weight-Bearing Exercises).

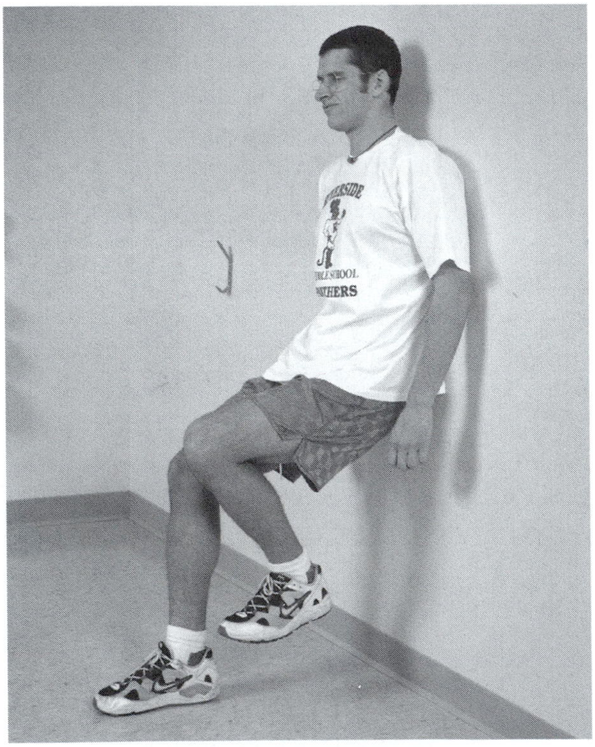

FIGURE 21-19 Single-leg wall slides.

The final phase of rehabilitation helps return the patient to her premorbid level of function in ADLs, work, or recreation. Because the activity level and functional goals are different for each patient, the rehabilitation program must be tailored to individual needs. For the individual returning to sedentary work and recreational walking, discharge to an independent program may be considered after motion, strength, endurance, and impairments and functional limitations have been normalized. The patient should demonstrate a thorough understanding of the home management of impairments, including inflammation, pain, ROM, and strength. For individuals returning to a higher level of physical functioning, such as physical labor or sports activities, reconditioning to that level is necessary. This may require advanced work related activities such as lifting, pushing, pulling, and carrying objects over uneven surfaces. A functional capacity evaluation may be performed to determine restrictions or precautions affecting a return to work.

Running, cutting, jumping, and sports skill activities can help ensure a safe return to to sporting activities (Fig. 21-21). A running program or sport-specific drills may be used to test readiness to return to play. Completion of an appropriate functional progression can ensure a safe return to sports. Although this program does not need to be under the direct supervision of the physical therapist, it should be constructed with and guided by the clinician in conjunction with the pa-

Patient-Related Instruction

Performing Weight-Bearing Exercises

When performing exercises in weight-bearing, the following important points should be reviewed:

1. Be sure that your knee is at the correct angle, as directed by your clinician.
2. Avoid hyperextending your knee (bending it backward).
3. Keep your knee in line with your toes and your hips. Avoid letting your knees "roll in" (ie, being "knock-kneed").
4. Tighten your buttocks muscles together, and use the muscles in the front of your thigh, as directed by your clinician.
5. Hold each exercise for the amount of time specified by your clinician. Be sure to breathe in and out slowly while performing each exercise.

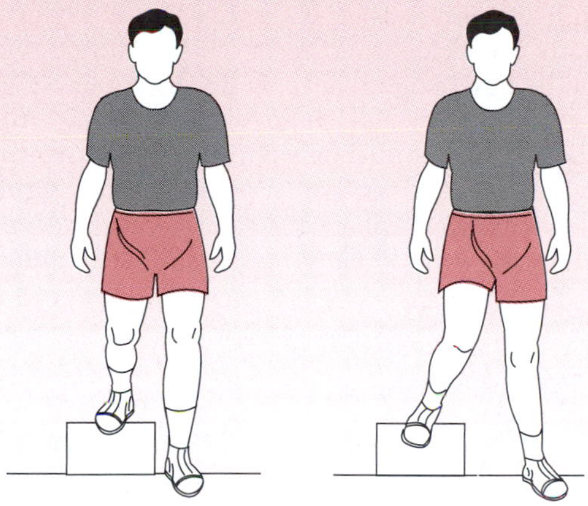

tient. Any deficits in movement patterns should have been corrected by the clinician in the earlier therapy stages and should not be an issue at the functional progression stage.

Fractures

Knee fractures can involve the patella, distal femur, or proximal tibia. These fractures generally occur as a result of trauma such as a fall or motor vehicle accident but can also result from osteoporosis.

The rehabilitation issues associated with knee fractures include the effects of immobilization, surgical procedures, and the original trauma. A trauma significant enough to fracture a bone also causes substantial soft tissue damage, which is frequently overlooked. Damage to articular cartilage and fractures extending through the articular cartilage to the joint surface have the potential to affect the long-term health of the joint, and these issues should be considered in the rehabilitation program.

PATELLAR FRACTURES

Patellar fractures account for approximately 1% of all skeletal injuries and occur most frequently in persons between the ages of 40 and 50 years.[37] Falls account for the greatest percentage of patellar fractures, followed by motor vehicle accidents. Fractures can occur as a result of a forceful quadriceps contraction. Traumatic fractures usually produce comminuted fractures, and transverse fractures result from quadriceps contractions. However, the degree of knee flexion, the patient's age, presence of osteoporosis, and the velocity of injury can affect the type and location of fracture.[37]

Treatment of patellar fractures can be conservative, such as casting, or surgical, such as open reduction with internal fixation (ORIF) or partial patellectomy. Because of the morbidity associated with immobilization, ORIF is often the treatment of choice for medically sound candidates. A

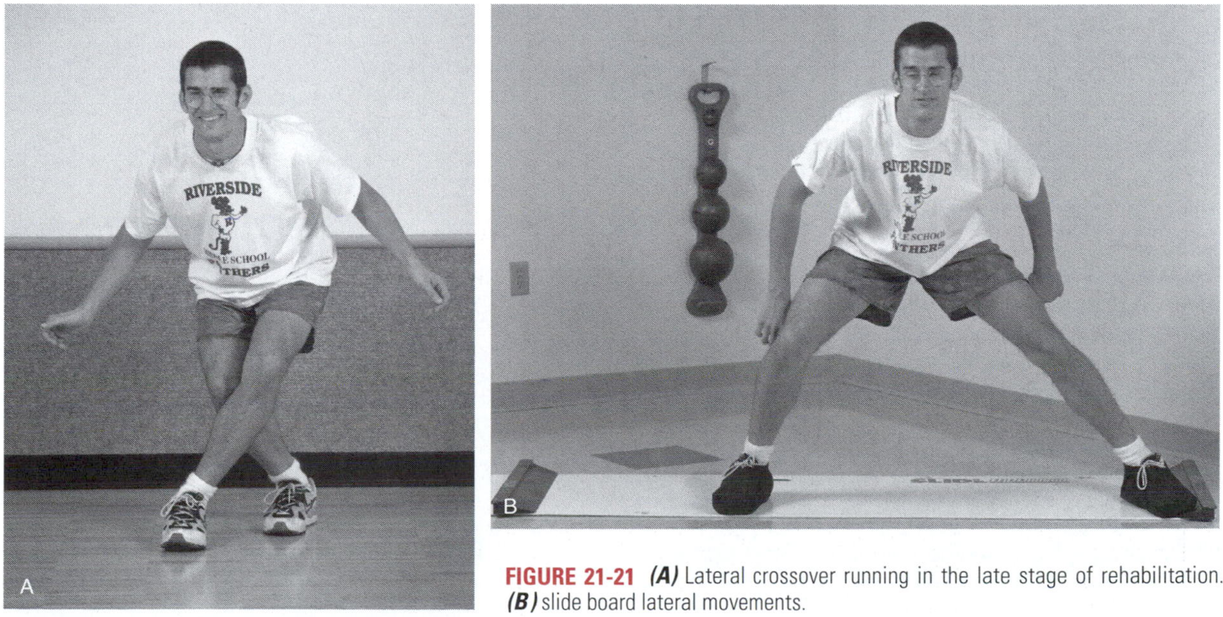

FIGURE 21-21 ***(A)*** Lateral crossover running in the late stage of rehabilitation. ***(B)*** slide board lateral movements.

transverse fracture is distracted by quadriceps activation and is best treated by fixation. Tension cerclage wiring is frequently used, particularly for comminuted and transverse fractures. Because of the superficial nature of the patella, the hardware is frequently removed after healing is ensured. Occasionally, a small fragment or fragments are removed rather than fixated (ie, partial patellectomy). The prognosis after patellar fracture is good if patellofemoral pain, muscular atrophy, and loss of motion are addressed. These impairments occur regardless of treatment method. With conservative management, the clinician must also be aware of the effects of immobilization on the soft tissues.

DISTAL FEMUR FRACTURES

Distal femur fractures are the consequence of trauma in most cases, although spiral fractures may occur in the elderly as the result of a twisting injury. Motor vehicle accidents and falls account for most fractures. Associated fractures are common and include those of the patella, tibial plateau, foot, ankle, and hip. Distal femur fractures can be classified as pure supracondylar, supracondylar and intercondylar, or monocondylar, each with subclassifications.[37] Fractures through the growth plate occur in children and adolescents and are classified as Salter types I through V.[38]

As for patellar fractures, treatment of distal femur fractures is categorized as conservative or surgical. Nondisplaced, minimally displaced, stable, or impacted fractures or fractures in individuals who are not surgical candidates may be treated with immobilization. Because of the morbidity associated with lengthy immobilization, surgical ORIF is the treatment of choice in most cases. Reduction of distal femur fractures requires restoration of the anatomic alignment and mechanical axes in the sagittal, frontal, and transverse planes. The specific surgical procedure and fixation choice depend on factors such as the type and location of fracture, quality of bone, associated injuries, and the patient's age and lifestyle. Complications after ORIF include deep vein thrombosis, infection, and delayed union or nonunion.

TIBIAL PLATEAU FRACTURES

Tibial plateau fractures occur almost exclusively as the result of trauma such as motor vehicle accidents, pedestrians hit by cars, accidental falls, or twists or direct blows to the knee. Fractures are produced by a varus, valgus, or compressive force, resulting in lateral plateau, medial plateau, or bicondylar fractures. Tibial plateau fractures are classified morphologically[37]:

1. Split fracture, in which the margin of the tibial plateau is separated from the rest of the plateau
2. Compression fracture, in which the subchondral bone is crushed but the margins are spared
3. Combination split-compression fracture

Compression fractures are the most difficult to diagnose, because the depressed fragments are often missed on standard radiographs. These fractures also are the most difficult to treat, because adequate reduction requires the elevation and stabilization of depressed fragments. Compression fractures are seen most commonly after falls from heights and in elderly individuals with osteoporosis.

Treatment of tibial plateau fractures depends on the location and type of fracture. Compression fractures with depressed fragments require surgical elevation and stabilization of the fragments. These fragments usually are supported with bone grafts, and split fractures are stabilized with screws, wires, or plates and lag screws. Conservative management with or without traction and immobilization is an option that must be considered in light of the deleterious effects of immobilization. Postoperative or postimmobilization rehabilitation depends on the numerous factors outlined previously.

TREATMENT OF FRACTURES

Treatment programs for individuals with fractures at the knee may begin early after the fracture or after healing has taken place. Persons with fractures surgically fixated generally begin mobility and strengthening exercises soon after the operation (see Self-Management: Straight-Leg Raises). Active and passive ROM for flexion and extension and functional mobility exercises for the entire kinetic chain are initiated early. Quadriceps setting and hamstring setting exercises can be initiated early to retrain these muscle groups. When permitted, closed chain weight-bearing exercises should be initiated, even if only partially weight bearing (see Patient-Related Instruction: Walking With Crutches). These activities can enhance articular cartilage nutrition throughout the kinetic chain and provide a stimulus for

SELF-MANAGEMENT: *Straight-Leg Raises*

Purpose: To increase the strength of the quadriceps and hip flexor muscles and to improve control of the knee

Position: Lying on your back, with your opposite knee bent and foot flat on the floor; stomach muscles are tightened.

Movement technique: This is a four step process.

1. Perform a quadriceps set, tightening the quadriceps muscles.
2. Slowly raise the leg until it is even with the opposite thigh.
3. Slowly lower the leg back to the floor.
4. Relax the quadriceps set. Be sure to relax the quadriceps muscle between each repetition.

Repetitions: _______ ***times***

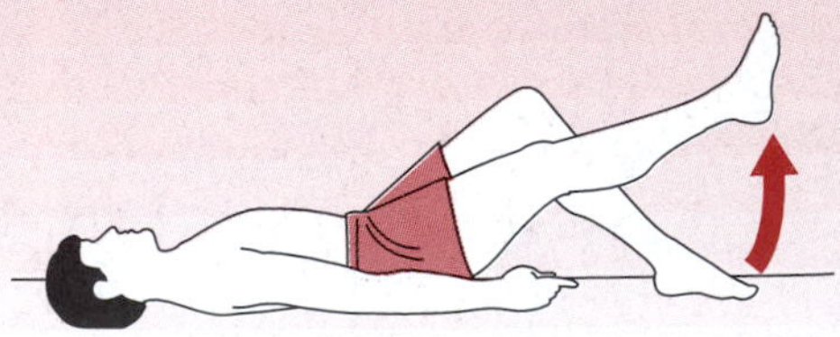

Patient-Related Instruction

Walking With Crutches

When walking with crutches and some of your weight on the involved knee, several guidelines should be followed:

1. Make sure your weight is on your hands, not under your arms. Your arms should be slightly bent when your crutches fit properly.
2. When walking, place your crutches out first, followed by your involved leg and then your uninvolved leg.
3. Place your involved heel down first, let your knee bend slightly, and allow your foot to roll toward your toes as you begin to bring your uninvolved leg forward.
4. As you bring your uninvolved foot through, bend your involved knee, and pick it up behind you. Straighten the involved knee as you bring it past your crutches to place it on the floor in front of you. Your knee should be straight just before your heel contacts the ground.
5. When using a single crutch, be sure to use it on the side *opposite* your injured knee.
6. Check with your clinician to ensure that your gait with crutches is correct.

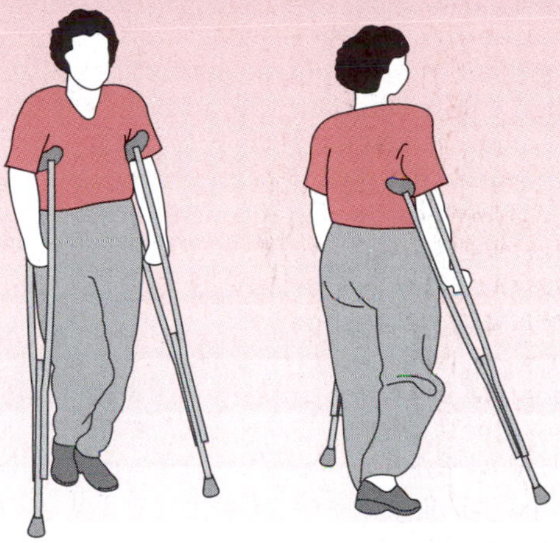

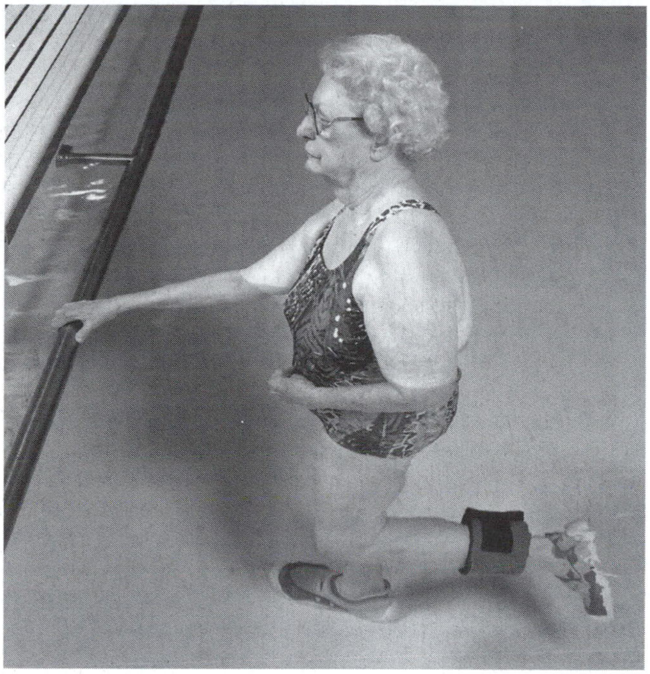

FIGURE 21-22 Buoyancy-assisted knee flexion using a buoyant strap. The return motion (to extension) is buoyancy resisted, eliciting a concentric quadriceps muscle contraction.

muscle activation. An exercise bicycle with little or no resistance can enhance nutrition and muscle activity in the area while improving mobility.

Pool exercise is excellent for the individual with a knee fracture. Weight bearing may be limited while muscle activation and mobility exercises are performed with assistance from buoyancy. Passive motion assisted by buoyancy or active motion can improve ROM about the knee (Fig. 21-22). Gait can be normalized with or without railing assistance.

Meniscal Injuries

The menisci were originally thought to be useless remains of leg muscles.[39] As the importance of the meniscus to the long-term health of the knee became better understood, preserving the meniscus after injury became a high priority. The menisci are composed primarily of type I collagen and are more fibrous than articular cartilage. The herringbone arrangement on the surface allows for shear forces that occur with normal joint arthrokinematics; the deeper major fiber orientation is circumferential. The menisci receive their blood supply from the medial and lateral superior and inferior geniculate arteries and have variable vascularity. The vascular supply penetrates 10% to 30% of the width of the medial meniscus and 10% to 25% of the width of the lateral meniscus. The peripheral one third is often called the red zone, the middle one third is the red-white zone, and the central one third is the white (avascular) zone. The meniscus receives its nutrition by diffusion, and it has a low metabolic rate and a low reparative response. Repair of the meniscus considers this low reparative response and often uses the peripheral blood supply to assist the healing process.

The menisci have many functions, underscoring the importance of maintaining their structure. In addition to enhancing joint congruity and stability, the menisci also function to transmit load across the knee joint, with approximately 40% to 50% of the compressive load transmitted through the meniscus in full extension and 85% at 90 degrees of flexion.[16,40] Partial meniscectomy with a 10% decrease in contact area increases peak local stresses by 65%, whereas total meniscectomy decreases the contact area by 75% and increases peak local stresses by 235%.[41] Total meniscectomy is no longer routinely performed because of the Fairbanks changes seen postoperatively. These changes include marginal femoral osteophyte ridging, flattening of the medial femoral condyle, and narrowing of the joint space.[42] The menisci also work as shock absorbers, although the subchondral bone is the main static shock absorber at the knee. Some of the most important functions of the menisci are joint lubrication and articular cartilage nutrition. The biphasic properties of the meniscus assist in providing a lubricant film across the joint surface with loading and unloading of the knee.[39]

The meniscus may be acutely injured traumatically or chronically injured, as with a degenerative tear. Traumatic tears usually occur in individuals between the ages of 13 and 40 who are involved in physical activities or in those who sustain trauma in a fall or motor vehicle accident. Degenerative tears occur with increasing frequency with advancing age and are often complex tears. A degenerative tear can be precipitated by a specific stress, although it may seem to be minor, such as turning to walk a different direction.

TREATMENT

Degenerative tears associated with articular cartilage lesions often require surgery to remove loose fragments and to stimulate a healing response in the articular cartilage. Acute traumatic tears may heal without intervention if the tear is longitudinal and peripheral. Some tears may not heal but remain asymptomatic.[43] Tears producing mechanical symptoms such as catching, locking, and effusion are treated by partial meniscectomy or by meniscal repair. The treatment of choice depends on the type and location of the tear and on the associated injuries. For example, a meniscal repair in the posterior horn of the medial meniscus in an ACL-deficient knee does not heal well. However, if the ACL is reconstructed simultaneously, the meniscal repair has an opportunity to heal if provided a blood supply. Complex degenerative tears are nearly impossible to repair and probably will fail in the setting of articular cartilage degeneration.

The interventions chosen for patients with partial meniscectomy correlate with the changes in load distribution and increases in peak local stresses associated with this procedure. The knee has been distributing and dispersing loads during normal activities based on the patient's anatomy for many years. Suddenly, the load distribution is changed, and other structures must shoulder the burden of the load previously carried by the intact meniscus. The joint's ability to adapt to this change in loading pattern depends on many factors, including lower extremity alignment, quadriceps function, comorbidities, and the response to the stresses placed on it (ie, Wolff's law). The body must have time to adapt to the changing loading pattern, and although some individuals adapt quickly, others may develop symptoms of overload such as inflammation, effusion, or pain. Any activity that produces significant shear forces with compressive loading (eg, squatting, steps) may overwhelm the load-bearing capabilities in some knees. Individuals with suboptimal alignment, degenerative joint disease, poor quadriceps function or neuromuscular control, or limited ROM probably will have the most difficulty.

Issues associated with meniscal repair are related to the normal meniscal motion during knee flexion and extension, the shear forces across the repair, and the location and type of tear repaired. The meniscus moves posteriorly up to 12 mm during knee extension to flexion, with most motion occurring between 0 and 15 degrees and beyond 45 degrees.[16,44] Although motion up to 80 to 90 degrees is permitted in the early phase actively and passively, weight-bearing activities through a large range should be avoided. Early partial weight bearing or weight bearing as tolerated is often permitted depending on the tear size, type, and location. The knee goes through a limited ROM in a weight-bearing position during normal gait. Repairs in the white zone, repairs with additional vascular access, or repairs of complex or radial tears are protected longer, and progression is dictated by the procedure.

Degenerative Arthritis Problems

ARTICULAR CARTILAGE LESIONS

Articular cartilage is a unique tissue that has remarkable properties, including an ability to be deformed and regain its original shape, exceptional durability, and an unparalleled low-friction surface.[45] These are just a few of the properties that make articular cartilage so difficult to reproduce. Despite the prevalence of artificial joint replacements, the average life of an artificial joint is much shorter than that of native articular cartilage. This comparison highlights the unique characteristics of this material, which functions optimally in the presence of adequate ROM, joint stability, and an equitable load distribution.[39]

Articular cartilage is composed primarily of water, type II collagen, and proteoglycans.[45,46] Water is approximately 60% to 85% of the weight of articular cartilage and is responsible for its biphasic properties.[39,45,46] The water content decreases with age, increasing the stiffness and deformation of cartilage and decreasing its biphasic material properties. This decrease contributes to the changes seen in the normal aging process. Every joint has its own pattern or "footprint" on the surface, reflecting the specific shear forces across that joint.[39] The articular cartilage in adults receives its nutrition by diffusion, and the cartilage in children receives some nutrition from the underlying subchondral bone.[46]

Articular cartilage responds to loads in a time-dependent manner like any other viscoelastic material; it creeps under a constant applied load and relaxes under a constant deformation. When an external load is applied to the cartilage surface, an instantaneous deformation occurs, and approximately 70% of the water within the cartilage may be moved, until the compressive stress within the articular cartilage matches the applied stress, and equilibrium is reached. Stress and relaxation also occur, depending on the length of time the cartilage is loaded. Cartilage also increases the congruity of the surfaces, distributing loads over a greater surface area.[45] The ability to withstand compressive loads (based on these properties) varies from joint to joint and within the same articular surface.[46]

From a mechanical perspective, the requirements for a healthy joint include freedom of motion, stability, and an equitable load distribution.[39] These necessities form the basis for some of the treatments for articular cartilage lesions. Adequate lower extremity strength to absorb loads during the loading response of the gait cycle, and normal movement patterns help minimize excessive loads on the articular cartilage. Partial-thickness articular cartilage lesions in adults do not heal, but they may not get any worse in a joint with freedom of motion, stability, and an equitable load distribution. However, in an ACL-deficient knee or a knee with a significant varus alignment, the lesion may progress to become a full-thickness lesion. When this lesion degrades far enough, bleeding occurs, and the healing process begins. This is the rationale for abrasion arthroplasty, in which an articular cartilage lesion is treated with perforations, drilling, or "punctating" the underlying bone to stimulate a healing response. However, the replacement tissue is fibrocartilage, which is a lesser-quality tissue than the original articular cartilage. The fibrocartilage may be adequate in the presence of adequate motion, joint stability, and equitable load distribution.

The rehabilitation program must consider the fundamental requirements for a healthy joint when determining the appropriate mode and progression of therapeutic exercise. Activities that minimize shearing forces while increasing stability and mobility provide the foundation for the therapeutic exercise program (see Patient-Related Instruction: Tips to Maintain the Long-term Health of Your Knee).

OSTEOTOMY

The high tibial osteotomy or tibial varus osteotomy is performed in cases of unicompartmental osteoarthritis and varus alignment; the supracondylar (femoral) osteotomy is used to treat unicompartmental osteoarthritis and valgus alignment.[47,48] The rationale behind high tibial osteotomy for varus alignment is that the alignment excessively loads the medial tibiofemoral compartment, which promotes osteoarthritis.[49] Conversely, the valgus alignment loads the lateral tibiofemoral compartment, leading to subchondral sclerosis, loss of cartilage space, and osteophyte formation, indicative of osteoarthritis. The tibial osteotomy is generally performed on patients wishing to delay total joint replacement. Despite the short-term success of tibial osteotomy, most results can be expected to deteriorate over time.[50]

The technique of tibial osteotomy includes making a wedge cut in the tibia at least 1.5 cm distal to the joint line. For a varus alignment, the lateral osteotomy is inclined medially and distally, and the tibia is fixated with hardware. A fibular osteotomy is performed as well. The results of this procedure depend on proper patient selection, accurate measurements, and adequate correction. Patients who are poor candidates for this procedure include those with tricompartmental degeneration, significant ligamentous laxity, or markedly restricted motion.[51] Correction of varus deformities to at least 5 degrees of valgus produce the best results.[52–54] Two-plateau weight bearing is the ultimate goal, and excessive bone loss, inaccurate measurements, or inadequate correction can interfere with achieving this goal. Patients with preoperative low adduction moment at the knee maintained better clinical results that those with high adduction moment, suggesting that adaptive gait mechanics play a role in outcome.[55]

Rehabilitation after tibial osteotomy is guided by the requirements for a healthy joint and the sudden change in loading patterns across the joint. The individual has been loading the joint in an established pattern until the realignment procedure changed the loading pattern. The soft tissues need adequate time to remodel and adapt to the change. How well the tissues adapt varies significantly from individual to individual, accounting for the variation in intervention choices, treatment frequency, and treatment duration. Restoration of normal ROM is essential to ensure distribution of loads over as large a range as possible. Normalization of movement patterns to minimize impact loads and excessive compartmental loading can prolong the life of the osteotomy. Quadriceps strengthening for shock absorption during the loading response of the gait cycle can minimize loads on the articular cartilage and subchondral bone.

TOTAL KNEE ARTHROPLASTY

Individuals with significant bicompartmental (medial and lateral) or tricompartmental (medial, lateral and anterior) osteoarthritis and associated impairments, functional limitations, and disability are candidates for total knee arthroplasty (TKA). These individuals may have undergone previous osteotomies that subsequently deteriorated and may present with impairments such as pain, joint instability, or loss of motion. Pain is one of the chief indications for TKA; stability, bone integrity, and age are additional considerations. Patients generally present for evaluation when the pain becomes disabling, affecting their ability to participate in community, work, leisure, or basic ADLs. The materials

Patient-Related Instruction

Tips to Maintain the Long-Term Health of Your Knee

The following tips can help you maintain the long-term health of your knee:

1. Maintain the mobility of your knee. With your clinician's help, choose a couple of simple exercises to be done daily to maintain your ability to fully bend and straighten your knee.
2. Keep the muscles around your knee strong, especially the muscles in the front of your thigh and your hip muscles. With your clinician's help, choose a couple of simple exercises to be done daily to maintain the strength of your leg.
3. Maintain a healthy body weight.
4. Wear good supportive shoes that provide some shock absorption.
5. Use a supportive device (eg, cane, crutch) when walking long distances.

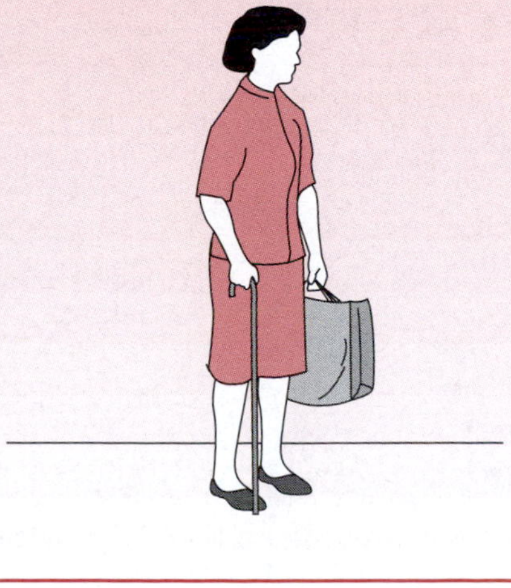

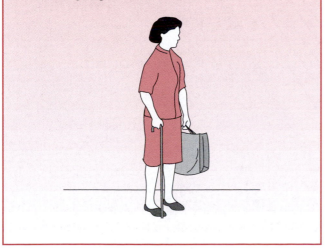

and techniques used in TKA have advanced significantly in the past decade, thereby increasing the patient pool, minimizing complications, and decreasing disability.

The prostheses used are classified in many ways, including the number of compartments replaced (ie, unicompartmental, bicompartmental, or tricompartmental), the degree of constraint (ie, unconstrained, partially constrained, or fully constrained), and the type of fixation (ie, cemented, cementless, or hybrid). The prosthesis choice depends on the status of the bone and any soft tissue deformities (eg, ligament laxity, absence of PCL). Most prostheses are tricompartmental and partially constrained with hybrid fixation. However, other prostheses are used in special cases, and this information should be obtained before initiating treatment.

Several factors affect the rehabilitation approach after TKA. The type of prosthesis provides an indication of the underlying stability, bone quality, and ultimately the prognosis. Fixation choice also affects rehabilitation, with noncemented components protected longer to allow biologic ingrowth. Patellar instability is a problem in 5% to 30% of TKAs, and the clinician should be alert to signs of patellar subluxation or dislocation.[56] Ligamentous stability, particularly varus and valgus stability should be assessed after TKA. Most prosthetic designs assume that no ACL exists and that the PCL is variably intact. The medial and lateral ligaments and joint capsule provide most of the stability. The overall status of the patient's condition and the lower extremity can affect rehabilitation. Individuals with osteoarthritis at the knee may have concurrent changes in other lower extremity joints. Limitations in ROM at the hip and ankle can affect the function and prognosis at the knee. It is reasonable to attempt knee flexion ROM from 0 to 120 degrees or more. Patients with less than 120 degrees of flexion after TKA use compensatory movements of the hip, trunk, and ankle during daily activities.[57]

TREATMENT OF DEGENERATIVE ARTHRITIS PROBLEMS

Interventions used by physical therapists should address the impairments, functional limitations, and disabilities identified during the initial and subsequent evaluations. Impairments should be treated if they are associated with a functional limitation or disability or if continued impairment could lead to disability in the future. For example, limited ROM after abrasion arthroplasty may not be immediately disabling, but it could lead to future functional limitations or disability by overloading focal areas of articular cartilage or by damaging other joints because of compensatory movements. Individuals with articular cartilage damage cannot expect to be cured of their problem, but they must learn to manage their symptoms and maintain the long-term health of their joint. Individuals with joint surface damage must demonstrate an understanding of the home management of impairments, including inflammation, pain, and mobility and strength loss.

After surgery, physical therapy interventions are generally aimed at the immediate impairments of pain, effusion, and loss of motion and neuromuscular control. Physical agents, mechanical and electrotherapeutic modalities, and gentle mobility can minimize pain and facilitate resorption of an effusion. Therapeutic exercise in the form of active and passive mobility, physiologic stretching, or joint mobilization facilitate normal osteokinematics and arthrokinematics. After the surgical incisions are healed or with the use of a bioclusive dressing, many of these impairments can be treated in the pool. The hydrostatic pressure of the water minimizes effusion, and the water's buoyancy limits weight bearing to a comfortable level. If progressive loading of the joint surface is the goal, gradually decreasing the water's depth can slowly increase the joint load. Isometric setting exercises for the quadriceps, hamstrings, and gluteal muscles help re-educate these muscles while facilitating circulation.

In the subacute phase, rehabilitation continues to focus on residual impairments, functional limitations, and disabilities identified during reexamination. Ambulation training and progressive weight bearing advance according to the specific injury and therapeutic procedure. The rehabilitation should continue to focus on restoring full mobility, normalizing gait, and re-establishing full function to the individual. Mobility activities should emphasize activities that enhance articular cartilage nutrition, such as gentle active and passive ROM or compressive loading and unloading. Combining these two modes should be approached with caution to avoid overloading developing or remodeling fibrocartilage or articular cartilage. Closed kinetic chain exercises with significant weight bearing through a ROM should be incorporated judiciously (Fig. 21-23). Strengthening exercises must respect the changes in loading patterns after some surgical procedures. Eccentric strengthening of the quadriceps and gluteals facilitates shock absorption during the loading response phase of gait, stair and incline descent, and lowering into a chair. Strengthening can be initiated in an open kinetic chain and progressed to a closed kinetic chain as the joint allows. Similar exercises must be performed on a daily basis as part of the home exercise program to continue the advances made in the clinic.

The final rehabilitation phase emphasizes return to the previous activity level or higher. For the individual under-

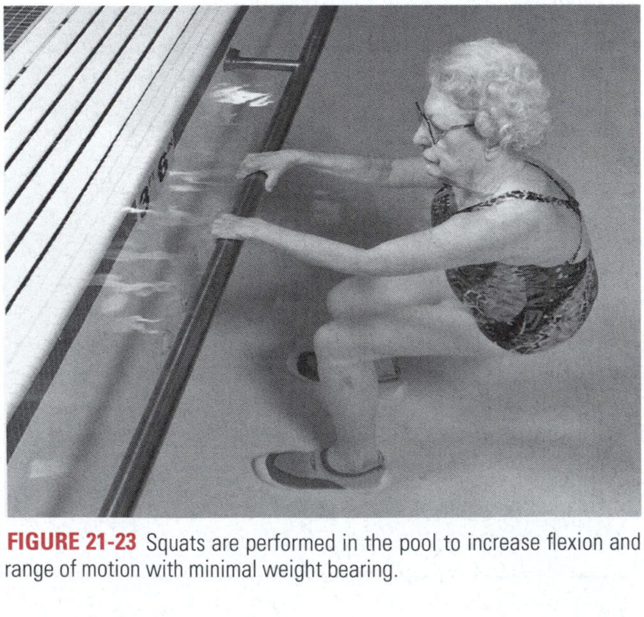

FIGURE 21-23 Squats are performed in the pool to increase flexion and range of motion with minimal weight bearing.

going a tibial osteotomy or TKA, the expectation is return to a higher level of function because of a decrease in pain. Each person should be provided with a functional retraining program tailored to the activities to which she will be returning. Moreover, the importance of continuing an exercise program incorporating activities to maintain the long-term health of the joint must be emphasized. Demonstration of the ability to home manage an exacerbation of symptoms is fundamental to safe and cost-effective long-term management of the knee.

Tendinopathies

Tendinopathies about the knee occur most frequently in the patellar tendon but can also be found in the hamstring tendons and pes anserine tendon. Iliotibial band friction syndrome can be considered a type of tendinopathy. Although tendinopathies can result from an acute injury, they usually are caused by microtrauma or overuse. Repetitive loading without adequate recovery time prevents the normal adaptations to occur. Although single loads do not exceed the strength of the tendon, the cumulative loads exceed the reparative capabilities. Intrinsic factors contributing to tendinopathies include malalignment, limb length discrepancies, and muscular imbalance or insufficiency. Extrinsic factors include training errors, surfaces, environmental conditions, and footwear.[58]

PATELLAR TENDINOPATHIES

Patellar tendinopathy occurs at the distal pole of the patella, and is distinct from Sinding-Larsen-Johanssen disease, which is apophysitis of the distal patellar pole, and from Osgood-Schlatter disease, which is apophysitis at the tibial tubercle. Both of these syndromes occur in adolescents before closure of the growth plates. Patellar tendinopathy has also been called *jumper's knee* because of its high prevalence in jumping and impact sports. The eccentric nature of jumping places tremendous loads on the patellar tendon, often resulting in overuse. The patellar tendon attaches one of the strongest muscles in the body, the quadriceps femoris, to its insertion using the patella as a "balance." The loads generated by the quadriceps mechanism are transmitted through the tendon to its bony attachments. Areas of increased stress such as transitional zones are susceptible to overuse. In the adult with closed epiphyses, the transition zone on the undersurface of the patella's distal pole is the most vulnerable area.

Tendinopathies of the patellar tendon can take various forms. All tendinopathies tend to demonstrate a normal macroscopic appearance without any gross degeneration of the tendon, but microscopic abnormalities at the bone-tendon junction most always exist.[59] Necrosis and fragmented tissues with mucoid degeneration usually involve the deep central fibers at the tendinous insertion and can be palpated at the undersurface of the patella's distal pole.[60]

Individuals with patellar tendinopathies present with various degrees of impairments, functional limitations, and disabilities. The person often reports a history of pain and stiffness in the anterior knee that improves as the knee is warmed, gets sore as the activity continues, and gets stiff and sore after completion of the activity. Point tenderness is experienced on the undersurface of the distal pole of the patella and is best palpated by tipping the inferior border anteriorly to allow access to the undersurface. Functional limitations may include abnormal walking or running gait, pain with jumping or kneeling, or pain when ascending and descending stairs. Disabilities can include an inability to participate in community, work, or leisure activities, depending on the individual's lifestyle and functional limitations. Blazina[61] categorized patellar tendinitis in athletes in four stages, based on the pain history (Display 21-3). Poor postural habit, such as standing with the knees hyperextended, can contribute to patellar tendinitis because of a shortening of the quadriceps and patellar tendon.

Treatment

Rehabilitation for the individual with patellar tendinopathies focuses on the patellar tendon's role in decelerating knee flexion in gait, jumping, descending stairs, and many other functional activities. The role of tendon length and speed relative to deceleration activities forms the foundation for the rehabilitation program. Stretching exercises to ensure adequate tendon length are combined with eccentric quadriceps contractions of progressively increasing velocity up to the speeds used in daily activities. Before an individual can perform an eccentric muscle contraction, she must be able to preset isometric tension in the muscle. The rehabilitation program may begin with isometric contractions before progressing to eccentric contractions. To create an optimal healing environment, adjuncts to the therapeutic exercise program are used and typically include forms of cryotherapy. Deep-heat modalities should be used judiciously in highly active individuals, because simple ADLs can perpetuate an acute inflammation. Postural retraining should be incorporated with appropriate patellar mobilization and soft tissue stretching.

ILIOTIBIAL BAND SYNDROME

Iliotibial band syndrome is a common cause of lateral knee pain in individuals who regularly jog, bicycle, or walk for exercise. Postural problems such as anterior pelvic tilt or knee hyperextension along with poor mechanics such as decreased gluteus medius or VMO activity can be predisposing factors.

DISPLAY 21-3

The Blazina Classification for Functional Limitations Associated With Patellar Tendinitis

Stage 1: Pain after sports activity
Stage 2: Pain at the beginning of sports activity, disappearing with warm-up and sometimes reappearing with fatigue
Stage 3: Pain at rest and during activity; inability to participate in sports
Stage 4: Rupture of the patellar tendon

Blazina ME, Kerlan RK, Jobe FW. Jumper's knee. Orthop Clin North Am. *1973;4:665–678.*

These factors should be identified during the examination process to ensure comprehensive treatment.

The individual presenting with iliotibial band syndrome often complains of a sharp, stabbing pain at the lateral epicondyle that begins with the onset of activity and worsens as the activity progresses. Palpable tenderness over the lateral epicondyle can confirm the diagnosis. Predisposing factors such as poor postural habit or muscle imbalance should be identified during the examination. Hamstring, gluteal, quadriceps, and iliotibial band flexibility should be assessed. Any impairments or functional limitations identified during the examination should form the basis for the rehabilitation program. In many cases, a combination of predisposing factors, activity choices, and impairments converge to produce iliotibial band syndrome.

Treatment

Rehabilitation focuses on the identification and treatment of predisposing factors, impairments, and functional limitations. Patient education regarding these factors and conscientious participation in self-managing this problem contribute to a successful outcome. Postural education and identification of the underlying impairments (eg, hip rotator weakness) provide the foundation for appropriate stretching or strengthening exercises. Stretching for the hip and knee musculature with emphasis on good posture is the mainstay of treatment. These stretches may be performed on land or in the pool (see Figs. 21-8 through 21-11). Iontophoresis and ice may be used to treat pain and inflammation associated with this problem.

Patellofemoral Pain

The continuum of patellofemoral pain can arise from trauma (eg, blow, fall, dislocation) or overuse (eg, continued activity, kneeling position, excessive squatting). True chondral degeneration, or chondromalacia, can occur on the patellar or femoral surfaces. This degeneration can be a result of lateral patellar tracking and excessive compressive forces at the patellofemoral joint. Habitual areas of noncontact, such as the medial odd facet, are common areas of degeneration. Early degeneration can be worsened by prolonged immobilization or inactivity. Active individuals are at risk of cartilage damage when going from low levels of stress to high levels of stress. A gradual transition in activity level is the key to rehabilitation, because it progressively stresses the articular cartilage to stimulate growth. Patients should be advised of the need for activity modification in preparation for activity level changes.

Lateral patellar tracking can be caused by static or dynamic forces. Static patellar tracking refers to the patellar position at rest and during passive ROM, and it is influenced primarily by the length of the lateral structures, including the lateral retinacula and the iliotibial band. With static lateral tracking, the patella laterally tilts or glides excessively throughout the ROM. Because of the dynamic relationships between the hip and knee soft tissues, the patellar position changes with different hip and knee positions. For example, the gluteus maximus portion of the iliotibial band tightens with increasing hip flexion, adduction, or medial rotation, and the tensor fascia lata component tightens with increasing hip extension, adduction, or lateral rotation.

Dynamic lateral tracking refers to the patellar position under the influence of muscle contraction. The patellar position may remain the same or be worsened with a quadriceps contraction. If it remains the same, dynamic structures are balanced, whereas a worsening indicates an imbalance of the VMO and VL. Most often, a combination of static and dynamic components influences patellar position and tracking.

In addition to medial-lateral balance, malalignments can occur in rotation and in posterior positioning of the inferior pole. The rotation component is designated by the inferior pole, and external rotation refers to a lateral alignment of the inferior pole relative to the line of the femur. Although internal rotation can also occur, external rotation is most common. These rotations are influenced by which part of the lateral retinaculum is tight and therefore spins the patella like a wheel. Rotations are discussed relative to the static position because a quadriceps contraction makes this component difficult to evaluate.

The posterior displacement of the inferior pole (ie, anteroposterior component) can cause pain and often occurs in individuals with knee hyperextension in standing or gait patterns. Posterior displacement may be found statically because of lateral retinacular shortening or dynamically because of VMO and VL imbalance. For rehabilitation, controlling the amount of hyperextension in standing and gait is critical to managing the symptoms related to the anteroposterior component of maltracking.

Symptoms of patellofemoral pain can be confused with and may coexist with other knee disorders. Generally, individuals with patellofemoral pain complain of a diffuse ache around the knee. Inferiorly, pain is often caused by irritation of the infrapatellar fat pad, and anteromedial pain may result from a stretched medial retinaculum caused by lateral tracking. Pain in the anterolateral aspect of the knee may be produced by a shortened lateral retinaculum, possibly producing a neuroma. Pain with activity such as ascending or descending stairs is a common complaint, and pain with prolonged sitting (ie, movie goer's sign) is common in those with a tight lateral retinaculum.

Swelling may or may not be detectable in patients with patellofemoral pain. Swelling is usually mild, although even small quantities of fluid can result in VMO atrophy. Spencer and Hayes[24] found inhibition to occur with only 30 to 40 mL of fluid in the knee joint, an amount barely detectable by observation. This finding may explain why those with ACL reconstructions have difficulty recruiting the VMO in the presence of mild effusion.

Locking and giving way are are common complaints of patients with patellofemoral pain. Giving way can be confused with cruciate ligament injury, and symptoms of locking can be confused with meniscal injuries. However, those with cruciate ligament injuries tend to experience instability during rotational activities, and those with patellofemoral pain experience instability during straight-plane motions. Meniscal injuries tend to require passive movements to unlock the knee, and patellofemoral locking can be unlocked with active movement. A careful history and evaluation can exclude other causes of knee pain.

Normal patellar tracking requires a delicate balance of soft tissues and proper bony alignment. Patellar dynamics can be influenced by the quadriceps angle, tight lateral structures, muscle shortening, excessive pronation, patella alta, and VMO insufficiency. These factors must be considered in the overall evaluation process. The more complex cases resolve slowly because of the severity or multiplicity of influences on joint biomechanics.

The Q angle represents the line of pull of the quadriceps muscle, and alterations have been implicated in the development of patellofemoral pain.[25] The normal Q angle is considered to be 12 to 15 degrees for males and 15 to 18 degrees for females.[25] Because patellar complaints typically involve weight bearing, it is important to observe the Q angle during dynamic activities such as standing, walking, and descending stairs. The dynamic Q angle is rarely the same as the static Q angle and is strongly influenced by muscle recruitment patterns and by hip and foot structural alignment (eg, foot pronation, hip anteversion, tibial torsion).

Excessive foot pronation can influence patellar alignment and alignment of the entire lower extremity. Many foot types can produce symptomatic pronation (see Chapter 22). In the closed chain, pronation causes internal rotation of the tibia, which causes internal rotation of the femur. Rotation increases the dynamic Q angle, and subsequent lateral vector forces contribute to lateral tracking.

Other structural faults at the hip, knee, and foot may influence patellar alignment directly or indirectly. A shallow lateral femoral condyle, femoral anteversion or retroversion, and coxa valgus or varus in addition to foot pronation influence the static and dynamic Q angles. These findings are important in determining the individual's prognosis. Although the clinician may have little influence over these structural factors, they should be considered during the exercise and education program.

Because of the multitude of factors influencing patellofemoral mechanics, the assessment should include a complete examination of all potentially contributing factors. The overall alignment of the lower extremity in standing and during movement is the most important component to consider when examining and treating the individual with patellofemoral pain (see the Examination and Evaluation section of this chapter). The relative importance and interactions of these components influence the treatment chosen by the clinician.

TREATMENT

Treatment must correlate with the significant findings of the examination. Therapeutic exercise components of the rehabilitation program most often include VMO re-education using surface EMG, hip and foot muscle re-education, stretching, EMG-triggered electrical stimulation, and work-, ADL-, or sport-specific retraining. Other adjunctive treatment components are taping, soft tissue mobilization or myofascial release, mobilization of peripatellar soft tissues, cryotherapy, and orthotics. Because of the chronic nature of patellofemoral pain, specific treatment phases (eg, acute, subacute) are not included in the treatment program.

TREATMENT METHODS

Vastus Medialis Obliquus Re-education

VMO re-education provides a foundation for advanced functional activity progressions. Examination and treatment of VMO insufficiency is simplified with the use of surface EMG. Use of the 1:1 ratio for the VMO and VL contributions is helpful for patient training and goal setting. The positions for training vary according to specific impairments or functional limitations, activity levels, and the irritability of the condition. Because the purpose of the activity is muscle re-education, a few repetitions are performed several times throughout the day. The short duration also minimizes VMO fatigue and resultant VL dominance. Prolonged training beyond VMO fatigue can promote muscle imbalance. As muscle endurance improves, training should increase in intensity and duration. The training should address functional limitations as much as possible, and exercises are often performed in a closed kinetic chain.

In a sitting position, the VMO may be retrained in multiple positions of knee flexion with the foot firmly fixed on the ground at all times. Isometrics should be performed at 10- to 15-degree intervals between 5 and 90 degrees of flexion. Because the VMO arises from the adductor magnus, simultaneous hip adduction may help some individuals to fire the VMO. Careful attention to this activity can prevent hip internal rotator substitution. The hip, patella, and second toe should be aligned and respond to verbal cues such as "pull the patella up and in" or "pull the knee inward without allowing any movement" (Fig. 21-24).

In a standing position, VMO training becomes more difficult but also more functional. With the knee in full or nearly full extension, the patella is unsupported by the trochlear groove. The VL is quite active in this position. Training should begin with good postural alignment, with the individual standing with the knees slightly unlocked. The hip, knee, and foot should remain in good alignment,

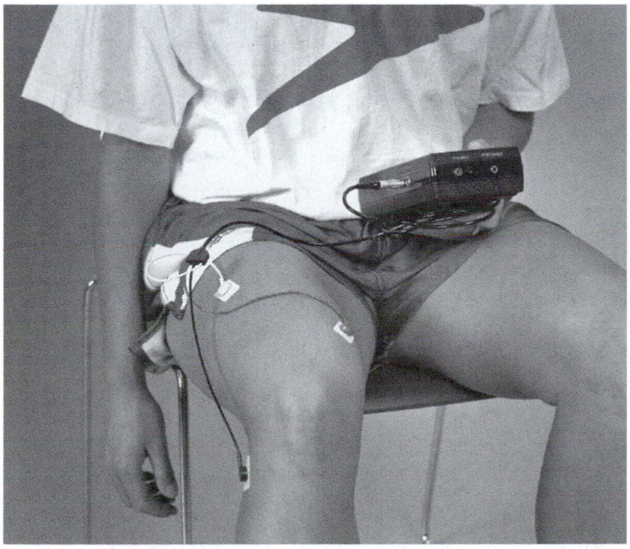

FIGURE 21-24 VMO training in a sitting position.

and the same verbal cues used in the sitting position may be used in the standing position (Fig. 21-25). These standing isometric exercises should be performed frequently throughout the day for short intervals.

The partial squat position can be used to train the VMO isometrically at 10- to 15-degree intervals. Individuals with patellofemoral pain often find this position less challenging because of the bony stability provided by the patella in the trochlear groove. As VMO control at the various angles improves, the exercise may be progressed to a fluid, dynamic motion, starting in the extended position and flexing. The activity may also be started in a position in which producing a strong contraction is easy and then move into the more challenging parts of the ROM (Fig. 21-26).

The wall slide is useful for those having difficulty with VL dominance in the standing position. The VL seems to be less active in this position and therefore allows greater VMO recruitment. With the back against the wall, the feet well away from the wall, and the hip, knee, and foot in good alignment, the individual can perform isometrics at multiple angles or can slide dynamically, as with the partial squat exercise. The individual should be positioned such that the tibia remains vertical and the knees remain posterior to the feet. An adductor squeeze can also be used in this position by those having difficulty with VMO recruitment.

The walk stance or single-leg stance position is used to begin retraining for gait. Full weight should be placed on the involved leg, and the toe of the uninvolved leg may be used for balance. The knee should be positioned in a few degrees of flexion, but the concepts of training in the partial squat position can be carried over to this position. This exercise can be progressed by rocking back and forth in the in the sagittal plane to practice VMO recruitment simultaneously with weight acceptance (Fig. 21-27).

Step-down exercises are important as stairs are a problem for most individuals with patellofemoral pain. Many individuals have poor eccentric control during stair descent and drop off the step and catch their body weight with the uninvolved leg. When asked to control the step-down motion, many are unable to do so because of pain or inadequate muscle control. Initially, a small step should be used if a larger step causes pain or loss of control. The individual

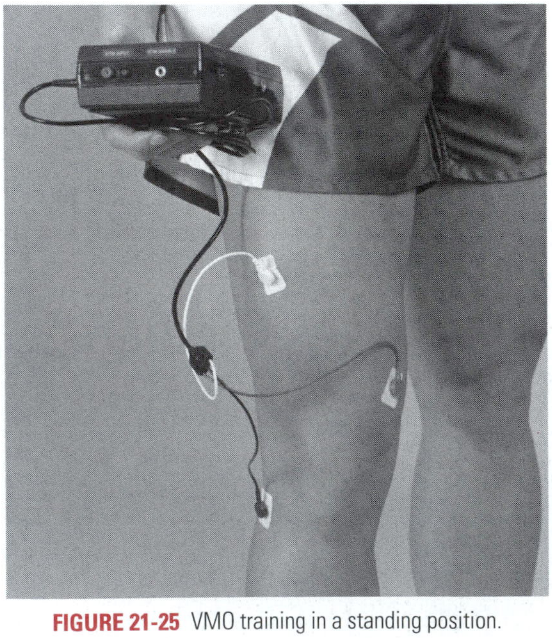

FIGURE 21-25 VMO training in a standing position.

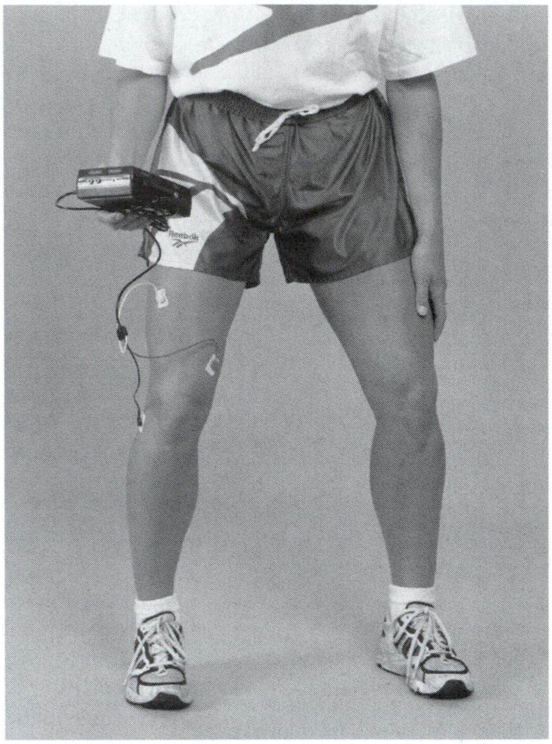

FIGURE 21-26 VMO training in a partial squat position.

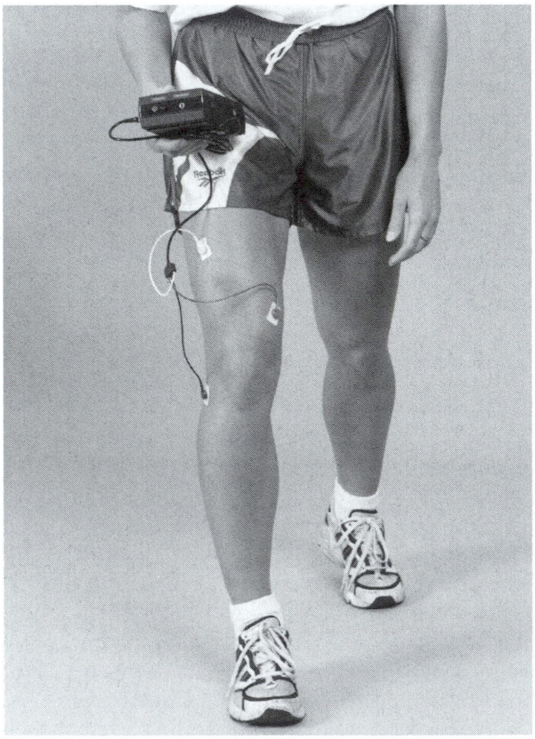

FIGURE 21-27 VMO training in a walk stance position.

should move slowly enough to be able to stop at any point during the motion. Close observation can detect poor alignment of the hip, knee, and ankle or substitution at the hip. At later stages, the speed and step height should be increased to approximate normal function.

As the individual demonstrates continuing control over the VMO in static positions, more challenging dynamic activities such as gait should be encouraged. Starting from the walk stance position, a VMO contraction should be elicited and held while slowly shifting the weight forward as in gait. The VMO should be relaxed during the swing phase of gait. With improvement, the speed can be increased until a normal gait pattern is assumed. Success with slow movement must be ensured before speed is increased.

The vastus medialis can be added to many exercise regimens with leg presses, jumping, squats, lunges, resistive cord exercises, stairstepping, and balance and agility drills. These training exercises should be specific for the functional activities to which the patient will return. Someone returning to bowling should be trained in the lunge position, and a freight truck driver should be trained during lifting (Fig. 21-28).

Adjunctive Interventions

Patellar taping is a useful adjunct to the training program. Taping can reduce pain and is specific to each patellar orientation. Taping can be used to correct the components of lateral tilt, lateral glide, rotation, and anteroposterior tilt and to treat patellar tendinitis, unload the fat pad, and inhibit the VL. The tape should be adjusted to provide immediate relief of symptoms, and it is worn all day and in conjunction with training and activity. As the individual gains control of the VMO, taping should be eliminated. Patellar taping can enhance VMO recruitment and quadriceps torque production.[62]

Mobilization should address the tightness of the lateral retinaculum. Although the clinician should mobilize the lateral retinaculum, the patient should be instructed in a self-mobilization technique. This procedure is performed in the sitting position, with the patient's hand on the medial aspect of the patella while a posteriorly directed force is applied. This force produces a patellar tilt and stretch of the deep fibers of the lateral retinaculum. Like re-education exercises, this mobilization should be performed several times throughout the day and can be performed at multiple angles of knee flexion.

Stretching exercises for the hamstrings, gastrocnemius, and iliotibial tract should be incorporated based on the examination findings. A simple active hamstring and gastrocnemius exercise that can be performed in sitting is appropriate and convenient for most patients. In a sitting position, the patient should support the low back with a firm hand support to maintain the lumbar lordosis. She slowly extends the lower leg while maintaining this lumbar lordosis. At the end of the comfortable ROM, she dorsiflexes the foot and holds for 15 to 30 seconds. This exercise can be performed frequently throughout the day (see Self-Management: Hamstring and Gastrocnemius Stretching While Maintaining a Lumbar Neutral Position).

Surface EMG can be used as an adjunct to all of the aforementioned exercises, with the exception of the patellar mobilization. EMG-triggered electrical stimulation can be useful for patients with severe atrophy or poor recruitment of the VMO despite efforts with surface EMG. The same exercises or positions can be used as with the VMO training outlined previously.

Postoperative Rehabilitation

The three common types of surgical procedures for the patellofemoral joint are chondroplasties for debridement

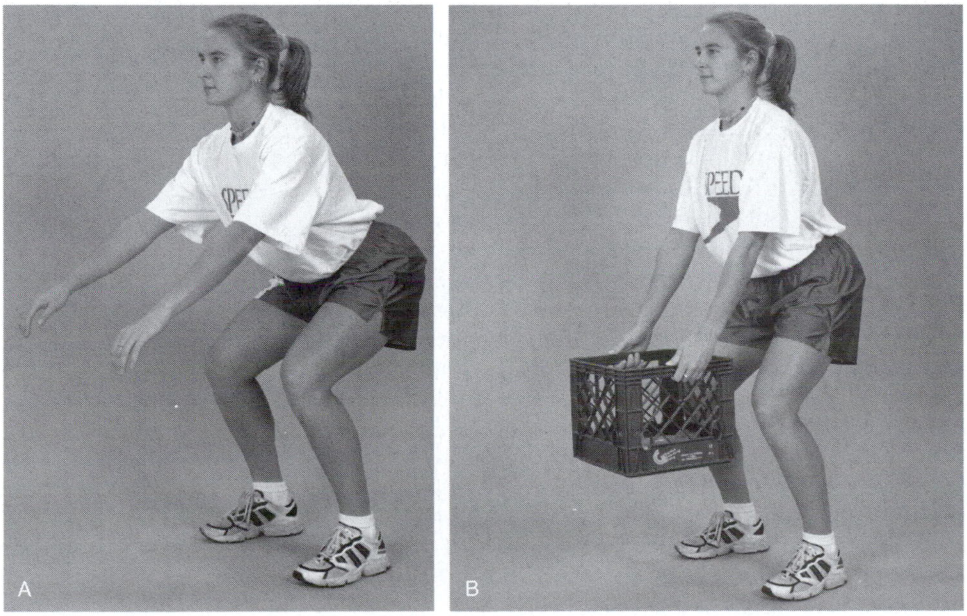

FIGURE 21-28 ***(A)*** Patient performing a squat exercise. ***(B)*** Progressing to a lifting exercise.

SELF-MANAGEMENT: Hamstring and Gastrocnemius Stretching While Maintaining a Lumbar Neutral Position

Purpose: To increase the flexibility of the hamstring and calf muscles

Position: In a sitting position, place one hand behind your back to maintain the proper position of your lower back.

Movement technique: Maintaining this position, slowly straighten the knee until you feel a gentle stretch behind your thigh. While holding this position, pull your toes up, flexing your ankle until you feel a gentle stretch behind your calf. Hold for 15 to 30 seconds.

Repetitions:_______ times

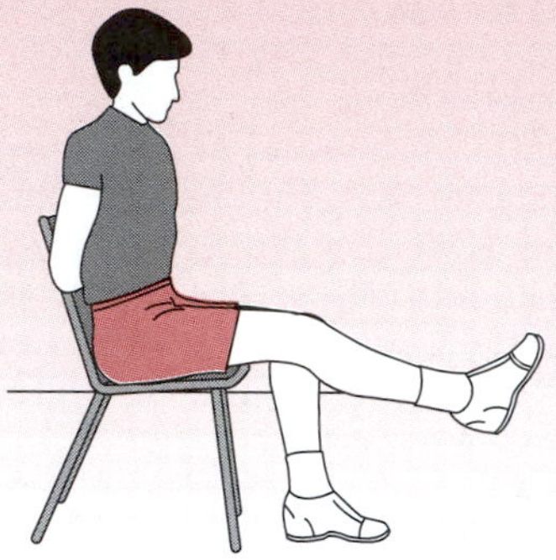

of patellar or femoral chondral degeneration, lateral retinacular release for the severely restricted lateral retinaculum, and realignment procedures for those with more complicated biomechanical problems. Rehabilitation after any of these procedures should follow the program as previously outlined. With simple chondroplasties, the program should progress without problems unless significant pain or swelling exists. If more progressive chondral damage has occurred, more caution should be placed on gradual and careful reintroduction of activity and exercise to allow the accommodation of the chondral surfaces. With lateral retinacular releases, care should be taken to ensure the lateral retinaculum does not adhere to surrounding soft tissues. Aggressive releases must be progressed much more slowly than conservative releases, because postoperative pain and large amounts of edema are common. The time for recovery and the length of rehabilitation may also be prolonged as a result of aggressive surgery. Realignment procedures can be complex. The same principles of rehabilitation apply, with VMO reeducation and alignment training as critical components of a successful program.

Re-education at Adjacent Joints

Hip muscle re-education is often overlooked during patellofemoral joint rehabilitation. Contraction of the gluteus medius posterior and the hip lateral rotators can dramatically improve the hip, knee, and foot alignment. Individuals with patellofemoral pain often demonstrate gluteus medius weakness that increases the demand on the iliotibial tract to support the hip. Eventually, the iliotibial tract can lose extensibility and displace anteriorly, contributing to lateral tracking of the patella. Gluteus medius and hip lateral rotator function is important to maintain balance at the hip and optimal lower quadrant kinetics and kinematics. Gluteus medius retraining is best performed in the positions mentioned earlier and in conjunction with VMO contraction. Ultimately, it is crucial to use this muscle properly during gait.

The foot position can also influence the lower extremity alignment and should be observed during the exercise program. Foot muscle training is best performed in the positions used for the VMO exercises and requires the individual to improve the alignment of the foot in relation to the leg and subtalar joint. This approach includes educating and training the individual to recognize a position close to the neutral position of the foot for all standing activities. As the individual lifts the arch, it is important to observe for anterior tibialis substitution. The tibialis posterior should lift the subtalar joint while the peroneus longus stabilizes the great toe. Pressing down through the great toe is often a beneficial cue to facilitate correct alignment and appropriate muscle recruitment.

Key Points

- The relationships among the lumbopelvic, hip, knee, ankle, and foot necessitate a thorough examination and an integrated approach to treatment.
- The major anatomic impairments at the knee are genu valgum and genu varum. These postures predispose the lateral and medial compartments, respectively, to excessive loads.
- Physiologic impairments such as mobility loss at the knee can be compensated by motion at other joints. For example, increased ankle, hip, or lumbar motion can compensate for decreased knee flexion.
- Because of these compensations and the relationships among joints, therapeutic exercises may be performed incorrectly, allowing substitution to occur.
- Palpation, education, and biofeedback are techniques to ensure proper muscle firing patterns without substitution during rehabilitative exercises.
- Examination of the patellofemoral joint must include muscle length at the hip, knee, and ankle and the patellar position relative to glide, tilt, and rotation.
- Loss of the meniscus can lead to degenerative joint disease. Treatment after meniscectomy should focus on preservation of articular cartilage and joint protection techniques.
- The major function of the quadriceps muscle in the long-term health of the knee is its ability to absorb shock eccentrically in the loading phase of the gait cycle. A focus

LAB ACTIVITIES

1. Demonstrate the likely gait pattern if your quadriceps strength was 3/5.
2. Demonstrate three strengthening exercises to treat quadriceps strength impairment, given a strength grade of 3/5.
3. Demonstrate two exercises to treat the functional limitations seen in the gait pattern.
4. Is an assistive device necessary? If so, what would you choose for this patient if she had no other impairments? Fit and instruct the patient in use of the device.
5. Demonstrate the likely gait pattern if the patient's quadriceps strength was 2/5.
6. Demonstrate three strengthening exercises to treat the quadriceps strength impairment, given a strength grade of 2/5.
7. Refer to Case Study #2 in Unit 7. Instruct your patient in the first phase of the exercise program. Have your patient demonstrate all exercises.
8. Identify (palpate or point out the location of) the following structures:
   a. Medial tibial plateau
   b. Tibial tuberosity
   c. Medial femoral condyle
   d. Adductor tubercle
   e. Lateral tibial plateau
   f. Fibular head (which nerve?)
   g. Medial and lateral patellar facets
   h. Pes anserine tendon
   i. Medial and lateral joint lines
   j. MCL and LCL
   k. Semitendinous tendon
   l. Semimembranosus tendon
   m. Biceps femoris tendon
9. Determine your patient's 10 repetition maximum for a straight-leg raise with the weight.
   a. At the ankle
   b. Above the knee
10. Teach your patient how to check VMO firing during the following activities:
   a. Isometric quadriceps contraction while
      i. Sitting with the knee at 90 degrees
      ii. Sitting with the knee at 70 degrees
      iii. Sitting with the knee at 45 degrees
      iv. Sitting with the knee at 30 degrees
      vi. sitting with the knee at 0 degrees
   b. Wall slide
   c. Sit to stand
   d. Lunge
   e. Gait

on eccentric, closed chain quadriceps exercise in the first 0 to 15 degrees of flexion is essential to maintain the health of articular cartilage.

- Patellar tendinitis results from the tendon's inability to withstand eccentric forces during impact activities. The rehabilitation program must eventually progress to eccentric impact activities if the patient is to return to this type of activity.

Critical Thinking Questions

1. Read Case Study #6 in Unit 7.
   a. List the patient's impairments and functional limitations.
   b. Describe the relationship between this patient's impairments and functional limitations.
   c. Describe the relationship between this patient's impairments, functional limitations, and any disability.
   d. Identify and prioritize short- and long-term goals.
   e. Choose a specific goal, and describe five different exercises used to achieve that goal. Include posture, mode, and movement.
   f. This patient is returning to work as a delivery truck driver. Describe three functional exercises that can prepare him for this activity.
   g. Presume that this same patient is returning to work as a basketball referee. Describe three functional exercises that can prepare him for this activity.
2. Read Case Study #3 in Unit 7.
   a. Describe three exercises to address her difficulty with stairs. Include posture, mode, movement, and precautions.
   b. Given her history, describe three exercises to increase the endurance of her quadriceps muscles. Include posture, mode, movement, and precautions.
   c. Describe three exercises to increase the endurance of her calf muscles. Include posture, mode, movement, and precautions.
   d. The patient no longer feels any muscle fatigue when performing the exercises outlined in questions b and c. Describe how you would progress each of these exercises. Include dosage parameters.

REFERENCES

1. Beynnon BD, Fleming BC, Johnson RJ, et al. Anterior cruciate ligament strain behavior during rehabilitation exercises in vivo. *Am J Sports Med.* 1995;23:24.
2. Yack HJ. Comparison of closed and open kinetic chain exercise in the ACL-deficient knee. *Am J Sports Med.* 1993;21:49.
3. Yack HJ. Anterior tibial translation during progressive loading of the ACL-deficient knee during weight bearing and nonweight-bearing exercise. *J Orthop Sports Phys Ther.* 1994; 20:247.
4. Parker MG. Biomechanical and histological concepts in the rehabilitation of patients with anterior cruciate ligament reconstructions. *J Orthop Sports Phys Ther.* 1994;20:44–50.

5. Ciccotti MG, Kerlan RK, Perry J, Pink M. An electromyographic analysis of the knee during functional activities: the normal profile. *Am J Sports Med.* 1994;22:645–650.
6. Moore KL. *Clinically Oriented Anatomy.* Baltimore: Williams & Wilkins; 1980.
7. Pratt NE. *Clinical Musculoskeletal Anatomy.* Philadelphia: JB Lippincott; 1991.
8. Norkin CC, Levangie PK. *Joint Structure and Function: A Comprehensive Analysis.* 2nd ed. Philadelphia: FA Davis; 1992.
9. Insall JN. Anatomy of the knee. In: Insall JN, ed. *Surgery of the Knee.* New York: Churchill Livingstone; 1984:1–20.
10. Williams PL, Warwick R, Dyson M, Bannister LH, eds. *Gray's Anatomy.* 37th ed. New York: Churchill Livingstone; 1989.
11. Fulkerson J, Hungerford D. *Disorders of the Patellofemoral Joint.* 2nd ed. Baltimore: Williams & Wilkins; 1990.
12. Dye SF. Patellofemoral anatomy. In: Fox JM, Del Pizzo W, eds. *The Patellofemoral Joint.* New York: McGraw-Hill; 1993:1–13.
13. Hutchinson MR, Ireland ML. Knee injuries in female athletes. *Sports Med.* 1995;19:222–236.
14. Lund-Hanssen H, Gannon J, Engebretsen L, Holen KJ, Anda S, Vatten L. Intercondylar notch width and the risk for anterior cruciate ligament rupture. *Acta Orthop Scand.* 1994;65:529–532.
15. Harner CK, Xerogeanes JW, Givesay GA, et al. The human posterior cruciate ligament complex: an interdisciplinary study. *Am J Sports Med.* 1995;23:736–745.
16. Fu F, Thompson WO. Biomechanics and kinematics of meniscus. In: Finerman GAM, Noyes FR, eds. *Biology and Biomechanics of the Traumatized Synovial Joint: The Knee as Model.* Rosemont, IL: American Academy of Orthopaedic Surgeons; 1992:153–184.
17. Kendall FP, McCreary EK, Provance PG. *Muscles Testing and Function.* 4th ed. Baltimore: Williams & Wilkins; 1993.
18. Torzilli PA. Biomechanical analysis of knee stability. In: Nicholas JA, Hershman EB, eds. *The Lower Extremity and Spine in Sportsmedicine.* St. Louis: CV Mosby; 1986:728–764.
19. Peterson L, Frankel VH. Biomechanics of the knee in athletes. In: Nicholas JA, Hershman EB, eds. *The Lower Extremity and Spine in Sportsmedicine.* St. Louis: CV Mosby; 1986:695–727.
20. Hungerford DS, Barry M. Biomechanics of the patellofemoral joint. *Clin Orthop.* 1979;144:11.
21. Reilly DT, Martens M. Experimental analysis of the quadriceps muscle force for various activities. *Acta Orthop Scand.* 1972;43:126–137.
22. Voight ML, Weider DL. Comparative reflex response times of vastus medialis obliquus and vastus lateralis in normal subjects with extensor mechanism dysfunction. *Am J Sports Med.* 1991;19:131–137.
23. Mariani P, Caruso I. An electromyographic investigation of subluxation of the patella. *J Bone Joint Surg.* 1979;61:169–171.
24. Spencer J, Hayes K, Alexander I. Knee joint effusion and quadriceps reflex inhibition in man. *Arch Phys Med.* 1984;65:171–177.
25. Magee D. *Orthopedic Physical Assessment.* 3rd ed. Philadelphia: WB Saunders; 1997.
26. Karst G, Willett G. Onset timing of electromyographic activity in the vastus medialis oblique and vastus lateralis muscle in subjects with and without patellofemoral pain syndrome. *Phys Ther.* 1995;75:813–823.
27. Witvrouw E, Sneyers C, Lysens R, Victor J, Bellemans J. Reflex response times of vastus medialis oblique and vastus lateralis in normal subjects and in subjects with patellofemoral pain syndrome. *J Orthop Sports Phys Ther.* 1996;24:160–165.
28. Galloway MT, Grood ED. Posterior cruciate ligament insufficiency and reconstruction. In: Finerman GAM, Noyes FR, eds. *Biology and Biomechanics of the Traumatized Synovial Joint: The Knee as Model.* Rosemont, IL: American Academy of Orthopaedic Surgeons; 1992:531–550.
29. Butler DL, Noyes FR, Grood ES. Ligamentous restraints to anterior-posterior drawer in the human knee: a biomechanical study. *J Bone Joint Surg Am.* 1980:62:259–270.
30. Fukubayashi T, Torzilli PA, Sherman MF, Warren RF. An in vitro biomechanical evaluation of anterior-posterior motion of the knee: tibial displacement, rotation, and torque. *J Bone Joint Surg Am.* 1982:64:258–264.
31. Clancy WG, Shelbourne KD, Zoellner GB, et al. Treatment of knee joint instability secondary to rupture of the posterior cruciate ligament: report of a new procedure. *J Bone Joint Surg Am.* 1983:65:310–322.
32. Zarins B, Boyle J. Knee ligament injuries. In: Nicholas JA, Hershman EB, eds. *The Lower Extremity and Spine in Sportsmedicine.* St. Louis: CV Mosby; 1986:929–982.
33. Fetto JF, Marshall JL. Medial collateral ligament injuries of the knee: a rationale for treatment. *Clin Orthop.* 1978;132:206–218.
34. Woo SL-Y, Newton PO, MacKenna DA, Lyon RM. A comparative evaluation of the mechanical properties of the rabbit medial collateral and anterior cruciate ligaments. *J Biomech.* 1992;25:377–386.
35. Woo SL-Y, Inoue M, McGurk-Burleson E, Gomez MA. Treatment of the medial collateral ligament injury: II. Structure and function of canine knees in response to differing treatment regimens. *Am J Sports Med.* 1987;15:22–29.
36. Woo SL-Y, Ohland KJ, McMahon PJ. Biology, healing and repair of ligaments. In: Finerman GAM, Noyes FR, eds. *Biology and Biomechanics of the Traumatized Synovial Joint: The Knee as Model.* Rosemont, IL: American Academy of Orthopaedic Surgeons; 1992:241–274.
37. Aglietti P, Chambat P. Fractures of the knee. In: Insall JN, ed. *Surgery of the Knee.* New York: Churchill Livingstone; 1984:395–412.
38. Salter RB. *Textbook of Disorders and Injuries of the Musculoskeletal System.* 2nd ed. Baltimore: Williams & Wilkins; 1983.
39. Arnoczky S, Adams M, DeHaven K, et al. Meniscus. In: Woo SL-Y, Buckwalter JA, eds. *Injury and Repair of the Musculoskeletal Soft Tissues.* Park Ridge, IL: American Academy of Orthopaedic Surgeons; 1988:487–537.
40. Ahmed AM, Burke DL. In vitro measurement of static pressure distribution in synovial joints: Part I. Tibial surface of the knee. *J Biomech Eng.* 1983;105:216–225.
41. Baratz ME, Fu FH, Mengato R. Meniscal tears: the effect of meniscectomy and of repair on intraarticular contact areas and stress in the human knee. *Am J Sports Med.* 1986;14:270–275.
42. Fairbank TJ. Knee joint changes after meniscectomy. *J Bone Joint Surg Br.* 1948;30:664–670.
43. Fitzgibbons RE, Shelbourne KD. "Aggressive" nontreatment of lateral meniscal tears seen during anterior cruciate ligament reconstruction. *Am J Sports Med.* 1995;23:156–165.
44. DeHaven KE, Arnoczky SP. Meniscal repair. In: Finerman GAM, Noyes FR, eds. *Biology and Biomechanics of the Traumatized Synovial Joint: The Knee as Model.* Rosemont, IL: American Academy of Orthopaedic Surgeons; 1992:185–202.
45. Buckwalter J, Hunziker E, Rosenberg L, et al. Articular cartilage: composition and structure. In: Woo SL-Y, Buckwalter JA, eds. *Injury and Repair of the Musculoskeletal Soft Tissues.* Park Ridge, IL: American Academy of Orthopaedic Surgeons; 1988:405–426.

46. Mow V, Rosenwasser M. Articular cartilage: biomechanics. In: Woo SL-Y, Buckwalter JA, eds. *Injury and Repair of the Musculoskeletal Soft Tissues*. Park Ridge, IL: American Academy of Orthopaedic Surgeons; 1988:427–463.
47. Coventry MB. Proximal tibial varus osteotomy for osteoarthritis of the lateral compartment of the knee. *J Bone Joint Surg Am*. 1987;69:32–38.
48. Coventry MB. Proximal tibial osteotomy. *Orthop Rev*. 1988;17:456–458.
49. Noyes FR, Barber SD, Simon R. High tibial osteotomy and ligament reconstruction in varus angulated, anterior cruciate ligament-deficient knees. *Am J Sports Med*. 1993;21:2–12.
50. Hernigou P, Medeviell D, Deberyre J, Goutallier D. Proximal tibial osteotomy for osteoarthritis with varus deformity. *J Bone Joint Surg Am*. 1987;69:332–354.
51. Kettelkamp DB, Leach RE, Nasca R. Pitfalls of proximal tibial osteotomy. *Clin Orthop*. 1975;106:232–241.
52. Kettelkamp DB, Wenger DR, Chao EYS, Thompson C. Results of proximal tibial osteotomy. *J Bone Joint Surg Am*. 1976;58:952–960.
53. Keene JS, Dyreby JR. High tibial osteotomy in the treatment of osteoarthritis of the knee. *J Bone Joint Surg Am*. 1983; 65:36–42.
54. Insall JN, Joseph DM, Msika C. High tibial osteotomy for varus gonarthrosis. *J Bone Joint Surg Am*. 1984;66:1040–1047.
55. Wang JW, Kuo KN, Andriacchi TP, Galante JO. The influence of walking mechanics and time on the results of proximal tibial osteotomy. *J Bone Joint Surg Am*. 1990;72:905–909.
56. Menkow RL, Soudry M, Insall JN. Patella dislocation following knee replacement. *J Bone Joint Surg Am*. 1985;67: 1321–1327.
57. Keays S, Mason M. The benefit of increased range of motion following total knee replacement. Platform presentation at the 12th International Congress of the World Confederation for Physical Therapy; June 25–30, 1995; Washington, DC.
58. Jarvinen M. Epidemiology of tendon injuries in sports. *Clin Sports Med*. 1992;11:493–504.
59. Puddu G, Cipolla M, Cerullo G, DePaulis F. Non-osseous lesions. In: Fox JM, Del Pizzo W, eds. *The Patellofemoral Joint*. New York: McGraw-Hill; 1993:177–192.
60. Leadbetter WB. Cell-matrix response in tendon injury. *Clin Sports Med*. 1992;11:533–578.
61. Blazina ME, Kerlan RK, Jobe FW. Jumper's knee. *Orthop Clin North Am*. 1973;4:665–678.
62. McConnell JS. The management of chondromalacia patellae: a long term solution. *Aust J Physiother* 1986;32:215–223.

RECOMMENDED READINGS

Buckwalter J, Rosenberg L, Coutts R, et al. Articular cartilage: injury and repair. In: Woo SL-Y, Buckwalter JA, eds. *Injury and Repair of the Musculoskeletal Soft Tissues*. Park Ridge, IL: American Academy of Orthopaedic Surgeons; 1988:465–483.

Buckwalter JA. Mechanical injuries of articular cartilage. In: Finerman GAM, Noyes FR, eds. *Biology and Biomechanics of the Traumatized Synovial Joint: The Knee as Model*. Rosemont, IL: American Academy of Orthopaedic Surgeons. 1992:83–95.

Mow VC, Ateshian GA, Ratcliffe A. Anatomic form and biomechanical properties of articular cartilage of the knee. In: Finerman GAM, Noyes FR, eds. *Biology and Biomechanics of the Traumatized Synovial Joint: The Knee as Model*. Rosemont, IL: American Academy of Orthopaedic Surgeons. 1992: 185–202.

CHAPTER 22

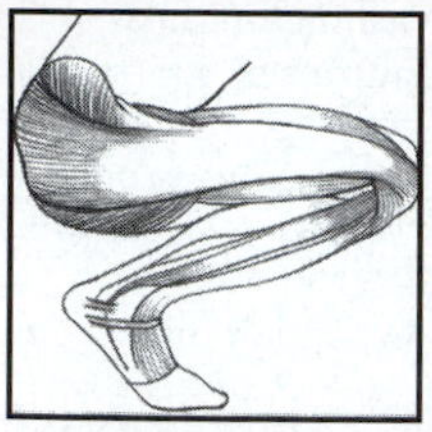

The Ankle and Foot

Stan Smith, Carrie Hall, and Lori Thein Brody

The key to developing a successful therapeutic exercise program for the ankle and foot is to understand the interactions among the lower extremity joints. Anatomic impairments (eg, coxa vara, anteversion, forefoot varus), physiologic impairments (eg, hypomobility, hypermobility, loss of force or torque production, loss of balance and coordination), or trauma at one joint can lead to dysfunction at other joints in the kinetic chain. For example, excessive pronation, a faulty movement pattern of the foot and ankle, can lead to compression of the medial tibiofemoral compartment because of excessive pronatory forces up the kinetic chain. The patient experiences medial knee pain with gait. If left untreated, the medial compartment of the knee may undergo degenerative changes caused by abnormal and excessive forces. Treatment of the faulty ankle and foot movement patterns can relieve abnormal forces in the medial knee compartment.

Impairments are rarely isolated. Typically, appropriate treatment of the complex interplay of impairments throughout the kinetic chain alleviates the impairments and results in return of function to the ankle and foot. Effective examination, diagnosis, and exercise intervention are essential for long-term resolution of symptoms, impairments, functional loss, and disability.

REVIEW OF ANATOMY AND KINESIOLOGY

A thorough knowledge of the anatomy and kinesiology of the foot and ankle is necessary to understand the functional effects of impairments of the kinetic chain. Structure for the unique kinematic relationships among lower extremity joints is provided by the local anatomy.

Osteology

The talocrural joint is composed of the distal fibula, tibia, and the talus bones. The distal fibula, or lateral malleolus, projects distally and posteriorly. It extends farther distally than the medial malleolus, the distal projection of the tibia. The distal flat end of the tibia articulating with the talus is wider anteriorly, allowing dorsiflexion mobility. Of the seven tarsal bones, the talus provides the link between the leg and the foot. The talus is composed of a head, a neck, and a body (Fig. 22-1). The largest talar bone, the calcaneus, is an irregularly shaped cuboid bone. It contains several muscle attachments and grooves for tendons passing distally. Its plantar surface serves as the attachment of the plantar fascia. Together, the talus and the calcaneus comprise the hindfoot.[1] The midfoot consists of the navicular, cuboid, and three cuneiform bones.[1] The navicular bone is most medial and articulates between the talar head proximally and the cuneiform bones distally. The navicular plays an important mechanical role in maintenance of the longitudinal arch. It contains a tuberosity for distal attachment of the posterior tibialis muscle. The cuboid is the most lateral bone in the distal tarsal row, and it sits between the calcaneus proximally and the fourth and fifth metatarsals distally. It contains a groove for the tendon of the peroneus longus muscle. The three cuneiform bones are wedge shaped and articulate with the navicular proximally and the bases of the first to third metatarsal bones distally. Of

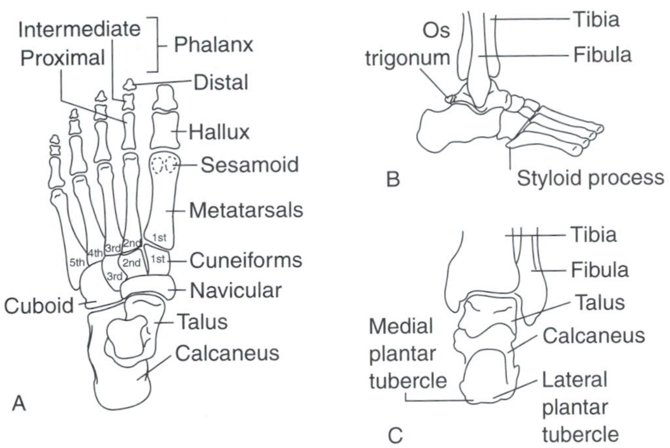

FIGURE 22- 1 Osteology of the foot and ankle. ***(A)*** Superior view. ***(B)*** Lateral view. ***(C)*** Posterior view.

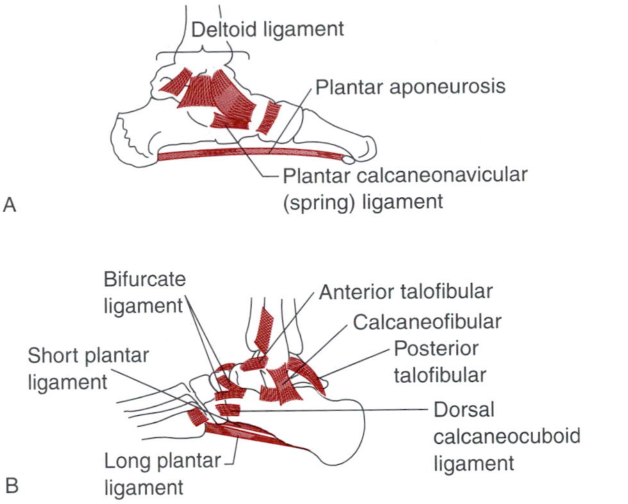

FIGURE 22-2 Ligaments of the ankle. ***(A)*** Medial aspect. ***(B)*** Lateral aspect. (From Norkin CC, Levangie PK. *Joint Structure and Function: A Comprehensive Analysis.* 2nd ed. Philadelphia: FA Davis; 1992).

these bones, the medial cuneiform is the largest, and the middle cuneiform is the smallest.

The forefoot consists of the five metatarsals and the phalanges. The first metatarsal bone is the shortest and thickest, and the fifth contains a styloid process on the lateral side of its base. The phalanges are similar to the those of the hand, and each consists of a shaft, base, and head.[1]

An understanding of bony relationships can clarify the terminology used throughout this chapter. The talocrural joint is the articulation of the tibia and fibula with the talus. The subtalar joint is a composite joint formed by three distinct planar articulations between the talus and the calcaneus. The midtarsal joint, or transverse tarsal joint, is a complex articulation formed by the talonavicular and calcaneocuboid joints.

Arthrology

TALOCRURAL JOINT

The capsule of the ankle joint is fairly thin and weak anteriorly and posteriorly, and the stability of the ankle joint depends on an intact ligamentous structure. The two major ligaments are the medial collateral ligament and the lateral collateral ligament.[2]

The medial collateral ligament is commonly referred to as the deltoid ligament, a fan-shaped ligament with superficial and deep fibers (Fig. 22-2*A*). This ligament is quite strong; stress on the medial joint line may avulse the tibial malleolus before tearing the deltoid ligament. This ligament controls medial joint stability and controls extremes of plantar flexion and dorsiflexion.

The lateral collateral ligament is far weaker than the medial collateral ligament and is composed of three separate bands: the anterior and posterior talofibular and the calcaneofibular ligaments (Fig. 22-2*B*). The anterior talofibular ligament is the weakest of the lateral collateral ligament complex. The lateral collateral ligament controls lateral joint stability and checks extremes of range of motion (ROM). The anterior talofibular and the calcaneofibular ligaments are the most frequently injured when the ankle is sprained, which usually is an inversion injury while the ankle is in its most unstable position of plantar flexion.

SUBTALAR JOINT

The subtalar joint is a stable joint that rarely dislocates. Its ligamentous support consists of the medial and lateral collateral ligaments, the interosseous talocalcaneal ligament, and the posterior and lateral talocalcaneal ligaments (Fig. 22-3).

MIDTARSAL JOINT

The calcaneocuboid joint has its own capsule that is reinforced by several major ligaments: the lateral band of the bifurcate ligament, the dorsal calcaneocuboid, the plantar calcaneocuboid (short plantar), and the long plantar ligament. The long plantar ligament is the most important of these ligaments, because it extends from the calcaneus and cuboid to the bases of the second through fourth metatarsals. It contributes significantly to midtarsal joint stability and support of the lateral longitudinal arch of the foot. Important support for the midtarsal joint is also provided by the extrinsic muscles passing medially and laterally and the intrinsic muscles inferiorly.

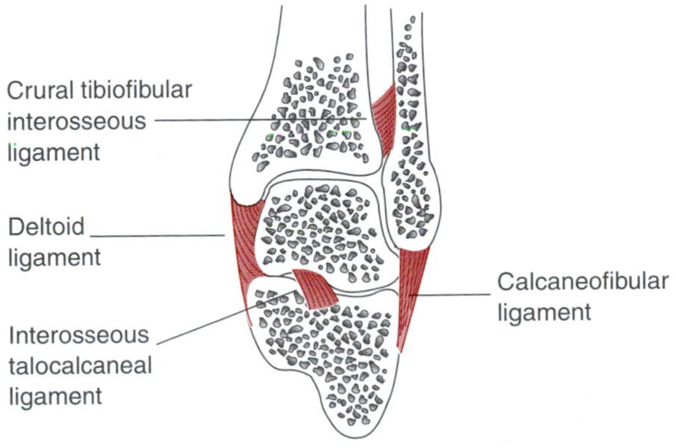

FIGURE 22-3 Cross-sectional posterior view of the ligaments of the subtalar joint.

The talonavicular joint is enclosed by the same capsule that encloses the anterior and middle facets of the subtalar joint. Ligamentous support for this joint is provided by the ligaments supporting the subtalar joint, the spring ligament, the medial band of the bifurcate ligament, and the dorsal talonavicular ligament. The triangular spring ligament arises from the sustentaculum talus and inserts on the inferior navicular. The central portion supports the talar head. Medially, it is continuous with the deltoid ligament, and laterally, it joins the medial band of the bifurcate ligament. The spring ligament is the primary support of the medial longitudinal arch. As it spans and supports the talocalcaneonavicular joint, it checks joint motion that contributes to flattening of the arch. Additional support is supplied from the ligaments that reinforce the adjacent calcaneocuboid joint.

The plantar aponeurosis, also known as the plantar fascia, spans and supports the longitudinal arch (see Fig. 22-2).[3] It begins posteriorly on the calcaneus and continues anteriorly to attach to the proximal phalanx of each toe. Its strong fibrous structure provides protection to the underlying muscles, vessels, and nerves. The plantar fascia participates in longitudinal arch support during the propulsion phase of gait. Dorsiflexion of the toes causes traction on the plantar fascia, which elevates the longitudinal arch through the windlass mechanism (Fig. 22-4).

Myology

The musculature of the foot and ankle can be categorized into four major groups: anterior, lateral, posterior, and intrinsic. This section lists the muscles of the ankle and foot by these four major groups and describes their open chain function. However, to prescribe exercise with precision, the practitioner should know the unique function of each muscle. The Recommended Reading section provides sources for more information on muscle function. Closed chain function is described later in the Gait Kinematics section.

The anterior muscle group consists of the tibialis anterior, extensor hallucis longus, extensor digitorum longus, and peroneus tertius. They form a functional complex for open chain dorsiflexion. The lateral muscle group consists of the peroneus longus and brevis, which function as evertors in the open kinetic chain. The posterior group can be further divided into superficial and deep layers. The superficial layer consists of the gastrocnemius, soleus, and plantaris, and the deep layer consists of the tibialis posterior, flexor hallucis longus, and flexor digitorum longus. The posterior group functions as plantar flexors in the open kinetic chain.[2]

The intrinsic muscle group can be divided into four layers. The superficial layer consists of abductor hallucis, flexor digitorum brevis, and abductor digiti minimi. These muscles extend from the calcaneus to the toes and comprise a functional group that assists longitudinal arch maintenance. The second layer consists of the quadratus plantae and four lumbricals, which are closely associated with the flexor digitorum longus. The third layer comprises the shorter intrinsic muscles of the great and fifth toes. It includes the flexor hallucis brevis, adductor hallucis, and flexor digiti minimi brevis. The deepest layer consists of seven interossei—three plantar and four dorsal. They are similar to the interossei in the hand, except that they are arranged to abduct and adduct around the second rather than the middle toe.

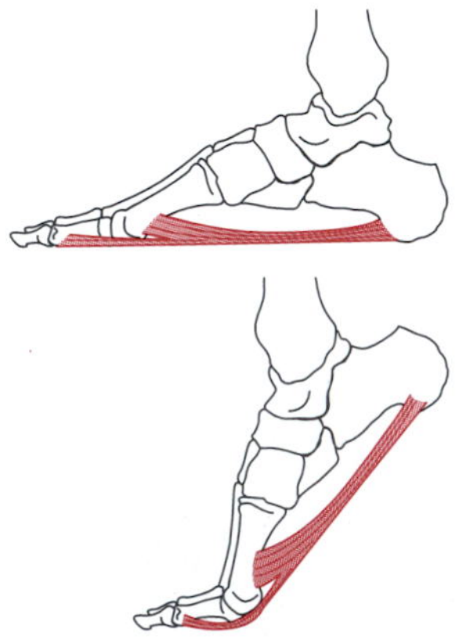

FIGURE 22-4 As the toes are extended, the windlass effect of the plantar fascia assists passive elevation of the heel. (From APRN When the feet hit the ground everything changes, In *Program Outline and Prepared Notes-A Basic Manual.* Toledo, Ohio: 1984).

Neurology

The primary motor and sensory nerve supply to the foot are the tibial and common peroneal nerves. The motor portion of the tibial nerve innervates the gastrocnemius, soleus, plantaris, popliteus, flexor hallucis longus, flexor digitorum longus, and tibialis posterior muscles. It further divides into the medial and lateral plantar nerves. The medial plantar nerve innervates the flexor digitorum brevis, abductor hallucis, flexor hallucis brevis, and first lumbrical. The lateral plantar nerve innervates the quadratus plantae, abductor digiti minimi, flexor digiti minimi brevis, adductor hallucis, dorsal and plantar interossei, and second to fourth lumbricals. The sensory supply from the tibial nerve, the medial sural cutaneous, joins the lateral sural cutaneous from the common peroneal to form the sural nerve, which supplies the skin on the dorsolateral surface of the lower leg and the lateral side of the foot. The medial plantar nerve supplies the medial side of the sole and the medial three and one-half toes. The lateral plantar nerve innervates the lateral side of the sole and the lateral one and one-half toes.

The common peroneal is divided into the deep and superficial peroneal nerve. The deep peroneal nerve innervates the tibialis anterior, extensor hallucis longus, extensor digitorum longus, peroneus tertius, and extensor digitorum brevis. The superficial peroneal nerve innervates the peroneus longus and brevis. The sensory portion, the lateral sural cutaneous nerve, joins the medial sural cutaneous nerve from the tibial nerve as stated previously. The deep peroneal nerve ends as a cutaneous branch to the adjacent sides of the great and second toes. The superficial peroneal nerve supplies the skin on the front of the lower leg, dorsum of the foot, medial side of the great toe, and adjacent sides of the second to the fifth toes.

Foot and Ankle Kinesiology

The foot and ankle have several fundamental functions:

- Adapting to uneven terrain
- Absorbing shock
- Absorbing lower extremity rotation
- Providing a rigid lever for effective propulsion

Three joints of the multiple joints in the foot and ankle complex are chiefly responsible for these functions: the talocrural joint, the subtalar joint, and the midtarsal joint.[4,5] Motion at the talocrural, subtalar, and midtarsal joints occur around triplane axes, which run from a posterior lateral plantar position to an anterior medial dorsal position. The resulting triplane motion is called pronation and supination (Display 22-1). *Pronation* is movement in the direction of eversion, abduction, and dorsiflexion; *supination* is movement toward inversion, adduction, and plantar flexion.

TALOCRURAL JOINT

The talocrural joint axis is pitched close to the frontal and transverse plane, with minimal angulation in the sagittal plane (Fig. 22-5).[6] Technically, the talocrural joint pronates and supinates. During pronation, dorsiflexion is the most dominant component motion, with minimal components of eversion and abduction. Talocrural joint supination is dominated by plantar flexion, with minimal components of inversion and adduction. Clinically, the dorsiflexion and plantar flexion components are so dominant that pronation and supination terms are rarely used to describe the movement. During closed kinetic chain talocrural joint function, the foot and talus are stabilized by weight bearing forces and motion is in the form of the tibia and fibula moving over the foot.[7]

SUBTALAR JOINT

Subtalar joint axis is pitched midway between the sagittal and transverse planes, with minor angulation in the frontal plane (Fig. 22-6).[8] Closed chain weight-bearing forces at the subtalar joint differ from open chain forces; however, the joint still follows triplane motion. During closed chain subtalar joint pronation, the calcaneus everts, but because of weight-bearing forces, the foot does not abduct or dorsiflex. The talus completes the triplane motion by adducting and plantar flexing (Fig. 22-7).[8] This motion of the talus results in lowering of the medial longitudinal arch, and it influences internal rotation of the tibia and fibula. During closed kinetic chain subtalar joint supination, the calcaneus inverts, and the talus adducts and dorsiflexes (Fig. 22-8). Subtalar joint supination elevates the medial longitudinal arch and influences external rotation of the tibia and fibula.[5]

MIDTARSAL JOINT

The midtarsal joint has two independent axes (Fig. 22-9).[1,7] The longitudinal midtarsal joint axis falls close to the sagittal plane, and during pronation, it has a large component of eversion and small components of dorsiflexion and abduction. The oblique midtarsal joint axis crosses the frontal and transverse plane with minimal angulation toward the sagittal plane. This axis gives rise to large components of

---

DISPLAY 22-1
Planar Motion

General Principles of Planar Motion

- Joint motion occurs perpendicular to an axis.
- Joint motion is often described by the cardinal plane in which it occurs.
- The three cardinal planes are frontal, sagittal, and transverse.
- An axis that lies in two planes will give rise to a single plane motion in the third plane.

Planar Motion of the Ankle and Foot

- In the foot and ankle, an axis that lies in the frontal and transverse plane gives rise to plantar flexion and dorsiflexion in the sagittal plane.
- An axis falling in the sagittal and transverse planes gives rise to inversion and eversion in the frontal plane.
- An axis running in the frontal and sagittal planes gives rise to abduction and adduction in the transverse plane.
- An axis that obliquely crosses the three cardinal planes gives rise to motion in all three planes, or triplane motion.

General Principles of Triplane Motion

- Triplane motion is often described by the component motions from each cardinal plane.
- The angulation or pitch of an axis determines the amount of each component motion.
- A triplane axis that is pitched evenly across all three planes gives rise to motion with equal components from each plane.
- If the axis is pitched closer to one plane, there is a larger or dominant component motion. For example, if a triplane axis lies close to the sagittal plane, the dominant component motion is inversion or eversion. Abduction or adduction and plantar flexion or dorsiflexion are less significant.

Triplane Motion of the Ankle and Foot

- Motion at the talocrural, subtalar, and midtarsal joints occur around triplane axes.
- These axes run from a posterior lateral plantar position to an anterior medial dorsal position.
- Triplane motion at the foot and ankle that occurs around an axis in the previously described angulation is called pronation and supination.
- Pronation is movement in the direction of eversion, abduction, and dorsiflexion.
- Supination is movement toward inversion, adduction, and plantar flexion.
- The axis of each joint has a different pitch and therefore has different degrees of component motions from the cardinal planes.
- Triplane motion at the foot and ankle during open chain motion is readily apparent by observing the plantar surface of the forefoot.
- During closed kinetic chain function, weight-bearing forces provide some element of distal fixation, which limits motion distal to the axis and promotes motion above the joint axis.
- Triplane motion under load is less apparent because of the motion occurring distal and proximal to the joint axis.
- It is important to understand triplane motion in the open and closed kinetic chain to duplicate the ideal biomechanics during range of motion exercise and functional retraining of the ankle and foot complex and its relationships to the talofibular, tibiofemoral, and hip joints.

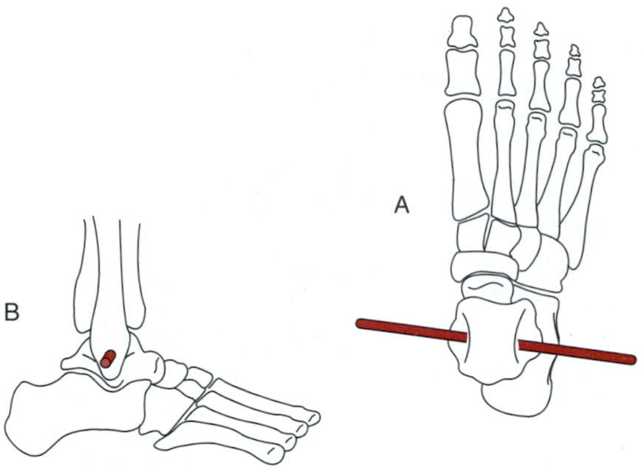

FIGURE 22-5 The axis of the talocrural joint is rotated laterally 25 degrees in the transverse plane and inclined distolaterally 10 degrees in the frontal plane. ***(A)*** Superior view. ***(B)*** Lateral view.

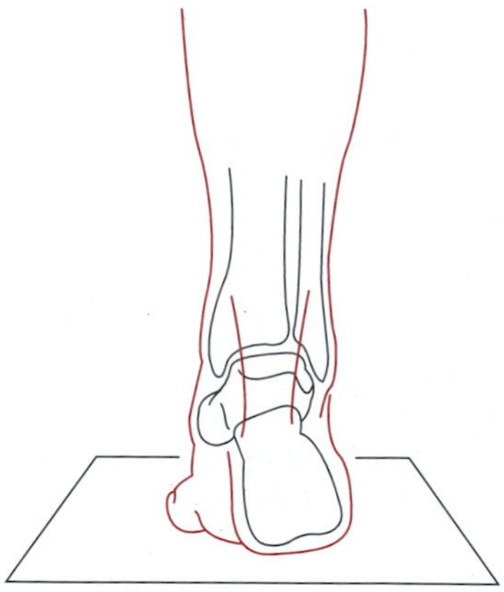

FIGURE 22-7 Posterior view of the right foot showing subtalar joint pronation. Pronation is a triplane motion consisting of calcaneal eversion, talar abduction, and dorsiflexion. (From APRN When the feet hit the ground everything changes, In *Program Outline and Prepared Notes-A Basic Manual.* Toledo, Ohio: 1984).

dorsiflexion and abduction and a small component of eversion during pronation. Although complex, the biomechanics of the midtarsal joint can be thought of as depending on subtalar joint biomechanics. In a subtalar joint pronated position, the talar head moves medially and plantarly. In this position, the axes of the midtarsal joint are parallel, which promotes mobility in the midtarsal joint and forefoot. As the subtalar joint supinates toward a neutral and then supinated position, the axes of the midtarsal joint progressively converge. The converging axes promote stability in the midtarsal joint and forefoot (Fig. 22-10). Subtalar joint pronation and supination is said to "unlock and lock" the midtarsal joint.[4,5]

Gait Kinetics

Ambulation is a primary functional goal for most patients. A thorough understanding of the kinesiology of gait is crucial for developing a therapeutic exercise program promoting functional return. This section describes the phases of gait, the relationship of gait to ankle and foot biomechanics, the relationship of gait to hip and knee biomechanics (see Chapters 20 and 21), and muscle function during the gait cycle.

A normal gait cycle includes a stance phase and a swing phase. Stance phase is further broken down into initial contact, loading response, midstance, terminal stance, and preswing. The swing phase is divided into initial swing, midswing, and terminal swing. Kinetics are discussed relative to the gait phase (Table 22-1).[9,10]

STANCE PHASE

At initial contact, the talocrural joint is in neutral position, and the subtalar joint is slightly supinated. As the foot passes into loading response, the talocrural joint plantar flexes from 0 to 15 degrees, and the subtalar joint pronates. This pronation "unlocks" the midtarsal joint, creating mobility throughout the foot. Shock absorption results from a com-

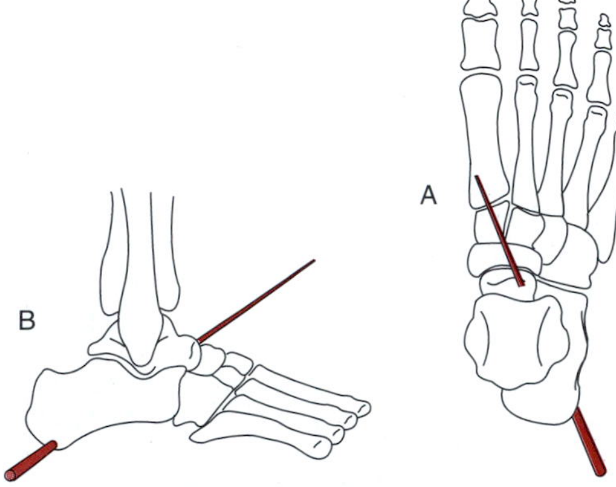

FIGURE 22-6 The axis of the subtalar joint is inclined 42 degrees anterosuperiorly from the transverse plane and inclined medially 16 degrees from the sagittal plane. ***(A)*** Superior view. ***(B)*** Lateral view.

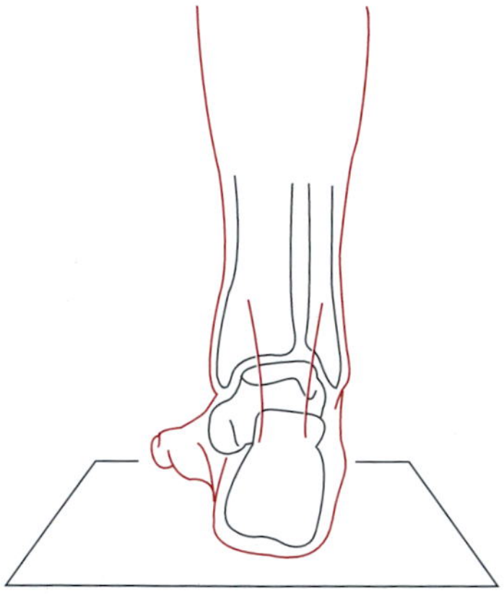

FIGURE 22-8 Posterior view of right foot showing subtalar joint supination. Supination is a triplane motion consisting of calcaneal inversion, talar adduction, and plantar flexion. (From APRN When the feet hit the ground everything changes, In *Program Outline and Prepared Notes-A Basic Manual.* Toledo, Ohio: 1984).

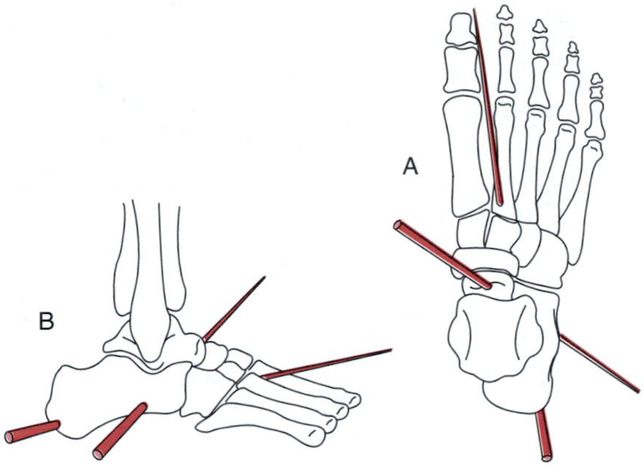

FIGURE 22-9 Midtarsal joint axes. The two axes are the ***(A)*** longitudinal midtarsal joint axis and ***(B)*** oblique midtarsal joint axis.

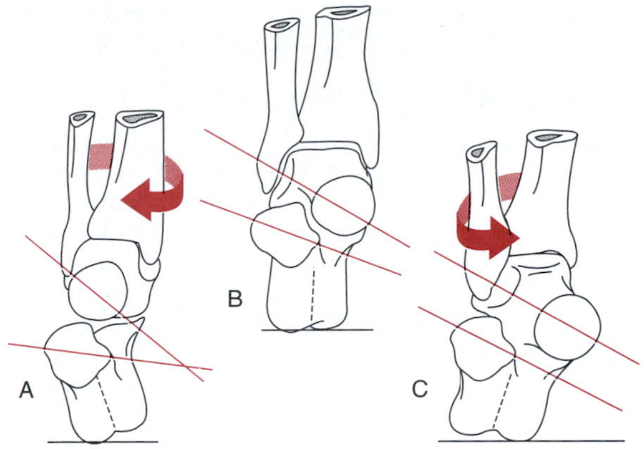

FIGURE 22-10 Locking and unlocking of the midtarsal joint. ***(A)*** When the axes are divergent, the midtarsal joint is locked producing a rigid foot. ***(B)*** The axes in the neutral, resting position of the foot. ***(C)*** When the axes are parallel, the midtarsal joint is unlocked, producing a flexible foot.

bination of subtalar pronation, calcaneal eversion, talar plantar flexion, knee flexion, and tibial and femur medial rotation. Biomechanically, the knee requires medial tibial rotation for effective knee flexion. Talar plantar flexion and adduction during subtalar joint pronation allows the required tibial medial rotation. At the midfoot, midtarsal pronation occurs, and the forefoot has a compensatory supination twist. This twist is relative to the position of the rearfoot.[4,5] As the leg moves into midstance, the lower extremity moves forward over the foot by way of talocrural joint dorsiflexion. Ideally, the talocrural joint moves to a position of 10 degrees of dorsiflexion before heel rise. Loss of talocrural dorsiflexion is a common physiologic impairment, which can lead to further intrinsic and extrinsic physiologic impairments (see Patient-Related Instruction: Ankle Mobility and Walking Patterns). As the lower extremity moves forward, the subtalar joint supinates from a pronated position and passes from neutral to slight supination before heel rise. This supination progressively "locks" the midtarsal joint and promotes stability throughout the foot, creating a

Table 22-1. KINETICS AND KINEMATICS OF THE FOOT AND ANKLE DURING GAIT

PHASE OF THE GAIT CYCLE	JOINT	RANGE OF MOTION	MOMENT	MUSCLE ACTIVITY	MUSCLE CONTRACTION TYPE
Initial contact	**TCJ**	0 deg dorsiflexion	Plantar flexion	Dorsiflexors	Isometric
	STJ	STJ supination	Varus	Evertor muscles	Isometric
Loading response	**TCJ**	Plantar flexes from 0–15 deg PF	Plantar flexion	Dorsiflexors	Eccentric
	STJ	STJ begins pronating	Moving to valgus	Invertors	Eccentric
Midstance	**TCJ**	Dorsiflexes to 10 deg DF	Moving to dorsiflexion	Plantar flexors	Eccentric
	STJ	STJ begins resupinating	Valgus moving to varus	Invertors	Eccentric to concentric
Terminal stance	**TCJ**	Dorsiflexes to 15 deg DF	Dorsiflexion	Plantar flexors	Eccentric to concentric
	STJ	STJ continues supinating	Varus	Evertors	Isometric
Preswing	**TCJ**	Plantar flexes to 20 deg PF	Dorsiflexion		
	STJ	STJ remains supinated	Varus		
Initial swing	**TCJ**	Dorsiflexes to 10 deg PF		Dorsiflexors	Dorsiflexors
Midswing	**TCJ**	Dorsiflexes to 0 deg		Dorsiflexors	Dorsiflexors
Terminal swing	**TCJ**	Stays at 0 deg		Dorsiflexors	Dorsiflexors

STJ, subtalar joint; TCT, talocrural joint; PF, plantar flexion; deg, degrees of; DF, dorsiflexion.

Patient-Related Instruction

Ankle Mobility and Walking Patterns

To restore the most ideal walking pattern, you must have adequate ankle mobility. You will be asked to perform a specific exercise or series of exercises frequently throughout the day to improve your ankle mobility. The pictures show what your walking pattern should look like. Half-way through the step, you need the most ankle mobility. Be sure that your foot remains pointed forward and does not toe-out (Fig. A). Be sure that you do not allow your arch to flatten (Fig. B).

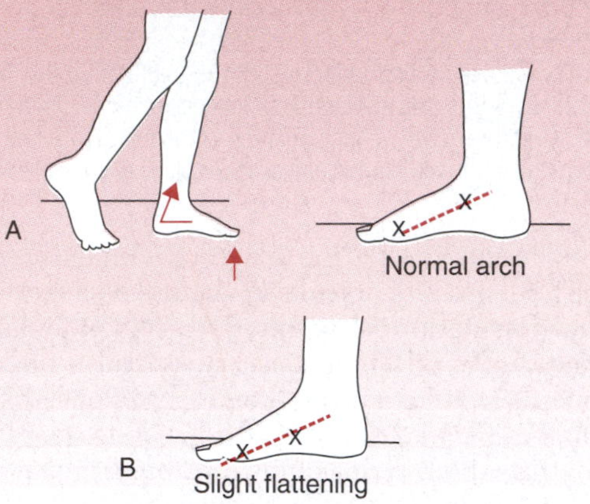

rigid lever for propulsion. At the forefoot, weight is progressed distally to the metatarsal heads. The knee and hip are extending throughout midstance, and the tibia and femur are laterally rotating. This lateral rotation is augmented by talar abduction and dorsiflexion and by subtalar joint supination.

As the heel is lifted during terminal stance, the talocrural joint flexes an additional 5 to 15 degrees of dorsiflexion. The talocrural joint then plantar flexes to 20 degrees during terminal stance. The subtalar joint and midtarsal joints remain supinated during these phases, maintaining a rigid lever at the foot. A relative pronation twist occurs at the forefoot. Moving into the swing phases, the talocrural joint plantar flexes, the knee flexes, and the lower extremity continues to laterally rotate until the toe has left the ground.[4,5]

SWING PHASE

Swing phase begins with preswing and ends with initial contact. The swing phase of gait is in part responsible for effective propulsion. As the lower extremity moves forward during swing, developing momentum provides much of the energy for propulsion on the opposite extremity. If the lower extremity biomechanics are sound, ambulation is performed with a low expenditure of energy. During swing phase, the lower extremity prepares itself for upcoming initial contact. By terminal swing, the femur has medially rotated to near neutral, the knee is near extension, and the ankle is dorsiflexed to the neutral position. The subtalar joint is slightly supinated and prepared for initial contact just lateral to midline of the calcaneus.[9]

Gait Kinematics

A thorough understanding of muscle function during gait is necessary to provide specificity to exercise prescription and functional retraining. To be efficient and effective in exercise prescription, it is important to restore the type of muscle contraction and the precise phase of gait in which the muscle functions. In terms of closed kinetic chain biomechanics, the muscles of the foot and ankle function eccentrically to decelerate motion, isometrically to stabilize motion, and concentrically to accelerate motion. Muscles often have double functions at two or more joints during the different periods of stance.

STANCE PHASE

At initial contact, the anterior tibialis and toe extensors fire to maintain the neutral talocrural position opposing a plantar flexion moment.[11] As the foot moves into loading response, these same muscles work eccentrically to lower the foot to the ground in opposition to the plantar flexion moment. At the subtalar joint, the peroneus longus and brevis fire to evert the calcaneus and initiate pronation.

As the foot moves from loading response to midstance, the tibia advances over the stationary foot, necessitating eccentric gastrocnemius and soleus activity to decelerate the advancing tibia. At the subtalar joint, the tibialis posterior, flexor digitorum longus, and flexor hallucis longus also work eccentrically to control the pronating foot. This eccentric work is minor during slow walking, but it significantly increases during fast walking and running. The tibialis posterior functions to accelerate resupination and provides medial longitudinal arch stability during midstance. When moving from midstance through preswing, the gastrocnemius-soleus complex continues firing eccentrically until preswing, when heel lift is a relatively passive event. The peroneus longus also functions to plantarly stabilize the first cuneiform and first metatarsal during these phases. Plantar stability of the first metatarsal is important for normal push off and weight distribution across the metatarsal heads during late midstance and preswing phases (see Patient-Related Instruction: Maintaining the Long Arch in Standing and Walking).[4,5]

Ideal Alignment

Alignment of the ankle and foot is an important component of function because of the interplay of alignment and movement and the relationships among kinetic chain components. Deviation from ideal alignment occurs in the form of anatomic or physiologic impairments.

Ideal alignment of the foot must be assessed from a subtalar neutral position. Controversy surrounds the idea of *subtalar joint neutral*. The traditional concepts are presented, followed by information questioning the validity of this ideal position. Subtalar neutral is the position in which the subtalar joint is neither pronated nor supinated and the position in which the subtalar joint optimally functions. Subtalar neutral is assessed in the prone position and is found by palpating congruency of the talonavicular joint with one hand and loading the lateral side of the foot with the opposite hand. An ideal rearfoot alignment is a perpen-

Patient-Related Instruction

Maintaining the Long Arch in Standing and Walking

While walking, attempt to maintain the long arch of your foot during the weight-bearing period of the step. Avoid rolling onto the outside portion of your foot by attempting to keep your big toe firmly against the floor as you keep your long arch elevated. Exercises in sitting or standing positions can help you to feel this action (Fig. A). After you can feel this action during static postures, try to incorporate it into walking (Fig. B).

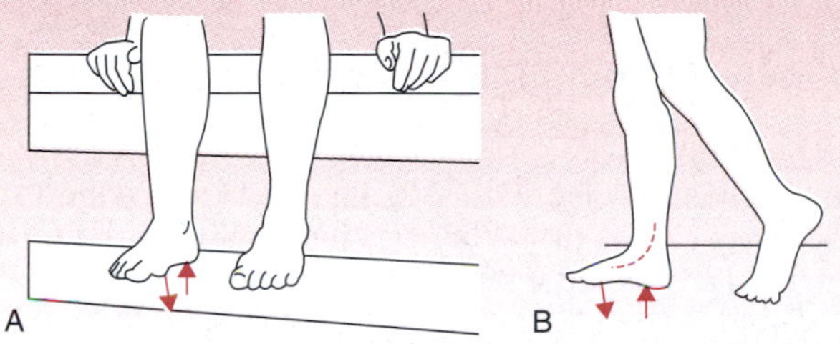

dicular relationship between the bisection of the posterior calcaneus and the bisection of the distal tibia and fibula (Fig. 22-11). Ideal forefoot alignment is determined by a perpendicular relationship between the posterior bisection of the calcaneus and a plane made by the plantar surface of the metatarsal heads. The rearfoot and forefoot relationships are independent of each other and must be assessed separately.

The findings assessed in non–weight-bearing subtalar neutral must be compared with the standing position. The relaxed alignment of the longitudinal and transverse arches, tibia, talus, calcaneus, and toes demonstrate the compensation (or lack thereof) for abnormal forefoot to rearfoot relationship assessed in a non–weight-bearing position. Ideal alignment of the tibia, foot, and ankle in a standing position should be as follows for the sagittal plane:

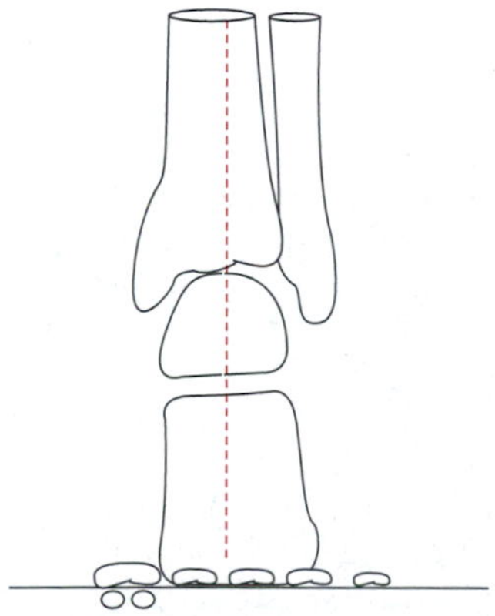

FIGURE 22-11 Ideal rearfoot alignment. The plumb line bisects the calcaneus and talus. (From Gould JA. *Orthopaedic and Sports Physical Therapy*, 2nd ed. St. Louis: C.V. Mosby; 1990:298–301).

- Plumb line alignment is slightly anterior to a midline through the knee and lateral malleolus and through the calcaneocuboid joint.
- The navicular tubercle is on a line drawn from the medial malleolus to the point where the metatarsophalangeal joint of the great toe rests on the floor.

Ideal alignment of the tibia, foot, and ankle in a standing position should be as follows for the frontal plane:

- The distal one third of the tibia is in the sagittal plane.
- The great toe is not deviated toward the midline of the foot (ie, hallux valgus).
- The toes are not hyperextended.

Although lower extremity problems have been treated for many years on the basis of this subtalar neutral concept, the scientific and clinical foundations for this concept are questionable. The original classification system and criteria for subtalar neutral were developed by Root and colleagues.[12] There are several concerns about the Root approach:

- The reliability of the measurement techniques to assess normal and abnormal foot posture
- The criteria for normal foot alignment
- The proposition that the subtalar joint reaches neutral between midstance and preswing[13]

Measurements of weight-bearing and non–weight-bearing calcaneal and subtalar joint positions have shown low reliability.[14–17] Clinicians are unable to arrive at the same measurements when evaluating patients. Because treatment is based on these measurements, variability must exist in the treatment as well. Moreover, on the basis of Root's criteria for normal foot alignment, most of the population (68% ± 27.5% based on a normal distribution) should have normal feet. Studies of foot alignment in normal populations have found Root's normal alignment in only 15% to 31% of subjects studied.[15,17]

Another area of dispute is the position of the subtalar joint during gait. Root and colleagues[12] have asserted that the subtalar joint reaches its neutral position at or just after midstance. They based this assertion on the findings of Wright and coworkers,[18] who studied two patients with external potentiometers applied to their feet during gait. They found that the subtalar neutral position was achieved at or shortly after midstance. However, their definition of subtalar neutral was significantly different from Root's interpretation.[12] Wright defined subtalar neutral as the resting calcaneal stance position, or the resting position with the subject in relaxed standing. This position is significantly different from the current posture purported to be the ideal subtalar neutral position. The clinician should consider the posture of subtalar joint neutral during exercise prescription, although this posture may be the patient's resting calcaneal stance position rather than the ideal position described.

Descriptions of ideal alignments of the spine, pelvis, femur, and tibia can be found in Chapters 18 through 22. Alignment of the entire lower extremity must be assessed and treated because of the structural and functional relationships of the knee, hip, foot, and ankle (see Patient-Related Instruction: Ideal Alignment of the Lower Extremity).

Patient-Related Instruction

Ideal Alignment of the Lower Extremity

You should practice good alignment of your hips, legs, ankles, and feet. Good alignment of your lower extremities helps to achieve normal movement. Your physical therapist will instruct you in exercises to help overcome problems that make it difficult for you to achieve normal alignment. The picture below can assist in understanding ideal alignment of the hips, knees, ankles, and feet. Practice this alignment frequently throughout the day. Soon, it will feel normal, and your old posture will feel abnormal.

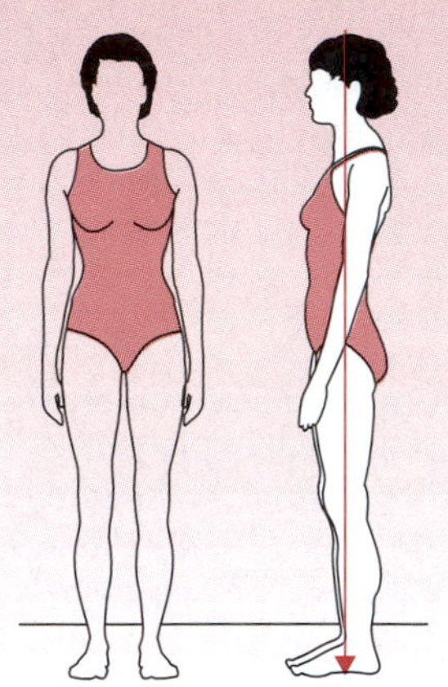

ANATOMIC IMPAIRMENTS

Anatomic impairments throughout the lower extremity can lead to abnormal alignment and movement patterns of the foot and ankle. Conversely, anatomic impairments of the foot and ankle can lead to abnormal alignment and movement patterns up the kinetic chain at the knee, hip, pelvis, and spine. Abnormal alignment and movement patterns (see Chapter 8) can result in excessive stress and strain on soft tissue and bony structures, leading to cumulative microtrauma and musculoskeletal pain. If left untreated, microtrauma can result in pathology, evidenced radiologically or neurologically, of the musculoskeletal system that can impair function and lead to disability.

When ideal alignment is lacking, the clinician must decide whether the alignment fault results from an anatomic impairment or a physiologic impairment. An anatomic impairment cannot be altered with manual therapy or exercise intervention, because it is a fixed structural abnormality. However, it can be treated with orthotic therapy and exercise to prevent associated physiologic impairments from developing within or extrinsic to the foot. A physiologic impairment can be altered with appropriate intervention, such as joint mobilization, soft tissue stretching, muscle strengthening. It is beyond the scope of this text to describe the tests for differentiating anatomic from physiologic impairments. The following impairments are described as if structural, and they are therefore listed as anatomic impairments. Physiologic impairments are discussed in the context of therapeutic exercise intervention.

Anatomic impairments within the foot and ankle are called *intrinsic impairments.* The most common intrinsic anatomic impairments are subtalar varus, forefoot varus, and forefoot valgus. Anatomic impairments above the ankle are known as *extrinsic impairments.* Because of the close interplay between foot and ankle function and knee and hip function, extrinsic anatomic impairments may produce physiologic impairments at the foot and ankle. The most common extrinsic anatomic impairments are femoral anteversion and retroversion, coxa vara and coxa valga, tibial varum and valgum, and tibial torsion.

Intrinsic Anatomic Impairments

SUBTALAR VARUS

Subtalar varus is defined as an inverted twist within the body of the calcaneus.[5] While the foot is held in the subtalar neutral position, the bisection of the posterior calcaneus is inverted relative to the bisection of the distal tibia and fibula (Fig. 22-12). The typical physiologic impairment resulting from subtalar varus is excessive pronation during loading response and midstance. The subtalar joint may resupinate in midstance; however, if the excessive pronation is significantly large, the subtalar joint may not reach the desired neutral to slightly supinated position before heel rise. This may result in decreased stability at the midtarsal joint during propulsion, thereby increasing the shearing forces in the forefoot and causing potential strain on supportive soft tissue structures. Further up the kinetic chain, excessive pronation may produce excessive medial rotation patterns of the tibia and femur, which may affect function of the sacroiliac joint and lumbar spine with excessive rotational forces.

FOREFOOT VARUS

Forefoot varus is an inversion deviation of the forefoot relative to the bisection of the posterior calcaneus (Fig. 22-13).[4] The physiologic impairment resulting from forefoot varus is excessive pronation during midstance. Excessive

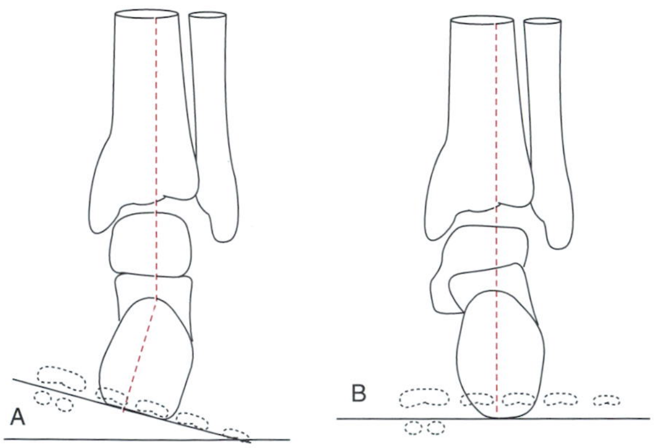

FIGURE 22-12 Posterior view of right foot subtalar varus. ***(A)*** Uncompensated subtalar varus. ***(B)*** Compensation for this impairment is usually excessive pronation. (From Gould JA. *Orthopaedic and Sports Physical Therapy,* 2nd ed. St. Louis: C.V. Mosby; 1990:298–301).

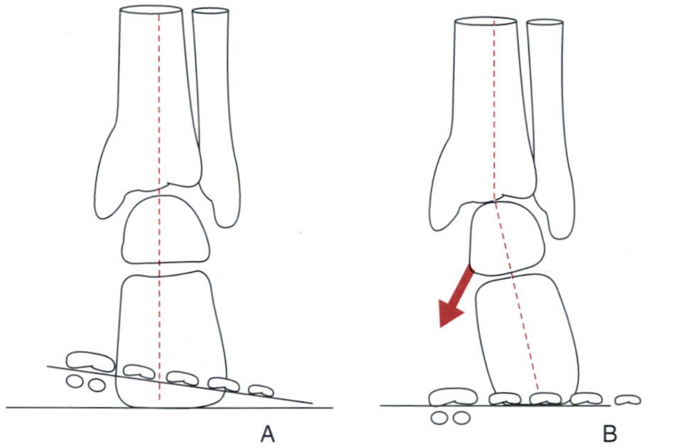

FIGURE 22-13 Posterior view of right foot forefoot varus. ***(A)*** Uncompensated forefoot varus. ***(B)*** Compensation for this impairment is usually excessive pronation. (From Gould JA. *Orthopaedic and Sports Physical Therapy*, 2nd ed. St. Louis: C.V. Mosby; 1990:298–301).

pronation during midstance produces excessive forefoot mobility during push off. Supporting structures of the foot are strained, and lower extremity medial rotation takes place when lateral rotation is normally occurring. This rotational fault can contribute to physiologic impairments up the kinetic chain in the knee, hip, pelvis, and lumbar spine.

FOREFOOT VALGUS

Forefoot valgus is an eversion deviation of the forefoot relative to the bisection of the posterior calcaneus (Fig. 22-14).[4] The typical physiologic impairment resulting from a forefoot valgus is early and excessive supination in midstance phase. Functionally, this compensation creates a rigid lever for propulsion, and adaptation to the terrain and shock absorption may be compromised. There may also be a lateral weight shift, creating greater forces at the fifth metatarsal and potential lateral instability.

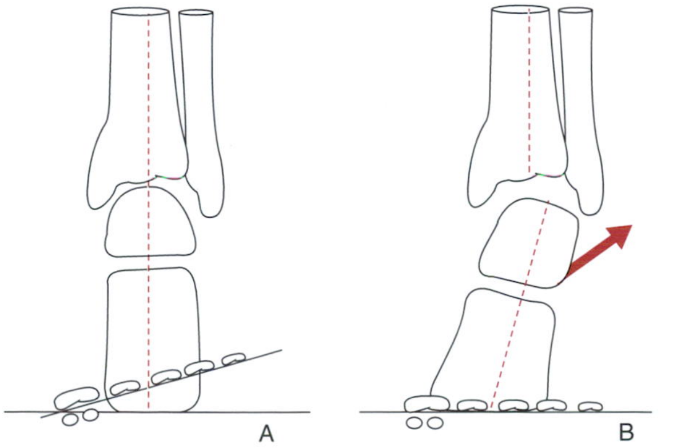

FIGURE 22-14 Posterior view of right foot forefoot valgus. ***(A)*** Uncompensated forefoot valgus. ***(B)*** Compensation for this impairment is usually excessive supination. (From Gould JA. *Orthopaedic and Sports Physical Therapy*, 2nd ed. St. Louis: C.V. Mosby; 1990:298–301).

EQUINUS

Equinus is a lack of 10 degrees of talocrural joint dorsiflexion. Equinus may not be a true anatomic impairment; it is rarely a structural fault. This abnormality may result from a short gastrocnemius muscle or from talocrural joint hypomobility, which can be treated with exercise or manual therapy. However, in the case of talocrural immobility caused by long-term immobilization or surgical stabilization, equinus is considered an anatomic impairment.

The physiologic impairment resulting from equinus is excessive pronation during midstance or early terminal stance. The position of the subtalar joint and consequently the degree of foot stability at end range of talocrural dorsiflexion determine which type of compensation occurs. If the subtalar joint is pronated, the foot is in a relatively flexible state. The body's momentum carries the tibia through the end range of talocrural dorsiflexion and forces the subtalar joint into greater pronation. Compensatory dorsiflexion occurs at the oblique axis of the midtarsal joint, which produces a medial rotation on the lower extremity in late midstance and a mobile foot at preswing. If the subtalar joint is near neutral and the talocrural joint is relatively hypomobile, early heel rise occurs, which may affect the kinetic chain proximally because of the sudden rise in the center of gravity in the gait cycle.

Extrinsic Anatomic Impairments

Anatomic impairments extrinsic to the ankle and foot are described in Chapters 20 and 21. This section describes the relationship of extrinsic impairments to the biomechanics of the ankle and foot.

COXA VALGUM–GENU VARUM

Coxa valgum–genu varum is a frontal plane anatomic impairment in which the angulation of the femoral neck is greater than normal, resulting in a relative valgus position of the femoral shaft. The knee typically develops a varus attitude, giving the individual a bow-legged appearance.[19]

Coxa valgum–genu varum affects the subtalar joint in the contact phase by setting up heel strike in a greater varus angle. The subtalar joint usually compensates by excessively pronating to bring the calcaneus to a vertical position.

COXA VARUM–GENU VALGUM

Coxa varum–genu valgum is a frontal plane anatomic impairment in which the angulation of the femoral neck is less than normal, resulting in a greater varus attitude of the femoral shaft. The knee develops a valgus attitude, giving the individual a knock-knee appearance.[19]

The normal mechanical weight-bearing line runs from the acetabulum through the center of the knee and into the foot. With coxa varum–genu valgum, the mechanical weight-bearing line falls medial to the foot, and the subtalar joint is forced into pronation throughout stance. Impairments in muscle length, strength, and patterns of recruitment around the pelvic girdle can enhance the coxa varum–genu valgum dysfunction. Insufficient abdominal and gluteal recruitment can result in an anterior pelvic tilt and medial rotation of the femur. This proximal orientation may result in hyperextension and valgum of the knee, medially shifted weight-bearing forces, and excessive subtalar joint pronation.

FEMORAL TORSION

The medially rotated position of the femoral shaft in relation to the position of the head and neck creates an angulation in the transverse plane called the *angle of torsion.* The angle is normally around 12 degrees, but it can range from 8 to 25 degrees. An abnormal increase in the angle of torsion is called *anteversion,* and a decrease is known as *retroversion.*[20] Anteversion may result in excessive subtalar joint pronation because of the medial forces at the hip and knee imposed by the increased angle of torsion. Compensation for anteversion is usually tibial lateral rotation, and combined with the proximal medial forces from the hip, this rotation leads to further pronatory forces at the subtalar joint.[20] Retroversion creates lateral forces at the hip and knee that may result in foot abduction. Foot abduction brings weight-bearing forces over the medial arch, and the foot is subjected to pronatory forces throughout late midstance phase.

OBESITY

Obesity may be considered a quasi-extrinsic anatomic impairment because it is a structural fault. The difference between obesity and other anatomic impairments is that obesity can be altered with individualized exercise prescription and with nutritional and behavioral modification. The body's center of mass falls between the feet and, with obesity, has an excessive pronatory effect on the foot. Obesity is a critical impairment to address when treating the patient with biomechanical concerns and must be dealt with on an individual basis. Referral to the appropriate health care professionals frequently is necessary to treat the problem in a comprehensive manner.

EXAMINATION AND EVALUATION

Examination and evaluation of the foot and ankle must consider the findings related to the foot and ankle and the relationships of the knee, hip, pelvis, and spine. The tests described in this section are primarily for the ankle and foot and should be considered in any foot and ankle examination. However, examination of the knee and hip may need to be included to assess extrinsic impairments contributing to foot and ankle dysfunction. The tests listed also may be included in a knee or hip examination to assess foot and ankle impairments contributing to knee or hip dysfunction. The clinician is assumed to have the knowledge and skill to perform the tests necessary to diagnose impairments and functional loss of the foot and ankle.

History

The patient's history is obtained first. This data guides the overall examination and provides the clinician with important information about functional limitations and disability. In addition to the medical history, questions should focus on the signs and symptoms that caused the patient to seek treatment. Key questions focus on which symptoms are most disabling for the patient, including pain, instability, mobility loss, weakness, catching, or other aggravating symptoms. The clinician should inquire about usual footwear and daily activities. Using this information, the clinician chooses tests to match the patient's symptoms and designs a treatment program to address the impairments, functional limitations, and disabilities described by the patient.

General Observation and Clearing Tests

Observation of posture and position of the limb and screening tests for the lumbopelvic and hip regions are important aspects of the examination and evaluation.[19,21,22] Any of these areas may refer pain along the kinetic chain. Listed are several important aspects of this part of the assessment:

- Plumb line landmarks anteriorly, posteriorly, and laterally
- Genu recurvatum, flexion, valgum, or varum
- Hip anteversion or retroversion
- Subtalar neutral
- Hallux and toe alignment
- Integrity of longitudinal and transverse arches
- Rearfoot to forefoot relationship in subtalar joint neutral
- Relaxed calcaneal stance position
- Muscle tone of lower extremities
- Ecchymosis, swelling, or redness
- Ability to place weight on the limb
- Assessment of footwear

Mobility Examination

Mobility examination of the foot and ankle includes osteokinematic and arthrokinematic testing. The examination must include all joints throughout the kinetic chain. These joints work in unison to produce smooth, coordinated movement through the limb. The following tests of mobility should be performed:

- Hip and knee ROM
- Hip and knee muscle flexibility
- Calcaneal inversion and eversion ROM
- Midtarsal joint motion
- First ray position and mobility
- Hallux dorsiflexion ROM
- First to fifth ray position and mobility
- Ankle dorsiflexion and plantar flexion ROM with the knee flexed and extended

Impaired Muscle Performance Examination

Muscle functioning at the hip, knee, foot, and ankle should be tested in a logical order and based on patient history information and clinician's impression. Functioning of all ankle and foot muscles should be tested. Any proximal muscles that may affect the foot and ankle should be tested as well. Proximal muscle weakness can contribute to mechanical faults distally.

Pain and Inflammation Examination

The pain and inflammation examination is performed as part of the subjective examination and is further clarified during the objective examination. Complaints of warmth, swelling, and local tenderness indicate pain and inflammation. Palpable tenderness and warmth over specific anatomic structures are objective indications of pain. This objective information is correlated with subjective information to guide the remaining examination and treatment planning.

Special Tests

A variety of special tests are used to assess the integrity of foot and ankle structures. Many of the specific tests are used to more closely assess the mechanics of the foot and ankle. Magee[22] provides a complete listing and description of special tests, but these are some of the most common:

- Leg length discrepancy
- Neutral position of the subtalar joint
- Ligament stress testing
- Sensory testing
- Reflex testing
- Circumferential measurements
- Pulse assessment
- Gait analysis

SELF-MANAGEMENT: Toe and Ankle Active Range of Motion

Purpose: Increased mobility in the foot and ankle after an injury

Position: Lying on your back with your foot elevated above chest level

Movement technique: Repeatedly flex and extend your toes. Move your ankle up and down or write the alphabet with your ankle.

Repeat ____ times

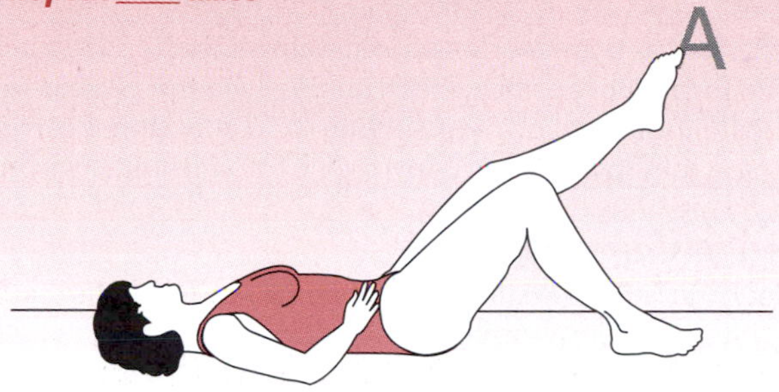

THERAPEUTIC EXERCISE INTERVENTION FOR COMMON PHYSIOLOGIC IMPAIRMENTS

Therapeutic exercise is an invaluable clinical tool for treatment of physiologic impairments of the ankle and foot. This section provides examples of therapeutic exercise for the treatment of pain and swelling, hypomobility or hypermobility, force or torque production, balance and coordination, alignment, and movement.

The clinician may need to make appropriate modifications based on individual signs and symptoms. Exercise recommendations for specific diagnoses of the ankle and foot are addressed in a later section.

Pain and Swelling

Swelling can become a chronic problem in the foot and ankle, because the ankle is the most dependent weight-bearing joint in the body. Early intervention is critical to efficiently treat this impairment. Low-level dynamic exercise and compression in conjunction with frequent elevation can be effective for control of swelling. Emphasis is placed on high-repetition, low-intensity dynamic exercise for adjacent noninjured joints. For example, a patient with swelling at the rearfoot and pain on subtalar joint supination may be instructed how to perform elevated active toe flexion and extension and to perform midrange talocrural joint plantar flexion and dorsiflexion (see Self-Management: Toe and Ankle Active Range of Motion). High-repetition exercise can be prescribed as multiple repetitions at one sitting, but it is probably more effective if prescribed as moderate repetitions completed frequently throughout the day (eg, every 2 hours). The latter approach is most beneficial for the more irritable symptoms.

The key for an effective exercise prescription for treating pain is in prescribing the appropriate intensity of exercise. Severity, irritability, and nature of pain must be assessed and used in the development and progression of exercise. For example, exercise for the involved joint should be initiated in pain-free range in the acute stage, just up to the painful range in the subacute stage, and slightly into the painful range in the chronic stage. Active assisted exercise may be required if the patient demonstrates poor active control.

Exercise for the involved side's hip and knee may be indicated to prevent disuse weakness and can decrease pain (ie, Gate theory of pain). In many situations, stationary biking is tolerated well and can maintain cardiovascular and musculoskeletal health of all tissues exercised. Biking with the heels on the pedal is less stressful to the foot and ankle than pedaling with the forefoot. Biking with a high seat position requires less ankle dorsiflexion, which may be indicated in the acute phase. Soft tissue mobilization, cryotherapy, electrical stimulation, and a variety of other therapeutic modalities may be beneficial in conjunction with exercise for the control of pain and swelling.

Mobility Impairment

The talocrural, subtalar, and midtarsal joint have triplane axes and therefore demonstrate triplane motion. Passive and active assistive ROM exercise for treatment of hypomobility should follow the triplane concept. Accessory joint mobility should be assessed, and joint mobilization techniques should be initiated if indicated. Open chain active stretch can be progressed to passive stretch and eventually progressed to use of the new mobility during function.

Certain guidelines should be followed in addressing hypermobility impairments:

- In the acute phase, the hypermobile segment must be protected from excessive motion by taping, bracing, casting, or more stable footwear.
- Adjacent hypomobile segments should be mobilized with manual therapy or mobility exercise to prevent excessive motion from being imposed on the hypermobile segment.
- Dynamic stabilization exercise should be initiated at the hypermobile segment.

At the foot and ankle, dynamic stabilization exercise can be in the form of proprioception training (see the Balance and Coordination Impairment section) and functional retraining (see the Posture and Movement Impairment section).

TALOCRURAL JOINT

Talocrural joint dorsiflexion is a common ROM limitation after injury or immobilization of the foot and ankle. This limitation can result from a short or stiff gastrocnemius muscle, from talocrural joint hypomobility, or from both conditions. The clinician must rely on the examination to determine the source of hypomobility. Complaints of anterior ankle discomfort during dorsiflexion suggest talocrural joint hypomobility. Gastrocnemius stretching can be performed in a long-sitting position with a towel or similar object positioned around the forefoot. The patient is instructed to actively dorsiflex the talocrural joint and then apply graded overpressure into dorsiflexion using the towel (Fig. 22-15*A*). Care must be taken to prevent subtalar pronation while dorsiflexing at the talocrural joint. If the patient is using the long-sitting position, the clinician must ensure proper patient positioning, avoiding posterior pelvic tilt and lumbar flexion due to short hamstrings. A cushion under the pelvis shortens the hamstrings and improves the patient's position (Fig. 22-15*B*). The supine position is an alternative to the long-sitting position and can accommodate short hamstrings, maintaining better lumbopelvic alignment. It has the added benefit of stretching the hamstrings without overstretching the lumbar spine.

Talocrural joint dorsiflexion ROM can be performed in a long-sitting position, but a pillow is placed under the knee to minimize the gastrocnemius and hamstring stretch. The soleus is stretched in this position if the talocrural joint has adequate dorsiflexion mobility (Fig. 22-15*C*). Lower extremity biomechanics must be considered when progressing dorsiflexion ROM exercises to a weight-bearing position. If the subtalar joint is pronated in stance, talocrural joint or gastrocnemius stretching will increase the pronatory forces.

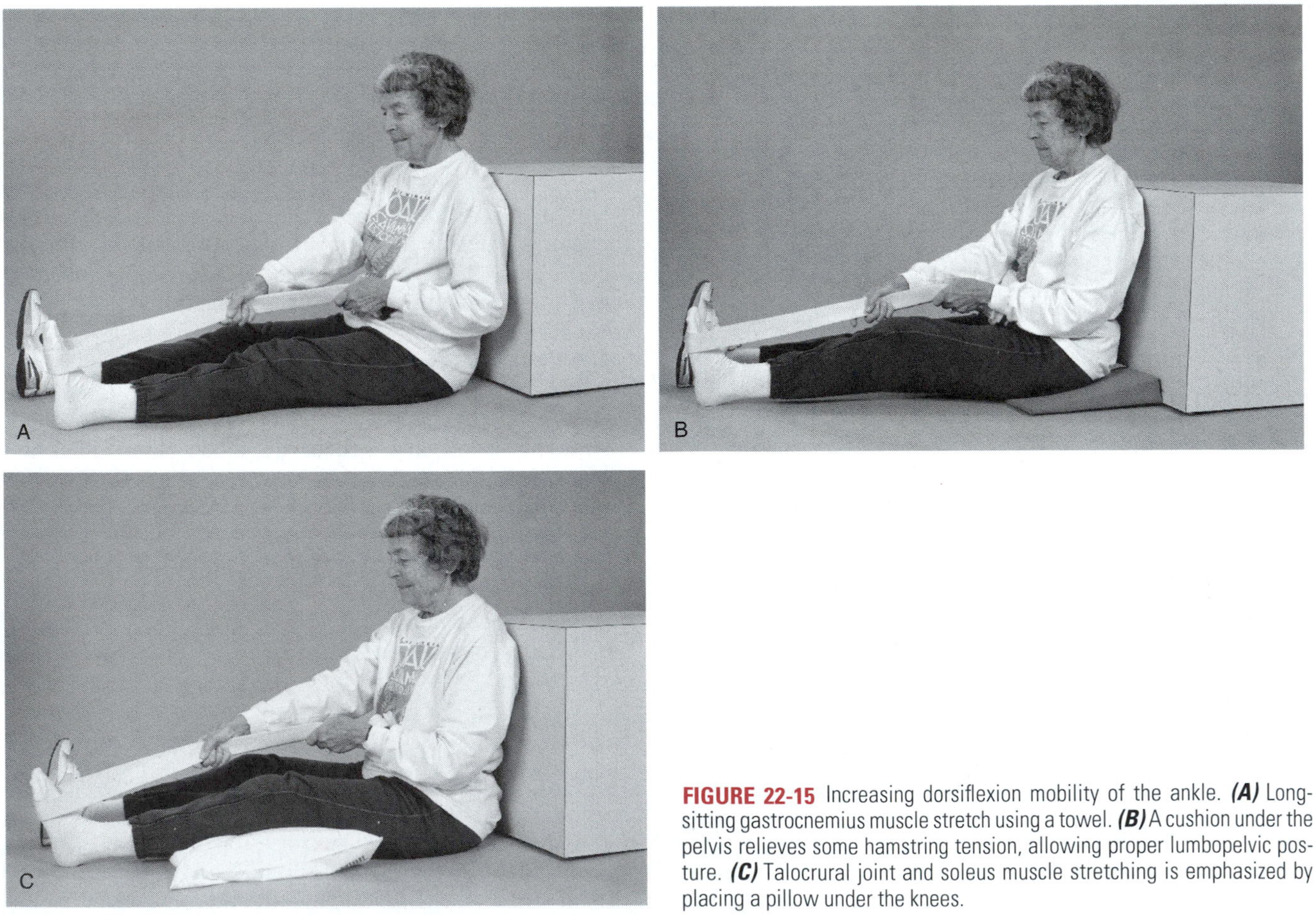

FIGURE 22-15 Increasing dorsiflexion mobility of the ankle. ***(A)*** Long-sitting gastrocnemius muscle stretch using a towel. ***(B)*** A cushion under the pelvis relieves some hamstring tension, allowing proper lumbopelvic posture. ***(C)*** Talocrural joint and soleus muscle stretching is emphasized by placing a pillow under the knees.

Stretching should be completed with the subtalar joint in a neutral to slightly supinated position. The gastrocnemius can be passively stretched with the patient standing arm's length plus approximately 6 inches away from the wall. The involved foot is positioned with its lateral border perpendicular or slightly toe-in to the wall. It is important to be in this position, because gastrocnemius stretching in a toe-out position causes weight-bearing forces to cross the medial longitudinal arch and promote increased subtalar joint pronation. The patient moves the uninvolved foot to the wall and then leans toward the wall while maintaining a vertically oriented trunk position. The involved knee is maintained in full extension, and the heel is held flat on the floor (Fig. 22-16). The use of a small hand towel folded under the medial longitudinal arch may help support the subtalar joint and midtarsal joint during stretching. Weight-bearing talocrural joint dorsiflexion ROM is completed in a similar position, however, but the involved knee is flexed while the heel is held on the floor. A soleus stretch is performed in the position if ROM at the talocrural joint is adequate.

These exercises should be incorporated into a patient's functional activities throughout the day (Fig. 22-17). An active exercise, such as small knee bends from a standing position, may reinforce functional mobility of talocrural dorsiflexion instead of subtalar pronation. Progressing small knee bends to a walk stance position reinforces gastrocnemius lengthening as the knee is in extension. Attention must focus on maintaining a subtalar neutral position and avoiding a toe-out position (see Patient-Related Instruction: Ideal Alignment During Walking). Therapeutic exercise progression must involve functional retraining of the new mobility during the swing phase of gait and during late midstance, when maximal dorsiflexion is required. During the late midstance phase, care must be taken to ensure a subtalar neutral position is maintained and that the foot is progressed without toeing-out. These compensations avoid talocrural dorsiflexion and produce subtalar pronation and midtarsal abduction.

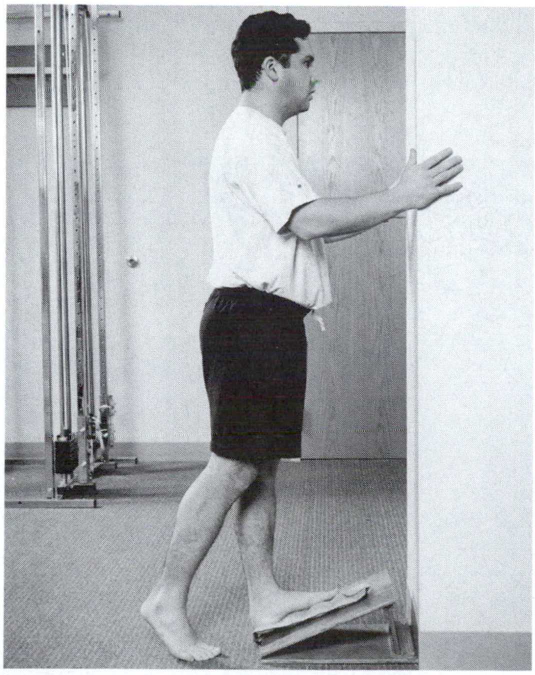

FIGURE 22-16 The gastrocnemius muscle can also be stretched by leaning against a wall or using a stretching board. Support under the longitudinal arch can prevent excessive pronation compensation.

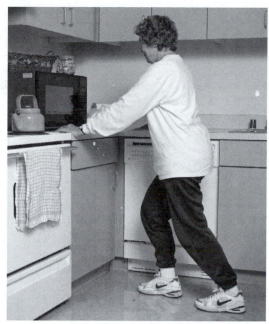

FIGURE 22-17 Stretching exercises should be incorporated into the patient's functional activities. Talocrural and soleus muscle stretching is done with the knee slightly flexed.

Patient-Related Instruction

Ideal Alignment During Walking

You should attain ideal alignment during walking. The most difficult phase to control is during the weight-bearing period of the step. Place the heel, ball of the foot, and toes down on the floor as three distinct areas. The heel should hit slightly on the outside border without turning the entire foot out. The weight line should progress from the outside of the foot toward the big toe. Attempt to maintain the knee over the toes, with the foot progressing straight ahead and the long arch of the foot held upward. If these alignments are maintained throughout the weight-bearing period, the foot should feel stable for push-off.

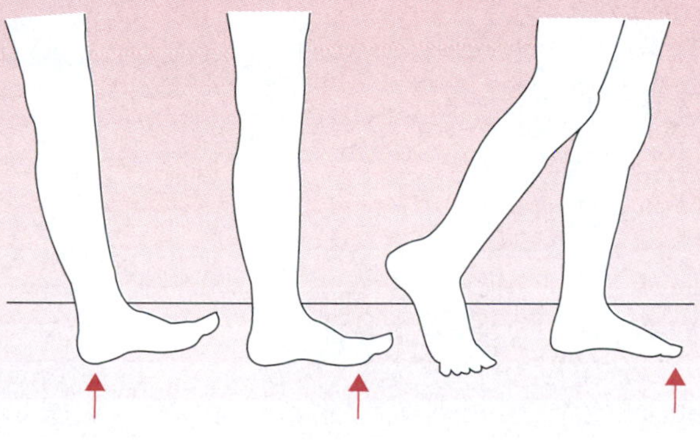

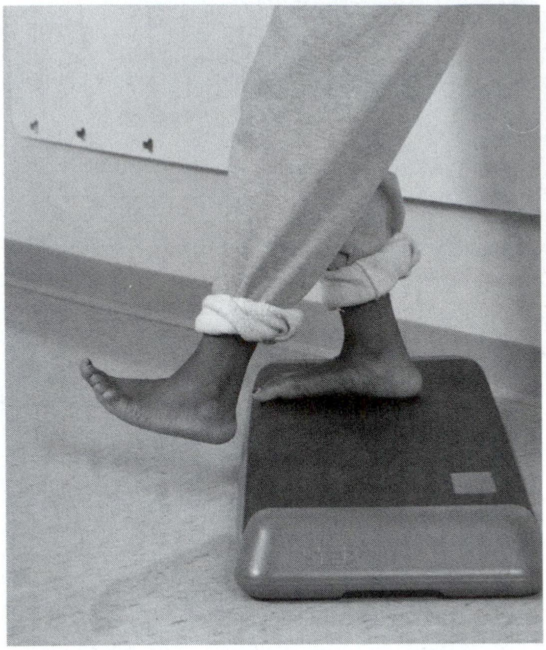

FIGURE 22-18 A step-down exercise is used to improve functional dorsiflexion. The patient must be able to control the pronation component of this motion.

Step-down training can be used to facilitate controlled eccentric lengthening of the calf muscle group and the knee and hip extensors. A patient stands on a 2- or 4-inch box and is instructed to maintain involved side heel contact while lowering the uninvolved heel to the floor (Fig. 22-18). This exercise is progressed by increasing the step height.

SUBTALAR JOINT

Subtalar joint supination mobility can be addressed with the patient sitting with the involved distal leg placed on the opposite knee. Full active supination is performed, followed by the patient using his hands to progressively pull the calcaneus and foot into greater supination (Fig. 22-19*A*). If combined with dorsiflexion, this exercise also stretches the peroneal musculature. Subtalar joint pronation ROM can be completed in a similar position by the patient actively pronating and applying graded overpressure (Fig. 22-19*B*). If combined with dorsiflexion, this exercise also stretches the tibialis posterior muscle. Therapeutic exercise progressions involve functional retraining of the new pronation and supination mobility during the appropriate phase of the gait cycle.

Impaired Muscle Performance

Resisted exercise is used to restore muscular force or torque production lost because of muscle strain, neurologic deficit, or disuse. Although open chain exercise is useful to improve physiologic strength parameters and patient awareness of muscle function (ie, muscle re-education), it is critical to progress the exercise to weight-bearing activities as soon as tolerated. In many cases, closed chain activity can be broken into simple steps and serve as a starting point for exercise prescription.

INTRINSIC MUSCLES

Intrinsic muscle strengthening can be performed in a sitting position with the patient's feet placed on the end of a towel lying on the floor. The patient flexes his toes, attempting to draw the towel under the foot. Using the toes to pick up marbles and other small objects also exercises the intrinsic musculature. Standing with a resistive band along the bottom of the foot and pulling the toes into extension can be used to resist toe flexion (see Self-Management: Resisted Toe Flexion). These exercises are low intensity and may require high repetitions to achieve a training effect. Maintenance of the longitudinal and transverse arches during closed chain exercises such as small knee bends, the walk stance position, stair stepping, and gait use the intrinsic musculature in a functional manner.

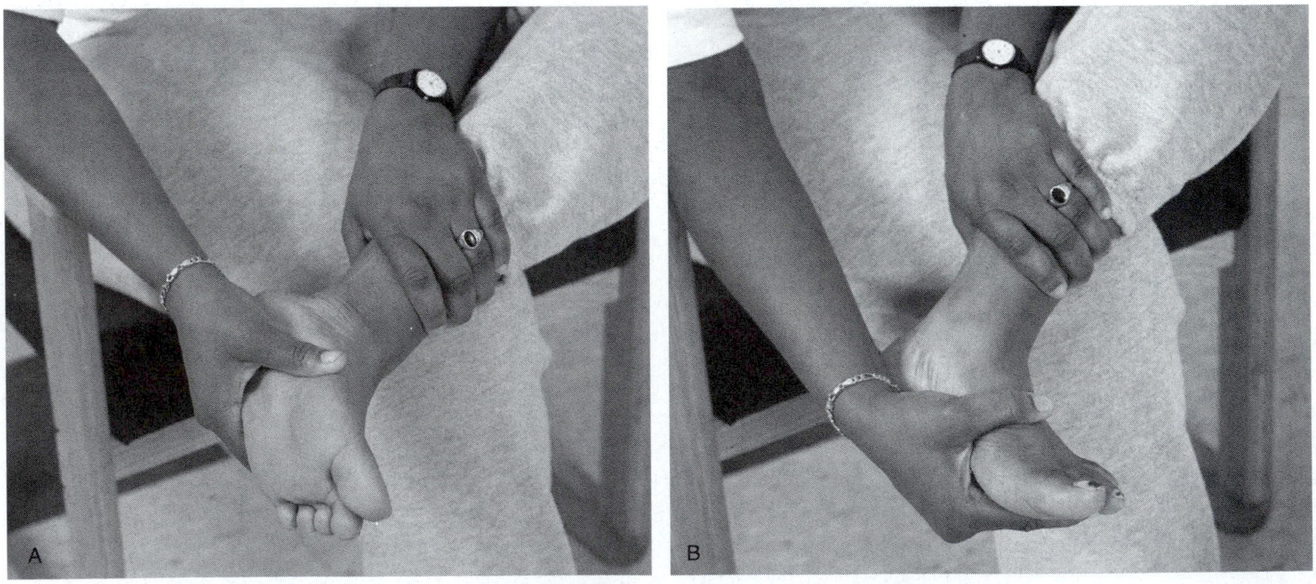

FIGURE 22-19 Passive stretching for triplane motion of the foot. ***(A)*** Subtalar joint supination. ***(B)*** Subtalar joint pronation.

SELF-MANAGEMENT: Resisted Toe Flexion

Purpose: Increased strength in toe flexor and intrinsic foot muscles

Position: Standing with your foot along the length of the resisted band and with the band in one hand, pull up to pull toes up.

Movement technique: Holding the band in this position, curl your toes down against the resistance of the band.

Repeat ___ times

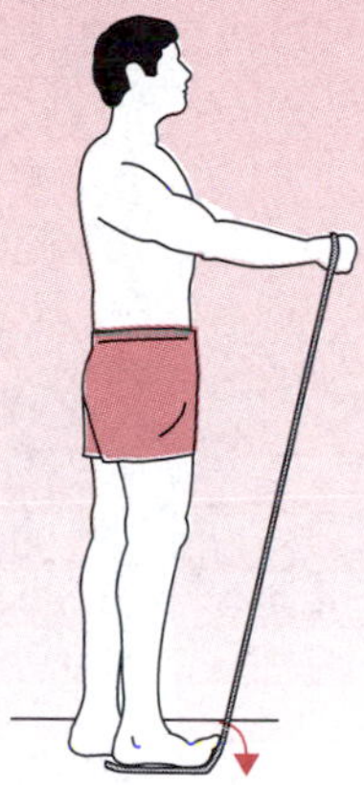

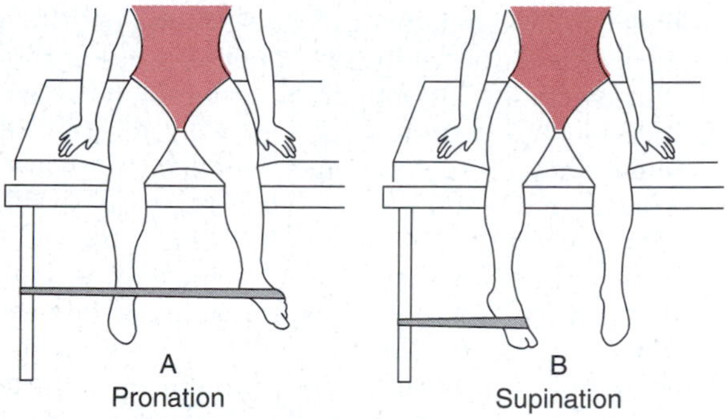

FIGURE 22-21 Resisted supination and pronation with the knee flexed. Flexing the knee minimizes hip rotation substitution. ***(A)*** Resisted pronation. ***(B)*** Resisted supination.

EXTRINSIC MUSCLES

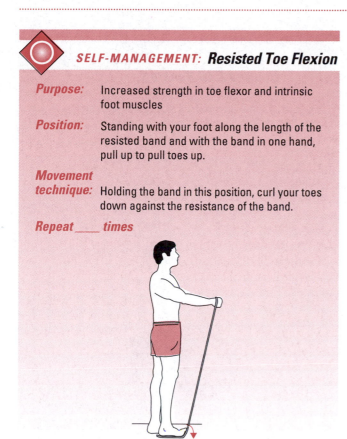

Open chain strengthening exercises for extrinsic musculature can be performed with elastic bands or tubing. Care must be taken not to overload weak muscle groups, which may cause unwanted substitution patterns and abnormal joint shearing and pain.

Resisted talocrural plantar flexion can be achieved in a long-sitting position with the elastic band wrapped around the plantar surface of the forefoot. While holding the opposite end of the band, the patient plantar flexes against the resistance of the band (Fig. 22-20). Slow, eccentric lengthening to a dorsiflexed position should be emphasized because of the gastrocnemius muscle's deceleration function during gait. A towel roll or small pillow placed under the leg, proximal to the talocrural joint, is helpful in providing heel clearance. Resisted talocrural dorsiflexion and subtalar joint pronation and supination can be completed with an elastic band looped around a table leg or similar secure structure. The patient performs the intended movement against the resistance of the band (Fig. 22-21). Care must be taken when performing pronation and supination to ensure the motion is at the subtalar joint and not at the tibiofemoral or hip joint. A pulley and weight stack system can be used for resistance. Slow, eccentric lengthening should be emphasized because of the deceleration function during gait.

Closed chain, weight-bearing strengthening exercises are a natural progression toward return to functional activity. Talocrural joint plantar flexors can be strengthened by performing double-leg toe stands off the end of a stair step. Emphasis is placed on eccentrically controlling a descent to end-range talocrural dorsiflexion without excessive pronation or eversion (Fig. 22-22). This is followed by concentric lifting to a neutral or slightly plantar-flexed position without excessive supination or inversion. The exercise is progressed by shifting weight toward the involved extremity and eventually performing a single-heel rise.

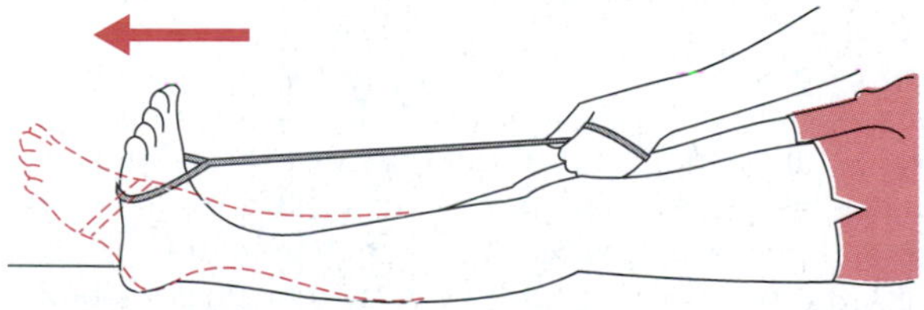

FIGURE 22-20 Resisted plantar flexion with a resistive band should emphasize plantar flexor–controlled eccentric dorsiflexion.

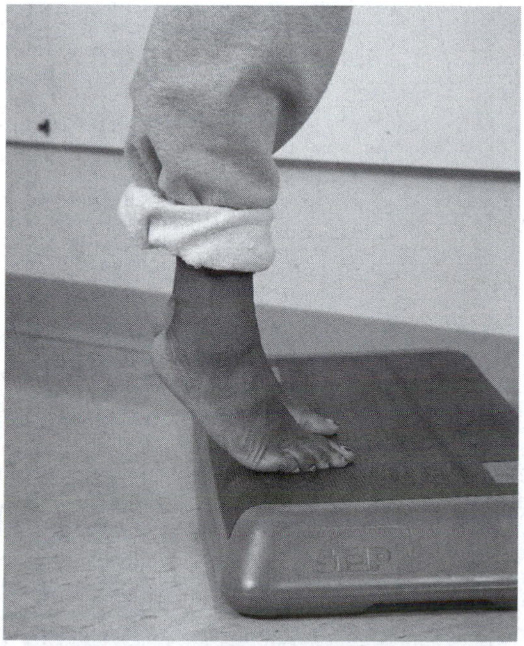

FIGURE 22-22 A standing toe raise will strengthen a number of muscles throughout the foot and ankle as medial, lateral, and intrinsic muscles stabilize the foot and ankle while the gastrocnemius and soleus muscles plantar flex the ankle.

Subtalar joint supinators can be strengthened by performing double-leg arch lifts. In a standing position, the patient is instructed to lift both arches, thereby rocking outward to the lateral portion of the feet. Care must be taken to maintain the great toe in contact with the floor to involve the peroneals and their role in stabilizing the first ray. Slow, controlled lowering to a neutral position is emphasized. Exercise intensity is increased by progressing body weight toward the involved extremity. Finger touch may be needed for balance.

Commercial equipment designed to objectively unload body weight (ie, pool or treadmill with traction unloading device) allows weight-bearing exercise to be performed early in the rehabilitation process (Fig. 22-23). Early intervention can decrease the effects of prolonged lack of weight bearing and promote a faster return to function (see Self-Management: Partial–Weight-Bearing Ball Rocking).

Balance and Coordination Impairment

The specific adaptations to imposed demands (SAID) principle means that the involved joint structures must be sufficiently prepared to assume the loads required for the patient's chosen activities. A well-conditioned and neurologically trained ankle is necessary to enable balance and function in a variety of directions as the center of gravity fluctuates. The patient must be able to control the ankle at extremes of motion while performing simultaneous activities in other extremities. The level of activity (eg, walking to the mailbox compared with playing competitive basketball) should be considered when designing proprioceptive training activities.

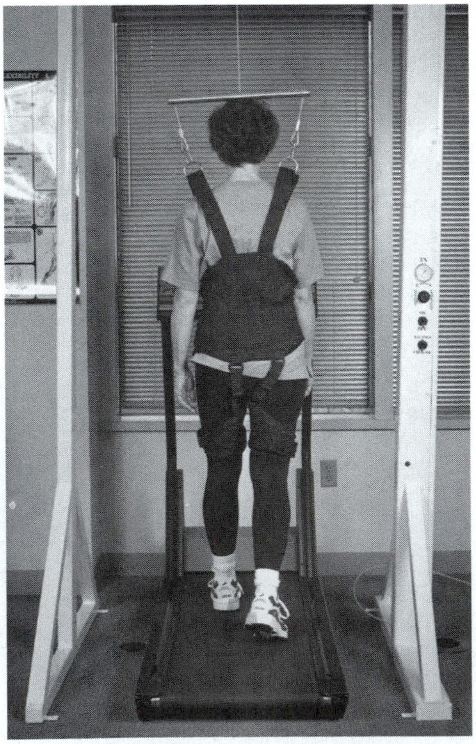

FIGURE 22-23 Unloading the lower extremity is performed on a treadmill with unloading equipment.

SELF-MANAGEMENT: Partial–Weight-Bearing Ball Rocking

Purpose: Increased mobility and calf muscle control in a partial–weight-bearing position

Position: Sitting on a therapeutic ball, feet flat on the floor, and weight equal on both feet

Movement technique: Slowly roll forward on the ball, bending your ankle as far as is comfortable.

Repeat ____ times

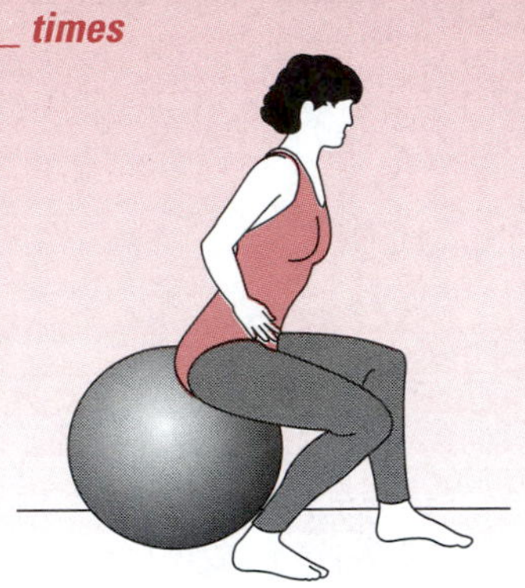

An elderly person recovering from an ankle fracture should be able to balance on one leg for 30 seconds with his eyes closed during a mild external perturbation (ie, with a balance board, a balance machine, or another person providing an external force). This prepares the elderly person to regain balance if he trips over a rug in a dark hallway during the night. Another patient may need to return to high-level gymnastics, and drills designed on a low balance beam would be appropriate. Plyometric exercises in the form of progressive height jump-down activities prepare the ankle to balance during high-impact activities.

Restoration of balance and coordination requires position sense, or proprioception. With an ankle sprain or muscle strain, these proprioceptive nerve fibers are often injured. The proprioceptive sense can also become deconditioned after a period of immobilization. The proprioceptors must be trained in a controlled, progressive manner in a weight-bearing position. Use of a balance board can provide proportionate and progressive stress. The following exercise progression can be used at home without special equipment:

- Balancing on one leg with eyes open
- Balancing on one leg with eyes closed
- Standing on one leg on a pillow with eyes open
- Standing on one leg on a pillow with eyes closed

Single-leg balance can also be progressed by swinging the uninvolved lower extremity first in flexion and extension and then in abduction and adduction (see Self-Mangement: Balance Activities). The faster and greater excursion of the swing, the more the static stance is challenged.

Elastic bands can be used for the advanced patient. An elastic band is tied in a circle and looped around a table leg or similar secure structure. Standing toward the table leg, the pa-

SELF-MANAGEMENT: Balance Activities

Purpose: Increased balance on a single leg

Position: Standing on one leg, near a counter or in a doorway to provide a surface to stabilize if necessary

Movement technique:
Level 1: Practice standing on a single leg with your eyes open for 30-second periods.
Level 2: Eyes closed
Level 3: Standing on a pillow with your eyes open
Level 4: Standing on a pillow with your eyes closed

Repeat ____ times

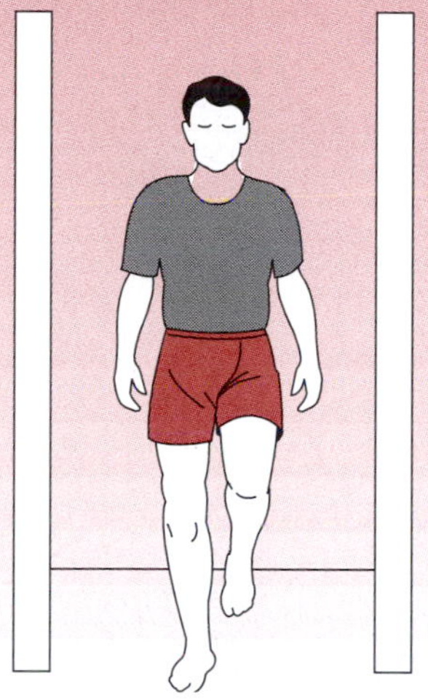

tient puts the uninvolved ankle inside the circled elastic band. While balancing on the involved foot, the patient is instructed to extend his hip against the elastic band. The patient performs a predetermined number of repetitions of extension-flexion oscillations before returning to double-limb support. The patient then turns 90 degrees and performs adduction-abduction oscillations into the band (Fig. 22-24). The rotating continues until the patient returns to the initial starting position. The exercise can be progressed by increasing oscillation repetitions, oscillation speed, or upgrading the tension of the elastic band.

The proprioceptors are essential in preventing recurrent injury, but they are often overlooked in many ankle rehabilitation programs. Creative prescriptions and following the SAID principle ensure proper training of this crucial element of the movement system.

Posture and Movement Impairment

The most common faulty movement patterns affecting the ankle and foot complex are excessive pronation and excessive supination. These abnormal patterns should not be reinforced in prescribed exercise. The impairments responsible for excessive pronation (eg, short gastrocnemius, stiff talocrural joint, forefoot varus, weak posterior tibialis) or supination (eg, hypomobile dorsiflexed first ray, hypomobile supinated talus post immobilization, short posterior tibialis) must be treated specifically and ultimately dealt with during a functional activity. Numerous repetitions of exercise developed from components of gait (eg, walk stance, single-limb stance, step-through) should be employed frequently throughout the day to alter neuromuscular function and change a habitual faulty movement pattern.

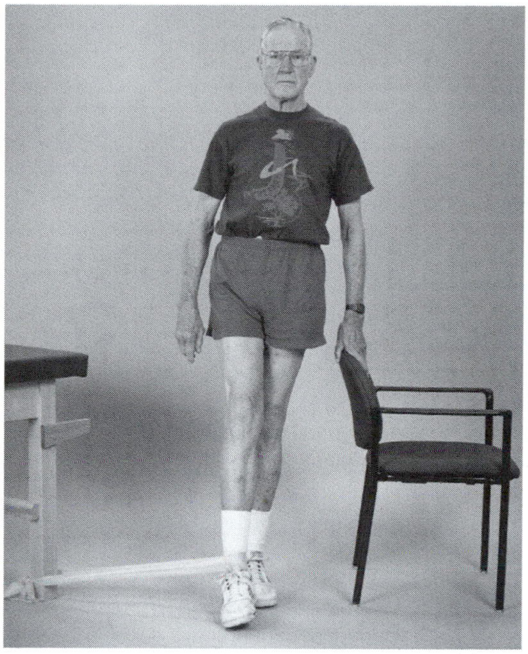

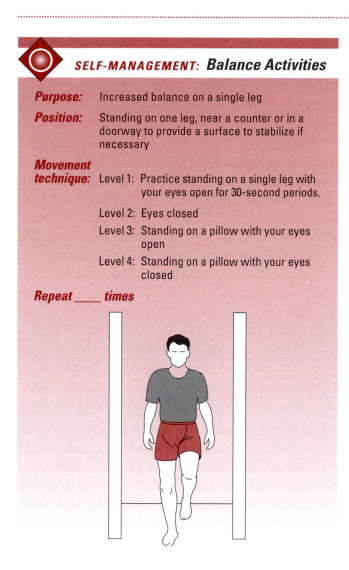

FIGURE 22-24 Resisted hip adduction retrains balance and proprioception on the weight-bearing limb. A chair or other stable surface must be available to ensure patient safety.

Posture and movement impairments are often treated simultaneously in the foot and ankle. Exercises combining these elements are sometimes referred to as *functional exercises*. Functional exercises have already been discussed as final progressions for treating impairments. Ideal alignment and movement should be emphasized, regardless of what impairment or combination of impairments are being addressed. A functional exercise program's goal is progression from the ability to maintain a static position to control of motions into and out of the static position and to accelerated motion in a smooth functional movement. The functional exercise program should be consistent with the patient's activity level and functional goals. Trunk and lower extremity alignment, strength, mobility, and movement patterns must be assessed and treated during a functional exercise program.

Functional exercise can begin early in the rehabilitation process, depending on the nature of the injury. Because gait is a primary functional goal, the patient is encouraged to use a three-point gait pattern with walker or two axillary crutches in conjunction with controlled partial weight bearing and a near-normal gait pattern (ie, heel to toe pattern). Ambulation on a painful foot without an assistive device results in compensations and abnormal gait biomechanics.

These abnormal biomechanics can lead to cumulative stress affecting the involved extremity, trunk, and uninvolved extremity. These compensations can develop into habits that are difficult to alter.[11]

Assistive devices are valuable in performing static and dynamic weight-shifting drills in preparation for weight bearing. Static weight-shifting drills are completed by progressively shifting weight toward the involved foot. A bathroom scale, indicating the amount of weight bearing, can be used for objectivity, control, and motivation. Dynamic weight-shifting drills are performed with the patient's involved foot stable on the floor and the uninvolved extremity stepping forward and backward. This drill can increase weight-bearing tolerance, promote heel to toe weight transfer, and facilitate talocrural dorsiflexion.

Medial-lateral weight shifting can be facilitated through a circular weight-shifting drill. The patient uses an assistive device for balance and stands with weight equally distributed over both feet. The patient is instructed to shift weight in a slow circular pattern, beginning at the fifth metatarsal head. The patient should then progress posteriorly to the lateral heel, medially to the medial heel, and anteriorly to the first metatarsal head. The drill can be performed clockwise and counterclockwise. It may be easier for the patient to perform this drill with both lower extremities simultaneously. As weight-bearing tolerance improves, the drill can be progressed by increasing body weight toward a single-leg stance.

Functional drills such as retrowalking, side stepping, cross-over stepping, and resisted walking are also beneficial for upgrading the patient's level of function. These drills are progressed by distance, speed, and adding resistance through elastic tubing or a pulley and weight-stack system. Jumping down may be a critical functional demand for athletes and persons returning to medium and heavy occupations. This task can be initiated bilaterally on a 2- to 4-inch box.

Ultimately, exercise must be progressed to higher levels of function (eg, stair stepping, running, jumping, cutting) that are appropriate for each patient's goals. Ideal alignment and movement patterns must be reinforced with each repetition. Orthotic prescription or counseling about proper footwear may be necessary to promote ideal function (see Patient-Related Instruction: Purchasing Footwear). However, exercise in bare feet may be appropriate in lower-level activities to ensure foot muscle function is providing the ideal alignment and movement pattern instead of the orthotic or footwear providing external support. An exception is a severe anatomic impairment (eg, significant forefoot varus), for which the use of a custom orthotic during all exercise is recommended.

THERAPEUTIC EXERCISE INTERVENTION FOR COMMON ANKLE AND FOOT DIAGNOSES

Although rehabilitation intervention is based on the impairments, functional limitations, and disability of each patient, some generalizations can be made about common medical diagnoses. Certain impairments are commonly associated with certain diagnoses, and these are highlighted.

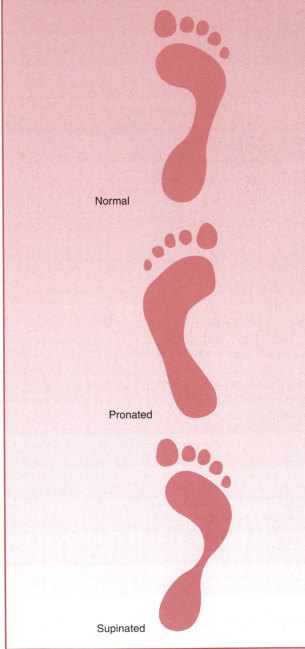

Patient-Related Instruction

Purchasing Footwear

Know your foot type. Your shoe size and width give a two-dimensional picture of your foot, but your foot is a three-dimensional object. Your foot's arch height affects the fit of your shoe. You can gauge your foot's arch height with a "wet test." Wet the soles of your feet, and then stand on a dry surface, such as a piece of cardboard, to leave an imprint of your foot. The imprint shows whether you have a flat (pronated), normal, or high-arched (supinated) foot. Match the bottoms of the shoes you're considering with your foot type.

This section is not exhaustive, but it addresses the most common conditions encountered.

Heel Pain Syndrome and Plantar Fascitis

ORIGIN AND DIAGNOSIS

The plantar fascia originates posteriorly at the medial tubercle of the calcaneus and runs anteriorly to multiple attachments throughout the midfoot, forefoot, and first phalanx of the toes. The plantar fascia provides stability to the foot by increasing the longitudinal arch during the propulsion phase of gait by means of the windlass mechanism.

Injury to the plantar fascia can result from trauma, such as an awkward step onto a ladder rung or an excessive amount of sports-like activity. More commonly, the mechanism of injury is cumulative stress from faulty lower extremity biomechanics. Excessive traction on the origin of the fascia on the calcaneus can cause microtears and result in heel pain syndrome (HPS). Excessive subtalar pronation and medially shifted weight-bearing forces fatigue supportive structures and can sprain the plantar fascia or result in plantar fascitis. The HPS symptoms are associated with stress to the plantar fascia where it arises from the medial calcaneal tuberosity on the anteromedial aspect of the heel. A common symptom is sharp pain at the medial aspect of the heel. Because of the proximity of the medial calcaneal tuberosity and the origin of the plantar fascia, it is not possible to clinically differentiate a fascial from a bony source of pain. Both structures are usually involved, and the term HPS is used to describe pain arising from this region. HPS is similar to plantar fascitis in that symptoms are worse in the morning with initial weight bearing, the pain gradually decreases with further weight bearing, but the pain is intensified by athletic activity, especially running or jumping.

Tenderness over the plantar fascia in the midfoot is true plantar fascitis. This condition manifests with tenderness over the midportion of the plantar fascia. Dorsiflexion of the toes almost always exacerbates the patient's symptoms because of the windlass mechanism stretching the fascial fibers.

The differential diagnosis of plantar fascitis and tendinitis of the flexor hallucis longus tendon can be made with selective tissue tension testing. Resisted flexion of the toes is painful with involvement of the flexor hallucis longus tendon.

TREATMENT

The cornerstone of conservative treatment for HPS and plantar fascitis is modification of activity. For the running athlete, for example, mileage reduction, alternate activities, work reduction, and shortened workouts should be considered. Low-resistance cycling and swimming pool running are effective alternatives to running on land. The goal of treatment of plantar fascitis in the acute stage is the control of inflammation through the use of nonsteroidal anti-inflammatory medications, steroid injection, iontophoresis, or ultrasound. Circumferential taping of the foot is usually beneficial as an initial intervention to unload the plantar fascia and reduce inflammation. Temporary relief of pain may be achieved by soft tissue mobilization with trigger point pressure to the intrinsic musculature and calf. In the subacute phase, progressive cross-friction massage and stretching of the plantar fascia helps guard against abnormal scar formation and can improve plantar fascia extensibility (see Self-Mangement: Plantar Fascia Step Stretch).

Stretch of the gastrocnemius-soleus complex is often indicated in HPS, because limited dorsiflexion mobility places increased stress on the plantar fascia at its origin. Surprisingly, no clear correlation between HPS and pes planus (ie, low-arch foot alignment) has been established. However, a positive correlation between HPS and obesity exists, and appropriate intervention for obesity is therefore indicated.

Treatment of structural or functional leg length discrepancy is also indicated. HPS is seen more frequently in shorter legs. A functional short leg may result from running on the same tilt of road or in the same direction on the track. By using both sides of the road or intermittently changing directions on a track, stress between both heels can be equalized.

Long-term resolution of symptoms of HPS and plantar fascitis can only be achieved by addressing the physiologic impairments directly affecting the biomechanics of the plantar fascia. For example, if pronation is causing stress to the plantar fascia and a short gastrocnemius muscle and stiff talocrural joint are contributing to the pronation, calf stretching should be performed regularly throughout the day. If intrinsic muscle weakness is contributing to loss of longitudinal and transverse arch support, intrinsic muscle strengthening can be initiated to promote dynamic stability against excessive pronation. Lower extremity alignment, muscle flexibility, strength, and movement patterns must be assessed for extrinsic pronatory factors. Functional exercise and proprioceptive training should be initiated to reduce pronatory forces and improve talocrural dorsiflexion.

SELF-MANAGEMENT: **Plantar Fascia Step Stretch**

Purpose: Increased flexibility of the plantar fascia

Position: Standing with the toes extended against the vertical part of a step and the heel on the floor

Movement technique: Slowly bend the knee above the toes you are stretching back. Keep your arch from rolling in.

Duration ____

Repeat ____ times

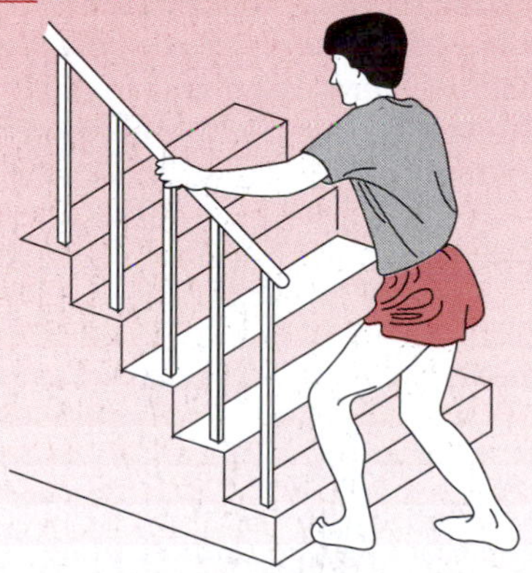

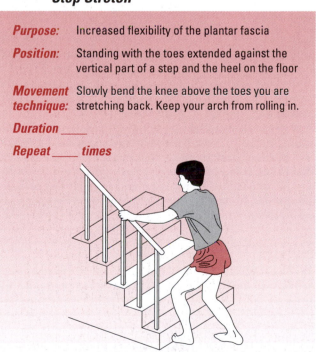

Abnormal intrinsic rearfoot and forefoot alignment must be assessed for potential orthotic therapy. Longitudinal arch support is often not tolerated by patients with plantar fascitis, because it pushes up on the plantar fascia and increases tension on the fibers. However, proper orthotic prescription with appropriate forefoot and rearfoot posting can support the plantar fascia without direct pressure on the soft tissue underneath the longitudinal arch. A small heel lift can be beneficial in treating HPS resistant to appropriate exercise intervention.

Tibialis Posterior Tendinitis

ORIGIN AND DIAGNOSIS

The tibialis posterior muscle originates at the posterior tibia and interosseous membrane. It runs posterior and inferior to the medial malleolus to an insertion at the navicular, first and second cuneiforms, and the base of the second, third, and fourth metatarsals. With open chain mechanics, the tibialis posterior inverts and plantar flexes the foot. With closed chain mechanics, it decelerates subtalar joint pronation in the loading response phase and supinates the subtalar joint in the midstance and terminal stance phases. The mechanism of tibialis posterior tendon injury is usually excessive subtalar joint pronation. However, the tendon can be strained because of poor physical condition or by excessive physical activity. The least common mechanism of injury is an eversion ankle sprain. Symptoms are commonly located at the distal one third of the medial tibia or inferior and posterior to the medial malleolus. Symptoms include tenderness to palpation along the tendon, pain with resisted inversion and plantar flexion, and pain with closed chain pronation. Walking can become painful if accompanied by excessive pronation. Running, cutting, or jumping can become painful because of recruitment of the posterior tibialis during deceleration activities.

TREATMENT

As in plantar fascitis, a primary goal in the acute phase is to control inflammation with appropriate medications and therapeutic modalities. Arch strapping is beneficial for controlling end-range pronation, which decreases the strain on the tibialis posterior muscle. Pain-free, low-intensity, high-repetition, open chain plantar flexion and inversion exercises should be initiated early in the rehabilitation process to control pain and inflammation. Open and closed chain strengthening exercises are initiated as tolerated in the subacute phase. Intrinsic and extrinsic pronatory factors should be assessed and treated with orthotic therapy and functional exercise as indicated for long-term resolution of symptoms.

Achilles Tendinitis

ORIGIN AND DIAGNOSIS

Achilles tendinitis is one of the more common tendon injuries of the lower extremity. It is particularly prevalent among persons participating in running and jumping sports. The Achilles tendon functions eccentrically to lower the heel to the floor when landing from a jump. The tendon is also stressed during the late midstance phase of gait, when it elongates to slow the advancing tibia. This stress is particularly high when walking or running uphill, when the tendon must slow the tibia eccentrically but propel the body uphill concentrically. The tendon is particularly susceptible to injury approximately 2 to 5 cm above its insertion into the calcaneus. A one-fourth turn compromises the vascular supply, predisposing this area to injury.

The Achilles tendon is also susceptible to rupture in the same area. The typical patient sustaining a rupture is a middle-aged, competitive man involved in intermittent athletic activities. Chronic degeneration is observed in most ruptured tendons, although most ruptures occur without any preexisting complaints. The patient complains of feeling as if he had been kicked in the back of the leg, although most ruptures are noncontact injuries. A defect may be palpated, and the Thompson test result is positive.

TREATMENT

Treatment of Achilles tendinitis should follow the guidelines set forth in Chapter 10. Stretching is essential to increase the length over which the tendon loads can be dispersed. Stretching should be performed with the knee straight and the knee bent, ensuring neutral foot position. This stretching should not produce pain; only a pulling sensation is felt. Strengthening exercises are an important intervention, with the focus on progression to eccentric exercise. Controlled lowering from a plantar-flexed to dorsiflexed position challenges the plantar flexors eccentrically. The speed should be gradually increased to progressively challenge this muscle group (see Self-Management: Hop-Down Drills). Achilles tendon ruptures are treated conservatively with immobilization in a cast or cast boot for as long as 12 weeks, followed by progressive rehabilitation as outlined for Achilles tendinitis. The effects of immobilization and the damage to the Achilles tendon must be considered in planning activities. Mobility activities to restore the length of the gastrocnemius-soleus complex and restore the mobility of the talocrural joint are necessary. Surgical treatment is common after rupture and is discussed in the Surgical Procedures section.

Ligament Sprains

ORIGIN AND DIAGNOSIS

Ligament sprains are the most common injuries to the foot and ankle. Between 70% and 80% of the sprains involve the anterior talofibular ligament (ATFL), calcaneal fibular ligament (CFL), or posterior talofibular ligament (PTFL).[21,23–25] Ligaments of the midfoot, including the dorsal calcaneal cuboid and the bifurcate ligament, may also be involved. The mechanism of injury is usually an inversion and plantar flexion twist. Isolated injuries of the ATFL constitute 65% of ankle sprains, and a combination injury involving the ATFL and CFL comprise 20% of the cases. Isolated injury of the CFL or PTFL is rare.

Ligament sprains are generally classified as one of three grades:

- Grade I represents minor tearing with no functional loss of ankle stability.

SELF-MANAGEMENT: Hop-Down Drills

Purpose: Increased balance and coordination during dynamic movement, impact loading, and controlled lengthening of the Achilles

Position: Standing on a small step of about 4 inches

Movement technique: Level 1: Hop down onto both feet, controlling the landing.

Level 2: Hop down, landing on a single leg.

Repeat ____ times

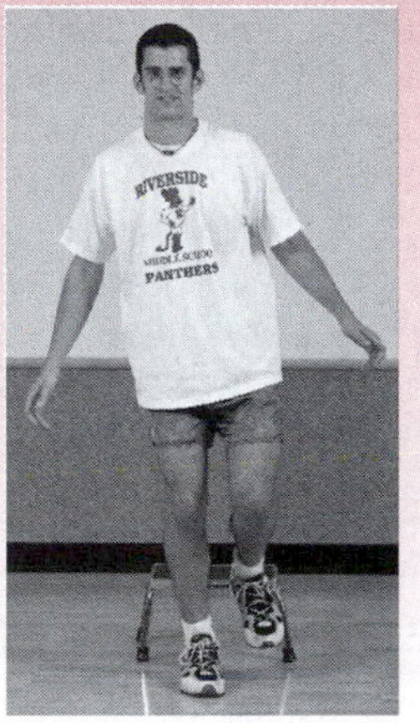

LEVEL 2

- Grade II represents partial tearing of the ligament with moderate instability.
- Grade III describes a complete rupture with significant functional instability.

Grade III sprains are further classified by degrees of injury. First-degree sprains suggest complete rupture of the ATFL. A second-degree sprain is a complete rupture of the ATFL and CFL. A third-degree sprain suggests a dislocation in which the ATFL, CFL, and PTFL are ruptured.[23]

The patient can usually recall the mechanism of injury, and there is usually a specific site of pain and tenderness. A sprain ultimately has edema of the area. Ecchymosis may occur, indicating injury to blood vessels in the area. Specific stability testing of the affected ligaments may produce guarding and pain.

Syndesmosis sprains are common and often occur in combination with other injuries. A syndesmosis sprain is a disruption of the distal tibiofemoral ligaments, resulting in diastasis, or widening of the mortise at the talocrural joint. The mechanism for syndesmosis disruption is external rotation on a fixed foot or extreme dorsiflexion. These mechanisms force the talus into the mortise formed by the tibia and fibula, widening this space and disrupting the distal tibiofibular ligaments. If missed on initial evaluation, the patient may subsequently complain of posterior ankle pain, particularly when trying to push off of the involved ankle. Failure to recognize and treat a significant syndesmosis sprain can produce widening of the mortise and severe degenerative joint disease. Weight-bearing radiographs are necessary to assess the integrity of the tibiofibular joint in a suspected syndesmosis sprain.

TREATMENT

Healing of a ligament sprain, as in most soft tissue injuries, follows a process of inflammation, repair, and remodeling. These events are sequential, but each phase of healing overlaps another. Optimal healing occurs when the introduction of exercise and functional activity is appropriate for each phase. Controlled stress promotes healing and results in a stronger repair, but excessive loading can interrupt healing and prolong the inflammatory process. The time needed for healing depends on the grade of injury, and clinical decisions should be based on signs, symptoms, and functional assessments.

The initial treatment goals focus on controlling inflammation and associated pain and swelling. Treatment of grade I and II ankle sprains during the first 1 to 4 days includes protection, rest, ice, compression, and elevation (PRICE). Early weight bearing is allowed and encouraged, but the injury must be protected with an external support in the form of a brace or tape. Severe grade I and grade II sprains may need axillary crutches for additional protection during ambulation. Patients are instructed to elevate the foot higher than the heart in conjunction with ice applications. Compression with an elastic wrap is beneficial, especially when the foot is in a dependent position. Elevated edema massage and vasopneumatic compression are also helpful in controlling pain and swelling. Midrange active dorsiflexion and plantar flexion ROM exercises are initiated early, with care not to elongate the injured ligament.

Exercise is progressed as pain and swelling are controlled and weight-bearing tolerance increases. Open chain inversion ROM is progressed as tolerated. Dorsiflexion ROM and calf flexibility can be treated more aggressively. Weight-shifting drills performed with full or partial weight bearing and with an external support help to maintain muscle tone and promote balance reactions. Proprioception boards are helpful, but exercise must be controlled to prevent interruption of the repair process. Toe raises off of a step help maintain strength and flexibility of the calf. Trunk, hip, and knee exercises are helpful in preventing the obvious effects of inactivity.

Remodeling of new collagen is under way 3 to 6 weeks after an injury. Restoration of proprioception and strength are key treatment goals to prevent recurrent hypermobility impairments. Reinjury may occur during this phase, because many patients have false confidence in the ankle. Return to a high level of activity should be controlled. Running at slow speeds in straight lines must precede fast speeds and cutting. Slow running in a large figure-eight pattern can be progressed to faster speeds in a smaller figure-eight pattern. An external support should be used during high-level activity for 6 to 8 weeks after injury.

Immediate treatment of grade III sprains is somewhat debated. One school of thought suggests surgical repair followed by immobilization and then rehabilitation. Others suggest immobilization followed by rehabilitation. Subotnick[24,25] thinks that surgical repair is indicated if there has been history of other disabling sprains; otherwise, conservative treatment should be attempted. The rehabilitation approach for grade III sprains, whether treated with surgical repair or immobilization, is similar to that for grade I and II sprains. A clinician should expect greater deficits in ROM, flexibility, and muscle strength throughout the lower extremity. External supports are important until full strength and proprioception have been obtained.

Chronic recurrent sprain or functional loss is usually related to insufficient recovery of proprioception and strength, hypomobility related to abnormal scarring, or hypermobility due to insufficient ligamentous healing. A patient with ankle dysfunction related to hypomobility usually demonstrates limitation and pain with inversion and plantar flexion stress testing. Cross-friction massage, joint mobilization, and mobility exercises are usually beneficial. Recurrent sprains due to hypermobility may require long-term use of external supports or surgical repair. Progressive proprioception and functional strength training is usually needed in cases of chronic ankle dysfunction.

Syndesmosis sprains are treated conservatively with cast immobilization for 4 to 6 weeks. An unstable and widened mortise is often treated with surgical fixation. Subsequent rehabilitation is similar to that for medial or lateral ankle sprains.

Ankle Fractures

ORIGIN AND DIAGNOSIS

Talocrural fractures are the most common fractures in the lower extremity. Excessive talar external rotation, abduction, or adduction within the malleoli can result in shearing or avulsion fractures of the malleoli. Ligament sprains are frequently associated with malleolar fractures. Talocrural joint fractures are commonly classified by the position of the foot (pronated or supinated) and by the direction of force exerted on the malleoli by the talus. Symptoms are similar to those of ankle sprains, although more severe in nature. The following is a description of common talocrural fractures using the Lauge-Hansen classification system.[26]

Supination Adduction Injury. Extreme lateral loading of the foot results in excessive supination and potential avulsion fracture of the distal fibula in addition to lateral collateral ligament strain. If the force continues, the talus is adducted in the distal tibiofibular joint, which results in a shearing fracture of the distal medial malleolus at the joint line.

Supination External Rotation Injury. Forced external rotation of the talus with a supinated foot can result in tearing of the anterior inferior tibiofibular ligament, followed by fracture of the distal fibula. Continued external rotation force may result in a deltoid ligament rupture or avulsion fracture of the distal medial malleolus. Because the deltoid ligament is very strong, the avulsion fracture of the medial malleolus is more common.

Pronated Abduction Injury. Excessive abduction of the talus in the distal tibiofibular joint while the foot is pronated results in avulsion fracture of the medial malleolus. Continued abduction of the talus can rupture the anterior and posterior tibiofibular ligament. Separation of the distal tibiofibular joint is referred to as joint diastasis. The final stage of this fracture pattern is shearing off of the lateral malleolus at the level of the joint line.

Pronated External Rotation Injury. Forced external rotation of the talus on a pronated foot can result in a avulsion fracture of the medial malleolus, followed by tearing of the anterior tibiofibular ligament and fracture of the fibula. The fibular fracture is usually in the fibular shaft above the talocrural joint. Tibiofibular diastasis may exist.

TREATMENT

The key element in the acute treatment of talocrural joint fractures is the restoration of tibiotalar anatomic alignment. Fractures can be treated with closed reduction or with open reduction and internal fixation (ORIF). Fibular fractures without loss of tibiotalar alignment are usually treated with closed reduction. Fractures of both malleoli or one malleolus and a ligament rupture usually result in malalignment and therefore require ORIF. Patients are usually immobilized in a plaster cast for 6 to 10 weeks after ORIF.

The initial phase of rehabilitation should include instruction in elevation and active exercise of the noninjured joints. Edema massage, surgical scar mobilization, and modalities for edema reduction are beneficial. Talocrural accessory joint motion must be assessed and joint mobilization techniques initiated as indicated. Active ROM begins in midrange with low intensity and high repetition. Controlled, partial–weight-bearing ambulation with an assistive device (ie, walker or axillary crutches) is often preferred to ambulation with no assistance. Unprotected ambulation may increase pain and swelling at the foot and ankle and result in undue strain at the lumbopelvic region and opposite lower extremity. Early stationary biking provides a gentle exercise for both lower extremities. Patients are initially instructed to pedal with the heel and progress to pedaling with the forefoot.

As swelling is controlled, treatment emphasis swings toward aggressive ROM, strengthening, and functional exercise. Involved knee and hip biomechanics should be assessed and treated. The key structural deficit seen in ankle fractures is usually lack of talocrural joint dorsiflexion. Common gait compensations for limited dorsiflexion include the following:

- Abduction and external rotation of the lower extremity
- Genu recurvatum
- Excessive subtalar joint pronation

Early use of heel lifts can help eliminate these compensations (see Heel and Full Sole Lifts section). As function normalizes, ROM exercise is generally more tolerable, and progress is usually accelerated. The goal is to remove the heel lifts as soon as ROM is improved. If trauma was extreme and the structural impairment is deemed permanent, heel lifts can be fabricated externally on the shoe for long-term use.

Excessive subtalar joint pronation as a compensation for limited talocrural joint dorsiflexion can create midfoot hypermobility and dysfunction. Foot orthotics may be indicated for the current condition and future foot health. Heel lifts in conjunction with foot orthotics are an adjunct to functional strengthening and proprioceptive training. These supportive devices should be considered early in the rehabilitation process and may be needed for long-term function.

Functional Nerve Disorders

Assessment of impairments associated with nerve dysfunction affecting muscles of the lower leg, ankle, and foot should always begin with screening of the lumbar spine. Paresis or paralysis of muscles innervated by the posterior tibial or common peroneal nerves can be the result of a spine impairment. After the spine has been excluded as the source of the nerve disorder, other entrapment sites in the hip (eg, piriformis syndrome) should be ruled out.

Many nerve disorders are considered to be functional, which means that the nerve is compressed during functional activity. Nerves can be compressed by bony impingements, compartment syndromes, or as a result of joint hypermobility or instability. Occasionally, a nerve can be compressed in multiple locations. It is important to understand the anatomy and innervation patterns to diagnose and treat nerve disorders appropriately. Nerve compression or entrapment may resolve with shoe changes, orthotics, or alteration of impairments in alignment, mobility, and movement patterns through the application of therapeutic exercise. The following sections describe selected sites for injury, compression, or entrapment of the posterior tibial and common peroneal nerves and branches.

TIBIAL NERVE

The tibial nerve is injured less frequently than the common peroneal nerve because of its deep and protected position within the popliteal fossa. If a lesion or entrapment occurs in the popliteal fossa, all of the calf muscles and plantar muscles of the foot are affected. A complete lesion in the popliteal fossa results in a shuffling gait and difficulty raising the heel during propulsion because of the loss of ankle plantar flexors. The unopposed action of the muscles innervated by the common peroneal nerve can lead to an increased concavity of the longitudinal arch of the foot (ie, pes cavus) and clawing of the toes. Sensory loss occurs on the sole of the foot and the plantar surfaces of the toes. Painful disorders, such as causalgia, are common with incomplete or irritative lesions.

If entrapment is suspected, the muscles surrounding the popliteal fossa must be assessed for length. If the popliteus, plantaris, and gastrocnemius are short, the tibial nerve may be compressed. Appropriate stretching and changes in alignment and movement patterns that perpetuate muscle shortening may alleviate the pressure and reduce nerve compression.

A more common disorder affecting the tibial nerve is tarsal tunnel syndrome. The tarsal tunnel is a fibro-osseous tunnel formed by the flexor retinaculum, the medial wall of the calcaneus, the posterior portion of the talus, the distal tibia, and the medial malleolus. The tibial nerve travels through this tunnel and may be compressed behind the medial malleolus under the retinacular ligament. Compression results in weakness of toe flexion, abduction, and adduction and in sensory changes of the medial and lateral side of the sole of the foot and toes.

With a hypermobile subtalar joint, the posterior tibial nerve is stretched by a prominence of the posteromedial talus. Intervention for compression or entrapment in this region should include treating the impairments associated with subtalar pronation. This may involve stretching a short gastrocnemius, strengthening a weak posterior tibialis, educating the patient regarding altered postural habits, and instructing the patient in proper foot biomechanics during components of gait. Improved biomechanics during gait and other functional activities are the goal. In conjunction with exercise, the use of appropriate footwear alone or with orthotics to control excessive pronation may be necessary for complete resolution of symptoms related to nerve compression.

PERONEAL NERVE

The common peroneal is the most commonly injured nerve in the lower limb, primarily because of its exposed position as it winds around the neck of the fibula. Injury causes paresis or paralysis of all the muscles supplied by the deep and superficial peroneal nerves. The result is a loss of dorsiflexion and eversion of the foot and extension of the toes, producing footdrop and a steppage gait. An accompanying loss of sensation occurs in the front of the lower leg, dorsum of the foot, and adjacent sides of all toes. Recurrent ankle sprains may also result from peroneal weakness. A thorough knowledge of anatomy, innervation patterns, and function of the affected muscles during gait is necessary to develop an appropriate exercise program during the stages of nerve recovery. Care must be taken to prevent fatigue of a muscle recovering from a nerve injury. An external support (ie, dorsiflexion assist splint) is usually necessary during the early phases of recovery, when the muscles are weakest.

The deep peroneal nerve may become entrapped distally under the extensor retinaculum, a condition known as anterior tarsal tunnel syndrome. Trauma often plays a role. Recurrent ankle sprain places the deep peroneal nerve on maximal stretch as the foot plantar flexes and supinates. Tight-fitting shoes or ski boots have also been implicated. Compression of the deep peroneal nerve usually results in pain radiating into the first web space. The extensor digitorum brevis may be weak or atrophied.

For patients with anterior tarsal tunnel syndrome, ensure that nerve compression is not caused by poorly fitting footwear. If the ankle is hypermobile or unstable, associated impairments should be treated with appropriate therapeutic exercise, footwear, bracing, taping, or orthotics to reduce excessive stretch of the deep peroneal nerve. Exercise may include strengthening the peroneals, combined with drills to train ankle proprioceptors and help prevent recurrent ankle sprains.

Surgical Procedures

Therapeutic exercise interventions for selected postoperative diagnoses are presented in this section. Complete discussion of the cause and treatment of each diagnosis is not provided, but guidelines for postoperative therapeutic exercise management are presented. Some surgeons may have established intervention protocols for specific surgical techniques, and these should take precedence.

GENERAL PRINCIPLES OF POSTSURGICAL REHABILITATION

The first 72 hours after surgery is a critical time to prevent and decrease postoperative swelling by elevation, compression, and icing. Postoperative immobilization with a cast should be done when indicated, but the immobilization time should be minimized to prevent stiffness and atrophy. Isometric exercises during the immobilization period can retard muscle atrophy. Use of a splint or cast-brace to allow early mobility and strengthening should be used whenever possible.

Cross-training of unaffected limbs or joints should be initiated early, even when the patient is restricted to upper extremity exercise. A comprehensive rehabilitation plan, including dates for weight-bearing changes, suture removal, and exercise progression, should be developed by the surgeon so that the patient and therapist know what to expect. The exercise program must be progressed gradually with close supervision to increase activity demands without compromising healing or exposing the patient to postoperative complications or reinjury.

ACHILLES TENDON REPAIR

If the decision has been made to perform surgery in the case of an acute rupture, a tendon repair is usually performed. Rehabilitation after surgical repair of an acute rupture of the Achilles tendon requires a regimented program to allow time and protection of soft tissue healing while preventing muscle atrophy and regaining gastrocnemius-soleus complex strength and length.

An intermediate approach to postoperative rehabilitation is described. A short-leg cast is applied with the foot in equinus. Initially, only touch-down weight bearing is allowed. At 3 to 4 weeks, the cast is changed to a cast-brace, with the ankle locked at 10 to 15 degrees. The patient is encouraged to remove the brace for unrestricted plantar flexion exercises and for gentle kicking and plantar flexion exercises in a swimming pool. Dorsiflexion beyond neutral is avoided by using a Plastizote dorsiflexion block splint in the pool. Partial weight bearing is allowed at 4 weeks. At 6 weeks, progressive weight bearing is allowed as tolerated in a modified shoe with a heel lift. Over the next 6 weeks, the heel lift is reduced as dorsiflexion ROM returns to normal. Cycling and swimming are encouraged to restore cardiovascular fitness. At 3 months, jogging and sport-specific training are allowed. A full return to vigorous sport can take 5 to 6 months.

Therapeutic exercise intervention should focus on pain and swelling, hypomobility, loss of force or torque, loss of balance and coordination, and alignment and movement impairments. Each of these impairments usually is present to some extent. In the initial stages, pain, inflammation, and hypomobility are the most critical impairments to address. As these impairments resolve, strength, proprioception, and functional return become more critical. During the later stage of rehabilitation, repeat rupture must be prevented. Progression of resisted exercise should err on the conservative side. The temptation to shorten the period of protection must be resisted to minimize the possibility of repeat rupture.

Tendon transfer procedures are used in late Achilles tendon repairs. The flexor digitorum longus and flexor hallucis longus are the most commonly used tendons. The transfer is sutured onto the Achilles, with the ankle in about 5 to 10 degrees of plantar flexion. Postoperative immobilization for 6 to 10 weeks is accomplished in a progression of casts and cast-braces, followed by a well-directed rehabilitation program. Tendon transfer requires more recovery time and a slower progression of rehabilitation. Full return to vigorous activity can occur within 3 to 6 months. Consultation with the surgeon is necessary to develop the appropriate, tailored program, because only the physician knows the extent of tendon damage and the complexity of the resultant repair or reconstruction.

ANKLE LIGAMENT RECONSTRUCTION

Ankle ligament reconstruction is performed after all conservative treatment fails and when the patient has continued complaints of ankle sprains despite taping or bracing. Appropriate ligament surgery is performed, followed by immobilization in a weight-bearing, short-leg cast for 3 weeks and a removable cast-brace for an additional 3 weeks. During the first 3 weeks, isometric exercises for the dorsiflexors and evertors are performed. During the second 3 weeks, Achilles tendon stretching and peroneal strengthening are initiated. Plantar flexion ROM exercises are avoided. Proprioceptive training is initiated in a partial–weight-bearing mode with the use of parallel bars. At 6 weeks postoperatively, a functional rehabilitation program is initiated. For example, agility exercises are progressed from straight jogging to running to figure-eight jogging to cutting. Other agility exercises, such as hopping from side to side without resistance and then with resistance, are incorporated into the program as the athlete gains confidence in the ankle (see Self-Management: Agility Drills).

HALLUX VALGUS REPAIR

The postsurgical regimen after a hallux valgus repair (ie, bunionectomy) must ensure adequate immobilization of the

SELF-MANAGEMENT: **Agility Drills**

Purpose: Increased agility in high level activity

Position: Standing sideways along the length of a gym or hallway

Movement technique:
Level 1: Run sideways using a grapevine step (cross in front, step to the side, cross in back, step to the side, and repeat).
Level 2: Add a skill activity such as catching a ball.

Repeat ____ times

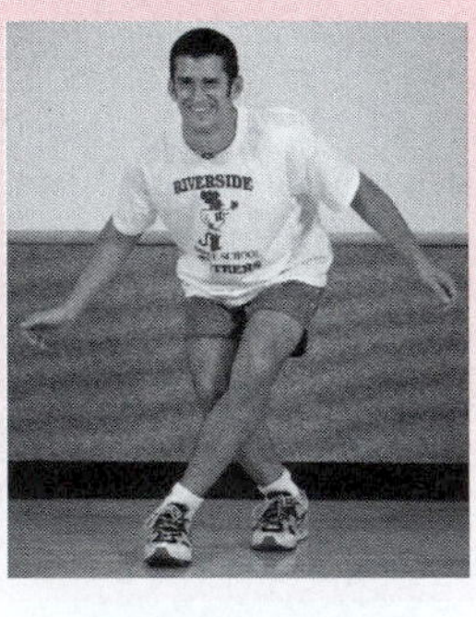

first metatarsophalangeal joint and osteotomy for satisfactory healing of tissues. Usually, 6 to 8 weeks of immobilization is required. During this period of immobilization, patients can carry out nonimpact activities such as riding a stationary bike and weight lifting, but stress across the surgical site should be avoided. After 6 to 8 weeks of immobilization, gentle ROM exercises can be initiated along with progressive reconditioning. Return to athletic activity can take an additional 6 to 8 weeks.

Hallux valgus may be caused by excessive forces along the medial side of the great toe. This condition can occur as a result of intrinsic or extrinsic impairments contributing to pronatory forces at the foot. Long-term resolution of hallux valgus requires treatment of ankle and foot impairments related to pronation. If pronation is not addressed postoperatively, the hallux valgus deformity may return.

ADJUNCTIVE INTERVENTIONS

A therapeutic exercise program for the ankle and foot can be enhanced by the use of supportive devices. Adhesive strapping, wedges and pads, biomechanical foot orthotics, and sole or heel lifts can help control excessive compensation and promote a faster return to functional activity. The supportive devices are an adjunct to a thorough exercise program and, if used independently, may be less successful. In many situations, the converse is also true.

Adhesive Strapping

The use of adhesive strapping is beneficial in controlling the end range of joint motion. Longitudinal arch strapping is valuable when excessive pronation is deemed a primary stressor. Caution must be taken in supportive strapping if the foot is swollen. Strapping should improve the patient's symptoms, and if symptoms increase, the strapping should be removed immediately. The patient must be instructed to remove the strapping slowly by pulling the tape backward on itself. Avoid quick jerking movements and excessive skin distraction when removing the tape, because this could pull superficial skin layers off the body. The foot must be properly prepared before adhesive strapping is applied to enhance support and decrease the risk of skin irritation Display 22-2 provides guidelines for preparing the foot for adhesive strapping.

DISPLAY 22-2

Preparing the Foot for Adhesive Strapping

1. The foot must be clean and dry. Soap and water or alcohol wipes are used to remove perspiration and skin oils, which decreases the tape adherence to the skin.
2. Hair should be shaved to avoid irritation to hair follicles and the pain associated with pulling hair out during tape removal.
3. Skin should be sprayed with a skin preparation or "toughener" that improves tape adherence.
4. Thin foam prewrap used before taping helps protect the skin, but when maximal support is necessary, the tape should be applied directly to the skin. Prewrap has been used successfully when patients are limited to a medium or low activity level.

DISPLAY 22-3

Longitudinal Arch Strapping Technique

Tape: 1-inch athletic tape.
Taping position: Patient is supine on the treatment table, with his foot over the edge.
Taping technique: Place two anchor strips circumferentially just proximal to the metatarsal heads (apply lightly). Begin the first diagonal strip of tape on the medial side of the foot, just proximal to the head of the first metatarsal. Tape posteriorly and around the heel. Angle the tape under the foot, crossing the plantar surface, and return medially near the origin of this strip (A). Place the second diagonal strip of tape on the lateral side of the foot, just proximal to the head of the fifth metatarsal. Tape under the foot, around the heel, and up the lateral side toward the origin of this strip (B). Continue alternating strips in the same pattern until the "fan" is filled in (C). Tie down the entire procedure by placing plantar strips over the previous strips by starting on the dorsolateral aspect of the foot; continue under the arch, and finish on the dorsomedial aspect of the foot. Leave a gap on the top of the foot; bridge this by placing short strips of tape across the gap (D) and (E). Each strip of tape should overlap the previous strip by approximately ¼ inch.

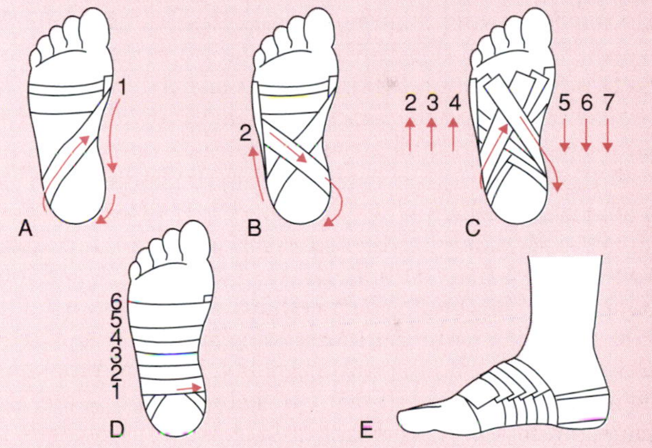

The longitudinal arch strapping technique presented in Display 22-3 is designed to decrease soft tissue strain caused by excessive subtalar joint pronation. Many additions and variations of supportive foot strapping can be explored.

Wedges and Pads

Medial heel wedges, longitudinal arch pads, and metatarsal pads can be placed in a shoe or on a flat insole to decrease soft tissue strain. Medial heel wedges or varus wedges are thick medially and taper laterally. They are made of firm rubber and used with the philosophy of controlling calcaneal eversion and thereby decreasing the degree of subtalar joint pronation. Metatarsal and longitudinal arch pads are made of felt or foam rubber. The metatarsal pad is placed directly proximal to the symptomatic metatarsal head. Medial wedges, longitudinal arch pads, and metatarsal pads are most successful when used in conjunction with adhesive strapping. Longitudinal arch and metatarsal pads can be taped on top of an arch strapping for precise positioning. The medial wedge can be secured in a shoe with the use of double-faced tape. If symptoms are relieved and performance is improved through adhesive strapping and supportive pads, a biomechanical orthotic may be indicated.

Biomechanical Foot Orthotics

It is beyond the scope of this text to provide a detailed description of orthotic evaluation and prescription. This section describes the purpose of orthotic devices, the general fabrication method, the concept of posting, and therapeutic exercise prescription to augment orthotic prescription.

A biomechanical foot orthotic is a device that attempts to control dysfunction by controlling the subtalar joint near its neutral position. A foot orthotic is composed of a shell, which conforms to the contours of the foot, and posting material, which tilts the shell according to the angulation and degree of control desired.

The shell is fabricated from an impression of the foot taken while the subtalar joint is held in a neutral position. The shell encompasses the heel, fits closely to the arch, and ends immediately proximal to the metatarsal heads. The shell can be made of a variety of materials, ranging from a flexible foam to a semirigid thermoplastic. Generally, the more rigid shells are indicated for the hypermobile foot requiring motion control. Flexible accommodative shells are used for arthritic conditions, diabetes, and the hypomobile foot. Body weight is also a deciding factor when choosing a shell's rigidity. A heavy individual may require a more rigid shell for more adequate motion control.

Orthotic posting is prescribed from the findings of a biomechanical evaluation of the entire lower extremity. Posting material is added to the undersurface of the shell. Rearfoot posting is placed under the heel of the shell, and forefoot posting runs under the metatarsal area to the end of the shell. Medial or varus rearfoot posting is indicated for a subtalar varus or a genu varus abnormality. Varus forefoot posting is indicated for a forefoot varus abnormality. Lateral or valgus forefoot posting is indicated for a forefoot valgus abnormality. Posting brings the shell up to the foot and supports the structural abnormality of the foot. The foot orthotic therefore decreases the compensation caused by the structural abnormality.

Foot and ankle exercises such as calf stretching, arch lifts, toe claws, and single-leg standing balance drills can help prepare the foot before orthotic therapy. Foot orthotic therapy requires a break-in period of 1 to 6 weeks. During the break-in period, the orthotics are worn intermittently, perhaps as little as 1 to 2 hours per day, with a 1-hour progression each day. The break-in period can be accelerated based on orthotic tolerance and nature of the injury. Open chain exercises established before orthotic wear should continue. Closed chain exercise in the orthotics should be progressed slowly. Initially, patients can be instructed to actively supinate off of the orthotic and slowly lower onto it. Static weight-shifting drills can be progressed to exercise involving higher ground reaction forces. Athletic activity should not begin until light activity is tolerated well.

Foot orthotics must be reassessed for wear and breakdown. Refurbishment or upgrading may be necessary. During the orthotic reassessment, the patient's foot and function should also be reassessed. Alignment due to anatomic impairments does not change, but the patient's ability to control his compensation may improve. Alignment due to physiologic impairments may change. Day-to-day orthotic wear and wear for various activities may be adjusted. The reassessment schedule varies with each individual, ranging from 1 week to 1 year after the break-in period.

Heel and Full Sole Lifts

Heel lifts are commonly used for correction of leg length discrepancies. However, full sole lifts are more appropriate for the treatment of leg length discrepancies, because the heel is in contact with the ground for only a short period in the gait cycle. After the loading response phase is completed and the foot enters the midstance phase, the forefoot is in contact with the ground. If the lift is only in the heel, the foot functions as if it is descending a small step after the forefoot contacts the ground. The full sole lift eliminates this problem. However, the disadvantage of the full sole lift is that it can occupy excessive room within the shoe. Typically, if a lift beyond ⅛ inch is recommended, it should be added to the outside of the shoe. The prescription of a sole lift should be considered carefully, because an apparent leg length discrepancy often is functional and not structural.

A functional leg length discrepancy occurs with alignment impairments about any axes at any joints within the spine, pelvis, hip, knee, ankle, or foot (eg, functional scoliosis, pelvic obliquity, hip flexion, tibial varum, foot pronation). Structural leg length discrepancy usually is accompanied by a history of trauma (eg, tibial fracture) or congenital anatomic impairment (eg, structural scoliosis). A functional leg length discrepancy often can be treated with therapeutic exercise intervention, especially focusing on alignment and movement impairments throughout the kinetic chain. The use of a lift for a functional leg length discrepancy can capture and reinforce the alignment impairment rather than resolve the impairment.

Heel lifts can be helpful in the treatment of foot and ankle dysfunctions related to limited motion of the talocrural joint. A lack of 10 degrees of talocrural joint dorsiflexion can result in compensatory subtalar joint pronation during midstance and propulsion. A heel lift places the talocrural joint in a few degrees of plantar flexion at midstance (Fig. 22-25). This increases the available range of dorsiflexion and decreases the abnormal compensation.

Heel lifts can be used in the acute phase to decrease strain on the Achilles tendon, talocrural joint, and subtalar joint.

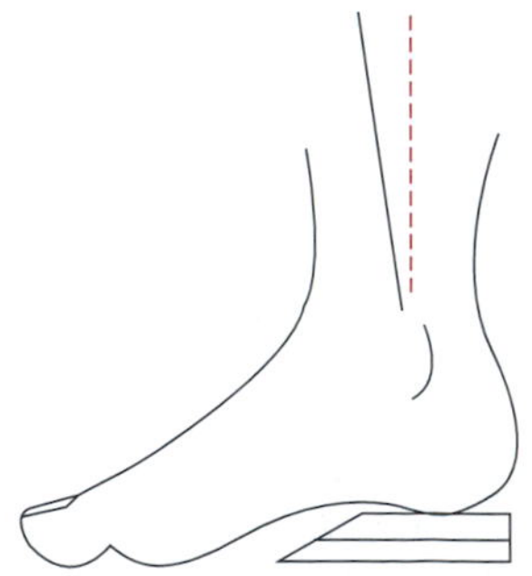

FIGURE 22-25 A heel lift is used to increase the range of dorsiflexion at midstance.

LAB ACTIVITIES

1. Perform resisted ankle dorsiflexion, plantar flexion, inversion, and eversion using a variety of resistive bands. Perform exercises in long-sitting and short-sitting positions and while standing on one leg. What are the most likely substitutions in each position?
2. Instruct a laboratory partner in correct lower extremity standing posture.
3. Perform the following exercises, maintaining subtalar neutral position and exaggerating pronation. Observe the differences in alignment throughout the lower extremity:
   a. Wall slide
   b. Single-leg wall slide
   c. Step down
   d. Standing on a minitramp
   e. Stair stepper, forward and backward
4. Consider the patient in Case Study #1 in Unit 7. Design a rehabilitation program for this athlete in the early, intermediate, and late phases. Instruct your patient in the exercise program, and have your patient perform all exercises.

Early ambulation with less pain increases independent function and enhances the effects of an exercise program. The goal is to normalize the impairment and remove the heel lifts.

If a heel lift is necessary, the following information can guide the proper amount of lift to prescribe. A patient with 0 degrees dorsiflexion may require a ¾- to 1-inch heel lift. Less severe limitations can be treated with smaller lifts. A ¼- to ⅜-inch lift can be placed inside the shoe. The lift depends on shoe style and fit. All or some portion of the lift can be added to the sole of the shoe by a shoe repair service. A lift of the same height should be added to the uninvolved extremity to avoid creating a leg length discrepancy.

Key Points

- The three main joints of the ankle and foot are the talocrural, subtalar, and midtarsal, which is further subdivided into the calcaneocuboid and talonavicular.
- The medial collateral ligament controls medial joint stability and controls the extremes of plantar flexion and dorsiflexion in the ankle and foot. The lateral collateral ligament controls lateral joint stability and checks extremes of ROM along with the medial collateral ligament.
- The extrinsic muscles consist of the anterior, lateral, and posterior groups. The anterior group allows dorsiflexion, the lateral group functions as evertors, and the posterior group functions as plantar flexors. The intrinsic muscle group is composed of four layers.
- The functions of the foot during gait are shock absorption, load transmission, surface adaptation, and propulsion.
- The foot and ankle examination must include a subjective history and evaluation of the weight-bearing and non–weight-bearing foot. Relationships of the lower extremity joints must be evaluated.
- Common lower extremity anatomic impairments include subtalar varus, forefoot varus, and forefoot valgus.
- The common physiologic impairments at the foot are mobility loss, loss of force or torque production, impaired posture and movement, pain, and impaired balance and coordination.
- The therapeutic exercise program must consider the kinetics and kinematics of the foot during gait.
- Adjunctive agents may be necessary to treat the structural impairment or to prevent secondary problems associated with physiologic impairments.

Critical Thinking Questions

1. Consider Case Study #1 in Unit 7. How would the treatment program differ if the patient was
   a. A competitive swimmer
   b. A landscaper walking on uneven surfaces
   c. An elderly individual who is a community walker
   d. A recreational golfer
2. Consider Case Study #9 in Unit 7. Theorize about potential relationships between this patient's plantar fascitis, her thigh pain, and other symptoms. Describe a comprehensive treatment program for this individual.

REFERENCES

1. Cailliet R. *Foot and Ankle Pain.* Philadelphia: FA Davis; 1968.
2. Sarrafian SK. *Anatomy of the Foot and Ankle.* Philadelphia: JB Lippincott; 1983.
3. Kessler RM, Hertling D. *Management of Common Musculoskeletal Disorders.* New York: Harper & Row; 1983.
4. Donatelli RA, ed. *The Biomechanics of the Foot and Ankle.* Philadelphia: FA Davis; 1990.
5. Hunt GC, ed. *Physical Therapy of the Foot and Ankle.* New York: Churchill Livingstone; 1988.
6. LeVeu B. *Biomechanics of Human Motion.* Philadelphia: WB Saunders; 1977.
7. Norkin C, Levangie P. *Joint Structure and Function.* 2nd ed. Philadelphia: FA Davis; 1992.
8. Nordin M, Frankel VH. *Basic Biomechanics of the Musculoskeletal System.* 2nd ed. Philadelphia: Lea & Febiger; 1989.
9. Inman VT, Ralston HJ, Todd P. *Human Walking.* Baltimore: Williams & Wilkins; 1981.
10. Smidt GL. *Gait in Rehabilitation.* New York: Churchill Livingstone; 1990.
11. Bampton S. *A Guide to the Visual Examination of Pathological Gait.* Philadelphia: Temple University Rehabilitation and Training Center #8; 1979.

12. Root ML, Orien WP, Weed JH. *Normal and Abnormal Function of the Foot,* vol 2. Los Angeles: Clinical Biomechanics Corp.; 1977.
13. McPoil TG, Hunt GC. Evaluation and management of foot and ankle disorders: present problems and future directions. *J Orthop Sports Phys Ther.* 1995;21:381–388.
14. Lattanza L, Gray GW, Kantner RM. Closed versus open kinematic chain measurements of subtalar joint eversion: implications for clinical practice. *J Orthop Sports Phys Ther.* 1988; 9:310–314.
15. Smith-Oricchio K, Harris BA. Interrater reliability of subtalar neutral, calcaneal inversion and eversion. *J Orthop Sports Phys Ther.* 1990;12:10–15.
16. Diamond JE, Mueller MJ, Delitto A, Sinacore DR. Reliability of a diabetic foot evaluation. *Phys Ther.* 1989;69:797–802.
17. McPoil TG, Cornwall MW. The relationship between subtalar joint neutral position and rearfoot motion during walking. *Foot Ankle.* 1994;15:141–145.
18. Wright DG, Desai SM, Henderson WH. Action of the subtalar and ankle-joint complex during the stance phase of walking. *J Bone Joint Surg Am.* 1964;46:361–382.
19. Hoppenfeld S. *Physical Examination of the Spine and Extremities.* New York: Appleton-Century-Crofts; 1976.
20. Sgarlato TE. *A Compendium of Podiatric Biomechanics.* San Francisco: California College of Podiatric Medicine; 1971.
21. Gould JA, Davies GJ. *Orthopedic and Sports Physical Therapy.* St. Louis: CV Mosby; 1985.
22. Magee DJ. *Orthopedic Physical Assessment.* 3rd ed. Philadelphia: WB Saunders; 1997.
23. Roy S, Irvin R. *Sports Medicine: Prevention, Evaluation, Management and Rehabilitation.* Englewood Cliffs, NJ: Prentice-Hall; 1983.
24. Subotnik SI, ed. *Sports Medicine of the Lower Extremity.* New York: Churchill Livingstone; 1989.
25. Subotnik SI. *Podiatric Sports Medicine.* Mount Kisco, NY: Futura Publishing; 1975.
26. Lauge-Hansen N. Fractures of the ankle: genetic roentgenologic diagnosis of fracture of the ankle. *Am J Roentgenol Radium Ther Nucl Med.* 1954;71:456.

RECOMMENDED READING

D'Ambrosia R, Drez D. *Prevention and Treatment of Running Injuries.* Thorofare, NJ: Slack; 1989.
Kendall FP, McCreary EK, Provance PG. *Muscles Testing and Function.* Baltimore: Williams & Wilkins; 1993.
Langer S, Wernick J. *A Practical Manual for a Basic Approach to Biomechanics.* Wheeling, IL: Langer Biomechanics Group; 1989.
Magee D. *Orthopedic Physical Assessment.* 3rd ed. Philadelphia: WB Saunders; 1997.
McPoil TG, Cornwall MW. The relationship between static measurements of the lower extremity and the pattern of rearfoot motion during walking [abstract]. *Phys Ther.* 1994; 74:S141.
McPoil TG, Knecht HG, Schuit D. A survey of foot types between the ages of 18 to 30 years. *J Orthop Sports Phys Ther.* 1988; 9:406–409.
Root ML, Orien WP, Weed JH. *Neutral Position Casting Techniques.* Los Angeles: Clinical Biomechanics Corporation; 1971.

SELECTED INTERVENTION
For the Lower Quadrant

See Case Study 1. Although this patient requires comprehensive intervention as described in previous chapters, only one exercise prescribed in the final stage of recovery is described.

ACTIVITY: Lunging ball drill

PURPOSE: Improve balance, proprioception, and agility

RISK FACTORS: 10 weeks after second-degree sprain of the right calcaneofibular ligament

ELEMENT OF THE MOVEMENT SYSTEM: Modulator

STAGE OF MOTOR CONTROL: Skill

POSTURE: Standing in "ready" position with knees flexed

MOVEMENT: Step forward, and lunge as ball is tossed toward you.

SPECIAL CONSIDERATIONS: Be sure foot lands in a good position and that it is in good alignment with respect to the knee, hip, pelvis, and spine.

DOSAGE

Special Considerations

Anatomic: Calcaneofibular ligament
Physiologic: Late-stage recovery from grade 2 sprain
Learning capability: Good body awareness and coordination, should be no trouble

Repetitions/sets: To form fatigue, pain, or 20–30 repetitions, up to three sets

Frequency: Every other day

Sequence: Following warm-up of light activity and stretching

Speed: Functional speed

Environment: Home with a partner

Feedback: Initially in clinic with mirror and verbal feedback, tapered to no mirror in home environment

FUNCTIONAL MOVEMENT PATTERN TO REINFORCE GOAL OF SPECIFIC EXERCISE: Play basketball with same form

EXPLANATION OF CHOICE OF EXERCISE: Chosen as skill-level activity to prepare patient for return to basketball. She will require excellent balance, proprioception, and agility to return to basketball without recurrent ankle sprain. High repetitions of this exercise for 2 to 3 weeks should prepare her for basketball without recurrent injury.

Functional Approach to Therapeutic Exercise for the Upper Extremities

CHAPTER 23

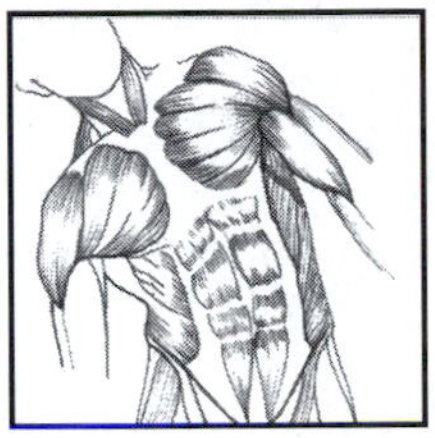

The Temporomandibular Joint

Darlene Hertling and Lisa Dussault

The temporomandibular joint (TMJ) cannot be viewed in isolation. Its relationships with the cranium, jaw, and cervical spine are important in function and dysfunction and should be acknowledged in assessment and management strategies. TMJ dysfunction can be the result of a problem anywhere along this kinetic chain. The TMJ is unique because its function is directly related to dentition and the contacting tooth surfaces. Problems with the TMJ can directly influence occlusion and vice versa. A comprehensive approach to the treatment of the TMJ addresses the person as a whole by taking into account these relationships, the performance of functional activities, and the influence of physical and emotional stress on this system.

This chapter provides a brief review of TMJ anatomy and kinesiology and supplies guidelines for the basic examination and evaluation. It covers treatment interventions for common physiologic impairments and common diagnoses affecting the TMJ.

REVIEW OF ANATOMY AND KINESIOLOGY

In referring to the TMJs, the masticatory system, its component structures, and all the tissues related to it, the term *stomatognathic system* is used. This system has several components:

- Bones of the skull, mandible, maxilla, hyoid, clavicle, sternum, shoulder girdle, and cervical vertebrae
- TMJ and dentoalveolar joints (ie, joints of the teeth)
- Teeth
- Cervical spine
- Area vascular, lymphatic, and nervous systems
- Muscles and soft tissues of the head and neck and muscles of the cheeks, lips, and tongue

Kinematically, the joints and muscles of this system interact to influence the alignment and function of the mandible in the TMJ. Functional activities such as talking and eating are affected by the kinematics of this system.

Bones

The mandible, the largest and strongest bone of the face, articulates with the two temporal bones and accommodates the lower teeth. It is composed of a horizontal portion, called the body, and two perpendicular portions, called the rami, which unite with the end of the body nearly at right angles. Each ramus has two processes: the coronoid process and the condylar process. The coronoid process serves as an insertion for the temporalis and masseter muscles. The condylar process consists of the neck and the condyle. The condyle, which is convex, articulates with the disk (Fig. 23-1). The two condyles form the floor of the TMJ.

The roof of the TMJ consists entirely of the squamous part of the temporal bone, and it is divided into four descriptive parts:

1. Articular tubercle
2. Articular eminence

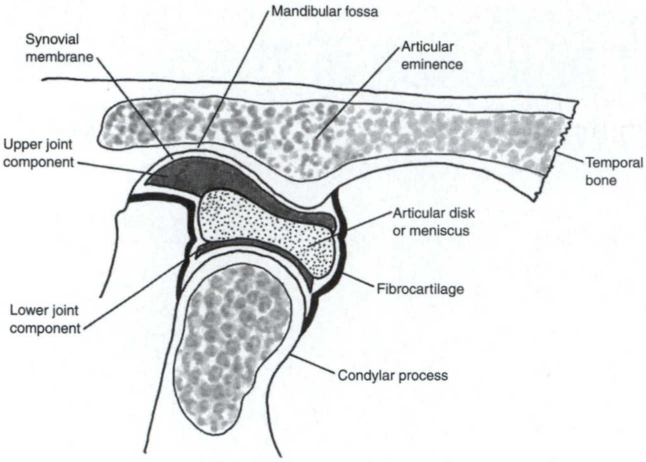

FIGURE 23-1 Articular structures of the temporomandibular joint in the closed position.

3. Mandibular fossa
4. Posterior glenoid spine

The hyoid bone is a horseshoe-shaped bone at the level of C3 and acts as an attachment for the suprahyoid and infrahyoid muscles (Fig. 23-2). The greater wings of the sphenoid bone join into the pterygoid plates that serve as attachment for the medial and lateral pterygoid muscles (Fig. 23-3).

Ostoekinematically, three basic movements exist within the mandible: depression, protrusion, and lateral excursion. These three basic movements can be combined to produce an infinite variety of mandibular motions.

Joints

There are two TMJs, one on either side of the jaw. Both joints must be considered together with the teeth (ie, the trijoint complex) in an examination.[1] The TMJ is a synovial, condyloid joint found between the mandibular fossa of the temporal bone and the condylar process of the mandibular bone (see Fig. 23-1). The two bony surfaces are covered with collagen fibrocartilage rather than the hyaline cartilage found in most synovial joints of the body. The presence of fibrocartilage is significant because of its ability to repair and to remodel.[2]

The articular disk, or meniscus, also consists of pliable collagen fibrocartilage, but it lacks the ability to repair or remodel. This biconcave disk divides each joint into two cavities (an upper and a lower joint cavity) and compensates functionally for the incongruity of the two opposing joint surfaces (see Fig. 23-1). During opening and closing, the convex surface of the condylar head must move across the convex surface of the articular eminence.

Kinematically, the mandible may be considered a free body that can rotate in angular directions. It has three degrees of freedom. The basic accessory movements required for functional motion are rotation, translation, distraction, compression, and lateral glide.[3] Accessory movements most often restricted because of periarticular tissue tightness and disk displacement are lateral glide, translation, and distraction. According to Kraus,[4] of these accessory movements, translation causes the most limitation of osteokinematic movement of the mandible and is more difficult to restore. Gliding movements occur in the upper cavity of the joint, whereas rotation or hinge movements occur in the lower cavity. Gliding and rotation are essential for opening and closing the mouth.

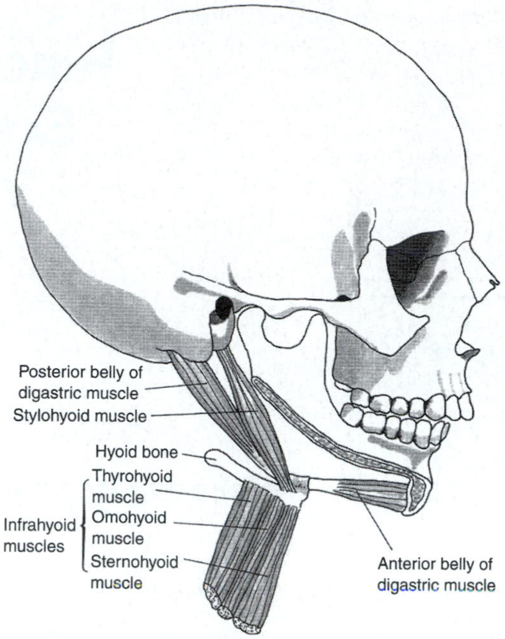

FIGURE 23-2 Hyoid bone and the digastric, stylohyoid and infrahyoid muscles.

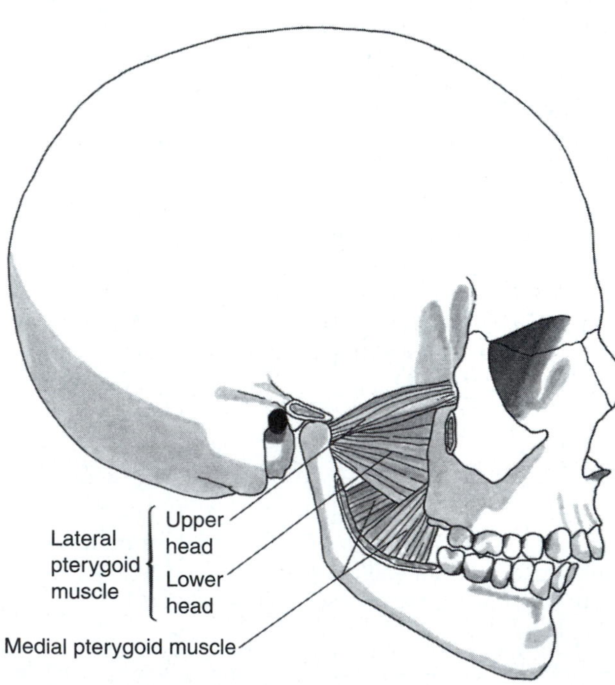

FIGURE 23-3 Medial and lateral pterygoid muscles.

The capsule of the TMJ is thin and loose. The capsule and the disk are attached to one another anteriorly and posteriorly but not attached medially or laterally. Because there are no medial and lateral attachments of the disk and capsule, translation (anteriorly) of the disk can occur within the capsule. The posterior ligament attaches the disk to the posterior aspect of the neck of the mandible, in the bilaminar zone, and the posterior portion of the TMJ.[1–6]

The strongest ligamentous attachments are on the medial side, such as the mediodisco ligament (ie, Tanaka's ligament).[5,6] The TMJ has no capsule on the medial half of the anterior aspect, which allows excessive translation of the condyle, leading to joint pathology.[7] The TMJ can actively displace anteriorly and slightly displace laterally.[2]

The rest position, or loose packed position, for the TMJ is with the mouth slightly open so the teeth are not in contact. The rest position of the tongue, often referred to as the postural position, is with the first half of the tongue against the hard palate of the mouth.[8,9] Tongue up, teeth apart, and lips closed (TUTALC) is the functional rest position that should be taught to the patient.

There are two closed packed positions: maximal anterior position of the condyle with maximal opening and maximal retrusion in which the ligaments are taut and the condyle cannot go farther back. The mouth is closed, and the teeth are clenched. In bilateral restriction, the capsular pattern of restriction produces significant loss of lateral movements and limits opening of the mouth and protrusion. In unilateral capsular patterns of restriction, contralateral excursions are most limited. During mouth opening, the mandible deviates toward the restricted side.

The normal range of mandibular opening is 40 to 50 mm. The range of motion (ROM) is considered functional for most jaw activities if 40 mm of opening is possible. This motion should be composed of 25 mm of rotation and 15 mm of translation.[10] To achieve the initial 25 mm opening, rotation occurs between the mandibular condyle and the inferior surface of the disk. The last 15 to 25 mm is the result of anterior translation between the superior surface of the disk and the temporal bone.

Muscles

Function of all the muscles of the upper quadrant need to be understood because of their impact on TMJ function and dysfunction. The movements of the mandible are the result of the action of the cervical and jaw muscles:

- Elevation
- Depression
- Protraction
- Retraction
- Lateral gliding

All of these movements are used to some extent when chewing. Because the TMJ is bilateral, the muscles of mastication must activate and relax in a regular pattern and in perfect synchronization with the muscles on the contralateral side. Muscles often need to be re-educated after trauma, surgical procedures, and long-standing parafunctional activity, including habitual excessive use of biting force, such as clenching, nail biting, and forced mandibular opening on an unstable occlusion. Muscles can be re-educated by the use of exercise, biofeedback, and functional electrical stimulation.

MAIN MUSCLES OF TEMPOROMANDIBULAR JOINT MOTION

Five main muscles contribute to TMJ motion:

1. Temporalis
2. Masseter
3. Medial pterygoid
4. Lateral pterygoid
5. Digastric

These muscles also connect the cranium to the mandible along with the buccinator and superior pharyngeal constrictor.[11]

The three major elevator muscles of the mandible are the temporalis, the masseter, and the medial pterygoid. All of the fibers of the temporalis (Fig. 23-4 and Table 23-1) contribute to elevation for closure, particularly for positioning of the condyle at the end of closure.[5] The masseter (Fig. 23-5 and see Table 23-1) is composed of the deep and superficial bellies. The superficial fibers protract the jaw to some degree, and the deep portion acts as a retractor. The medial pterygoid's function (see Fig. 23-3 and Table 23-1) is similar to the masseter's function, although it is less powerful than the masseter.

The primary muscle responsible for mandibular depression is the digastric (see Fig. 23-2 and Table 23-1).[2,12] The lower portion of the lateral pterygoid and the other suprahyoids are active during forced opening of the mandible, when the hyoid bone is fixed by the infrahyoid muscle group.

The lateral pterygoid inserts into the mandibular condyle and articular disk and plays a large role in stabilization of the TMJ (Fig. 23-6). The inferior fibers are active in conjunction

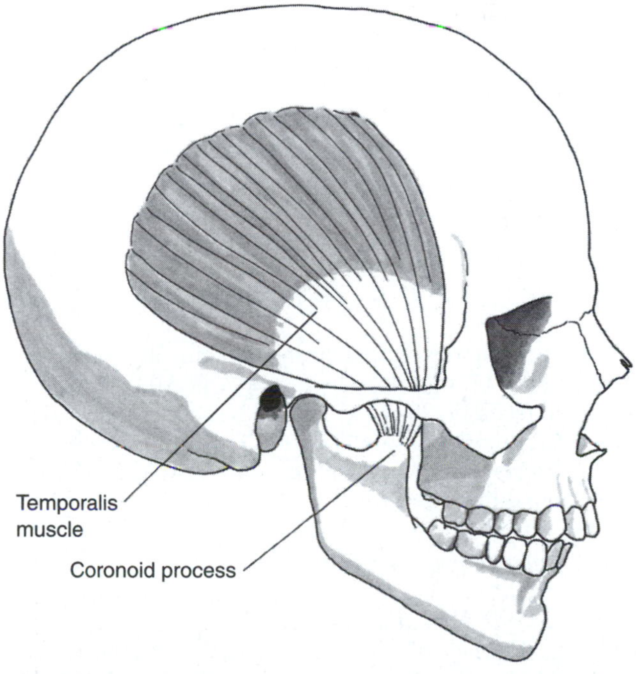

FIGURE 23-4 Temporalis muscle.

Table 23-1. MUSCLES AND NERVES OF THE MANDIBLE

MUSCLE AND NERVE (N)	ORIGIN	INSERTION	FUNCTION
Digastric N: trigeminal and facial	Anterior belly: depression on inner side of inferior border of mandible Posterior belly: mastoid notch of the temporal bone	Common tendon to the the hyoid bone	Mandibular depression and elevation of hyoid (in swallowing)
Temporalis N: mandibular division of trigeminal nerve	Temporal fossa and deep surface of temporal fascia	Medial and anterior coronoid process and anterior ramus of mandible	Elevates mandible to close the mouth and approximates teeth (biting motion); retracts the mandible and participates in lateral grinding motions
Masseter N: mandibular division of trigeminal nerve	Superficial: zygomatic arch and maxillary process Deep portion: zygomatic arch	Angle and lower half of lateral ramus Lateral coronoid and superior ramus	Elevates the mandible; active in up and down biting motions and occlusion of the teeth in mastication
Medial pterygoid N: mandibular division of trigeminal nerve	Greater wing of sphenoid and pyramidal process of palatine bone	Medial ramus and angle of mandibular foremen	Elevates the mandible to close the mouth; protrudes the mandible (with lateral pterygoid). Unilaterally, the medial and lateral pterygoid rotate the mandible forward and to the opposite side.
Lateral pterygoid N: mandibular division of trigeminal nerve	Superior: inferior crest of greater wing of sphenoid bones Inferior: lateral surface of pterygoid plate	Articular disk, capsule, and condyle Neck of mandible and medial condyle	Protracts mandibular condyle and disk of the temporomandibular joint forward while the mandibular head rotates on disk; aids in opening the mouth. Joint action of the medial and lateral pterygoid rotates the mandible forward and to the opposite side.
Mylohyoid N: mylohyoid branch of the trigeminal nerve	Medial surface of mandible, entire length	Body of the hyoid bone (floor of the mouth)	Elevates the hyoid bone and tongue for swallowing; depresses the mandible when fixed
Geniohyoid N: ventral ramus of C1 through hypoglossal nerve	Mental spine of mandible	Body of the hyoid bone	Assists in depression of the mandible; elevates and protracts the hyoid bone; moves the tongue forward
Stylohyoid N: facial	Styloid process of temporal bone	Body of the hyoid bone	Draws the hyoid bone upward and backward in swallowing; assists in opening the mouth and participates in mastication

with mandibular depressors during mandibular opening and protraction. The superior fibers (upper head) of the lateral pterygoid (see Fig. 23-3 and Table 23-1) act in concert with the elevator muscles during closing. Their role is to decelerate and prevent invagination of the joint capsule with closure of the mandible.[5] Because the attachment of the superior and inferior fibers are mostly medial, they pull the condyle and disk in a medial direction.

SUPRAHYOID AND INFRAHYOID MUSCLES

The lingual surface of the mandible, anterior to the muscles of mastication, is composed of the suprahyoid muscles. These muscles influence jaw position and play an important role in tongue mobility, speech, mandibular depression, manipulating boluses of food, and swallowing.[11] The suprahyoids consist of the mylohyoid, geniohyoid (Fig. 23-7 and see Table 23-1), and the paired digastric and stylohyoid muscles (see Fig. 23-2).

The infrahyoid muscles (ie, sternohyoid, thyrohyoid, sternothyroid, and omohyoid) act together to stabilize the hyoid bone. This provides the suprahyoids with a stable base from which to contract and move the mandible (see Fig. 23-2).

TONGUE

The tongue is composed of various intrinsic and extrinsic muscles. The genioglossus is the main muscle responsible

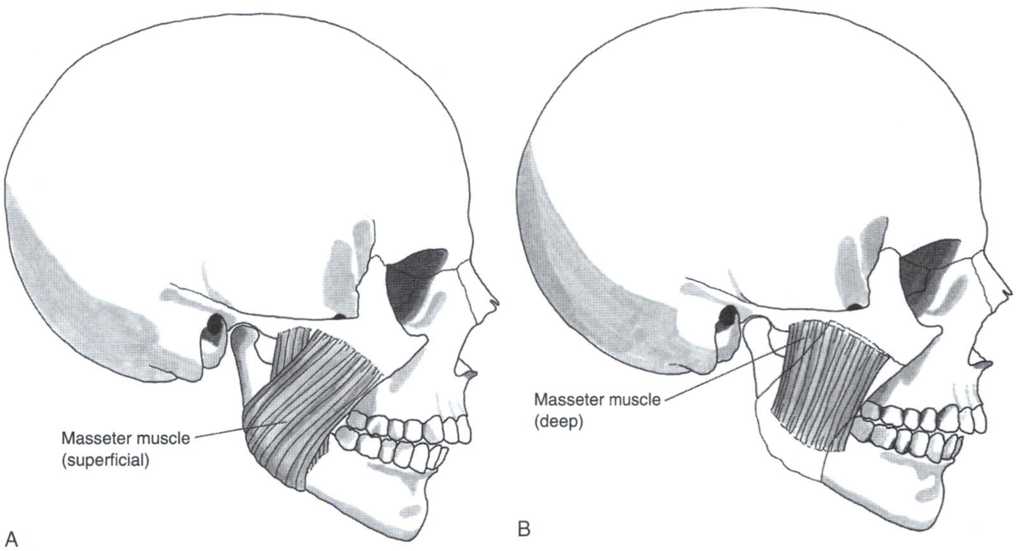

FIGURE 23-5 *(A)* Superficial and *(B)* deep layers of masseter muscle.

for positioning of the tongue in the oral cavity.[4] It is primarily responsible for establishing and maintaining the rest position of the tongue and is active in protracting and elevating the tongue. The resting position of the tongue provides the foundation for the resting muscle tone of the mandibular elevators (ie, temporalis, masseter, and medial pterygoid) and establishes resting activity of the tongue musculature itself (ie, jaw-tongue reflex).[4,13–17]

Tongue thrust and other parafunctional habits are often accompanied by an abnormal tongue position against the lingual surface of the mandibular incisors rather than the normal palatal tongue posture.[14–16] Excessive masticatory muscle activity is thought to occur in patents who acquire an altered sequence of swallowing in which tongue thrust occurs.[4] The most frequently cited signs of tongue thrust activity during swallowing include protraction of the tongue against or between the anterior teeth and excessive muscle activity.[15] As a result, the masseter muscles contract incompletely, and there is a concomitant variable state of tension of the orbicularis oris and buccinator muscles.[15] Although tongue thrust is more common in children, it also occurs in adults and is referred to as an acquired adult tongue thrust.[4] It is theorized that tongue movement and positioning in the oral cavity are influenced by dysfunctional mobility and positioning of the cervical spine.[18]

Nerves and Blood Vessels

The region is supplied by cranial and cervical nerves. Overlapping of the branches from both types of nerves complicates the neurologic analysis of this region and may account for the extensive range of symptoms in head, TMJ, and cervical dysfunctions.

The innervated tissues of the TMJ are supplied by three nerves that are part of the mandibular division of cranial nerve V. The posterior deep temporal and masse-

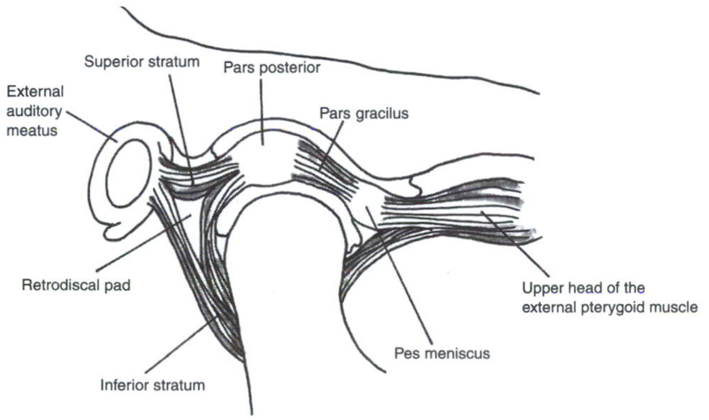

FIGURE 23-6 Sagittal section of the temporomandibular joint. The lateral pterygoid inserts into the mandibular condyle and the disk. The disk has three parts: (1) a thick anterior band (pes meniscus), (2) a thicker posterior band (pars posterior), and (3) a thin intermediate zone (pars gracilis) between the two bands.

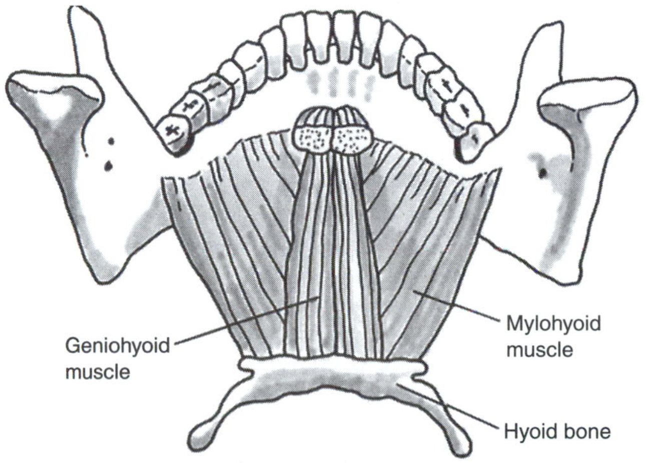

FIGURE 23-7 Mylohyoid and geniohyoid muscles viewed from above and behind the floor of the mouth.

teric nerves supply the medial and anterior regions of the joint, and the auriculotemporal nerve supplies the posterior and lateral regions of the joint. The auriculotemporal nerve is the major nerve innervating the capsular blood vessels, the retrodiskal pad, the posterolateral capsule, and the TMJ ligament of the TMJ. These tissues have an abundant supply of type IV receptors (ie, articular pain receptors). Because branches of the auriculotemporal nerve supply the tragus, external acoustic meatus, and tympanic membrane, temporal mandibular dysfunction is often associated with hearing problems, tinnitus, and vertigo.

The external carotid arterial system provides the main vascular supply to the TMJ, masticatory muscles, and associated soft tissues. This vessel divides at the level of the neck of the condyle into the superficial temporal and internal maxillary arteries. The internal maxillary artery and its branches supply the maxilla and mandible, the teeth, and the muscles of mastication. The arterial supply and venous and lymphatic drainage can be clinically significant in patients with head and neck pain. Theses circulatory systems can be compromised by trauma, disease, changes of the head and neck positions, and muscle spasm.

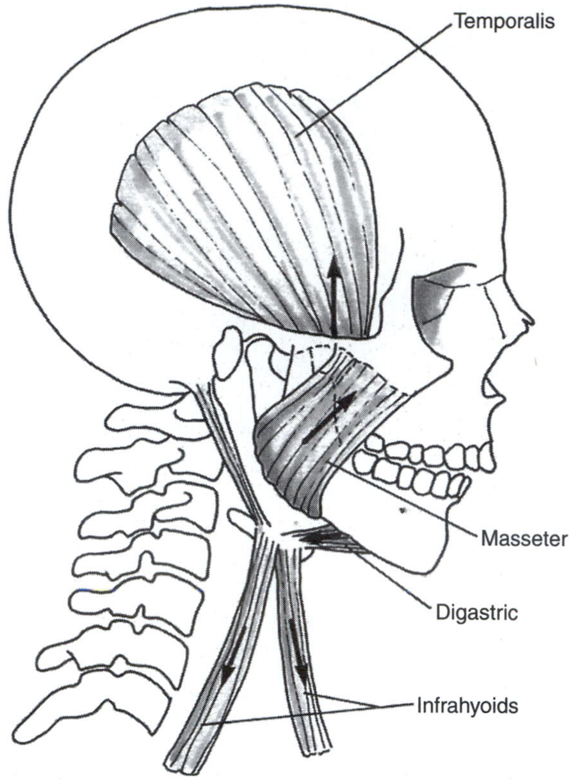

FIGURE 23-8 A lateral view of the head, neck, and mandible showing the muscular forces that flex the head. The infrahyoid muscles pull downward on the hyoid bone. The suprahyoids pull down on the mandible, and the muscles of mastication stabilize the jaw.

Kinetics

An overview of the management of the cervical spine muscle imbalances and the relationship of head posture and the rest position of the mandible are included because of the frequently associated muscle hyperactivity and accompanying symptoms observed in the mandibular and cervical spine areas. Functionally, the TMJ, the cervical spine, and the articulations between the teeth are intimately related (Fig. 23-8). Muscles attach the mandible to the cranium, the hyoid bone, and clavicle. The cervical spine is, in essence, interposed between the proximal and distal attachments of some of the muscles controlling the TMJ.[2] The balance between the flexors and extensors of the head and neck is affected by the muscles of mastication and the suprahyoid and infrahyoid muscles.[19] Dysfunction in the muscles of mastication or the cervical musculature can easily disturb this balance. The neuromusculature of the cervical and masticatory regions actively influences the function of mandibular movement and cervical positioning.[20–22]

Cervical posture change affects the mandibular path of closure, the mandibular rest position, masticatory muscle activity,[20,21,23] and the occlusal contact patterns. A forward head posture (FHP) is a common postural defect that increases the gravitational forces on the head and often leads to hyperextension of the head (ie, posterior cranial rotation [PCR] on the neck) (Fig. 23-9*A*). When the head is held anteriorly, the line of vision extends downward if the normal angle at which the head and neck meet is maintained. To correct for visual needs, the head tilts backward, the neck flexes over the thorax, and the mandible migrates posteriorly.[24] The posterior cervical muscles are shortened and forced to contract excessively to maintain the head in this position while the anterior submandibular muscles are stretched, resulting in a retraction force on the mandible and an altered occlusal contact pattern. The contracted posterior cervical muscles may entrap the greater occipital nerve and refer pain to the head.[25] Excessive mandibular shuttling (ie, excursions) between opening and closing, which are necessary for functional activities such as chewing and eating, may lead to hypermobility of the TMJ from overstretching of the capsule.[26]

In the presence of a FHP with no significant PCR (Fig. 23-9*B*), the suprahyoids shorten, and the infrahyoids lengthen, consequently decreasing or eliminating the freeway space, a space that exists between the upper and lower arch of the teeth when the mandible is in the rest position.[27,28] The hyoid bone is repositioned superiorly, and the degree of elevation is proportional to the decrease in the cervical lordosis or increase in the FHP.[27,28] Hyperactivity of the suprahyoids produces a depressive force on the mandible. According to Mannheimer,[28] when combined with hyoid anchoring by means of the infrahyoids, the net mandibular repositioning effect is one of retraction and depression with increased contact in the molar region. The tonic neck reflex plays a primary role in an individual's ability to achieve correct head-neck posture. FHP is often assumed if tonic neck reflexes or cervical proprioceptive afferents are injured (eg, whiplash, direct trauma) or are overused (eg, sports activities, daily postures). The proprioceptive afferents may lose their ability to position the head and neck.[7]

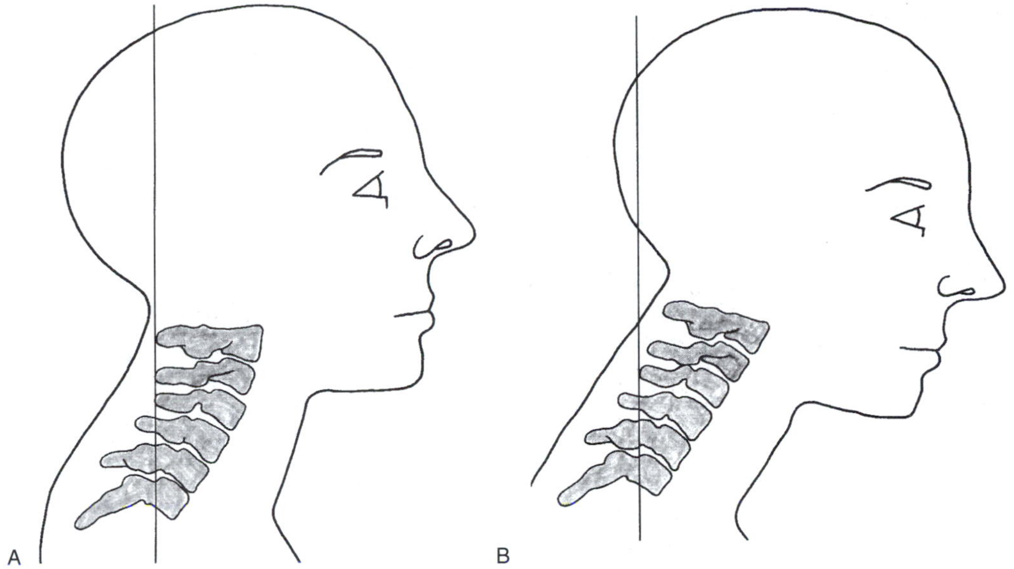

FIGURE 23-9 Types of forward head: ***(A)*** increased cervical lordosis with posterior cranial rotation, and ***(B)*** total flattening out of the cervical lordosis without posterior cranial rotation.

The FHP is exacerbated by many occupations and activities of daily living (ie, improper home, work, or driving postures) that require the upper extremities and the head to be positioned more anterior to the trunk than is normal or comfortable.[13,27–29] Another contributing factor is the effect of mouth breathing. The dysfunctional patterns of the mouth-breathing syndrome constitute a chain reaction of body adaptation to abnormal breathing patterns. Various investigations have shown that postural relationships change to meet respiratory needs.[16,29] Breathing through the mouth facilitates FHP, a low and forward tongue position (as a result of this pattern, abnormal swallowing ensues), and increased activity of the accessory muscles of respiration (ie, sternocleidomastoids, scaleni, and pectorals).[7,16,30] This pattern is perpetuated by decreased activity of the diaphragm and hypotonicity of the abdominal musculature.[16] Consequently, many abnormal force vectors are created by abnormal swallow.

EXAMINATION AND EVALUATION

A thorough evaluation of the TMJ includes all components of the stomatognathic system. This assessment assists the therapist in determining the cause of the dysfunction and the influence of other factors and in designing an effective treatment plan.

History

A comprehensive history is essential and helps to direct the objective evaluation. The client should provide detailed information about the onset of symptoms, incidence of joint locking, presence of joint noise, history of surgery and trauma, and medical history. Pain should be described in terms of location, intensity, frequency, time of day, and activities that reproduce it. Functional limitations should be addressed along with parafunctional habits. Clients should be asked about their level of psychosocial, environmental, and postural stress, noticing if they sense an increase in clenching or other parafunctional habits when under stress. The type of job a patient has can provide information about posture. Use of a functional outcome questionnaire is helpful in evaluating these patients.

Mobility Impairment Examination

Mobility testing at the TMJ should look at the quality and symmetry of the motions performed to determine the type of dysfunction:

- ROM
- TMJ: vertical opening, lateral excursion, protrusion
- Cervical and upper quadrant
- Joint function
- Rotation and translation
- Joint play
- TMJ muscles
- Cervical and postural muscles (if indicated)

Pain Examination

Subjective complaints of pain should be evaluated. The client should be asked to point to the site of greatest pain while the therapist notices whether the pain is in the joint or muscular region. Tenderness, warmth, and inflammation should be assessed during palpation and especially when examining several areas:

- Posterior and lateral joints
- Oral facial muscles
- Cervical and upper quadrant muscles

Special Tests and Other Assessments

Several tests address the functional component of the TMJ complex:

- Oral function
- Occlusion pattern
- Swallowing pattern
- Breathing pattern

The therapist also should evaluate the patient's posture and screen for systemic hypermobility.

THERAPEUTIC EXERCISE INTERVENTIONS FOR COMMON PHYSIOLOGIC IMPAIRMENTS

A treatment plan is implemented after a thorough examination and determination of the diagnosis, functional limitations, and prognosis. Therapeutic exercise interventions should address specific impairments and seek to increase functioning of the TMJ.

Mobility Impairment

HYPOMOBILITY

Etiology

Mandibular hypomobility (ie, limitation of functional movements) may result from disorders of the mandible or cranial bone, which include aplasia, dysplasia, hypoplasia, hyperplasia, fractures, and neoplasms.[31] Temporomandibular dysfunctions that can contribute to mandibular hypomobility are ankylosis (fibrous or bony); arthritides, especially polyarthritides involving the periarticular tissue (capsule) and structural bony changes; disk displacement (ie, acute disk displacement that does not reduce); and inflammation or joint effusion. Also contributing to hypomobility are masticatory muscle disorders such as myofascial pain, muscle splinting, myositis, spasm, contracture, and neoplasia.[31]

Hypomobility may lead to capsular fibrosis (a result of the intermolecular cross-linking adhesions of collagen fibers). It most commonly accompanies one or some combination of three situations:

1. Resolution of an acute articular inflammatory process
2. A chronic, low-grade articular inflammatory response
3. Immobilization in which the capsule may be partially or totally involved

This condition may or may not be painful. If painful, the pain is felt over the side of involvement, with possible reference into areas innervated by cranial nerve V. Pain increases during functional and parafunctional movements of the mandible. If complete capsular shortening exists, the mandibular opening is less than functional, and the patient presents with a capsular pattern of restriction. Lateral movements of the mandible to the opposite side are decreased. With bilateral restriction, lateral movements are most restricted; opening of the mouth and protrusion are limited, but closing is free.

Treatment

Therapeutic modalities such as ice or heat can help to decrease pain and muscle guarding. Ultrasound in conjunction with active motion or prolonged static stretch is used to increase extensibility of the capsular tissues.[32] Joint mobilization techniques are used to further enhance capsular extensibility. Joint mobilization procedures for the TMJ include distraction, medial glide, and translation (Fig. 23-10).[4,19,24,33] In each case, the manual hold is performed over the mandible or over the inner aspect of the lower molars. Direct joint mobilizations may also be used, with contact of the therapist's thumbs over the lateral or posterior surface of the condyle of the mandible.[32] Mobilization of the involved soft tissues can facilitate stretching techniques and joint mobilization procedures, making them more tolerable and effective.

Most patients with hypomobility impairment require a home program of active ROM exercises, self-mobilization, and a passive stretching program with tongue depressors or the Therabite (Therabite Inc, Bryn Mawr, PA) to maintain and facilitate capsular extensibility along with instructions on proper posture and avoidance of aggravating factors.[34] As part of their home program, they are educated about

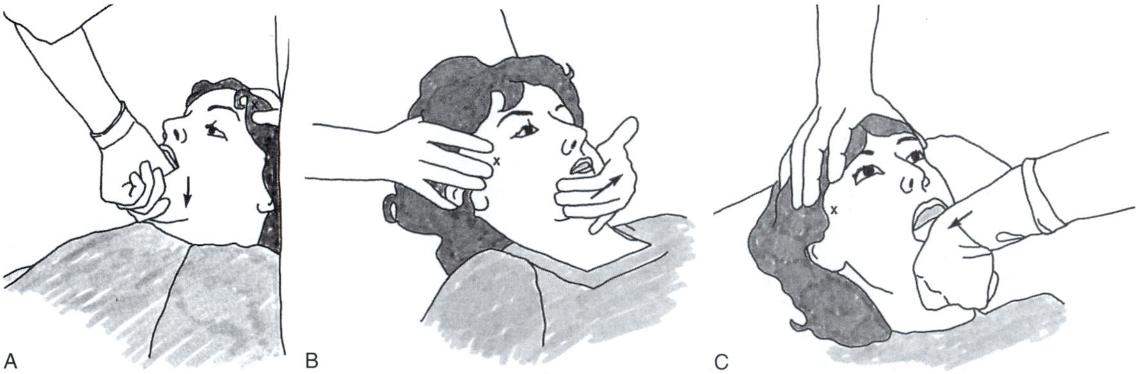

FIGURE 23-10 ***(A)*** Interoral distraction. The clinician's thumb is positioned to apply a distraction force. ***(B)*** Lateral glide. The clinician's thumb is positioned to apply a lateral glide force. ***(C)*** Intraoral translation (ventral glide). The clinician's index and third fingers are positioned to apply translation.

maintaining the normal rest position of the tongue and mandible (ie, TUTALC).

Limited mandibular movement can be corrected by a number of self-treatment techniques. Frequent active stretch (ie, active opening and closing of the mandible) during the day should be encouraged. The therapeutic value of this exercise is to develop mandibular movement in a controlled manner. The tongue-up exercise can control translation. Active protrusion and lateral excursions (with or with out tongue blades positioned between the teeth) can be used to actively mobilize the mandible (Fig. 23-11).

Passive stretch (ie, prolonged static stretch) may be used by placing a number of stacked tongue blades horizontally between the upper and lower incisors to increase the mandibular opening. The stretch position is maintained for 5 to 10 minutes or until the muscles relax. As the ROM increases, the patient can gradually increase the number of tongue depressors until she can open far enough to insert the knuckle of her index and middle fingers between the anterior teeth. Normal translation begins after 11 mm, or about six tongue blades.[13]

The simplest method of self-stretch is to use the thumb crossed over the index finger. The index finger is placed on the lower teeth, as far posteriorly as possible, and the thumb is placed on the upper teeth. The patient actively opens the jaw and applies gentle pressure in opening until a stretch is felt (Fig. 23-12). This technique should be performed bilaterally to avoid compression of one joint while trying to stretch the other side.

Techniques used for mandibular opening may be helpful in joint restrictions caused by anterior disk displacement with and without reduction. In the case of a nonreducing disk, it is important to limit intracisal opening to approximately 30 mm to protect the retrodiskal tissue from being overstretched.[13]

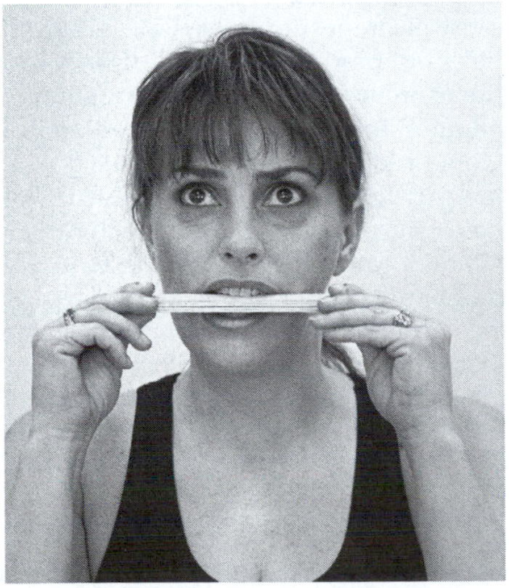

FIGURE 23-11 Active exercise to increase mandibular lateral excursions and protrusion. The patient is given enough tongue blades to place between the teeth to allow for approximately 10 to 11 mm of opening. The patient is then asked to protrude the mandible at this opening to improve translation. The patient may also be instructed to protrude and glide the mandible to one side to improve translation of one side.

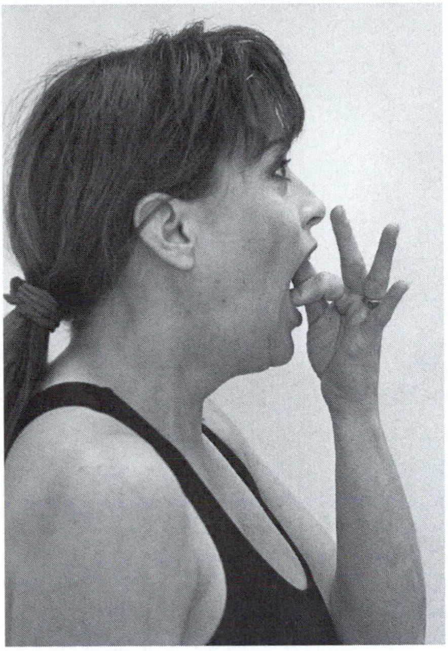

FIGURE 23-12 Active–passive mandibular exercise. The patient is instructed to actively open the mouth. Then finger pressure is applied to the maxillary and mandibular dentitions with one or both hands.

Postisometric relaxation techniques (PIRs) use active muscle contractions at various intensities from a precisely controlled position in a specific direction against a counterforce to facilitate motion.[35] For one PIR technique for mandibular opening, the patient sits at a table, with one elbow on the table and with the hand propping her forehead; the fingers of the other hand are on the mandibular dentition.[35] After opening her mouth to take up the slack, she breathes out; during inhalation, she opens her mouth as wide as possible, as if yawning (Fig 23-13). This is followed by closing the mouth against isometric resistance with minimal force, and the exercise then is repeated. Deviation of the mandible to the side during the relaxation phase may be introduced as a separate exercise.

For PIR self-treatment for relief of tension of the lateral pterygoid, the patient assumes a supine position. Using her thumbs on the mandible, she presses her chin forward against the isometric resistance of her thumbs with minimal force while breathing. She next holds her breath and then breathes out while relaxing and letting the chin drop back (Fig. 23-14).[35] The exercise should be done with minimal effort; the relaxation phase is most important.

Tension of the digastric is best diagnosed by trying to shift the hyoid from side to side. When tightness or tension is marked on one side, deviation of the thyroid cartilage to the ipsilateral side may be evident. For self-treatment using PIR, the thumb of one hand lies lateral to the hyoid on the restricted or tense side. During the resistance phase, the patient slightly opens her mouth and breathes in, holds her breath, and then relaxes while breathing out. She closes her mouth while her thumb moves the hyoid very gently to the opposite side (Fig. 23-15).[35]

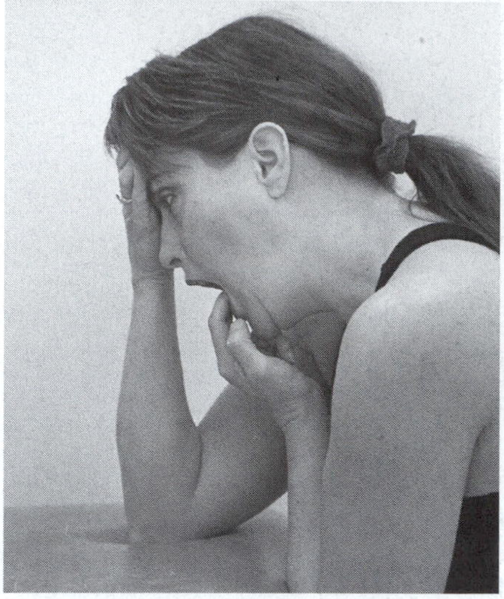

FIGURE 23-13 Postisometric relaxation self-exercise for mandibular opening (temporal, masseters and medial pterygoid muscles). The patient sits at a table, with one elbow on the table and with the hand propping her forehead; the fingers of the other hand are on the maxillary teeth. After taking up the slack of mouth opening, she breathes out. During inhalation, she opens her mouth as wide as possible. The hand on her forehead should prevent flexion, which would interfere with maximum opening.

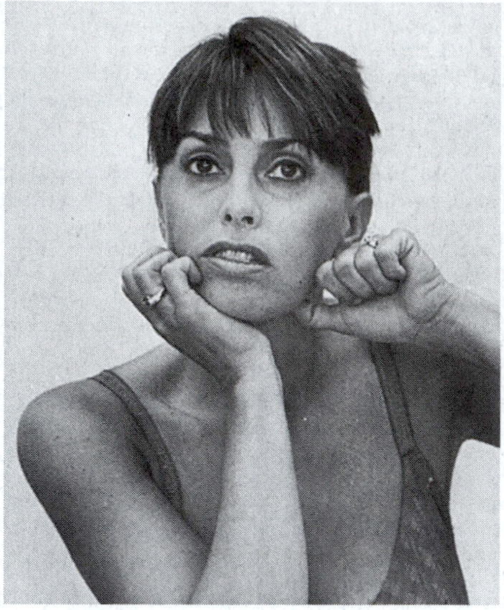

FIGURE 23-15 Postisometric relaxation self-exercise for the digastric muscle. While sitting, one hand is placed under the chin, and the other hand contacts the lateral aspect of the hyoid bone (tense side) with the thumb. After the resistance phase, the thumb gently moves the hyoid medially.

The goal of functional kinetic exercises developed by Klein-Vogelbach[36,37] is for the patient to learn to move the TMJs freely and with precision in all directions. In normal TMJ activity, it is the mandible that moves while the head remains stationary. If movement at the TMJ is restricted, it is often helpful to reverse these roles. Normally, jaw elevation, depression, protraction, retraction, and lateral gliding are initiated at the mandible (ie, distal lever). To facilitate increased motion and to functionally circumvent and break faulty habit patterns, the levers are reversed; the head (ie, proximal lever) initiates the motion. The head moves but not the mandible. These movements are transmitted to the upper cervical spine joints (ie, atlanto-occipital and atlantoaxial joints).

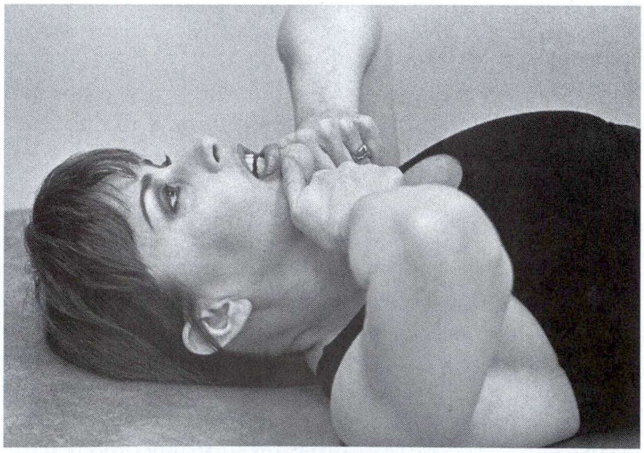

FIGURE 23-14 Postisometric relaxation self-exercise of the lateral pterygoid. The patient is supine, with her mouth slightly open. She places both thumbs on the mandible and is instructed to press her chin forward against her thumbs while breathing in. She holds her breath, then breathes out, letting the chin drop back.

While the patient sits with good vertical alignment, the therapist or patient provides fixation of the mandible; the fingers of both hands should grasp the mandible. Exercises include opening and closing of the mouth, lateral deviations, and protrusion and retrusion (Fig. 23-16). These precise and unfamiliar movements of the TMJ must be performed at low intensity and slowly, because the body is learning movement that it does not need in normal motor behavior but that can be used effectively to reduce restriction.[37] These exercises are followed with normal mandibular motions to assess progress and maintain function. A sensory awareness exercise tape, using these same principles of initiating motion of the jaw with the head and other neuromuscular learning techniques based on the Feldenkrais Method, has been developed by Wildman[38] for home use.

A variation of Klein-Vogelbach's kinetic exercises for opening and closing the jaw freely and with precision is an exercise with the head in the inverted position (for patients who can assume the position) (Fig. 23-17). Opening of the mouth in this position must be performed against gravity, providing eccentric isotonic work of the masseter muscle in opening and concentric work in closing. The reverse is true of the jaw-opening muscles, the suprahyoids.

HYPERMOBILITY

Etiology

The cause of TMJ hypermobility is unknown. Potential predisposing factors range from joint laxity to psychiatric disorders to skeletal disorders.[39] Investigations suggest that systemic hypermobility (ie, ligament laxity) may be closely related to TMJ hypermobility, and other investigations suggest disk displacement and osteoarthrosis.[39–41] Parafunctional habits that contribute to hypermobility of the TMJ in-

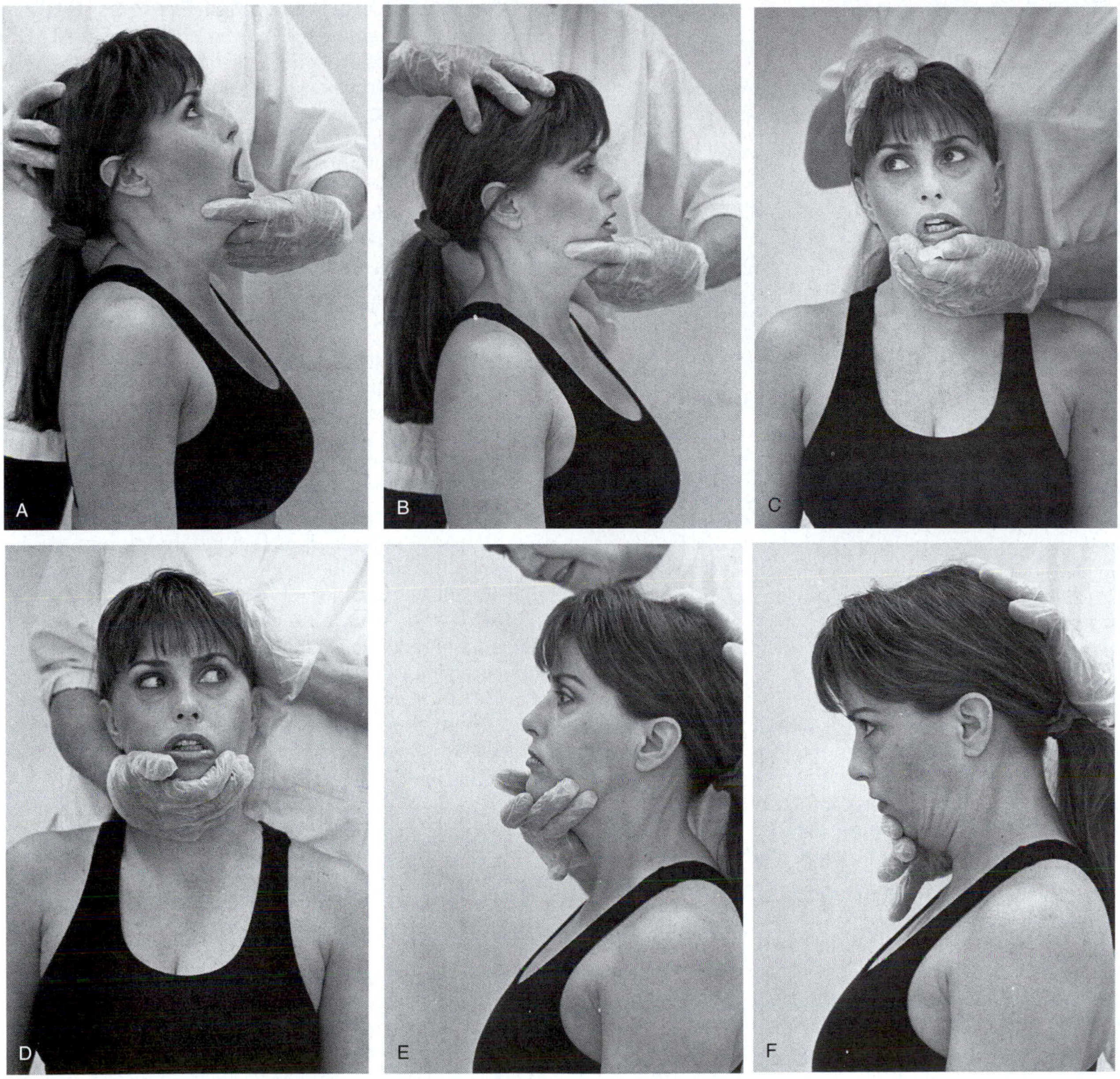

FIGURE 23-16 Functional kinetic exercises using the proximal lever for ***(A)*** opening. With the mandible stabilized; the patient extends the head (the tip of the nose moves cranially and dorsally). As the mouth opens, the joints of the upper cervical spine extend, and the TMJs open. ***(B)*** Closing. The patient flexes the head (the tip of the nose moves caudally and ventrally) as the mouth closes; the joints of the upper cervical spine flex and the TMJs close. ***(C)*** Functional kinetic exercises using the proximal lever for lateral movements to the right. With the mandible silized, the right upper teeth slide laterally to the right of the silized mandible and ***(D)*** to the left (the opposite applies for movement to the left). The movement is one of rotation of the atlanto-occipital and atlanto-axial joints of the cervical spine and lateral translation in the TMJ. ***(E)*** Functional kinetic exercises using the proximal lever for protrusion. With the mandible stabilized the upper teeth slide dorsally in relation to the lower teeth. ***(F)*** Retrusion. With the upper teeth moving ventrally to the lower. The movement is one of dorsal or ventral glide of the cervical spine and dorsal or ventral translation of the TMJs.

clude prolonged bottle feeding, thumb sucking, and pacifier use in children.[16] Many adult patients present with a history of habitually opening their mouths excessively wide when yawning or eating. Both joints usually are involved, but unilateral hypermobility can occur as a compensatory reaction to hypomobility of the contralateral side.

Believed to be the most common mechanical disorder of the TMJ, hypermobility of the TMJ is characterized by early or excessive anterior translation or by early and excessive anterior translation of the mandible.[42] In cases of hypermobility, translation occurs within the first 11 mm of opening, rather than the last 15 to 25 mm. Excessive anterior translation results in laxity of the surrounding capsule and ligaments. The breakdown of these structures allows disk derangement in one or both TMJs. Ultimately, impairments such as functional loss and arthritic changes may occur.

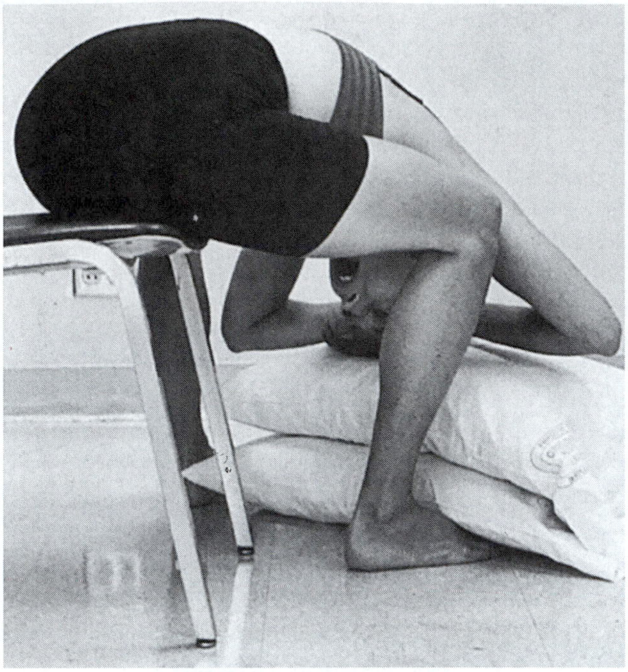

FIGURE 23-17 Opening the mouth exercise with the long axis of the body inverted.

Treatment

Therapeutic modalities such as heat and ice are beneficial if the condition is painful. An important step is to educate the patient regarding the functioning of her joints, the reason for her symptoms, and how to modulate these symptoms. The following sections describe treatment options for hypermobility impairment.

Temporomandibular Joint Rotation and Translation Control. For the therapist to teach control of the jaw muscles, the patient must first recognize the resting position of the mandible: lips closed, teeth slightly apart, and the tongue on the hard palate. The patient should breath in and out through the nose and use diaphragmatic breathing.

The initial exercise limits TMJ mechanics to condylar rotation through an active assistive technique using the index finger and thumb to assist the movement. While maintaining the tongue on the roof of the mouth, one index finger is placed on the involved TMJ, and the other index finger is placed on the chin. The lower jaw is allowed to drop down and back with the guidance of the index finger and thumb (Self-Management: Concentric and Eccentric Exercises). The use of a mirror to monitor motion is helpful in achieving normal tracking and to ensure that the tongue stays up and the jaw does not deviate.

The exercise is progressed by placing both index fingers on the TMJs (Fig. 23-18). The lower jaw is allowed to drop down and back, bringing the chin to the throat, as in the first exercise but without the guidance of the index finger on the mandible. As the patient learns to control movement by proprioceptive feedback, she may then attempt rotation on opening without the tongue on the palate (without condylar translation), first with the guidance of the index finger and thumb on the mandible, as shown in Self-Management: Concentric and Eccentric Exercises, and then with both index fingers on the TMJs (see Fig. 23-18).

Strengthening and Stabilization Exercises. After or concurrently with an exercise program to develop TMJ rotation and translation control, a mandibular stabilization program should be started to strengthen the jaw muscles and balance the strength and function of the right and left TMJs. These strengthening exercises are also used to control excessive translation and establish a normal jaw position at rest and in the open-mouth position. Isotonic exercises may be used in the management of painless clicking, after a painful episode is resolved, and when the click is not caused by a displaced articular disk.[43] Strengthening exercises are also indicated after TMJ operations and for a variety of other TMJ dysfunctions and disorders.

Isometric or Static Exercises. Proprioceptive neuromuscular techniques (PNF), such as the contract-relax exercise and rhythmic stabilization technique are used. Light pressures are applied to the jaw with the index finer and thumb on either side of the mandible. The patient is asked to place the tip of the tongue up against the palate, with the teeth slightly apart. Gentle pressures are applied for a short time. Pressure is applied as the patient attempts to open and close the mandible, glide it to the left or right, and glide it ventrally and dorsally or in diagonal direction back toward or away from either ear (see Patient-Related Instruction: Mandibular Stabilization Instructions). Motion in each direction is repeated several times to exercise various muscles and stimulate neuromuscular awareness. These exercises may then be performed with the jaw in a position with the teeth one knuckle apart and then two knuckles apart (Fig. 23-19).

PNF techniques of resisted isometric opening contractions of the lateral pterygoids and suprahyoids promote relaxation of the primary closing muscles of the mandible (ie, temporalis and masseter) through reciprocal inhibition. This technique can also facilitate maximum interincisal distance.[44,45]

Isotonic or Dynamic Exercises. Isotonic exercises are performed against the manual resistance of the patient's or therapist's hand on the mandible. The amount of chin resistance allows controlled jaw movements over a restricted ROM, allowing full activity of all the muscles operating about the joint. Exercises include resisted opening and closing and lateral movements (Fig. 23-20). Open-close movements are limited to about 15 mm of opening (ie, width of one knuckle). The patient should be reminded not to push the jaw forward during the opening movement and to allow the jaw to open in an arc toward the chest. Resistance to closing should be done slowly. Lateral movements are limited to about 5 mm. These exercises should never be performed so that pain or clicking sounds occur. ROM should stop before the onset of pain or clicking.

Posture and Movement Impairments

SIGNS AND SYMPTOMS

FHP with resultant rounding of the shoulders can produce dysfunction of the craniocervical and temporomandibular system. Symptoms associated with the FHP can be extremely variable. Patients complain of stiffness, tiredness, tingling, aching, numbness, and vertigo. A patient may also

SELF-MANAGEMENT: Concentric and Eccentric Exercises

Purpose: To restore proper "tracking" to the temporomandibular joint (TMJ), to limit TMJ mechanics to rotation through an active assisted technique (the patient's thumb and finger of one hand are needed to assist the movement), and to decrease or eliminate clicking, cracking, popping, or excessive movement occurring in the TMJ.

Precautions: Carefully monitor the axis of rotation of the TMJ joint, eliminating any subsequent translatory motion.

Monitor this trial jaw opening in a mirror to ensure a straight opening (ie, tongue stays on roof of the mouth).

Exercise must be done slowly and rhythmically within the pain limits.

Position: The patient sits on a firm chair, close to the front edge, with feet on the floor about 12 inches apart.

Instruct the patient to maintain, neutral pelvis, lumbar thoracic, and cervical spine alignment.

Instruct the patient to think of the head leading up and the torso lengthening and widening to achieve full spinal length. The cervical spine should remain in neutral (eyes focused to horizontal).

Assistive positioning devices may be used.

The patient can sit with the back and cervical spine supported against a wall (towels behind the head to maintain neutral cervical spine if forward head posture is stiff or rigid).

Movement technique: Instruct patient to:

Keep the tongue on the roof of mouth.

Place one index finger on the TMJ.

Place the opposite thumb and index finger lightly on the tip of the chin.

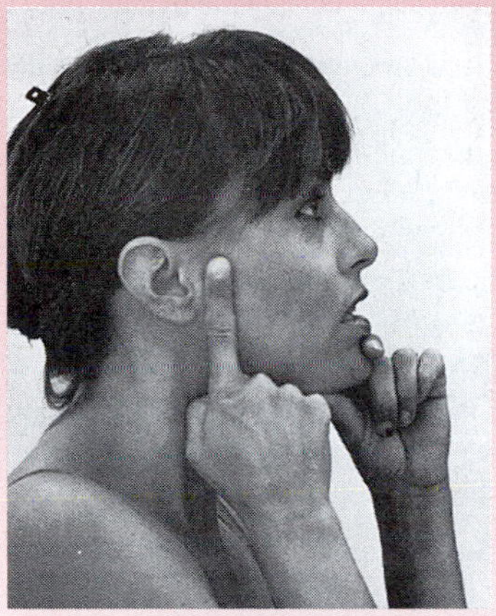

Allow the lower jaw to drop down and back with guidance from the thumb and index on the chin.

After learning to control movement by proprioceptive feedback, rotation-controlled movement without the tongue on the roof of the mouth may be attempted.

Dosage: **Repeat** this exercise 5 times, 5 times per day. The patient is instructed to use this pattern of movement frequently during the day or whenever she observes herself in a mirror.

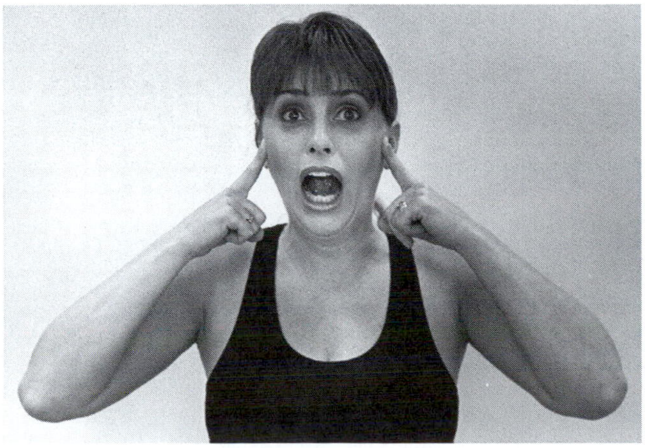

FIGURE 23-18 Neuromuscular re-education for rotation and translation control. The patient starts with the tongue on the roof of the mouth and index fingers on both TMJs. The mandible is allowed to drop down and back; the tongue is dropped from the roof of the mouth and opening is completed. A mirror is used to monitor complete opening and to ensure a straight opening.

complain of limitation of neck motion and various pain referrals to the head, arms, and upper thoracic spine.

To restore balance to the system, patients must address excess tension, head and shoulder girdle alignment, jaw and tongue position, and breathing. Postural re-education exercises; manual therapy techniques applied to tight muscles, soft tissue, and joints; and neuromuscular relaxation training may be needed. In general, treatment should begin by developing a home program of relaxation training and postural correction programs monitored jointly by the patient and therapist. Ergonomic advice and spinal supports should be provided as needed. Ultimately, management should become the patient's responsibility. The therapist assists with reinforcement and periodic follow-up visits for adapting programs based on the patient's changes and progress.

TREATMENT

Neuromuscular Relaxation Training

Effective self-regulatory and neuromuscular relaxation training involves development of more flexible habits of at-

Patient-Related Instruction

Patient-Related Instruction: Mandibular Stabilization Instructions

The objectives are to strengthen the jaw muscles and to establish a normal jaw position at rest and in the open-mouth position. The following exercises require the application of light pressure to the jaw with your index fingers. The intensity of pressure should be 2 on a scale of 1 to 10 (10 = highest force). The jaw should not move during the application of pressure. Monitor this exercise in front of a mirror.

Maintain the following mouth and jaw position:

1. Keep your teeth apart. Let your jaw and mouth drop open slightly and remain in that position.
2. The tip of the tongue remains on the roof of the mouth, just behind the upper two front teeth.

Maintain good head, neck, and back posture. It is helpful to imagine two strings. One string pulls straight up from the top and back of the head to the ceiling; the second string pulls up from the breast bone.

1. Place the index fingers and thumbs of your hands on either side of your jaw.

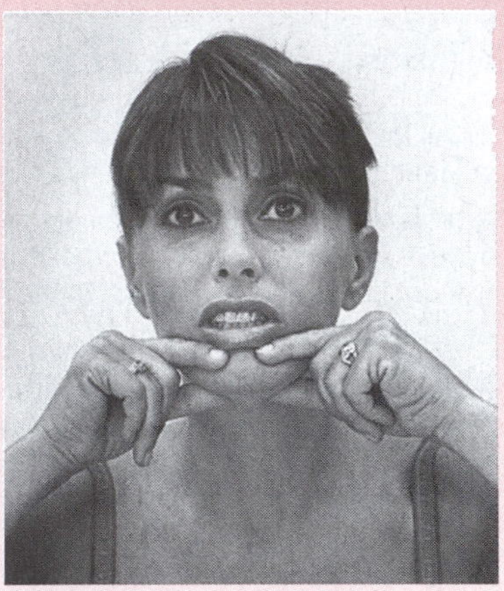

2. Apply gentle pressure (2 on a scale of 1 to 10) in the following directions
   a. To the left side of the jaw
   b. To the right side of the jaw
   c. Up to the ceiling
   d. In toward the neck
   e. Diagonally back toward left ear
   f. Diagonally back toward right ear
3. Hold each pressure for 2 seconds.
4. Repeat each direction ___ times, ___ times per day.

tention, which must be fully transferred by the trainee to everyday activities. Various relaxation procedures that employ physical and mental exercises and exercises called therapeutic awareness have been devised.[46–48] Relaxation therapies may be integrated into biofeedback-assisted attention training.

Progressive relaxation involves a structured isometric approach that asks the patient to contract the muscles and then relax.[49,50] Another form of progressive relaxation uses a reverse approach in which the muscles are passively stretched and then relaxed.[51,52]

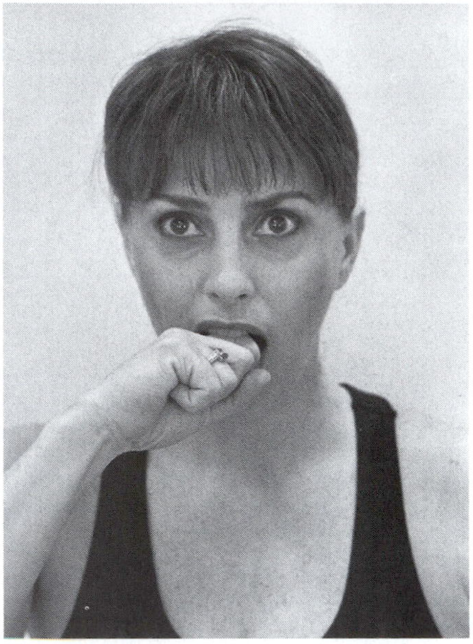

FIGURE 23-19 Isometric stabilization exercises (one- and two-knuckle-width opening). First one and then two knuckles are placed between the upper and lower teeth. The knuckle or knuckles are removed, keeping the teeth apart. Apply gentle pressure to the lower jaw as in Patient-Related Instruction: Mandibular Stabilization Instructions. These exercises build on the exercise shown in the Patient-Related Instruction. The earlier stabilization exercise is continued as these exercises are added. Not all patients are progressed automatically to the two-knuckle-width opening exercise.

Autogenic training employs adaptive mental imagery.[53,54] The verbal content of the standard exercises is focused on the neuromuscular system (eg, heaviness of the limbs), the vasomotor system (eg, warmth of the limbs, coolness of the forehead), and slowing of the cardiovascular system and respiratory mechanisms.

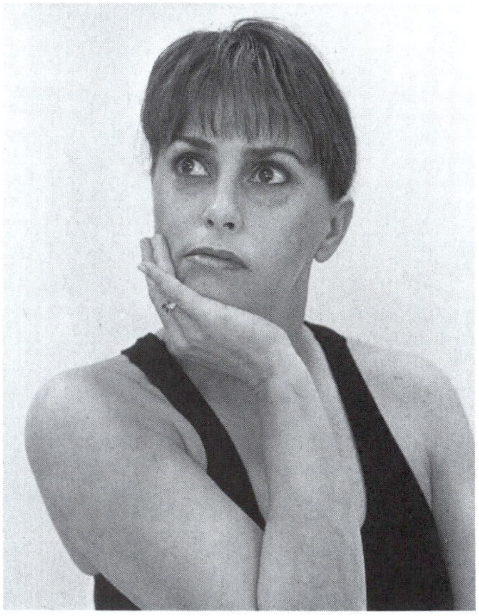

FIGURE 23-20 Isotonic strengthening exercise. Resistive exercise strengthens the left lateral pteryoids against a right lateral force provided by the patient's right hand. Resistance is provided by placing the palm against the chin with the arm stabilized (ie, elbow resting against a firm surface or with the arm held firmly against the chest).

Yoga, meditational mantra, and diaphragmatic breathing techniques are adapted from Eastern disciplines.[55–58] Particularly valuable approaches, which focus on integrated functions of the tongue, jaw, and breathing, include the use of sensory awareness techniques[56,59–62] and sensory-motor learning exercises.[38,63–67]

Head, Neck, and Shoulder Postural Exercises

A significant aspect of the therapy for the head, neck, and shoulder is a postural exercise program. The principles proposed by Kendall and coworkers[68] and Sahrmann[69,70] are most beneficial for these patients (see Chapters 18, 24, and 26). Therapists may also use a variety of movement reeducation approaches to attain balanced posture, alignment, structure, and function. Therapeutic approaches include a variety of methods, such as Aston Patterning,[71,72] the Alexander Technique,[59,60,73] the Feldenkrais Method,[63–67] tai chi,[74–76] and Trager Psychophysical Integration,[72] which use sensory, kinesthetic, and proprioceptive feedback to the body-mind system (see Chapter 16).

A useful method of achieving good postural alignment in sitting and standing is to imagine two "strings" attached to the body: one to the sternum and the other to the top of the head posteriorly. As these strings are pulled up to the ceiling, head posture is made more axial, with increased opening of the suboccipital space. As the sternum becomes elevated, the shoulder girdle becomes more retracted and depressed. However, flattening of the cervical curve should be avoided. According to Rocabodo,[24] cranial flexion should not exceed 150 degrees.

The sternum must be lifted without hyperextension of the thoracic or lumbar spine. The concept of allowing the neck to release so the head can balance "forward and up" should be used to encourage length in the spine.[59] The forward instruction does not mean that the head moves forward of the rest of the body; it is implemented only to undo the backward pull or PCR on the neck. In a patient with PCR, the distance between the occiput and atlas is decreased, narrowing the suboccipital region. This pulls the occiput posteriorly and inferiorly, resulting in upward and backward displacement of the mandible in the fossa. The Alexander use of the word *up* means away from the top of the spine, with the purpose of eliminating any muscle tension that pulls the head down into the neck. The head *forward and up* movement is allowed to happen by releasing tension in the posterior neck muscles (Fig. 23-21).[59]

Mandibular and Tongue Postural Exercises

Proper resting position of the tongue, in addition to helping maintain normal posturing of the mandible and axial spine, enhances normal swallowing patterns and makes daytime clenching more difficult.[77] The correct resting position of the tongue (ie, comfortably resting against the hard palate) should be discussed with the patient and demonstrated.[8] The most anterosuperior tip of the tongue should lie in an area against the palate just posterior to the back side of the upper central incisors. Instructing the patient to maintain TUTALC helps to achieve the resting position of the jaw and tongue and overcome parafunctional and functional muscle hyperactivity.[16]

Tongue push-ups may be used as an initial exercise to strengthen the tip of the tongue and familiarize the patient with the correct placement of the tongue.[15] The tongue tip is pointed and pressed against the hard palate (just above the upper teeth), then released, and the exercise is repeated.

One exercise involves instructing the patient to "cluck" the tip of the tongue against the hard palate and leave it there.[24] Another requires the patient to practice certain sounds, such as those made by the letters T, D, L, and N, that raise the tip of the tongue to the incisal papilla. Words such as Ted, dad, love, and nut can be practiced with added force to activate the tongue muscles.[15]

Neuromuscular control can be achieved by practicing tongue-up exercises along with opening and closing the

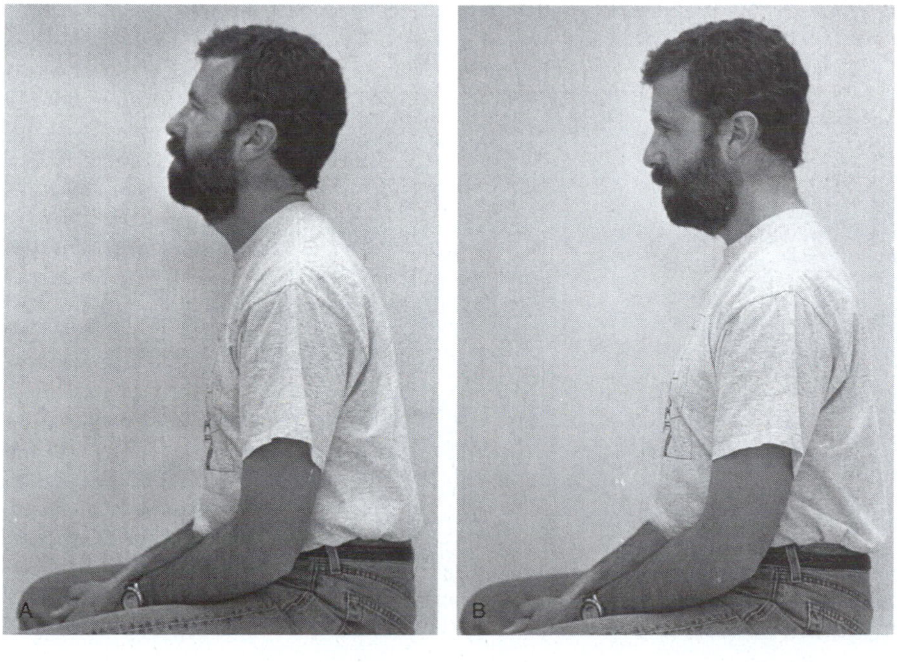

FIGURE 23-21 Head and neck release. ***(A)*** Incorrect: head pulled back and down. ***(B)*** Correct: head releasing forward and up.

mouth with speed.[4] This exercise involves having the patient open and close the mouth wide with the tongue in its resting position. The patient should be instructed to stop short of a "click" with no deviations of the mandible or excessive anterior translation. After controlled opening is achieved, the patient increases the speed of movement. Kraus[4] found this a useful technique in reducing symptoms associated with inflammatory disorders such as synovitis and capsulitis and when inflammation coexist with hypermobility, hypomobility, or excessive parafunctional activities.

Exercises to Correct Dysfunctional Swallow Sequence and Breathing Patterns

A commonly overlooked problem in patients presenting with TMJ and craniocervical disorders is an altered swallowing sequence, which is most often associated with tongue thrust swallow or abnormal breathing. In abnormal breathing, such as mouth breathing, the tongue is usually depressed, and the upper and lower part of the teeth are apart during swallowing. Persons who swallow abnormally usually bring their tongues forward to meet the glass or cup when taking a drink, and excessive lip activity may be evident. Because of the FHP, the hyoid bone may elevate on swallowing and abnormal contraction of the suboccipital musculature may occur.[13] One of the methods, according to Funt and colleagues,[15] of changing this pattern when drinking from a cup or glass is to instruct the patient to bite the back teeth together, put the tongue to "the spot" on the anterior palate directly behind the upper incisors, siphon the water in between the teeth, and swallow (Fig. 23-22).[15] As water is siphoned during the initial phase of swallowing, the tip of the tongue should return to its resting position without putting pressure on the posterior teeth. When this is accomplished, many sips of water are taken and swallowed without any movement of the facial muscles. Because a tongue thrust habit is usually well rooted, this exercise should be practiced several times daily. After the patient can use the new swallowing pattern for all eating and drinking activities and has learned proper posturing, she must apply (at a subconscious level) what she has learned to all swallowing activities and become aware of the rest position of the tongue throughout the day.

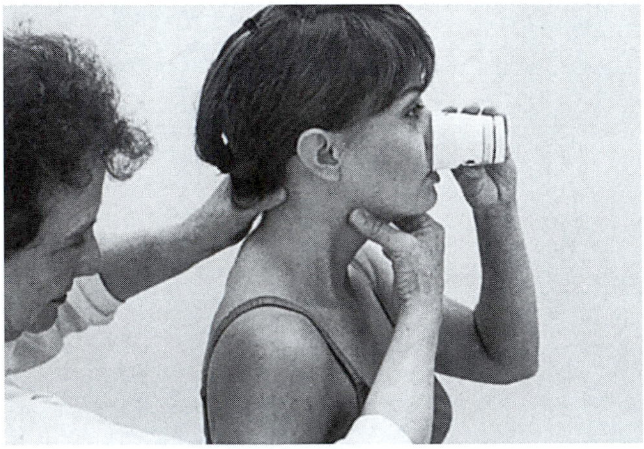

FIGURE 23-22 Swallowing exercise. As water is siphoned during the initial phase of swallowing, the tip of the tongue should return to its resting position. When this is accomplished, many sips of water are taken and swallowed without any movement of the facial muscles.

Proper diaphragmatic breathing is also important to normal TMJ function.[55,59,61,78–80] The mouth breathers, patients with allergies, or patients with nasal obstruction often breathe with increased activity of the accessory muscles of respiration (ie, scaleni, sternocleidomastoids, and pectoralis minor), leading to the FHP with PCR.[81] The patient should be instructed in nasodiaphragmatic breathing (see Patient-Related Instruction: Diaphragmatic Breathing). Diaphragmatic breathing occurs more easily by breathing through the nose and with correct positioning of the tongue. A correct rest position of the tongue forces nasodiaphragmatic breathing. Diaphragmatic breathing is best learned in supine, followed by practice during sitting, standing, and activity. Diaphragmatic breathing controls stress, promotes general relaxation of the body, strengthens the diaphragm, improves oxygenation with increased depth of respiration, and decreases the use of the accessory muscle of respiration. This is an important technique taught to patients with dysfunctional involvement of other regions, such as the pelvic floor, lumbar spine, thorax, and cervical spine.

Attempts to alter breathing patterns are often difficult. However, a more normal breathing pattern can be facilitated by altering the head and neck posture. This may be facilitated by an exercise proposed by Fielding.[82] A soft ball (eg, old tennis ball) or equivalent is placed behind the patient's back at the level of the scapula as she sits in a straight-back chair (Fig. 23-23). The mechanism for improvement is not clear, but observation of the patient reveals a slower rate of breathing, improved spinal alignment, mouth closure, and relaxation of the shoulder girdle. The patient should be encouraged to make a conscientious effort to keep the tongue on the roof of the mouth and to practice diaphragmatic breathing.

To fully transfer these ideas to other activities on a subconscious level, it is often helpful for the trainee to practice awareness exercises directed at restoration of the neutral resting position of the head, neck, jaw, and shoulder girdle throughout the day. The RTTPB system (relaxation, teeth apart, tongue on the palate, posture, and breathing) proposed by Ellis and Makofsy[77] is one way to help the trainee remember and practice frequently. This helpful acronym addresses the common imbalance seen in the upper quadrant.

THERAPEUTIC EXERCISE INTERVENTIONS FOR COMMON DIAGNOSES

In an average clinical setting, the most common disorder of the TMJ is dysfunction involving the capsule and intra-articular structures. TMJ dysfunction can occur as a separate entity or can be a complication of disease, trauma, or developmental abnormalities. Some of the more common diagnoses of the TMJ are reviewed in the following sections.

Patient-Related Instruction

Diaphragmatic Breathing

- Initially, assume a comfortable position on the floor with your hands on your stomach.
- Relax your belly as much as possible.
- During the first third of inhalation, the belly should expand slightly (on its own) in an outward direction as the diaphragm pushes down on the contents of the abdomen.

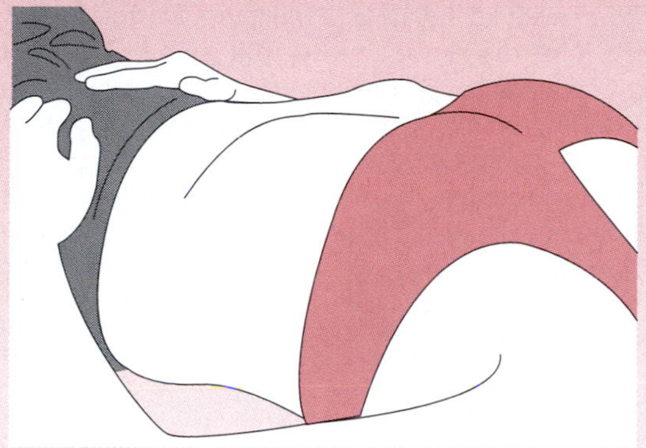

- Next, the air should move into the middle portion of the lungs, causing the area of the lower and middle ribs to expand. Complete inhalation means filling the lungs forward, sideways, and backward.

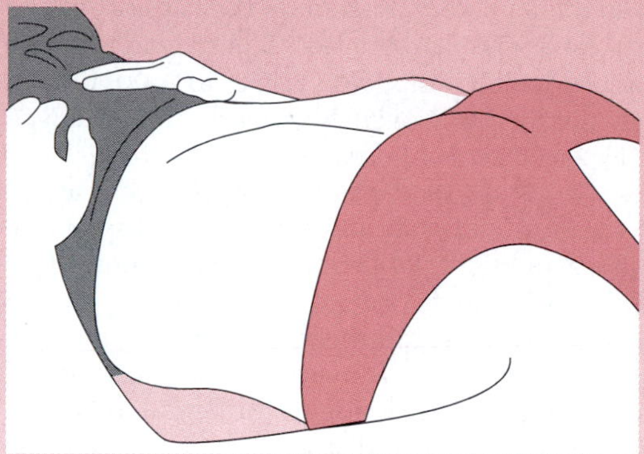

- The dimension of breathing often neglected is sideways intercostal breathing.
- Exhalation is largely a passive occurrence. The chest muscles and diaphragm relax, the ribs drop back close together, and the lungs recoil as air is quickly expelled.

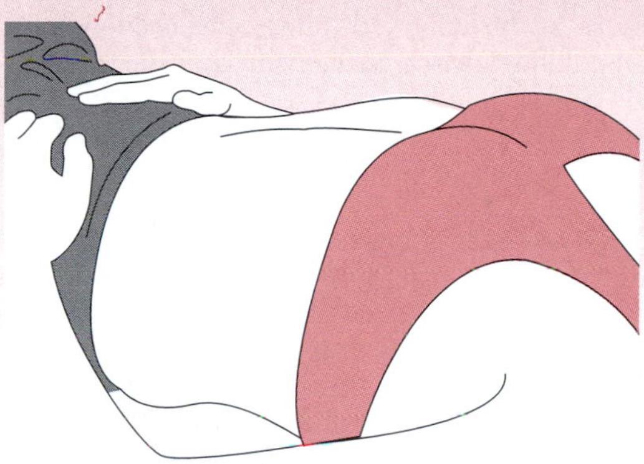

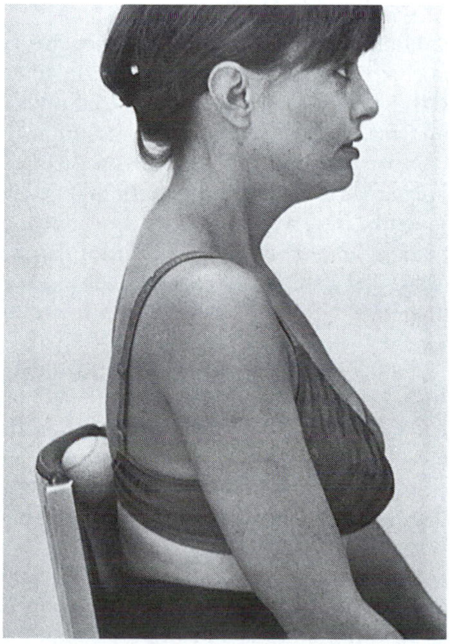

FIGURE 23-23 Posterior cocontraction using a ball behind the back at the level of the scapula to facilitate a more normal breathing pattern.

Capsulitis and Retrodiskitis

SIGNS AND SYMPTOMS

Overloading of the joint from bruxism, excessively hard chewing, trauma, strain, or infection may cause an inflammatory response in the fibrous capsule, synovial membrane, and retrodiskal tissues. The condition is called capsulitis. Habits such as bruxing, tongue thrusting, gum chewing, and pencil chewing can offset the normal pattern of masticatory behavior and lead to asymmetric muscle activity and mandibular malalignment. Overload problems are often related to emotional stress causing excessive muscular activity.

Retrodiskitis occurs with encroachment of the condyle on the articular disk. This causes inflammation or exacerbation of an existing inflammatory condition. It can occur gradually, as the result of chronic repetitive microtrauma when the condyles are displaced posteriorly because of anterior disk displacement, or by acute external trauma to the chin, forcing the condyles posteriorly into the tissues.

Persistent, subtle changes in joint kinematics may cause muscular imbalance between the elevators and depressors and produce abnormal stresses sufficient to result in improper loading of the articular cartilage. This pattern can lead to potential fatigue failure and possible arthritic changes in the articular cartilage. Repeated overload leads to microtrauma and an inflammatory reaction in the capsule, the peripheral parts of the disk, and the lateral pterygoid insertion. The overfatigued lateral pterygoid's ability to move the disk harmoniously during jaw movements can be upset and result in disk displacement and damage.[7]

Signs and symptoms of capsulitis include pain at rest (intensified during functional maximum intercuspation of the teeth) and parafunctional (bruxism) movements of the mandible. Pain occurs on the side of involvement in the area of the TMJ, with possible reference of pain into areas innervated by cranial nerve V. Impairment due to capsulitis ranges from minor joint restriction to total immobilization.

Signs and symptoms of retrodiskitis include constant pain and palpable tenderness posterior and lateral to the joint. Pain is usually increased by clenching or by moving the mandible to the affected side, which permits the condyle to press against the inflamed tissue. With swelling, the condyle may be forced anteriorly, resulting in acute malocclusion. Because chewing on the contralateral side can increase pressure in the inflamed joint, causing more pain, the patient should be advised to chew on the side of the involved joint.[12,83]

TREATMENT

Treatment depends in large part on the cause. If caused by a single traumatic event, a program of limited mandibular function, mild analgesics, ice, and moist heat or ultrasound may be effective. To decrease pain and muscle guarding, use of phonophoresis, ionophoresis, or laser therapy may be indicated.[13,16,84] The most commonly used therapeutic modality after trauma or surgical intervention is cryotherapy.[13] Cold is used to reduce inflammation, muscle spasm, and edema. Cold packs, ice massage, or vapocoolant sprays are used. Massage, biofeedback, relaxation techniques, and electrical stimulation of the mandibular elevators can help promote muscle relaxation. If minor tenderness persists unduly, judicious use of ultrasound with exercises to extend translatory movement may be needed. Because hemarthrosis may occur in an acutely traumatized joint, measures should be taken to prevent ankylosis. As soon as the occlusion remains stabilized, cautious movement of the joint should be encouraged until resolution is complete.

When the inflammation is related to chronic microtrauma or disk displacement, more definitive therapy may be indicated. Placement of a joint-stabilization splint may reduce bruxism and decrease pressure on the joint.[85] Surface electromyography is often beneficial in the treatment of diurnal parafunction.[86,87] When retrodiskitis is caused by disk displacement, anterior repositioning therapy is indicated to reestablish the normal disk-condyle relationship. Maintaining the mandibular rest position by adapting to the normal rest position of the tongue against the palate with normal lip closure also reduces joint pressure.

After inflammation, pain and muscle guarding are under control, a program of stretching and muscular re-education should be instituted. The stretching and PIR techniques discussed in the Hypomobility section help to increase capsular extensibility and restore muscle length. Functional kinetic exercises and strengthening and stabilizing exercises can assist in muscular re-education and relaxation.

Degenerative Joint Disease

SIGNS AND SYMPTOMS

Osteoarthritis, often referred to as degenerative joint disease, of the TMJ is considered primarily a disease of middle or older age. Osteoarthritis alters the force-bearing surfaces of the TMJ, often leading to secondary inflammation of the capsular tissue. The joint space narrows with spur formation and marginal lipping of the joint. There is often erosion of the condylar head, articular eminence, and fossa.[7] Advanced joint disease may lead to atrophy of associated muscles. Some causes of this degenerative process include internal derangement of the disk, an anterior placed disk, and repetitive overloading.

The clinical features of osteoarthritis are similar to those of other forms of joint dysfunction. Typically, pain and crepitation occur during mandibular motions. Usually, crepitation remains after the other symptoms disappear. Most persons experience restriction of the mandible.

TREATMENT

The primary therapy is directed at symptoms and may involve surgery, drug therapy, and physical therapy. Active ROM exercises, mobilization techniques, and stretching, as discussed in the Hypomobility section, may be used during the chronic phase. Graded exercises involving a few simple movements performed frequently during the day are often prescribed as a home treatment. Joint protection techniques, such as avoidance of excessive opening and parafunctional habits, and proper resting position of tongue and mandible should be taught. Advanced bony changes within the joint may necessitate arthroplasty and joint debridement.

Derangement of the Disk

Two general classifications of this disorder are recognized: the anteriorly displaced disk that reduces during joint translation and the anteriorly displaced disk that does not reduce during joint translation.[88] These two conditions may exist indefinitely or may be one of the stages in the continuum of a disease process that leads to degenerative joint disease.[89]

Malocclusion (ie, overclosure of the mouth with backward displacement of the condyle) or trauma may cause derangement of the disk. Trauma to the disk may cause a partial tearing of the disk from its capsular attachment. Among the various theories regarding the cause of disk derangement are excessive pressure on the joint from clenching or trauma; incoordinate contraction of the two bodies of the lateral pterygoid so that the disk snaps over the condyle rather than following the movement smoothly and coordinately when the mouth is open; deterioration of the disk and cartilaginous surfaces; and stretching of the joint ligaments by frequent subluxation.[85,90,91]

Joint sounds such as clicking are considered one of the hallmarks of disk derangement. The frequency and quality of clicking or other sounds and their association with specific functional movements and pain often helps to provide important clues regarding the condition of bony and soft tissues within the joint. Clicking may occur as one or more clicks in one or both joints, and it may or may not be associated with pain. Various types of clicking noises have been observed during sagittal opening, including a opening click, an intermediate click during the opening phase, and an end range click at full opening.

An opening click is believed to be caused by an anterior displacement of the disk, with the condyle displaced posteriorly and superiorly. As the mandible opens, the condyle must pass over the posterior band of the disk and fall into its normal position in the concave articular surface beneath the disk (Fig. 23-24).[91] Clicking during various parts of opening is probably caused by ruptures or rents of the disk or anteroposterior displacement.[92] A click occurring early in jaw opening indicates a small degree of anterior disk displacement; a click occurring near maximal opening suggests farther anterior displacement.

On closing, a soft closing click may also be detected as the condyle slips behind the posterior edge of the band of the disk, leaving the disk displaced anteriorly and medially. The opening click occurs as the disk snaps back into its normal position, and the closing click results in disk displacement. Clicking can worsen with time as the posterior ligamentous attachments become further stretched and damaged. In addition to clicks produced during mandibular opening, clicks may be produced by eccentric movements. These clicks may result from structural changes in the disk or incoordinate function of the parts of the joint.

ASSOCIATED IMPAIRMENTS

The classic signs of the type of anterior disk dislocation with reduction is a distinguished, somewhat loud click or pop on opening accompanied by a coincident palpable jarring of the joint. This signifies that the disk has relocated itself with respect to the condyle. The opening click is followed by a more subtle click, usually occurring during closing and signifying that the disk has displaced anterior to the mandibular condyle. Mandibular ROM is usually normal in disk displacement with reduction, and the amount of vertical opening may be greater than normal.[85]

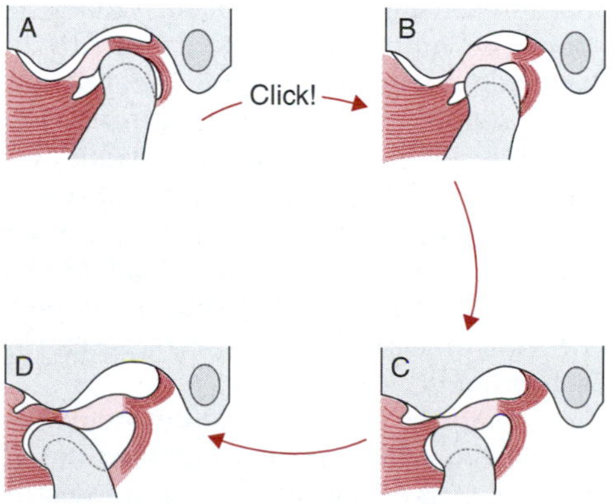

FIGURE 23-24 Mandibular depression with disk displacement. ***(A)*** TMJ with the mouth closed. ***(B)*** Early in the translatory cycle, the condyle is unable to pass under the posterior aspect of the disk. It overrides the posterior disk material and clicks. ***(C*** and ***D)*** Normal joint motion allows complete opening.

The sign of an anterior disk dislocation that does not reduce is the absence of joint noises with a series of reproducible restrictions during mandibular movements. These restrictions are caused by the disk blocking translatory glide. This results in limited condylar translation in the affected joint, and the disorder is often referred to as a closed lock.[93–95] A restricted maximum opening of 20 to 25 mm is the most obvious sign of an acute anterior disk displacement without reduction. The mandible is sharply deflected to the affected side at the end of opening. Lateral excursion to the contralateral side is limited. Over time, a more normal range is achieved because of elongation of the posterior attachment and continued stretching and tearing of the diskal attachments.[84,90,96]

Pain may be felt in the region of the TMJ on the side of involvement, with possible reference of pain into areas innervated by the trigeminal nerve. Pain increases or is altered during functional and parafunctional movements of the mandible. Most patients with chronic anterior disk displacement without reduction report a history of clicking and occasional locking. The most common sound is crepitus, which represents degenerative changes in the articular surfaces. Moffett and coworkers demonstrated that perforation of the disk is usually followed by osteoarthritic changes on the condylar surface, which is followed by similar bony alterations on the opposing surface of the fossa.[97]

TREATMENT

Anteriorly Dislocated Disk With Reduction

A common treatment for an anteriorly dislocated disk with reduction is to use an anterior repositioning appliance or a nonrepositioning appliance applied by a dentist specializing in the treatment of TMJ. Physical therapy modalities such as heat and ice help to decrease pain and muscle guarding, enhancing the effectiveness of the appliance. Instituting a home program to decrease the incidence of parafunctional activity is a first step in management. After parafunctional activities such as gum chewing, nail biting, clenching, excessive opening, and overuse are identified, the client is instructed to avoid these habits. With clenching, the client should be instructed in self-cuing techniques to decrease frequency. The client should check the position of the tongue and mandible frequently throughout the day. A visual cue, such as as clock, in her environment should be used as a reminder. When she notices clenching, a deep breath is taken, and the tongue and mandible are restored to their normal resting positions. Education and exercises in facilitating relaxation of muscle tone of the jaw and cervical muscles are often beneficial; these exercises were discussed in previous sections.

Temporomandibular Joint Clicking

In the absence of obvious malocclusion, simple exercises designed to allow controlled joint movement under load with simultaneous activity of the extensor and flexor muscles operating about the joint have been found to alleviate the annoying problem of TMJ clicking. Gerschmann[98] found that simple exercises, such as lower jaw thrust exercises in a forward, backward, or anterior direction with the teeth disengaged with a pencil and performing chewing exercises with the pencil, could decrease clicking in about 2 weeks (Fig. 23-25).

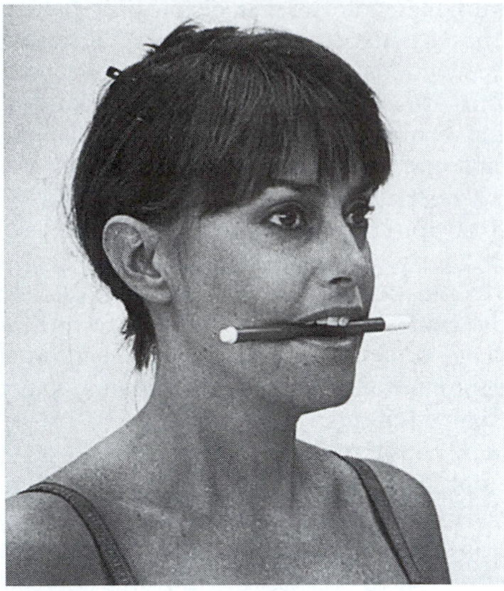

FIGURE 23-25 Chewing the pencil exercise. A soft cylindrical rod (1.5 to 2 mm) is placed horizontally at the back of the mouth so that the object thrusts forward with the mandible. The patient is instructed to bite on the rod with a grinding movement.

Au and Klineberg,[43] in a study of young adults, found that clicking was a reversible condition that could be treated successfully with noninvasive isometric exercises (ie, jaw opening as a hinge movement and lateral deviations) (see Patient-Related Instruction: Mandibular Stabilization Instructions), which suggests that there is a neuromuscular cause for many TMJ clicking problems.

Anteriorly Dislocated Disk Without Reduction

Joint mobilization techniques of distraction (ie, caudal glide) and translation (ie, protrusion) to the involved side may be beneficial when hindrance in function warrants treatment (see Fig. 23-10). Therapeutic modalities and soft tissue mobilization techniques, such as myofascial release and massage, can be used to decrease pain and increase tissue extensibility. If articulation techniques in relocating the disk are successful, proceed immediately with the treatment discussed for an anterior disk dislocation that reduces.

Management in disk derangements may best be accomplished by normalization of muscle tone and function. When pain or hindrance of function is significant and therapeutic intervention and appliances are unsuccessful, consultation with an oral surgeon is indicated.

Surgical Procedures

Postoperative rehabilitation can take 6 months to 1 year. A preoperative physical therapy evaluation should include obtaining a complete medical history and conducting a craniomandibular evaluation, which includes assessment of posture, tongue position, and swallowing sequence. Patient education and patient compliance are critical to successful postoperative treatment. At the preoperative visit, patients should be made aware of the surgical procedure and what to expect postoperatively. Patients should be instructed in techniques of pain control and the reduction of swelling (eg, cryotherapy, transcutaneous electrical nerve stimulation, diaphragmatic breathing) to be used immediately after surgery. Active and passive exercises that may be indicated after surgery should be explained before surgery. Physical therapy procedures after surgery consist of modalities to decrease inflammation, edema, reflex muscle guarding, and pain. The patient's diet is often limited to soft foods for up to 3 months, depending on the extent of surgery and possible scar growth. It is important to emphasize that the home program is the most significant part of the patient's rehabilitation program.

POSTOPERATIVE ARTHROSCOPIC SURGERY

Arthroscopic surgery is indicated for diagnosis and treatment of intracapsular derangement and joint adhesions.[99] Before the advent of TMJ arthroscopy, physical therapy referrals were made usually no earlier than 2 weeks and as late as 6 weeks postoperatively.[100] Arthroscopy has changed this course dramatically. Patients are seen in physical therapy 24 to 48 hours after surgery.

The patient should be reevaluated postoperatively. Changes in pain patterns, sensation, occlusion, and active motions should be recorded along with evidence of intracapsular or extracapsular swelling. In most postoperative procedures, an immediate goal is to maintain the interincisal opening achieved under anesthesia by the surgeon.[13] Postoperative adhesions between the articular surfaces and the disk may occur if mobility is not maintained. Intraoral joint mobilization techniques include distraction and lateral glides (see Fig. 23-10). These techniques are designed to inhibit reformation of adhesions, decompress the TMJ, enhance synovial lubrication, promote muscle relaxation, and restore functional ROM.[4,101] Joint mobilization techniques must be performed gently and slowly within the pain-free range and usually to both TMJs to prevent hypomobility from long-standing dysfunction on the nonsurgical side.

One of the most important exercises postoperatively is teaching the patient to open her mouth with the tip of the tongue on the hard palate to inhibit early translation (see Self-Management: Concentric and Eccentric Exercises). Studies by Osborne[102,103] and Salter[104] have shown that constant mobility after joint trauma or surgery usually lyses blood clots, forestalling organization into connective tissue. Active isometric and isotonic exercises are performed as previously described (see Patient-Related Instruction: Mandibular Stabilization Instructions and Figs. 23-19 and 23-20). Time and effort should be spent on achieving normal tracking and balancing lateral movements. Self-distraction (Fig. 23-26) and gentle active-passive mandibular opening exercises (see Figs. 23-12 and 23-18 and Self-Management: Concentric and Eccentric Exercises) and lateral deviation of the mandible (see Fig. 23-11) should be performed without causing pain.

If hypomobility develops as healing progresses and the problem is attributed to capsular constriction, ultrasound treatment (under the constant force of tongue blades or a Therabite unit) and more vigorous joint mobilization techniques may be considered. Emphasis should be placed on lateral and medial gliding and on protrusive movements. If hypomobility is attributed to fascial restriction or muscle dysfunction, myofascial release techniques, PNF tech-

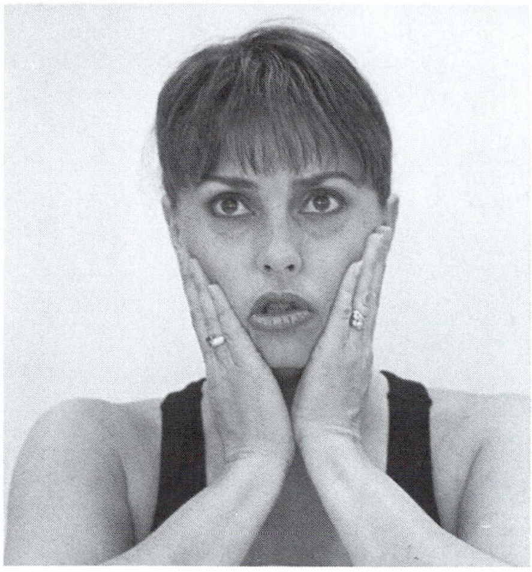

FIGURE 23-26 Self-distraction may be performed by the patient gently squeezing the face and pulling forward and downward on the mandible. The elbows should rest on a firm surface, or the patient should hold the forearms firmly against the chest. To enhance the mobilization techniques, active participation by the patient is encouraged. The patient actively opens or closes using minimal muscle contraction, and after relaxing, additional distraction can be applied.

niques (ie, contract-relax exercises, rhythmic stabilization), PIR techniques (see Figs. 23-12 through 23-15), and isotonic exercises may be used increase mandibular motion and promote relaxation.

At all times, the therapist must consider the cervical spine and any abnormal forces that the exercise may place on the TMJs. The therapist must consider the suprahyoid-infrahyoid length-tension relationship and its influence on tongue physiology and the resting position of the jaw.[17,105] Treatment of the cervical spine, based on the evaluation findings, may be directed at postural corrective exercises for the head and neck, releasing myofascial restrictions, restoring joint mobility, or providing segmental stabilization exercises for hypermobile segments.[106] The typical postarthroscopic surgical patient is followed for 5 to 7 weeks.[13]

POSTARTHROTOMY SURGERY

The most common indication for postarthrotomy surgery is a derangement of the disk that has not responded to nonsurgical management. Arthrotomy (ie, open joint) procedures vary, depending on the existing pathology and the technique of the maxillofacial or oral surgeon. Surgical options include disk plication and partial or total diskectomy with grafts or without replacement. The degree of disk deformation and health of the intercapsular disk attachments dictate the feasibility of plication.

The patient should be seen within the first 3 to 4 days postoperatively to administer appropriate anti-inflammatory modalities and to begin active or passive ROM.[107] Most surgeons request that only active motion without resistance be used during the first 3 postoperative days.[13] They believe passive mobilization can disrupt healing and cause surgical failure.

Physical therapy after a disk plication procedure is based on an understanding of revascularization and healing of the involved tissues. The greatest change in vascularity and healing occurs in the second and third week after surgery, and complete healing occurs in 6 weeks.[108] If a disk has been reconstructed or retrodiskal tissue repair performed, motion may be quite limited, initially allowing only condylar rotation. Splint therapy is usually an integral part of the patient's overall treatment.

After the fifth or sixth week postoperatively, condylar rotation is allowed. Careful early mobilization prevents the potential loss of mandibular movement associated with immobilization. The method of choice is extraoral medial glides, protrusion (Fig. 23-27), and distraction, which can also be done by the patient (see Fig. 23-26).[13] The patient should be instructed in active and passive mandibular exercises (see Fig. 23-12; Self-Management: Concentric and Eccentric Exercises; and Patient-Related Instruction:

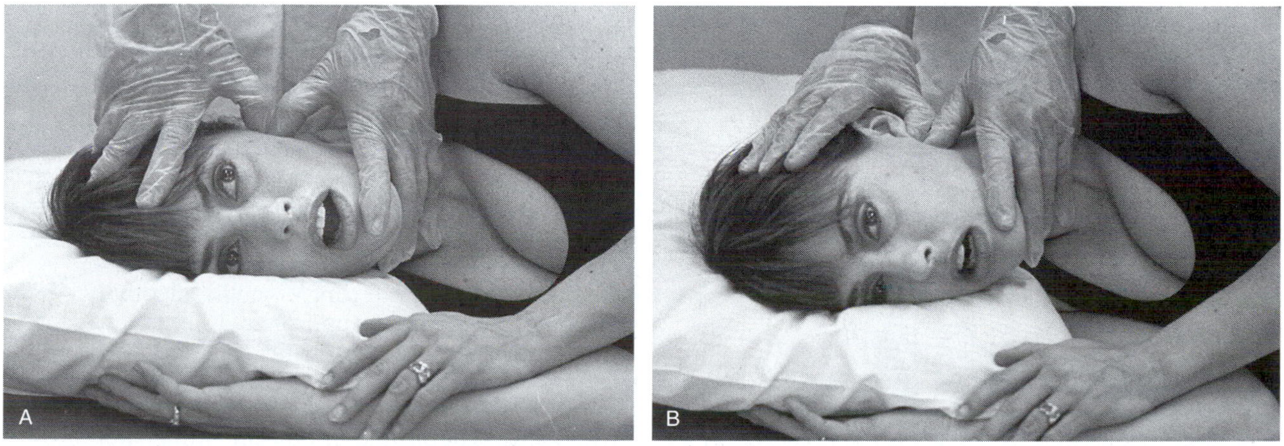

FIGURE 23-27 Extraoral articulation techniques are performed with the patient in sidelying on the noninvolved side with the head supported on a pillow. ***(A)*** Extraoral medial glide. Gentle oscillatory mobilization are performed over the lateral pole of the condyle in a medial direction with the thumbs. ***(B)*** Extraoral protrusion. Gentle oscillatory mobilizations are performed over the posterior aspect of the condyle in an anterior direction.

Diaphragmatic Breathing). Re-education of the masticatory muscles is usually started in the third or fourth week. Resisted opening (Fig. 23-28) and active lateral glide with tongue blades (see Fig. 23-11) or surgical tubing is first initiated on the contralateral side (Fig. 23-29). Lateral glide exercises may then be performed with submaximal isometrics. Lateral deviations are usually limited to 5 mm on the side opposite the surgery.

Massage of the temporalis and inferior to the masseter in particular permits a better stretch.[103] Soft tissue mobilization techniques may include deep pressure-point massage,[109] friction massage,[110] acupressure,[111] strain-counterstrain,[112] craniosacral therapy,[113–115] and myofascial release or manipulations.[13,116,117]

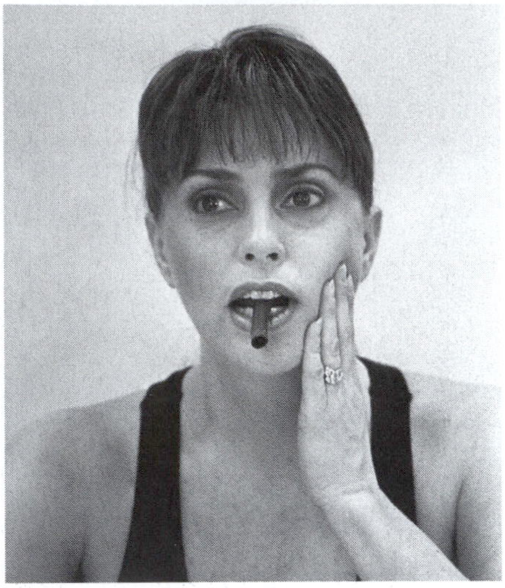

FIGURE 23-29 Lateral deviation of the mandible. Tubing is maintained with the frontal incisors at an end-to-end position. Active exercises are performed by rolling it side to side. A mirror should be used for visual feedback to ensure that no retrusion occurs.

ADJUNCTIVE THERAPY

Surface electromyography (EMG) of the muscles of mastication is used routinely by some dentists and therapists as part of the diagnosis and treatment of TMJ disorders. Muscle hyperactivity, spasms, and imbalance have been suggested in the literature for many years to be major features of TMJ disorders, but evidence to support such concepts is lacking.[118–120] The use of surface EMG is based on the assumption that various dysfunctional or pathologic conditions can be discerned from records of EMG activity of the masticatory muscles, including muscle imbalances,[85,121–123] functional hyperactivity and hypoactivity,[124–128] postural hyperactivity,[85,126,129–131] muscle spasm,[125,126,132,133] fatigue,[134,135] and abnormal occlusal positions.[123,136–139]

Records of EMG activity before and after therapeutic intervention have been used to document changes in muscle function and have been cited as proof that the treatment was successful.[121,122,133] Most researchers agree that surface EMG can measure a behavioral event such as bruxism or clenching.[138,141] With portable EMG devices, relaxation of the masticatory muscles may be attained by the patient through biofeedback at home or work. Nocturnal biofeedback exercise can produce a significant decrease in the frequency and duration of nighttime bruxism.[142–146] However, the benefits of this treatment did not last long, and a return to pretreatment EMG levels was observed as soon as biofeedback stopped.[143,144] A few controlled studies have shown significant reduction of diurnal masseter muscle activity by using diurnal biofeedback.[65,86]

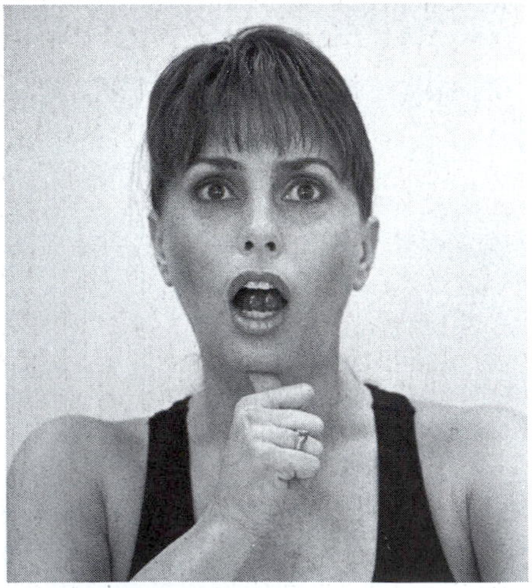

FIGURE 23-28 Resisted concentric opening at the midline is performed by the closing force provided by the therapist's or patient's hand. Emphasis is placed on straight, midline mandibular depression and protrusion with the tongue on the hard palate. To avoid provoking pain or clicking, opening should be restricted to less than 20 mm inter-incisor separation.

Key Points

- The relationships of the stomatognathic system, in terms of structure and function, require a thorough evaluation and integrated treatment approach.
- FHP affects the position if the mandible, tongue, and hyoid, altering mandibular rest position, swallowing function, breathing pattern, and muscle balance.
- Proper positioning of the tongue on the roof of the mouth helps to maintain normal resting position of the mandible and promotes normal swallowing function.
- Hypomobility of the TMJ may result from various conditions involving the bones, muscles, joint capsule, retrodiskal tissue, or disk. Treatment seeks to decrease inflammation and pain and increase motion and function.
- In the case of a nonreducing disk, it is important to limit interincisal opening to approximately 30 mm to protect the retrodiskal tissue from being overstretched.
- Hypermobility of the TMJ is characterized by early and excessive translation of the mandible. Treatment seeks to increase joint proprioception and retrain motion, limiting translation through controlled motions and stabilization exercises.
- Hypermobility is usually bilateral; however, it occurs unilaterally when the contralateral joint is hypomobile.

LAB ACTIVITIES

1. Outline a conceptual model of musculoskeletal TM joint dysfunction and its sequelae.
2. List nine generic treatment goals appropriate for treatment of a patient with musculoskeletal pain and dysfunction of the TMJ.
3. Provide a sequential treatment plan using the goals identified in question #2 for the following:
   a. A soft tissue lesion without a mechanical deficit
   b. A soft tissue restriction without an articular deficit
   c. An articular deficit with soft tissue lesions or length and flexibility deficit

- Postoperative rehabilitation can take 6 months to 1 year. Therapeutic intervention should begin as soon as possible to administer appropriate anti-inflammatory modalities and to begin active or passive ROM. One of the most important exercises postoperatively is teaching the patient to open the mouth with the tip of the tongue on the hard palate to inhibit early translation.
- It is important to involve patients actively in their treatment plan and to emphasize that the home program is the most significant part of their rehabilitation program.

Critical Thinking Questions

1. Describe the following:
   a. The rest position of the tongue
   b. The motions available to the TMJ
   c. The relationship of the cervical spine and the TMJ
   d. The muscular control necessary for normal TMJ motion
2. Differentiate
   a. Between the motions available in the upper and lower joint components of the TMJ.
   b. Between the classic sign of anterior disk location with reduction and anterior disk location that does not reduce.
3. What are the major elements of the exercise prescription after
   a. Postoperative arthroscopic surgery.
   b. Postarthrotomy surgery.

REFERENCES

1. Magee DJ. Temporomandibular joints. In: Magee DJ, ed. *Orthopedic Physical Assessment.* 2nd ed. Philadelphia: WB Saunders; 1992:71–89.
2. Norkin CC, Levangie PK. The temporomandibular joint. In: Norkin CC, Levangie PK, eds. *Joint Structure and Function: A Comprehensive Analysis.* 2nd ed. Philadelphia: FA Davis; 1992:193–206.
3. Moss M. The functional matrix concept and its relationship to temporomandibular joint dysfunction and treatment. *Dent Clin North Am.* 1983;27:445–455.
4. Kraus S. Physical therapy management of TMD. In: Kraus S, ed. *Temporomandibular Disorders.* 2nd ed. New York: Churchill Livingstone; 1994:161–216.
5. Eggleton TM, Langton DP. Clinical anatomy of the TMJ complex. In: Kraus SL, ed. *Temporomandibular Disorders.* 2nd ed. New York: Churchill Livingstone; 1994:1–40.
6. Tanaka TT. *Advanced Dissection of the Temporomandibular Joint.* Chula Vista, CA: Instructional Video, Clinical Research Foundation; 1988.
7. Hartley A. Temporomandibular assessment. In: Hartley A, ed. *Practical Joint Assessment: Upper Quadrant.* 2nd ed. St Louis: Mosby; 1995:1–41.
8. Fish F. The functional anatomy of the rest position of the mandible. *Dent Pract.* 1961;11:178.
9. Sauerland EK, Mitchell SP. Electromyographic activity of intrinsic and extrinsic muscles of the human tongue. *Tex Rep Biol Med.* 1975;33:445–455.
10. Pertes RA, Attanasio R, Cinotti WR, Balbo M. The temporomandibular joint in function and dysfunction. *Clin Prev Dent.* 1988;10:23–29.
11. Assael LA. Functional anatomy. In: Kaplan AS, Assel LA, eds. *Temporomandibular Disorders: Diagnosis and Treatment.* Philadelphia: WB Saunders; 1991;2–10.
12. Bell WE. *Temporomandibular Disorders: Classification, Diagnosis, Management.* 3rd ed. Chicago: Year Book Medical Publishers; 1990.
13. Dunn J. Physical therapy. In: Kaplan AS, Assael LA, eds. *Temporomandibular Disorders.* Philadelphia: WB Saunders. 1991:455–500.
14. Fricton JR, Kroening RJ, Hathaway KM. *TMJ and Craniofacial Pain: Diagnosis and Management.* St Louis: Ishiyzku EuroAmerica; 1988.
15. Funt LA, Stack B, Gelb S. Myofunctional therapy in the treatment of the craniomandibular syndrome. In: Gelb H, ed. *Clinical Management of Head, Neck, and TMJ Pain and Dysfunction: A Multi-Disciplinary Approach to Diagnosis and Treatment.* 2nd ed. Philadelphia: WB Saunders; 1985:432–470.
16. Racabado M, Iglarsh ZA. *Musculoskeletal Approach to Maxillofacial Pain.* Philadelphia: JB Lippincott; 1991.
17. Moumoto T, Kawamura Y. Properties of tongue and jaw movements elicited by stimulation of the orbital gyrus of cat. *Arch Oral Biol.* 1973;18:361–372.
18. Kraus SL. Influences of the cervical spine on the stomatognathic system. In: Donatelli R, Wooden M, eds. *Orthopaedic Physical Therapy.* 2nd ed. New York: Churchill Livingstone; 1993.
19. Racabado M. *Advanced Upper Quarter Manual.* Tacoma, WA: Rocabado Institute; 1981.
20. Halbert R. Electromyographic study of head position. *J Can Dent Assoc.* 1958;23:11–23.
21. Perry C. Neuromuscular control of mandibular movements. *J Prosthet Dent.* 1973;30:714–720.
22. Wyke BD. Neuromuscular mechanisms influencing mandibular posture: a neurologist's review of current concepts. *J Dent.* 1972;2:111–120.

23. Prieskel HW. Some observations on the postural position of the mandible. *J Prosthet Dent.* 1965;15:625–633.
24. Racabado M. Diagnosis and treatment of abnormal cranioiomandibular mechanics. In: Solberg W, Clark G, eds. *Abnormal Jaw Mechanics: Diagnosis and Treatment.* Chicago: Quintessence Publishing; 1984.
25. Cailliet R. *Neck and Arm Pain.* 3rd ed. Philadelphia: FA Davis; 1991.
26. Friedman MH, Weisberg J. *Temporomandibular Joint Disorders: Diagnosis and Treatment.* Chicago: Quintessence Publishing; 1985.
27. Mannheimer JS, Dunn J. Cervical spine. In: Kaplan AS, Assael LA, eds. *Temporomandibular Disorders.* Philadelphia: WB Saunders; 1991:50–94.
28. Mannheimer JS, Rosenthal RM. Acute and chronic postural abnormalities as related to craniofacial pain and temporomandibular disorders. *Dent Clin North Am.* 1991;35:185–208.
29. Darnell M. A proposed chronology for events for forward head posture. *J Craniomandib Pract.* 1983;1:50–54.
30. Proffit W. Equilibrium theory revisited: factors influencing position of the teeth. *Angle Orthod.* 1978;48:175–186.
31. McNeill C, ed. *Temporomandibular Disorders: Guidelines for Their Classification and Management.* Chicago: Quintessence Publishing; 1993.
32. Maitland GDP. *Peripheral Manipulations.* 3rd ed. Boston: Butterworth; 1991.
33. Hertling DM. The temporomandibular joint. In: Hertling DM, Kessler R, eds. *Management of Common Musculoskeletal Disorders.* 3rd ed. Philadelphia: JB Lippincott; 1995;444–485.
34. Mannheimer J. Physical therapy modalities and procedures. In: Pertes RA, Gross SG, eds. *Clinical Management of Temporomandibular Disorders and Orofacial Pain.* Chicago: Quintessence Publishing; 1995:227–244.
35. Lewit K: Therapeutic techniques. In: Lewit K, ed. *Manipulative Therapy in Rehabilitation of the Locomotor System.* 2nd ed. Oxford, UK: Butterworth-Heinemann; 1991:143–230.
36. Klein-Vogelback S. *Functional Kinetics: Observing, Analyzing, and Teaching Human Movement.* Berlin: Springer-Verlag; 1990.
37. Klein-Vogelback S. *Therapeutic Exercises in Functional Kinetics: Analysis and Instruction of Individually Adaptive Exercises.* Berlin: Springer-Verlag; 1991.
38. Wildman F. *The TMJ Tape for Jaw, Head and Neck Pain.* The Intelligent Body Tape Series. Berkeley, CA: Institute of Movement Studies; 1993.
39. Keith DA. *Surgery of the Temporomandibular Joint.* 2nd ed. Boston: Blackwell Scientific Publications; 1992.
40. Buckingham RB, Braun T, Harinstein DA, et al. Temporomandibular joint dysfunction: A close association with systemic joint laxity (the hypermobile joint syndrome). *Oral Surg Oral Med Oral Pathol.* 1991;72:514–519.
41. Westling L, Mattiasson A. General joint hypermobility and temporomandibular joint derangement in adolescents. *Ann Rheum Dis.* 1992;51:87–90.
42. Morrone L, Makofsky H. TMJ home exercise program. *Clin Management.* 1991;11:20–23.
43. Au AR, Klineberg JJ. Isokinetic exercise management of temporomandibular joint clicking in young adults. *J Prosthet Dent.* 1993;70:33–38.
44. Carstensen B. Indications and contraindications of manual therapy for TMJ. In: Grieve G, ed. *Therapy of the Vertebral Column.* New York: Churchill Livingstone; 1986.
45. Plante D. Postoperative physical therapy. In: Keith DA, ed. *Surgery of the Temporomandibular Joint.* Chicago: Blackwell Scientific Publishers; 1988.
46. Benson H, Stuart EM. The Wellness Book: *The Comprehensive Guide to Maintaining Health and Treating Stress-Related Illness.* New York: Simon & Schuster; 1992.
47. Cannistraci AJ, Fritz G. Biofeedback—the treatment of stress-induced muscle activity. In: Gelb H, ed. *Clinical Management of Head, Neck and TMJ Pain and Dysfunction: A Multi-Disciplinary Approach to Diagnosis and Treatment.* 2nd ed. Philadelphia: WB Saunders; 1985:414–431.
48. Davis M, Robbins Eshelmann E, McKay M. *The Relaxation and Stress Reduction Workbook.* 3rd ed. Oakland, CA.: New Harbinger Publishers; 1988.
49. Jacobson E. *Progressive Relaxation.* 4th ed. Chicago: University of Chicago Press; 1962.
50. Jacobson E. *Anxiety and Tension Control.* Philadelphia: JB Lippincott; 1964.
51. Carlson CR, Collin FL, Nitz AJ, et al. Muscle stretching as an alternative relaxation training procedure. *J Behav Ther Exp Pschiatry.* 1990;21:29–83.
52. Carlson CR, VenTrella MA, Sturgia ET. Relaxation training through muscle stretching procedures: a pilot case. *J Behav Ther Exp Psychiatry.* 1987:18:121–123.
53. Luthe W, ed. *Autogenic Therapy,* vols 1–6. New York: Grune & Stratton; 1969–1972.
54. Schultz JH, Luthe W. *Autogenic Training: A Psychophysiological Approach in Psychotherapy.* New York: Grune & Stratton; 1959.
55. Jenks B. *Your Body: Biofeedback at Its Best.* Chicago: Nelson, Hall; 1977.
56. Iyengar BKS. *Light on Yoga.* New York: Schocken; 1979.
57. Proctor J. *Breathing and Meditative Techniques,* tape 12. New York: Bio-Monitoring Applications; 1975.
58. Schatz MP. *Back Care Basics: A Doctor's Gentle Yoga Program for Back and Neck Pain Relief.* Berkeley, CA: Rodmell Press; 1992.
59. Caplan D. *Back Trouble.* Gainesville, FL: Triad Publishing; 1987.
60. Alexander FM. *The Use of Self.* London: Re-education Publications; 1910.
61. Barlow W. *The Alexander Technique.* New York: Alfred A Knopf; 1973.
62. Masters R, Houston J. *Listening to the Body: The Psychophysical Way to Health and Awareness.* New York: Delta; 1978.
63. Feldenkrais M. *Body and Mature Behavior.* New York: International University Press; 1949.
64. Feldenkrais M. *Awareness Through Movement.* New York: Harper & Row; 1972.
65. Feldenkrais M. *The Master Moves.* Cupertino, CA: Meta Publishers; 1984.
66. Feldenkrais M. *The Potent Self.* Cambridge: Harper & Row; 1985.
67. Feldenkrais M. Bodily expressions. *Somatics.* 1988;4:52–59.
68. Kendall FP, McCreary, EK, Provance PG. *Muscle Testing and Function.* 4th ed. Baltimore: Williams & Wilkins; 1993.
69. Sahrmann S. A program for correction of muscular imbalances and mechanical imbalances. *Clin Manag.* 1983;3:23–28.
70. Sahrmann S. Adult posturing. In: Kraus S, ed: *TMJ Disorders: Management of the Craniomandibular Complex.* New York: Churchill Livingstone; 1988.
71. Low J. The modern body therapies. Part four: Aston patterning. *Massage.* 1988;16:48–52.
72. Miller B. Alternative somatic therapy. In: Anderson R, ed. *Conservative Care of Low Back Pain.* Baltimore: Williams & Wilkins; 1991.
73. Jones F. *Body Awareness.* New York: Schocken Books; 1979.
74. Crompton P. *The Elements of Tai Chi.* Shaftesbury, Dorset: Element; 1990.

75. Crompton P. *The Art of Tai Chi.* Shaftesbury, Dorset: Element; 1993.
76. Kotsias J. *The Essential Movements of Tai Chi.* Brookline, MA: Paradigm Publishers; 1989.
77. Ellis JJ, Makofsky HW. Balancing the upper quarter through awareness of RTTPB. *Clin Manag.* 1987;7:20–23.
78. Frownfelter DL. *Chest Physical Therapy and Pulmonary Rehabilitation.* 2nd ed. Chicago: Year Book Medical Publishers; 1987.
79. Kisner C, Colby LA. Chest therapy. In: Kisner C, Colby LA, eds. *Therapeutic Exercise: Foundation and Techniques.* Philadelphia: FA Davis; 1990:577–616.
80. Allen RJ, Leischow SJ. The effect of diaphragmatic and thoracic breathing on cardiovascular arousal. In: *Proceedings of the VIIth International Respiratory Psychophysiology Symposium.* The Nobel Institute for Neurophysiology, Stockholm Sweden, 1987.
81. Tallgren A, Solow B. Hyoid bone position, facial morphology and head posture in adults. *Eur J Orthod.* 1987;9:1–8.
82. Fielding M. Physical therapy in chronic airway limitation. In: Peat M, ed. *Current Physical Therapy.* Toronto: BC Decker; 1988:12–14.
83. Okeson JP. *Management of Temporomandibular Disorders and Occlusion.* 3rd ed. St Louis: Mosby; 1993.
84. Mannheimer JS. Physical therapy concepts in evaluation and treatment of the upper quarter. In: Kraus SL, ed. *Disorders: Management of the Craniomandibular Complex.* New York: Churchill Livingstone; 1988:311–337.
85. Pertes RA, Gross SG. Disorders of the temporomandibular joint. In: Pertes RA, Gross, eds. *Clinical Management of Temporomandibular and Orofacial Pain.* Chicago: Quintessence Publishing; 1995.
86. Dohrmann RJ, Laskin DM. An evaluation of electromyographic biofeedback in the treatment of myofascial pain and dysfunction. *J Am Dent Assoc.* 1978;96:656–662.
87. Gale EN. Biofeedback treatment for TMJ pain. In: Igersoll BD, McCutcheon WR, eds. *Clinical Research in Behavioral Dentistry: Proceedings of the Second National Conference on Behavioral Dentistry;* 1979; University School of Dentistry; Morgantown, WV.
88. Farrar W, McCarty W Jr. *Outline of Temporomandibular Joint Diagnosis and Treatment.* 6th ed. Montgomery, AL: Normandy Study Group; 1980.
89. Lawrence ES, Razook SJ. Nonsurgical management of mandibular disorders. In: Kraus S. ed. *Temporomandibular Disorders.* 2nd ed. New York: Churchill Livingstone; 1994: 125–160.
90. Ross JB. Diagnostic criteria and nomenclature for TMJ arthrography in sagittal section. Part 1: Derangement. *J Craniomand Disord Facial Oral Pain.* 1987;1:185–201.
91. Shore MA. *Temporomandibular Joint Dysfunction and Occlusal Equilibration.* Philadelphia: JB Lippincott; 1976.
92. Whinery JG. Examination of patients with facial pain. In: Alling C, Mahan P, eds. *Facial Pain.* Philadelphia: Lea & Febiger; 1977.
93. Farrar WB, McCarty WL, Normandie Study Group For TMJ Dysfunction. *A Clinical Outline of Temporomandibular Join Diagnosis and Treatment.* 7th ed. Montgomery, AL: Normandie Publications; 1982:52–89.
94. Schwartz HC, Kendrick RW. Internal derangement of the temporomandibular joint: description of clinical syndromes. *Oral Surg Oral Pathol.* 1984;58:24–29.
95. Westesson PL. Clinical and arthrographic findings in patients with TMJ disorder. In: Moffett BC, ed. *Diagnosis of Internal Derangement of the Temporomandibular Joint,* vol 1. Seattle: University of Washington; 1984:59–71.
96. Eriksson L, Westesson PL. Clinical and radiological study of patients with anterior disc displacement of the temporomandibular joint. *Swed Dent J.* 1983;7:55–61.
97. Moffett BC, Johnson LC, McCabe JB, Askew HC. Articular remodeling in the adult human temporomandibular joint. *Am J Anat.* 1964;115:10–130.
98. Gerschmann JA. Temporomandibular dysfunction. *Aust Fam Physician.* 1988;17:274.
99. Vriell P, Bertolucci L, Swaffer C. Physical therapy in the postoperative management of temporomandibular joint arthroscopic surgery. *J Craniomandib Pract.* 1989;7:27–32.
100. Mannheimer JS. Postoperative physical therapy. In: Kraus SL, ed. *Temporomandibular Disorders.* New York: Churchill Livingstone; 1994;277–297.
101. Racabado M. Physical therapy management for the post surgical patient. *J Craniomandib Disord Facial Oral Pain.* 1989;3:75–82.
102. Osborne JJ. A physical therapy protocol for orthognathic surgery. *J Craniomandib Pract.* 1989;7:132–136.
103. Osborne JJ. Postorthognathic surgery. In: Kraus SL. ed. *Temporomandibular Disorders.* 2nd ed. New York: Churchill Livingstone; 1994:308–322.
104. Salter RD. Regeneration of articular cartilage through continuous passive motion: past, present and future. In: Stab R, Wilson PH, eds. *Clinical Trends in Orthopedics.* New York: Thieme Stratton; 1982.
105. Daly P, Preston CD, Evans WG. Postural response of the head to bite opening in adult males. *Am J Orthod.* 1982; 82:157–160.
106. Blakney M, Hertling D. The cervical spine. In: Hertling D, Kessler R, eds. *Management of Common Musculoskeletal Disorders.* Philadelphia: JB Lippincott; 1995;528–558.
107. Keith T. Postarthrotomy surgery. In: Kraus SL, ed. *Temporomandibular Disorders.* 2nd ed. New York: Churchill Livingstone; 1994;298–307.
108. Satko C, Blaustein D. Revascularization of rabbit temporomandibular joint after surgical intervention: histological and micro-angiographic study. *J Oral Maxillofac Surg.* 1986;44: 871–876.
109. Travell JG, Simons DG. *Myofascial Pain and Dysfunction: The Trigger Point Manual.* Baltimore: Williams & Wilkins; 1983.
110. Cyriax J. *Text of Orthopedic Medicine: Diagnosis of Soft Tissue Lesions,* vol 1. 8th ed. London: Bailliere Tindall; 1982.
111. Bradley JA. Acupuncture, acupressure, and trigger point therapy. In: Peat M, ed. *Current Physical Therapy.* Toronto: BC Decker; 1998:228–234.
112. Jones LH. *Strain and Counterstrain.* Colorado Springs, CO: The American Academy of Osteopathy; 1981.
113. Lay EM. The osteopathic management of temporomandibular joint dysfunction. In: Gelb H, ed. *Clinical Management of Head, Neck and TMJ Pain and Dysfunction: A Multi-Disciplinary Approach to Diagnosis and Treatment.* Philadelphia: WB Saunders; 1985:500–524.
114. Upledger JE. Temporomandibular joint. In: Upledger JE, ed. *Craniosacral Therapy II: Beyond the Dura.* Seattle: Eastland Press; 1987:151–208.
115. Upledger JE. *The Workbook of Craniosacral Therapy.* Palm Beach Gardens, FL: The Upledger Institute; 1983.
116. Manheim CJ, Lavett DK. *The Myofascial Release Manual.* Thorofare, NJ: Slack; 1989.
117. Cantu RL, Grodin AJ: *Myofascial Manipulations: Theory and Clinical Application.* Gaithersburg, MD: Aspen Publications; 1992.
118. Lund JP, Widmer CG. An evaluation of the use of surface electromyography in the diagnosis, documentation, and treatment of dental patients. *J Craniomand Disord.* 1989;3: 125–137.

119. Mohl ND, Lund JP, Widmer CG, McCall WD Jr. Devises for the diagnosis and treatment of temporomandibular disorders. Part II: electromyography and sonography. *J Prosthet Dent.* 1990;63:332–335.
120. Widmer CG. Evaluation of diagnostic tests for TMD. In: Kraus SL, ed. *Temporomandibular Disorders.* 2nd ed. New York: Churchill Livingstone; 1994:99–114.
121. Festa F. Joint distraction and condyle advancement with a modified functional distraction appliance. *J Craniomand Pract.* 1985;3:344–350.
122. Jankelson B, Pulley ML. *Electromyography in Clinical Dentistry.* Seattle: MyoTronic Research; 1984.
123. Moyers RE. Some physiologic considerations of centric and other jaw relations. *J Prosthet Dent.* 1956;6:183–194.
124. Moller E. Muscle hyperactivity leads to pain and dysfunction: position paper. In: Klineberg I, Sessle BJ, eds. *Oro-facial Pain and Neuromuscular Dysfunction.* Oxford, UK: Pergamon; 1985:69–92.
125. Moller E, Sheikoleslam A, Louis I. Response of elevator activity during mastication to treatment of functional disorders. *Scand J Dent Med.* 1984;92:64–83.
126. Sheikoleslam A, Moller E, Lous I. Postural and maximal activity in elevators of mandible before and after treatment of functional disorders. *Scand J Dent Res.* 1982;90:37–46.
127. Stohler C, Yamada Y, Ash MM. Antagonistic muscle stiffness and associated reflex behavior in the pain–dysfunction state. *Helv Odont Acta.* 1985;29:13–20.
128. Yemm R. A neurophysiological approach to the pathology and aetiology of temporomandibular dysfunction. *J Oral Rehabil.* 1985;12:343–353.
129. Cooper BC, Rabuzzi DD. Myofascial pain dysfunction syndrome: a clinical study of asymptomatic subjects. *Laryngoscope.* 1984;94:68–75.
130. Dolan EA, Keefe FJ. Muscle activity in myofascial pain-dysfunction patients: a structural clinical evaluation. *J Craniomand Disord.* 1988;2:101–105.
131. Lous I, Sheikoleslam A, Moller E. Postural activity in subjects with functional disorders of the chewing apatus. *Scand J Dent Res.* 1970;78:404–410.
132. Gordon TE. The influence of the herpes simplex virus on jaw muscle function. *J Craniomand Pract.* 1983;2:31–38.
133. Ramfjord SP. Bruxism, a clinical and electromyographic study. *J Am Dent Assoc.* 1961;62:21–44.
134. Naeije M, Hansson TL. Electromyographic screening of myogenous and arthrogenous TMJ dysfunction patients. *J Oral Rehabil.* 1986;13:433–441.
135. Van Boxtel A, Goudswaard P, Janssen K. Absolute and proportional resting EMG levels in muscle contraction and migraine headache patient. *Headache.* 1983;23: 223–228.
136. Frank AST. Masticatory muscle hyperactivity and temporomandibular joint dysfunction. *J Prosthet Dent.* 1965;15: 1122–1121.
137. Funakoshi M, Fujita N, Takehana S. Relations between occlusal interference and jaw muscle activities in response to changes in head position. *J Dent Res.* 1976;55:684–689.
138. Michler L, Moller E, Bakke M, et al. On-line analysis of natural activity in muscles of mastication. *J Craniomand Disord.* 1988;2:65–82.
139. Mongini F. *The Stomatognathic System.* Chicago: Quintessence Publishing; 1984.
140. Gelb M. Diagnostic tests. In: Kaplan AS, Assael LA, eds. *Temporomandibular Disorders: Diagnosis and Treatment.* Philadelphia: WB Saunders; 1991:371–385.
141. Rivera-Morales WC, McCall WD. Reliability of a portable electromyographic unit to measure bruxism. *J Prosthet Dent.* 1995;73:184–189.
142. Kardachi BJ, Clarke NG. The use of biofeedback to control bruxism. *J Periodontol.* 1977;48:639–642.
143. Pierce CJ, Gale EN. A comparison of different treatments for nocturnal bruxism. *J Dent Res.* 1988;67:597–601.
144. Rugh JD, Johnston RW. Temporal analysis of nocturnal bruxism during EMG feedback. *J Periodontol.* 1981;52:233–235.
145. Rugh JD, Solberg WK. Electromyographic studies of bruxist behavior before and during treatment. *J Calif Dent Assoc.* 1975;3:56–59.
146. Solberg WK, Rugh JD. The use of biofeedback to control bruxism. *J South Calif Dent Assoc.* 1972;40:852–853.

RECOMMENDED READINGS

Bell WE. *Temporomandibular Disorders, Classification, Diagnosis, Management.* 3rd ed. Chicago: Year Book Medical Publishers; 1990.

Bush FM, Dolwick MF. *The Temporomandibular Joint and Related Orofacial Disorders.* Philadelphia: JB Lippincott; 1994.

Cohen S. A cephalometric study of rest position in edentulous persons: influence of variations in head position. *J Prosthet Dent.* 1957;7:467–472.

Kaplan AS, Assel LA. *Temporomandibular Disorders: Diagnosis and Treatment.* Philadelphia: WB Saunders; 1991.

Kraus SL ed. *Temporomandibular Disorders.* New York; Churchill Livingstone; 1994.

Okeson JP. *Bell's Orofacial Pains.* 5th ed. Chicago: Quintessence Publishing; 1995.

Rocabado M, Iglarsh ZA. *Musculoskeletal Approach to Maxillofacial Pain.* Philadelphia: JB Lippincott; 1991.

Vitti M, Basmajian JV. Integrated actions of masticatory muscles: simultaneous intramuscular electrodes. *Anat Rec.* 1977;187: 173–189.

CHAPTER 24

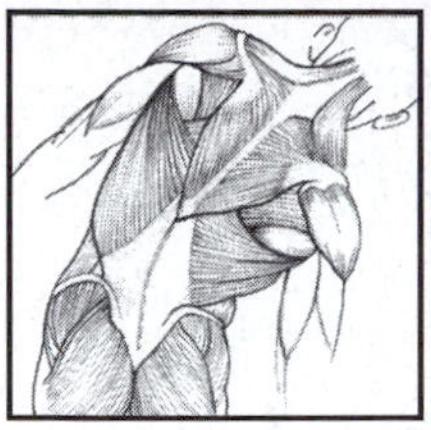

The Cervical Spine

Carol N. Kennedy

Therapeutic exercise interventions are crucial in the rehabilitation of any cervical spine disorder, particularly those of a recurrent or chronic nature. However, exercise programs designed for the treatment of the cervical spine cannot stand alone. Because of the close relationship between the neck, thoracic spine, shoulder girdle, and temporomandibular joint (TMJ), a complete and successful exercise program must also deal with impairments found in these regions. This chapter reviews cervical spine anatomy and kinesiology and provides guidelines for the examination and evaluation. Exercise treatment interventions are described for common physiologic impairments and common diagnoses affecting the cervical spine.

REVIEW OF ANATOMY AND KINESIOLOGY

The cervical spine is composed of two functional units: the craniovertebral (CV) complex and the middle to lower cervical spine. The two units are different in structure and biomechanics, but they act together to enable the large range of motion (ROM) available in the cervical spine. They also support and protect the vital structures found in this region. One important function of the cervical spine is to place the head in space for the vital functions of sight, hearing, and feeding. The coordinated movements permitted by the involved articular structures, ligaments, and muscles allow the cervical spine to perform this function.

Craniovertebral Complex

The CV complex includes the bony structures of the occiput, atlas, and axis and therefore includes the atlanto-occipital (AO) and atlantoaxial (AA) joints. Important ligaments of the CV complex include the alar ligaments, the transverse ligament, the tectorial membrane, the anterior and posterior AO membranes, and the posterior AA ligament. The biomechanics of the CV complex are governed by the articular surfaces, the complex ligamentous system, and to a large degree, the intricate muscular system.

ATLANTO-OCCIPITAL JOINT

The AO joint is formed by the convex occipital condyles articulating with the reciprocally concave superior atlantal facets of the lateral masses (Fig. 24-1). The long axis of the articulation runs anteromedially. The occipital condyles face inferolaterally to meet the laterally banked atlantal facet. The joint is inherently stable. The joint capsule is thickened anteriorly and laterally, but it is thin and deficient medially, where it may communicate with the median AA joint. Mercer and Bogduk[1] describe two types of intra-articular inclusions at this joint: intra-articular fat pads and capsular rims. These structures contribute to joint stability and, if injured, may be a cause of posttraumatic joint pain.

The AO joint is classified as a modified ovoid, bicondylar joint, with two degrees of freedom of motion: flexion-extension and combined side flexion–rotation. Flexion and extension should be a pure and relatively free motion at the AO joint (Fig. 24-2). Its ROM is 20–30 degrees, and the range of extension is greater than that of flexion. The ROM occurs about a transverse axis located approximately through the external auditory meatus. Because of the convex occipital condyles, the occiput glides posteriorly during flexion and anteriorly during extension. If one of the two joints is not free to move, the chin deviates. During extension, it deviates toward the side of restriction, and in flexion, it deviates away from the restricted side. High tension is developed in the anterior capsule during extension and to a much lesser degree in the posterior capsule during flexion.[2] Side flexion occurs about a sagittal axis that runs approximately through the nose. The occiput glides to the contralateral side, and because of the joint architecture, side flexion is coupled with a contralateral conjunct rotation (see Fig. 24-2*C and D*). The ROM is 5–10 degrees of side flexion and 3–5 degrees of rotation in one direction.

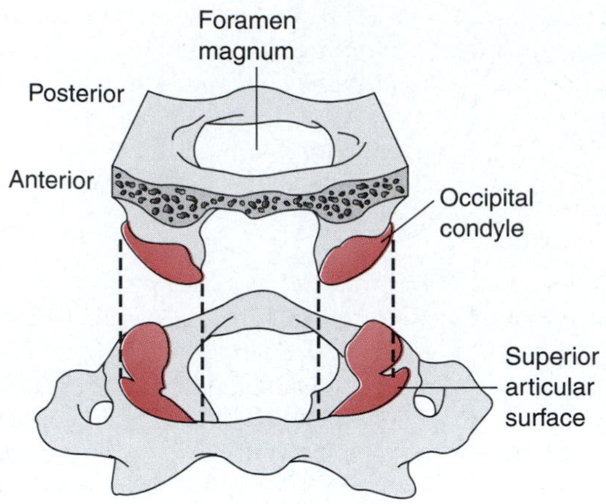

FIGURE 24-1 Atlanto-occipital joint architecture. White A, Panjabi M. *Clinical Biomechanics of the Spine*. Philadelphia: JB Lippincott; 1990:284.

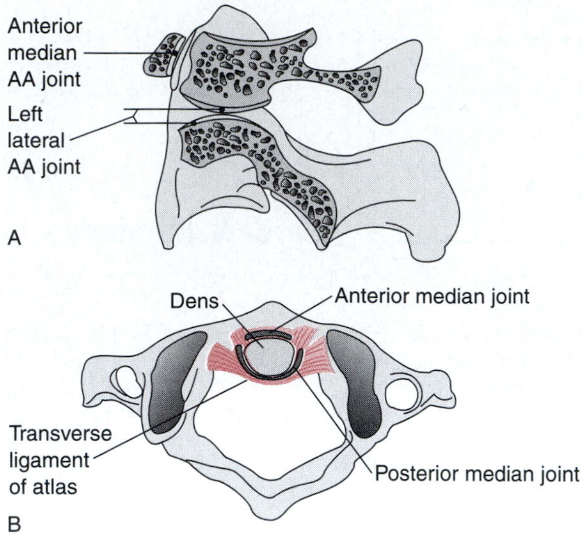

FIGURE 24-3 Atlantoaxial joint architecture. ***(A)*** Left lateral joint. ***(B)*** Median joint complex.

ATLANTOAXIAL JOINT

The AA joint is composed of two lateral joints and a median joint complex (Fig. 24-3). The lateral joints are the articulations between the inferior facets of the atlas and the superior facets of the lateral masses of the axis. With the articular cartilage intact, the surface is biconvex in the anteroposterior plane.[3] This architecture produces the unique biomechanics of this joint. In the transverse plane, the surfaces are more flattened, sloping inferolaterally. Congruency of the joint surfaces is improved by the presence of fibroadipose meniscoids, which extend well into the joint cavity.[1] These structures may be implicated in cases of acute restriction of joint mobility. Bruising of the AA joint meniscus was a common finding in Schonstrom and colleagues' study[4] of post-traumatic cervical spines. Although described as thin and loose, the AA capsule is a major restraint to rotation and assists in restricting extension more than flexion.[2,5,6]

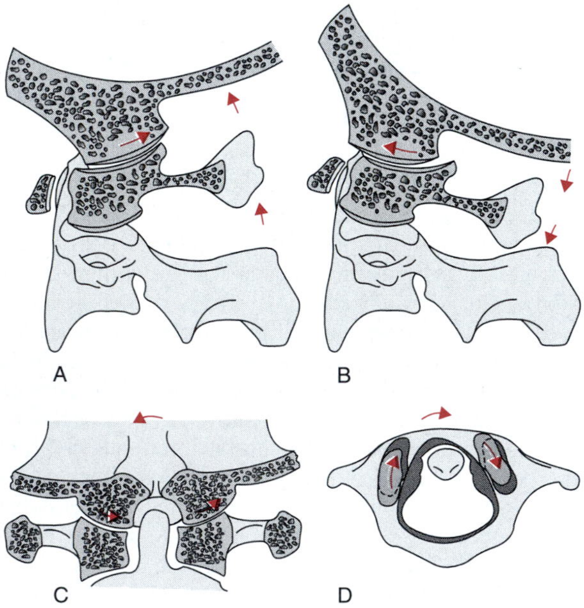

FIGURE 24-2 Atlanto-occipital joint movement. ***(A)*** Flexion. ***(B)*** Extension. ***(C)*** Left side flexion. ***(D)*** Conjunct right rotation.

The median joint complex is the articulation between the dens of the axis and the osseoligamentous ring of the atlas. There is an anterior portion between the arch of the atlas and the dens. The posterior portion is formed by the dens articulating with the cartilage-covered anterior surface of the transverse ligament. Both portions of the joint have a synovial membrane and capsule, which often communicate with the AO joint.

The AA joint is difficult to classify anatomically because it is a multijoint complex. It has two degrees of motion: flexion-extension and combined rotation–side flexion. Flexion and extension (Fig. 24-4*A* and *B*) occurs about a transverse axis through the osseoligamentous ring. It has 10 to 15 degrees of motion. At the lateral biconvex joints, the flexion-extension movement is primarily a rocking motion. With an intact transverse ligament, there should be minimal anteroposterior glide, with posterior translation occurring during flexion and anterior translation during extension.[7] At the median joint, there is a superior glide of the arch of the atlas on the dens during extension and an inferior glide during flexion.

Rotation (Fig. 24-4*C*) is the primary motion of the AA joint, and it contributes 50% to 70% of the rotational range of the entire cervical spine. The motion occurs about a vertical axis through the dens and has been reported as 35–45 degrees in one direction. At the lateral joints, the ipsilateral atlantal facet glides posteriorly, and the contralateral facet glides anteriorly. The motion at the median joint is primarily a spin. Because of the biconvex lateral joint surfaces, vertical translation is associated with rotation, which may decrease tension in the articular capsule of the lateral joint and allow greater ROM.

Studies have shown side flexion at this joint of up to 11 degrees (Fig. 24-4*D*). Several studies[8–10] have shown the coupling of rotation and side flexion to be contralateral at this joint.

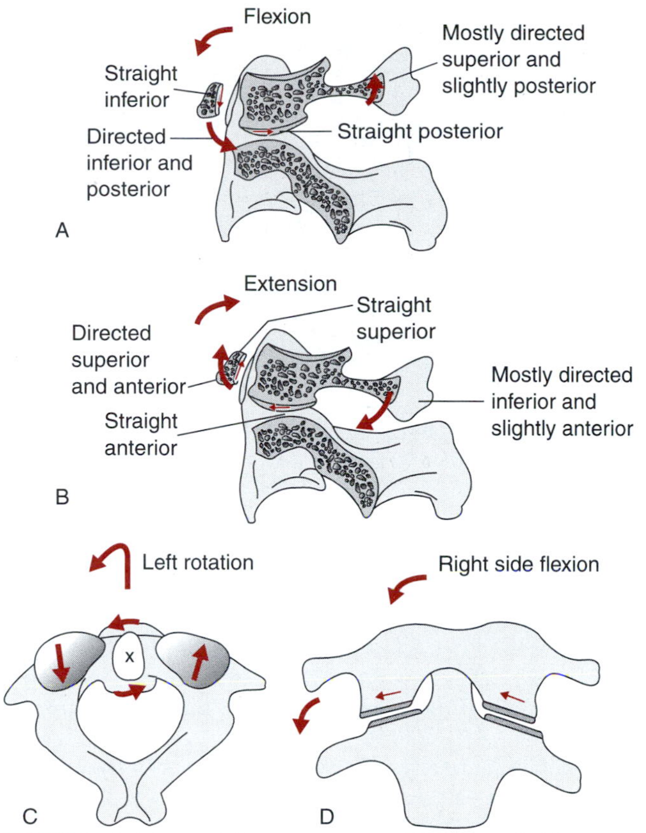

FIGURE 24-4 Atlantoaxial joint movement. ***(A)*** Flexion. ***(B)*** Extension. ***(C)*** Left rotation (x marks the axis of rotation). ***(D)*** Right side flexion.

LIGAMENTS OF THE CRANIOVERTEBRAL COMPLEX

The ligaments of the CV complex are illustrated in Figure 24-5. The transverse ligament is a component of the cruciform ligament. With an intact transverse ligament, the space between the dens and the anterior arch of the atlas, the atlantodental interval (ADI), is a maximum of 3 mm in adults and 4 mm in children. This structure is the major contributor to posteroanterior plane stability at the AA joint level. The most common causes of laxity of this ligament are rheumatoid arthritis, ankylosing spondylitis, Down syndrome, hyperemic softening (ie, Grisel's syndrome), and trauma.

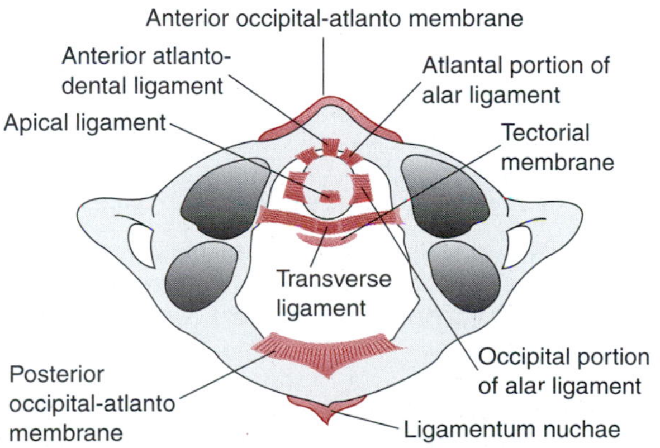

FIGURE 24-5 Craniovertebral ligamentous system, coronal view.

The alar ligament consists of three components: occipital, atlantal, and anterior atlantodental.[11] The occipital portion of the alar ligament limits contralateral more than ipsilateral rotation,[12] contralateral side flexion, and flexion at the AO and AA joints.[13] The atlantal portion limits ipsilateral side flexion.[14] Along with the articular capsule, the alar ligament is the primary restraint for rotary stability of the CV complex as a unit.

The tectorial membrane is a continuation of the posterior longitudinal ligament. According to Werne,[15] the membrane contributes to vertical stability of the CV complex. When the membrane is transected, vertical translation increases by 2.7 mm. When injured, this structure can cause pain and possibly laxity, as determined by manual traction tests. Studies have found this structure to be more important in stabilizing for flexion, rather than extension, at the AO and AA joints.[13,16]

The anterior AO membrane is composed of dense tissue and binds the foramen magnum with the anterior arch of the atlas. It blends with the AO joint capsules laterally. The posterior AO membrane attaches the occiput to the posterior arch of the atlas. It is closely associated with the vertebral artery traveling in an osseoligamentous tunnel as it wraps around the posterior AO joint. Its lateral edge is occasionally ossified, creating a bony foramen. This is a potential site of impingement. The posterior AA ligament, often referred to as the first ligamentum flavum, lacks the elastic fibers common to that ligament. These structures may be involved in vertical and rotary stability of the CV complex.[6,16]

Laxity of the CV ligamentous system results in increased translation, rotation, or distraction of the complex. Signs and symptoms are those related to pressure on the cervical cord, vertebral artery insufficiency, or overreactivity of the articular structures themselves.

Midcervical Spine

The midcervical spine consists of the region from the C2-C3 intervertebral segment to the C7-T1 segment. The axis (C2) is also included in the CV region and is the transitional bone between the two units. Each mobile intervertebral segment of the midcervical spine includes several joints, including the paired zygapophyseal and uncovertebral (UV) joints and the interbody (disk) joint. Each segment of the midcervical spine has two degrees of motion: flexion-extension and combined rotation–side flexion. Important ligaments in this area include the anterior and posterior longitudinal ligaments (ALL and PLL), the ligamentum flavum, the interspinous ligaments, and the ligamentum nuchae.

ZYGAPOPHYSEAL JOINT

The zygapophyseal joints are composed of the inferior articular facet of the cranial vertebra and articulate with the superior facet of the caudal vertebra. The surfaces are planar. The joint orientation gradually changes from approximately 60 degrees from the vertical in the upper levels to 30 degrees from the vertical in the lower spine, affecting the relative amounts of angular and translatory motion during flexion and extension. The articular capsule is relatively lax, allowing free mobility, but it is also very strong, controlling motion in the end range. It is reinforced by the ligamentum flavum and slips of the deep cervical muscles. Fibroadipose meniscoids are commonly found in the cervical zygapophyseal joints.[1] Injury to this structure resulting in restricted articular glide can cause acute torticollis (ie, wry neck).

UNCOVERTEBRAL JOINTS

The UV joints are nonsynovial clefts between the uncinate processes of adjacent vertebral bodies (Fig. 24-6*A*). They are located at the posterolateral corners of the superior aspect of the C3 to C7 vertebrae. The uncinate process is present by the end of the first decade, and the joint is fully developed by the end of the second decade. The UV joints limit the lateral translation component of side flexion, limit posterior translation, and guide the motion of flexion and extension in the cervical spine. More details about the development and function of these joints are provided in other sources.[17–19]

INTERBODY JOINT

The vertebral body–disk–vertebral body joint, or interbody joint, is classified as a synchondrosis. The nucleus of the cervical disk is initially very small and exists as a gel for only the first decade. The UV joint concentrates translational forces onto the posterior disk, resulting in medial extensions of the UV joint cleft, and by the end of the first decade, horizontal fissuring of the disk is evident. The fissuring often extends through the posterior disk and, by late adult life, may completely divide the posterior two thirds of the disk, leaving the anterior disk intact.[20] Transverse clefting of the posterior disk increases the amount of rotation and side flexion range available in the cervical spine. It may also explain the more common occurrence of lateral translation hypermobility found in the cervical region (Fig. 24-6*B*).

MOTION AT THE MIDCERVICAL SPINE

Movement of the midcervical spine involves the coordinated motion of each of the three joints described previously. It is therefore more functional to discuss the movement as a whole unit, instead of breaking down the motion for each joint. Each intervertebral segment of the midcervical spine has two degrees of freedom of motion: flexion–extension and combined rotation–side flexion.

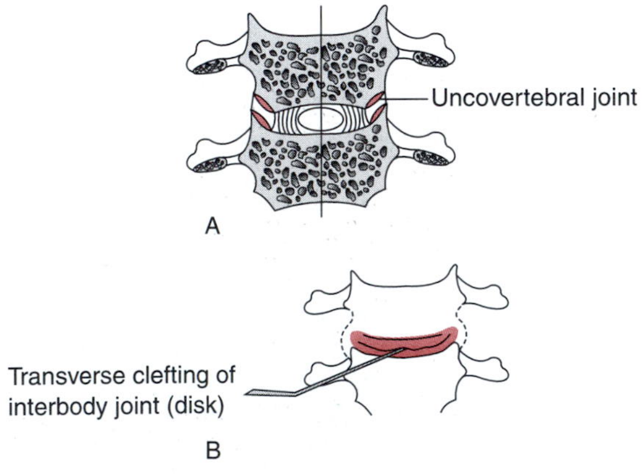

FIGURE 24-6 ***(A)*** Uncovertebral joint. ***(B)*** Transverse clefting of the interbody joint (disk).

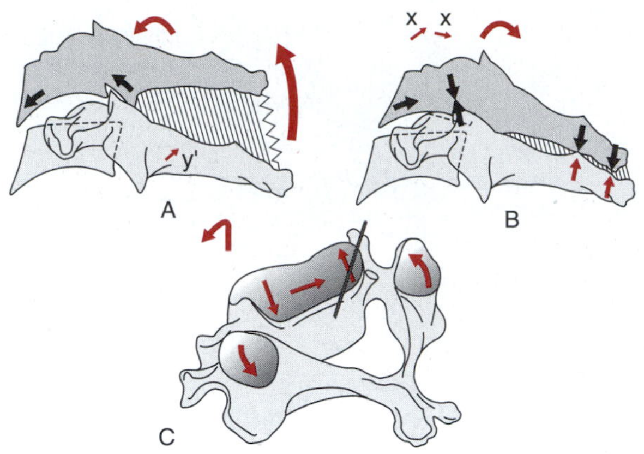

FIGURE 24-7 ***(A)*** Midcervical flexion. ***(B)*** Midcervical extension. ***(C)*** Midcervical rotation left and side flexion.

Flexion and extension (Fig. 24-7*A*) is a sagittal-plane motion about a transverse axis. This axis is located in the caudal vertebra of the segment, moving from a posteroinferior position at the C2-C3 level to a midsuperior position at the C6-C7 level.[21] There is more ROM at the middle vertebral segments than at the upper levels or at the cervicothoracic junction.

Osteokinematically, the two components of the motion of flexion and extension are rotation, or angular motion, and translation. There is a larger amount of rotation in the lower segments, but relative to ROM, translation is greater in the upper levels. Flexion consists of an anterior rotation of the vertebra with anterior translation. This movement pattern can also be found in hypermobile vertebral segments.[14] Arthrokinematically, there is an anterior superior glide at the zygapophyseal joint and an anterior glide at the UV joint during flexion. In extension, the zygapophyseal joint glides posteriorly and inferiorly, and the UV joint glides posteriorly. A paradoxical motion sometimes occurs in patients with hyperlordosed, forward head posture (FHP); the posterior vertebral rotation of extension is associated with anterior, rather than posterior, translation.

Rotation and side flexion should be considered as a single, combined motion about an oblique axis. This axis was originally described by Penning[22] as running perpendicular to the plane of the zygapophyseal joint in the midsagittal plane. Because of the orientation of the zygapophyseal joint surfaces, rotation and side flexion are always coupled ipsilaterally. Arthrokinematically, the ipsilateral zygapophyseal joint glides posteriorly, inferiorly, and medially. The ipsilateral UV joint also glides in a similar direction. The contralateral zygapophyseal joint and UV joint glides anterior, superior, and laterally (Fig. 24-7*B*). Panjabi[23] divided the full ROM of an intervertebral segment into two parts:

Neutral zone: portion of the ROM that produces little resistance from the articular structures

Elastic zone: portion of the ROM from the end of the neutral zone up to the physiologic limit of motion

The entire cervical spine, particularly the CV region, has a large neutral zone of motion. Because of the lack of tension in the capsular or ligamentous system in this part of the range, there is less passive control of this motion compared with other regions of the spine. The muscular system must be recruited to actively control the motion in the neutral zone. If there is damage to the ligamentous system, resulting in an increased neutral zone, muscular control becomes even more important (Fig. 24-8).

LIGAMENTS OF THE MIDCERVICAL SPINE

The ALL and PLL bind the anterior and posterior aspects of each vertebral body. In the cervical region, the PLL is broad and has uniform width throughout. It is continuous with the tectorial membrane. The ligamentum flavum connects adjacent laminae and reinforces the zygapophyseal joint capsule laterally. The yellow elastic tissue in the ligament helps prevent buckling of the ligament into the spinal canal on extension. The interspinous ligaments are only slightly developed in the neck, the supraspinous ligament is absent, and the intertransverse ligament is replaced by the intertransversarium muscle.[24] The ligamentum nuchae, although not well developed in humans, decreases the cervical lordosis when tightened during CV flexion.[25] It may also have a proprioceptive function for the cervical erector spinae muscles, which are closely related to it.[14]

Vascular System

An important aspect of cervical spine anatomy is the vertebral artery. It provides vital blood supply and is close to various structures of the cervical spine that could impede its flow.

The vertebral artery supplies the cervical spinal cord, the cervical spinal column, and the posterior cranial fossa. Intrinsic factors affecting arterial flow are atherosclerosis and thrombus formation. Flow in the artery can be compromised by various anomalies of the artery itself or the muscles through which it passes. Swelling, degenerative thickening, and osteophytic formation of the UV and zygapophyseal joints can encroach on the artery. These processes should be considered in the patient with a history of degenerative disk disease, cervical osteoarthritis, or trauma. Excessive ROM at the CV joints, as in cases of hypermobility, can kink the artery during rotation. Decreased arterial flow may occur during rotation of the neck, and the addition of extension and traction may further reduce flow. Some of the signs and symptoms of vertebral artery insufficiency include dizziness, drop attacks, diplopia, dysarthria, dysphasia, and nystagmus. Vertebral artery tests should be performed for each patient before using these motions during treatment.

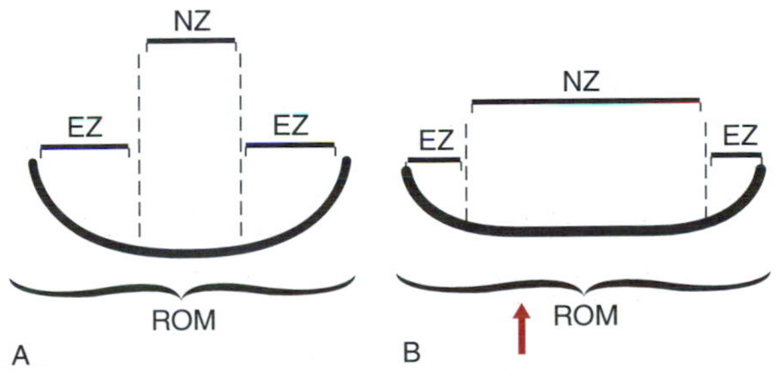

FIGURE 24-8 Neutral zone. ***(A)*** Normal. ***(B)*** Hypermobile. NZ, neutral zone; EZ, elastic zone; ROM, range of motion.

Nerves

The cervical nerve roots exit from the intervertebral foramen above the vertebra. The C1 nerve root exits through the osseoligamentous tunnel formed by the posterior AO membrane, which puts it at risk for impingement. As the cervical nerve roots exit the intervertebral foramen, they are surrounded by several structures:

- Zygapophyseal joint
- UV joint
- Cervical disk
- Bony pedicle

Degenerative changes affecting any of these structures may diminish the foramen size and alter nerve function. Cervical roots 4 through 6 have strong attachments to the transverse processes. The dural sleeve at each level forms a plug that protects the nerve and cord from traction forces. Tension in the neuromeningeal structures may produce a pull on the cervical vertebrae.

Muscles

The musculature of the cervical spine is complex, and anatomy texts[24] should be consulted for descriptions of origins and insertions. Table 24-1 lists the muscles of the CV complex and their actions (Fig. 24-9). These muscles enable the specific, fine movements of this region that are required for sight, hearing, and balance. They are richly supplied with mechanoreceptors, which are integral to the muscles' strong proprioceptive function and implicated in the production of dizziness in patients with dysfunctions of this region. The upper cervical flexors are crucial in obtaining and maintaining optimal postural balance of the head on the neck. Several long muscles, such as the sternocleidomastoid, link the head directly to the trunk.

The muscles of the midcervical spine, arranged as elsewhere in the spine, consist of slips traversing a various number of segments. Table 24-2 lists these muscle groups and their actions. In individuals with FHP, the deep anterior cervical musculature lengthens and becomes functionally weak, but the posterior group tends to shorten.

Table 24-1. CRANIOVERTEBRAL REGION MUSCULATURE

MUSCLE	ACTION
Rectus capitis posterior minor	Atlanto-occipital joint extension
Rectus capitis posterior major	Craniovertebral complex extension and ipsilateral rotation
Superior oblique	Atlanto-occipital joint ipsilateral side flexion and extension
Inferior oblique	Atlantoaxial joint ipsilateral rotation
Rectus capitis lateralis	Atlanto-occipital joint ipsilateral side flexion
Rectus capitis anterior	Atlanto-occipital joint flexion

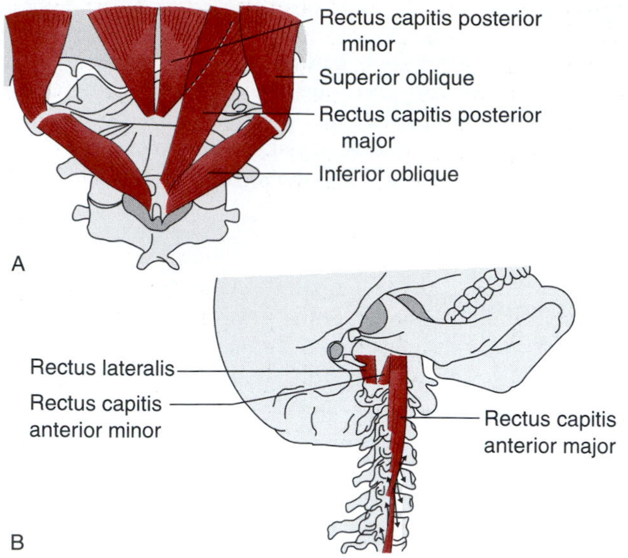

FIGURE 24-9 Craniovertebral muscles. ***(A)*** Posterial suboccipitals muscles. ***(B)*** Short upper cervical flexor muscles.

SCALENE MUSCLE GROUP

Of particular clinical interest is the scalene muscle group (Fig. 24-10). These muscles have a tendency to become dominant, often being overused during a poor pattern of apical respiration. Because of the angle of pull, increased muscle activity creates compressive and lateral forces on the intervertebral segment. Because of its insertion onto the first and second ribs, the increased activity elevates these ribs. This elevation decreases the space available in the thoracic outlet, which can eventually lead to the symptoms of thoracic outlet syndrome. Adaptive shortening of this group also can impinge on the cervical nerve roots as they travel between the scalenes.

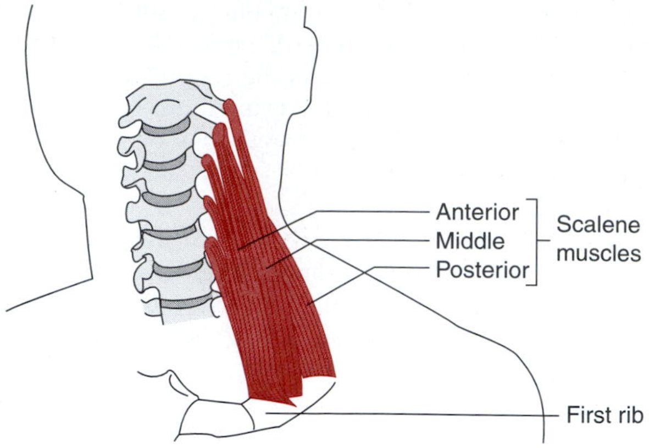

FIGURE 24-10 Scalene muscles.

STERNOCLEIDOMASTOID MUSCLE

With FHP, the sternocleidomastoid muscle tends to shorten, increasing the compression load on the cervical spine. It is a prime mover of head on trunk flexion, but the movement pattern it produces causes substantial amounts of anterior translation. When flexing the head forward on the trunk, it

Table 24-2. MIDCERVICAL MUSCULATURE

	ACTION			
MUSCLE	Flexion	Extension	Rotation	Ipsilateral Side Flexion
Longus colli	X	NA	Ipsilateral	MC
Longus capitis	X	NA	Ipsilateral—MC	NA
Scalenes (elevates 1st or 2nd rib)				
Anterior	X	NA	Contralateral—MC	X
Medius	MC	NA	Contralateral—MC	X
Posterior	MC	NA	Contralateral	X
Sternocleidomastoid	X	X	Contralateral	X
Trapezius upper fibers	NA	X	Contralateral	X
Levator scapula	NA	X	Ipsilateral	X
Splenius, capitis and cervicis	NA	X	Ipsilateral	X
Spinalis, capitis and cervicis (inconsistent—blends with semispinalis)	NA	X	NA	NA
Semispinalis, capitis and cervicis	NA	X	Contralateral	NA
Longissimus, capitis and cervicis	NA	X	Ipsilateral	X
Iliocostalis cervicis	NA	X	NA	X
Interspinalis (most distinct in cervical spine)	NA	X	NA	NA
Multifidus	NA	X	Contralateral	NA
Rotatores (inconsistent)	NA	X	Ipsilateral	UI
Intertransversarii (most distinct in cervical spine)	NA	NA	Contralateral	NA

NA, no action; MC, minimal contribution; X, active.

may increase cervical lordosis. A study by deSousa[24] demonstrated sternocleidomastoid involvement in cervical extension and flexion.

LEVATOR SCAPULA AND UPPER FIBERS OF TRAPEZIUS

Several muscles can be classified as cervical or shoulder girdle muscles. The levator scapula and the upper fibers of the trapezius have broad insertions into the cervical spine that originate at the scapula. Alterations in the shoulder girdle resting position and function change the length of these muscles, affecting the cervical spine as well. For example, a depressed scapular resting position lengthens the upper fibers of the trapezius muscle and produces a lateral translation and compression force on the cervical spine. Continuous translational forces on the cervical spine can lead to hypermobility in various planes, depending on the angle of pull.

SUPRAHYOID AND INFRAHYOID MUSCLE GROUPS

The suprahyoid and infrahyoid muscle groups are primarily involved with the functions of swallowing, speech, mastication, and the TMJ. These muscle groups are discussed in Chapter 23. Dysfunction of these muscle groups can have a profound effect on cervical posture, and they should be assessed in persons with chronic neck conditions.

EXAMINATION AND EVALUATION

Examination of the cervical spine should include evaluation of the entire spine, particularly the thoracic region, the TMJ, and shoulder girdle complex. These regions directly influence the posture and mobility of the cervical spine. The clinician must have the knowledge and skills necessary to perform all the appropriate tests to diagnose impairments and functional losses of the cervical spine.

History and Clearing Tests

In addition to the questions included in any musculoskeletal subjective examination, some questions specifically address the cervical region. These questions are detailed in Grieve's *Common Vertebral Joint Problems.*[26] Functional questionnaires provide an excellent baseline determination and can be used to monitor the progress of treatment over time. For example, the Neck Disability Index was developed by Vernon and Mior[27] to provide a reliable and valid measure of cervical spine disability.

Shoulder girdle tests should be performed on the patient if indicated by the subjective history and outcomes of alignment tests.

Posture and Movement Examination

Standing alignment should be assessed in all three planes. The examination includes the spinal curves (ie, CV region, midcervical region, and cervicothoracic junction), pelvic alignment, and the scapular resting position.

Sitting alignment should be evaluated in all three planes. The examiner should look for changes that occur from standing to sitting. Supine alignment also is evaluated. The examiner should assess the resting position of each vertebral segment through palpation.

Various motion tests are used to assess the patient's flexibility and ability to move in certain ways:

- Movement assessments
  - Active ROM
  - Combined movements
- Assessment of cervical spine passive mobility
  - Passive intervertebral movements
  - Passive accessory vertebral movements
- Assessment of myofascial extensibility
  - Muscle lengths
- Assessment of neuromeningeal extensibility
  - Upper limb tension test
    - Median nerve bias
    - Radial nerve bias
    - Ulnar nerve bias

Muscle Performance, Neurologic, and Special Tests

Assess the patient's cervical musculature by performing manual muscle tests for strength and for endurance. Neurologic tests of sensation, motor activity (ie, key muscle strength), and reflexes are performed to detect any nerve root conduction signs in the cervical region.

Stability tests, vertebral artery tests, and the foraminal compression test are performed to exclude pathology of the cervical spine.

THERAPEUTIC EXERCISE INTERVENTIONS FOR COMMON PHYSIOLOGIC IMPAIRMENTS

Any comprehensive therapeutic exercise program for the cervical spine must address various physiologic impairments. This section describes exercise interventions for impairments of muscle performance (including endurance), mobility (ie, hypomobility and hypermobility), and posture. Appropriate modifications may be necessary for some patients, depending on their signs and symptoms.

Impaired Muscle Performance

ETIOLOGY

Janda has suggested that certain muscles in the cervical spine tend to weaken; the most common of these are the deep, anterior cervical flexors. Studies of patients with cervicogenic headache symptoms have found decreased maximal isometric strength and isometric endurance of the short upper cervical flexor muscles compared with those of normal subjects.[28] A group of patients with mechanical neck pain also showed significant weakness of the neck flexor muscles compared with controls.[29] A study of patients with osteoarthritis showed more pronounced fatigue curves for anterior and posterior neck muscles than for the muscles of normal subjects.[30]

Many articles in the literature describe cervical strengthening protocols, mainly for the prevention of athletic injuries.[31–34] However, few controlled studies have measured the effectiveness of cervical strengthening programs in obtaining strength gains for injury prevention or as a component of treatment of the painful neck. A program that may be safe for training the healthy neck of an athlete may have little application to the injured neck and particularly to the hypermobile cervical spine. In a study of 90 patients with cervical pain, the subjects participated in an 8-week strengthening program that involved concentric-eccentric and variable resistance cervical extension exercises. As a group, the patients gained strength and range, and they experienced a reduction in pain.[35]

Exercise dosage should be determined on an individual basis, depending on the variables of strength, endurance, and irritability. A better response seems to occur when loads are initially very low (less than the weight of the head) and progressed slowly. An exercise is considered too difficult or stopped when it produces pain, muscle tremors occur because of fatigue, or the exercise cannot be executed correctly. The endurance function of many of these cervical postural muscles should be emphasized by encouraging longer, sustained contractions.

TREATMENT

Short, Deep Cervical Flexors

The most common muscles to become weak with neck dysfunction are the deep, single segment cervical flexors, particularly of the upper cervical spine. The primary exercise to recruit these muscles is the head nod exercise of CV flexion, continuing segmentally down into midcervical flexion. It is important to control the tendency to excessively translate anteriorly during this exercise. If done initially while sitting, the exercise is gravity assisted. It can be progressed from supported sitting against the wall to unsupported sitting to ball sitting. The effects of the assistance of gravity can be decreased by performing the exercise supine on an incline board. The board is progressively tilted backward.

When performed while the patient is supine, the muscles work against the resistance of gravity, making the exercise more difficult. The head is supported on a pillow, and at first, the head nod is performed with no lifting of the head off the pillow. To progress, a small rolled towel can be placed under the hollow of the midcervical spine to support the normal cervical lordosis; the head nod uses the towel roll as a fulcrum, and the back of the head may lift just off the pillow during the motion (Fig. 24-11). The neck should not lose contact with the towel, because this is a sign of excessive anterior translation and recruitment of other cervical flexors (eg, sternocleidomastoid) to substitute for the weaker deep neck flexors. The ROM allowed depends on the muscle strength and the ability to continue the head nod without excessive anterior translation. A head nod into a flexion quadrant (eg, flexion, side flexion, rotation to the same side) emphasizes contraction of the deep flexors more unilaterally and can be used in cases of asymmetric weakness.

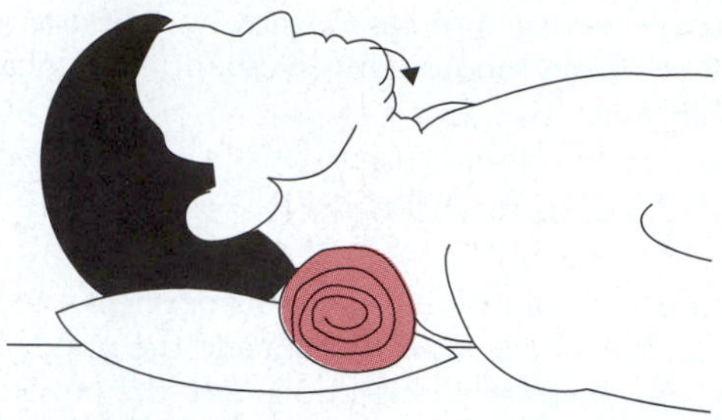

FIGURE 24-11 Short flexor muscle strengthening over a towel roll.

The exercise is also more difficult when done in a prone position over an exercise ball than done while sitting. In this position, gravity draws the head forward into a position of upper cervical extension, which is countered by the head nod motion into upper cervical flexion. The four-point kneeling (FPK) position can be used to simulate the prone ball position at home (Fig. 24-12). These two exercises recruit the upper cervical flexors only; gravity is assisting the lower cervical flexors in this position. Using the supine position on the ball, with the head unsupported, the exercise is difficult to accomplish properly and must be supervised with care.

In many of the previous positions, autoresistance can be applied to the head nod motion to increase the load on the muscle. Resistance must be applied at such an angle to appropriately resist the head nod motion and not encourage a head forward movement. The proper movement can be encouraged by resistance under the chin rather than at the forehead.

Cervical Extensor Muscles

Few studies have investigated the effects of cervical spine dysfunction on the extensor muscle group. A study of patients with cervical osteoarthritis did find more pronounced fatigue curves for the cervical flexors and extensors compared those of controls.[30] Studies on the lumbar spine have shown a tendency for the multifidus to atrophy in cases of spinal dysfunction, and a similar process may occur in the cervical spine.[36]

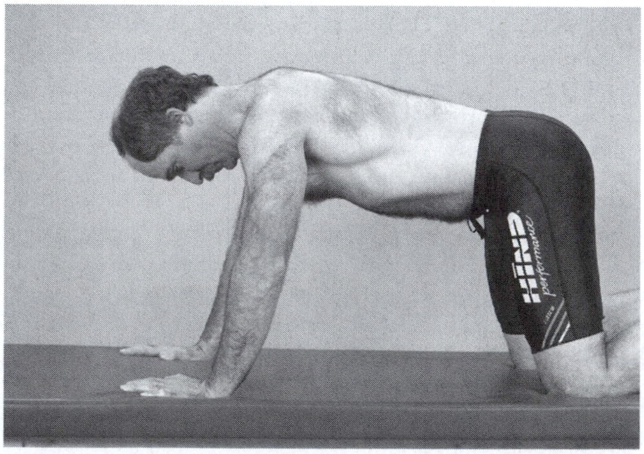

FIGURE 24-12 The four-point kneeling position can be used at home to simulate the prone ball position.

The use of electrical muscle stimulation is effective in the initial stages of retraining, especially when the patient has a high level of pain that precludes resisted exercise. With the patient lying supine with the head supported, small electrodes are placed over the extensor muscles bilaterally at the vertebral level with poor segmental recruitment.

The patient can be taught to apply autoresistance to the contraction of a specific muscle determined to be weak on assessment. For example, a weak superior oblique muscle can be retrained by applying autoresistance to AO joint side flexion into extension on the same side (Fig. 24-13). Contraction of the multifidus at the C4-C5 level can be obtained by pressure applied to the C4 lamina as the patient attempts side flexion and rotation to the same side into extension.

Multisegmental extension exercises for more generalized weakness can be performed in a supine position with pillow support. The cervical lordosis should be further supported with a foam roll or rolled towel. While the patient squeezes the roll by the extension movement, the therapist must ensure that the motion remains angular and no shearing occurs. The exercise can be made more specific in cases of asymmetric weakness by working into the extension quadrant (ie, combined extension, side flexion, and rotation to the same side). The roll is then squeezed between the head and the shoulder on the affected side (Fig. 24-14).

In the prone position over an exercise ball, midcervical extension exercises can be performed against gravity. The position tends to encourage the poking-chin posture of CV extension. The patient should be taught to control the upper cervical flexion while working the middle and lower cervical spine into extension. The exercise can be done into the quadrant position to target the muscles unilaterally. The same exercise can be performed in the FPK position at home.

With any exercise into cervical extension or an extension quadrant, it is important to consider the following effects:

- Effects on the vertebral artery
- Compression load on the zygapophyseal joints
- Foraminal compression and its effect on the neurologic structures
- Risk of encouraging the cervical lordosis of the FHP

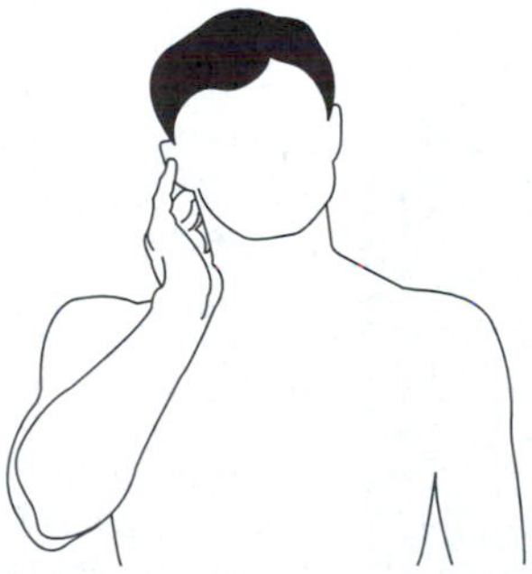

FIGURE 24-13 Retraining a weak right superior oblique muscle by applying autoresistance to atlanto-occipital joint side flexion into extension on the same side.

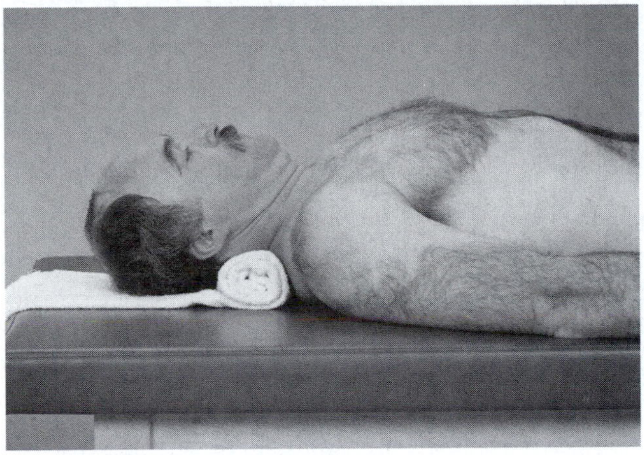

FIGURE 24-14 Concentric muscle contraction into the extension quadrant over a foam roll or rolled towel.

Rotation and Side Flexion Component

By exercising into a quadrant position, the muscles that are primarily side flexors and rotators are also recruited. A foam wedge can be used to apply resistance to combined flexion, side flexion, and rotation of the cervical spine. In supine lying, the head is positioned just to one side of the peak of the wedge. As the patient rotates the head down the wedge slope, the opposite side musculature controls the motion eccentrically. The movement back to center uses the same muscle group concentrically to bring the weight of the head back up the slope (Fig. 24-15). The head can then be positioned to the other side of the wedge peak, and the same exercise can be repeated to train the muscles of the other side of the neck. In the sidelying position with the head supported on a pillow and a foam or towel roll under the neck, these muscles can also be trained more specifically and intensely. The roll can be squeezed between the head and shoulder to apply resistance to muscles on the same side as the patient is lying while gravity assists the movement. The muscles opposite to the side the patient is lying on can be contracted against gravity as the head is lifted off the pillow. The roll is used as the fulcrum, and the deeper muscles can be emphasized by ensuring that the neck remains in contact with the roll, decreasing the amount of translation taking place (Fig. 24-16). By shifting the roll slightly up or down, some localization to a specific

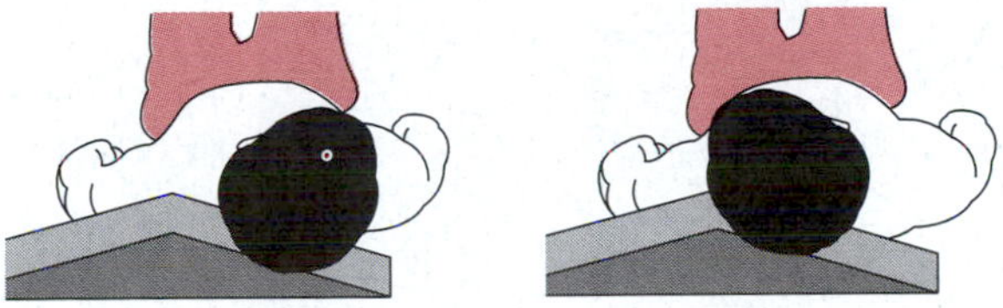

A B

FIGURE 24-15 Recruiting the side flexor and rotator muscle using a foam wedge. ***(A)*** As the patient rotates the head down the wedge slope, the opposite side musculature controls the motion eccentrically. ***(B)*** The movement back to center uses the same muscle group concentrically to bring the weight of the head back up the slope.

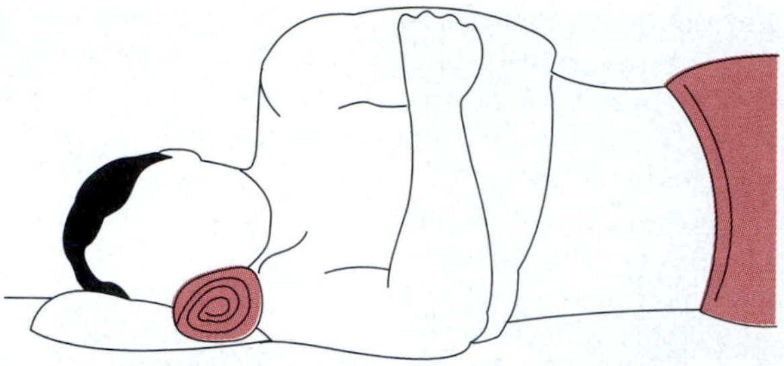

FIGURE 24-16 Recruiting the side flexors and rotators more specifically. The patient is in the sidelying position, with the head supported on a pillow with a towel roll under the neck. The roll is used as the fulcrum, and the deeper muscles can be emphasized by ensuring the neck remains in contact with the roll decreasing the amount of translation taking place.

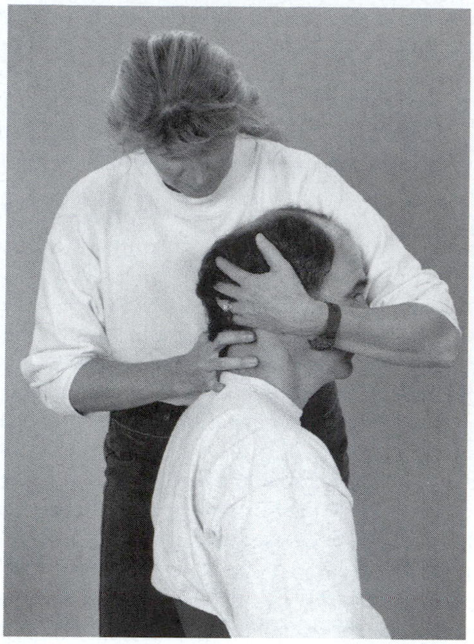

FIGURE 24-17 Strengthening in functional movement patterns. With the patient sitting, the therapist palpates at the affected level as the patient performs the motion against the resistance of the therapist.

segmental level can be obtained. A flexion or extension component can also be included.

Strengthening Functional Movement Patterns

Several strengthening exercises use combined movements. Because many of the movement patterns required for functional activity are multiplanar, it is beneficial to train the muscle group using these movements. The movement patterns chosen for a particular patient depend on the assessment findings (ie, specific weakness or reproduction of pain) and on the requirements of work and leisure activities.

The patient can be taught the correct movement pattern by using a modified muscle energy technique for muscle recruitment rather than mobilization. With the patient sitting, the therapist palpates at the affected level as the patient performs the motion against the resistance of the therapist (Fig. 24-17). The recruitment of the muscles at that segment and any excessive translation can be monitored. Concentric or eccentric muscle contractions can be used.

After the patient can perform these movements correctly (without excessive translation), autoresistance throughout the range can be applied by the patient. Heavy resistance should be avoided, because it tends to encourage faulty movement patterns, as does static maximal isometric contractions. Concentric contractions can be used first through short-arc movements, progressing to full-arc motion and then to eccentric contractions (Fig. 24-18).

Pulley systems can be used to apply graded resistance. Head pieces can apply resistance to the weak cervical muscles as determined at assessment. The pulley height is important in providing the correct angle of pull to encourage an optimal movement pattern of the neck. The weights must be kept low enough to allow the patient to perform the motion smoothly and without substitution of unwanted muscle groups. Supervision is important, because there is a tendency to use a translation motion against the resistance, which often exacerbates the problem, especially in cases of hypermobility.

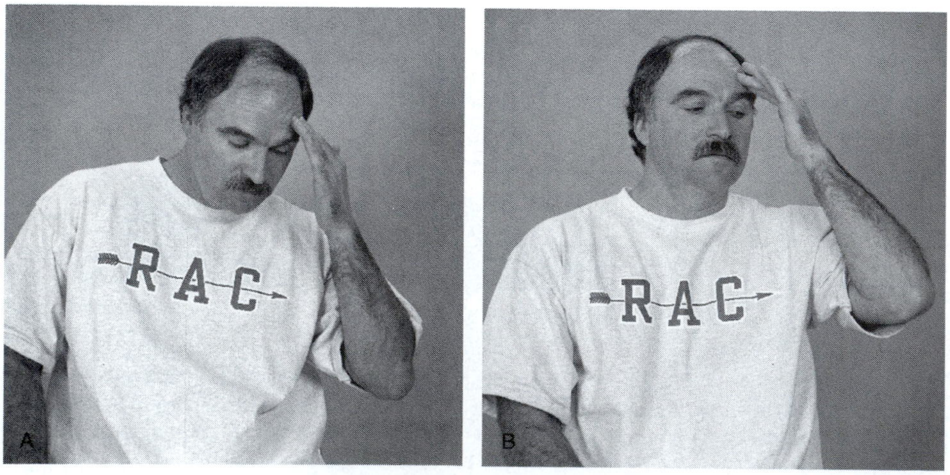

FIGURE 24-18 Strengthening in functional movement patterns using autoresistance. ***(A)*** Concentric contractions into the left flexion quadrant. ***(B)*** Eccentric contractions back into the right extension quadrant (early in range).

Mobility Impairment

Impairment of mobility can be classified as hypomobility (ie, reduced motion) or hypermobility (ie, increased motion). In the case of hypomobility, exercises are given to regain and maintain motion. For hypermobility, a stabilization exercise program is used to regain control of the excessive motion.

HYPOMOBILITY

Etiology

Cervical mobility can be reduced for several reasons:

- Segmental articular mobility restriction
- Capsular thickening and contracture
- Degenerative bony changes
- Segmental muscle spasm
- Myofascial extensibility
- Adverse neuromeningeal tension

Cervical mobility also can be affected by syndromes involving the shoulder girdle, and treatment may need to include interventions for impairments in that region.

Treatment

Even in the early stages of treatment for an acute neck problem, ROM exercises can be taught for each of the restricted planes of motion. Care must be taken in teaching these exercises to ensure that the normal movement pattern is performed and that this pattern is reinforced with repetition. With the patient lying supine with the head supported on a pillow, the weight of the head is eliminated, decreasing the compression load. This position can be helpful for patients with painful neck motion. The use of rhythmic respiration during the exercise can aid in relaxation of the scalene muscles and create a pumping action to help reduce swelling. This activity can be progressed to rotation exercises with the head positioned on the peak of a foam wedge (Fig. 24-19). The amplitude of motion obtained is increased, and there is some extension incorporated with the movement on rotation and flexion on return to midline. ROM exercises can also be performed in the upright position.

If a mobility exercise into extension or the extension quadrant is being considered, the effects on vascular and neurologic tissue should be tested. Keep in mind that a considerable weight-bearing force is sustained by the articular facet in these positions.

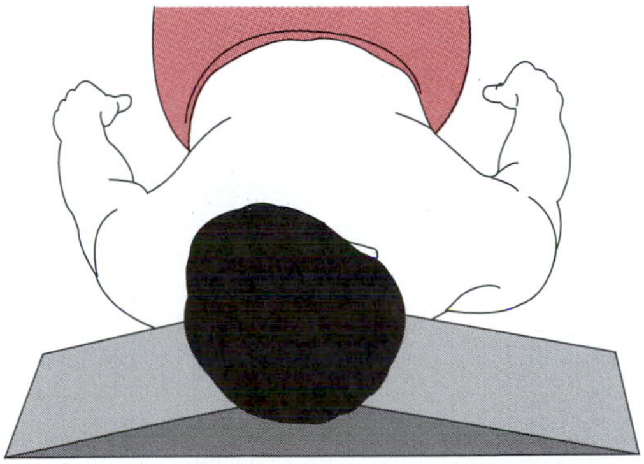

FIGURE 24-19 Range of motion exercises on a foam wedge. Allows non–weight-bearing motion, combining rotation and side flexion with flexion–extension.

Segmental Articular Restrictions. Segmental articular restrictions generally respond well to manual therapy mobilization techniques unless there is excessive degeneration of the bony structures. Self-mobilization exercises are a useful adjunct to this treatment. The patient is taught to localize to the involved segment with his fingers or a towel support and perform a specific, sometimes multiplanar motion to mobilize the joint restriction as determined by mobility testing.

AO joint fixation is obtained by clasped hands behind the neck, just under the occiput. Care is taken to not drag the neck into a forward head position. To gain unilateral flexion, the chin is tucked and deviated toward the same side. To gain unilateral extension, the chin is poked forward toward the opposite side (Fig. 24-20*A and B*).

AA joint fixation is obtained in the same manner as for the AO joint, but the hands slide down to the C2 level. To gain rotation, the head is rotated over the hand fixation with eyes maintained level. To encourage ipsilateral facet motion, add slight flexion (Fig. 24-20*C*). To encourage contralateral facet motion, add slight extension (Fig. 24-20*D*).

For addressing the midcervical joint, the patient is taught to locate the affected joint, sometimes through palpation of segmental muscle tenderness. To gain flexion, the patient fixes the caudal vertebra with inferior pressure by the fingers and performs flexion and side flexion and rotation away from the affected side about the appropriate axis (Fig. 24-20*E*). To gain extension, the patient fixes the caudal lamina

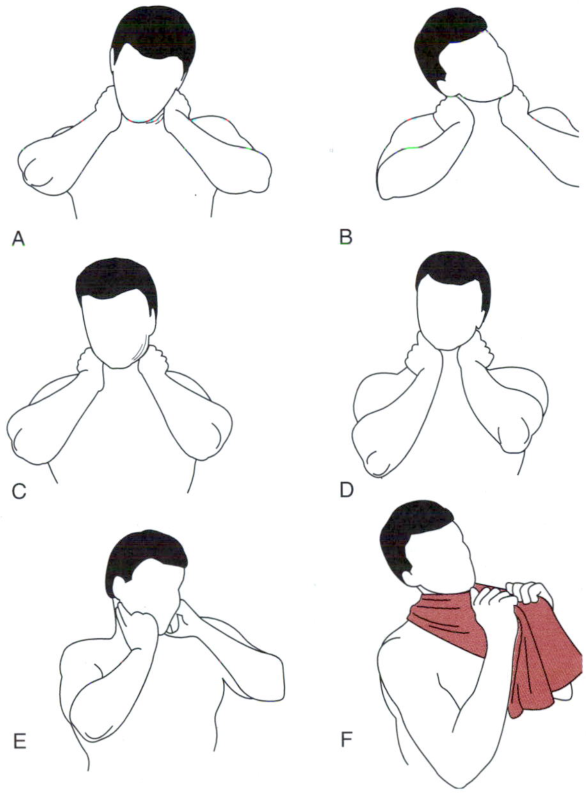

FIGURE 24-20 Self-mobilization exercises. ***(A)*** Unilateral flexion of right AO joint. ***(B)*** Unilateral extension of right AO joint. ***(C)*** Ipsilateral facet posterior motion of AA right joint. ***(D)*** Contralateral facet anterior motion of left AA joint. ***(E)*** Flexion of the midcervical joint. ***(F)*** Extension of the right midcervical joint.

with anterosuperior pressure and performs extension, side flexion, and rotation over the fixation point (Fig. 24-20*F*).

Muscle Extensibility. Assessment of muscle lengths is necessary because of muscle imbalances and postural asymmetries that are unique to each individual. Janda[37] states that certain muscle groups in the cervical spine have a greater tendency to shorten. This may be related to the effect of the limbic system on these muscles, the large percentage of afferent fibers supplying these muscles, and the more tonic rather than phasic properties of these muscles. Some muscles tend to shorten:

- Posterior suboccipital muscles
- Cervical erector spinae muscles
- Scalenes (anterior, medius, posterior)
- Sternocleidomastoid
- Levator scapula
- Trapezius, upper fibers

A study of cervical musculoskeletal function in postconcussional headache[38] showed a higher incidence of moderate muscle tightness compared with controls. This finding of tightness was not isolated to any one of the muscles tested (eg, upper fibers of the trapezius, levator scapula, scalenes, upper cervical extensors), but it was most frequent identified in the upper cervical extensors. Alterations in resting posture may cause a muscle that is of normal length to be placed on tension because of the increased distance between the origin and insertion caused by the posture. For example, a depressed scapular resting position puts tension on the levator scapula, potentially reducing opposite-side flexion and rotation of the cervical spine. The motion can be regained immediately on elevating the scapula, confirming that the length of the levator scapula muscle was normal. Other muscles may adaptively shorten because of longstanding changes in posture. The sternocleidomastoid, for example, tends to adaptively shorten in response to FHP. When the head is brought back into a more normal position, the muscle may appear to be a tight band, inhibiting attempts to retrain optimal posture. Treatment of both cases consists of postural correction exercises.

The posterior suboccipital muscle group can be lengthened by using the CV flexion head nod exercise (Fig. 24-21). The stretch can be localized by supporting the rest of the neck with clasped hands and further localized by side flexion away and rotation toward the tighter side. The localization can also be obtained using a folded towel placed just below the level to be stretched.

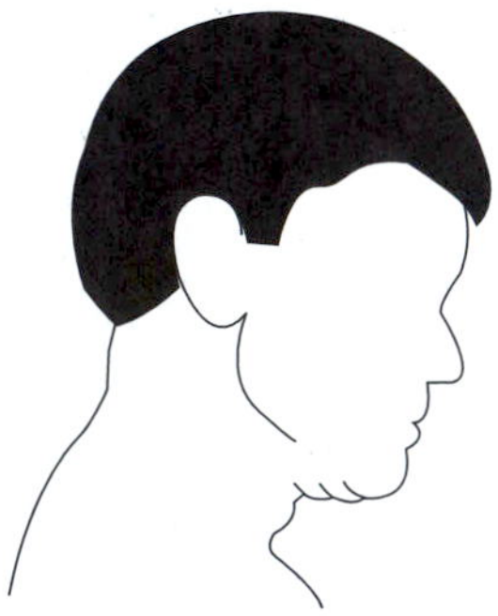

FIGURE 24-21 Stretching the posterior suboccipital muscles using the craniovertebral flexion head nod exercise.

Further neck flexion must be incorporated to obtain a stretch into the middle to low cervical erector spinae. CV flexion must be maintained throughout the exercise. If any anterior translation is allowed, cervical lordosis is produced, which results in a shortening of these muscles. Adding side flexion and rotation to the opposite side biases the stretch to the right or left side (Fig. 24-22).

The scalene muscle group also tends to shorten and become overactive because of improper breathing patterns. Teaching proper diaphragmatic breathing can decrease recruitment of this group as a secondary muscle of inspiration. Exercises designed to stretch this muscle must allow for adequate fixation of the first and second ribs, which can be achieved through manual or belt fixation. The scalene group is lengthened by side flexion away and slight rotation toward the affected side (Fig. 24-23). The anterior scalene muscle may be further stretched by the addition of slight extension. The patient must be instructed to stop at the point of tension, because the muscle pull can produce a lateral translation force on the cervical spine.

An effective method of regaining normal sternocleidomastoid muscle length is to correct the FHP. Retraining the use of the deep cervical flexors for the habitual movement pattern of neck flexion also decreases overuse tightness of the sternocleidomastoid. If the muscle has become shortened by posttraumatic adhesions, it may be necessary to stretch the muscle. This can be achieved by extension side flexion away from and rotation toward the side being treated. Lordosis must be controlled, because that position shortens the muscle. This effect can be achieved by bringing the head on a straight neck back behind the line of the trunk (Fig. 24-24). When attempting to lengthen the levator scapula muscle, it is important to fix the scapula into de-

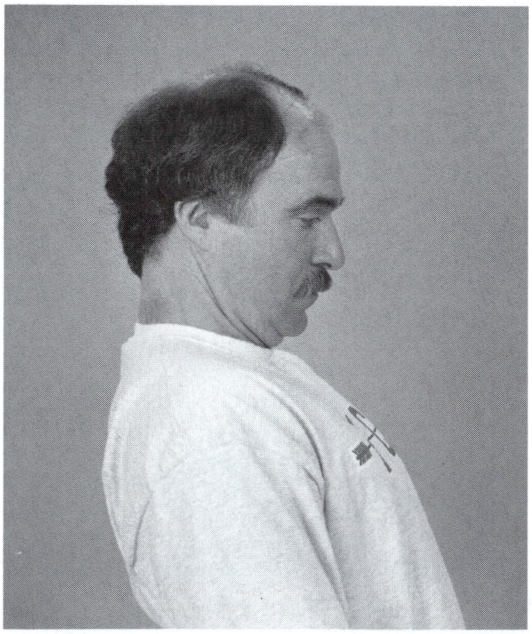

FIGURE 24-22 Stretching into the middle to low cervical erector spinae.

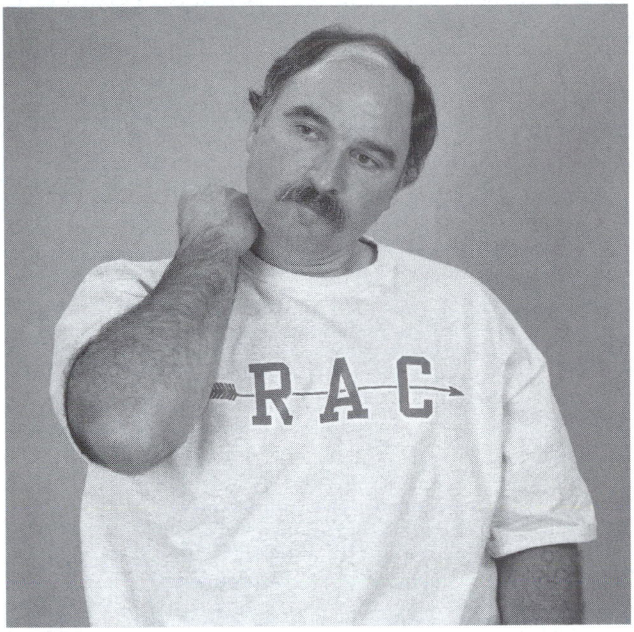

FIGURE 24-23 Stretching the scalene muscles—first rib fixed, side flexion away, and slight rotation toward the affected side.

pression, upward rotation, or both. Upward rotation of the scapula can be achieved by arm elevation, but this position may be difficult for patients with pain on arm elevation. In the sitting position, depression can be maintained by holding the underside of a chair. The muscle is then stretched by cervical side flexion and rotation to the opposite side and stretched by cervical flexion (Fig. 24-25).

To stretch the upper fibers of the trapezius, the scapula must be fixed into depression, downward rotation, or both. Scapular depression can be achieved while sitting by holding the underside of the chair, and by reaching the arm down and behind the back, a position of downward rotation is obtained. The stretch is then performed into neck flexion, with side flexion away from and rotation toward the affected side (Fig. 24-26).

The concern about the latter two stretches is the resultant forces on irritable zygapophyseal joints from the end-range combined movements. These two muscles and the scalene muscles, because of their angle of pull, also produce

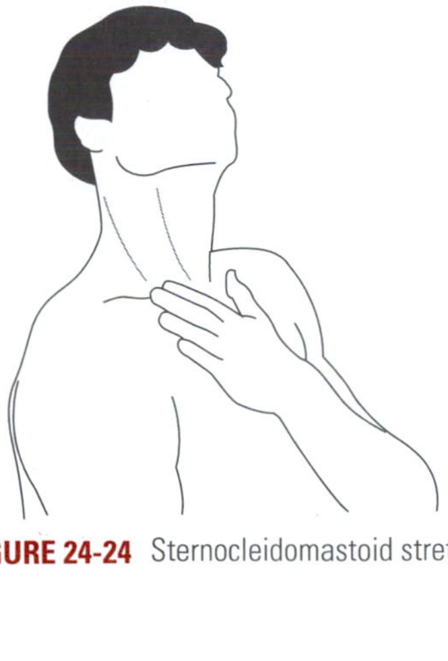

FIGURE 24-24 Sternocleidomastoid stretch.

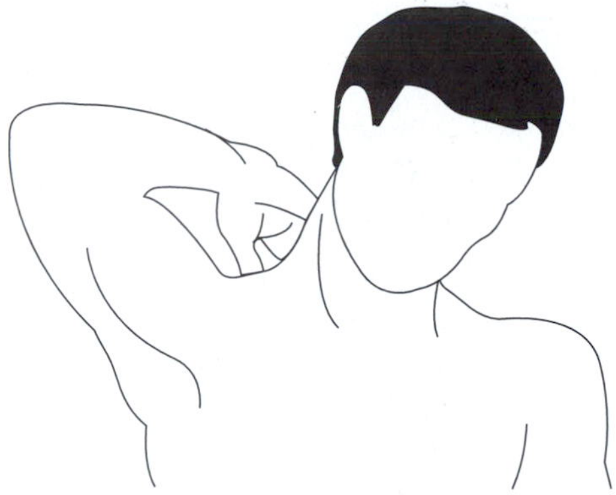

FIGURE 24-25 Stretching the levator scapula—arm overhead (scapular upward rotation), scapular depression, side flexion away, rotation away from affected side, and flexion.

a lateral translation force on the vertebrae when stretched. An alternative exercise is to have the patient face the wall, with the ulnar border of the hands and forearm in contact overhead, and perform a wall slide. The arms are slid downward, creating scapular depression. The cervical spine can then be moved into flexion. From this position, contralateral rotation lengthens the levator scapula muscle, and ipsilateral rotation lengthens the upper fibers of the trapezius muscle (Fig. 24-27).

Adverse Neuromeningeal Tension. Adverse tension in the neuromeningeal structures of the cervical spine can affect the mobility of the neck, thoracic spine, shoulder girdle, and upper extremity.[39] Signs of decreased extensibility of these structures are found on the Upper Limb Tension Tests, with a median, radial, or ulnar nerve bias. When prescribing an exercise designed to improve neuromeningeal extensibility, the effect on the cervical spine should be

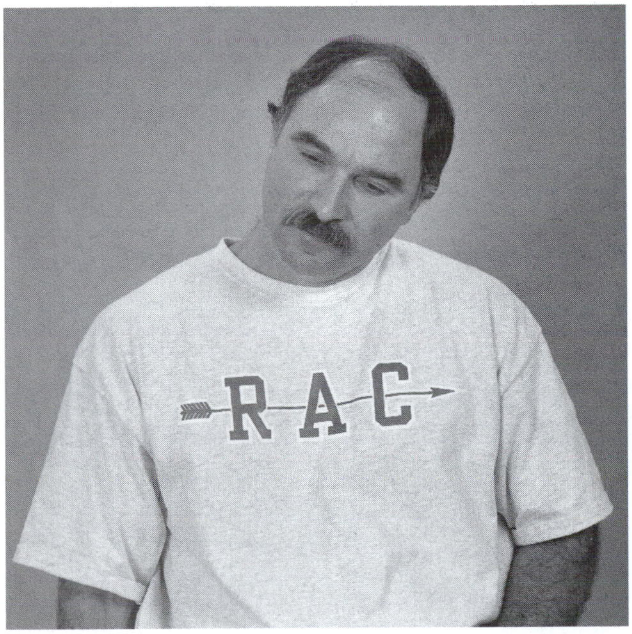

FIGURE 24-26 Stretching the upper fibers of the trapezius—scapular depression, neck flexion, side flexion away, and rotation toward the affected side.

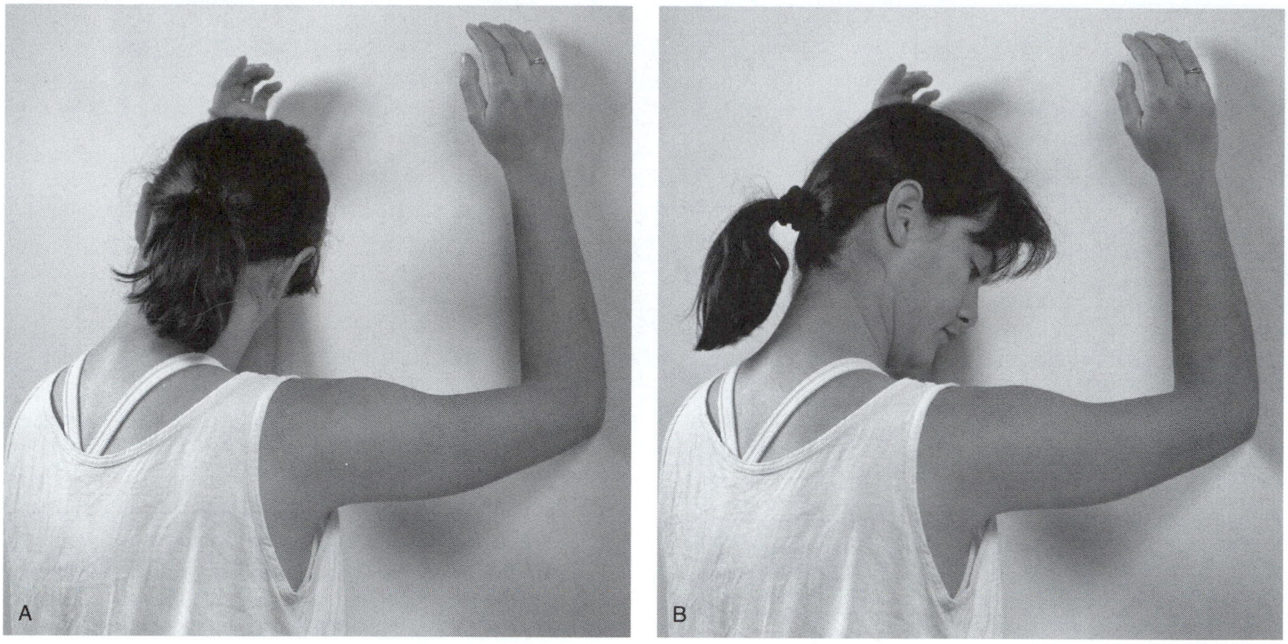

FIGURE 24-27 Alternative wall slide exercise. ***(A)*** Contralateral rotation lengthens the levator scapula muscle. ***(B)*** Ipsilateral rotation lengthens the upper fibers of the trapezius muscle.

considered. Because of direct attachment of dural structures into the cervical vertebrae, tightness in the neuromeningeal system may cause lateral translation of the vertebrae with each attempt to stretch the structures, which can lead to hypermobility of the segment. The affected segment should be manually fixated by the opposite hand supporting under the neck so that the fingers wrap around to the affected side and prevent the lateral translation (Fig. 24-28).

The stretch can be performed by the patient lying supine with a belt wrapped over the shoulder and around the knee to maintain the scapular depression:

For median nerve bias, the arm, flexed at the elbow, is abducted to the tension point and externally rotated, with the forearm supinated and the wrist and fingers extended. The elbow is then slowly extended to produce the stretch (Fig. 24-29*A*).

For radial nerve bias, the arm, flexed at the elbow, is internally rotated, pronated, and abducted with the wrist flexed. The stretch is produced by slowly extending the elbow (Fig. 24-29*B*).

For ulnar nerve bias, the arm, flexed to a right angle at the elbow, is abducted, externally rotated, and supinated with the wrist extended. The stretch is produced through further flexion of the elbow (Fig. 24-29*C*).

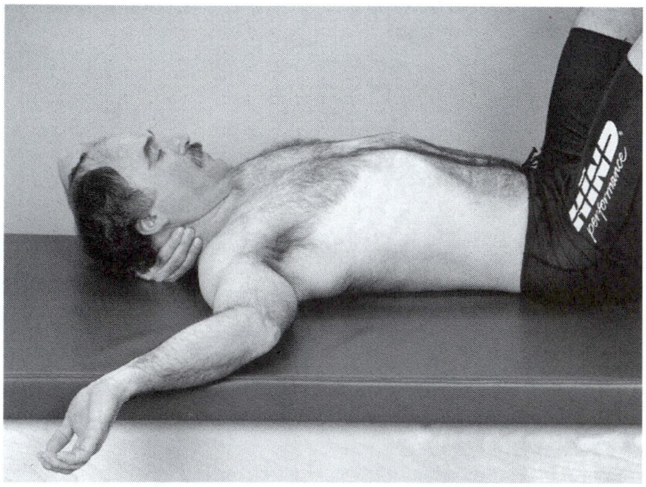

FIGURE 24-28 Dural stretch with manual stabilization and fixation of lateral shear.

Similar stretches can be performed by the patient while standing and using the opposite hand to maintain the depression of the scapula. With each of these exercises, a more intense stretch can be obtained by the addition of contralateral side flexion or rotation of the neck. A study by Edgar and coworkers[40] showed a relationship between

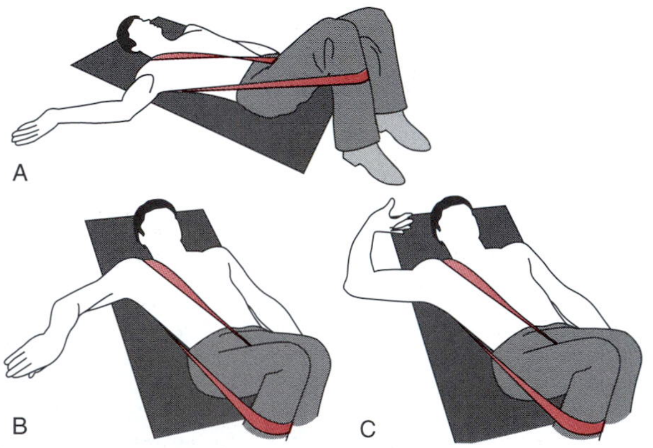

FIGURE 24-29 Dural stretch in supine lying with a belt wrapped over the shoulder and around the knee to maintain scapular depression. ***(A)*** median nerve bias. ***(B)*** Radial nerve bias. ***(C)*** Ulnar nerve bias.

decreased neuromeningeal extensibility and decreased length of upper fibers of the trapezius.

HYPERMOBILITY

Etiology

Hypermobility is excessive motion of the intervertebral segment. As hypothesized by Panjabi,[23] spinal stability is obtained through three subsystems:

- Passive musculoskeletal subsystem: inert osseoligamentous column, including the vertebra, disk, capsule, and ligament
- Active musculoskeletal subystem: the muscle and tendon units
- Control subsystem: the neural and feedback mechanisms

The role of the spinal stability system is to provide sufficient stability through all three subsystems to match the demands made on the spine. Deficiencies in one subsystem can be compensated for, within certain limits. Gross instability, as documented by functional radiographs, may require surgical fixation. Hypermobilities are best addressed by conservative measures, including a progressive exercise program. Exercise programs can be used to enhance the active and control subsystems.

Specific stability testing is performed to determine the degree and planes of laxity. Special attention is given to the amount of translation and the end feel. This assessment determines the structural integrity of the passive subsystem of the spine. To determine the dynamic stability of the cervical spine, the hypermobile segment is palpated during active motion of the neck or upper extremity. The clinician is able to detect excessive amounts or inappropriate directions of translation during the particular motion while the spine is under active control (Fig. 24-30). Because of the large neutral zone in the cervical spine, much of the stability in this region is imparted by the dynamic control of the active muscular system. In the case of loss of integrity of the inert stabilizing structures, training of neuromuscular control may result in a functionally stable spine.

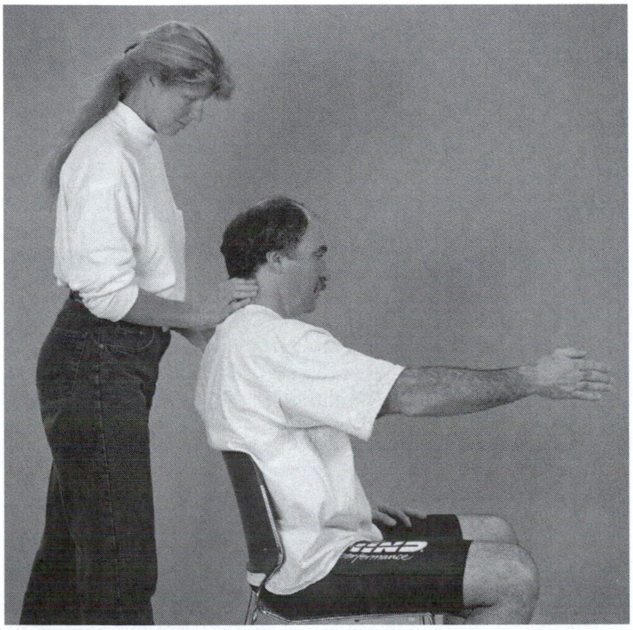

FIGURE 24-30 Palpation of cervical spinal segment stability during arm motion.

Treatment

For the hypermobile cervical spine, care must be taken in prescribing ROM or stretching exercises that may exaggerate the excessive translation. The neck must be passively fixed at the affected segment during the stretch, or another exercise should be chosen that does not incorporate the unwanted motion. For example, a patient may have a tight levator scapula muscle but also be hypermobile into right lateral translation at the C3-C4 intervertebral segment. Attempts to stretch the levator scapula muscle by left side flexion encourage right lateral translation. The patient can control the right lateral translation with the left hand cupping behind the neck, offering a counteracting left translation at the C4 vertebra (Fig. 24-31). It may be more appropriate in this case to choose the wall slide exercise described in the Hypomobility section, using contralateral rotation rather than side flexion.

For the patient with lateral translation hypermobility, attempts to incorporate dural stretch exercises cause repetitive lateral translation at the affected joint. A stretch can be performed effectively by first stabilizing that segment for lateral translation (see Fig. 24-28).

Postural correction exercises are an integral component in unloading the hypermobile segment in the cervical spine. Any deviation from the optimal posture of the cervical spine increases the translational forces that the spine is subjected to. The resting posture of the shoulder girdle also plays a role in imparting translational forces to the cervical spine. For example, weakness or poor recruitment of the upper fibers of trapezius leads to a depressed and downwardly rotated scapula, which places the muscle in a lengthened position. Constant pull on the insertion into the cervical spine may eventually lead to hypermobility into lateral translation. In cases of pre-existing lateral hypermobility, the continuous lateral force exacerbates symptoms arising from that segment. Exercise should focus on correcting the impairments found on assessment of the shoulder girdle. Taping to reposition the scapula into elevation and upward rotation can reduce this force, allow a more normal movement pattern of the cervical spine, and relieve the increased dural tension caused by the abnormal resting position (see Chapter 26).

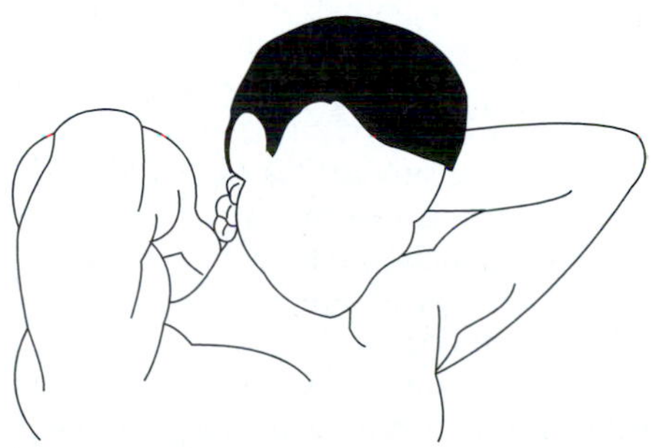

FIGURE 24-31 Levator scapula stretch: fixing C4 to prevent right lateral translation.

Cervical hypermobility can also be addressed through training to facilitate neuromuscular control of the cervical spine with graduated exercise. A series of cervical strengthening exercises can be implemented as determined by specific muscle testing. These exercises, as described in the Impaired Muscle Performance section, enhance the active subsystem of the spinal stability system. Another approach is to determine the direction of the hypermobility and to design exercises that can control those particular motions by recruiting muscles that move the spine out of that direction. For example, for hypermobility into the right extension quadrant, strengthening exercises can be done for left side flexion and rotation and flexion. Although an isometric contraction produces higher force values, it is easiest for the patient to control and therefore may be the first exercise taught. Concentric contractions, initially short-arc motion and then progressing to full-arc motion, are taught before eccentric contractions.

Simultaneously, a cervical stabilization program can be developed to focus on the control subsystem. Throughout the stabilization program, motion at the hypermobile segment must be controlled, particularly for the excessive translation component. In many cases, the patient can be taught to palpate the translation motion of the vertebra and stop moving when it begins. The patient can also be taught to stabilize the affected level manually or through muscle cocontraction as an exercise is performed. Progressing regardless of translation of the affected level does not succeed in developing stability, and through increased stresses on the capsule and ligaments, it may result in painful exacerbation to the point that the program has to be discontinued.

Stage I. The first stage of the stabilization program is to isolate the short neck flexors. The head nod exercise and progressions for strengthening this muscle group are described in the Impaired Muscle Performance section. The ability to cocontract the deep neck flexors with the cervical extensors muscles and the scapular stabilizer muscles is also a goal for this stage. Early training can be accomplished in supine lying with the cervical lordosis supported over a towel roll. The extensors are recruited using the electrical muscle stimulator while the patient prevents the extension motion by simultaneously performing the head nod exercise such that the cervical spine remains in neutral. With the patient prone over the exercise ball or in FPK, the head nod motion is performed concurrently with lower cervical extension. The cervical lordosis should straighten (see Fig. 24-12).

Stage II. After the patient is able to maintain the cocontraction of the anterior and posterior muscles of the cervical spine, exercises can be progressed by integrating arm motion while ensuring cervical stabilization. Because the most stable position is supine, it is used as the starting position. Various movements of the upper extremity (eg, flexion, abduction, diagonals) are tested while palpating the affected segment for translation to determine the effect of the arm motion (see Fig. 24-30).

Bilateral arm motions below 90 degrees often are the least challenging, but unilateral, overhead movements place higher demands on the stabilization system. However, these effects depend on factors such as the plane or direction of the hypermobility, dural tension, and shoulder or thoracic mobility.

The exercises consist of initial cocontraction of the cervical musculature, which is maintained while the patient performs repetitive motion of the upper extremity using the pattern chosen during assessment. The amplitude of the arm motion depends on the point at which the patient is no longer able to maintain cervical stabilization. Progression includes adding hand weights, which increases the resistance, or lying on a half roll, which produces a more unstable base (Fig. 24-32).

These same exercises can be progressed by having the patient perform them in a sitting or standing position. These positions are more challenging to spinal stability. Upper extremity motion can be altered in direction, amplitude, and pattern. They can be bilateral or unilateral, and weights can be added to increase the demands on the spinal stability system. Ball sitting and the use of pulley systems are beneficial at this stage (Fig. 24-33). The use of proprioceptive neuromuscular facilitation patterns or sport- and work-specific movements introduce a more functional approach.

The therapy ball can be used at all levels of the stabilization program. Prone, progressed to supine on the ball, the patient can be taught to maintain a controlled cervical spine position while performing simple rocking motions. Increased demands can be made on the cervical spine by adding unilateral or bilateral arm motions, with or without weights. This can be progressed to more complicated arm and leg patterns (Fig. 24-34).

Because of the importance of the role of muscles in dynamic stability of the spine, it can be deduced that, despite the presence of hypermobility, functional stability can be regained through neuromuscular retraining. The key is gradually challenging the cervical musculature over some months while preventing excessive motion at the involved segment.

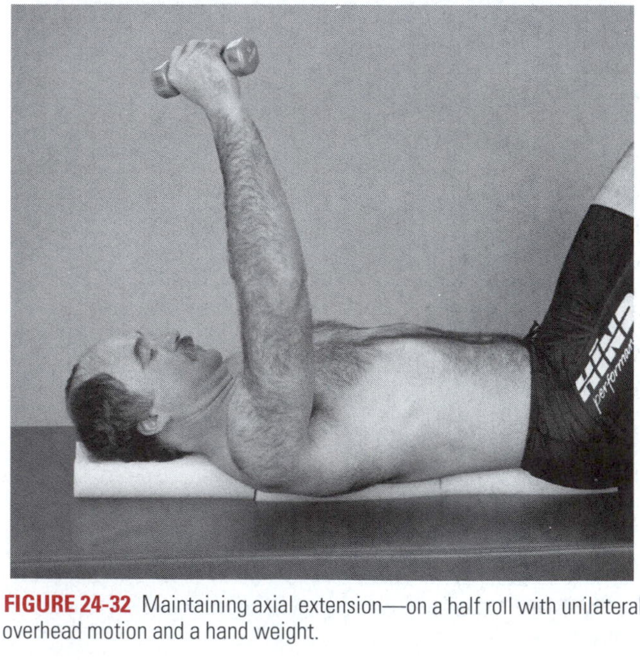

FIGURE 24-32 Maintaining axial extension—on a half roll with unilateral overhead motion and a hand weight.

Posture Impairment

ETIOLOGY

Although posture is affected by the whole of the axial skeleton, the cervical spine plays an important role in the control of posture. The rich supply of mechanoreceptors in the articular capsules and muscles of the cervical spine provide proprioceptive input and feed into the vestibular system.[41] Any attempt to alter cervical spine posture must include an evaluation of the thoracic spine, shoulder girdle, and pelvis. Many of the involved muscles are multijoint muscles, spanning the first three of these related regions. Changes in the lengths of muscles such as the levator scapula, trapezius, pectoralis major and minor, or rhomboids have profound effects on the shoulder complex and the cervical spine. Changes in the strength of these scapular stabilizers also alters the resting posture of the neck. Alterations of the pelvic base in any plane have effects throughout the spinal column, including the cervical spine. The optimal posture for the cervical spine is the position of axial extension (see Patient-Related Instruction: Optimal Posture of the Neck). This can be defined as (Fig. 24-35A)

- CV flexion
- Midcervical spine neutral (slight cervical lordosis)
- Cervicothoracic extension
- Upper thoracic extension

In axial extension, minimal muscle work is required to maintain the position, the spine is in an elongated state, and compressive and translatory forces on the spinal structures are reduced compared with those in the FHP. The most common postural impairment of the cervical spine is the FHP, which includes

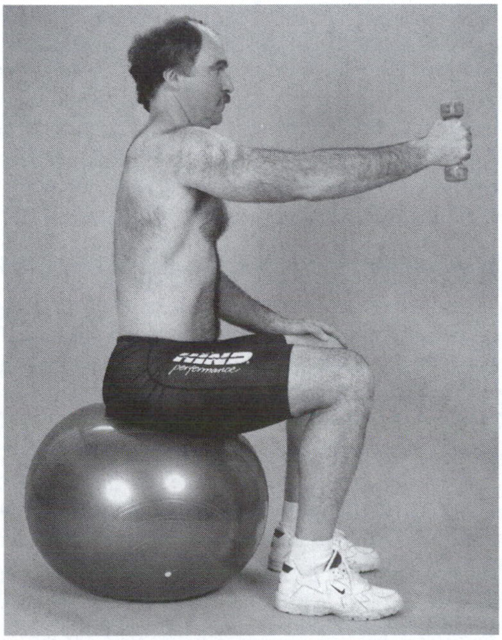

FIGURE 24-33 Maintaining sitting axial extension on a ball—arm motion with a weight.

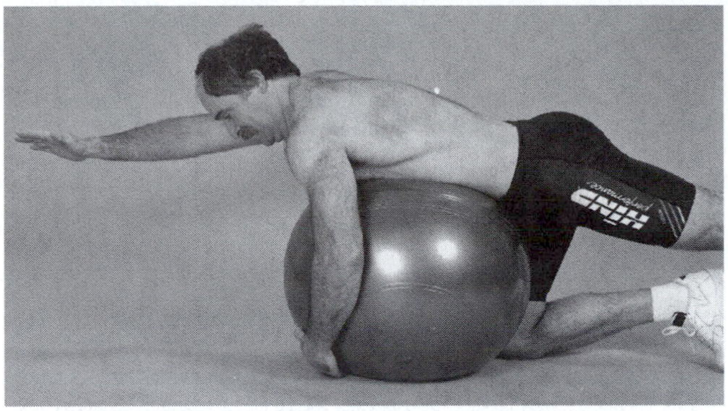

FIGURE 24-34 Maintaining axial extension—opposite arm and leg pattern.

- CV extension
- Midcervical lordosis
- Low cervical and upper thoracic flexion
- Thoracic kyphosis

A patient with FHP can present with several variations. In some individuals, the lower cervical spine flexion juts the whole cervical spine forward above that level, and extension

Patient-Related Instruction

Optimal Posture of the Neck

It is important to practice proper posture of the head and neck. Good posture decreases the stresses on muscles, joints, and ligaments of the cervical spine, which can reduce pain and prevent wear and tear on these structures. Your therapist will instruct you in additional exercises to enable you to achieve and maintain this posture.

The upper back should be straightened, the shoulder blades pulled back together, and the chin brought back so that the head is centered over the trunk. A useful guideline is that the ear should be over the midline of the shoulder. Do not over correct, because a slight curve in the neck is normal. Proper posture must be practiced frequently throughout the day so that this position becomes habitual. This posture must also be adopted during exercise for the neck and upper extremity.

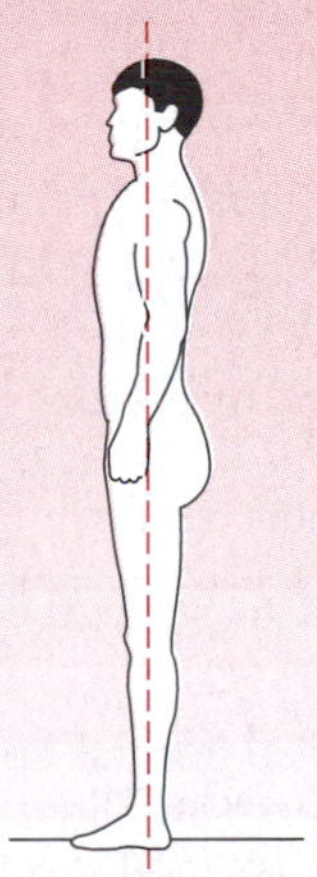

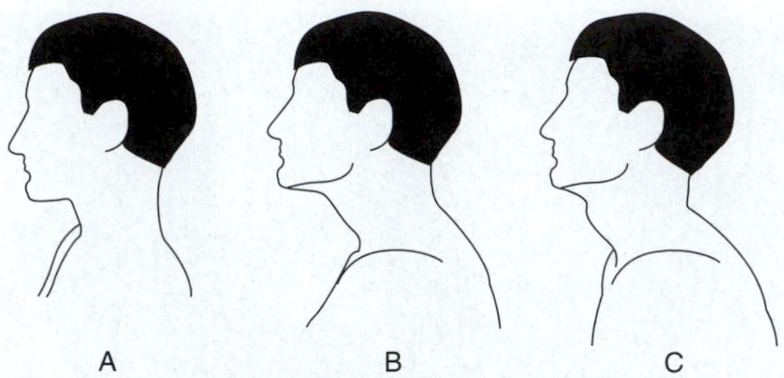

FIGURE 24-35 (***A***) Axial extension. (***B***) Forward head position: minimal midcervical lordosis. (***C***) Forward head position: excessive midcervical lordosis.

mainly occurs at the CV region with little increase in the midcervical lordosis (Fig. 24-35*B*). In others, the lower cervical spine flexion is compensated for by an exaggerated cervical lordosis that may start abruptly, sometimes as low as the C6-C7 segment. In these cases, the midcervical lordosis tends to be accompanied by an excessive anterior translation that is an unphysiologic coupling of motion, because extension (ie, lordosis) should couple with posterior translation (Fig. 24-35*C*). Each individual should be assessed to determine the exact components of his abnormal posture, the levels at which changes in the spinal curves are taking place, and what the emphasis of the postural correction should be.

Reversal of the normal cervical lordosis is a less common postural impairment. In this situation, the patient presents with a very straight cervical spine or even a kyphosis. Treatment focuses on regaining extension in the cervical spine to encourage the normal cervical lordosis.

Postural abnormalities may be observed in the frontal plane with the head and neck tilted to one side. This posture can be caused by factors such as muscle imbalance, articular hypomobilities, habitual work or leisure positions, and hearing or other sight deficits necessitating altered head position. Treatment should be directed at the cause of the asymmetry.

TREATMENT

Treatment for FHP should address muscle imbalance, neuromeningeal extensibility, articular hypomobility, and proprioception.

Muscle Imbalance

The following short muscles should be lengthened:

- Posterior cervical extensors
- Scalene muscles
- Upper fibers of the trapezius
- Levator scapula
- Pectoralis major and minor

It also is important to strengthen the following weak muscles:

- Deep, short cervical flexors (upper and midcervical)
- Scapular stabilizers (middle and lower fibers of the trapezius, rhomboids, and serratus anterior)
- Upper thoracic erector spinae

Neuromeningeal Extensibility

Abnormal cervical postures may be caused by an attempt to decrease stretch on shortened neuromeningeal structures. Side flexion of the cervical spine and elevation of the scapula decrease tension in these structures. Exercises designed to alter these postures without first addressing the adverse neural tension can exacerbate the pain and possibly amplify the neurologic symptoms.

Articular Hypomobility

Manual therapy techniques may be indicated in conjunction with mobility exercises to regain the restricted motions of

- Upper cervical flexion
- Cervicothoracic junction extension
- Upper thoracic extension

Proprioception

The patient must be taught how to maintain the improved cervical posture during various activities, especially during upper extremity motion. Many of the exercises used to address these impairments have been described in the preceding sections. The primary exercise for achieving many of the goals of postural correction is the head nod exercise. It corrects the upper cervical extension, and because it also tightens ligamentum nuchae, it simultaneously reduces cervical lordosis. In patients with excessive lordosis of the midcervical spine, continuing the head nod into further cervical flexion stretches the posterior structures that have become shortened by the lordotic position. The head nod exercise can be modified to include posterior displacement (retraction) of the head and neck complex to encourage extension at the lower cervical spine and cervicothoracic junction.

One study on the effect of repeated neck retractions in normal subjects found that there was a significant change in resting posture toward a more retracted position after two sets of repeated retractions.[42] It is important to control the amount of flexion and retraction motion to prevent overcompensation into a kyphotic cervical spine position. Supine is a good position for for the patient learning this exercise, because there is more proprioceptive feedback from the contact of the head. Lying lengthwise along an Epifoam roll, with the roll directly under the spine, encourages the thoracic extension component of postural correction (Fig. 24-36). In this position, the patient controls the lumbar curve with a sustained contraction of transversus abdominis and then performs the head nod exercise. Sitting and standing against wall support are natural progressions of the exercise (Fig. 24-37). The patient must maintain a neutral lumbar spine position, and a towel may have to be used behind the head initially to support the forward head or later to to maintain a neutral neck position.

Exercises must be included to help regain thoracic extension. Chapter 25 provides descriptions of these exercises.

Maintaining this axial extension posture while incorporating upper extremity motion is the next progression; the exercise is done first with wall support and then in free standing (Fig. 24-38). Resisted upper extremity exercises can be added through the use of free weights, elastic tubing, or pulley systems. Exercises can be chosen to address

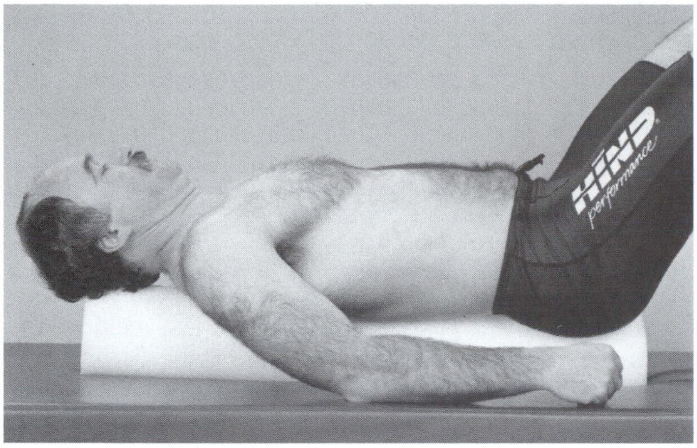

FIGURE 24-36 Lying on an Epifoam roll.

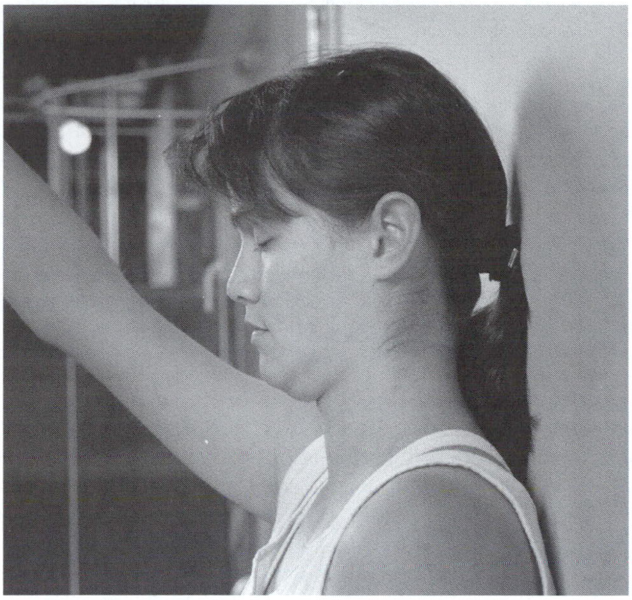

FIGURE 24-38 Wall posture with unilateral arm elevation.

strength impairments found on assessment or to simulate work or leisure movement patterns (Fig. 24-39). Various wobble board systems can be used; the unstable base can further challenge the control of posture as the patient performs various upper or lower extremity movements. Because many daily activities require a bent-forward position, maintaining proper axial extension while prone over the exercise ball can simulate this position, and upper extremity movements can be incorporated as described previously (see Fig. 24-34).

THERAPEUTIC EXERCISE INTERVENTIONS FOR COMMON DIAGNOSES

Some of the more common diagnoses of cervical spine disorders are discussed in the following sections. The impairments that occur with each diagnosis are identified, and examples of exercises for treatment of that condition are given.

Disk Dysfunction

ETIOLOGY

Although disk herniation is less common in the cervical spine than in the lumbar spine, various dysfunctions of cervical disks do occur. The term *disk dysfunction* could be used whenever changes in the disk alter its biomechanical properties and prevent normal function. Included in this

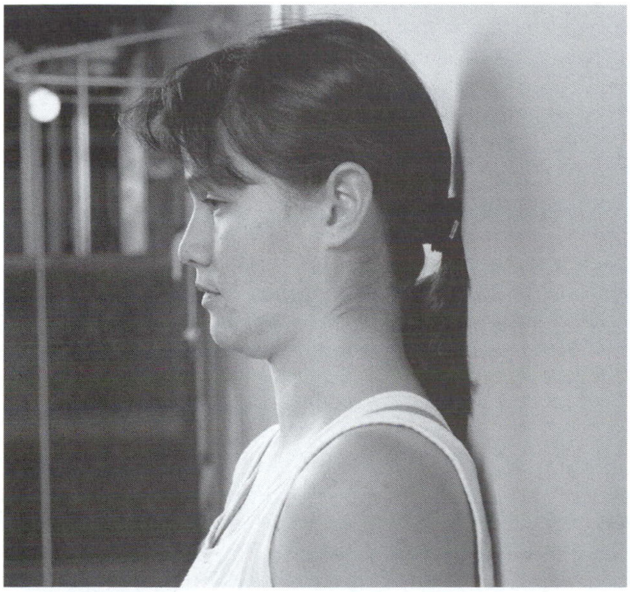

FIGURE 24-37 Head nod exercise performed against a wall.

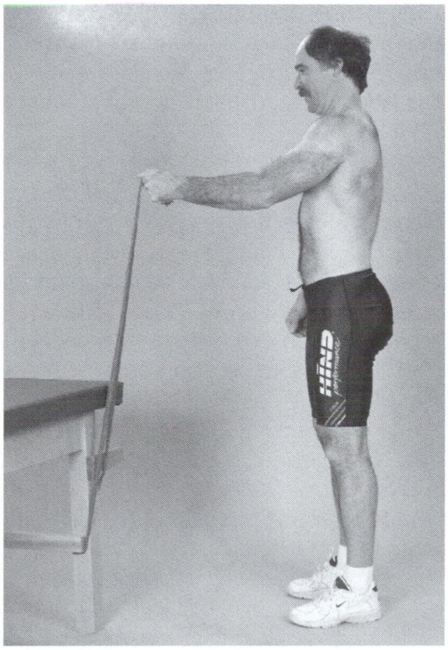

FIGURE 24-39 Maintaining axial extension with proprioceptive neuromuscular facilitation pattern against tubing resistance.

grouping are degenerative disk disease, excessive disk clefting, and rim lesions (ie, separation of the disk from the end plate).[43,44] In the acute stages, disk dysfunction can manifest as an irritable condition, with painful limitation of active ROM in all planes, particularly flexion; pain on cough or sneeze; painful cervical muscle contraction due to compression loading; and difficulty in maintaining upright postures because of the compression load of the head on the neck. There may or may not be associated neurologic signs, depending on the degree of foraminal encroachment by the disk and the condition of other structures surrounding the foramen, such as the Z joint capsule, ligaments, and bone.

TREATMENT

Treatment initially is aimed at resting the neck, which is achieved through education about proper resting positions to unload the compressive and translatory forces on the cervical spine. Therapeutic modalities may be useful to help alleviate the inflammatory response and decrease associated muscle spasm. Manual therapy techniques can be used to mobilize the involved segment if segmental hypomobility is found during mobility testing. Muscle energy techniques can also be used to mobilize and alter muscle activity at that segment.

Manual traction techniques help to decompress the disk and increase intervertebral foramen size. Breathing pattern re-education is a good exercise during the acute stages, because excessive use of the secondary muscles of inspiration, such as the scalenes, can add a compression load to the cervical spine and should be avoided. Instruction in diaphragmatic breathing encourages an optimal breathing pattern and unloads the cervical spine. Using postural correction exercises reduces translational forces. Supine exercises, such as gentle head nod (ie, CV flexion) may be tolerated at this stage.

As the condition improves, impairments can be identified and addressed. After a period of protected function, the patient probably may exhibit signs of hypomobility impairment. Degenerative changes at that vertebral segment may also decrease its mobility. Care must be taken in selecting and teaching ROM exercises to minimize compressive or translatory forces.

Because muscle extensibility may be decreased as a result of muscle guarding during the acute phase, stretching exercises should be implemented. Neuromeningeal extensibility should also be assessed at later stages, particularly in cases of neurologic involvement. Exercises to increase the mobility of these structures should not be started when there are still signs of decreased nerve conduction, because the movements can easily exacerbate the condition. The disk is an important structure in the control of motion of the intervertebral segment, and hypermobility impairment may occur as a result of disk dysfunction. Stability testing at the affected segment may detect increased motion because of the loss of the disk's ability to control translational forces in the spine. This impairment must be addressed with a progression of stabilization exercises. The Hypermobility section describes these exercises.

To prevent further disk degeneration and reduce the incidence of recurrence of an acute episode, it is important to correct all postural impairments of the cervical spine, thoracic spine, and shoulder girdle. Postural asymmetry of the pelvic girdle also influences the cervical spine, and impairments should be addressed as previously discussed.

Cervical Sprain and Strain

ETIOLOGY

Any traumatic incident can produce a sprain or strain of the cervical spine. The most common incident is the acceleration-deceleration injury after a motor vehicle accident.

The complex injuries sustained can involve many different tissues. The soft tissue structures involved can include muscle, ligament, capsule, articular cartilage, and the disk (including rim lesions). Concurrent bony injuries can include fractures of the articular subchondral bone, transverse and spinous processes, lateral masses of the atlas, and the vertebral body,[43] and suspicion of these injuries requires referral to the physician for management. Patients exhibiting signs of instability from traumatic injury should also be referred to the physician for further diagnostic tests and appropriate medical intervention. The severity of these injuries varies widely, and the irritability of the condition must be assessed individually.

TREATMENT

During the acute inflammatory stage, treatment is aimed at reducing pain and inflammation and promoting optimal healing. Education about proper resting positions, limitations of activity, and the use of ice can assist in reaching these goals. If segmental hypermobility is suspected, bracing should be considered to reduce stresses on the healing structures. Exercise at this time involves the use of breathing exercises and ROM exercises within the pain-free range. The supine position is often best tolerated at this stage, because it unloads the weight of the head. Rhythmic neck rotation movements performed in a supine position in conjunction with breathing can increase mobility and assist vascular flow. Therapeutic modalities such as ice, interferential current, ultrasound, or transcutaneous electrical nerve stimulation may also be indicated at this stage to reduce inflammation, decrease muscle spasm, and assist in pain control.

In the subacute stage, it is important to continue to protect the injured structures and to introduce stresses that encourage optimal healing. Grade I and II manual therapy mobilization techniques are effective in pain relief, and grade III and IV mobilizations can help restore motion of the involved segments. Impairment of mobility may continue to be the primary dysfunction. Mobility exercises may be progressed into larger-arc movements, more specific to the multiplanar articular restrictions found on manual mobility testing. Specific muscle length tests may also indicate that certain muscles are stretched. However, the effect on the whole spine (eg, dural stretch, disk compression) must be taken into consideration when choosing exercises. It is also prudent to begin postural re-education, progressing through the exercises as tolerated. Overhead arm motions are often too stressful on the cervical spine at this stage because of increased translation and compression forces.

During the remodeling phase or as the condition becomes more chronic, other impairments can be addressed. The muscles strained at the time of injury and the segmental muscles related to levels of articular dysfunction often show impairment of force production. A specific strengthening program can be designed to improve muscle function. Depending on the degree of ligamentous or disk injury, there may be a mobility impairment of hypermobility. Development of a stabilization program must take into consideration the direction, severity, and irritability of the hypermobility and progress with exercises as tolerated (see the Hypermobility section). Postural impairments continue to be a concern, and treatment interventions should include dynamic exercises that encourage movement patterns that incorporate optimal posture.

Neural Entrapment

ETIOLOGY

The cervical nerve roots can become entrapped at their exit at the intervertebral foramen. The foramen is bounded by the zygapophyseal joint, the UV joint, the disk, and the pedicle. Any pathologic condition increasing the size of these surrounding structures can lead to narrowing or stenosis of the foramen, potentially entrapping the nerve root. Foramen size is also reduced by the movements of extension and ipsilateral side flexion and rotation. Any muscle imbalance producing this resting position of the cervical spine would further aggravate the problem. The FHP can place the upper and midcervical spine into a posture of increased cervical lordosis, decreasing the intervertebral foramen size. Any scapular resting position that encourages this cervical position (eg, elevated scapula) or stretches the nerve root (eg, depressed or protracted scapula) would also aggravate the condition. Changes in neural conduction depend on the degree of pressure or traction on the nerve root.

The term double or multiple crush syndrome has been used to describe the syndrome in which the nerve is affected at multiple sites along its course from the cervical spine to the hand. Common sites of entrapment are the cervical intervertebral foramen, the thoracic outlet, the elbow, and the carpus. Pressure at any one of these sites in isolation may be insufficient to produce symptoms, but there can be a summation effect as subsequent sites add their "crush" to the nerve.

A common example of crush syndrome is carpal tunnel syndrome. There may be decreased space in the carpal tunnel locally, but it may not be as marked as the symptoms suggest. There may be additional proximal symptoms that are unexplained by pressure at the carpal tunnel alone. In the cervical spine, there may be some mild degenerative changes involving the zygapophyseal joint and uncinate process that decrease the intervertebral foraminal dimensions. A superimposed FHP places the upper and midcervical spine into a resting position of extension, further compromising intervertebral foramen size. A short scalene muscle on the same side, because of a faulty respiratory pattern or the habitual crooking of a phone between head and shoulder, causes a side-flexed posture of the cervical spine and further decreases the intervertebral foramen space. At the thoracic outlet, a shortened scalene muscle can also elevate the first rib, decreasing the size of the thoracic outlet and creating another potential site of neural entrapment. A depressed scapular resting position places a traction force on the brachial plexus, which can also decrease neural conduction, and increases tension in the neuromeningeal system in the upper quadrant, which can aggravate the condition.

TREATMENT

Thorough assessment at each of the sites of entrapment can identify the impairments contributing to the condition. Treatment interventions address the impairments found at the cervical spine, thoracic spine, shoulder girdle, and wrist. If wrist dysfunction is treated in isolation, the symptoms tend to recur or change, often working their way proximally. Exercise treatment interventions for the impairment of posture are particularly useful, as is addressing the findings of neuromeningeal hypomobility.

Cervicogenic Headache

ETIOLOGY

Cervicogenic headache can be caused by two mechanisms. First, the posterior aspect of the skull, as far forward as the vertex, is supplied by the greater occipital nerve (a branch of the C2 and C3 posterior rami). Any structure supplied by the second or third cervical nerve can refer pain into that distribution. Second, the spinal nucleus of the trigeminal nerve descends into the spinal cord to at least the level of C3. Branches of the trigeminal nerve supply the mandibular, maxillary, and frontal areas of the face. Afferents from the first three or four cervical nerves converge with afferents of the trigeminal nerve. Any structure supplied by these neurologic segments can refer pain into the head and face, causing headache of cervical origin.[41]

A study by Watson and Trott[28] found an increased incidence of FHP and weakness and decreased endurance of upper cervical flexor muscles in subjects with cervical headaches compared with controls. Several studies[28,45–47] have found involvement of the upper four cervical zygapophyseal joints in patients presenting with cervicogenic headache. In another study, patients with postconcussional headache were found to have significant differences from the control group, including a trend toward a more FHP, symptomatic segmental hypomobility of the upper cervical spine, decreased endurance of the upper cervical flexor muscles, and a higher incidence of moderate muscle tightness, most commonly of the upper cervical extensor muscles. Jaeger[47] found a significant number of myofascial trigger points on the symptomatic side compared with the asymptomatic side in patients presenting with cervicogenic headache.

TREATMENT

Treatment interventions should mainly target impairments of posture and mobility. Mobility exercises may be performed as generalized ROM exercises or designed as specific articular mobilization exercises to address the segmental mobility restrictions found on manual mobility testing, most often of the upper cervical intervertebral levels (see the Hypomobility section). Specific muscle stretches, particularly for the upper cervical extensor muscles, can address the myofascial tightness and trigger points that may be contributing to the headache. Exercises to increase muscle performance and endurance of the deep upper cervical flexor muscles should be included in the exercise program.

Key Points

- The craniovertebral (CV) complex includes the atlanto-occipital (AO) and atlantoaxial (AA) joints. Ligaments include the alar, transverse, tectorial membrane, anterior and posterior AO membranes, and posterior AA ligament.
- The AO joint is a bicondylar, modified ovoid joint. It has two degrees of motion: flexion-extension and combined side flexion–rotation. The AA joint is a multijoint complex and has two degrees of motion: flexion-extension and rotation combined with a small amount of conjunct side flexion.
- The joints of the midcervical spine include the paired zygapophyseal joints, the uncovertebral (UV) joints, and the interbody joint. The important ligaments of the midcervical spine include the anterior longitudinal ligaments (ALL) and posterior longitudinal ligaments (PLL), the ligamentum flavum, the interspinous ligaments, and the ligamentum nuchae.
- Coordinated motion occurs among the joints of the midcervical spine. Each segment of the midcervical spine has two degrees of motion: flexion-extension and combined rotation–side flexion. Each joint participates in any motion.
- The cervical spine examination and evaluation consists of a patient report (subjective history) and the physical (objective) examination. The patient report should include information about the client's job, sitting position, and type of exercise performed. The physical examination includes visual observation; active and passive movement tests, including myofacial and neuromeningeal extensibility tests; manual muscle testing; neurologic tests; various special tests; and clearing tests of the thorax, shoulder girdle, and TMJ.
- Common physiologic impairments affecting the cervical spine include muscle performance impairment, posture impairment, and mobility impairment (ie, hypomobility and hypermobility).
- A therapeutic exercise program is developed to address each impairment and improve overall function of the individual.
- Disk dysfunction is a common diagnosis of the cervical spine. Impairments that are often associated with this diagnosis include mobility (ie, hypomobility and hypermobility) and posture. Another diagnosis is sprain or strain. Impairments associated with this diagnosis include mobility, posture, and muscle performance. Neural entrapment is another common diagnosis of the cervical spine, and the impairments associated with this diagnosis include mobility and posture. Cervical headache is another common diagnosis of the cervical spine, and associated impairments include mobility, posture, and muscle performance production, particularly endurance.
- For any patient presenting with a particular diagnosis, the associated impairments are identified. They must then be prioritized according to their relative importance as those requiring immediate attention and those most likely to be tolerated by the patient.

LAB ACTIVITIES

1. Consider a 35-year-old female nurse with FHP and a history of trauma to the cervical spine who presents with signs and symptoms of decreased conduction of the right C5 nerve root, deltoid weakness, decreased biceps reflex, decreased sensation of the radial aspect of forearm, and decreased ROM, most notably of right rotation and right side flexion and extension. Her right quadrant tested positive for paraesthesia of the base of the thumb. The Upper Limb Tension Test results were positive for decreased motion on right compared with the left (paraesthesia to the base of the thumb) Traction eases and compression aggravates her symptoms. A slight increase in right lateral translation at the C4-C5 intervertebral level was detected by stability testing.
   a. List some of the possible causes of the C5 root palsy.
   b. Identify the physiologic impairments that may be contributing to this problem.
   c. Design a therapeutic exercise program to improve the hypermobility impairment described for this patient. Teach your partner these exercises.
   d. What are your criteria for discharging this patient?
   e. Prescribe a home program for this patient.
2. List the posterior suboccipital muscles and state their actions. Test the strength of these individual muscles on your partner. Be aware of the recruitment of other more dominant muscles during testing.
3. Your partner plays the role of a patient at 1 week after an acceleration-deceleration injury from a skiing accident.
   a. Educate this very active patient about appropriate activity.
   b. Teach the patient appropriate breathing exercises to retrain an optimal respiratory pattern.
   c. Teach the patient the initial exercises for improvement of a postural impairment.
4. Have your partner hold the position of right scapular depression, and then test cervical rotation and side flexion ROM in each direction. Repeat the same tests with the scapula held in a position of elevation.
   a. Is there any difference in ROM between the two scapular positions?
   b. Which muscles may be implicated in restrictions of which movements?
   c. Teach your partner an exercise to increase the length of each of the muscles you have identified.

Critical Thinking Questions

1. Using the intervention model, describe at least two activities or techniques that would address the posture impairments contributing to neck pain in Case Study #7 in Unit 7. You may need to include therapeutic exercise for other physiologic impairments to resolve posture impairments related to neck pain.
2. Could neck pathology contribute to lateral forearm and interscapular pain in Case Study #8 in Unit 7?
   a. Describe this mechanism.
   b. If neck pain does contribute to lateral forearm and interscapular pain, would you expect complete resolution of pain in these regions without resolution of neck dysfunction?
   c. Using the intervention model described in Chapter 2, develop a comprehensive therapeutic exercise program for the patient's functional limitations and related impairments caused by neck dysfunction. You may need to include exercise for the shoulder girdle and thoracic spine.

REFERENCES

1. Mercer S, Bogduk N. Intra-articular inclusions of the cervical synovial joints. *Br J Rheum.* 1993;32:705–710.
2. Goel V, et al. Development of a computer model to predict strains in the individual fibres of a ligament across the ligamentous occipito-atlanto-axial (CO-C1-C2) complex. *Ann Biomed Eng.* 1992;20:667–686.
3. Koebke J, Brade H. Morphological and functional studies on the lateral joints of the first and second cervical vertebra in man. *Anat Embryol.* 1982;164:265–275.
4. Schonstrom N, et al. The lateral atlanto-axial joints and their synovial folds: an in vitro study of soft tissue injury and fractures. *J Trauma.* 1993;35:886–892.
5. Goel V, et al. Moment-rotation relationships of the ligamentous occipito-atlanto-axial complex. *J Biomech.* 1988;21:673–680.
6. Goel V, et al. Ligamentous laxity across CO-C1-C2 complex, axial torque-rotation characteristics until failure. *Spine.* 1990; 15: 990–996.
7. Oda T, et al. Three-dimensional translational movements of the upper cervical spine. *J Spinal Disord.* 1991;4:411–419.
8. Penning L, Wilmink JT. Rotation of the cervical spine. *Spine.* 1986;12:732–738.
9. Mimura M, et al. Three-dimensional motion analysis of the cervical spine with special reference to axial rotation. *Spine.* 1989;14:1135–1139.
10. Iai H, et al. Three-dimensional motion analysis of the upper cervical spine during axial rotation. *Spine.* 1993;18:2388–2392.
11. Dvorak J, Panjabi M. Functional anatomy of the alar ligaments. *Spine.* 1987;12:183–189.
12. Panjabi M, et al. Effects of alar ligament transection on upper cervical spine rotation. *J Orthop Res.* 1991;9:584–593.
13. Panjabi M, et al. Flexion, extension, and lateral bending of the upper cervical spine in response to alar ligament transections. *J Spinal Disord.* 1991;4:157–167.
14. White A, Panjabi M. *Clinical Biomechanics of the Spine.* Philadelphia: JB Lippincott; 1990.
15. Werne S. The possibilities of movement in the cranio-vertebral joints. *Acta Orthop Scand.* 1957;28:165–173.
16. Harris M, et al. Anatomical and roentenographic features of atlantooccipital instability. *J Spinal Disord.* 1993;6:5–10.
17. Hyashi K, Yabuka T. Origin of the uncus and of Luschka's joint of the cervical spine. *J Bone Joint Surg Am.* 1985;67: 788–791.
18. Milne N. The role of zygapophyseal joint orientation and uncinate processes in controlling motion in the cervical spine. *J Anat.* 1991;178:189–201.
19. Tondury G. The behaviour of the cervical disc during life. In: *Proceedings of the International Symposium on Cervical Pain.* 1971; Wennergreu Centre, Stockholm.
20. Twomey L, Taylor J. Functional and applied anatomy of the cervical spine. In: Grant R, ed. *Physical Therapy for the Cervical and Thoracic Spine.* Melbourne: Churchill Livingstone; 1994:1–25.
21. Dvorak J et al. In vivo flexion/extension of the normal cervical spine. *J Orthop Res.* 1991;9:828–834.
22. Penning L. Normal movements of the cervical spine. *Am J Roentgenol.* 1978;130:317–326.
23. Panjabi M. The stabilizing system of the spine. Part 1: Function, adaptation, and enhancement. Part 2: Neutral zone and instability hypothesis. *J Spinal Disord.* 1992;5:383–397.
24. Williams P, Warwick R. *Gray's Anatomy.* 36th ed. Philadelphia: Churchill Livingstone; 1980.
25. Jirout J. The dynamic dependence of the lower cervical vertebra on the atlanto-occipital joints. *Neuroradiology.* 1974; 7:249–252.
26. Grieve G. *Common Vertebral Joint Problems.* Edinburgh: Churchill Livingstone; 1981.
27. Vernon H, Mior S. The neck disability index: a study of reliability and validity. *J Manipulative Physiol Ther.* 1991;14, 409–415.
28. Watson D, Trott P. Cervical headache: an investigation of natural head posture and upper cervical flexor muscle performance. *Cephalgia.* 1993;13:272–282.
29. Silverman J, et al. Quantitative cervical flexor strength in healthy subjects and in subjects with mechanical neck pain. *Arch Phys Med Rehabil.* 1991;72:679–681.
30. Gogia P, Sabbahi M. Electromyographic analysis of neck muscle fatigue in patients with osteoarthritis of the cervical spine. *Spine.* 1994;19:502–506.
31. Stump J, et al. A Comparison of two modes of cervical exercise in adolescent male athletes. *J Manipulative Physiol Ther.* 1993;16:155–160.
32. Deange J. Strengthening the neck for football. *Athlet J.* 1984; Sept:46–48.
33. Leggett S, et al. Quantitative assessment and training of isometric cervical extension strength. *Am J Sport Med.* 1991; 19:653–659.
34. Pollack M, et al. Frequency and volume of resistance training: effect on cervical extension strength. *Arch Phys Med Rehabil.* 1993;74:1080–1086.
35. Highland T, et al. Changes in isometric strength and range of motion of the isolated cervical spine after eight weeks of clinical rehabilitation. *Spine.* 1992;17(suppl 6):S77–S82.
36. Hides J, et al. Evidence of lumbar multifidus muscle wasting ipsilateral to symptoms in patients with acute/subacute low back pain. *Spine.* 1994;19:165–172.
37. Janda V. Muscles and motor control in cervicogenic disorders: assessment and management. In: Grant R, ed. *Physical Therapy for the Cervical and Thoracic Spine.* Melbourne: Churchill Livingstone; 1994:195–216.
38. Treleavan J, et al. Cervical musculoskeletal dysfunction in post-concussional headache. *Cephalgia.* 1994;14:273–279.
39. Butler DS. *Mobilization of the Nervous System.* Melbourne: Churchill Livingstone; 1991.

40. Edgar D, et al. The relationship between upper trapezius muscle length and upper quadrant neural tissue extensibility. *Aust Physiother J.* 1994;40:99–103.
41. Bogduk N. Cervical causes of headache and dizziness. In: Grieves,G, ed. *Modern Manual Therapy of the Vertebral Column*. Edinburgh: Churchill Livingstone; 1986:289–302.
42. Pearson N, Walmsley R. Trial into the effects of repeated neck retractions in normal subjects. *Spine.* 1995;20:1245–1251.
43. Taylor J, et al. Road accidents and neck injuries. *Proc Australas Soc Hum Biol.* 1992;5:211–231.
44. Taylor J, Twomey L. Acute injuries to the cervical joints. *Spine.* 1993;18:1115–1122.
45. Jull G. Headaches of cervical origin. In: Grant R, ed. *Physical Therapy for the Cervical and Thoracic Spine*. Melbourne: Churchill Livingstone; 1994:261–281.
46. Jull GA. Headaches associated with the cervical spine—a clinical review. In: Grieves G, ed. *Modern Manual Therapy of the Vertebral Column*. Edinburgh: Churchill Livingstone; 1986:322–329.
47. Jaeger B. Are “cervicogenic” headaches due to myofascial pain and cervical spine dysfunction? *Cephalgia.* 1989;9:157–163.

CHAPTER 25

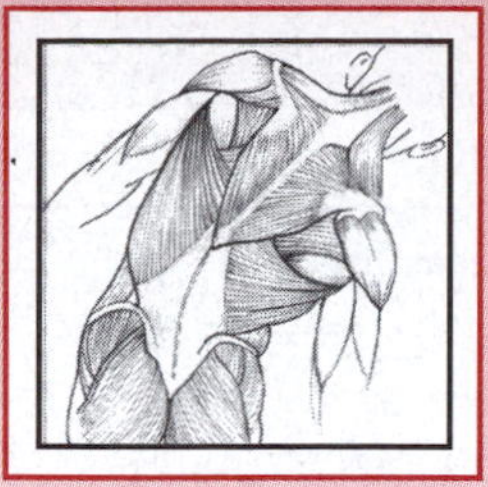

The Thoracic Spine

Sandra Rusnak-Smith and Marilyn Moffat

The thoracic spine is unique in its structure and function from the remainder of the spine because of its articulations with the sternum and ribs and its critical role in ventilation. Because the thoracic spine is located between the cervical and lumbar spine, impairments in these regions affect function of the thoracic region, and impairments in the thoracic region affect function of the surrounding spinal regions. The thoracic spine is a critical link in the kinematic chain. As a result, functions of other regions of the body (eg, shoulder girdle, hip, foot, ankle) affect function of the thoracic spine and vice versa. This chapter reviews basic anatomic and biomechanical features and presents principles and examples of therapeutic exercise prescription for common impairments and medical diagnoses affecting the thoracic region.

ANATOMY

Like the cervical and lumbar regions, the thoracic spine contains centrally placed vertebrae, each composed of a body, two pedicles, two laminae, two transverse processes, and one spinous process. Two vertebrae articulate through two zygapophyseal joints and one interbody joint. Table 25-1 describes a typical thoracic vertebra (Fig. 25-1).[1–5] In the thoracic region, 5 of the 12 vertebrae are considered atypical: T1 and T9 through T12. Each of these atypical vertebra possesses certain characteristics, as listed in Table 25-2.

The sternum is another unique feature of the thoracic region. It is composed of a manubrium, body, and xiphoid process (Fig. 25-2). The suprasternal notch is located at the center of the uppermost border of the manubrium. A clavicular notch on each side of the manubrium is where the sternal end of the clavicle joins the manubrium. Immediately below the clavicular notch, the costal cartilage of the first rib is fused to the manubrium. The point where the manubrium joins the body is the manubriosternal joint, and it is at this level where the second ribs articulate with the sternum. The third through sixth costal cartilages articulate with the side of the body of the sternum. The lower end of the body joins with the xiphoid process.

The most apparent difference of the thoracic region from the remainder of the spine is the group of 12 ribs and their articulations. The 12 pairs of ribs have several functions:

- To protect the heart, lungs, and great vessels against trauma
- To provide attachment for skeletal and respiratory muscles
- To facilitate postural alignment and upper extremity function

Ribs 3 through 9 are considered typical, and ribs 1, 2, and 10 through 12 are considered atypical. Each rib has a head, neck, tubercle, and body (ie, shaft) (Fig. 25-3). The head of the rib has two articular facets for articulation with the numerically corresponding vertebra and superior vertebra. The typical rib has two costovertebral articulations that join the typical rib with the bodies of the vertebrae above and below by means of demifacet joints. The rib is also connected to the intervening annulus of the intervertebral disk through a strong ligamentous attachment (Fig. 25-4). The costotransverse articulation joins the tubercle of the rib with the transverse process of the numerically corresponding vertebra. For example, rib 3 attaches by its

- Upper facet to the inferior demifacet (costovertebral joint) of T2
- Lower facet to the superior demifacet (costovertebral joint) of T3
- Strong ligamentous attachment to the intervertebral disk between T2 and T3
- Costotransverse articulation to the transverse process of T3

The anterior articulations of the ribs are called the costochondral joints. The costal cartilages, composed of hyaline cartilage, greatly enhance mobility of the ribs.[6,7] Ribs 1 through 7 are called true ribs because they articulate

Table 25-1. TYPICAL THORACIC VERTEBRAE

ANATOMIC SITE	DESCRIPTION	CLINICAL SIGNIFICANCE
Body and intervertebral joint	The ratio of disk height to vertebral body height is less in the thoracic spine than in the cervical or lumbar regions. The ratio of disk diameter to disk height is two to three times higher in the thoracic spine than in the lumbar spine. There is an acute angular orientation of the lamellae of the anulus and a relatively small nucleus pulposus.	Creates stiffness and stability
Spinous processes	Slope inferiorly and overlap the spinous processes of the adjacent inferior vertebrae	Limit extension
Transverse processes	On the ventral aspect, a facet articulates with the tubercle of the rib to form the costotransverse joint. In the upper and middle thoracic spine (T1-T6), this facet is concave, corresponding to a convex tubercle on the neck of the rib. In the lower thoracic region (T7-T10), this facet is planar.	The shape of the upper and middle thoracic costotransverse joints restricts motion of the rib in rotation about an axis parallel to and through the neck of the rib. The shape of the lower thoracic costotransverse joint allows the rib greater flexibility of motion during respiration and motion of the thorax.
Facets	Orientation of the zygapophyseal facets depends on the region of the thorax. Except for T1, T11, T12, the posterolateral corners of the superior and inferior aspects of the vertebral body contain an ovoid demifacet.	Zygapophyseal facet orientation guides and restricts mobility. Demifacets articulate with the head of the rib at the costovertebral joint. Development of the costovertebral joint is delayed until early adolescence, contributing to the flexibility of the young thorax.

with the sternum through their costal cartilage. Rib length increases from rib 1 through 7. Ribs 8 through 10 are classified as false ribs because they are attached to the sternum through the costal cartilage of the rib immediately above.[8–10] Rib length decreases from rib 8 through 10. Ribs 11 and 12 are classified as floating ribs because they do not attach to the sternum or costal cartilages at their distal ends.

Numerous ligaments stabilize the thoracic vertebral segment and rib articulations (see Fig. 25-4). Other sources can provide more information about the function of each ligamentous structure, which are critical in contributing to stability of the respective articulation.[2,6,7,11]

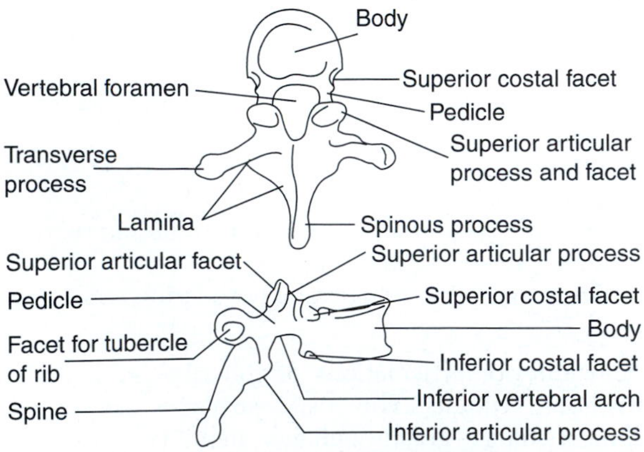

FIGURE 25-1 A typical thoracic vertebra.

Numerous muscles control movement of the thoracic spine and the process of respiration. The movements that they produce or assist with are categorized in Table 25-3.[6,8,12]

BIOMECHANICS

The thoracic region is less flexible and more stable than the cervical region because of the limitations imposed by structural elements such as the rib cage, spinous processes, zygapophyseal joints, and the dimensions of the vertebral bodies (see Table 25-1). Ribs 1 through 10 articulate with the vertebral column by two synovial joints posteriorly, the costovertebral and the costotransverse, and with the manubriosternum anteriorly. The joints therefore form a closed kinematic chain. The closed chain relationship means the segments are interdependent, and motion is more restricted. Ribs 11 and 12 form an open kinematic chain and are less restricted. These ribs are free to move in any direction because they have no anterior articulations. All motions are possible in the thoracic region, but the magnitude depends on the segmental level.

Range of Motion

The range of motion (ROM) for the thoracic spine is given in Table 25-4.[13]

Table 25-2. CHARACTERISTICS OF THE FIVE ATYPICAL THORACIC VERTEBRAE

VERTEBRAL LEVEL	CHARACTERISTICS
First thoracic vertebra	Superior costal facets are circular to articulate with the entire head of the first rib. Spinous process is horizontal and is as long and prominent as C7.
Ninth thoracic vertebra	The inferior costal facets are absent, and there is no direct articulation with the 10th ribs.
Tenth thoracic vertebra	The inferior costal facets are absent, and there is no direct articulation with the 11th ribs.
Eleventh thoracic vertebra	It articulates only with the heads of the 11th ribs. The transverse processes are small and do not have articular facets for the tubercles of the ribs.
Twelfth thoracic vertebra	It possesses only two costal facets for the 12th ribs. The body, transverse processes, and inferior facets are similar to those of the lumbar vertebrae.

- Flexion and extension are more limited in the upper thoracic region, where the facets lie closer to the frontal plane.
- Lateral flexion remains similar throughout but increases in the lower thoracic region.
- Rotation is more limited in the lower thoracic region, where the facets lie closer to the sagittal plane.

Osteokinematics and Arthrokinematics of Thoracic Motion

Flexion occurs in the sagittal plane during forward bending of the trunk and during the exhalation phase of respiration. The total osetokinematic range of flexion is 20 to 45 degrees.[13] During flexion, the articular facets of the superior vertebra glide upward and forward on the inferior partner.[14] Flexion is coupled with anterior translation. The posterior longitudinal ligament, ligamentum flavum, interspinous ligament, supraspinous ligament, and the capsular ligaments limit flexion.

The ROM of extension in the thoracic spine is 20 to 45 degrees.[13] Extension also occurs in the sagittal plane, but with backward bending, elevation of both arms, and during the inspiration phase of respiration. Extension is coupled with posterior translation. The articular and spinous processes limit extension. During extension, the anterior longitudinal ligament is taut, and the posterior longitudinal ligament, ligamentum flavum, and the interspinous ligament are relaxed.

Lateral flexion of the thoracic spine occurs in the frontal plane and is approximately 20 to 40 degrees.[13] As the thorax bends toward the right, the ribs on the right approximate, and the ribs on the left separate at their lateral margins. Rotation occurs about the transverse plane and is approximately 35 to 50 degrees in each direction.[13] Although lateral flexion and rotation are coupled motions in the thoracic spine, the coupled motions depend on which motion is introduced first. Lee[2] states that, if lateral flexion is performed about the frontal plane, it is accompanied by contralateral rotation, whereas if rotation is performed about the transverse plane, it is accompanied by ipsilateral rotation. Lee[1] explained these proposed mechanics elsewhere. The in vivo osteokinematics and arthrokinematics of the ribs have not been well studied. Clinical hypotheses about the specific mechanics of these joints are beyond the scope of this text, but other sources can provide information on the topic.[1] The mechanics of the articulations of the ribs follow certain principles[6,7,15]:

- Rotation of the neck of the rib about its long axis occurs at the costotransverse articulations of the upper six or seven ribs.
- Gliding occurs at the costotransverse articulations of the seventh or eighth to tenth ribs.
- A hinge type of movement occurs at the manubriosternal joint, which is a symphysis.
- Movement occurs at the xiphisternal joint until about age 40, when it usually becomes a synostosis, but it can remain ununited.

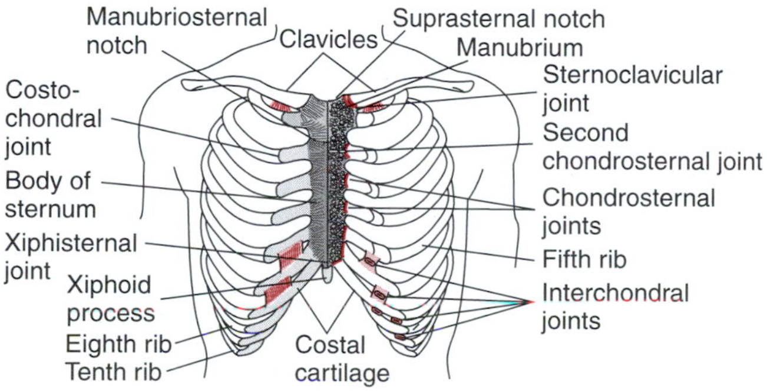

FIGURE 25-2 An anterior view of the articulations of the rib cage. The shaded areas indicate costal cartilage. The costal cartilages join the ribs at the costochondral joints. Interchondral joints may also exist between the fifth through ninth costal cartilages. (From Norkin CC, Levangie PK. *Joint Structure and Function: A Comprehensive Analysis*. 2d ed. Philadelphia: FA Davis; 1992.)

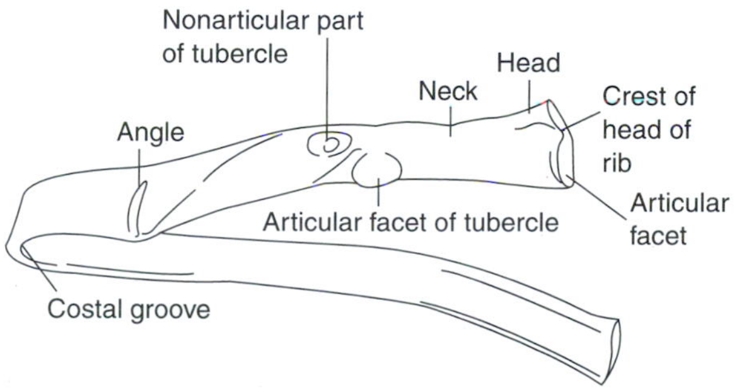

FIGURE 25-3 A typical rib.

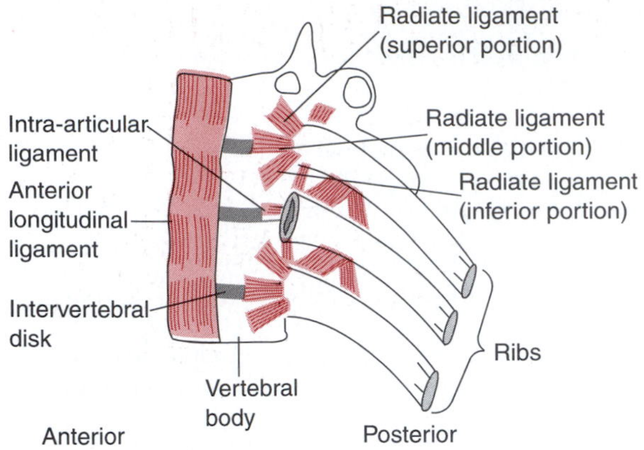

FIGURE 25-4 A lateral view of the costovertebral joint and ligaments. The three bands of the radiate ligament reinforce the costovertebral joint. The superior and inferior portions of the radiate ligament attach to the capsular ligament (removed) and to the vertebral body. The middle portion of the radiate ligament attaches to the intervertebral disk. The middle of the illustration demonstrates the costovertebral joint with the radiate ligament and capsule removed to show the intra-articular ligament, which attaches the head of the rib to the annulus.

- A small amount of movement occurs in the sixth to the eighth and, in some cases, the ninth and tenth interchondral joints, but they may become fibrous and fuse in later life.

Respiration

The rhythmic movements of respiration cause changes in the size and shape of the thorax.[6,16] The thoracic cavity may be increased in its transverse, anteroposterior, and vertical dimensions. The anteroposterior diameter of the thoracic cavity is increased by the elevation of the shaft of the rib, the forward and upward thrust of the rib, and the minimal movement occurring at the sternal angle. The transverse diameter is increased by the rib rotation and the elevation of the ribs posteriorly. Contraction of the diaphragm increases the vertical dimension of the thoracic cavity.

During inhalation and exhalation, the primary rib movements have been described as pump handle and bucket handle movements (Fig. 25-5). Pump handle movement is the result of the anterior aspect of a rib moving superiorly. Bucket handle movement is the result of the lateral aspect of the rib moving superiorly. During exhalation, the anterior and lateral aspect of the rib move inferiorly.

EXAMINATION AND EVALUATION

A comprehensive examination, including the history, systems review, and tests and measures, is to be performed for all patients; the findings enable the physical therapist to determine the diagnosis (based whenever possible on impairments, functional limitations, and disabilities), prognosis, and interventions.[2,17] The physical therapist must follow an organized, sequential approach to avoid omitting crucial information that may prevent an accurate interpretation of the findings.

History

For individuals with impairments, functional limitations, or disabilities related to the thoracic spine, a detailed history must be taken to determine the nature and extent of the dysfunction. Clinically relevant information must be obtained through this process, which necessitates good listening skills and skill in asking questions to promote open communication in an effective, efficient manner. Because the thoracic region is a referral site for many systemic problems (see Appendix 1), questions should be tailored to elicit information that may offer insight about the patient's condition. In obtaining the history, which in part can take place by questionnaire, the therapist should seek information about all of the following:

- Age
- Demographics
- Current condition
- Subjective report of pain, including location, description (eg, pain scales),[18,19] frequency and duration, and precipitating or alleviating factors
- Current and previous occupations
- Living environment
- Functional status or level of activity (eg, self-report measure of disability)[19]
- Social habits
- Family history
- Medical history, including general health status, nutritional status, medications, and pertinent surgical history
- Results of laboratory, radiographic, neurologic, or other tests

Systems Review

A systems review provides a quick screen of the pertinent systems. If problems are observed during this review, more detailed tests should be done as the next phase of the examination process.

Information about disorders of other systems (eg, cardiopulmonary, genitourinary, gastrointestinal) that may mimic thoracic musculoskeletal disorders should be obtained during the medical history portion of the examination. For example, a systems review of the cardiopulmonary system includes screens of the lungs (eg, respiratory rate, breath sounds), heart (eg, heart rate, heart sounds), and blood pressure.

A systems review of the skeletal system is also called a scan examination. The scan examination is a quick procedure that includes tests and measures listed in Display 25-1. Because the thoracic spine spans the upper and lower quadrants, screens of both regions are advisable, particularly as they relate to the transitional zones (ie, C7-T1 and T12-L1). Chapter 24 provides a more detailed explanation of the upper quadrant scan examination, and Chapter 18 explains the lower quadrant scan examination.

Tests and Measures

The next step in the examination process is the selection of one or more tests and measures to ascertain the impairments, functional limitations, and disabilities of the patient. This determination leads to the development of the diagnosis and the prognosis, which can guide the physical therapist's

Table 25-3. MYOLOGY OF THE THORACIC SPINE

MOVEMENT	MUSCLE
Extension	Spinalis capitis, cervicis, thoracic Longissimus thoracis (bilateral) Iliocostalis thoracis (bilateral) Semispinalis thoracis (bilateral) Rotatores thoracis (bilateral) Multifidus (bilateral) Interspinales
Flexion	Levatores costarum Rectus abdominis (bilateral) Internal obliques (bilateral) External obliques (bilateral)
Lateral flexion	Longissimus thoracic (unilateral, ipsilateral) Iliocostalis thoracis (unilateral, ipsilateral) Semispinalis thoracis (unilateral, contralateral) Multifidus (unilateral, contralateral) Intertransversarii (unilateral, ipsilateral) Levatores costarum
Rotation	Iliocostalis thoracis (unilateral, ipsilateral) Semispinalis thoracis (unilateral, contralateral) Rotatores thoracis (unilateral, ipsilateral) Multifidus (unilateral, contralateral) Intertransversarii (ipsilateral) Internal oblique (unilateral, ipsilateral) External oblique (unilateral, contralateral) Levatores costarum
Rib depression	Longissimus thoracis (bilateral) Iliocostalis lumborum (bilateral)—lower ribs
Rib elevation	Iliocostalis cervicis (bilateral)—upper ribs
Viscera compression	Transversus abdominis
Respiration	Diaphragm (inspiration) Intercostals (inspiration and expiration) Rectus abdominis (expiration) Internal/external obliques (expiration) Transversus abdominis (expiration)
Accessory muscles of respiration	
Inspiration	Levatores costarum Pectoralis major Pectoralis minor Rhomboids Anterior, medial, posterior scalenes Serratus anterior Serratus posterior superior Sternocleidomastoid Subclavius Thoracic erector spinae Trapezius
Expiration	Iliocostalis lumborum Transversus thoracis
Inspiration/expiration	Latissimus dorsi Quadratus lumborum Serratus posterior inferior
Maintenance of rib cage shape	Intercostals

Table 25-4. RANGE OF MOTION OF THE THORACIC SPINE

INTERSPACE	COMBINED FLEXION AND EXTENSION (LIMITS OF RANGE IN DEGREES)	UNILATERAL LATERAL FLEXION (LIMITS OF RANGE IN DEGREES)	UNILATERAL AXIAL ROTATION (LIMITS OF RANGE IN DEGREES)
T1-T2	3–5	5	14
T2-T3	3–5	5–7	4–12
T3-T4	2–5	3–7	5–11
T4-T5	2–5	5–6	5–11
T5-T6	3–5	5–6	5–11
T6-T7	2–7	6	4–11
T7-T8	3–8	3–8	4–11
T8-T9	3–8	4–7	6–7
T9-T10	3–8	4–7	3–5
T10-T11	4–14	3–10	2–3
T11-T12	6–20	4–13	2–3
T12-L1	6–20	5–10	2–3

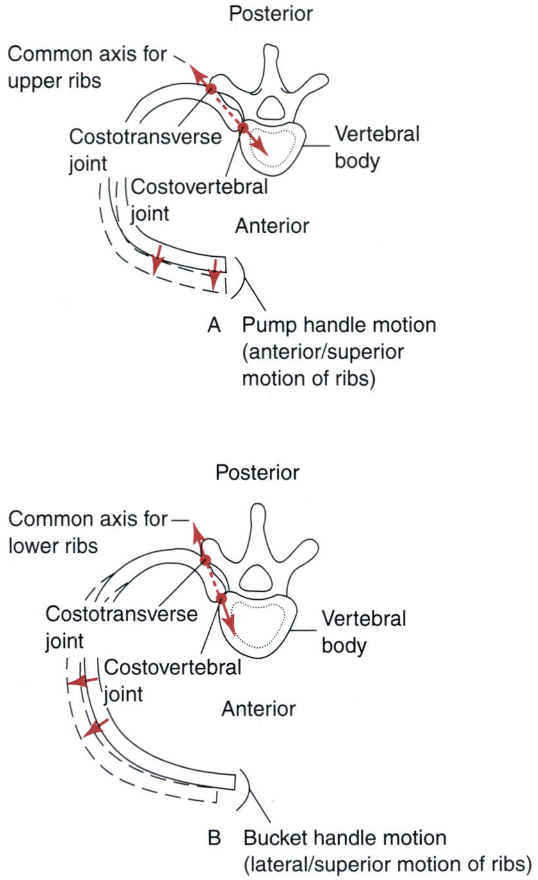

FIGURE 25-5 Pump and bucket handle motions of the ribs during inspiration. ***(A)*** The arrow represents the common axis of motion for the upper ribs, which is close to the frontal plane. The upper ribs move upward and forward in a pump handle motion. ***(B)*** The axis of the lower ribs lies closer to the sagittal plane. The upward and lateral motion of these ribs is referred to as bucket handle motion. (From Norkin CC, Levangie PK. *Joint Structure and Function: A Comprehensive Analysis*. 2d ed. Philadelphia: FA Davis; 1992:183.)

selection of interventions. The following tests and measures depend on the results of the history and systems review.

Posture Assessment

- Assess posture of the thoracic region, particularly as it relates to the head and neck and lumbar-pelvic-hip complex in standing, sitting, and recumbent positions. Often, improving posture of the associated regions improves the posture of the thoracic spine. If you make a correction in the thoracic posture, and the symptoms change, this result is an initial step in determining the pathomechanics correlating with symptoms.
- Detect signs of asymmetry because of the high incidence of acquired or structural scoliosis.

DISPLAY 25-1

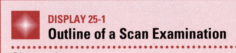

Outline of a Scan Examination

Observation
Range of motion
Motor assessment
Sensory assessment
Vascular status
Reflexes
Palpation
Clearing tests
- Upper quadrant (see Chapters 24 and 26)
  - Foraminal encroachment
  - Compression or distraction
  - Upper limb tension test (ulnar bias may indicate upper thoracic pathology)
  - Thoracic outlet syndrome tests
- Lower quadrant (see Chapters 18 and 20)
  - Prone knee bend (may indicate low thoracic pathology)
  - Straight-leg raising
  - Slump test
  - hip flexion, abduction, external rotation (FABER)
  - Scour test

- Assess the ergonomics of the work station(s), which can provide vital information regarding the pathomechanics of the condition.

Aerobic Capacity and Endurance Tests and Measures

- Assessment of vital signs may be necessary, particularly in working with patients with a diagnosis of cardiopulmonary disease.
- Assessment of respiration is of particular importance for thoracic spine patients. Although the rate of breathing is important, the quality of breathing is crucial in patients with thoracic spine dysfunction. In addition to observing for proper pump and bucket handle motions of the rib cage, specific testing of osteokinematic function of the ribs can be assessed during inhalation and exhalation.[2]

Gait and Balance Tests and Measures

- Assess movement of the thoracic spine and rib cage.
- Assess how movements of other regions of the kinematic chain are affecting movement of the thoracic spine and rib cage.

Mobility Tests and Measures

- Active osteokinematic movements include flexion, extension, lateral flexion, rotation, and combined movements of rotation with ipsilateral lateral flexion and lateral flexion with contralateral rotation. Assess for quality and quantity of motion in general and segmentally.
- Passive osteokinematic movement testing can be more sensitive for assessing restrictive barriers to movement or hypermobility and instability. In addition to cardinal-plane testing, coupled lateral flexion–rotation motion testing and three-dimensional testing (ie, lateral flexion coupled with contralateral rotation in flexion or extension) can be performed.
- Passive arthrokinematic testing for the zygapophyseal, costotransverse, sternocostal, and sternochondral joints is performed to detect hypomobility or hypermobility and to provoke symptoms.[2]
- Tests of muscle length should be included as needed. For example, if specific articular function is normal, and mobility is limited, muscular extensibility can affect mobility of the thoracic spine. A stiff or short right external and left internal oblique can limit right thoracic rotation.
- Unilateral upper extremity elevation can assess mobility of the upper thoracic region. For example, upper thoracic extension and rotation to the ipsilateral side should accompany upper extremity arm elevation.[2]
- Cervical spine, lumbar spine, and hip mobility should be tested to look for mobility impairments in associated regions that may affect thoracic function. For example, stiff hip and lumbar flexion may promote excessive thoracic flexion.

Muscle Performance Tests and Measures

- The upper and lower quadrant scan examinations test motor function of pertinent cervicothoracic and thoracolumbar innervated muscles. These scan examinations should exclude or confirm possible joint dysfunction or nerve root dysfunction as sources of impaired muscle performance.
- Motor function of the intercostal nerves is examined by observing and palpating the intercostal muscles.
- Assessment of the back extensor, abdominal, and shoulder girdle muscle performance should be included in a thoracic examination. Chapters 18 and 26 discuss trunk and shoulder girdle muscle performance testing. Tests should look for imbalances in muscle performance between synergists and agonist–antagonist relationships. Hypotheses can be generated about how impairments in muscle performance of these regions may impact the function of the thoracic region.

Pain Tests and Disability Measures

- Although there are no specific pain or disability tests or measures for the thoracic spine, those for the cervical and lumbar spine can be used as indicated (ie, upper versus lower thoracic regional involvement) to gain insight into the condition's effect on the patient's life (see Chapters 24 and 18).

Sensory Integrity Tests and Measures

- Sensory testing for the relevant cervicothoracic and thoracolumbar regions is performed during the upper and lower quadrant scan examinations.
- Sensory function of the intercostal nerves is examined by testing skin sensation in the intercostal spaces. Altered sensation may be found, although it is rarely a primary complaint.
- Special tests such as those for thoracic outlet syndrome and neural tension are performed during the upper and lower quadrant scan examinations.
- A modification of the slump test can detect segmental neural dysfunction of the thorax. At the end of the slump, the patient rotates the thorax to the right and left to relieve or increase neural tension in the thoracic region.[2]

Functional Movement Testing

- Observation of the activities of daily living and the patient's occupational and recreational movement patterns can reveal impairments in movement in the thoracic and related regions. For example, insufficient hip and thoracic rotation can promote excessive thoracic flexion and lateral flexion as compensatory movements when a person is reaching across the body.
- Alteration of impaired movement patterns and the associated change in symptoms is another stage of determining the pathomechanics of the symptoms. For example, in the case of compensatory thoracic flexion and lateral flexion because of reduced hip and thoracic motion, the movement should be altered by teaching the patient to rotate the hip and thoracic spine to the limit of mobility while thoracic flexion and lateral flexion are restricted. This is achieved manually by the therapist or by the patient who is able to make the change from verbal instruction. If the symptoms are reduced, the flexion or lateral flexion movement patterns are assumed to be contributing to the symptoms.

Other Tests and Measures

- Radiographic tests and measures may be necessary for the diagnosis and curve angle measurements of scol-

iosis, Scheuermann's disease, and kyphosis related to osteoporosis.
- Radiographic tests are necessary for the diagnosis of disk pathology. The findings of radiographic testing must be correlated with the findings of the clinical examination if the significance is to be understood.
- Additional medical screening may be necessary to exclude or confirm possible systemic or visceral sources of symptoms (see Appendix 1).

THERAPEUTIC EXERCISE INTERVENTIONS FOR COMMON PHYSIOLOGIC IMPAIRMENTS

Carrie M. Hall

Therapeutic exercise interventions for the thoracic spine include activities and techniques that address impairments directly related to the function of the thoracic spine and others that address impairments in related areas that indirectly affect the function of the thoracic spine. Related regions include the cervical spine, the shoulder girdle, and the lumbopelvic region. Comprehensive treatment of functional limitations and impairments of the thoracic spine requires treatment of these related regions.

Mobility Impairment

Impairment of mobility of the thoracic spine can span the continuum from hypomobility to hypermobility. Because of the unique structure of the thoracic spine, numerous joints and soft tissues influence mobility in this region. The thoracic region differs from the cervical and lumbar regions of the spine in that its spinal mechanics are directly influenced by the attachment of the ribs and sternum. The motion available in a particular region of the thoracic spine also is influenced by the changing orientation of facet planes. A more coronal facet orientation in the upper thoracic spine allows greater range of axial rotation, and a more sagittal orientation at the thoracolumbar junction allows a greater range of flexion and extension.

Myofascial tissues of the anterior and posterior trunk, rib cage, cervical spine, and shoulder girdle regions can also influence thoracic mobility. Disease and disorders such as osteoporosis, scoliosis, Scheuermann's disease, ankylosing spondylitis, and degenerative joint disease can influence thoracic mobility. The thoracic spine is located between the cervical spine, shoulder girdle, and lumbar-pelvic-hip region. Mobility of these related regions influences mobility of the thoracic spine.

HYPERMOBILITY

Macrotrauma to the thorax, such as a rotational injury or direct blow to the chest, can result in hypermobility or instability of the thoracic vertebrae or rib articulations or both. Impairments in habitual posture and repetitive movement can lead to hypermobility and, if left untreated, instability of the thoracic spine. Therapeutic exercise intervention for hypermobility of the thoracic spine must consider the mechanism or cause of the hypermobility. If the cause is impairments in habitual posture or repetitive movement, the clinician must consider the integrated relationship between the foot and ankle, pelvic girdle, trunk, and upper extremity in developing a plan of intervention. If the cause is macrotrauma and the expected healing time has been surpassed, the clinician must consider issues contributing to delayed or interrupted healing.

Regardless of the mechanism or cause of the hypermobility, central to the success of a program to improve stability of the thoracic spine is the concept that the trunk muscles must hold the vertebral column stable for independent upper and lower extremity movement to occur. This role must be executed regardless of the speed of movement and any additional load the individual may be carrying. Loads must be transferred from the ground upward in an efficient manner, and this can be done without cumulative microtrauma only if the forces are attenuated through an efficient kinematic chain from the foot and ankle upward through to the thoracic spine. The functions of the foot, ankle, knee, hip, pelvic girdle, and lumbar spine must be considered in optimizing ground reaction forces transmitted to the thoracic spine.

Intervention for hypermobility begins at the stability stage of motor control. The patient is instructed to hold the spine in ideal alignment during movements of the upper and lower extremity. The activity or technique chosen depends largely on the level of intensity the patient can sustain while maintaining ideal alignment with proper recruitment patterns. The prescribed direction of force imposed on the spine depends on the direction of the hypermobility. For example, a patient may present with difficulty in stabilizing against flexion forces such that, when the arm is lowered from a flexed position, the thoracic spine flexes instead of remaining in neutral alignment. A flexion force such as resisted (in some cases, from the weight of the arm) or rapid upper extremity extension (from an overhead start position) can be used to challenge the spinal extensors (Fig. 25-6). Standing is a high level of posture control, so the exercise can be modified to sitting with the back against the wall or supine (see Fig. 25-6). These latter positions require stabilization of fewer regions than standing (ie, sitting eliminates the need to stabilize the foot, ankle, knee, and hips), and the wall or floor provides proprioceptive feedback to enhance

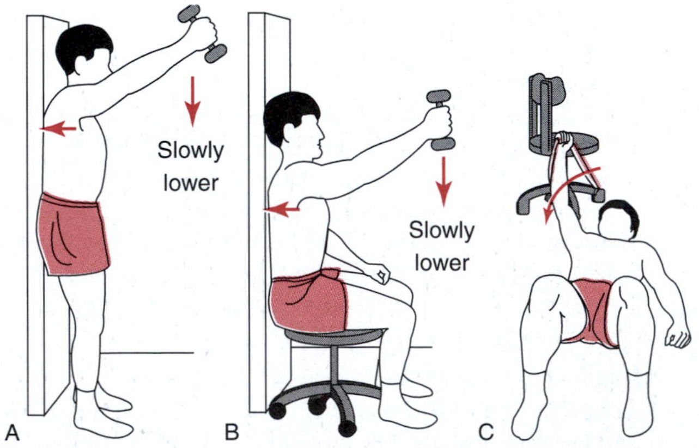

FIGURE 25-6 Activity promoting strength of the thoracic spine extensors in the short range in various start positions. ***(A)*** Standing upper extremity extension from a flexed position. ***(B)*** Sitting with back against a wall during upper extremity extension from a flexed position. ***(C)*** Supine, resisted upper extremity extension from a flexed position

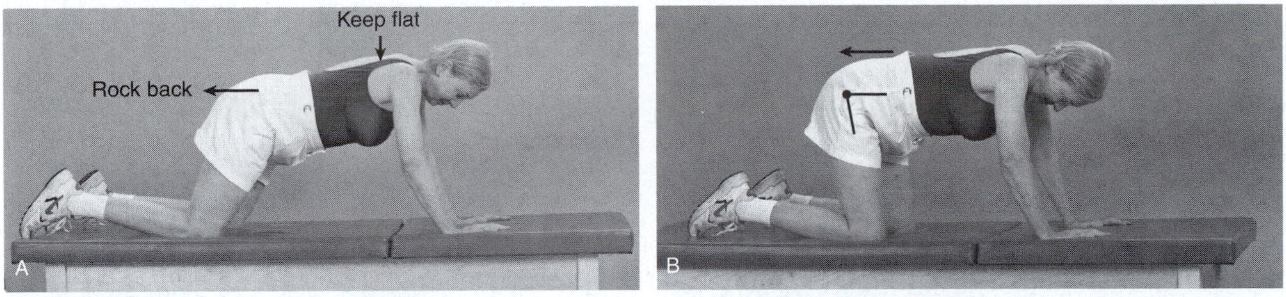

FIGURE 25-7 In four-point kneeling, the patient is instructed to maintain neutral spine position while rocking back toward the heels ***(A*** and ***B)***. At the point of hip flexion stiffness, the tendency is to flex in the lumbar or thoracic spine. The patient is instructed to stop at the onset of spine flexion.

stabilization. Similar principles can be used in creating exercises to stabilize against rotational or lateral flexion forces.

Difficulty stabilizing against flexion forces is a common problem for the thoracic spine. The therapist must consider that excessive thoracic flexion may occur because of lack of mobility in related regions. For example, decreased hip flexion mobility may be compensated for by thoracic flexion with forward-reaching or forward-bending movements. Four-point kneeling with a sit-back movement (Fig. 25-7) can promote hip flexion mobility and thoracic spine stability. This movement pattern must eventually be transferred to controlled mobility and skill level activities in sitting and standing positions, such as reaching forward with hip flexion while maintaining neutral spine position (Fig. 25-8).

Gymnastic balls, foam rolls, and balance boards can modify stabilization activities to provide a greater challenge by destabilizing the base of support (Fig. 25-9). The theory behind the use of these pieces of equipment is that the labile base of support stimulates balance and equilibrium reactions. Continuous postural adjustments are required, facilitating smooth coordination of posture and movement. Care must be taken to ensure that proper stabilization strategies are employed when using equipment that destabilizes the base of support.

Another common cause of excessive thoracic spine motion is lack of thoracic and hip rotation combined with excessive shoulder girdle protraction. For example, in cross-body reaching tasks, the elbow extends and the shoulder flexes and horizontally adducts until the full length of the arm has been reached. If further reach is required, the thoracic spine should rotate, followed by hip joint flexion and rotation, and if standing, a step toward the object can increase the reach span. A prevalent faulty movement pattern is to reach instead with scapular abduction and thoracic flexion (Fig. 25-10). The arm can effectively reach across the body if the scapula provides a stable base for arm movement and the thorax provides a stable base for the shoulder girdle. This movement requires appropriate recruitment and length-tension properties of the scapulothoracic, glenohumeral, spinal extensor, and deep abdominal muscles. There must be ample mobility in the glenohumeral joint for upper extremity horizontal adduction and in the thoracic spine and hip joints for rotation. Impairments in the shoulder girdle, thorax, and hips may need to be addressed separately to improve the movement pattern of cross-body reaching and thereby reduce the tendency toward excessive thoracic flexion. One useful activity to retrain independent motion among the upper extremity, thoracic spine, and hip

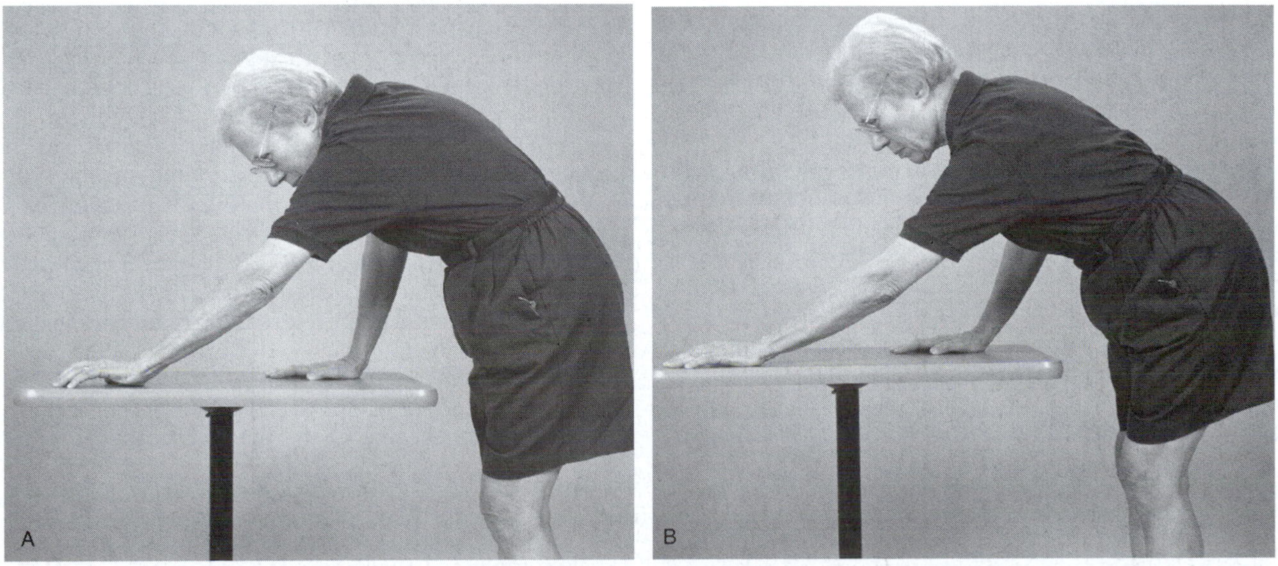

FIGURE 25-8 ***(A)*** The standing subject reaches forward with excessive thoracic flexion. ***(B)*** The movement pattern is altered such that flexion takes place at the hips, knees, and shoulder, and the thoracic spine remains in neutral.

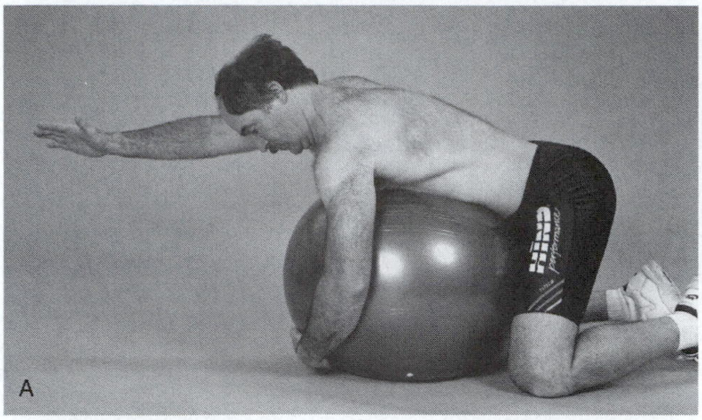

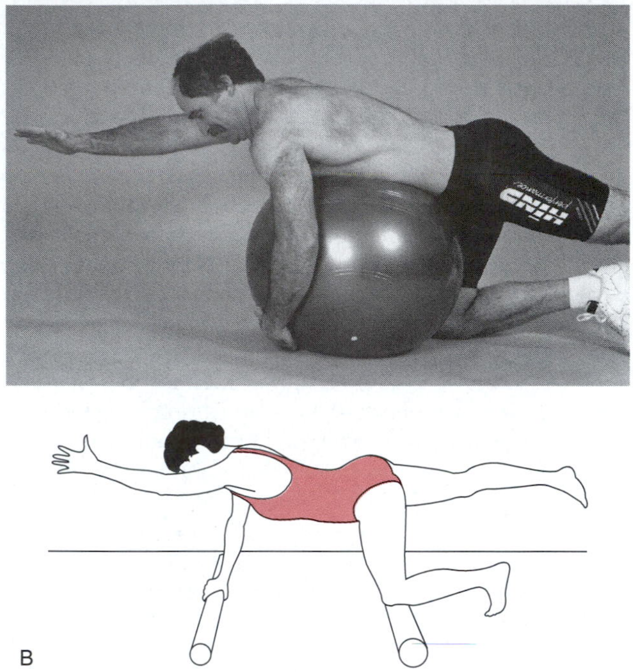

FIGURE 25-9 *(A)* These exercises use the labile surface of the gymnastic ball to stimulate balance and equilibrium reactions. *(B)* The foam rolls further destabilize the base of support.

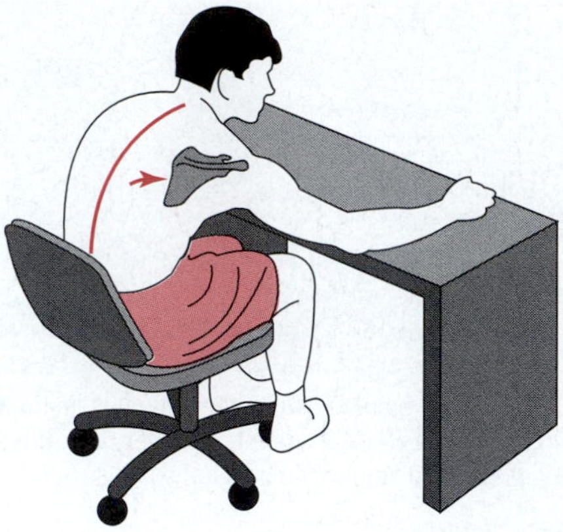

FIGURE 25-10 A prevalent movement pattern is to reach with scapular abduction and thoracic flexion.

joints is shown in Self-Management: Cross-body Reaching. The prerequisites for correct performance of this exercise are proper movement patterns at the scapulothoracic, glenohumeral, and hip joints (see Chapter 26).

Treatment of hypermobility in the thoracic spine may also include supportive devices such as a posture brace (to prevent thoracic flexion) (Fig. 25-11) and taping. Taping can be used to prevent excessive flexion and rotation (Fig. 25-12).

HYPOMOBILITY

Loss of mobility in the thoracic spine is most commonly found in the direction of extension and in one direction of lateral flexion and rotation, which, depending on which movement is introduced first, may be coupled in the same direction or opposite directions. Hypomobility can result from pain or altered tone, restrictions in neural or dural mobility, trauma inducing osteokinematic restriction, degenerative joint changes, disease processes, or generalized stiffness in the joints or myofascial tissues from self-induced or externally induced immobility. Self-induced immobilization can result from pain or repetitive altered movement patterns. Repetitive altered movement patterns can produce sites and directions of relative mobility and concurrent sites and directions of hypomobility. For example, the movement strategy of scapular abduction and thoracic flexion to reach across the body can lead to hypomobility in thoracic rotation.

When hypomobility in the thoracic spine results from osteokinematic restriction, the cause may be articular, myofascial, or both. If the joint is truly hypomobile, the associated arthrokinematic glide is restricted. If the myofascia is the source of the restriction, the joint glide is normal. Treatment of joint restrictions usually require joint mobilization techniques, and treatment of myofascial tissue requires passive stretching, active ROM exercises, or both. Patients with long-standing joint restriction are likely to develop myofascial restrictions, requiring concurrent types of intervention. To maintain mobility gained with joint mobilization techniques, it is important to teach the patient a self-management exercise that includes a passive stretch, active ROM exercise, or both. Functional movement patterns should be instructed to reinforce the mobility gained with the mobilization and specific exercise.

A clinical example may best illustrate this point. A patient presents with left rotation and left lateral flexion restrictions in the thoracic spine at the T7 segmental level. The examination determines that this restriction as articular. The appropriate joint mobilization technique is performed to restore the arthrokinematic glide.[2,17] To maintain the mobility gained, the patient is instructed to perform specific midthoracic lateral flexion, blocking motion at the relatively hypermobile segments below T7, to facilitate motion at the stiff segmental level (Fig. 25-13). Repeated thoracic left rotation can also be instructed (Fig. 25-14). The patient should be instructed to use left rotation of the thoracic spine frequently throughout the day to further facilitate maintenance of articular mobility. All exercises should be done with high repetitions (up to 20 times) and frequently throughout the day (up to 10 times) in the pain-free range to prevent aggravation of symptoms.

Restrictions in oblique abdominal muscle length can limit thoracic rotation. In the case of myofascial restriction in the absence of articular hypomobility, correlating articular glides are normal, but osteokinematic motion is limited in rotation. Restriction in right rotation can indicate short or stiff right

SELF-MANAGEMENT: Cross-body Reaching

Purpose: To promote independent motion of the shoulder joint from the shoulder blade, torso, and hip. You should not progress to the next level without mastering the previous level. Use the movement pattern acquired in Level 4 when reaching across the body for an object farther away than the span of the arm. Avoid reaching by moving your shoulder blade or flexing in your thoracic spine excessively.

Starting position: Stand with feet about 2 inches away from the wall and the pelvis and spine in neutral. If your hip flexors are short or stiff, you may need to flex your hips and knees to achieve a neutral spine and pelvis position.

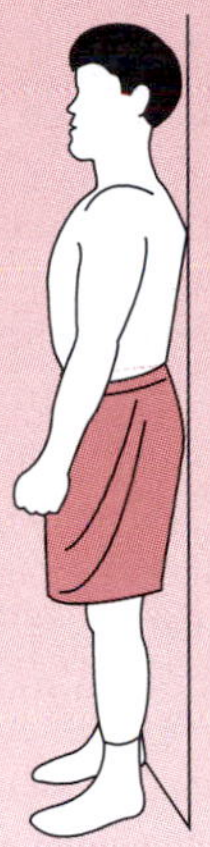

Movement technique: **Level 1:** Move your arm across your body to the midline without letting your shoulder blade move from its starting position. This may require a submaximal contraction of your interscapular muscles.

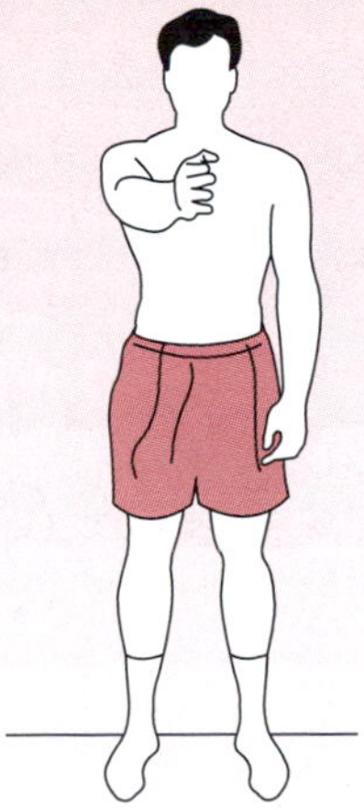

Level 2: After you can reach your arm to the midline of your body, rotate your torso as far as you can without moving at the hips, knees, ankles, or feet. Do not move your shoulder blade from its starting position. Do not let your thoracic spine flex; *rotate* it.

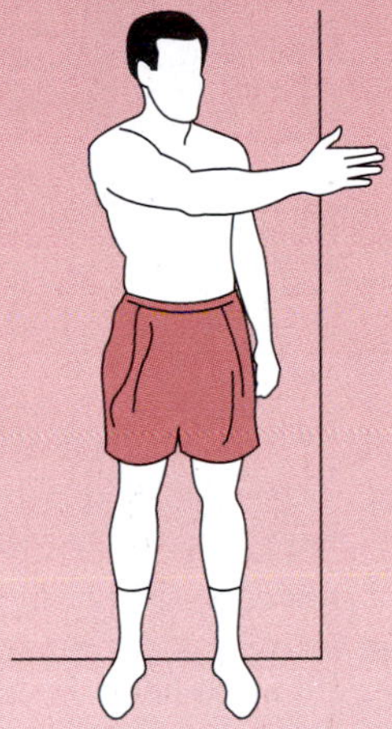

Level 3: After you have mastered independent rotation of your torso, add hip rotation to the movement. Do not move your feet from the starting position (ie, do not take a step forward, but allow your ankles and feet to rotate naturally with hip rotation). Do not move your shoulder blades from the original position or allow your thoracic spine to flex forward.

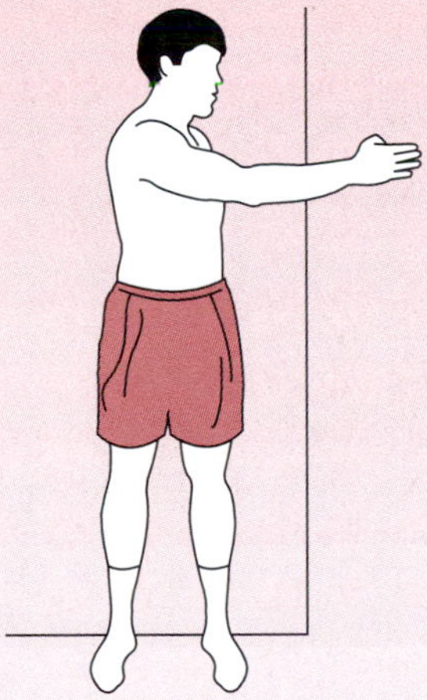

Level 4: After you have performed rotation sequentially at the torso and hips, take a step diagonally forward across midline of your body. Do not let your shoulder blade move from its starting position, but achieve a greater reach by stepping across your body.

(continued)

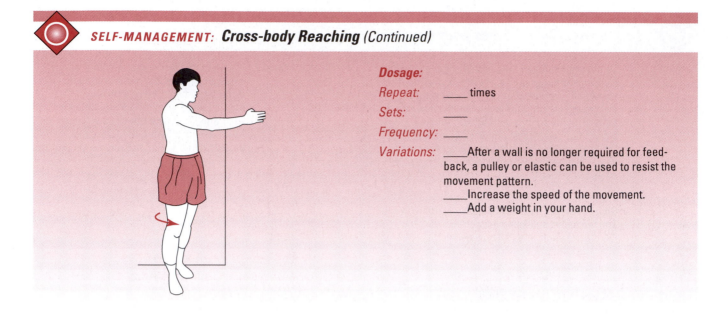

SELF-MANAGEMENT: ***Cross-body Reaching*** *(Continued)*

Dosage:

Repeat: ____ times

Sets: ____

Frequency: ____

Variations: ____After a wall is no longer required for feedback, a pulley or elastic can be used to resist the movement pattern.
____Increase the speed of the movement.
____Add a weight in your hand.

external and left internal oblique muscles. A passive stretch (Fig. 25-15) can be used in conjunction with diaphragmatic breathing (see Patient-Related Instruction: Diaphragmatic Breathing in Chapter 23) into the right thoracic rib cage. Postural habits and repetitive movement patterns must be analyzed for potential causes of myofascial restrictions. Comprehensive treatment may include changing the ergonomics of the workstation to reduce factors contributing to myofascial restrictions (eg, rearranging the workstation to reduce sustained and repeated left rotation and promote occasional right rotation). The patient's movement patterns and activities may need to be altered to limit repeated left rotation and promote more activities requiring symmetric rotation. For example, the patient should reduce the time spent playing tennis (an asymmetric activity) and begin walking, jogging, biking, or swimming (symmetric activities).

Hypomobility of the thoracic spine can also be found in relation to breathing, with reduced movement in pump or bucket handle breathing mechanics. The Patient-Related Instruction: Diaphragmatic Breathing in Chapter 23 describes proper diaphragmatic breathing, with emphasis on pump and bucket handle breathing. Proper diaphragmatic breathing is essential to the treatment of many impairments in the thoracic spine and related regions (see Chapters 18 and 23). After mastering diaphragmatic breathing in a supine position, the patient should progress to sitting and standing while applying the same breathing techniques.

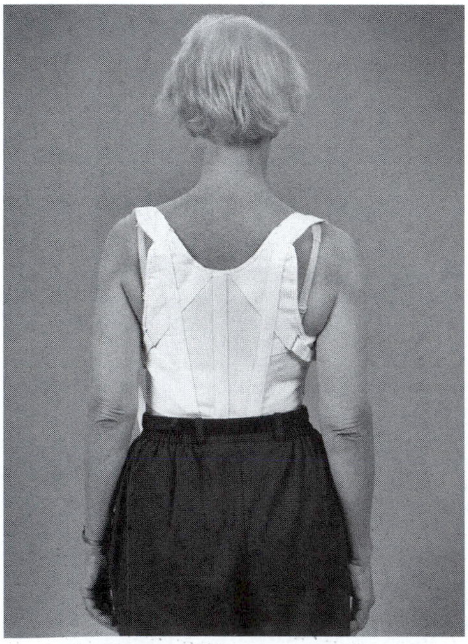

FIGURE 25-11 A posture brace can be used to prevent excessive thoracic flexion.

Impaired Muscle Performance

Impairments, functional limitations, or disabilities related to muscle performance in the thorax are those that result from

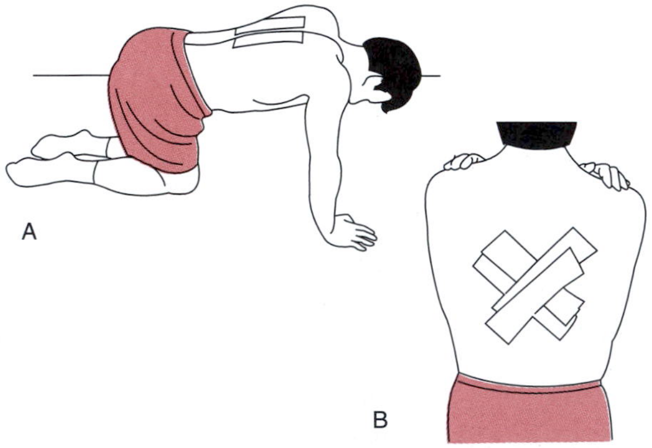

FIGURE 25-12 ***(A)*** Longitudinal tape spanning the kyphosis, applied in four-point kneeling to capture neutral spine alignment, can prevent excessive thoracic flexion. ***(B)*** Taping to prevent excessive thoracic flexion and rotation. Flexion and rotation can be controlled but not prevented by applying the tape obliquely across the hypermobile region.

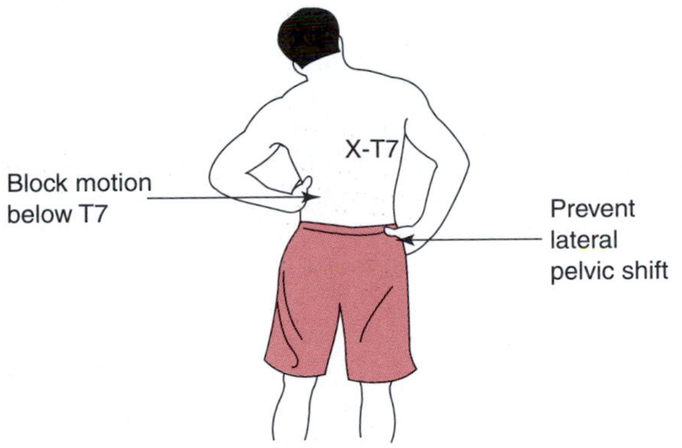

FIGURE 25-13 Left thoracic spine lateral flexion can be encouraged at T7 by blocking excessive lateral flexion below T7.

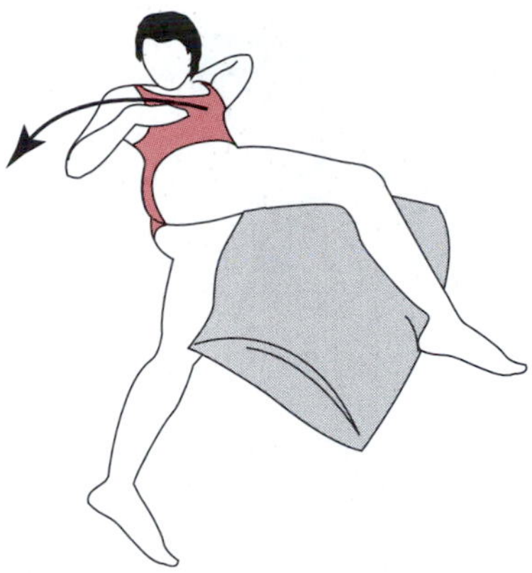

FIGURE 25-15 Rotation stretch for short or stiff right external and left internal oblique muscles.

changes in muscle force or torque production, power, or endurance of any of the muscles listed in Table 25-1. Patients with impairments, functional limitations, or disabilities related to impaired muscle performance require resistive exercise with dosage parameters specified toward a goal of increased force or torque production, power, or endurance (see Chapter 4).

The cause of the altered muscle performance must be determined to ascertain the appropriate intervention to treat the impairment. There are several possible sources of reduced force or torque production:

- Muscle injury or strain
- Neurologic impairment or pathology (eg, peripheral nerve injury, nerve root injury)
- Muscular or neuromuscular disease (eg, muscular dystrophy, cerebral palsy)
- Length-associated changes resulting in altered length-tension properties
- Disuse resulting in atrophy and general deconditioning

For therapeutic exercise intervention to improve muscle performance, the underlying source or cause of impaired muscle performance must be determined. The intervention plan developed is specific to the source or cause.

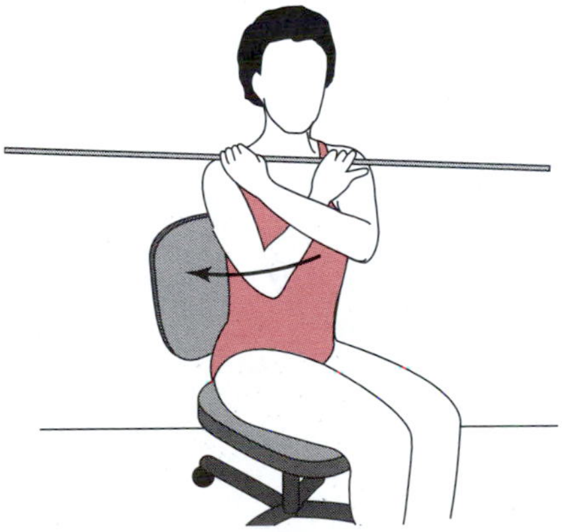

FIGURE 25-14 Holding onto a light dowel rod can encourage thoracic rotation by keeping the dowel rod level while rotating the torso. The patient is instructed to rotate at the sternum.

IMPAIRED MUSCLE PERFORMANCE FROM MUSCLE STRAIN OR INJURY

Although trauma, such as a blow to the chest resulting in soft tissue contusion or a sudden rotational injury, such as a motor vehicle accident, can lead to muscle injury or strain, an insidious-onset strain can also occur in muscles surrounding the thoracic region. Possible mechanisms of gradual insidious-onset muscle strain can include overuse or overstretch.

One example of overuse in the thoracic region is provided by the scalene muscle group, particularly the anterior scalene. The actions of the anterior scalene include cervical flexion, ipsilateral cervical lateral flexion, contralateral cervical rotation, and elevation of the first rib (ie, acting as an accessory muscle of respiration). Overuse of the anterior scalene can result from underuse of the deep cervical flexors (ie, longus colli and capitis and rectus capitis anterior), other contralateral cervical rotators (ie, deep cervical rotators, semispinalis cervicis, sternocleidomastoid, or upper trapezius), or primary muscles of inspiration (ie, diaphragm, levator costarum, and intercostals). Overuse of the anterior scalene can lead to stiffness or adaptive shortening, which can contribute to elevation of the first rib. Elevation of the first rib can disrupt cervicothoracic joint mechanics and contribute to thoracic outlet syndrome (see Chapter 26).

Treatment of overuse of the anterior scalene must address improved muscle performance of the underused synergists and the posture and movement patterns contributing to overuse. For example, instructing the patient in proper diaphragmatic breathing (see Patient-Related Instruction: Diaphragmatic Breathing in Chapter 23) rather than using accessory muscle strategies may be an important intervention to reduce the stress placed on the anterior scalene. Stretch of the anterior scalene should be performed with caution. Stabilization of the first rib is essential so that gentle active ROM of the cervical spine in ipsilateral rotation can stretch the scalene without rib elevation or cervical anterior shearing (Fig. 25-16). The patient should be instructed to avoid chronic postures of neck ipsilateral side bending and contralateral rotation to avoid overuse of the muscle in the short range (eg, talking on the phone for prolonged periods without use of a headset (Fig. 25-17).

Middle and lower trapezius strain refers to the painful upper back condition resulting from gradual and continu-

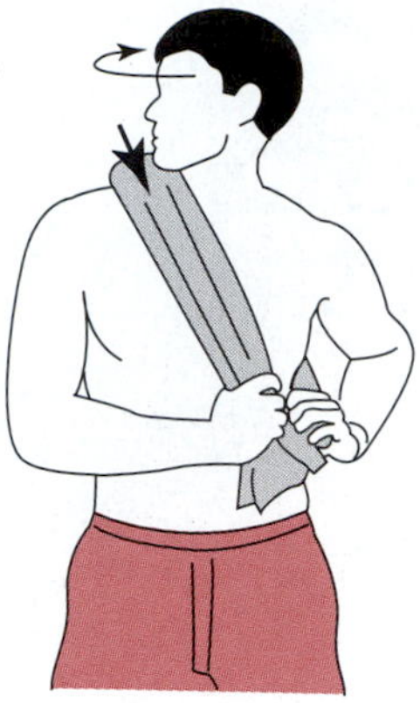

FIGURE 25-16 It is important to stabilize the first rib while stretching the anterior scalene. After the rib is stabilized, gentle active range of motion into ipsilateral rotation stretches to the same side anterior scalene without undue cervical shear or first rib elevation.

ous tension on the middle and lower trapezius muscles.[8] The strain in these muscles is caused by overstretch resulting from a habitual position of forward shoulders (see Chapter 26), kyphosis, or a combination of these two faults. Treatment of the thoracic region must include treatment of the impairments related to the kyphosis to reduce the habitual stretch on the tissues (see the Posture and Movement Impairment and Kyphosis sections).

MUSCLE PERFORMANCE IMPAIRMENT FROM NEUROLOGIC INJURY OR PATHOLOGY

One example of impaired muscle performance related to neurologic injury or pathology is reduced muscle force production in the diaphragm resulting in faulty breathing mechanics. Diaphragmatic breathing exercises cannot be effective until the source of the weakness is appropriately addressed. Because the diaphragm is innervated by the phrenic nerve (C3-C5), treatment of any cervical dysfunction at these levels may be necessary to improve diaphragmatic function.

When muscle performance is impaired because of neurologic injury or pathology, the neural input must be restored for muscle performance to improve. If the nerve injury or pathology is permanent and paresis or paralysis is the outcome, the clinician must consider the effect of the resulting muscle weakness and subsequent adaptive shortening or contracture in the opposing muscles. In the case of paresis, the clinician must consider the effect of stretch on the weak muscle because of pull of the unopposed strong muscle superimposed on the initial weakness caused by the nerve damage. If reinnervation is latent, these same considerations must be heeded during the recovery process. Weak muscles must be protected from overstretch with proper support and stimulated with appropriate-dosage resistive exercise in the short range. The strong muscles must be stretched to maintain proper extensibility and prevent contracture and deformity. In the example of the weak diaphragm caused by cervical dysfunction, appropriate diaphragmatic breathing must be instructed along with stretch of the lateral trunk and intercostal muscles (Fig. 25-18). The lateral trunk and intercostal muscles may become stiff because of the unilateral rib approximation that may result from inadequate rib expansion, causing weakness in the diaphragm.

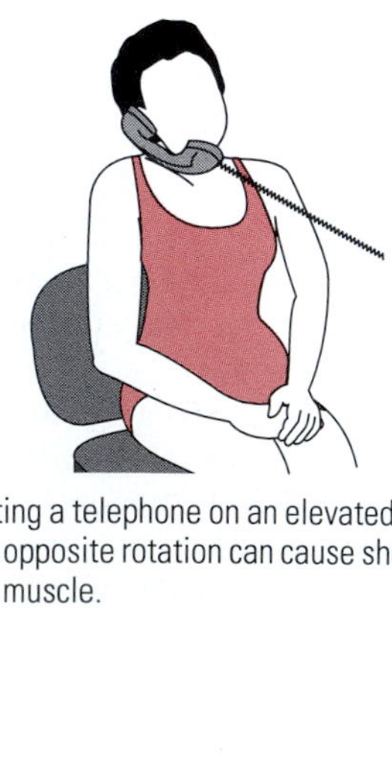

FIGURE 25-17 Resting a telephone on an elevated shoulder with the neck in lateral flexion and opposite rotation can cause shortening and overuse of the anterior scalene muscle.

MUSCLE PERFORMANCE IMPAIRMENT FROM LENGTH-ASSOCIATED CHANGES

Subtle imbalances in muscle length can lead to length-associated changes and positional weakness of one synergist compared with its counterpart or antagonist group. In the thoracic spine, the erector spinae and upper rectus abdominis are susceptible to length-associated changes from chronic kyphotic posture. The thoracic erector spinae are vulnerable to overstretch, and the upper rectus abdominis is susceptible to adaptive shortening. Overstretching and shortening can lead to conditions in the thoracic spine such as degenerative disk disease and middle and lower trapezius strain. The muscle imbalance can contribute to conditions in related areas such as cervical and lumbopelvic joints and soft tissue dysfunction from the kyphosis-lordosis or swayback posture (see the Kyphosis section).

Treatment of the muscle length imbalance requires a twofold approach of strengthening the thoracic erector spinae in the short range (see Fig. 25-6; Fig. 25-19) and stretching the upper rectus abdominis. Supportive taping (see Fig. 25-12*A*) can be used as an adjunctive measure to facilitate positive length-associated changes. Patient-related instruction in posture and movement patterns that

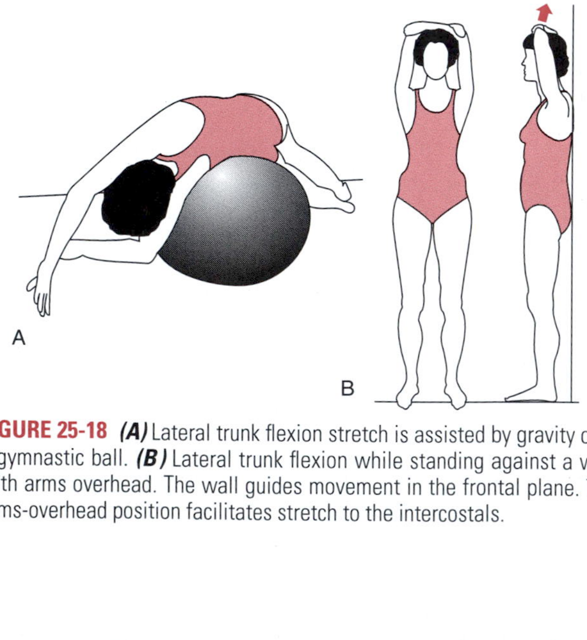

FIGURE 25-18 ***(A)*** Lateral trunk flexion stretch is assisted by gravity over a gymnastic ball. ***(B)*** Lateral trunk flexion while standing against a wall with arms overhead. The wall guides movement in the frontal plane. The arms-overhead position facilitates stretch to the intercostals.

perpetuate these length-associated changes is required to prevent recurrence of conditions caused by this muscle performance impairment.

MUSCLE PERFORMANCE IMPAIRMENT FROM DISUSE AND DECONDITIONING

Disuse and deconditioning can be caused by illness, immobilization, sedentary lifestyle, or subtle shifts in muscle balance from repetitive faulty movement patterns. Progressive resistive exercises for the upper body can address general disuse and deconditioning. Initially, the weight of the limb alone can provide enough stimulus for strength gains in the severely deconditioned individual. Progression in small increments is recommended because the upper body muscles are small compared with those of the lower body, and excessive resistance added prematurely may promote muscle imbalance by strengthening the dominant synergists or antagonists (see Chapter 26). Abdominal and back extensor strengthening (see Fig. 25-6) may be indicated to improve the alignment, movement, and stabilizing function of the thoracic region. Care must be taken to prevent the development or perpetuation of muscle imbalances when prescribing general resistive exercises for this region. Chapter 18 describes proper exercise prescription for the abdominal muscles.

Pain

Pain in the thoracic region has many possible causes or mechanisms. The onset of pain may be the result of joint dysfunction (ie, thoracic vertebrae or rib articulations), soft tissue injury, or strain or of nonvisceral (eg, osteoporosis, ankylosing spondylitis, Scheuermann's disease) or visceral diseases (see Appendix 1).

Treatment must focus on the cause or mechanism of the pain, not just the source. Earlier sections addressing individual impairments discussed theoretical strategies and provided clinical examples of exercises to alleviate impairments that could be contributing to the causes and mechanisms of musculoskeletal origin pain.

Because the thoracic region is a site of many visceral causes and sources of pain (eg, chest pain due to acute myocardial infarction, pain at the costovertebral angle of the lower thoracic segments due to renal origin pain), careful screening for mechanical sources of pain are necessary. The findings from a thorough history can indicate possible nonmechanical sources of pain (see Appendix 1). If the therapist suspects that the pain is derived from nonmechanical or visceral sources, the patient should be referred to the appropriate medical practitioner.

Posture and Movement Impairment

Treatment of impairment in posture and movement of the thoracic region must encompass related regions in the kinematic chain that may contribute to the impairments of this region.

POSTURE

Kyphosis is the most common posture impairment, followed by scoliosis and thoracic lordosis. Because the earlier discussion addressed kyphosis, this section focuses on the latter two postural faults.

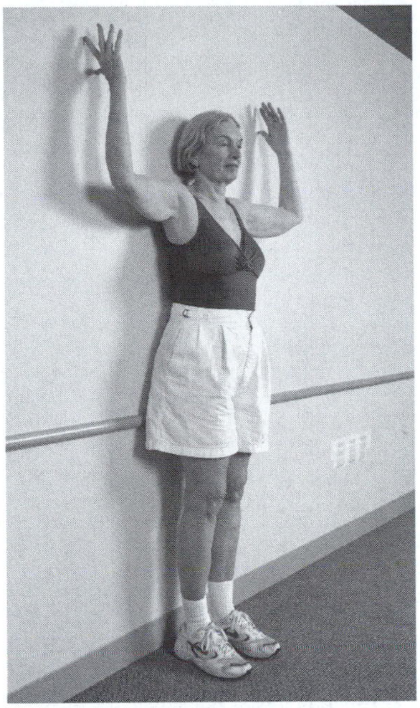

FIGURE 25-19 Standing with the back to the wall in a neutral spine position, the patient raises her arms raised in horizontal abduction. The elbows are forward of the wall to maintain the arms in scapular plane. Deep diaphragmatic breathing is performed in this position. The arms can slide up the wall as the length of the pectoralis major allows. Note: This exercise also stretches superior fibers of the external oblique muscle at the rib angle and the shoulder adductors, and it provides resistance to the spine extensors and scapular upward rotators in the short range. The lower abdominals contract to maintain the lumbar spine and pelvis in neutral alignment.

Scoliosis is a lateral curvature of the spine. Scoliosis involves lateral flexion and rotation of the vertebrae of the involved region. The known causes of scoliosis include congenital and acquired defects, disease, and injury. Many cases of scoliosis have no known cause, and these idiopathic cases are discussed later in this chapter.

Acquired scoliosis may result from highly repetitive, asymmetric activities related to hand dominance. A common pattern of muscle imbalance and alignment changes for right-handed individuals is pictured in Figure 25-20. The therapist should be aware of the postural habits of a child in the various positions of the body, such as sitting, standing, and lying, because habits developed in childhood can persist into adulthood. A right-handed child may sit at his desk to write with the upper body laterally flexed to the right. If this posture is also assumed in sidelying to perform homework (Fig. 25-21), sitting (Fig. 25-22), and to carry his homework in a backpack slung over the right shoulder, he is prone to develop muscle imbalance problems that can lead to acquired scoliotic deviations of the spine that persist into adulthood.

The pronation of one foot, standing on one hip, or standing with the same knee always bent (these habits often occur together) can contribute to the development of acquired scoliosis. The imbalances in hip musculature or faulty foot alignment or knee position that result in lateral

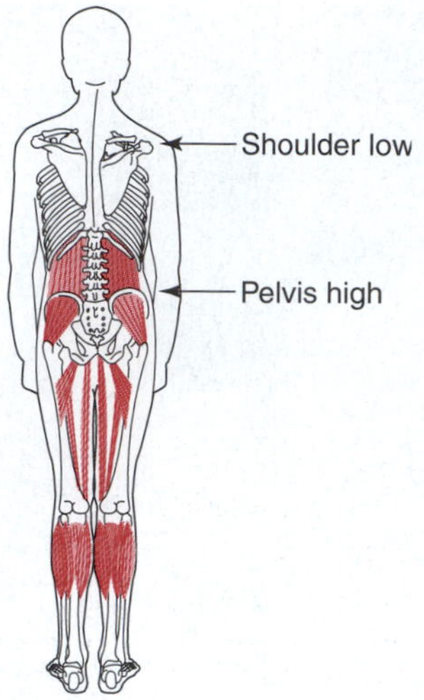

FIGURE 25-20 In a typical dominant right-hand pattern, the right iliac crest is high and the shoulder low. The darkly shaded muscles can develop adaptive shortening, while the lightly shaded muscles can develop adaptive lengthening. (From Kendall FP, McCreary EK, Provance PG. *Muscles: Testing and Function*. 4th ed. Baltimore: Williams & Wilkins; 1993:89.)

pelvic tilt are more closely related to primary lumbar or thoracolumbar curves than to primary thoracic curves.

Exercises should be carefully selected on the basis of thorough examination findings, and adequate instruction is needed to ensure that the exercises will be performed correctly and with precision. The object is to use asymmetric exercises to promote symmetry. To illustrate this point, consider the following case.

The patient is a gymnast with a right thoracic, left lumbar curve (Fig. 25-23). Along with other findings, right iliopsoas and right external oblique weaknesses are diagnosed. An example of an asymmetric exercise is resisted exercise to the right iliopsoas (Fig. 25-24). Because the psoas muscle attaches to the lumbar vertebrae, transverse processes, and the intervertebral disks, this muscle can pull directly on the spine. Figure 25-25*A* demonstrates the adverse effect of resisting the left iliopsoas, and Figure 25*B* illustrates the positive effect of resisting the right iliopsoas. A left upper extremity diagonal reaching movement pattern can facilitate right thoracic lateral flexion. Simultaneous right hip flexion and left upper extremity diagonal reaching should promote lateral deviation, correcting both curves (Fig. 25-26). If performed as a home program, someone should monitor this movement to ensure that the appropriate spine correction occurs.

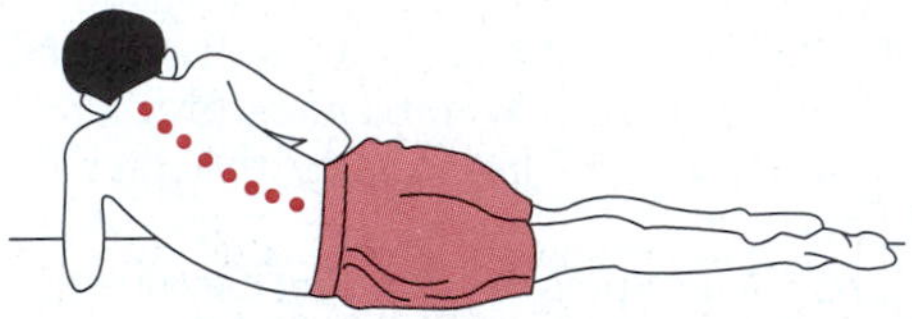

FIGURE 25-21 Children sometimes assume a sidelying position on the floor or bed to do their homework. A right-handed person lies on the left side so that the right hand is free to write or turn the pages in a book. Such a posture places the spine in a left convex curve.

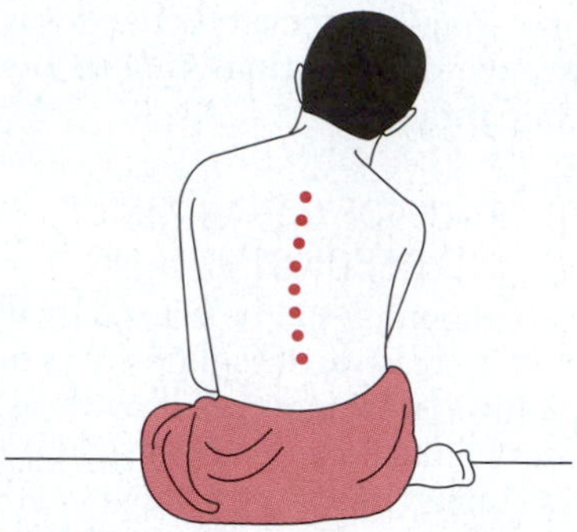

FIGURE 25-22 Sitting on one foot (the left in this illustration) causes the pelvis to tilt downward on the left and upward on the right. This places the spine in a left convex curve.

Kendall[2] describes an exercise in supine to address the weakness of the right external oblique:

> In the supine position, the subject places the right hand on the right lateral chest wall and the left hand on the left side of the pelvis. Keeping the hands in position, the object of the exercise is to bring the two hands closer by contraction of the abdominal muscles without flexing the trunk. It is as if the upper part of the body shifts toward the left, and the pelvis shifts toward the right. By not allowing trunk flexion and contracting the posterior lateral fibers of the external oblique, there will be a tendency toward some counterclockwise rotation of the thorax in the direction of correcting the thoracic rotation that accompanies a right thoracic curve.

Thoracic lordosis is a loss of the normal posterior curve of the thoracic spine, and it can be associated with abnormal posture correction strategies. For example, in an attempt to correct forward shoulders, the individual extends the thoracic spine. If this is done habitually, the thoracic spine becomes a site of relative flexibility. Attempts to improve impairments of the shoulder girdle with lower trapezius resistive exercises (Fig. 25-27*A*) cause thoracic extension instead of scapular adduction. Use of a support under sternum (Fig. 25-27*B*) can somewhat block the undesired thoracic extension to allow resistive exercises to transmit forces to the scapula instead of the thoracic spine. Patient-related instruction is necessary to alter the strategy of posture correction performed by the patient.

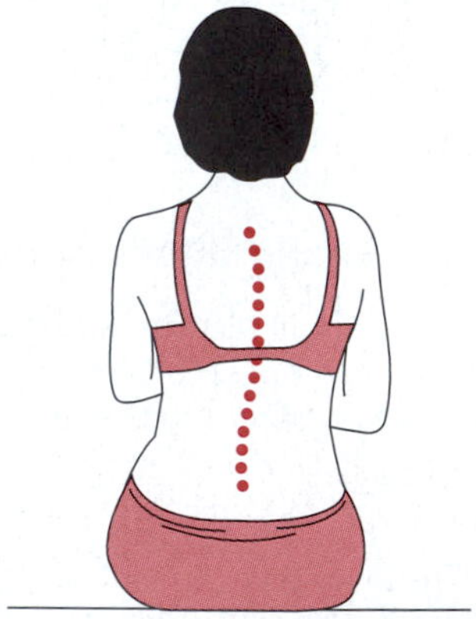

FIGURE 25-23 This person has a right thoracic and left lumbar curve.

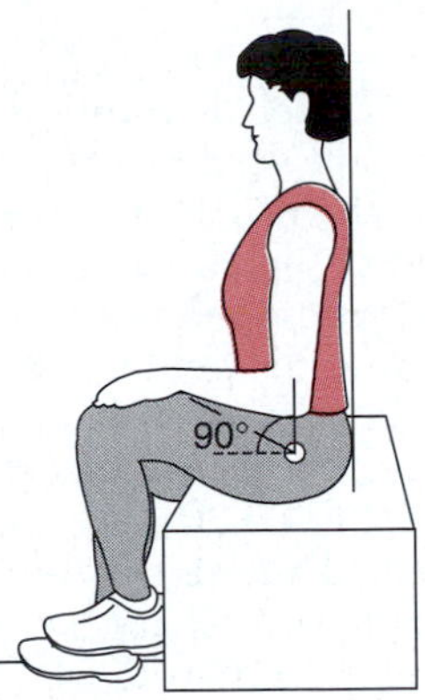

FIGURE 25-24 Resisted end-range hip flexion can isolate the iliopsoas from the other hip flexors that do not attach directly to the spine.

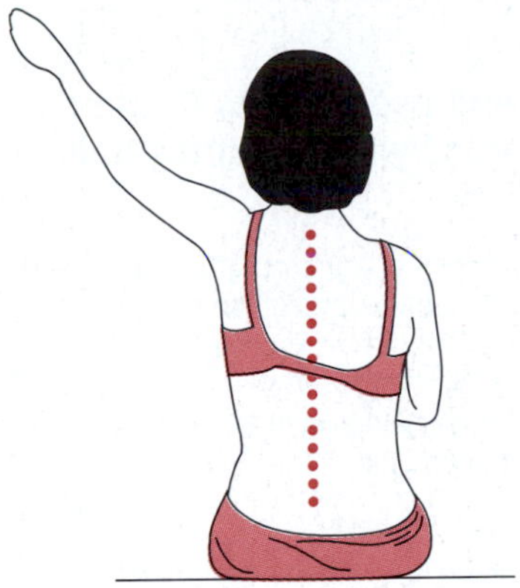

FIGURE 25-26 The dotted line shows the effect of reducing the right thoracic and left lumbar curve by simultaneously reaching diagonally upward with the left arm and resisting right hip flexion.

MOVEMENT IMPAIRMENT

The ultimate goal of all therapeutic exercise interventions should be to regain maximum pain-free function. This requires addressing component impairments contributing to the faulty movement that is related to the functional limitation and disability. Analysis of complex movements (eg, gait, forward bending, reaching, rising from sitting, ascending or descending stairs) requires division of the movement into component parts to analyze the contribution from each segment or region involved in the movement. The examination and evaluation can reveal specific regional physiologic impairments such as hypomobility in the hips or impaired muscle performance of the shoulder girdle. Combining the information obtained from movement analysis and specific examination of selected regions can determine which impairments need to be addressed to improve the strategy of movement for the given task. For example, a goal of maintaining a neutral spine while walking for an individual with pain related to thoracic kyphosis may require improving any one or all the impairments listed in Display 25-2.

Initially, addressing each related impairment with a specific exercise may be necessary to prepare the foundation for more functional exercises and eventually for specific movement pattern retraining. After component impairments are improved (eg, hip flexion and thoracic rotation mobility, hip flexor and spinal extensor or oblique abdominal muscle performance), exercises that integrate the movement patterns can be initiated. Figure 25-28 demonstrates an integrated movement in sidelying, which is gravity lessened for the hip flexors and gravity assisted for the oblique abdominals and spinal extensors. This movement pattern can be progressed to the upright position of the swing phase of step-up (Fig. 25-29), and eventually into the swing phase of gait after the stance phase of gait components have adequately improved through another set of exercises. Component impairments are first addressed, followed by integrated movements with relatively simple activities or techniques, progressed to more challenging activities or techniques, and then progressed to complex, integrated functional movement patterns.

Because the thoracic spine is between the shoulder girdle and lumbar-pelvic-hip complex, correction of movement impairments of these regions may be necessary to improve the movement pattern of the thoracic spine. Movement impairments at the foot and ankle also can contribute to impairments in the thoracic spine. The possible findings

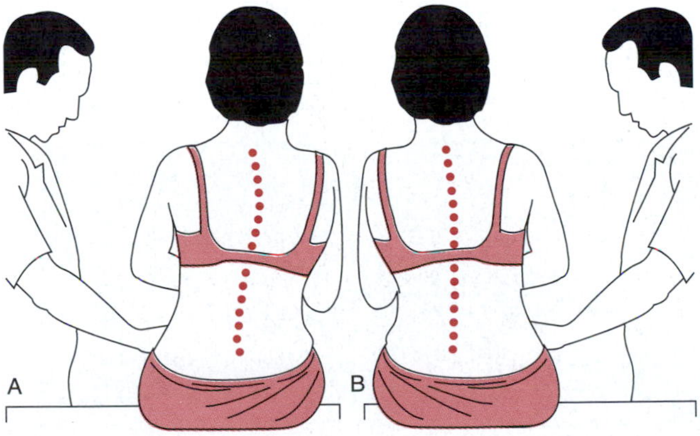

FIGURE 25-25 ***(A)*** The dotted line shows the adverse effect of resisting the left iliopsoas in a left lumbar curve. ***(B)*** The dotted line shows the positive effect of resisting the right iliopsoas in a left lumbar curve.

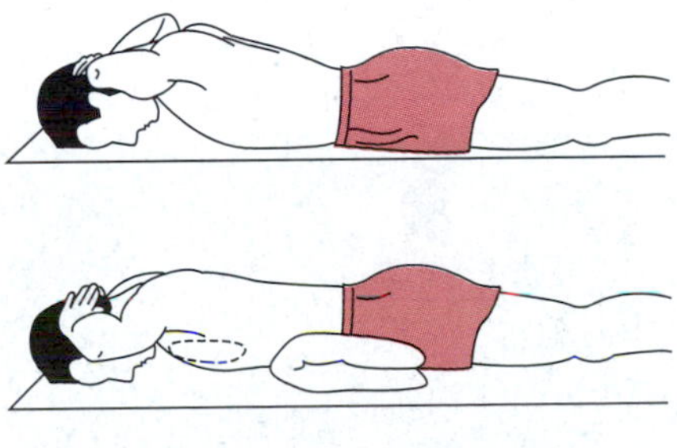

FIGURE 25-27 ***(A)*** In a person with thoracic lordosis, attempts at performing resisted lower and middle trapezius exercises promote thoracic extension instead of scapular adduction. ***(B)*** Use of a rigid cylinder placed under the sternum can stabilize the thoracic spine in flexion, allowing the force of the middle and lower trapezius to adduct the scapula instead of extending the thoracic spine.

DISPLAY 25-2

Component Impairments Related to Thoracic Kyphosis During Gait

Stance Limb

- **Initial contact:** Hip extensor strength is necessary to prevent backward lean by means of lumbar lordosis. Lumbar lordosis can lead to thoracic kyphosis.
- **Terminal stance:** Hip flexor length and hip joint extension mobility are necessary to prevent lumbar lordosis and secondary thoracic kyphosis.

Swing Limb

- Hip extensor length, hip joint flexion mobility, and hip flexor strength are necessary to perform proper hip flexion during swing and prevent backward lean by means of lumbar lordosis to advance the limb. Lumbar lordosis can lead to thoracic kyphosis.

Trunk

- Balance between length and performance of oblique abdominal or spinal extensor muscles is necessary to prevent thoracic kyphosis.
- Counterrotation between the pelvis and trunk is necessary to promote optimal trunk function during gait to prevent compensatory thoracic flexion.

associated with scoliosis are reviewed in a subsequent section and demonstrate the link between the foot and the thoracic spine. Chapter 22 details the exercise prescriptions for impairments in the foot and ankle.

THERAPEUTIC EXERCISE INTERVENTIONS FOR COMMON DIAGNOSES

This section contains selected medical diagnoses that have a bearing on the muscular, skeletal, and nervous systems as they relate to the thoracic region. Although there are numerous musculoskeletal diagnoses associated with the thoracic region, only a few are discussed to provide examples of therapeutic exercise prescriptions for the related functional limitations, disabilities, and related impairments.

Scoliosis

Scoliosis is a complicated deformity that is characterized by lateral curvature and vertebral rotation. On the concave side of the curve, the ribs approximate, and on the convex side, they are widely separated. As the vertebral bodies rotate, the spinous processes deviate toward the concave side, and the ribs follow the rotation of the vertebrae (Fig. 25-30). The posterior ribs on the convex side are pushed posteriorly, causing the characteristic rib hump seen in thoracic scoliosis (see Fig. 25-30). The anterior ribs on the concave side are pushed anteriorly (see Fig. 25-30). Scoliosis can also cause pathologic changes in the vertebral bodies and intervertebral disks (Fig. 25-31).

CLASSIFICATION OF SCOLIOSIS

The classification of scoliosis is given in Display 25-3.[20] Idiopathic scoliosis accounts for about 80% of all cases of scoliosis and has a strong female predilection (7 : 1).[20] It can be subclassified into infantile, juvenile, and adolescent types, depending on the age of onset. The adolescent type is the most common idiopathic scoliosis in the United States. Structural scoliosis can also result from congenital vertebral anomalies (Fig. 25-32). Discovery of these anomalies should prompt screening for associated cardiac, genitourinary, or other vertebral anomalies. Other causes of scoliosis include trauma, neurofibromatosis, and other neuromuscular disorders.[20]

CLASSIFICATION OF THE CURVE

The type of curve determines the most appropriate intervention. Scoliosis is generally described in terms of the location of the curve or curves (Fig. 25-33). The direction of the curve is named for the convexity of the curve, and each curve of a double curve must be named.

The most commonly used radiographic assessment of the magnitude of the curves is the Cobb method (Fig. 25-34). The first step is to decide which vertebrae are the end vertebrae of the curve. These end vertebrae are the upper and lower limits of the curve that tilt most severely toward the concavity of the curve. After these vertebrae have been selected, a line is drawn along the upper endplate of the upper body and along the lower endplate of the lower body. The angle if interest is the angle between these two lines. When reporting this angle, it is important to mention

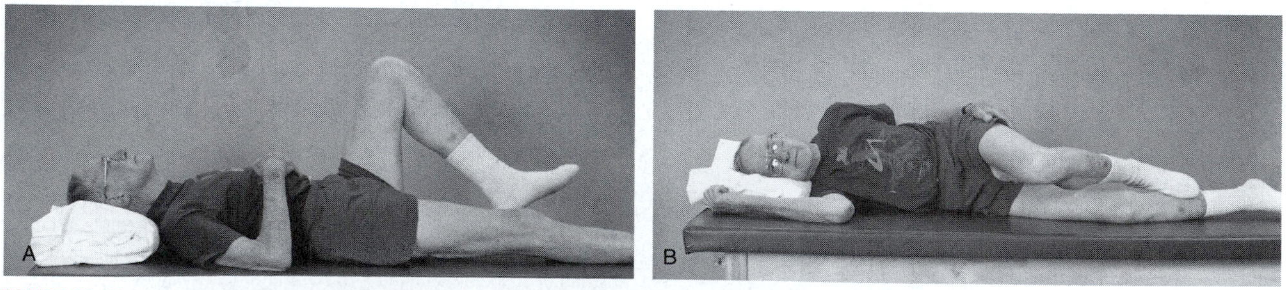

FIGURE 25-28 This exercise promotes simultaneous hip flexion and trunk counterrotation to prepare for the complex movement of the swing phase of gait on the left. ***(A)*** The start position is supine with hip and knee flexion. ***(B)*** The end position is sidelying with hip and knee flexion and left trunk rotation.

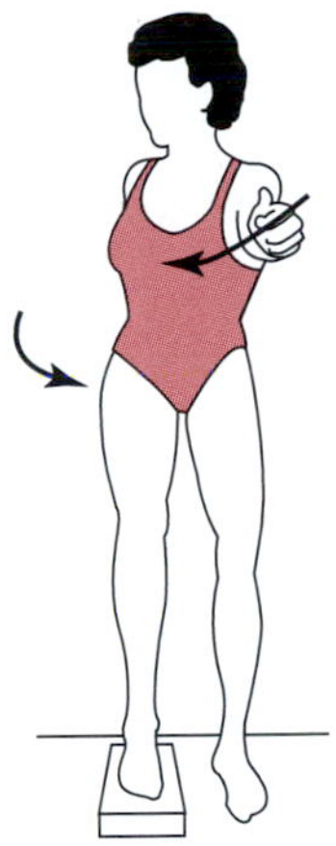

FIGURE 25-29 During the swing phase of the step-up, trunk counterrotation can be emphasized to facilitate the complex movement during the swing phase of gait.

that the Cobb method was used and to list which end vertebrae were chosen; this information allows the measurement to be consistent with follow-up radiographic studies.

Another goal of radiographic examination is to determine the physiologic or skeletal maturity of the patient. After skeletal maturity has been reached, a curvature of less than 30 degrees (by the Cobb method) typically does not progress.[20] Because the iliac crests are usually seen on a scoliosis study, they provide a convenient index of skeletal maturity. When the iliac crest apophyses meet the sacroiliac junction and firmly seal the ilium, maturation is nearly complete. The endplates of the vertebral bodies also provide evidence of skeletal maturation. When the plates blend in with the vertebral bodies to form a solid union, maturation is complete.

TREATMENT

Muscle imbalance that exists as a result of nonidiopathic scoliosis can be treated through the use of exercise to prevent further exaggeration of the scoliosis beyond that which the disease has caused. The message that exercise is of little or no value prevails in the literature, leaving individuals with scoliosis treatment the options of doing nothing, bracing, or surgery. In the American Academy of Orthopedic Surgeons 1985 lecture series, this statement appears:

> Physical therapy cannot prevent a progressive deformity, and there are those who believe specific spinal exercise programs work in a counterproductive fashion by making the spine more flexible than it ordinarily would be and, by so doing, making it more susceptible to progression.[21]

Kendall[8] warns that overemphasis on flexibility is the exercise approach that leads to the view that exercise is of

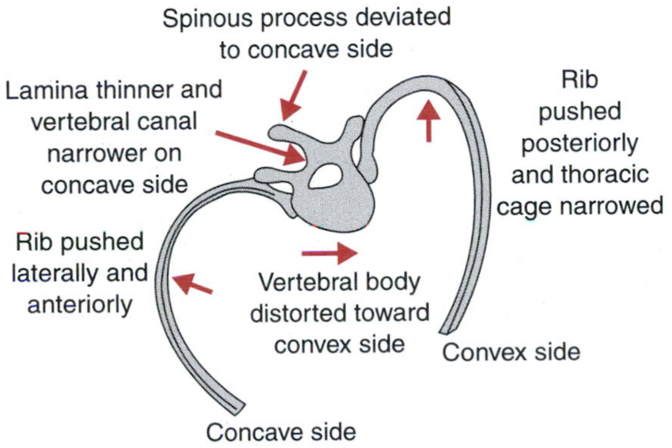

FIGURE 25-30 Typical distortion of the vertebra and ribs in thoracic scoliosis as seen from below.

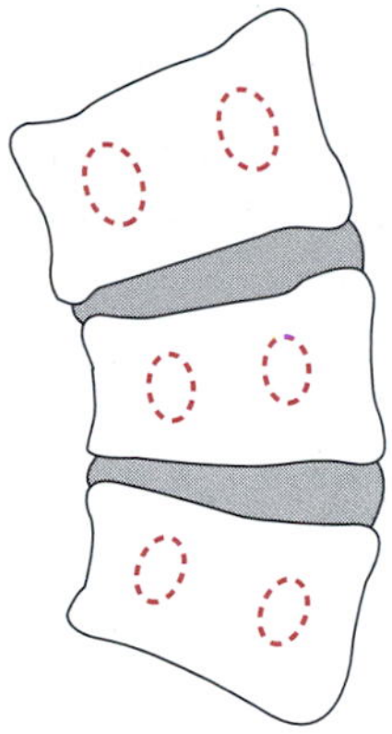

FIGURE 25-31 Coronal view of a scoliotic spine. The height of the vertebrae and intervertebral disks is decreased on the concave side.

DISPLAY 25-3

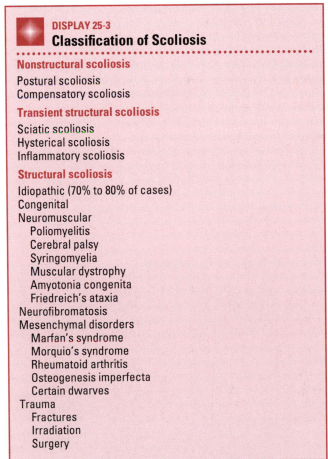

Classification of Scoliosis

Nonstructural scoliosis

- Postural scoliosis
- Compensatory scoliosis

Transient structural scoliosis

- Sciatic scoliosis
- Hysterical scoliosis
- Inflammatory scoliosis

Structural scoliosis

- Idiopathic (70% to 80% of cases)
- Congenital
- Neuromuscular
  - Poliomyelitis
  - Cerebral palsy
  - Syringomyelia
  - Muscular dystrophy
  - Amyotonia congenita
  - Friedreich's ataxia
- Neurofibromatosis
- Mesenchymal disorders
  - Marfan's syndrome
  - Morquio's syndrome
  - Rheumatoid arthritis
  - Osteogenesis imperfecta
  - Certain dwarves
- Trauma
  - Fractures
  - Irradiation
  - Surgery

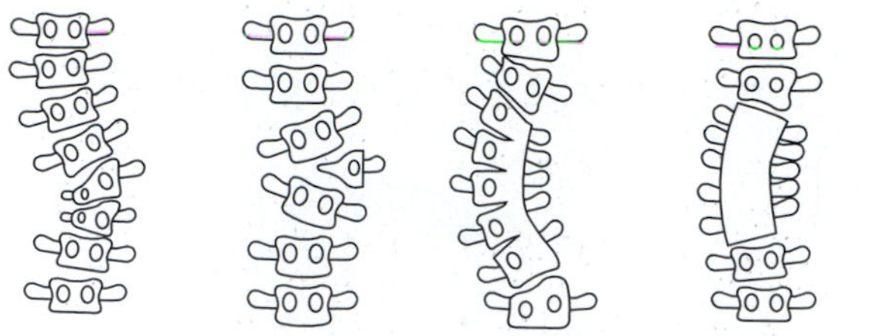

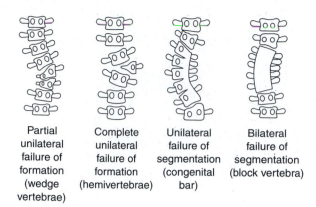

FIGURE 25-32 Vertebral anomalies causing scoliosis.

little value or even counterproductive in the treatment of scoliosis. She states that adequate musculoskeletal evaluation has been lacking, and as a result, there has been little scientific basis on which to justify the selection of therapeutic exercises. Kendall's premise for using therapeutic exercise is that scoliosis is a problem of symmetry and that restoring symmetry requires the use of asymmetric exercises along with appropriate support. Stretching of stiff or short muscles is desirable only if it is performed with simultaneous exercise and appropriate support to shorten and strengthen what is too long and relatively weak.

To develop a comprehensive approach to treatment, a comprehensive musculoskeletal evaluation must be performed. The evaluation should include the tests and measures described in Display 25-4. Exercises should be carefully selected on the basis of the examination findings. The general principles of exercise prescription for patients are listed in Display 25-5. Exercises to be avoided include those listed in Display 25-6. An alternative exercise is shown in Self-Management: Postural Exercise With Back to Wall. Exercises for muscle imbalances associated with acquired scoliosis were described previously.

Additional supports in the form of orthotics, lifts, and braces can be used to assist in the treatment of structural scoliosis. Correction of lateral pelvic tilt associated with a lumbar curve can be helped by proper lift on the side of the low iliac crest. However, no lift can help if the patient continues to stand in an asymmetric posture, such as with weight predominantly on the leg with the higher iliac crest and with the knee flexed on the side of the lift.

Unilateral pronation can also contribute to the asymmetry and muscle imbalance found in acquired and structural scoliosis. For example, the combination of left pronation, shortness of the left iliotibial band, and weakness of the right gluteus medius, left hip adductors, and left lateral abdominals can be seen in a person with a right thoracic curve and left lumbar curve. Along with specific exercises to improve the length of the left iliotibial band and strength of the right gluteus medius, left hip adductors, and lateral ab-

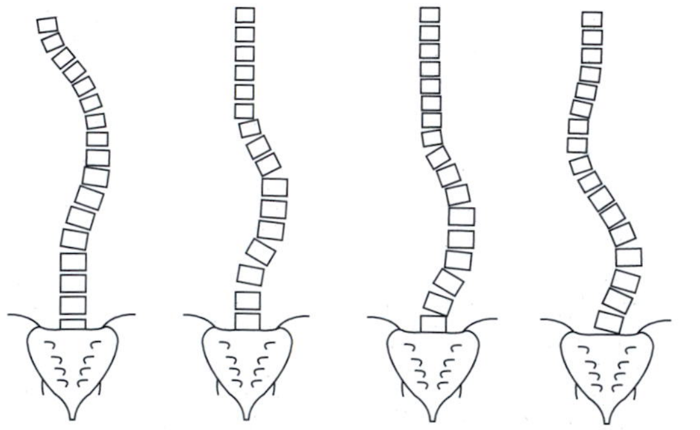

FIGURE 25-33 Patterns of scoliosis.

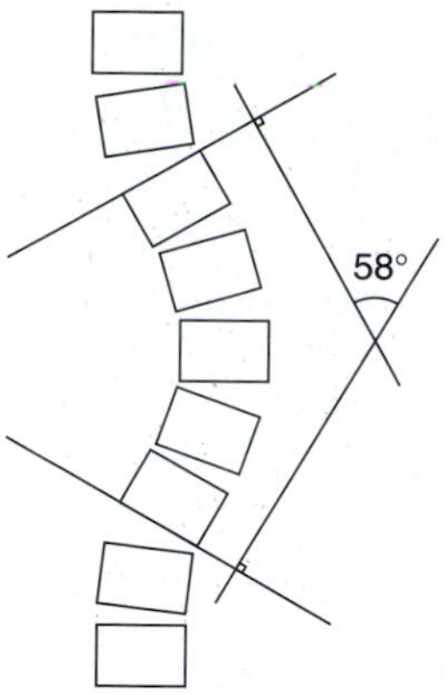

FIGURE 25-34 Cobb method for measurement of a scoliosis curve. (From Richardson M. (1994). Approaches to Differential Diagnosis in Musculoskeletal Imaging. [On-line]. Available: http://www.rad.washington.edu/Books/NewApproach/Scoliosis/CobbAngle7.gif).

DISPLAY 25-4

Tests and Measures Included in a Scoliosis Evaluation

Posture alignment
- Plumbline and segmental, in back, front, and side views

Muscle length tests
- Hip flexor (differentiating psoas from tensor fascia lata and rectus femoris)
- Hamstrings
- Forward bend for length of posterior muscles
- Tensor fascia lata–iliotibial band
- Teres major and latissimus dorsi

Muscle strength tests
- Back extensors
- Abdominal muscles (differentiating trunk curl from pelvic stabilization roles)
- Lateral trunk
- Oblique abdominals
- Hip flexors
- Hip extensors
- Hip abductors (differentiating posterior gluteus medius)
- Middle and lower trapezius

Movement
- Forward bending to determine a structural curve and the location of the curve

DISPLAY 25-5
Principles of Exercise Prescription for Scoliosis

- Symmetric exercises should not be attempted.
- If one group or one muscle within a group is too strong for its antagonist or synergist, that muscle or group should be stretched, and the weaker, longer antagonist or synergist should be strengthened and supported to provide balance to the region.
- The lateral and anterior abdominal muscles, pelvic girdle, and leg muscles usually have asymmetric strength, causing the body to deviate about all three planes of motion but primarily in the transverse and frontal planes. Because the posterior spinal muscles are relatively less affected, the program should emphasize promoting strength of the relatively weak muscle or groups of muscles in the anterior thoracolumbar region and the pelvic-hip complex.

DISPLAY 25-6
Exercises to Avoid in Treating Scoliosis

- Exercises that promote flexibility of the spine should be avoided without counterbalancing exercises or support promoting opposing shortening and strength to maintain corrections.
- A subject who is also developing kyphoscoliosis should avoid back extension exercises performed in prone because it promotes further lumbar extension (see Self-Management: Wall Sitting Postural Exercise for an alternative exercise. Trunk curl exercises or sit-ups should be avoided even if the rectus abdominis and internal oblique muscles are weak, because thoracic flexion promotes the kyphosis (see **Chapter 18** for alternative methods of abdominal strengthening).

SELF-MANAGEMENT: Postural Exercise With Back to Wall

Purpose: To reduce the tendency for excessive midback forward flexion and forward shoulder posture. After this exercise is mastered in sitting, it can be progressed to standing.

Starting position: Sit on a stool with the lower back nearly flat against the wall. You should be able to fit your hand behind your lower back if your spine is in optimal position. If you have an exaggerated upper and midback curve, you may have a larger space between the wall and your back. Try to reduce this space as much as possible by contracting your lower abdominal muscles. *Caution:* Do not let your upper and middle back forward flex more in an attempt to reduce the curve of your lower back.

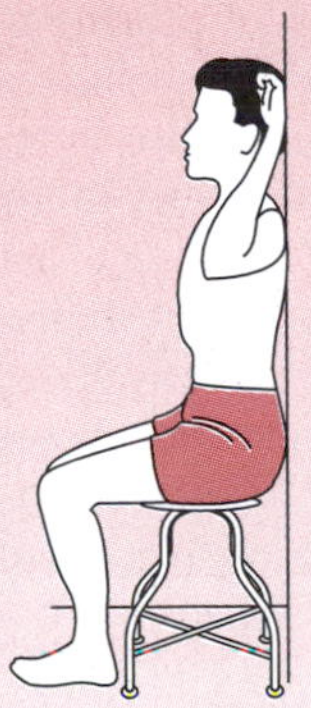

A.

Press your head back with your chin tucked down. If you have an exaggerated curve of your upper or middle back, you may not be able to get your head to the wall. Place one or two 1 or 2 towel rolls behind your head with your head as close to the wall as possible and with your eyes and nose positioned horizontally. *Caution:* Do not let your chin rise upward in an attempt to get your head closer to the wall.

Place your thumbs on the wall with your elbows pointing slightly forward. If you have an exaggerated curve of your upper or middle back, you may not be able to get your thumbs to the wall. (A)

Movement technique: Keep your thumbs in contact with the wall, keep your head and low back in the starting position, and slide your arms to a diagonal position overhead. When your head or low back deviate from the start position or your shoulders shrug excessively, stop the movement. (B)

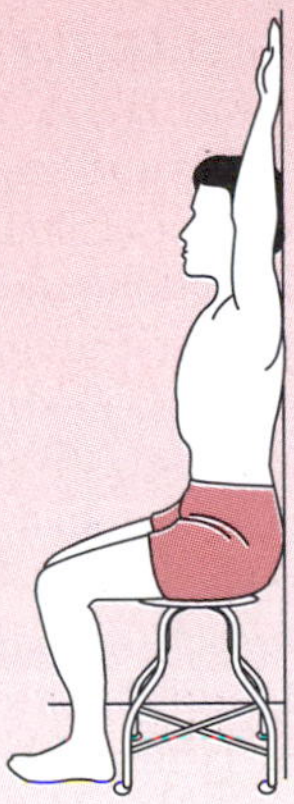

B.

Dosage:

Repeat:____ times

Sets:

Frequency:

dominal muscles (see Chapters 18 and 20), the use of an orthotic to support the left foot is indicated (see Chapter 22).

In addition to exercises and shoe correction, many scoliosis patients need some type of support. Bracing can prevent curves from getting worse. This treatment is reserved for children and adolescents in whom a rapid increase in the curve needs to be thwarted. A brace worn 16 or more hours each day has been shown to be effective in preventing 90% or more of the curves from getting worse, particularly mild curves (25 to 35 degrees).[22] Most authorities recommend wearing the brace for 23 hours each day, because using it part time can create compliance problems about when to take it off and put it on. When it becomes part of a daily routine, it becomes a standard function. However, the brace cannot correct a curve. At best, it can prevent it from worsening. In adults, the curve may progress slowly over the years, and bracing is not a practical solution.

Surgery is usually reserved for teens and preteens with curves of 40 degrees or more.[20] For adults, the reasons for doing surgery are less well defined but include increasing, disabling pain and documented increase in a curve.

Early detection and intervention are key to the treatment of scoliosis. A few carefully selected exercises that help to maintain muscle balance and a kinesthetic sense of good alignment are recommended over a vigorous, complex program. This means providing good patient-related education about how to avoid habitual positions and activities that can increase the curvature. It also means providing incentives that help keep the child, adolescent, or adult interested and cooperative in an ongoing program.

Kyphosis

Although kyphosis is considered to be a posture impairment and not a medical diagnosis, two medical diagnoses result in kyphosis: osteoporosis and Scheuermann's disease. The definitions, diagnoses, and general treatment recommendations for these two conditions are discussed in this section, followed by exercise guidelines for the treatment of kyphosis.

Osteoporosis

Osteoporosis is a major underlying cause of bone fractures in postmenopausal women and older persons in general.[23] It is a condition in which bone mass decreases, causing bones to be more susceptible to fracture. A fall, blow, or lifting action that would not bruise or strain the average person may cause fracture in a person with severe osteoporosis. Medical practitioners and patients alike are concerned with the optimum approach to the treatment and prevention of osteoporosis. The appropriate timing and proper use of agents such as calcium, vitamin D, estrogens, and fluorides and the role of exercise are issues that have generated major research efforts and considerable controversy. This discussion focuses on the effect of osteoporosis on the thoracic spine and the role of exercise in treatment of osteoporosis.

DIAGNOSIS

The clinical manifestations of osteoporosis include fractures of the vertebral bodies, the neck and intertrochanteric regions of the femur, and the distal radius.[23] Vertebral compression fractures occur more frequently in women than men and typically affect the T8-L3 region. These fractures may develop during routine activities such as bending, lifting light objects, or rising from a chair. Immediate, severe, localized back pain may accompany compression fracture. Pain usually subsides within several months. Some experience persistent pain from altered spinal mechanics. However, some vertebral fractures do not cause pain. Gradual, asymptomatic vertebral compression may be detected only on radiographic examination. The loss of height or the development of a kyphosis may be the only signs of multiple vertebral fractures. Discomfort, debility, and rarely, pulmonary dysfunction may accompany kyphosis. Abdominal symptoms may include early satiety, bloating, and constipation.

RISK FACTORS

Women are at higher risk than men because women have less bone mass, and for several years after natural or induced menopause, the rate of bone mass loss is accelerated. Early menopause is one of the earliest predictors for the development of osteoporosis. White women and men are at much higher risk than black women and men. Women who are underweight also have osteoporosis more often than overweight women. Cigarette smoking may be an additional risk, and calcium deficiency has been implicated in the pathogenesis of the disease.

Immobilization and prolonged bed rest produce rapid bone loss, but weight-bearing exercise can reduce bone loss and increase bone mass. Exercise sufficient to induce amenorrhea in young women may lead to decreased bone mass.

The relationship of osteoporosis to hereditary and dietary factors, such as alcohol, vitamins A and C, magnesium, and protein, is less firmly established. Some of these factors may act indirectly through their effect on calcium metabolism or body weight.

PREVENTION AND TREATMENT

Emphasis must be placed on measures that prevent, retard, or halt the progress of osteoporosis before irreversible structural defects occur. The mainstays of prevention and management of osteoporosis are estrogen and calcium, and exercise and nutrition are considered important adjuncts.

Inactivity leads to bone loss, but weight-bearing exercise can reduce bone loss and increase bone mass. The optimal type and amount of physical activity that can prevent osteoporosis have not been established, but moderate weight-bearing exercise such as walking is recommended. Resisted upper extremity exercise is also recommended to induce weight-bearing stress on the spine and wrist.

Strategies to prevent falls are important for elderly patients at risk for osteoporosis, because a fall in this population can lead to morbidity or death from the secondary effects of immobilization and reduced activity. Specific exercise techniques addressing impairments related to balance are addressed in Chapter 7 and Chapter 20. Further environmental interventions are indicated to minimize home hazards that can increase the risk of falling. Physicians treating fractures in osteoporotic patients should recognize the benefits of rapid return to function and avoidance of prolonged immobilization and bed rest.

Scheuermann's Disease

In 1920, Scheuermann first described the radiographic changes of anterior wedging and vertebral endplate irregularity in the thoracic spine associated with kyphosis in the preteen and adolescent population.[24] Scheuermann's disease is also known as juvenile kyphosis, vertebral osteochondritis, and osteochondritis deformans juvenilis dorsi. Scheuermann's disease of the thoracic spine is defined as an excessive thoracic kyphosis, with wedging of 5 degrees or more in at least three adjacent apical vertebrae with vertebral endplate irregularities.[17] A thoracic kyphosis greater than 45 to 50 degrees is usually considered abnormal, but there are individuals with normally shaped vertebrae that exceed this limit.[25]

Scheuermann's disease is a hereditary disorder transmitted in an autosomal dominant pattern.[26] The mechanism is unknown, but pathologic specimens exhibit abnormal cartilage with deficient bone growth under the areas of abnormal growth plates. Disk material herniated into the vertebral bodies (ie, Schmorl's nodes) is a common finding.

DIAGNOSIS

The typical patient is a preteen or adolescent presenting with excessive thoracic kyphosis, with or without pain at the apex of the curve or in the low back. The kyphotic deformity is usually acute, distinguishing it from acquired kyphosis. Associated lumbar lordosis is common, and 20% to 25% of patient s have associated scoliosis that does not progress.[17]

A thorough neurologic examination is indicated because cord compression can occur. Any degree of hyperreflexia or ataxia needs further investigation. Radiographic evaluation uses the Cobb method to measure the curve (see Fig. 25-34). The degree of anterior wedging and the number of vertebrae involved are documented. Decreased disk height, vertebral endplate irregularity, Schmorl's nodes, or persistence of a separate fragment of bone anterosuperior to the front edge of a vertebral body (limbus vertebra) may also be identified.

TREATMENT

Treatment is usually limited to patients with a painful deformity, documented progression, and at least 2 years of growth remaining. Younger children with a mild deformity can be initially treated with a program of exercise to strengthen spinal extensor muscles (see Fig. 25-12) and stretch the hamstring (see Fig. 20-25), pectoralis major (see Fig. 26-28), and superior fibers of the rectus abdominis muscles and anterior longitudinal ligament (see Self-Management: Prone Press-up Progression, level II, in Chapter 18).

In adolescents, Scheuermann's disease is effectively managed with bracing until skeletal maturity has been reached (see the Scoliosis section). Contraindications to brace treatment include curves greater than 70 degrees, severe apical wedging, and a rigid curve.

Surgery is considered as an option for patients with severe deformity and disabling pain and as necessary in cases of neurologic compromise. Spinal fusion is the recommended surgical technique.

EXERCISE MANAGEMENT OF KYPHOSIS

The posture impairment of thoracic kyphosis is a key characteristic of osteoporosis and Scheuermann's disease. Treatment of the kyphosis must consider the anatomic impairment and pathology in addition to the related physiologic impairments. Display 25-7 lists potential physiologic impairments associated with kyphosis, and Table 25-5 lists general exercise recommendations to address physiologic impairments associated with kyphosis.

Patient-related instruction is indicated to improve posture alignment and avoid positions that contribute to the kyphosis. Support to the lower back may be indicated to assist with the lordosis in the lordosis-kyphosis posture, and a shoulder support may be indicated for the kyphosis to help stretch the pectoralis minor and relieve strain on the middle and lower trapezius (see Fig. 25-11).

As illustrated by Table 25-5, exercise prescription for the treatment of kyphosis may need to go well beyond strengthening the thoracic erector spinae. The thoracic spine must function as part of a kinematic chain, and treatment of physiologic impairments in each region influencing the kyphosis is indicated. Ultimately, improved physiologic capabilities in each region can provide a good foundation for enhanced function and quality of life. Specific exercises must progress to functional movements meaningful to that patient. For example, a patient with Scheuermann's disease with a desk job needs to maintain his best neutral spine when working. He would benefit from learning to lean forward and backward

DISPLAY 25-7

Physiologic Impairments Associated With Kyphosis

Alignment

Forward head
Cervical lordosis
Abducted scapulae
Kyphosis-lordosis: Lumbar lordosis, anterior pelvic tilt, hip joint flexion, knee joint hyperextension, ankle plantar flexion
Swayback: Lumbar flexion, posterior pelvic tilt, hip joint hyperextension, knee joint hyperextension, neutral ankle

Kyphosis-Lordosis	**Swayback**
Short and Strong	
Neck extensors	Hamstrings
Hip flexors	Upper fibers of internal oblique
Lumbar spinal extensors	
Shoulder adductors	Shoulder adductors
Pectoralis minor	Pectoralis minor
Intercostals	Intercostals
Elongated and Weak	
Neck flexors	Neck flexors
Upper back spinal extensors	Upper back spinal extensors
External oblique	External oblique
Hamstrings	One-joint hip flexors
Middle and lower trapezius	Middle and lower trapezius

** Findings associated with short muscles must be tested by muscle length and manual muscle tests, because not all muscles held in short positions develop shortness.*

Table 25-5. THERAPEUTIC EXERCISE MANAGEMENT FOR KYPHOSIS

STRETCH	STRENGTHEN
Kyphosis	
Cervical spine extensors	Cervical spine flexors
Intercostals (see Figs. 25-18, 25-19)	Thoracic spine extensors (see Fig. 25-6)
Lumbar spine extensors (see Fig. 25-7)	
Pectoralis minor, shoulder adductors (see Fig. 25-19)	Middle and lower trapezius
Lordosis	
Lumbar spine extensors (see Fig. 25-7)	External oblique
Hip flexors	Hip extensors
Swayback	
Intercostals (see Figs. 25-18, 25-19)	External oblique
Hamstrings	Hip flexors

while maintaining a neutral spine. Thinking about the distance between the symphysis pubis and the base of the sternum and keeping this distance constant during forward and backward movements at the hip joints can be useful in changing movement patterns that promote thoracic flexion.

Although diseases such as osteoporosis and Scheuermann's cause anatomic changes in the vertebrae that create the kyphosis, postural habits and movement patterns can exaggerate the posture impairment. Although exercise cannot correct the anatomic changes that have occurred in the vertebrae, it can positively influence physiologic factors that exaggerate the kyphosis. Only through a comprehensive program of exercise and patient-related instruction can these contributing factors be properly addressed.

Key Points

- Stiffness and stability of the thoracic spine are facilitated by the rib cage, the low ratio of disk height to vertebral body height, the acute angular orientation of the lamellae of the anulus and the relatively small nucleus pulposus, and the orientation of the zygapophysial joints.
- Many muscles function about the thoracic spine to produce the primary movements of flexion, extension, lateral flexion, rotation, inspiration, and expiration. Imbalances in muscle length and performance can contribute to impairments in mobility and posture and movement of the thoracic spine.
- All motions are possible in the thoracic region, but the range of flexion and extension is limited in the upper thoracic region (T1-T6), where the facets lie closer to the frontal plane. In the lower part (T9-T12), the facets lie more in the sagittal plane, allowing an increased amount of flexion and extension. Lateral flexion is free in the upper thoracic region and increases in the lower region. Rotation, which also is free in the upper thoracic region, decreases caudally.
- During inhalation and exhalation, the primary movements of the ribs are called pump and bucket handle. To ensure proper breathing mechanics, both of these motions must be occurring during inhalation and exhalation.

LAB ACTIVITIES

1. Your patient has trouble stabilizing against rotational forces in the upper thoracic region. Develop and teach your partner three sequentially more difficult exercises to improve stabilization skills against rotational forces.
2. Refer to the Patient-Related Instruction: Diaphragmatic Breathing in Chapter 23. Assess your partner's breathing in the supine position. Does your partner have integrated pump and bucket handle rib motions? Are they symmetric? Teach your partner proper breathing mechanics.
3. Play the role of a person with Scheuermann's disease with a desk job at a visual display terminal. Teach your partner proper ergonomics at the workstation. Teach your partner to reach across the desk and into a file cabinet. Avoid exaggerating the kyphosis.
4. Design an exercise program for a patient with right thoracic and left lumbar scoliosis. Teach each activity to your partner. Can you see or feel the effect of asymmetric exercise on the spine?
5. Referring to Critical Thinking Question 4, what alternative exercise would you prescribe to your patient with osteoporosis if she had weak abdominal muscles? Teach your partner this activity. Which abdominal muscle would you expect to dominate in the exercise you instruct for someone with kyphosis?
6. Referring to Critical Thinking Question 5, what alternative exercise would you prescribe to your patient with osteoporosis if she had weak thoracic erector spinae? Teach your partner this activity. Be sure to role-play someone with moderate to marked kyphosis.

- A comprehensive examination of all patients, including the history, systems review, and tests and measures, must be performed to enable the therapist to determine the diagnosis (based on impairments, functional limitations, and disabilities), prognosis, and interventions.
- When considering therapeutic exercise interventions for common physiologic impairments of the thoracic region, the therapist must consider the role of the thoracic spine in the kinematic chain and how other segmental levels can affect the physiologic function of the thoracic spine.
- Although few exercises directly address the thoracic region, those that address respiration, mobility, and performance of the trunk, shoulder girdle, and cervical muscles are the most important.
- Thoracic spine function can be enhanced by treating the cervical and lumbar spine, shoulder girdle, pelvic-hip complex, and foot and ankle complex.
- Therapeutic exercise intervention is thought to affect the course of scoliosis if the disorder is treated through asymmetric exercises, patient-related instruction, and movement retraining.
- There are many causes of kyphosis. If the cause is a disease such as Scheuermann's or osteoporosis, exercise intervention cannot reverse the pathology, but it may be able to retard or prevent further exaggeration of the kyphosis.

Critical Thinking Questions

1. Describe how function of the foot and ankle, hip, and shoulder girdle could affect function of the thoracic spine. Provide one example for each region.
2. The client has Scheuermann's disease.
   a. What two posture types would this patient probably exhibit?
   b. List the possible shortened and lengthened muscles around the trunk and pelvis for each posture type.
3. The client has right thoracic and left lumbar scoliosis.
   a. What are the possible shortened and lengthened muscles in the anterior and posterior trunk and pelvic girdle?
   b. What foot and ankle alignment faults could contribute to this scoliosis?
4. Why would trunk curl exercises be contraindicated for someone with Scheuermann's disease or osteoporosis?
5. Why would prone hyperextension exercises be contraindicated for someone with Scheuermann's disease or osteoporosis?

REFERENCES

1. Lee DG. Biomechanics of the thorax: a clinical model of in vivo function. *J Manual Manipulative Ther.* 1993;1:13.
2. Lee DG. *Manual Therapy for the Thorax—A Biomechanical Approach*. Delta, British Columbia, Canada: DOPC; 1994.
3. Lee DG. Biomechanics of the thorax. In: Grant R, ed. *Physical Therapy of the Cervical and Thoracic Spine*. New York: Churchill Livingstone; 1994.
4. Edmondston SJ, Singer KP. Thoracic spine: anatomical and biomechanical considerations for manual therapy. *Manual Ther.* 1997;2:132–143.
5. Penning L, Wilmink JT. Rotation of the cervical spine—CT study in normal subjects. *Spine*. 1987;12:732.
6. Warwick R, Williams P. *Gray's Anatomy*. 35th ed. Philadelphia: WB Saunders; 1973.
7. Moore K. *Clinically Oriented Anatomy*. Baltimore: Williams & Wilkins; 1980.
8. Kendall FP, McCreary EK, Provance PG. *Muscles Testing and Function*. Baltimore: Williams & Wilkins; 1993.
9. Guide to physical therapy practice. *Phys Ther*. 1997;77: 1163–1650.
10. Maitland GD. *Vertebral Manipulation*. London: Butterworths; 1986.
11. Norkin C, Levangie P. *Joint Structure and Function*. Philadelphia: FA Davis; 1992.
12. Magee DJ. *Orthopedic Physical Assessment*. 2nd ed. Philadelphia: WB Saunders; 1992.
13. White AA, Panjabi MM. *Clinical Biomechanics of the Spine*. Philadelphia: JB Lippincott; 1990.
14. Panjabi MM, Brand RA, White AA. Mechanical properties of the human thoracic spine. *J Bone Joint Surg Am.* 1976;58: 642–652.
15. Schafer R. *Clinical Biomechanics: Musculoskeletal Actions and Reactions*. Baltimore: Williams & Wilkins; 1983.
16. Greenman P. *Principles of Manual Medicine*. 2nd ed. Baltimore: Williams & Wilkins; 1996.
17. Flynn TW. *The Thoracic Spine and Rib Cage: Musculoskeletal Evaluation and Treatment*. Boston: Butterworth-Heinemann; 1996.
18. Huskisson EC. Measurement of pain. *Lancet*. 1974;2: 1127–1131.
19. Westaway MD, Stratford PW, Binkley JM. The patient-specific functional scale: validation of its use in persons with neck dysfunction. *J Sports Phys Ther.* 1998;27:331–338.
20. Richardson ML. Scoliosis. Department of Radiology, University of Washington; 1994 [mrich@u.washington.edu].
21. American Academy of Orthopedic Surgeons Staff. Instructional Course Lectures. St. Louis, Missouri: CV Mosby, 1985; 34:103–104.
22. Blackman R, O'Neal K, Picetti G, Estep M. Scoliosis treatment. Oakland: Children's Hospital, Kaiser Permanente Hospital; 1998 [rgb@scoliosisrx.com].
23. *NIH Consensus Development Conference Statement* (online, April 2–4, 1984]. 1984;5:1–6.
24. Scheuermann HW. Kyfosis dorsalis juvenile. *Ugeskr Laeger*. 1920;82:385–398.
25. Stagnara P, deMauroy JC, Dran G. Reciprocal angulation of vertebral bodies in the sagittal plane: approach to references for the evaluation of kyphosis and lordosis. *Spine*. 1982;7: 335–342.
26. Halal F, Gledhill RB, Fraser FC. Dominant inheritance of Scheuermann's juvenile kyphosis. *Am J Dis Child*. 1978;132: 1105–1109.

RECOMMENDED READINGS

Ascani E, Bartolozzi P. Natural history of untreated idiopathic scoliosis after skeletal maturity. *Spine* 1986;11:784–789.

Brown C, Deffer P. The natural history of thoracic disc herniation. *Spine*. 1992;17(suppl 6):S97–S102.

Cantu R, Grodin A. *Myofascial Manipulation Theory and Clinical Application*. Gaithersburg, MD: Aspen Publishers; 1992.

Donatelli R, Wooden M. *Orthopaedic Physical Therapy*. New York: Churchill Livingstone; 1989.

Gould J, Davies G. *Orthopedic and Sports Physical Therapy*. St. Louis: CV Mosby; 1985.

Gross J, Fetto J, Rosen E. *Musculoskeletal Examination*. Cambridge, MA: Blackwell Science; 1996.

Irwin S, Tecklin J. *Cardiopulmonary Physical Therapy*. 3rd ed. St. Louis: Mosby; 1995.

Malone T, McPoil T, Nitz A. *Orthopedic and Sports Physical Therapy*. 3rd ed. St. Louis: Mosby–Year Book; 1997.

Mitchell FL, Moran PS, Pruzzo NA. *An Evaluation and Treatment Manual of Osteopathic Muscle Energy Procedures*. Valley Park, MO: Mitchell, Moran, and Pruzzo; 1979.

Pratt N. *Clinical Musculoskeletal Anatomy*. Philadelphia: JB Lippincott; 1991.

Richardson J, Iglarsh ZA. *Clinical Orthopaedic Physical Therapy*. Philadelphia: WB Saunders; 1994.

Winkel D. *Diagnosis and Treatment of the Spine*. Gaithersburg, MD: Aspen Publishers; 1996.

CHAPTER 26

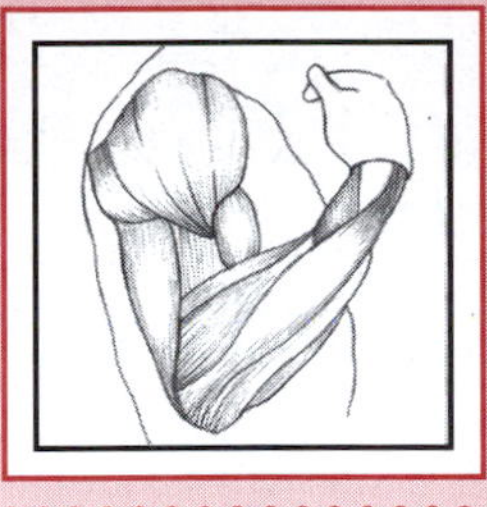

The Shoulder Girdle

Carrie Hall

Treatment of the shoulder girdle affects function of the scapula, the humerus, and the entire upper quadrant including the lumbar, thoracic, and cervical spine and the elbow, forearm, wrist, and hand. The shoulder girdle functions in a kinetic chain with the trunk and remainder of the upper extremity. Dysfunction of the shoulder girdle can affect function of related regions, and dysfunction of related regions can affect function of the shoulder girdle. For example, faulty movement patterns and associated impairments of the shoulder girdle can affect function of the cervical spine because of shared musculature (ie, levator scapula and upper trapezius). Faulty movement patterns and associated impairments of the spine and pelvis can affect function of the shoulder girdle. For example, asymmetric spine and pelvis alignment can contribute to faults in shoulder girdle alignment and movement patterns.

REVIEW OF ANATOMY AND KINESIOLOGY

The anatomy and kinesiology of the shoulder girdle are intricate. The combined coordinated movements of the four distinct articulations and the involved muscles and periarticular structures allow the arm and hand to be positioned in space for a variety of functions. The result is a range of motion (ROM) that exceeds that of any other joint complex in the body.

The shoulder girdle is composed of four distinct articulations: sternoclavicular, acromioclavicular, scapulothoracic, and glenohumeral. Each of these joints function interdependently and in synchrony.

Sternoclavicular Joint

The sternoclavicular joint is a synovial joint in which the clavicle articulates with the sternal notch and cartilage of the first rib (Fig. 26-1). It is the only bony attachment of the entire upper limb to the axial skeleton. An articular disk divides the joint cavity into two compartments (see Fig. 26-1). The disk blends with the joint capsule and is attached to the clavicle above and the sternum and first rib below.[1]

Binding to the clavicle, the disk prevents medial displacement and acts as a hinge and shock absorber on which the clavicle moves when the shoulder is moved up and down.[2] The movements allowed at the sternoclavicular joint are summarized in Table 26-1.

The major ligaments surrounding the sternoclavicular joint include the costoclavicular, the anterior and posterior sternoclavicular, and the interclavicular (see Fig. 26-1). The joint capsule is reinforced by these ligaments.[1] Although each of these ligaments provides a specific function, they function together to support the weight of the shoulder and arm. This support is so strong that, even with paralysis of the trapezius, the shoulder girdle remains supported.[3] Because the sternal end of the clavicle is well anchored and the ligaments are stronger than the bone, the middle clavicle often fractures before the sternoclavicular joint dislocates.[4]

Acromioclavicular Joint

The acromioclavicular joint is formed by the articulation of the acromion process of the scapula with the acromial end of the clavicle. The articular facets of the acromioclavicular joint are small, afford limited motion, and have a wide range of individual differences. For these reasons, studies

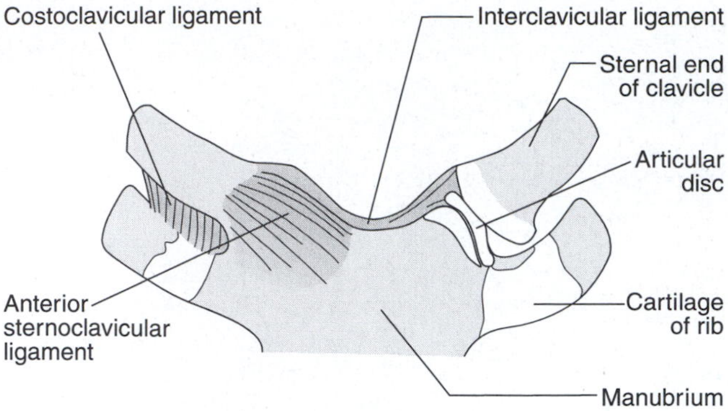

FIGURE 26-1 Sternoclavicular articulation, anterior view.

Table 26-1. STERNOCLAVICULAR JOINT MOTIONS

MOTION	DEGREES
Elevation	4–60
Depression	5–15
Protraction or retraction	15 (from resting position)
Rotation	30–50 (posteriorly about the horizontal axis)

Data from references 113, 114, and 115.

are inconsistent in identifying the movement and axes of motion for this joint. This text presents one theory of the biomechanics of the acromioclavicular joint described by Nordin and Frankel.[5] The movements are summarized in Table 26-2 and illustrated in Figure 26-2.

The three major ligaments that are important for proper functioning of the acromioclavicular joint are the superior and inferior acromioclavicular and coracoclavicular ligaments (Fig. 26-3). The superior and inferior acromioclavicular ligaments cover the superior and inferior aspects of the acromioclavicular joint, offer some protection to the joint, and assist horizontal joint stability. The coracoclavicular ligament provides much of the acromioclavicular joint stability and acts as the binding force between the clavicle and scapula. This ligament is divided into a lateral portion called the trapezoid and a medial portion called the conoid (see Fig. 26-3). The trapezoid lies in the sagittal plane, and the conoid lies essentially in the frontal plane. The most critical role played by this ligament is in producing longitudinal rotation of the clavicle, which is necessary for full ROM of the scapula during elevation of the upper extremity.[6]

The acromioclavicular joint is prone to degenerative changes,[113] which is significant for several reasons. Because scapular rotation is necessary for functional shoulder movement, disease or ossification of the acromioclavicular joint tends to encourage the scapula and clavicle to function as a unit. This pattern of use alters the scapular path of instant center of rotation (PICR). Because of its intimate association with the rotator cuff and bursa, changes in the PICR of the scapula can lead to microtrauma or macrotrauma of subacromial structures. Pathology of the subacromial structures can contribute to physiologic impairments, functional limitation, and disability. Evaluation of the function of the acromioclavicular joint is often critical to understanding causal determinants of several shoulder conditions.

Scapulothoracic Joint

The scapulothoracic joint is a functional joint (ie, not a true joint) of the concave ventral scapula and articulates with the convex rib cage. Surrounding this joint are the coracoacromial and superior transverse ligaments (see Fig. 26-3). The coracoacromial ligament forms a roof over the head of the humerus as it runs from the coracoid process to the acromion, helping to prevent upward displacement of the head of the humerus. This ligament provides a protective mechanism for the underlying bursa and supraspinatus tendon. It has a sharp lateral edge that may impinge on the underlying structures when the arm is elevated, particularly if the PICR of the glenohumeral or scapulothoracic joint is faulty or the tissues are inflamed.

The superior transverse ligament bridges the lesser scapular notch to form a foramen for the passage of the suprascapular nerve (see Fig. 26-3). Under ordinary circumstances the tunnel may offer protection to the nerve, but if there is injury, inflammation, or scarring in the region, the confined area becomes a source of entrapment.[7–9]

Scapulothoracic movement requires motion of the clavicle on the thorax at the sternoclavicular joint and motion of the scapula relative to the clavicle at the acromioclavi-

Table 26-2. ACROMIOCLAVICULAR JOINT MOTIONS

MOTION	AXIS	DESCRIPTION
Rotation	Sagittal axis through acromioclavicular joint	Scapular rotation cranially or caudally
Winging (medial rotation)	Vertical axis through conoid ligament	Vertebral border posterior, glenoid fossa anterior
Tilting (tipping)	Frontal axis through trapezoid ligament	Inferior border posterior, superior border anterior

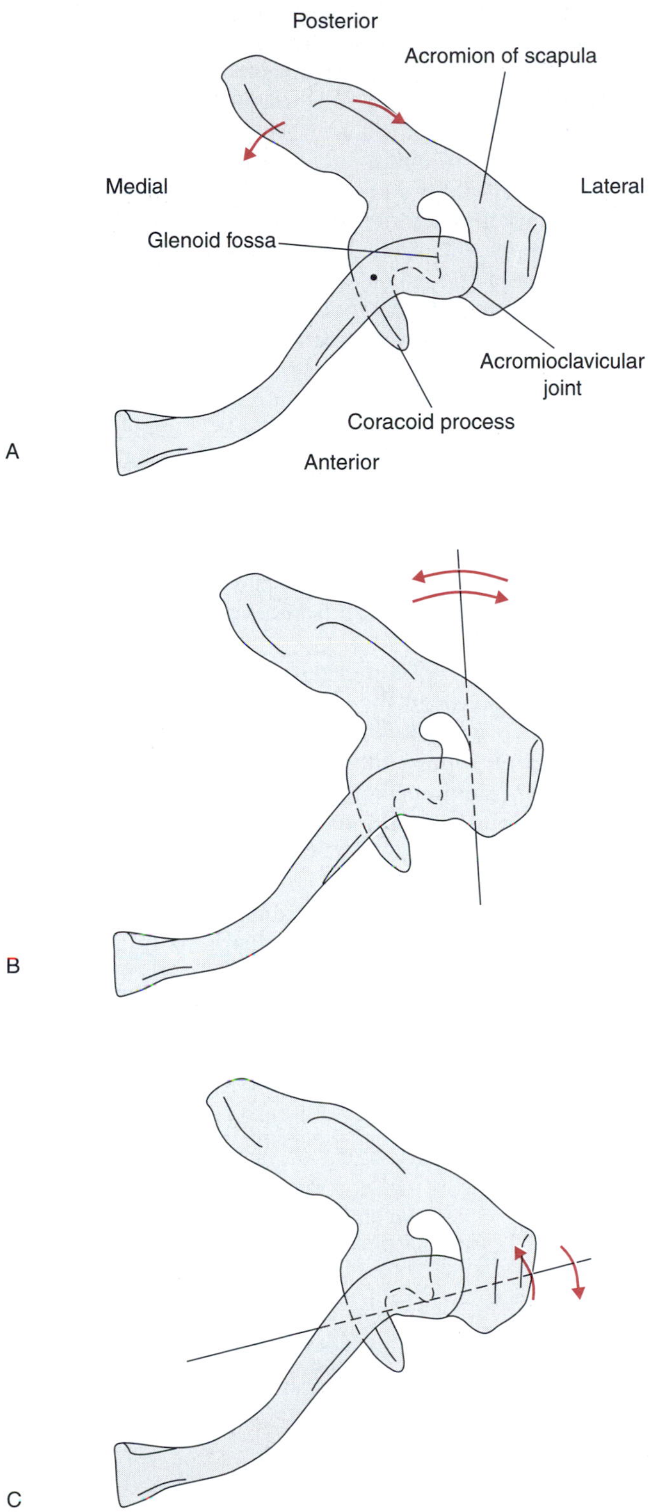

FIGURE 26-2 Top view of the scapula and clavicle, showing the axes of motion at the acromioclavicular joint. ***(A)*** Vertical axis (*solid dot*) for scapular medial rotation ("winging") and lateral rotation. ***(B)*** Transverse axis in the sagittal plane (*dotted line*) for scapular upward and downward rotation. ***(C)*** Transverse (horizontal) axis in the frontal (coronal) plane (*dotted line*) for scapular anterior and posterior tilting ("tipping"). (From Nordin M, Frankel VH. Basic *Biomechanics of the Musculoskeletal System*. 2d ed. Philadelphia: Lea & Febiger; 1989:232.)

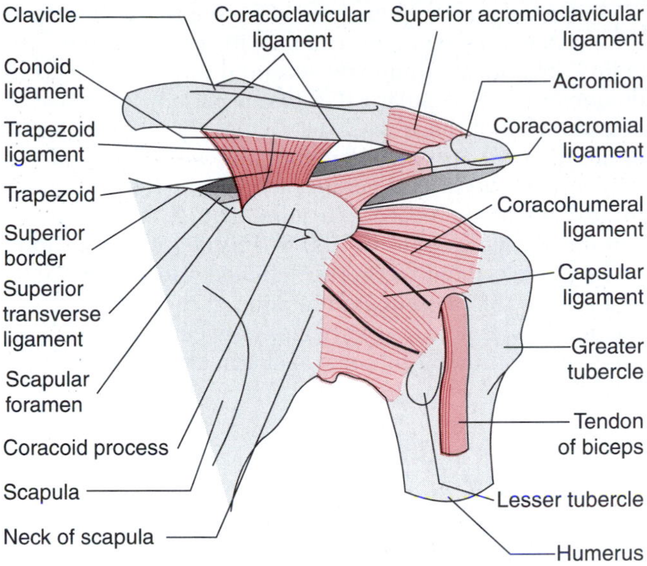

FIGURE 26-3 Acromioclavicular joint, anterior view.

ular joint. Traditionally, motions of the scapula are known as elevation and depression, abduction and adduction, and upward and downward rotation. These motions are described as if they occur independently, although linkage of the scapula to the sternoclavicular and acromioclavicular joints and the shape of the rib cage prevent such pure motions from occurring. For example, elevation is associated with upward rotation and anterior tilting (Fig. 26-4). During arm elevation, the scapula demonstrates a pattern of progressive upward rotation, decreased medial rotation (ie, winging), and movement from an anterior to a posterior tilted position.[11]

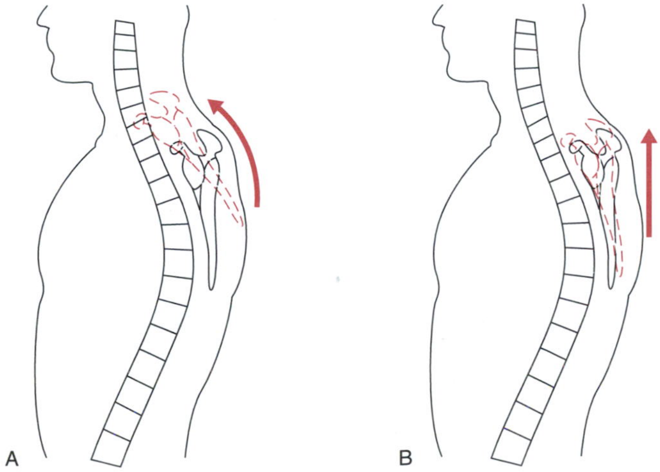

FIGURE 26-4. ***(A)*** Elevation of the scapula on the rib cage is accompanied by anterior tilting of the scapula. ***(B)*** If elevation were purely in a superior direction, the superior aspect of the scapula would come off the rib cage (*dotted lines*). (From Norkin CC, Levangie PK. *Joint Structure and Function: A Comprehensive Analysis*. 2d ed. Philadelphia: FA Davis; 1992.)

A two-dimensional analysis of scapular PICR reveals the existence of common trends with considerable variability. The most commonly accepted movement pattern demonstrates a scapular PICR that is initially located at or near the root of the scapula (ie, medial aspect of the spine of the scapula). As arm abduction progresses beyond 60 to 90 degrees, the instant center of rotation (ICR) migrates toward the acromioclavicular joint. The ICR reaches the acromioclavicular joint by 120 to 150 degrees. Elevation of the clavicle about the sternoclavicular joint occurs in the first 120 to 150 degrees, and rotation of the scapula about the acromioclavicular joint begins between 60 and 90 degrees and continues until maximal arm elevation has been completed.[11]

Glenohumeral Joint

The glenohumeral joint is a synovial joint composed of the head of the humerus articulating with the glenoid fossa of the scapula. With ideal postural alignment, the humeral head is oriented medially, posteriorly, and cranially, and the glenoid faces laterally, anteriorly, and cranially (Fig. 26-5).[12] However, variations in the alignment of the glenoid fossa occur. For example, an individual with a thoracic kyphosis does not have optimal alignment of the scapula. In most subjects, the fossa tilted slightly inferiorly, as would be expected with thoracic kyphosis.[13–18]

The glenoid is one half as long and one third as wide as the head of the humerus, but it is deepened somewhat by a fibrocartilage rim called the glenoid labrum. The glenoid labrum is attached to the margins of the glenoid cavity.[19] The functional significance of the glenoid labrum is questionable, because most authors agree that the labrum is a weak supporting structure.[20,21] Matsen and colleagues[22] described the glenohumeral joint as a "suction cup" because of the seal of the labrum and glenoid to the humeral head. These researchers illustrated the importance of an intact glenoid labrum in establishing a concavity compression. The muscles of the rotator cuff provide the compressive force in this stabilization mechanism.

Although the anatomic configuration of the glenohumeral joint allows significant motion, it makes the joint more susceptible to hypermobility and instability in any direction, particularly anteriorly and inferiorly. The glenohumeral joint capsule is reinforced anteriorly by three glenohumeral ligaments (superior, middle, and inferior), which appear as thickenings of the capsule (Fig. 26-6). The support that these ligaments offer is considered insignificant.[23] Superiorly, the capsule is reinforced by the coracohumeral ligament, which blends intimately with the rotator cuff tendons and fills in the space between the subscapularis and supraspinatus tendons (see Fig. 26-3). The inferior glenohumeral ligament is described as the thickest and most consistent structure (see Fig. 26-6).[24] At 90 degrees of abduction, external rotation is primarily restricted by the inferior glenohumeral ligament.[24] The subacromial bursa facilitates smooth passage of the humeral head and overlying rotator cuff beneath the acromial arch and coracoacromial ligament (Fig. 26-7).[1]

Glenohumeral joint flexion and extension is motion about a frontal axis in the sagittal plane. The total motion varies from 105 to 120 degrees of flexion and 30 to 55 degrees of extension.[6,12] Glenohumeral joint abduction and adduction is motion about a sagittal axis in the frontal plane. The total motion into abduction varies from 105 to 120 degrees abduction. Adduction is the return to anatomic position.[6,12]

Glenohumeral joint abduction in the plane of the scapula is also called scaption. This is motion about an oblique sagittal axis in the plane of the scapula—approximately 30 to 40 degrees anterior to the frontal plane—midway between flexion and abduction (Fig. 26-8).[25,26] Eleva-

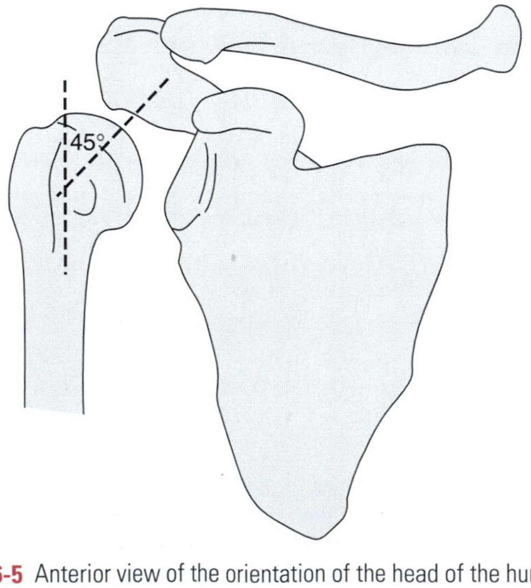

FIGURE 26-5 Anterior view of the orientation of the head of the humerus and glenoid fossa. (From Kessler, RM, Hertling, D. *Management of Common Musculoskeletal Disorders.* Philadelphia; Harper & Row; 1983: 275)

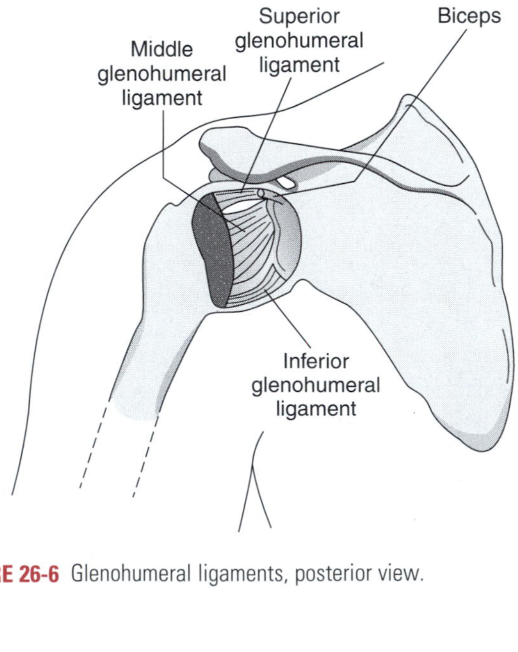

FIGURE 26-6 Glenohumeral ligaments, posterior view.

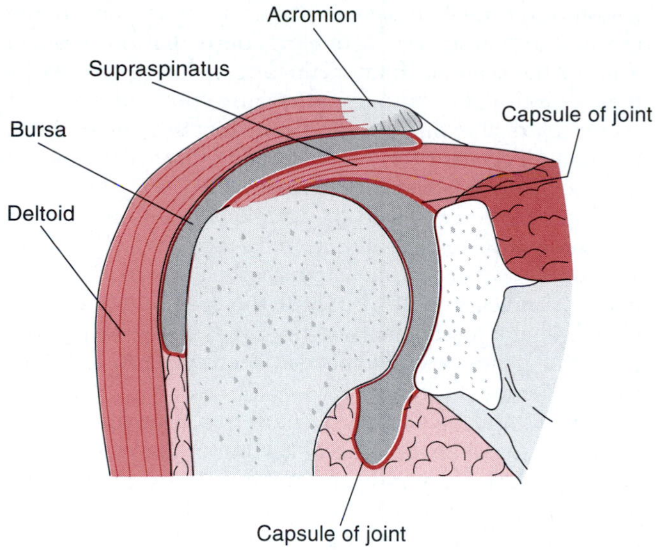

FIGURE 26-7 Subacromial bursa and capsule of the shoulder joint.

tion of the humerus in the scapular plane has a range of 107 to 112 degrees.[27]

The glenohumeral joint motions of lateral and medial rotation occur about the vertical axis and can be performed with the humerus in various degrees of elevation and planes of motion. With the humerus in adduction and the elbow flexed 90 degrees, medial rotation is stopped by the arm's contact with the body, whereas lateral rotation is limited by the anterior joint capsule, anterior glenohumeral ligaments, and the subscapularis muscle. Lateral rotation with the arm adducted is approximately 80 degrees.[28] As the arm abducts away from the body, lateral rotation increases to 90 degrees, and medial rotation increases to 70 degrees.[28]

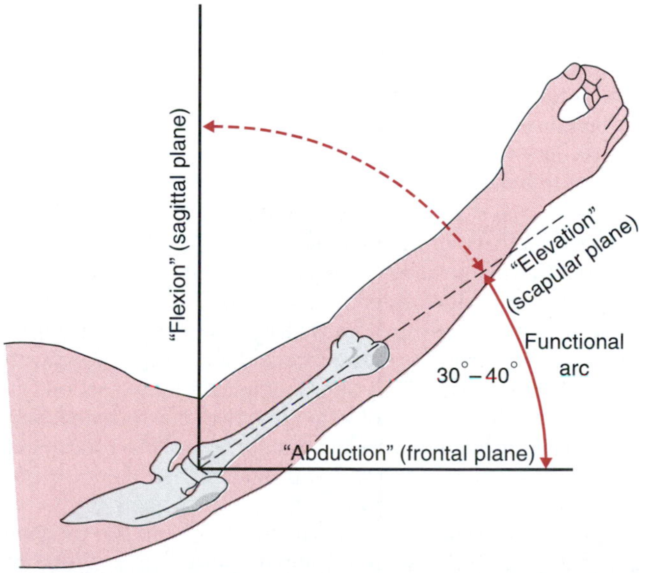

FIGURE 26-8 The scapular plane is approximately 30–40 degrees anterior to the frontal plane.[25,26]

Glenohumeral joint horizontal abduction and adduction are defined as movement of the arm in a horizontal plane. Measured from a starting position of 90 degrees of abduction, horizontal adduction is anterior movement toward the midline of the body of approximately 135 degrees (45 degrees past the midline of the body). Horizontal abduction is posterior movement of approximately 45 degrees. The glenohumeral joint is capable of about 180 degrees of motion about the horizontal plane.[29]

With conjunct rotation, simultaneous or conjunct rotation occurs at the glenohumeral joint during arm elevation. Lateral rotation of the humerus is required to elevate the arm in the frontal plane[6] to clear the greater tuberosity from the acromioclavicular joint during motion in the frontal plane. However, slight conjunct medial rotation occurs during motion in the sagittal plane because of ligamentous tension from the superior and inferior bands of the glenohumeral ligament, posterior band of the coracohumeral ligament, and the bony configuration of the glenohumeral joint.[30] When moving in the plane of the scapula, the humerus has less restricted motion. During scaption, there is less tension on the glenohumeral joint capsule, and lateral rotation of the humerus is not required to prevent the greater tubercle's impact on the acromion.[16]

The flexible glenohumeral joint also displays arthrokinematic motion, in which three types of surface motion may take place in any given plane—rotation, rolling, and translation (ie, gliding) (Fig. 26-9). Arthrokinematic motion at the glenohumeral joint is primarily rotational, but some combination of rolling and gliding take place. During shoulder elevation in the plane of the scapula, the humeral head moves slightly upward, indicating that rolling or gliding takes place, particularly in the early phases of arm elevation (0 to 30 degrees).[17] The average humeral head translates 3 mm initially when the deltoid vector of force is nearly perpendicular with the humerus. It then settles down to ride 1 mm superior to its initial rest position in the glenoid.[17] Conversely, measurements of patients with shoulder lesions indicate distinctly greater humeral head superior translations.[17]

Scapulohumeral Rhythm

The intricate interplay of the four articulations of the shoulder complex results in a coordinated movement pattern of arm elevation referred to as scapulohumeral rhythm.[31] The involved movements at each joint are continuous, although occurring at various rates and at different phases of arm elevation. Elevation of the arm involves glenohumeral and scapulothoracic motion; scapulothoracic motion is the result of motions at the acromioclavicular and sternoclavicular joints. Several investigators have attempted to correlate glenohumeral and scapulothoracic motion during arm elevation in various planes, and three of these studies deserve special mention.[6,12,16,17,27,32–37]

Inman and coworkers[6] reported that the humeral and scapular contributions to arm elevation were approximately 120 and 60 degrees, respectively, and that after a brief "setting" phase, a constant relationship exists, whereby for every 2 degrees of glenohumeral motion, 1 degree of scapular motion occurs. However, this belief has not been supported by

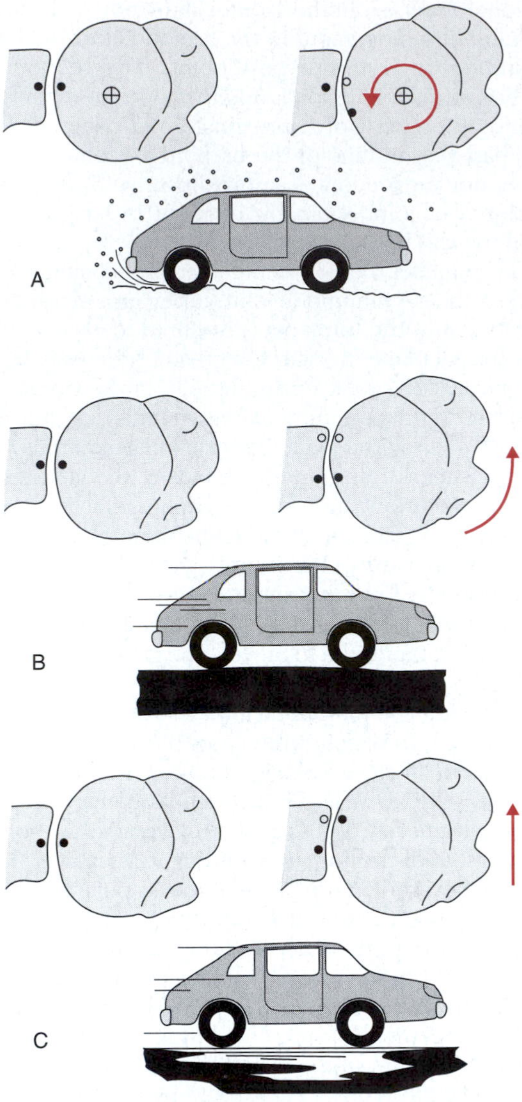

FIGURE 26-9 Surface motion at the glenohumeral joint. Three types of motion take place: rotation, rolling, and translation (gliding). ***(A)*** During rotation, the contact point on the glenoid surface remains constant, while the contact point on the head of humerus changes (analogous to the rear tires of a car spinning in the snow). ***(B)*** During rolling, the contact point on each surface changes (analogous with the tires on a car travelling down the road). ***(C)*** During translation (gliding), the contact point on the humeral head remains constant, while the contact point on the glenoid changes (analogous to the tires of a car skidding on ice). (From Nordin M. Frankel VH. Basic *Biomechanics of the Musculoskeletal System.* 2d ed. Philadelphia: Lea & Febiger; 1989:231.)

later investigations.[12,16,17,27,37] Bagg[12] reports that three distinct patterns of scapulohumeral rhythm exist and that each pattern is more complex than the 2:1 ratio proposed by Inman and colleagues.[6] The most common of the three patterns is characterized by three separate phases, each having different scapulohumeral rhythm ratios. During the middle phase, from approximately 80 degrees to 140 degrees of abduction, scapular rotation provides a greater contribution to arm elevation than glenohumeral motion. A possible explanation of the relative increase in the scapular contribution during the midrange of arm elevation is that the moment arms of the scapular rotators are larger during that period than those of the deltoid and rotator cuff muscles.[16,27] It seems reasonable that the greatest relative amount of scapular rotation occurs over the most difficult range of arm abduction.[12] The existence of three patterns of scapulohumeral rhythm may be explained by variations in anthropometric measures, postures, and muscle imbalances. We think it may be possible that one of the patterns is ideal and that the other patterns indicate faulty PICR at the scapulothoracic and glenohumeral joints. Faults in the PICR of the scapulothoracic and glenohumeral joints may predispose an individual to shoulder dysfunction.

It is helpful in diagnosing movement impairments to recognize that a disturbance of rhythm or loss of motion in any one phase may indicate impaired movement at the joint or joints that contribute the major share of movement during that phase or abnormal muscular force couples operating at any given phase at the glenohumeral or scapulothoracic joint. Muscular force couples are discussed later.

Myology

The muscles acting on the shoulder complex can be divided into three major groups: scapulohumeral, axioscapular, and axiohumeral. Table 26-3 provides a list of the muscles in each group and their primary functions.

The rotator cuff–deltoid force couple and scapular force couples deserve special mention because of the coordinated and integrated function of the muscles within and between each force couple. The rotator cuff–deltoid force couple requires the coordination of several muscles in the scapulohumeral group. The scapular force couple consists of an upward force couple and a downward force couple. The muscles necessary for these force couples are within the axioscapular group. Dynamic stabilization of the composite movement of the thoracic-scapular-humeral articulation requires coordinated function of the scapular and deltoid–rotator cuff force couples.

ROTATOR CUFF–DELTOID FORCE COUPLE

The rotator cuff consists of the supraspinatus, infraspinatus, teres minor, and subscapularis muscles. They terminate in short, flat, broad tendons that fuse intimately with the capsule of the shoulder joint to form a musculotendinous cuff. These muscles act as a force couple with the deltoid. The directional force of the deltoid is upward and outward with respect to the humerus, whereas the directional force of the rotator cuff is downward and inward. The deltoid acting alone elicits an upward translatory force on the humeral head, and the rotator cuff acting alone exerts a downward translatory force on the humeral head. If the two actions are combined, the motion of arm elevation is produced, with the deltoid providing the elevation force and the rotator cuff compressing the humeral head against the glenoid, preventing superior migration of the humeral head.[38]

The force couple is an essential principle in the mechanics of elevation; this same principle operates in scapular rotation. Impairment of either component of the force couple

Table 26-3. SHOULDER GIRDLE CATEGORIES AND MUSCLE FUNCTION

MUSCLE	FUNCTION
Scapulohumeral Group	
Supraspinatus*	Humeral abduction
Infraspinatus*	Lateral rotation (LR)
Teres minor*	LR
Subscapularis*	Medial rotation (MR)
Deltoid	
Anterior fibers	Flexion and MR
Middle fibers	Abduction
Posterior fibers	Extension and LR
Teres major	MR
Coracobrachialis	Flexion and MR
Axioscapular Group	
Trapezius†	
Upper fibers	Scapular elevation
Middle fibers	Scapular adduction
Lower fibers	Scapular depression and adduction
Serratus anterior†	Scapular abduction
Rhomboid major and minor‡	Scapular elevation and adduction
Levator scapula‡	Scapular elevation
Pectoralis minor anterior	Scapular depression and tilting
Axiohumeral Group	
Pectoralis major	MR extension and adduction, clavicular fibers flex to 90 degrees
Latissimus dorsi	MR and extension

* Part of the rotator cuff.
† Part of the scapular upward rotator force couple.
‡ Part of the scapular downward rotator force couple.

distorts the PICR and may cause microtrauma. Microtrauma can eventually cause macrotrauma to the soft tissue structures about the glenohumeral joint, particularly the rotator cuff (see the Impingement Syndrome section).

SCAPULAR FORCE COUPLE

The total motion of arm elevation is the result of motion at the glenohumeral and scapulothoracic joints. Although discrepancy exists in the literature about the exact ROMs occurring at each joint, upward scapular rotation usually is 50 to 60 degrees, and the range of glenohumeral elevation is 105 to 120 degrees. These motions combined achieve the 165 to 180 degrees of arm elevation necessary for function overhead.

Rotation of the scapula is provided by a force couple action from the trapezius (upper, middle, and lower fibers) and the serratus anterior. These muscles, working in combination, provide concentric control for upward rotation and eccentric control for the returning motion under slow, unresisted conditions. If working with optimal magnitude, direction, and timing, the PICR of the scapula migrates from the root of the scapula toward the acromioclavicular joint.[17,39,40] Understanding the timing of the onset of scapular muscle activity offers insights into the causes of abnormal PICRs of the scapula. This knowledge can help in the diagnosis and management of various shoulder conditions.

Participation of the middle trapezius, lower trapezius, and serratus anterior muscles varies with the plane of motion in which the arm is moving.[6] The middle and lower trapezius muscles are the more active component of the force couple during arm movement in the frontal plane, and the serratus anterior is the more active component of the force couple during arm movement in the sagittal plane.[6] The middle and lower trapezius muscles relax somewhat during movement in the sagittal plane, presumably to allow the scapula to abduct around the rib cage.[6]

If the onset of action of each scapular muscle in the course of scapular upward rotation in the scapular plane could be observed, the most optimal pattern[41] to create the expected PICR could be determined (Fig. 26-10). In the upper trapezius, increased activity occurs as soon as arm elevation begins. A plateau phase begins between 15 and 45 degrees and continues until an angle of 90 to 120 degrees arm elevation has been achieved. As the arm elevates beyond this point, the activity increases, reaching maximal activity at the termination of arm elevation; this pattern may result from the function of supporting the scapula against downward forces exerted by the weight of the arm in full elevation (see Fig. 26-10A).[41]

Minimal activity occurs in the lower trapezius until approximately 90 degrees of arm elevation. Early activity of the lower trapezius may interfere with elevation of the

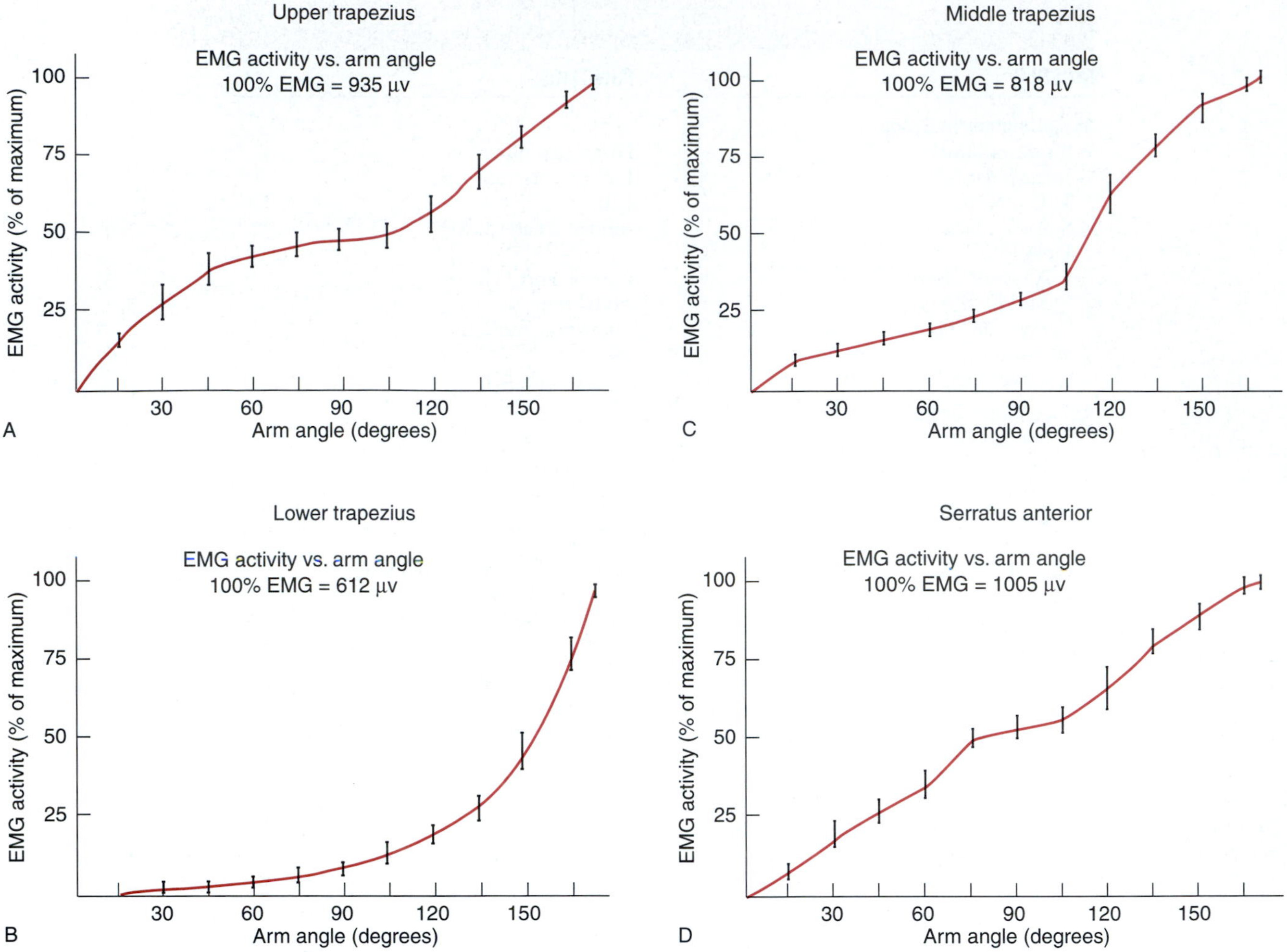

FIGURE 26-10 Commonly observed patterns of electrical activity for the trapezius and lower serratus anterior muscles. (Adapted from Bagg SD, Forrest WJ. Electromyographic study of the scapular rotators during arm abduction in the scapular plane. *Am J Phys Med.* 1986; 65:3.)

scapula at the sternoclavicular joint. As elevation increases beyond this point, activity increases quite rapidly until the termination of arm elevation; this pattern probably results from the improved mechanical advantage of the lower trapezius as the PICR migrates toward the acromioclavicular joint (see Fig. 26-10*B*).

Activity patterns vary markedly in the middle trapezius. There is a slight increase in activity initially, with a plateau phase occurring between 15 and 105 degrees. Beyond the plateau phase, the activity increases significantly until the termination of arm elevation. The middle trapezius most likely prevents excessive movement of the scapula into abduction from forces generated by the serratus anterior (see Fig. 26-10*C*).

The lower serratus anterior exhibits a gradual initial increase in activity, with a brief plateau phase occurring at approximately 90 degrees that is followed by a rise in activity until the termination of arm elevation. Relatively constant activity is found in the serratus anterior throughout scapular upward rotation. The abduction force provided by the serratus anterior may be kept in check by the middle trapezius (see Fig. 26-10*D*).

INTEGRATED ROTATOR CUFF–DELTOID AND SCAPULAR FORCE COUPLES

The integrated functions of the scapular and rotator cuff–deltoid force couples are essential for optimal function of the glenohumeral and scapulothoracic joints. Scapular rotation during arm elevation adds to the total ROM and enables the humeral head to clear the acromion process during arm elevation. Without adequate scapular rotation, the humerus may impinge against the acromion process (Fig. 26-11). Further importance is attached to scapular rotation when the length–tension relationship of the deltoid muscle is considered. When the arm is at the side, the deltoid muscle is at its resting length and is capable of generating maximum tension when contracting. As the arm is elevated, the deltoid contracts and shortens. If the scapula does not rotate sufficiently, the length–tension property of the deltoid is disrupted. Scapular rotation is necessary to keep the acromion moving away from the deltoid insertion to maintain the deltoid close to its resting length. If the scapula fails to rotate sufficiently, the deltoid functions in a relatively shortened length, which disrupts the deltoid–rotator cuff force couple, potentially leading to an excessive proximal force vector

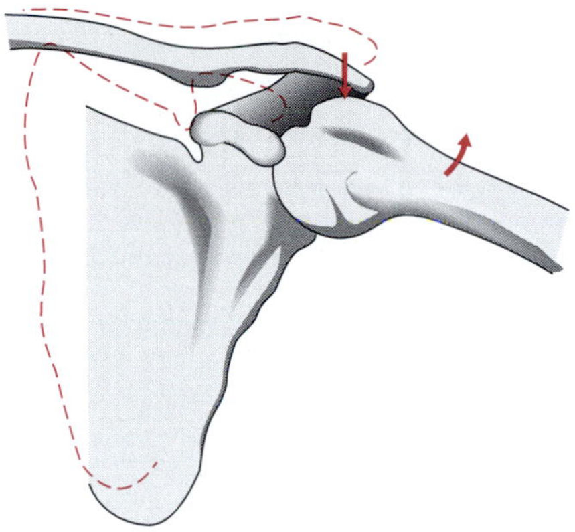

FIGURE 26-11 Decreased subacromial space due to lack of scapular rotation during arm elevation. This is a potential extrinsic cause of impingement syndrome. Dotted line shows a normal subachromial relationship.

from the deltoid. This disruption causes the head of the humerus to translate superiorly, leading to impingement of the subacromial structures.

Adequate movement of the scapula may also be necessary to assist in stabilization of the glenohumeral joint. Insufficient movement of the scapula may contribute to compensatory excessive movement of the glenohumeral joint to achieve the desired ROM. For example, during horizontal abduction movements, scapular adduction is necessary to move the arm posterior to the frontal plane. Failure of the scapula to adduct sufficiently may cause the humeral head to translate anteriorly to achieve the desired motion of the arm in a posterior direction. This motion is required in the cocking phase of pitching, the back-swing during a tennis ground stroke, or in reaching behind the back.

EXAMINATION AND EVALUATION

Examination and evaluation of the shoulder girdle should be performed for all shoulder-related functional limitations and associated impairments but should be considered for any upper quadrant dysfunction. The function of the shoulder girdle is intimately related to the functions of the cervical and thoracic spine. The shared musculature and joint articulations create this close relationship.[42] Functions of the elbow, forearm, wrist, and hand may be related to the function of the shoulder girdle, because they are part of the kinetic chain of the upper quadrant. Dysfunction in one segment of the chain affects the function of other segments. An example of this relationship is an individual with hypomobile forearm pronation. The compensation for this restriction during the activities of daily living (ADLs) requiring forearm pronation may be medial rotation of the shoulder. If this pattern is performed repetitively, particularly in elevated arm positions biased toward the frontal plane, impingement of the subacromial structures of the shoulder may develop.

The descriptive examination and evaluation information discussed in this section is not intended to be comprehensive or reflect any specific philosophical approach. It serves as a review of pertinent tests performed in most shoulder girdle examinations.

History

The history must attempt to establish several types of information:

- Onset and progression of the current condition
- Location, nature, and behavior of symptoms
- Past and current health status
- Effect of intraindividual and extraindividual interventions
- Effect the condition has had on ADLs and social roles

If an injury precipitated the condition, it is important to determine the mechanism of injury to aid in identification of the injured structures. A condition that has developed as the result of repetitive stress is probably characterized by an insidious onset. In this case, the clinician must attempt to identify the repetitive movements and prolonged postures the patient assumes to determine factors that may contribute to the current condition. Much of this information can be obtained through self-report forms, leaving the formal interview to clarify data. Display 26-1 illustrates a sample functional index questionnaire.

Cervical Clearing Examination

Routine screening for cervical involvement should be included during the examination of any patient with shoulder girdle signs and symptoms. One reason is the prevalence of cervical spine conditions in the general population, and another is the pain referral pattern of the cervical spine into the shoulder girdle region. Although this scan may seem extensive, it is pertinent to carefully exclude the cervical spine from involvement (see the Pain Impairment section). A cervical scan examination should include the following tests and measurements:

- General observation of cervical alignment
- Active movements of the cervical spine (followed by overpressure if no symptoms are elicited by active movements alone)
- Resisted cervical movements at end range
- General axial compression and specific foraminal compression (ie, cervical quadrant or Spurling test)
- Cervical traction
- Key muscle tests to determine if neurologically mediated strength deficits are present and, if so, what levels are affected
- Peripheral reflex testing
- Sensory testing
- Upper motor neuron tests
- Upper limb tension tests

Other Clearing Tests

The elbow-wrist-hand complex should be excluded as a source of pain, although it rarely refers pain proximally to the shoulder. Visceral structures can also be sources of pain

DISPLAY 26-1
Functional Index Questionaire

Functional Index
Part 1:

Answer all five sections in Part 1. Choose the one answer in each section that best describes your condition.

Walking
- ☐ Pain does not prevent me walking any distance.
- ☐ Pain prevents me walking more than 1 mile.
- ☐ Pain prevents me walking more than $^1/_2$ mile.
- ☐ Pain prevents me walking more than $^1/_4$ mile.
- ☐ I can only walk using a stick or crutches.
- ☐ I am in bed most of the time and have to crawl to the toilet.

Work

(Applies to work in home and outside)
- ☐ I can do as much work as I want to.
- ☐ I can only do my usual work, but no more.
- ☐ I can do most of my usual work, but no more.
- ☐ I cannot do my usual work.
- ☐ I can hardly do any work at all (only light duty).
- ☐ I cannot do any work at all.

Personal Care

(Washing, dressing, etc.)
- ☐ I can manage all personal care without symptoms.
- ☐ I can manage all personal care with some increased symptoms.
- ☐ Personal care requires slow, concise movements due to increased symptoms.
- ☐ I need help to manage some personal care.
- ☐ I need help to manage all personal care.
- ☐ I cannot manage any personal care.

Sleeping
- ☐ I have no trouble sleeping.
- ☐ My sleep is mildly disturbed (less than 1 h sleepless).
- ☐ My sleep is mildly disturbed (1–2 h sleepless).
- ☐ My sleep is moderately disturbed (2–3 h sleepless).
- ☐ My sleep is greatly disturbed (3–5 hrs. sleepless).
- ☐ My sleep is completely disturbed (5–7 h sleepless).

Recreation/Sports

(Indicate sport if appropriate ______________________)
- ☐ I am able to engage in all my recreational/sports activities without increased symptoms.
- ☐ I am able to engage in all my recreational/sports activities with some increased symptoms.
- ☐ I am able to engage in most, but not all of my usual recreational/sports activities because of increased symptoms.
- ☐ I am able to engage in a few of my usual recreational/sports activities because of my increased symptoms.
- ☐ I can hardly do any recreation/sports activities because of increased symptoms.
- ☐ I cannot do any recreational/sports activities at all.

Acuity

(Answer on initial visit.)

How many days ago did onset/injury occur? ________days

Part II:

Choose the one answer that best describes your condition in the sections designated by your therapist.

A. Upper Extremity
Carrying
- ☐ I can carry heavy loads without increased symptoms.
- ☐ I can carry heavy loads with some increased symptoms.
- ☐ I cannot carry heavy loads overhead, but I can manage if they are positioned close to my trunk.
- ☐ I cannot carry heavy loads, but I can manage light to medium loads if they are positioned close to my trunk.
- ☐ I can carry very light weights with some increased symptoms.
- ☐ I cannot lift or carry anything at all.

Dressing
- ☐ I can put on a shirt or blouse without symptoms.
- ☐ I can put on a shirt or blouse with some increased symptoms.
- ☐ It is painful to put on a shirt or blouse and I am slow and careful.
- ☐ I need some help but I manage most of my shirt or blouse dressing.
- ☐ I need help in most aspects of putting on my shirt or blouse.
- ☐ I cannot put on a shirt or blouse at all.

Reaching
- ☐ I can reach to a high shelf to place an empty cup without increased symptoms.
- ☐ I can reach to a high shelf to place an empty cup with some increased symptoms.
- ☐ I can reach to a high shelf to place an empty cup with a moderate increase in symptoms.
- ☐ I cannot reach to a high shelf to place an empty cup, but I can reach up to a lower shelf without increased symptoms.
- ☐ I cannot reach up to a lower shelf without increased symptoms, but I can reach counter height to place an empty cup.
- ☐ I cannot reach my hand above waist level without increased symptoms.

Adapted with permission from Therapeutic Associates Outcomes System, Therapeutic Associates, Inc. Sherman Oaks, CA.

referred into the shoulder girdle. Visceral referral of symptoms should be considered in cases refractory to physical therapy intervention. Appendix 1 lists specific visceral pain referral patterns into the shoulder girdle. A thorough health history can assist in identifying signs that may designate visceral sources of symptoms.

STANDING AND SITTING ALIGNMENT

Alignments of the clavicle, scapula, and humerus should be examined about all three planes with the client in a standing position. The clinician should observe the following:

- Total body alignment—particularly related to symmetry in limb lengths
- Head, thoracic, and lumbar spine alignment
- Pelvic position about all three planes, which directly affects alignment of the shoulder girdle and therefore is a recommended component of alignment testing
- Similar landmarks with the patient sitting, particularly if he spends prolonged periods in sitting

Mobility

Mobility testing of the shoulder girdle includes the following elements:

- Active and passive osteokinetic ROM of the scapulothoracic and glenohumeral joints, including mobility testing along the continuum of hypomobility to hypermobility
- Passive arthrokinematic mobility tests of the sternoclavicular, acromioclavicular, glenohumeral, scapulothoracic joints, and thoracic spine, including mobility testing along the continuum of hypomobility to hypermobility

Specific diagnostic information can be gained from careful active and passive ROM tests.[43] The therapist should notice whether pain is elicited and at what point in the range the pain occurs during active ROM (eg, painful arc, end range, on return from elevation). Passive ROM tests the status of noncontractile tissues, the presence of a capsular pattern of limitation, end feel, and the sequence of pain and end feel.

Visual observation and palpation of the PICR of the scapulothoracic and glenohumeral joints can be augmented by surface electromyography (SEMG). The use of SEMG can assist in determining patterns and timing of recruitment of the trapezius, serratus, deltoid, and infraspinatus muscles; the infraspinatus is the only rotator cuff muscle that can be examined with palpation or SEMG. SEMG can be useful in determining faulty motor control patterns responsible for many shoulder diagnoses. This type of qualitative testing is important, because active ROM may be within normal limits with an abnormal PICR. An abnormal PICR can contribute to shoulder dysfunction.

Tests of myofascial extensibility can also be performed. Muscle length testing should include muscles prone to reduced extensibility and those prone to adaptive lengthening. Examples of muscles that fall into each category are summarized in Display 26-2. Sarhmann[44] and Kendall[45] have described the appropriate muscle length testing procedures.

Functional movements should be examined, including reaching behind the back, touching the back of the head and neck, and reaching across to the opposite shoulder. Active functional movements test joint mobility, muscle extensibility, muscle strength, and willingness of the patient to complete the motion. Further testing can determine which impairments combine to alter the performance of the functional movement.

Impaired Muscle Performance

Impaired muscle performance can result from numerous sources:

- Muscle strain
- Neurologic injury (peripheral nerve or nerve root injury)
- General weakness from disuse because of muscle imbalance, deconditioning, or reduced force or torque production for a specific performance level (eg, high-level athlete in training)
- Altered length–tension relationships
- Pain

Tests can determine the presence and potential source of impaired muscle performance. Specific manual muscle testing (MMT) provides information regarding the amount of force or torque that a musculotendinous unit can generate. Display 26-3 provides a list of muscles that should be included in MMT of the shoulder girdle. MMT is traditionally done, but testing of muscle performance can be performed with a dynamometer, and both types of testing can be performed in conjunction with SEMG when appropriate. Texts on manual testing for specific protocols should be consulted.[45,46]

Some of the classic MMT positions have been modified in response to electromyographic studies that identified alternate positions for optimally recruiting a given muscle. Kelly and colleagues[47] have provided further information on this subject.[47]

Positional strength testing is a specialized form of MMT that specifically tests the muscle in the short range to obtain information regarding the length-tension properties of the muscle (see Chapter 4). Positional strength testing is particularly useful in determining whether a muscle is weak because of general disuse or deconditioning, neurologic deficits, or muscle strain or lengthening. If a muscle is lengthened, it tests weak in the short range but strong in a slightly more lengthened range. If a muscle is weak

DISPLAY 26-2
Shoulder Girdle Muscles Prone to Adaptive Length Changes[28]

Adaptive Shortening	Adaptive Lengthening
Rhomboid major and minor, levator scapulae	Middle trapezius
Upper trapezius	Lower trapezius
Subscapularis	Upper trapezius
Teres major	Subscapularis
Latissimus dorsi	Serratus anterior
Pectoralis major and minor	
Glenohumeral lateral rotators	

DISPLAY 26-3
Shoulder Girdle Muscles to Include in Manual Muscle Testing

- Upper, middle, and posterior deltoid
- Glenohumeral lateral rotators
- Glenohumeral medial rotators (with isolation of subscapularis)
- All portions of the trapezius
- Serratus anterior
- Rhomboids and levator scapula
- Pectoralis major
- Latissimus dorsi

because of other causes, it tests weak throughout the range. Sarhmann[44] has provided more information on positional strength testing of muscles in the shoulder girdle.[44]

Selective tissue tension tests combine active and passive ROM with resisted tests of muscles about the shoulder girdle.[43] The sum total of the results of each test assists the practitioner in determining what tissue is the probable source of the shoulder condition.

Resisted tests are used to determine the severity of a contractile lesion. If selective tissue tension test results are positive for a contractile lesion, the resisted test can diagnose the severity of the lesion. Table 26-4 highlights diagnostic findings of resisted tests.

Resisted tests can also be used to identify a neurologic deficit. Tests of shoulder girdle musculature, combined with elbow, forearm, wrist, and hand musculature, can indicate whether a nerve deficit is at the level of the cervical spine (ie, nerve root) or is a peripheral nerve lesion. The pattern of weakness indicates peripheral or nerve root involvement.

Pain, Altered Tone, and Inflammation

Examination of pain, altered tone, and inflammation is done throughout the examination process. Evaluation of the examination findings should determine which tissues are involved. If possible, the examination should reveal the postures and movements that are associated with the pain, altered tone, or inflammation.

Palpation of suspected tissues is used to determine which tissues are painful, have altered tone, or are inflamed. The clinician should use caution when palpating an area of tenderness outlined by the patient. The sensation of tenderness can be referred from other tissues or caused by radicular symptoms originating in the cervical spine.

Passive movement testing is another useful technique. Cyriax[43] and Maitland[48] advocate use of the sequence of pain and resistance during passive movement testing to establish the irritability level of a tissue. This information can guide the aggressiveness with which stretching and mobilization techniques are performed.

Because a subjective report of the pain associated with specific activities can help in the assessment, the clinician should question the patient about which activities are associated with pain. Pain often is latent (ie, experienced after the activity), which makes it difficult to relate a cause or source. The range of pain, from the least pain to the worst pain experienced, should be examined through some accepted method of pain assessment (eg, visual analog scale).[49]

The clinician must attempt to determine a mechanical cause of the pain or inflammation during the course of the examination. This is often quite challenging but necessary to ensure full recovery and prevention of recurrences. For example, although the supraspinatus tendon can be diagnosed as the source of pain through selective tissue tension testing and palpation, the cause of the pain may be insufficient scapular upward rotation. Insufficient upward scapular rotation can be the cause of pain because of mechanical impingement of the supraspinatus under the acromion process. Local treatment of the supraspinatus may resolve the pain in the short term. However, treatment of the faulty postures and movements and related impairments is essential to remedy the problem for the long term.

Table 26-4. DIAGNOSIS BASED ON RESISTIVE TESTS

FINDING OF RESISTIVE TEST	LESION
Strong and painless	Normal
Strong and painful	Minor muscle lesion Minor tendon lesion
Weak and painful	Gross macrotraumatic lesion such as fracture Partial rupture of muscle or tendon
Weak and painless	Muscle or tendon rupture Neurologic dysfunction

Special Tests

The following tests are considered special tests to confirm or exclude suspected shoulder girdle diagnoses. Details of specific examination procedures can be found in the supplied references.

Musculoskeletal unit tests are designed to identify the integrity of the musculotendinous unit. Tests specifically for bicipital tendinitis include Yergason's[50] and Ludington's tests.[51] The "empty can" or supraspinatus test examines the integrity of the supraspinatus.[52] The Gilcrest sign[53] and the drop arm test[51] assess the integrity of multiple muscles and tendons. Donatelli[54] has provided a comprehensive description of each of these tests.

Thoracic outlet tests,[55] neural tension testing,[56] and glenohumeral stability tests and glenoid labrum integrity tests[54] also can be performed. The thoracic outlet tests are discussed later, and details of the other tests can be found in the supplied references.

Impingement tests are designed to approximate the greater tubercle and soft tissues in the subacromial space under the acromion process. Common special tests that assist in the confirmation of a diagnosis of impingement syndrome include the locking test,[57] Neer test,[58] and the Hawkins and Kennedy[59] impingement tests. Donatelli[54] has provided descriptions of these tests.

Functional Limitation and Disability Testing

Functional testing, whether in the form of performance testing or subjective grading, should be included in the examination. Data on reliability and validity have been reported for only one health-related quality of life scale for the shoulder girdle, the Shoulder Pain and Disability Index (SPADI).[60,61] The SPADI is a self-administered questionnaire that consists of two dimensions, one for pain and the other for functional activities, and requires 5 to 10 minutes for a patient to complete. Display 26-4 lists the SPADI items. Roach and colleagues[60] and Williams and associates[61] have explained the administration of this test.

DISPLAY 26-4
Shoulder Pain and Disability Index

Pain dimension: How severe is your pain?

1. At its worst?
2. When lying on the involved side?
3. Reaching for something on a high shelf?
4. Touching the back of your neck?
5. Pushing with the involved arm?

Disability dimension: How much difficulty do you have?

1. Washing your hair?
2. Washing your back?
3. Putting on an underskirt or pullover sweater?
4. Putting on a shirt that buttons down the front?
5. Putting on your pants?
6. Placing an object on a high shelf?
7. Carrying a heavy object (eg, 10 lb)?
8. Removing something from your back pocket?

THERAPEUTIC EXERCISE INTERVENTIONS FOR COMMON PHYSIOLOGIC IMPAIRMENTS

After a thorough examination and evaluation of the shoulder girdle, the clinician should have a good understanding of the functional limitations affecting the patient and the related impairments. A diagnosis and prognosis are formulated, and an intervention is planned. After it is determined which impairments should be treated to restore function, a plan of care must be developed to remedy the appropriate impairments and functional limitations. Therapeutic exercise intervention is vital in the restoration of shoulder girdle function, primarily because exercise is important in restoring the precise coordinated muscular force couples acting on the four integrated joints in the shoulder girdle complex. The following sections provide information about therapeutic exercise interventions for common physiologic impairments.

Pain

Pain stemming from tissues in the shoulder girdle may be experienced locally or referred distally down the arm as far as the wrist and hand.[62] The shoulder girdle is a common region for referral from other musculoskeletal regions such as the cervical or upper thoracic spine or the elbow. Nonmusculoskeletal sources, such as the heart and diaphragm (see Appendix 1), also can refer pain into the shoulder girdle.

If the source of the pain is determined to be in the shoulder girdle, treatment may involve a combination of interventions, including manual therapy (eg, joint mobilization, soft tissue mobilization), physical agents or electrotherapeutic modalities, and therapeutic exercise. A clinical example can illustrate the use and interaction of physical therapy interventions. A common source of pain originating from the shoulder girdle is an inflamed supraspinatus tendon. Display 26-5 lists hypothetical examination and evaluation findings of a person diagnosed with supraspinatus tendinitis. Treatment of the source of the pain may include the following techniques:

- Transverse friction massage to the tenoperiosteal junction of the supraspinatus to assist in the formation of a strong and mobile scar[43]
- Effleurage massage of the belly of the muscle to enhance general blood flow to the region
- Active exercise, electrical stimulation in mid range, or both to broaden the muscle (serving a similar purpose to that of transverse friction massage)[43]
- Physical agents (eg, cryotherapy) or electrotherapeutic modalities (eg, phonophoresis, ultrasound) to treat the inflammatory process
- Activity modification in the form of reducing or eliminating the activities thought to cause or perpetuate the condition

DISPLAY 26-5
Examination Findings for Patient With Supraspinatus Tendinitis

Posture

Moderate forward head, moderate kyphosis, moderate scapular anterior tilt and downward rotation, slight humeral abduction and elevation

Active Movement Pattern

Excessive superior glide of the humerus in the glenoid fossa combined with insufficient scapular posterior tilt and upward rotation during middle- to end-range arm elevation and excessive anterior tilt during the return from elevation. Pain is experienced in the end range and on the return from elevation.

Manual Muscle Test

Subscapularis ($^{3+}/_5$)[44]
Infraspinatus/teres minor ($^{4}/_5$)
Supraspinatus—unable to test secondary to pain
Upper trapezius ($^{4-}/_5$)
Middle trapezius ($^{3+}/_5$)
Lower trapezius ($^{3-}/_5$)
Serratus anterior ($^{3-}/_5$)
Rhomboid major and minor, levator scapula ($^{5}/_5$)

Muscle Length

The pectoralis minor and rhomboid or levator are moderately short. Glenohumeral lateral rotators are slightly short.

Resisted Tests

The supraspinatus is weak and painful

Palpation

The supraspinatus tenoperiosteal junction is tender

Arthrokinematic Joint Mobility

Moderate hypomobility in inferior glide and lateral distraction of the head of the humerus. Slight pain is experienced with lateral distraction force in the region of the supraspinatus. Scapular posterior tilt is slightly hypomobile. Humeral head anterior translation is moderately hypermobile.

Treatment isolated to the source of the pain provides temporary relief, particularly if the cause of the pain is repetitive microtrauma from faulty postures or movement patterns. However, the clinician must address the cause of the pain for long-term resolution of the problem. A common cause of supraspinatus tendinitis is repetitive impingement under the acromion process of the scapula because of faulty movement patterns or postural habits. Display 26-5 lists the examination findings regarding the faulty posture, arthrokinematic and osteokinematic movements, and related impairments responsible for impingement in this case.

Treating the cause of the supraspinatus tendon pain requires retraining the common posture habits and active PICR in the repetitive movement patterns believed to contribute to or perpetuate the condition. This training is more specific than the basic activity modification described under treatment of the source of the pain. Optimal training of postural habits and movement patterns usually requires prior or simultaneous therapeutic exercise intervention focused on muscle force or torque production and endurance, joint mobility, and muscle extensibility. Improved physiologic capabilities provide a better foundation for precise posture and movement control. For example, lower trapezius and serratus anterior muscles with an MMT grade of 3−/5 cannot participate in a muscular force couple to upwardly rotate the scapula against gravity. Therapeutic exercise aimed at improving force or torque production of the upward rotators until they achieve a minimal MMT grade of 3 to 3+/5 is a prerequisite for retraining the coordinated muscular force couples required for functional movement patterns against gravity. Posture and movement education must be initiated as soon as possible, but premature introduction of functional activities can perpetuate the faulty postures and movement patterns causing the pain and inflammation.

In the case presented in Display 26-5, the following impairments must be addressed to promote optimal posture and movement patterns:

- Muscle force or torque and endurance of the rotator cuff (see Self-Management: Facelying Shoulder Rotation) and scapular upward rotators (see Self-Management: Facelying Arm Lifts and Self-Management: Serratus Anterior Progression)
- Muscle extensibility of the pectoralis minor (Fig. 26-12), rhomboids with levator scapula (Fig. 26-13), and glenohumeral lateral rotators (see Self-Management: Lateral Rotator and Posterior Capsule Stretch)
- Joint mobility of the acromioclavicular, sternoclavicular, scapulothoracic, and glenohumeral joints

Because of altered length–tension properties of the scapular upward rotators and the significant positional weakness, the exercises prescribed must be initiated at relatively low levels of intensity. For example, the patient should begin with level I of the lower trapezius (see Self-Management: Facelying Arm Lifts) and serratus anterior (see Self-Management: Serratus Anterior Progression) progressions. However, improving the force-generating capability of the lower trapezius, serratus anterior, and rotator cuff may not translate directly into improved function. Transitional exercises should be prescribed to train the muscle to function with the appropriate magnitude and timing during ADLs or instrumental ADLs. Examples of transitional exercises are shown in Figure 26-14.

If the source of the pain is not within the shoulder girdle, dysfunction in the shoulder girdle may still contribute to the cause of the pain despite treatment. For example, a patient may be diagnosed with radicular pain originating from an inflamed C5-C6 nerve root caused by a protruding nucleus pulposus at that level. However, it may be determined that faulty postures and movements of the shoulder girdle are contributing to faulty postures and movements of the cervical spine because of the shared musculature and joint articulations. An example is a person with a depressed scapula at rest (Fig. 26-15) and insufficient elevation of the scapula during movement. This person may experience excessive tension on the cervical spine because of overstretching of the upper trapezius and levator scapula. This excessive tension may compromise normal movement of the cervical spine and restrict cervical rotation with the arms at the side or simultaneously with movement of the shoulder girdle (eg, driving a car and needing to look behind the shoulder). In this case, treating the cervical spine in isolation may not result in full functional recovery. However, adding treatment of the posture and movement patterns of the shoulder girdle and the related shoulder impairments to the plan of care may remedy pain originating from the cervical spine. Intervention for this case could include the following features:

- Scapular taping into elevation and upward rotation
- Upper trapezius strengthening (Fig. 26-16)
- Education regarding posture habits (eg, do not allow the shoulder to assume a depressed position)
- Movement retraining (ie, exaggerating scapular elevation initially and retraining normal movement after the upper trapezius participates well in the scapular upward rotation force couple)

Mobility Impairment

Mobility impairments, including hypomobility and hypermobility, are common. An example of extreme hypomobility is adhesive capsulitis (ie, "frozen shoulder"), and an example of extreme hypermobility is glenohumeral dislocation. Mobility is a hallmark characteristic of the shoulder girdle. Even a minor loss of mobility at any of the four joints can disrupt the normal mechanics of the shoulder girdle.

Hypomobility can affect osteokinematic and arthrokinematic motions. Hypomobile osteokinematic motion causes a compensatory increase in motion at another joint in the complex (ie, scapular elevation as compensation for lack of glenohumeral motion). Hypomobile arthrokinematic motion causes an abnormal or excessive arthrokinematic motion in the opposite direction of the hypomobility (ie, a hypomobile posterior glenohumeral capsule may lead to excessive anterior glenohumeral translation and anterior hypermobility). Hypermobility and hypomobility impairments often coexist.

Because of its anatomic location and its locally unique anatomic features, the shoulder girdle is vulnerable to injury

SELF-MANAGEMENT: Facelying Shoulder Rotation

Purpose: To strengthen the shoulder rotators and train independent motion between the shoulder blade and the arm

Starting position: Kneel next to a weight bench; if at home, lie on your stomach adjacent to the edge of your bed. Place one or two rolled towels under your shoulder. Position your arm out to the side with the elbow bent to 90 degrees. Keep as much of your shoulder supported on the bench or bed as possible. Your arm should hang from your elbow down, not from your shoulder.

Movement technique:

Lateral rotation (target muscles: infraspinatous, teres minor)

- You may perform this exercise just by rotating your arm, or with weight. If you are to perform this with weight, see the amount of weight you have been prescribed under *dosage.*
- Slowly rotate your shoulder so that your forearm moves up toward your head. Stop just short of horizontal.
- Concentrate on letting your arm move independent from your scapula. Your shoulder should "spin" in the socket. There should be no movement of your scapula.

Dosage:

Weight _____

Sets/repetitions _____

Frequency _____

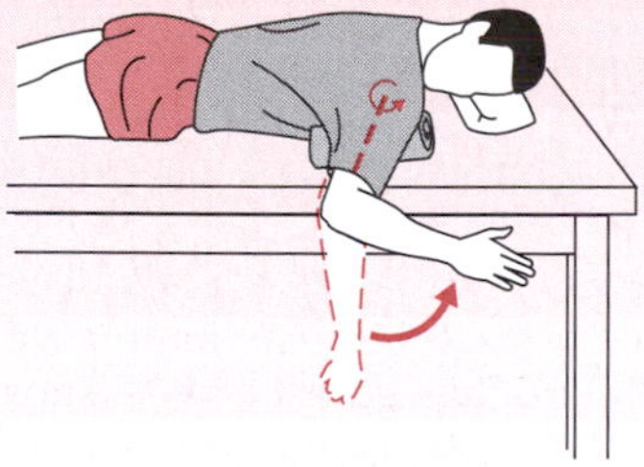

Lateral rotation

Medial rotation (target muscle: subscapularis)

- You may perform this exercise by rotating your arm with or without added weight. If you perform this with weight, see the amount of weight you have been prescribed under *dosage.*
- Slowly rotate your shoulder in the opposite direction so that your forearm moves backward.
- Do not let your shoulder displace into the towel roll. Think of keeping your shoulder "pulled away" from the towel roll.
- Your range of motion is more limited in medial rotation than lateral rotation (possibly only 10 to 20 degrees). Remember, it is *quality not quantity* that is important.

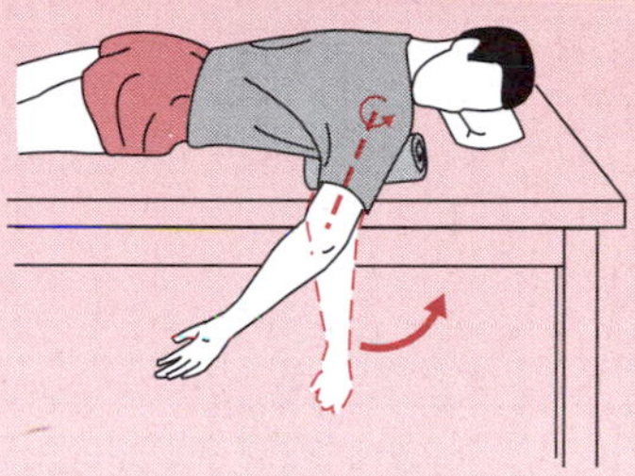

Medial rotation

Dosage

Weight _____

Sets/repetitions _____

Frequency _____

of stabilizing structures. Isolated hypermobility and instability impairments can occur as a result of trauma (eg, falling onto an outstretched arm).

HYPOMOBILITY

Hypomobility and hypermobility impairments can coexist in the shoulder girdle complex. For example, if the scapula does not fully upwardly rotate during arm elevation, arm elevation can be achieved by moving into excessive elevation, or the humerus may compensate by translating excessively inferiorly. When restoring balanced and coordinated motion to the shoulder girdle, mobility must be restored in the specific direction of the hypomobile joint; simultaneously, the hypermobile segments and direction within a segment must be trained to move less.

The method by which mobility is restored must be determined on a case by case basis. To choose the appropriate

text continues on page 593

SELF-MANAGEMENT: Facelying Arm Lifts

Purpose: To strengthen the muscles between your shoulder blades

Starting position: Lie on your stomach with a pillow under your abdomen. Place your hands on the back of your head. Use this position for levels I through III.

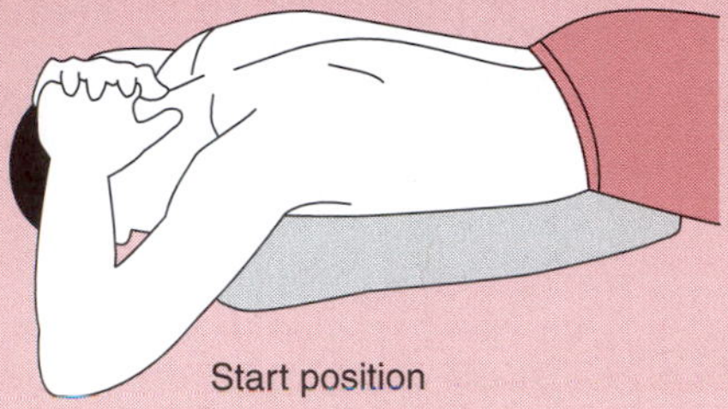

Start position

Movement technique:

Level I: Stomach-lying elbow lifts (target muscles: middle and lower trapezius)

- ***Barely*** lift your elbows. Keep your neck muscles (upper trapezius) relaxed, and contract the region between your shoulder blades (lower trapezius). Keep the contraction ***just enough*** to lift the elbows so as not to use rhomboids to adduct the shoulder blades.
- Hold the contraction for 5 seconds.
- Lower the elbows and repeat.
- Stop when your neck muscles become more tense; this is an indication that the middle and lower trapezius are fatiguing and that you should stop and rest.

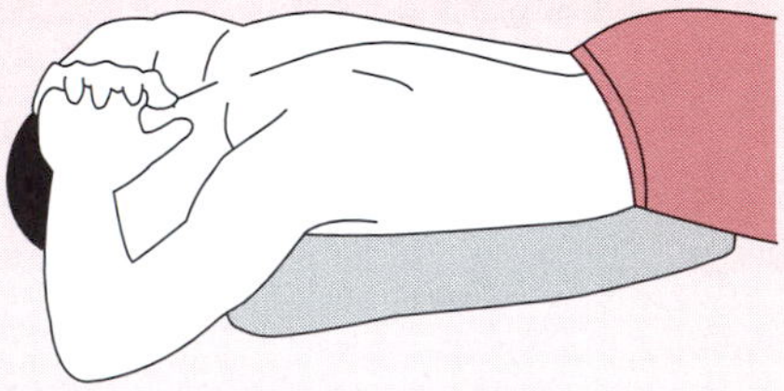

Level I

Dosage:

Sets/repetitions _____

Frequency _____

Level II: Stomach-lying elbow lift with arms extended (target muscles: middle and lower trapezius)

- ***Barely*** lift your elbows. Keep your neck muscles (upper trapezius) relaxed, and contract the region between your shoulder blades (lower trapezius). Keep the contraction just enough to lift the elbows so as not to use rhomboids to adduct the shoulder blades.
- Slowly extend your elbows so that your arms are straight. Bend your elbows so that the hands return to the position behind your head.
- Relax your elbows to the table.
- Stop when your neck muscles become more tense; this is an indication that the middle and lower trapezius are fatiguing and you should stop and rest.

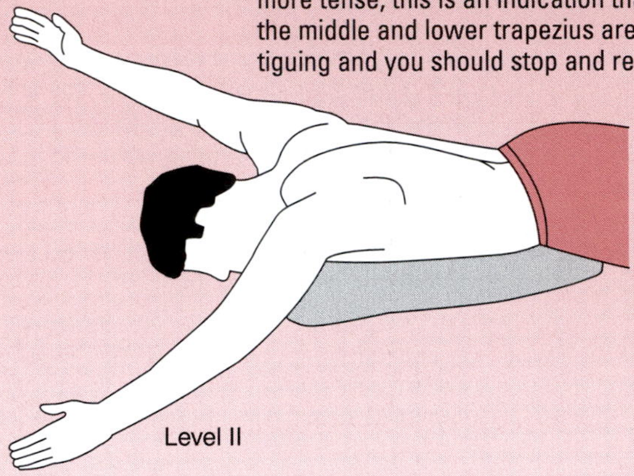

Level II

Dosage

Sets/repetitions _____

Frequency _____

Level III: Stomach-lying elbow lift with arm extension overhead (target muscles: middle and lower trapezius)

- ***Barely*** lift your elbows. Keep your neck muscles (upper trapezius) relaxed, and contract the region between your shoulder blades (lower trapezius). Keep the contraction just enough to lift the elbows so as not to use rhomboids to adduct the shoulder blades.
- As you extend your elbows while raising your arms overhead, be sure not to tense your neck muscles (upper trapezius) during this level. If you are unable to keep your neck muscles relatively relaxed, perhaps you are not ready for this level of exercise.

- Return your hands to your head, lower your elbows, and relax.

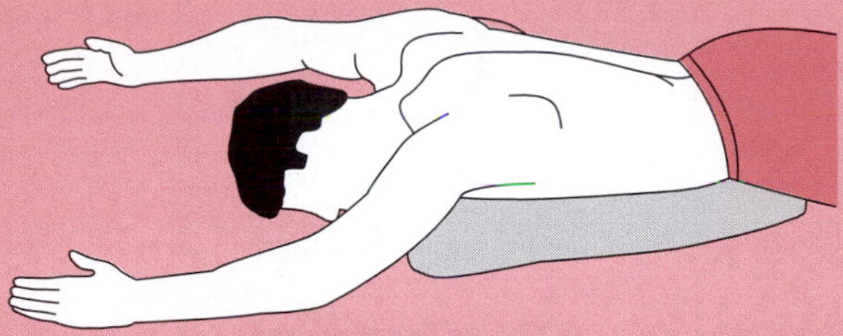

Level II

Dosage

Sets/repetitions _____

Frequency _____

Starting position:

- Lie on your stomach on a weight bench, piano bench, or low bed. Your chest should be suspended off the edge of the bench. Bend your knees if they extend too far off the bench. Pull your abdomen up and in. Your head should be in line with your spine with your chin tucked. Hold dumbbells with palms facing forward and ***thumbs up.*** Arms should be relaxed at chest level and resting on the floor or against the bench if the bench is tall. Keep elbows slightly bent.

Movement technique:

Level IVA: Stomach lying reverse horizontal fly (target muscle: middle trapezius)

- Raise the dumbbells in a semicircular motion to just below chest height. ***Do not*** lift beyond chest level.
- Lower to the starting position using the same path.
- Exhale up; inhale down.

Dosage

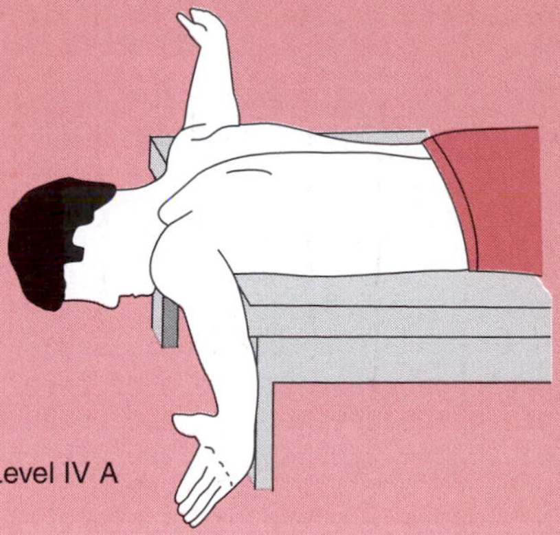

Level IV A

Weights _____

Sets/Repetitions _____

Frequency _____

Level IVB: Stomach-lying diagonal reverse fly (target (target muscles: lower trapezius)

- Raise your elbows in a semicircular motion, diagonally upward toward the head to just below the level of the head. ***Do not*** lift the elbows above the level of the head.
- Lower to the starting position using the same path.
- Exhale up; inhale down.
- Repeat in sets of 10 repetitions. Begin using a light weight when you can complete two sets of 10 repetitions maximum with proper technique.

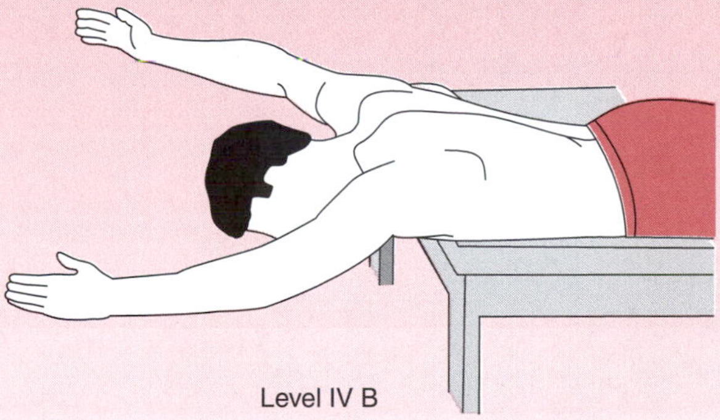

Level IV B

Dosage

Weight _____

Sets/repetitions _____

Frequency _____

SELF-MANAGEMENT: Serratus Anterior Progression

Purpose: To progressively strengthen your serratus anterior

Level I: Backlying isometric with arm overhead

Starting position: Lie on your back with 1 to 2 pillows positioned above (not under) your head.

Movement technique:

- Raise your arm overhead, close to your ear, until it reaches the pillow.
- Gently but consistently push your arm backward into the pillow and hold for 10 seconds.

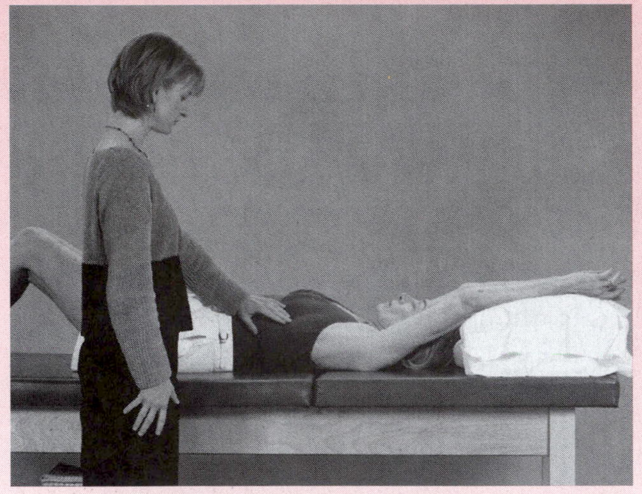

Level I

Dosage

Sets/repetitions _____

Frequency _____

Level II: Sidelying with dynamic arm slide

Starting position:

- Lie on your side with 2 to 3 pillows in front of your head and shoulders. Bend your hips and knees. Rest your arm on the pillows with your elbow bent. Grasp the prescribed color of elastic band in your hand and attach the other end to your top foot.

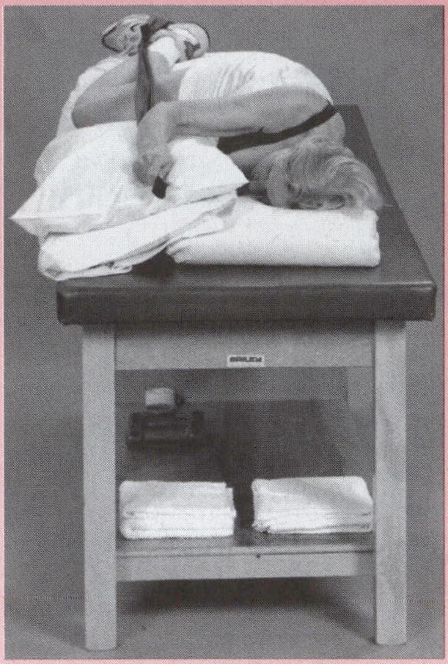

Level II—start position

Movement technique:

- Slide your arm upward toward your head, keeping it in contact with the pillows.
- Slowly lower the arm back down to the starting position. Do not pull the arm back down, but slowly lower it against the resistance of the elastic.

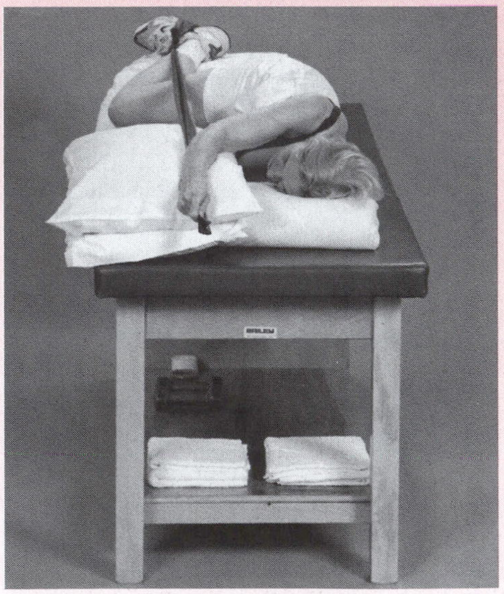

Level II—end position

Dosage

Color of elastic ____________

Sets/repetitions _____

Frequency _____

LEVEL III: Standing back to the wall and arm lift

Starting position: Stand with your feet about 2 to 3 inches from the wall. Your head should be against the wall. If you cannot bring your head against the wall, place 1 or 2 small, rolled hand towels behind your head. Pull in your stomach to rotate your pelvis backward and reduce the arch in your back. You should be able to place one hand between your lower back and the wall. If there is more space between your back and the wall, bend your hips and knees slightly to reduce the pull from your hip flexors. You should be able to reduce the arch of your back more easily.

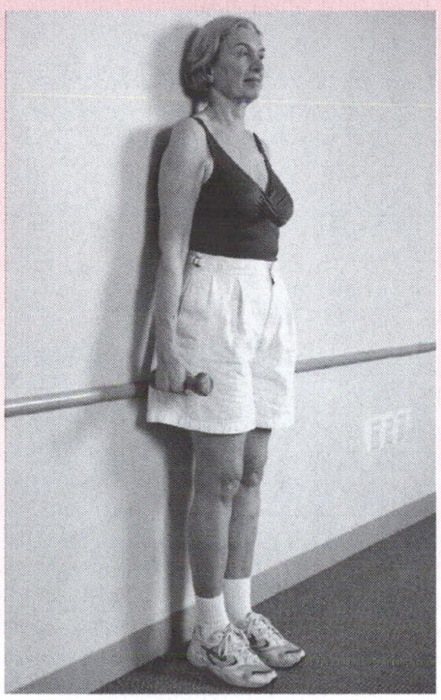

Level III—start position

Movement technique:

- Lift your arms in front of your body with your elbows straight.
- Try to bring the arms all the way back to the wall, but stop if you feel your back arching or your shoulders shrugging.
- Slowly lower your arms to your side, ensuring your shoulders stay back against the wall and do not roll forward.

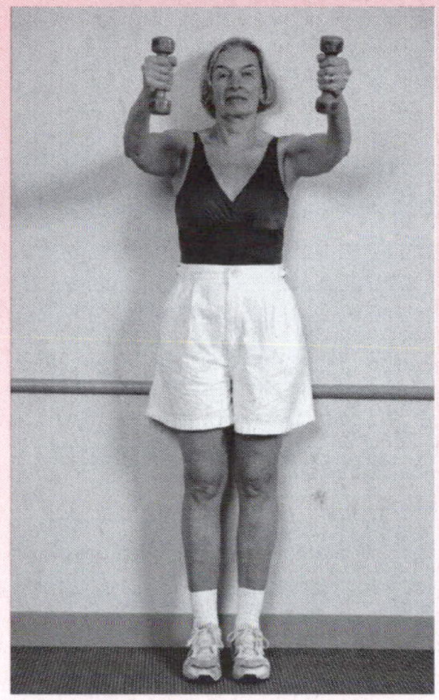

Level III—mid position

Dosage

Weight _____

Sets/repetitions _____

Frequency _____

treatment technique, it must be determined which structures are responsible for the loss of mobility, the direction of hypomobility, and the severity of restriction. Any one or a combination of the four joints may be restricted in one or numerous directions because of articular or periarticular soft tissue or bony restrictions or loss of extensibility or adaptive shortening of myofascial tissue. If the restrictions are mild and the compensatory movements can be minimized, self-stretching, self-mobilization, and active exercise may suffice. However, if the restrictions are significant (involving more than one segment) or affect a specific arthrokinematic motion, manual joint mobilization, soft tissue mobilization, or manual stretching may be indicated.

Stretching short muscles with an independent exercise program can be ineffective because of the complexity of the joint system and the ease of moving in compensatory patterns, especially in the shoulder girdle. For example, it is difficult to self-stretch a short rhomboid muscle that is limiting scapular upward rotation, because the compensatory motion may elevate the scapula, which does not stretch the rhomboids. Manual stretching (see Fig. 26-13) may be necessary to restore normal tissue extensibility to the rhomboids. Strengthening exercises for the scapular upward rotators (see Self-Management: Facelying Arm Lifts and Self-Management: Serratus Anterior Progression) may be necessary until normal scapular upward rotation mobility is restored during active motion.

The same challenge can occur in attempting to stretch a short pectoralis minor that is limiting scapular posterior tilt during arm elevation. The traditional corner stretch (Fig. 26-17) can be ineffective because the head of the humerus can compensate by moving anteriorly into the weak anterior capsule instead of stretching a short pectoral muscle. This action reflects a fundamental physical law: objects tend to move through the path of least resistance. The relatively lax anterior capsule is the path of least resis-

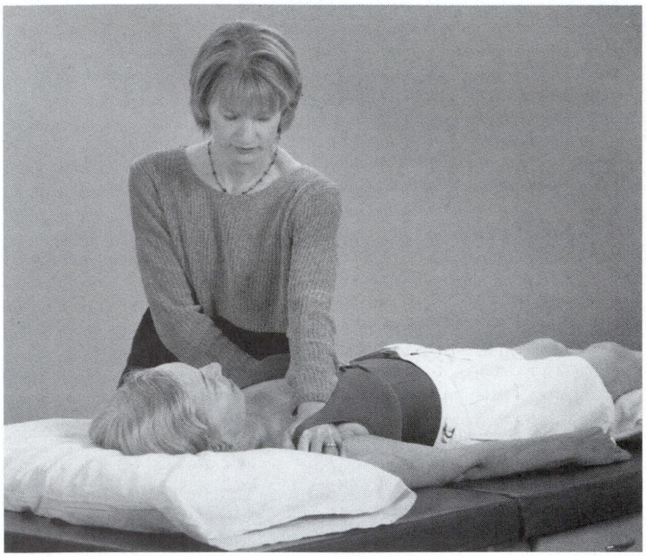

FIGURE 26-12 Manual stretch of the pectoralis minor. The hand applying the stretch force is placed over the coracoid process. A stabilizing hand can be placed over the rib cage. The force applied by the practitioner is a in posterior, superior, and lateral direction.

tance, and it stretches more readily than a short pectoralis minor. Manual stretching (see Fig. 26-12) may be necessary until normal extensibility of the pectoralis minor is achieved combined with strengthening of the lower trapezius (see Self-Management: Facelying Arm Lifts) and until posterior tilt is restored during active motion.

In these examples, stretching the short muscle was combined with strengthening an antagonist muscle. This principle is important to restore muscle balance (see Chapter 6). In this case, stretching the pectoralis minor, rhomboid, or both muscles can be complemented with active exercise of the middle and lower trapezius muscles in the shortened range.

Other common muscles in the shoulder girdle that require stretching include the glenohumeral lateral rotators and the medial rotator-adductor group. Although these often can be successfully self-stretched, special self-stabilization techniques should be employed to ensure compensatory motions do not occur. These exercises are illus-

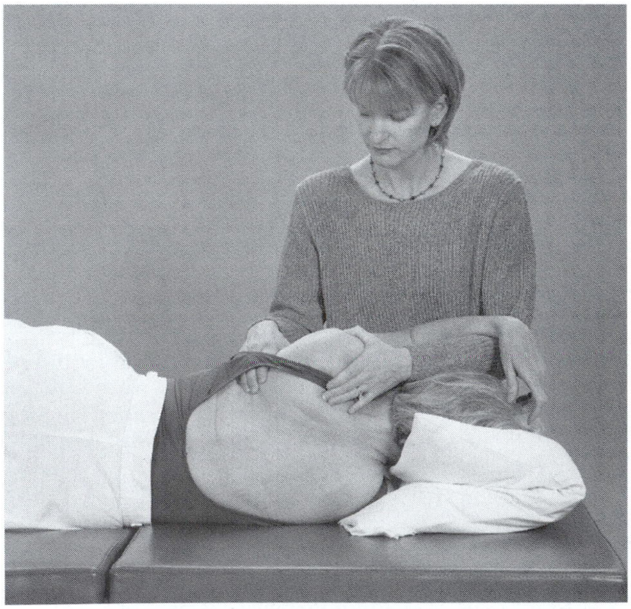

FIGURE 26-13 Rhomboid and levator stretch. The patient's elbow is resting on the practitioner's abdomen. The practitioner cups her hands around the scapula. By shifting the body weight from the caudal to the cranial positioned foot, a rotational force is transmitted to the scapula. The hands rotate the scapula upward like the scapular force couple.

SELF-MANAGEMENT: Lateral Rotator and Posterior Capsule Stretch

Purpose: To stretch the shoulder rotators and train independent movement between the shoulder blade and the arm

Starting position: Slide your arm out to the side, and bend your elbow to 90 degrees. Position your forearm so that the fingers point to the ceiling. Hold your shoulder down with the opposite hand.

Movement technique:

- *Relax* and let your shoulder joint rotate, allowing your forearm to move toward the floor.
- Do not let your shoulder come off the floor and move into your hand as your forearm gets closer to the floor.
- You may hold up to a 2-pound weight in your hand to assist in the stretch.

Dosage

Hold the stretch for _____ seconds

Sets/repetitions _____

Frequency _____

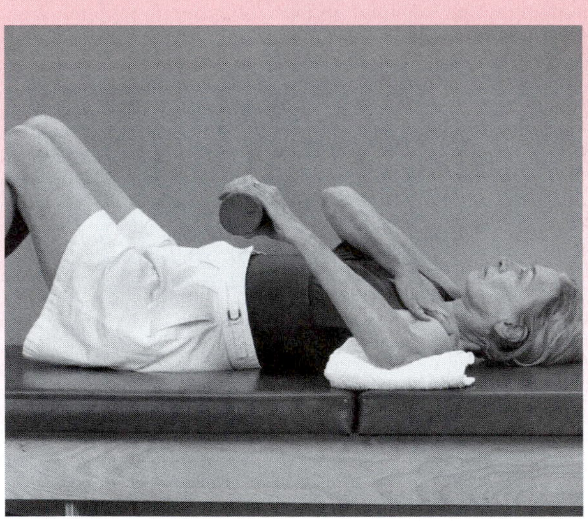

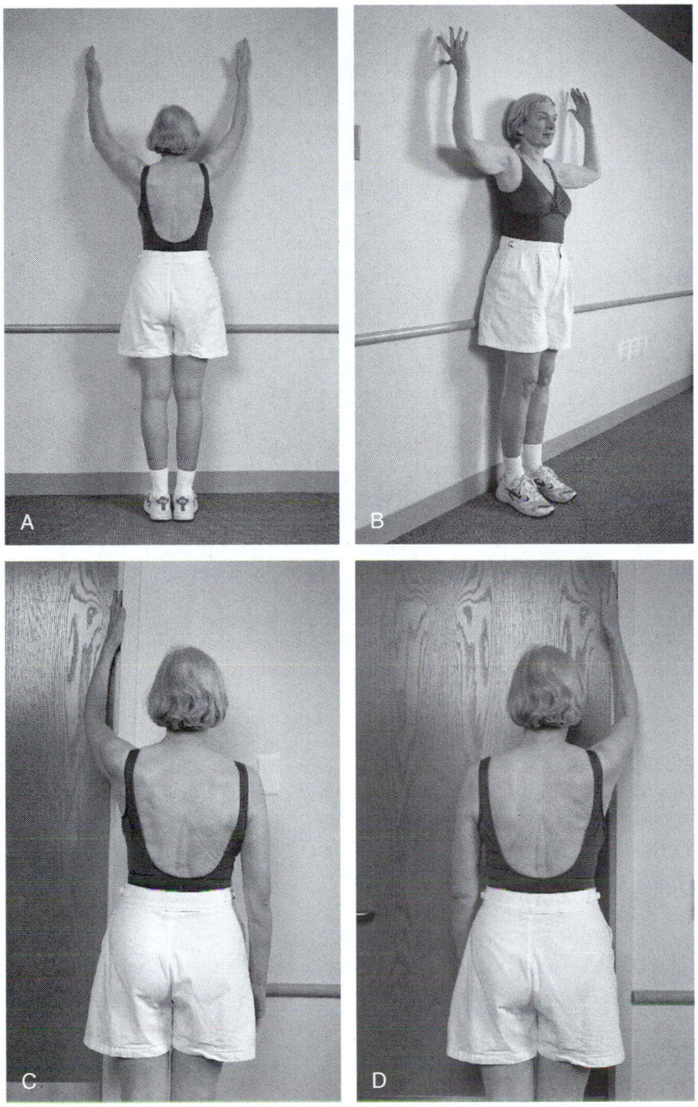

FIGURE 26-14 Wall slides. ***(A)*** The patient places the ulnar aspects of the hands on the wall and slides the hands up the wall in the sagittal or scapular plane, depending on whether the focus is on the serratus anterior or lower trapezius, respectively. ***(B)*** With the back to the wall, the elbows and humerus should be in the scapular plane. Thumbs can touch the wall to ensure that the humerus remains in the scapular plane. The patient slides the arms up the wall, and stops when the scapula deviates from the path of instant center of rotation (PICR) (ie., excessive elevation). The goal is to achieve full scapular plane elevation with the ideal PICR at the glenohumeral and sternothoracic joints. ***(C)*** Medial rotation bias. The patient places the palm of the hand against the door frame and slides the hand upward and downward while maintaining a mild pressure into medial rotation against the door frame. The patient must not push so hard that she recruits the pectoralis major, latissimus dorsi, and teres major. The goal is to use the subscapularis to encourage an increased rotator cuff force vector during arm elevation by facilitating subscapularis. ***(D)*** Lateral rotation bias. The patient places the dorsum of the hand against the door frame and slides the hand upward and downward while maintaining a mild pressure into lateral rotation against the door frame.

trated in Self-Management: Lateral Rotator and Posterior Capsule Stretch; Self-Management: Latissimus and Scapulohumeral Muscle Stretch; and Figure 26-18, respectively.

Stretching is futile if remediation of the impairment does not translate into an improved functional outcome. Posture education is another important aspect to consider when treating mobility impairment. The patient must be educated to avoid postures that adaptively shorten the target soft tissues and lengthen the opposing ones. In the case described previously, sitting or standing in kyphosis and forward head posture must be gradually reduced. Scapular taping can assist in improving postural habits. Figure 26-19 illustrates taping recommendations for maintaining a stretch of the pectoralis minor, and Figures 26-20 and 26-21 illustrate taping for the rhomboid.

Active exercise through a functional range must be instructed and performed precisely to stretch the short soft tissues and recruit the lengthened and weak muscles with the optimal length–tension relationships. Examples of active exercise for a patient with a short rhomboid is provided in Figure 26-14. Hypomobility can also occur as a result of immobilization; self-immobilization due to pain, fear, or a deconditioned state; or imposed immobilization after an injury to allow healing to occur. Immobilization should never be prolonged because of the tendency to develop myofascial shortening, loss of capsular extensibility, muscular atrophy, and disturbed motor control. Immobilization resulting in hypomobility can cause functional limitation and profound disability.

To prevent immobilization during painful periods or during the "rest" phase of healing, carefully prescribed ROM exercises can be initiated. Pain, lack of strength, and poor motor control can lead to further pain and injury during elevation against gravity. In the early phases of healing, a traditional gravity-lessened exercise in which glenohumeral motion is achieved is the Codman exercise, also called the pendulum exercise (Fig. 26-22). This exercise adds traction to the glenohumeral joint, stretches the capsule, avoids active abduction, and minimizes the common faulty movement pattern of scapular elevation during exercise against gravity. The rhythmic pendulum movements can modulate pain.

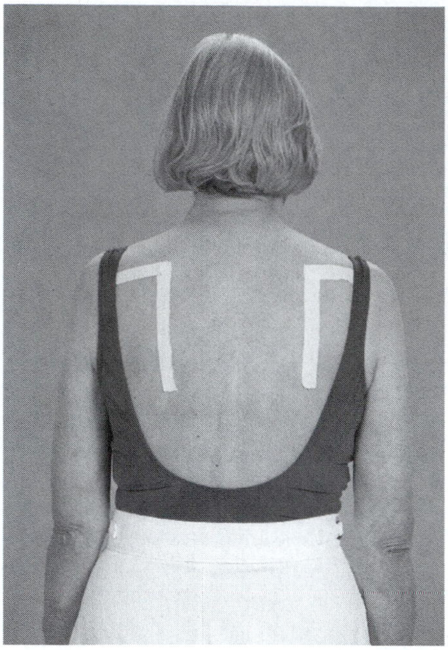

FIGURE 26-15 Depressed and downwardly rotated left scapula.

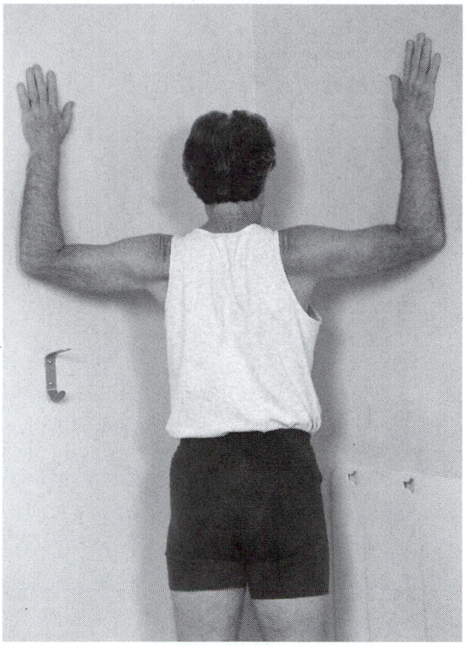

FIGURE 26-17 Traditional pectoralis major and minor stretch.

HYPERMOBILITY

To treat hypermobility in the absence of a traumatic onset, the hypomobile segments must be identified. Hypermobility does not improve despite aggressive exercise protocols if it is occurring in response to a hypomobile segment. For example, the glenohumeral joint may become hypermobile in the anterior direction in response to a hypomobile scapula in the direction of adduction. A functional scenario is reaching behind the back, which requires a combination of glenohumeral extension, medial rotation and adduction, and scapular downward rotation and adduction. If the scapula fails to adduct, it becomes a barrier to the head of the humerus. If the goal is to reach behind the back, the humerus may compensate by translating into the anterior capsule.

This is just one functional example of how the humerus may compensate with excessive anterior translation, but if this compensation is repeated throughout daily activities, hypermobility results in the glenohumeral joint in the anterior direction. Treatment must focus on the cause of the hypermobility by improving mobility of the hypomobile segments and subsequently reducing mobility at the hypermobile segments. Improving the force or torque capability, length–tension properties, and motor control of the dynamic stabilizers in the hypermobile direction is the recommended approach to decrease excessive or abnormal mobility. Specific exercise to remedy impairments associated with faulty movement patterns may be included in the plan of care. Ultimately, the functional movement patterns causing the hypermobility must be addressed (eg, retraining scapular adduction at the appropriate time in the coordinated horizontal adduction movement pattern).

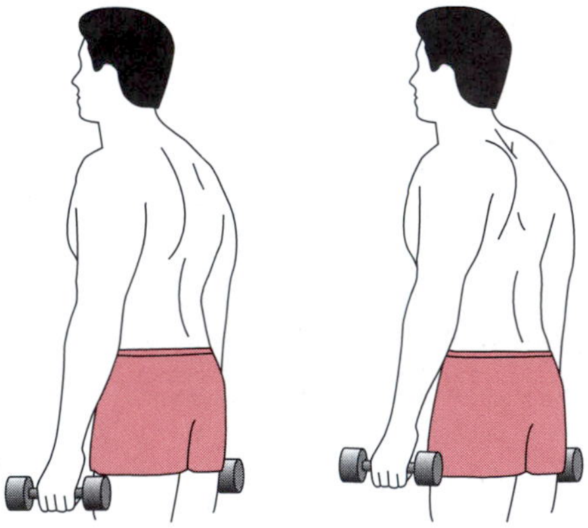

FIGURE 26-16 Upper trapezius strengthening into the short range.

An impairment commonly associated with a faulty movement pattern that contributes to an anterior glenohumeral hypermobility is reduced force or torque production and altered length–tension properties of the glenohumeral medial rotators. However, only one of the glenohumeral medial rotators is in an anatomic position to provide a dynamic anterior restraint to the glenohumeral joint: the subscapularis. To isolate subscapularis function from the other medial rotators (ie, pectoralis major, latissimus dorsi, and teres major), its unique function must be promoted by carefully prescribing the posture and movement parameters of the activity chosen. Because of its anterior insertion close to the axis of rotation, the subscapularis theoretically can prevent anterior translation during functional activities that require dynamic restraint against excessive glenohumeral anterior translation (ie, cocking phase of pitching).

An exercise to improve the force or torque capability and length–tension properties of a lengthened subscapularis is prone medial rotation (see Self-Management: Subscapularis Isometric Exercise). If the subscapularis can produce enough force or torque to rotate the arm against gravity, prone is the desired position for the patient to perform medial rotation. Prone medial rotation poses a greater challenge

SELF-MANAGEMENT: Latissimus and Scapulohumeral Muscle Stretch

Purpose: To stretch the trunk muscles that attach to your arm and the muscles that originate on the shoulder blade and attach to your arm.

Starting position: Lie on your back with your hips and knees bent and feet flat on the floor.

To stretch your scapulohumeral muscles, you need to prevent your shoulder blade from sliding out to the side. To do this, you need to hold the outside edge of your shoulder blade with the opposite hand.

Movement technique:

- Raise your arm over your head, keeping the arm close to your ear. When you feel your back arch or your shoulder blade slide out to the side, stop the movement.
- Rest your arm on the appropriate number of pillows so that your arm may relax in the position previously determined.
- Hold the stretch for the prescribed amount of time, and lower your arm back to your side. Keep your shoulder back as you lower your arm, and do not let it roll forward.

Dosage

Hold the stretch for _____ seconds

Sets/repetitions _____

Frequency _____

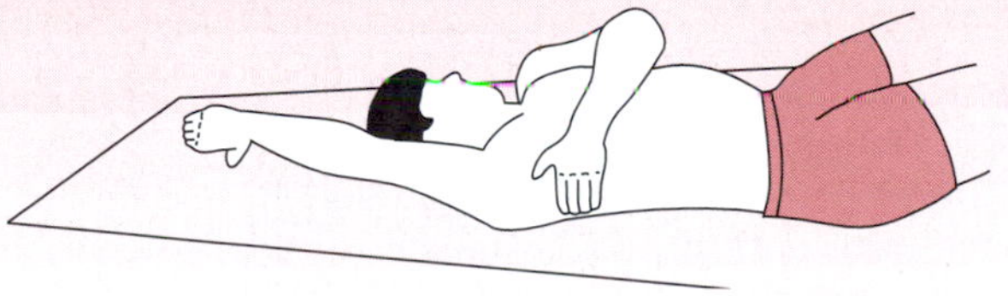

to the subscapularis to prevent the humerus from translating anteriorly than a supine position, in which gravity assists the humerus posteriorly. Theoretically, if the other medial rotators dominate the subscapularis during this exercise, anterior translation during medial rotation will occur.

The goal in this case is to strengthen the subscapularis to prevent abnormal or excessive anterior translation of the head of the humerus during glenohumeral medial rotation and during other functional movement patterns. Resolution of this impairment does not necessarily translate into a functional outcome unless the muscle is specifically trained during functional activities. The subscapularis muscle is kinesthetically limited, and it cannot be palpated or recorded with SEMG. The clinician's best indication that it is working is to observe or palpate movement of the head of the humerus during functional activities. Because movement occurs rapidly and the movement is difficult to observe, videotaping the movement can be useful for carefully analyzing movement.

If the humeral head appears to be translating excessively anteriorly, particularly if symptoms of hypermobility or pain are present, the clinician must determine whether the problem is caused by a base, modulator, or biomechanical element defect. A base element problem may be caused by insufficient subscapularis force or torque capability and length–tension properties and indicates that the introduction of functional retraining is premature. A modulator element problem may be caused by poor motor control of the subscapularis. Methods to improve motor control include verbal, visual (eg, patient views videotape to gain understanding of the movement pattern), or tactile feedback to provide knowledge of results. A biomechanical element problem may be caused by an increased thoracic flexion preventing adequate scapular adduction during horizontal glenohumeral adduction and thereby leading to excessive glenohumeral anterior translation. This condition requires work on the posture of the thoracic spine to ultimately improve the glenohumeral movement pattern.

Impaired Muscle Performance

Impaired performance of specific muscles or groups of muscles can contribute to nearly any functional limitation affecting the shoulder girdle. Examination and evaluation

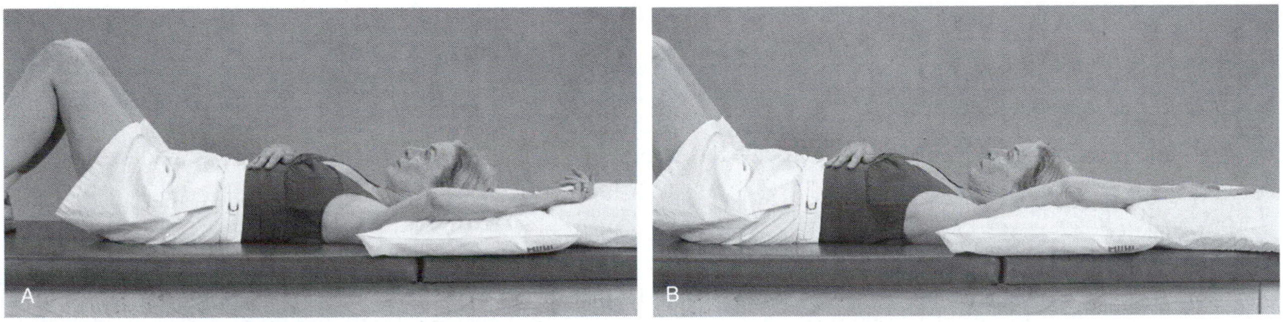

FIGURE 26-18 Active pectoralis major stretch. ***(A)*** The patient rests her abducted and laterally rotated arms on pillows in the scapular plane. The pillows should be of sufficient height to prevent glenohumeral anterior translation. ***(B)*** The patient slides her arms upward until she feels a stretch across the pectoralis region. A static stretch can be maintained at the end position.

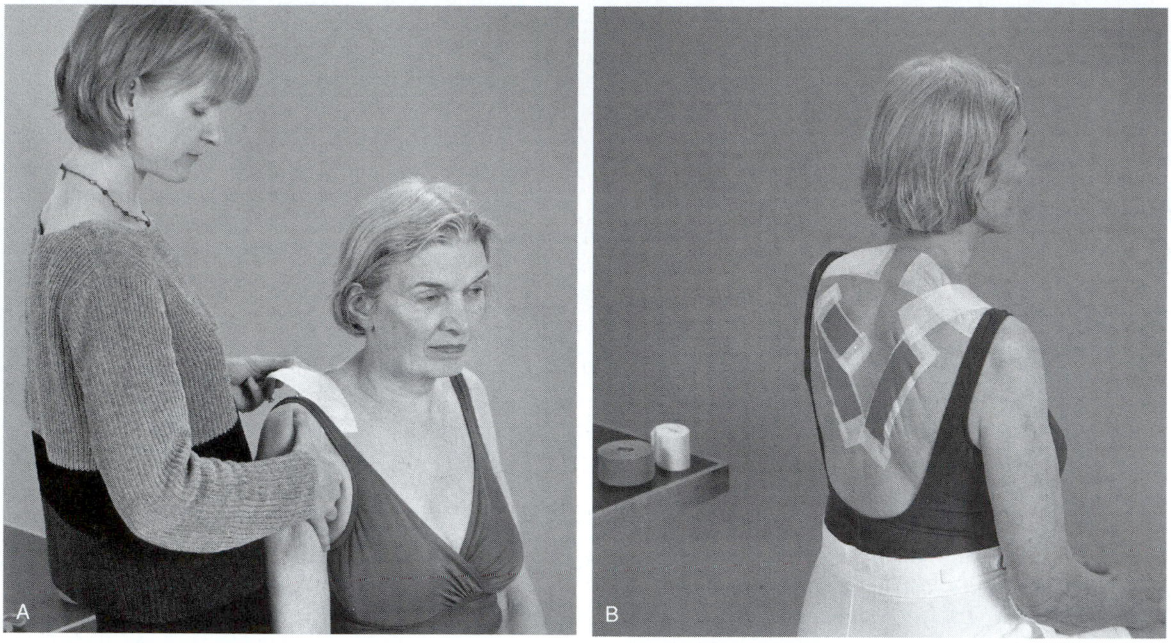

FIGURE 26-19 Taping the scapula into a posterior tilt. Use this technique to correct for scapular anterior tilt. ***(A)*** Anchor the tape to the coracoid process. ***(B)*** Pull the tape posteriorly, caudally, and medially (opposite to the direction of pull of the pectoralis minor). Anchor the tape to the spine of the scapula.

can detect impaired muscle performance and the potential cause of the impairment. The causes of impaired muscle performance are discussed in the Examination and Evaluation section. The following section provides examples of the causes of impaired muscle performance in the shoulder girdle and recommendations for therapeutic exercise interventions.

Impaired muscle performance can result from numerous causes:

- Neurologic injury (peripheral nerve or nerve root injury)
- Muscle strain
- General weakness from disuse due to muscle imbalance, deconditioning, or reduced muscle performance for a specific performance level (eg, a high-level athlete in training)
- Altered length–tension relationships
- Pain

NEUROLOGIC PATHOLOGY

Neurologic pathology can occur at the level of the nerve root or in the periphery. Thorough examination and evaluation can determine the anatomic site of the neurologic deficit.

Alterations in neurologic function at the nerve root level from cervical involvement can be a source of decreased force or torque production in the shoulder girdle musculature. For example, injury to the C5-C6 level after an acceleration injury to the neck can manifest as weakness in the glenohumeral lateral rotators. Strength-related activities do not improve force or torque deficits in the lateral rotators until the cause of the weakness has been resolved, which in this case mandates treatment of the neurologic deficit resulting from injury to the cervical spine.

Another common neurologic deficit involving the shoulder girdle is traction or compression injury of a peripheral nerve. Nerves that are vulnerable to injury are the supraspinatus nerve in the suprascapular notch, the axillary nerve between teres major and teres minor, the long thoracic nerve along the middle axillary line, and the brachial plexus in the thoracic outlet. Nerve injury often results in weakness of the innervated muscles. A stretched long thoracic nerve is discussed to demonstrate a peripheral nerve injury, the resulting force or torque deficits, and the related therapeutic exercise intervention.

The long thoracic nerve is particularly susceptible to stretch from postures or movements of depression of the shoulder girdle (eg, carrying a heavy bag with the strap over the shoulder). The injury manifests as weakness of the serratus anterior, a critical muscle for normal scapular mechanics. A hallmark sign for long thoracic nerve injury is scapular winging at rest that is exaggerated during arm elevation or pushing. The mechanism creating the injury must be rectified before strength-related activities can be effective. To alleviate the traction force imposed on the nerve, postures and body mechanics that cause depression of the shoulder girdle must be eliminated. Strength exercises for the scapular elevators may be necessary for long-standing cases and when the scapular elevators are weak because of disuse. Taping the scapula into elevation may be necessary to relieve the tension on the nerve (see Fig. 26-33).

After the impairments causing the traction injury to the nerve have been identified and intervention has been initiated, a progressive strengthening exercise program must be instructed. The exercise should duplicate the function of the serratus anterior. The most critical function of the serratus is to contribute to the scapular upward rotation force couple, particularly in the sagittal plan.[45] An activity

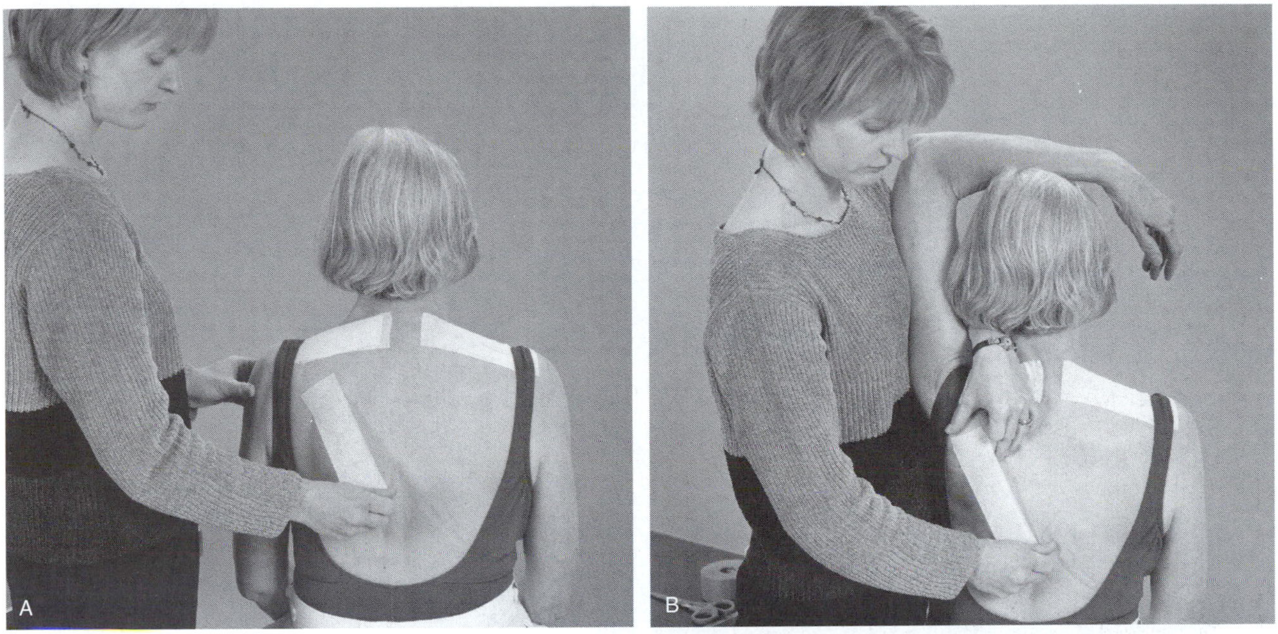

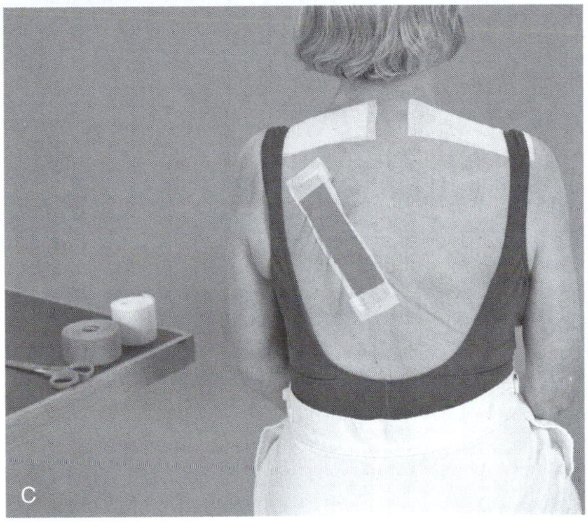

FIGURE 26-20 Taping the scapula into upward rotation. Use the following technique to correct for scapular downward rotation. ***(A)*** Anchor the tape slightly medial to the root of the scapula. ***(B)*** With the scapula in upward rotation, pull the tape medially and caudally toward the lower thoracic spine. ***(C)*** This piece provides a rotation point for scapular upward rotation.

simulating this function must be created. The posture, mode, movement, and dosage parameters depend on the strength of the muscle at the time of the examination and the expected functional outcome of the patient.

A clinical example can provide a platform for describing a therapeutic exercise intervention. A 39-year-old, female homemaker injured her long thoracic nerve from constantly carrying a diaper bag and her 25-pound toddler on her left side. The MMT grade of her serratus anterior at the time of initial examination is 3−/5. Her functional goals are to be able to perform ADLs and instrumental ADLs of a full-time homemaker. She is not involved in any upper extremity sports or recreational activities. A sample initial strengthening exercise for her serratus anterior is shown in Self-Management: Serratus Anterior Progression, level I. She is progressed from performing exercise in a gravity-assisted position, to a gravity-lessened position (see Self-Management: Serratus Anterior Progression, level II), to an against-gravity position (see Fig. 26-14*A*) and then to progressively more resisted exercises (see Self-Management: Serratus Anterior Progression—level III). The hand-knee position is an alternative position to provide resistance to the serratus anterior. Figure 26-23 illustrates an initial progression on hands and knees. The goal with this exercise is to support the body weight through the affected upper extremity without scapular adduction or winging. Rocking forward slightly increases the load the upper extremity must support (see Fig. 26-23*C* and *D*). This exercise can be progressed to a push-up position, first in the bent-knee position (see Fig. 26-23*E* and *F*) and then progressed to a straight-body position (see Fig. 26-23*G* and *H*) if higher levels of performance using the serratus anterior are required.

MUSCLE STRAIN

Muscle strain is defined as the effect of an injurious tension. Muscle strain can result from a sudden and excessive tension or from a gradual and continuous tension imposed on a muscle. Both types of muscle strain commonly occur in the shoulder girdle.

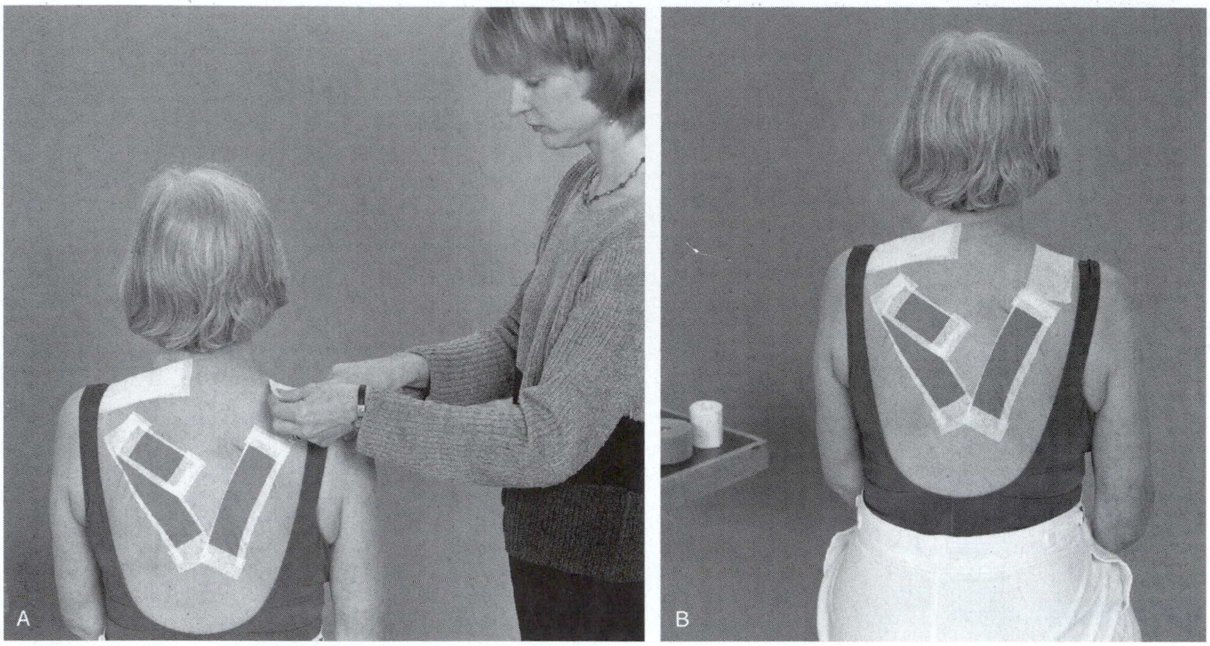

FIGURE 26-21 Taping the scapula into depression. Use this technique to correct scapular elevation. ***(A)*** Anchor the tape to the anterior border of the upper trapezius. ***(B)*** Pull the tape posteriorly, and anchor it to the spine of the scapula.

An example of a muscle strain caused by sudden and excessive tension imposed on a muscle is a sudden fall onto the shoulder or outstretched arm, resulting in a rotator cuff strain or complete tear. The examination may reveal weakness in some or all portions of the rotator cuff. Selective tissue tension tests may also reveal pain with resistive testing and stretch, depending on the severity of the strain.

Treatment should follow the guidelines for tissue healing outlined in Chapter 10. Low-load muscle contraction can be introduced in the repair-regeneration phase to impose a load on the healing tissue along lines of stress. Initially, submaximal isometric contractions at various positions within the pain-free range can be prescribed. Alternatively or in addition, concentric-eccentric dynamic exercise can be prescribed. Dosage parameters related to the load, starting and ending positions, and ROM through which the exercise is prescribed depend on the severity of the strain. More aggressive strength regimens can be gradually introduced in the later stages of the repair-regeneration phase to prepare the muscle for the final phase of healing (Fig. 26-24). The type of contraction and specific movement pattern required of the muscle should be trained as early as possible. For example, prevention of excessive humeral head superior translation is a specific and necessary function for the rotator cuff during arm elevation (concentric) and the return from arm elevation (eccentric). This function must be restored during the progression to functional activity (see Fig. 26-14*A,C,D*).

The final phase of healing should include activity-specific exercises related to the patient's functional goals. Complex functional movement patterns can be trained, and a gradual return to sport-specific activities, such as returning to a pitching program (Display 26-6),[54] can be accomplished. Quality of movement during exercise and functional activities must be emphasized and used as a guide for progression at any stage.

Another form of strain common in the shoulder girdle is the type resulting from gradual and continuous tension. For example, strain to the middle and lower trapezius often results from a habitual position of abducted and downwardly rotated scapulae and from kyphosis. This type of strain may produce certain physiologic impairments:

- Symptoms of "burning" pain along the course of the middle or lower trapezius may be experienced. If the strain is not accompanied by adaptive shortening of the anterior muscles, pain is not constant and can be relieved in the recumbent position. However, change of position does not affect the symptoms of a person with associated adaptive anterior shortness.
- Heavy breasts that are not adequately supported
- Shortened anterior shoulder girdle musculature
- Positional weakness in the middle and lower trapezius
- Adaptive shortening of the pectorals and other internal rotators

Treatment in the early healing phase should include support in the form of taping (see the Adjunctive Interventions: Taping section), bracing (Fig. 26-25), or supportive brassiere to relieve the tension on the middle and lower trapezius. If shortness affects the shoulder medial rotator and adductor group, gradual stretching (see Fig. 26-18 and Self-Management: Latissimus and Scapulohumeral Muscle Stretch) is indicated before strengthening the middle and lower trapezius. Stretching allows the middle and lower trapezius to be strengthened at the appropriate length.

Exercises to strengthen the middle and lower trapezius muscles should consider the length at which the muscles are being strengthened. The lengthened range must be avoided

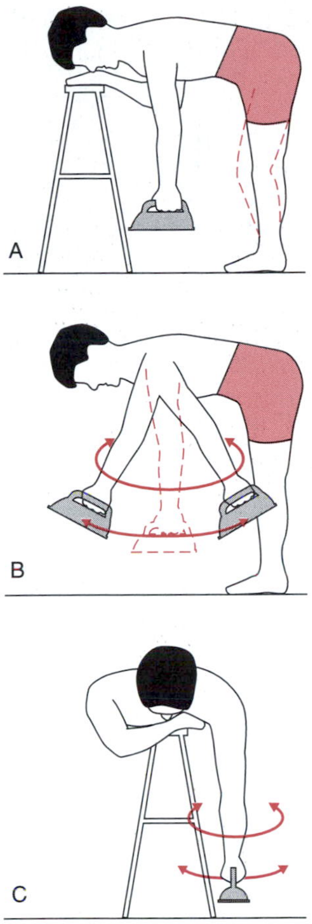

FIGURE 26-22. ***(A)*** The patient should bend forward at the hips approximately 90 degrees, and his knees should be slightly bent, to allow greater hip flexion and minimize stress to the low back. The patient should place the hand not being used in the exercise on a firm surface (eg stool) and place his head on the hand. This permits relaxed movement and concentration on the indicated movement of the involved shoulder. The involved arm should dangle freely, and a weight can be held in the hand. Use of an iron as a weight is suggested for home exercise. A weight adds traction to the glenohumeral joint and widens the pendulum arc. However, caution should be used, because the weight may tense the musculature and defeat the purpose of the exercise. ***(B*** and ***C)*** Pendulum exercises are done passively; no muscular action of the glenohumeral joint is required. Instead, muscular effort of the trunk and hips allow the body to sway and the arm to swing in sagittal, frontal, and transverse planes of motion. The exercise can be progressed to active exercise by actively swinging the arm in the same planes and arcs of motion. (From Cailliet R. *Shoulder Pain*. Philadelphia: FA Davis; 1966: 45.)

SELF-MANAGEMENT: *Subscapularis Isometric Exercise*

Purpose: To strengthen the subscapularis in the short range

Starting position: Kneel next to a weight bench; if at home, lie on your stomach adjacent to the edge of your bed. Place one or two towels rolled under your shoulder. Position your arm out to the side with elbow bent to 90 degrees. Keep as much of your shoulder supported on the bench or bed. Your arm should hang from your elbow down, not from your shoulder. Rotate your arm backward as far as you can before you feel the "ball" drop out of the socket. Position a garbage can or another object sufficient to support your arm.

Movement technique:

- Raise your hand ½ inch off the garbage can, and hold it for 10 seconds.
- Be sure the "ball" does not drop out of the socket.
- Lower your hand back to the garbage can.

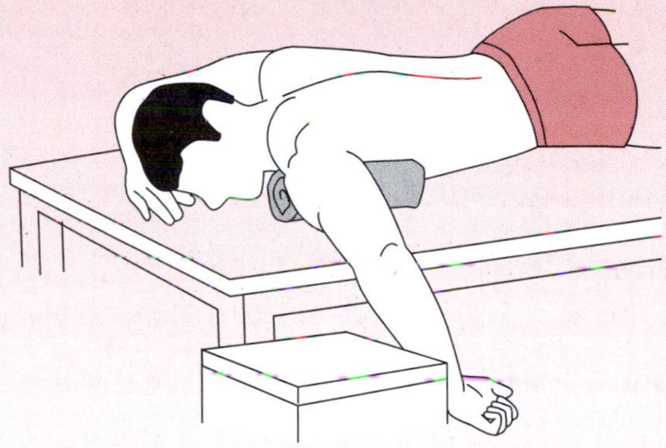

Dosage

Sets/repetitions _____

Frequency _____

to prevent further strain to the muscle. Lengthened muscles produce less force or torque in the short range, and initial exercises may need to be performed in gravity-lessened positions. The gravity-lessened position decreases the load on the lengthened muscle so it can produce sufficient force or torque in the short range. Figure 26-26 depicts a strengthening exercise for the lower trapezius in a gravity-lessened position. The progression exercises shown in Self-Management: Facelying Arm Lifts and Figure 26-14 should proceed when force or torque capability can be produced in the short range against the higher loads imposed by lengthening lever arms and gravity. The goal is to alter length–tension properties of lengthened and shortened muscles. New length–tension properties of the affected musculature (ie, the lengthened musculature adaptively shortens, and the shortened musculature adaptively lengthens) should be achieved if the following conditions are met:

- Strengthening in the shortened range is combined with proper support for the middle and lower trapezius.
- Stretch is applied to the anterior musculature.
- Education is provided regarding improved postures, movement patterns, workstation ergonomics, and body mechanics.

The strain is relieved, and the pathomechanics precipitating or perpetuating the strain are remedied.

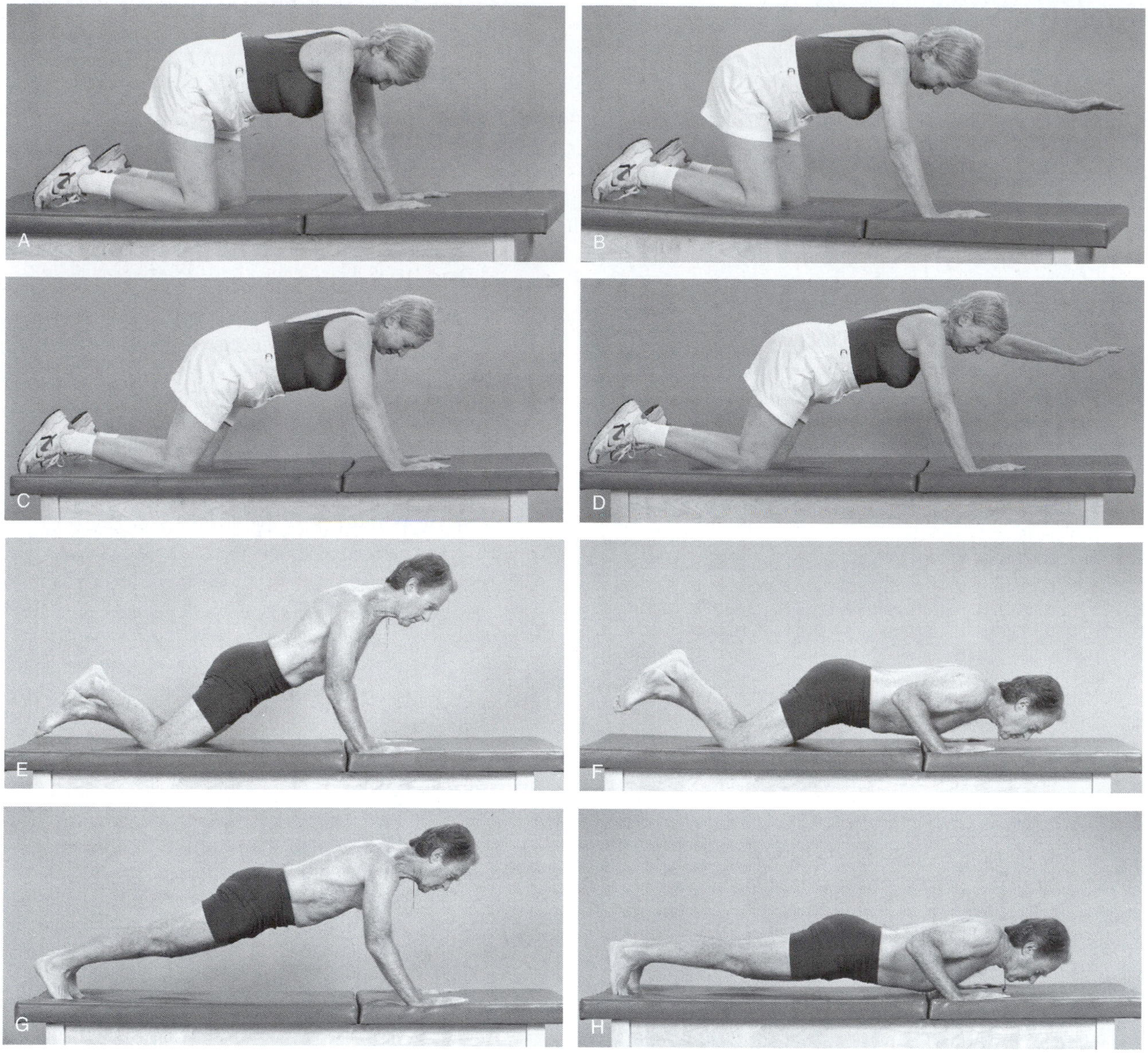

FIGURE 26-23 Progressive serratus strengthening exercises. ***(A)*** The patient assumes a quadruped position, with the hips directly over the knees and the shoulders directly over the hands. The scapula should be flat against the rib cage in neutral position. ***(B)*** The patient then lifts the opposite hand slightly off the ground. The supporting shoulder girdle should not demonstrate any alteration in scapular position. ***(C)*** The patient assumes a quadruped position, with the hips slightly in front of the knees and shoulders directly over the hands. The scapula should be flat against the rib cage in neutral position. ***(D)*** The patient then lifts the opposite hand slightly off the ground. The supporting shoulder girdle should not demonstrate any alteration in scapular position. ***(E)*** The patient assumes the position shown. The hips should be in neutral with respect to the sagittal plane. This subject is in more hip flexion than is desirable. The scapula should be resting against the rib cage in a neutral position. The elbows should be in the sagittal plane with the olecrenon process facing posteriorly and the antecubital fossa facing anteriorly. The fingers should be directed forward with the wrist in extension; a small towel roll may be placed under the palm of the hand to reduce the amount of wrist extension if full wrist extension is uncomfortable. ***(F)*** The patient slowly lowers his body toward the floor while maintaining neutral pelvis and spine alignment. The elbows should flex in the sagittal plane (sometimes called a triceps push-up). The scapula should abduct and adduct during the movement. Evidence of winging or lack of abduction indicates the load is too great or the muscle has fatigued. ***(G)*** The patient is positioned as in E and F, but the legs are straight. ***(H)*** The exercise proceeds as in E and F.

DISUSE, DECONDITIONING, AND REDUCED CONDITIONING

In some cases, muscles become weak because of disuse or deconditioning or may not be able to produce enough force or torque to enable an individual to achieve higher levels of performance (ie, reduced conditioning). Deficits in force or torque production because of disuse or lack of conditioning can manifest as alterations in performance of ADLs, instrumental ADLs, recreation, leisure activity, or sports. Strength deficits can be caused by many forms of disuse or deconditioning:

- Gradual development of subtle alterations in agonist–antagonist relationships caused by stereotypic pos-

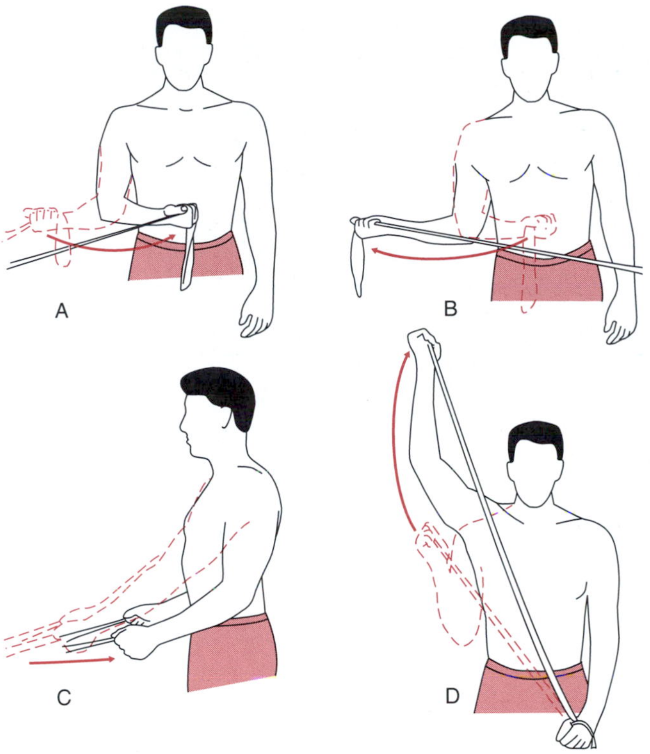

FIGURE 26-24 Higher-level rotator cuff exercise using elastic tubing. ***(A)*** Medial rotation. ***(B)*** Lateral rotation. ***(C)*** Extension. ***(D)*** Flexion.

tural habits or movement patterns, which can create problems related to muscle balance (eg, insidious onset of shoulder impingement without evidence of anatomic impairments as a precipitating factor)

- Generalized weakness from prolonged bed rest or reduction in activity because of illness, preventing performance of a ADLs and instrumental ADLs (eg, dressing, meal preparation, housework)

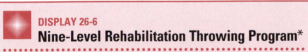

DISPLAY 26-6
Nine-Level Rehabilitation Throwing Program*

Level	Throws/Feet	Throws/Feet	Throws/Feet
One	25/25	25/60	
Two	25/25	50/60	
Three	25/25	75/60	
Four	25/25	50/60	25/90
Five	25/25	50/60	25/120
Six	25/25	50/60	25/150
Seven	25/25	50/60	25/180
Eight	25/25	50/60	25/210
Nine	25/25	50/60	25/240

** This program is designed for athletes to work at their own pace to develop the necessary arm strength to begin throwing from a mound. The athlete is to throw two days in a row and then rest for 1 day. It is not important to progress to the next throwing level with each outing. It is preferred that a number of outings at the same level be completed before progressing. It is important to throw with comfort, which may necessitate moving back a level on occasion.*
Data from reference 54.

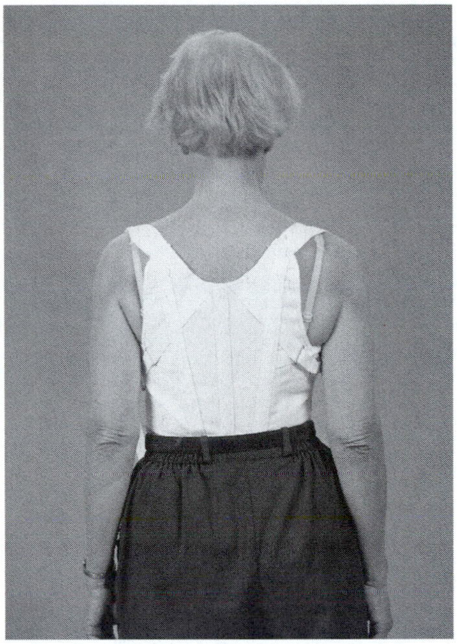

FIGURE 26-25 Posture brace.

- Decreased power output preventing maximal performance of a high-strength-demand sport, such as running, tennis, or figure skating

The shoulder girdle poses a challenge for the clinician prescribing a general strength-conditioning program because of the potential for creating muscle imbalances. A conditioning program should include exercises for all major muscle groups. The posture and movement of the technique are critical to a successful program. For example, if a biceps curl is done with poor technique (ie, anterior scapular tilt is increased during the elbow flexion motion) rather than optimal technique (ie, scapula remains at the optimal resting position during the elbow flexion motion), the patient risks development of impaired length properties of the scapular stabilizers, which could cause other impairments or pathology (eg, impingement syndrome from an anteriorly tilted scapula). This risk increases if the same faulty posture is used during a variety of techniques. Display 26-7 summarizes exercises that are recommended for inclusion in a general shoulder girdle conditioning program.

In the case of a high-level athlete or strenuous industrial worker, general conditioning exercises may not improve performance of the desired activity. The choice of what type of exercise (eg, dynamic, isokinetic, isometric) is used in training depends on the performance level and the specific activities to which the individual wishes to return. The prescription of high-level strength conditioning exercises must be specific for mode, contraction type, and velocity whenever possible. For example, when strength training the medial rotators in the pitching athlete, the type of contraction should duplicate the eccentric contraction used in the cocking phase to decelerate motion and a concentric contraction used in the acceleration phase to create pitching velocity.[63] Examples of techniques or activities that can pro-

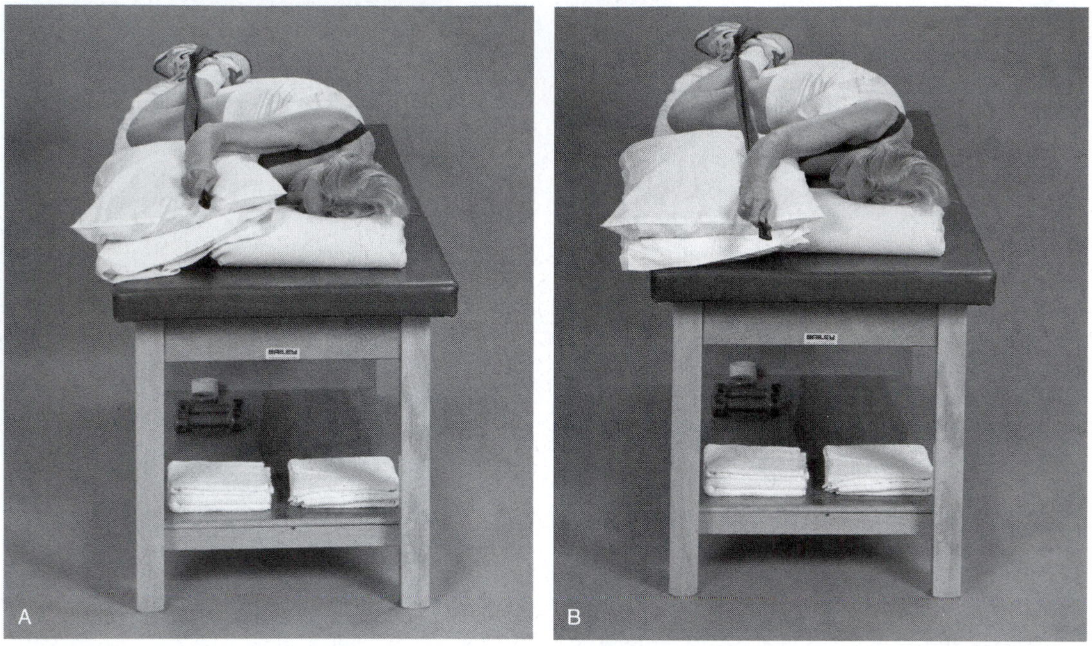

FIGURE 26-26 Sidelying active scapular upward rotation. ***(A)*** Position the patient in sidelying with as many pillows as necessary to support the arm in the sagittal or scapular plane. The arm rests on the pillow at 90 degrees of elevation with the elbow bent. To apply resistance for a self-management exercise, elastic can be held in the hand and secured to the foot. ***(B)*** Slide the arm upward toward full elevation and downward back to the rest position, maintaining the arm in contact with the pillows. The sternothoracic and glenohumeral joint path of instant center of rotation should be monitored for any deviations.

vide concentric and eccentric contraction training include manual resistance by the physical therapist in the clinic, plyometric equipment, and a home program using elastics (Fig. 26-27).

Prevention of injury is a major concern for the athlete or industrial worker. In designing a training program for these persons, the clinician should prescribe exercises to improve the force or torque capability of the muscles required for the sport or occupation and prescribe exercises to prophylactically strengthen opposing muscles to prevent muscle imbalances. For example, sports such as baseball may require training for the shoulder medial rotators. If strengthening for the opposing lateral rotators and scapular adductor and upward rotators is not performed, muscle imbalances may develop and lead to physiologic impairments and pathology.

Endurance Impairment

Postural faults in the upper quadrant often are attributed to lack of muscle endurance. However, little or no muscle activity has been found in upper quadrant muscles during relaxed standing posture.[64] Treating muscle endurance to correct a postural fault is of little value. Postural faults are commonly caused by alterations in muscle length whereby some muscles become adaptively lengthened and others adaptively shortened. The altered lengths of muscles do not provide the optimal support to the shoulder girdle structure.

Impairments in muscle endurance have been implicated in shoulder and neck symptoms. However, despite the methodologic problems associated with quantifying muscle fatigue,[65] most authorities agree that muscle fatigue is not associated with occupational neck and shoulder complaints.[66–67]

Research indicates that prevention and treatment of neck and shoulder symptoms require a multidimensional approach to reduce the workload on muscle.[71–74] Suggested interventions include ergonomic changes in the workstation and appropriate pacing of activity with rest, combined with measures to reduce stress and anxiety in the work place. In the case of recovery from injury, starting a new job with greater workload demands, or trying to improve performance levels in an upper extremity for a sport, endurance may need to be developed in the upper extremity musculature. Local muscle fatigue affects the PICR of the joints in the shoulder girdle complex.[75] When the ADLs or instrumental ADLs require more endurance than the muscles possess, endurance must be considered while making decisions about exercise dosage. Chapter 5 provides specific dosage recommendations.

Posture and Movement Impairment

Restoring optimal posture and movement patterns to the shoulder girdle complex and the entire upper quadrant (and in many cases, the lower quadrant) should be an integral component of any exercise prescription for the shoulder girdle. Attention to posture and movement patterns is a required component of exercise prescribed to remedy related impairments.

DISPLAY 26-7
Shoulder Girdle Conditioning Program

- Bench press (flat, incline, decline)

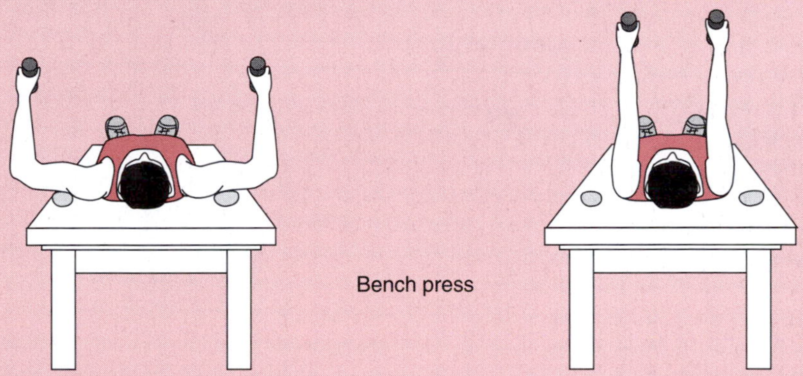

- Prone middle and lower trapezius

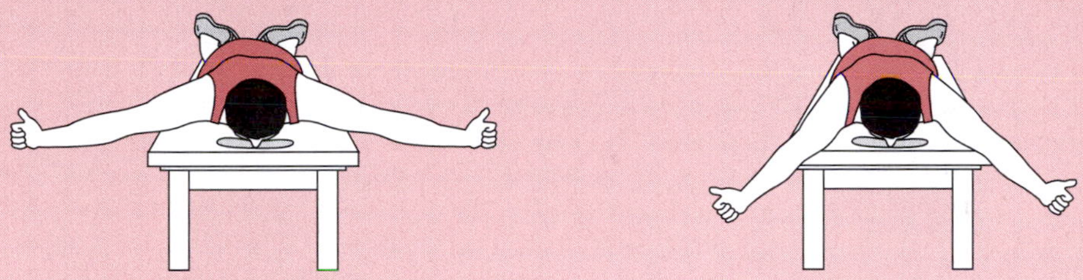

- Latissimus pulldown

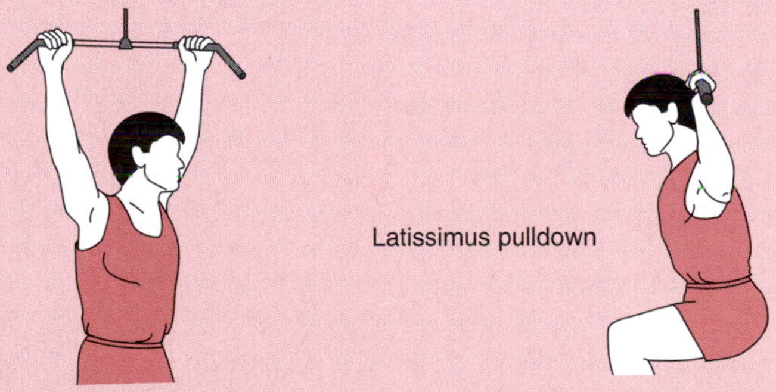

- Lateral deltoid raise—in frontal plane or scaption (through full range of motion) *or*

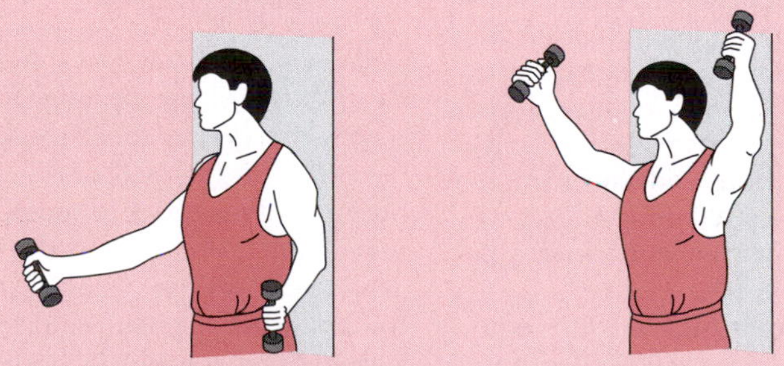

(continued)

DISPLAY 26-7

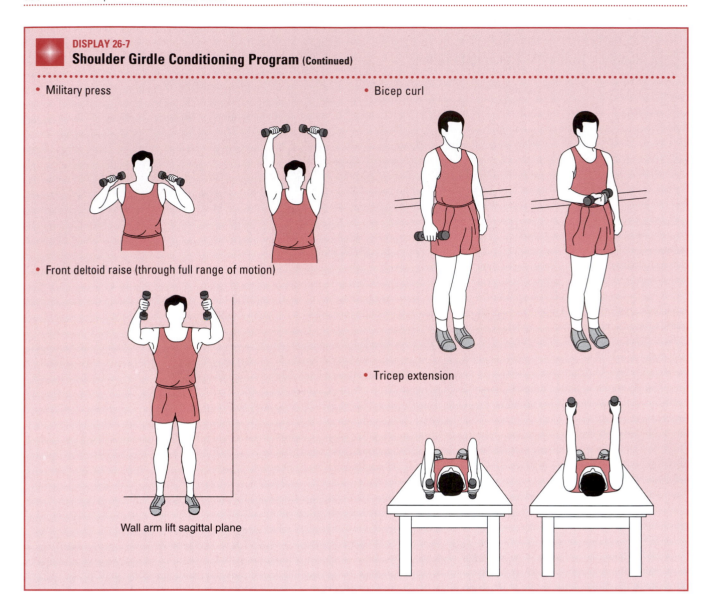

Shoulder Girdle Conditioning Program (Continued)

- Military press

- Front deltoid raise (through full range of motion)

- Bicep curl

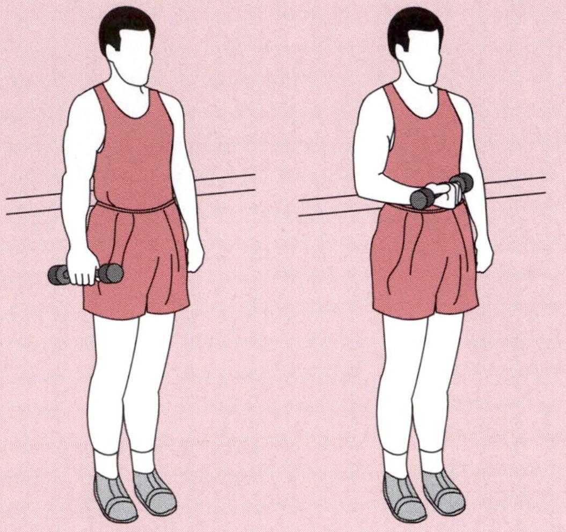

- Tricep extension

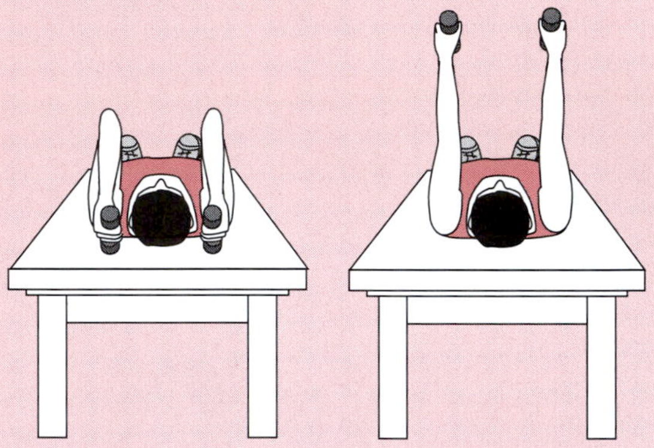

POSTURE

Optimal resting alignment of the shoulder girdle is described in Chapter 8. This alignment facilitates ideal joint positions and resting lengths of the axioscapular, scapulohumeral, and axiohumeral muscles. The resting length of a muscle can be a factor in its participation in active force couples.[28,44] Head, spinal, and pelvic alignment affects alignment of the shoulder girdle. For example, forward head, kyphosis, lordosis, and anterior pelvic tilt encourage abducted and downwardly rotated scapulae. Habitual faulty alignment such as this causes the middle and lower trapezius to adaptively lengthen. Adaptive lengthening affects the length–tension properties of these muscles and thereby affects their performance in scapular force couples.

Optimal alignment of the shoulder girdle requires education of preferred postural patterns during standing, sitting, and sleeping, and education of preferred postural patterns beginning and ending a frequently repeated movement. Posture is intimately related to movement. Altered ergonomics at the workstation (eg, factory assembly line, desk and chair, kitchen counter, car, baby changing table) is critical to successful postural changes. Support through bracing, taping, and supportive brassieres may be necessary to facilitate the re-education process and reduce strain on lengthened muscles.

MOVEMENT

Restoration of the optimal PICR during active motion requires knowledge about the kinesiology of the shoulder girdle complex. If the ideal is known, the clinician can devise a program of exercises to remedy the impairments and retrain movements to approach the ideal standard. The goal is to achieve movement as close to the ideal PICR as possible to enhance the health and longevity of the biomechanical system. The references and reading list at the end of the chapter provide sources for more information about electromyographic or cinematographic analysis of the shoulder girdle during common movement patterns, sport activities, and therapeutic exercises.

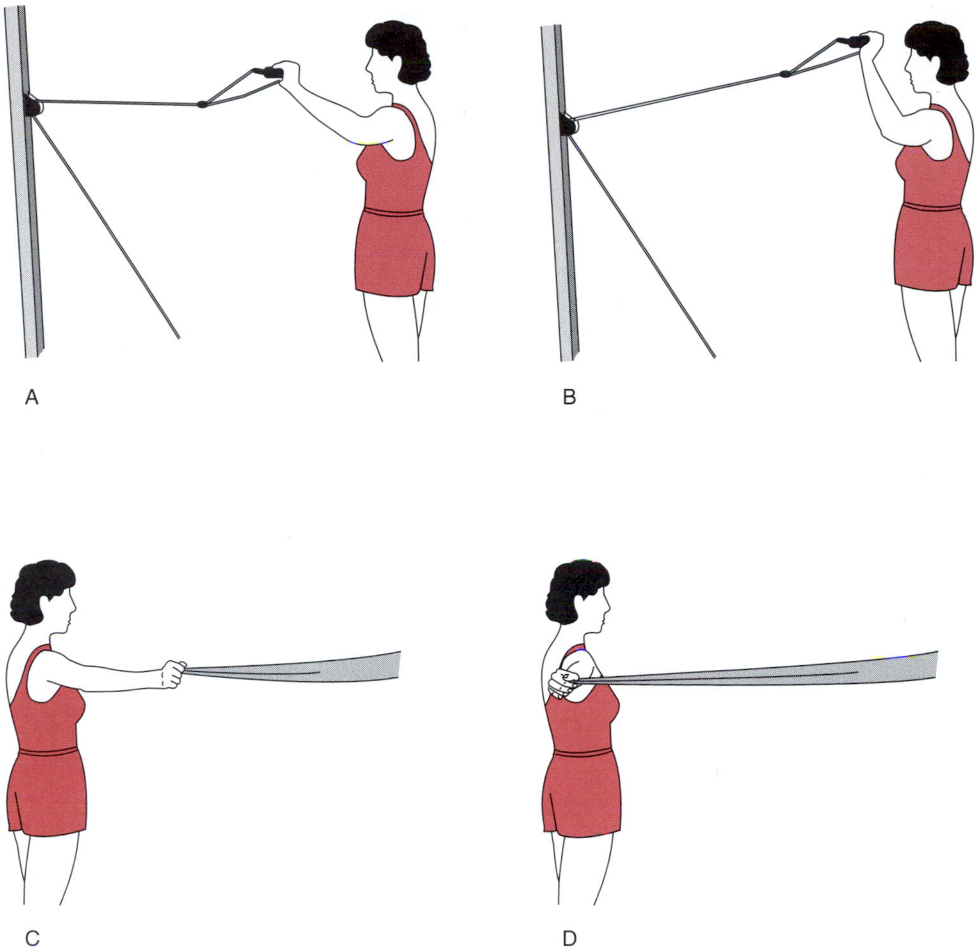

FIGURE 26-27 Plyometric exercise for rotator cuff. ***(A** and **B)*** Starting and ending positions for dynamic plyometric shoulder external rotation (using Impulse Inertial Exercise System). ***(C** and **D)*** Starting and ending positions for dynamic plyometric horizontal abduction using elastic tubing.

THERAPEUTIC EXERCISE INTERVENTIONS FOR COMMON DIAGNOSES

Although comprehensive descriptions and intervention plans for all diagnoses affecting the shoulder girdle are beyond the scope of this book, a few diagnoses are discussed. An overview of the pathogenesis or pathomechanics, examination findings, and proposed treatment plan, with an emphasis on exercise, is provided for each selected diagnosis.

Impingement Syndrome

Although impingement syndrome has often been associated with athletes, this syndrome commonly affects nonathletes. Impingement in the vulnerable avascular region of the supraspinatus and biceps tendons[76,77] occurs predominantly against the anterior or lateral edge of the acromion and coracoacromial ligament[78] during motions of the upper extremity into elevation. For example, chronic irritation from impingement in the avascular region of the supraspinatus leads to an initial inflammatory response in the form of tendinitis, which is difficult to heal. Impingement may also lead to inflammation in the biceps tendon and acromioclavicular joint. The inflammatory process often spreads to the subacromial region because of its intimate anatomic association with the rotator cuff. With time and attrition, microtears and partial-thickness rotator cuff tears may occur. If the process continues, there may be secondary bony changes in the acromioclavicular joint that may result in complete-thickness rotator cuff tears. This hypothesis is supported by cadaver studies that demonstrate bony changes consisting of roughness, erosion, and osteophyte formation on the anteroinferior surface of the acromion in older subjects who have been subjected to supraspinatus impingement.[59,79]

DIAGNOSIS

The condition of mechanical impingement of the supraspinatus and long head of the biceps underneath the acromial arch is often classified as primary impingement syndrome. Pathologic factors can be divided into intrinsic and extrinsic factors. Intrinsic factors can directly involve the subacromial space and include changes in vascularity of the rotator cuff,[31] degenerative changes in the acromioclavicular joint,[80] and anatomic impairments in the shape of the anteroinferior acromion.[81] Extrinsic factors include impairments in posture and movement during ADLs and instrumental ADLs and the related impairments in muscle force or torque capability, endurance, and mobility.

The cause of primary impingement is multifactorial and includes several intrinsic and extrinsic factors. The progressive pathologic process of primary impingement is commonly classified[82] into three stages:

1. Stage I: edema and hemorrhage
2. Stage II: fibrosis and tendinitis
3. Stage III: tendon degeneration and tendon rupture

Because primary impingement syndrome has three pathologic stages and may involve the supraspinatus, biceps tendon, subacromial bursa, and acromioclavicular joint, the presenting functional limitations and impairments can vary greatly. Table 26-5 describes the pathology, presenting and diagnostic signs, impairments, subjective complaints, and functional limitations based on the stage of the impingement.

Stage I can progress to stage II and ultimately to stage III disease if the condition is not appropriately treated. If the condition progresses to stage III, a minor injury to the shoulder (eg, overuse of the shoulder in raking leaves, loss of balance requiring a sudden upper extremity movement) may advance a degenerative or partial-thickness tear to a full-thickness tear. If this occurs, the individual experiences sudden weakness with diminished ability to raise the arm. For stage III, roentgenograms and arthrograms most often have positive findings of subacromial spurring, calcific deposits, and rotator cuff tear.

Impingement that results from glenohumeral hypermobility or instability is known as secondary impingement. Differentiating primary impingement from secondary impingement is crucial to proper management of the condition. Jobe and Pink[83] describe a four-level classification of the impingement-instability complex that focuses on instability as the central process. This classification is summarized in Display 26-8. Group I describes the individual with primary impingement as described in Neer's classification scheme (see Table 26-5). Examination findings for groups II through IV are summarized in Table 26-6.

PRIMARY IMPINGEMENT TREATMENT

Although the pathologic stage is commonly used to guide the physician's intervention, this information does not provide much guidance for the physical therapist's intervention. Physical therapy intervention should be guided by the impairments and functional limitations with which the individual presents at any given stage of pathology. Of particular interest to the physical therapist is treatment of the cause of the impingement. A clinical example and assessment of primary impingement syndrome and examples of exercises to treat the impairments of this patient are provided in Display 26-9. General treatment guidelines for impingement syndrome are presented in an algorithm in Display 26-10.

TREATMENT FOR SECONDARY IMPINGEMENT SYNDROME

As in treatment for primary impingement, the therapeutic exercise intervention should be based on the underlying pathology, presenting impairments, and functional limitations. Treatment should consider impairments related to impingement and to hypermobility and instability problems in the shoulder girdle. Treatment for hypermobility and instability is discussed later.

Anterior Glenohumeral Hypermobility and Subluxation

The anatomic and biomechanical features of the glenohumeral joint predispose it to hypermobility and instability problems. Because it is not within the scope of this text to

Table 26-5. DIAGNOSIS OF PRIMARY IMPINGEMENT

STAGE	PATHOLOGY	IMPAIRMENTS	FUNCTIONAL LIMITATIONS
I	Edema, hemorrhage	1. Pain with impingement test 2. Minimal to no weakness in biceps or supraspinatus 3. Minimal to no decrease in mobility 4. Altered PICR at GH and ST joints	Minimal pain with activity
II	Fibrosis, tendinitis	1. Pain with impingement test 2. Supraspinatus and/or biceps weak and painful 3. Moderate decrease in mobility at GH joint and probable compensatory motion at ST joint 4. AC joint tenderness	1. Toothache-like pain that disturbs sleep 2. Inability to participate in overhead activity without pain
III	Tendon degeneration or tendon rupture	1. Weakness (depends on pain level and integrity of rotator cuff and biceps) 2. Significant decrease in mobility at GH joint with obvious compensation at ST joint 3. Significant AC joint tenderness	1. Prolonged history of shoulder problems 2. Minimal pain (complete rotator cuff tear) or severe pain (partial rotator cuff tear) 3. Significant restriction in use of affected upper extremity

AC, acromioclavicular; GH, glenohumeral; PICR, path of instant center of rotation; ST, sternothoracic.
Adapted from *Neer CS, Walsh RP. The shoulder in sports. Orthop Clin North Am.* 1977;8:583–591.

DISPLAY 26-8

Classification of the Impingement-Instability Process

- Group I: Pure impingement without instability (primary impingement)
- Group II: Impingement with instability (secondary impingement)
- Group III: Impingement with multidirectional instability (secondary impingement)
- Group IV: Pure anterior instability without impingement (instability)

discuss diagnoses and treatments of the entire spectrum of glenohumeral joint conditions, the discussion focuses on anterior glenohumeral hypermobility leading to glenohumeral subluxation (ie, partial dislocation). Hypermobility and subluxation are difficult to diagnose and can best be understood if joint stability is considered in terms of a continuum of stability (Fig. 26-28).[84]

Glenohumeral hypermobility can lead to subluxation, dislocation, impingement, and rotator cuff tendinitis; the latter two are caused by stress or compression of anterior structures caused by excessive humeral head translations.[83] Certain physiologic impairments may contribute to this excessive translation, including inadequate muscle control secondary to weakness, poor endurance,[85] and altered kinesthetic sense.[86]

DIAGNOSIS

Early diagnosis and treatment of glenohumeral hypermobility can prevent serious pathology resulting from dislocation or impingement. However, glenohumeral hypermobility is difficult to diagnose, because it is caused by excessive translation of the humeral head during active movement without the signs or symptoms associated with subluxation or instability (ie, positive apprehension or relocation signs). Excessive passive joint mobility in specific directions combined with displaced PICRs of the glenohumeral joint during active arm elevation or glenohumeral rotation confirm the diagnosis of hypermobility. If positive impingement signs accompany glenohumeral hypermobility, this is classified as group II of the impingement-instability classification shown in Display 26-8. The most common abnormal glenohumeral motions are excessive superior translation during arm elevation, excessive anterior translation during lateral rotation, and abnormal anterior translation during medial rotation. Excessive translation can be confirmed by palpating the humeral head during active motions and comparing the motion to that on the unaffected side.

The diagnosis of glenohumeral subluxation is based on subjective complaints of pain or functional limitation and positive apprehension and relocation signs.[87,88] An excessive anterior translation of the humeral head in the glenoid usually can be clinically demonstrated, particularly during abduction and lateral rotation.

TREATMENT

Treatment for the hypermobile and subluxating shoulder is similar. The following sections highlight the physiologic impairments to be addressed in treating the hypermobile or subluxating shoulder.

Address All Mobility Impairments

Treatment of hypermobility and any hypomobility should occur simultaneously. For example, a common examination finding for the anterior hypermobile or subluxating shoulder is posterior capsular stiffness and an anteriorly displaced humerus at rest. The stiffness of the posterior capsule can restrain posterior translation, occurring primarily during the osteokinematic motions of medial rotation and flexion and causing an abnormal anterior translation during these osteokinematic motions. The posterior capsular stiffness can also contribute to an anteriorly displaced rest position of the humeral head. With the head of the humerus in an anteriorly displaced position at rest, it is vulnerable to moving into an

Table 26-6. EXAMINATION FINDINGS FOR IMPINGEMENT-INSTABILITY CLASSIFICATIONS

GROUP	PATHOLOGY	EXAMINATION FINDINGS
II	Arthroscopic findings of instability Labral damage Undersurface rotator cuff tear	Positive impingement sign Positive apprehensive and relocation signs
III	Arthroscopic findings of instability Attenuated, but intact labrum Undersurface rotator cuff tear Hyperelastic soft tissues	Positive impingement sign Positive apprehensive and relocation signs
IV	Arthroscopic examination reveals unstable shoulder without impingement	Positive apprehensive and relocation signs

From Jobe FW, Pink M. Classification and treatment of shoulder dysfunction in the overhead athlete. *J Orthop Sports Phys Ther.* 1993;18:427–432.

DISPLAY 26-9

Clinical Case of Primary Impingement Syndrome

Examination and Evaluation

History

A 35-year-old, right-handed man complains of right shoulder pain. His occupation requires him to sit at a visual display terminal (VDT) 8 to 10 hours each day, 5 days each week. He also engages in cross-country skiing, climbing, and kayaking. He is unable to sleep on his right shoulder and has pain at night that awakens hims briefly 2 to 3 times each week. He is unable to participate in any recreational acitivity using his right arm. Work is not disrupted at this time, although he does experience a fatiguing discomfort between his shoulder blades while working at the computer about two thirds into his workday.

Postural Alignment

Moderate forward head, moderate abducted, anterior tilted, and downwardly rotated scapulae, with the right scapula slightly depressed, bilateral humerus in moderate abduction (R > L), and moderate thoracic kyphosis

Cervical Clearing Examination

Slight stiffness in cervical rotation to the right, otherwise negative for shoulder girdle signs or symptoms

Passive Range of Motion

Elevation in the plane of the scapula—150 degrees
Lateral rotation at 90 degrees of abduction—90 degrees
Medial rotation at 90 degrees of abduction—40 degrees
Elbow, forearm, wrist, hand—within normal limits (WNL)

Active Range of Motion

Active arm elevation in flexion and abduction—WNL
Total scapular upward rotation is 45 degrees.
Glenohumeral (GH) lateral rotation with the arm adducted to the side is 60 degrees, but it improves to 80 degrees when the scapula is positioned in neutral instead of the patient's abducted rest position.

Scapulohumeral Rhythm

The scapula is slow to elevate in the early phase of elevation, is slow to upwardly rotate in the middle phase of elevation, and demonstrates excessive elevation in the final phase of elevation. The patient experiences pain from 100 degrees to the end range of elevation. Pain is decreased with assisted scapular elevation in the early phase of elevation and upward rotation in the middle to final phase of elevation.

Muscle Length

Moderate shortness in the GH lateral rotators and rhomboids and lengthened right upper trapezius, middle trapezius, lower trapezius, and serratus anterior

Joint Mobility

Hypomobile GH posterior and inferior glide, sternothoracic (ST) upward rotation, and acromioclavicular (AC) joint anteroposterior glide

Strength (tests performed on right only)

Unable to manually test deltoid and lateral rotators because of pain
Subscapularis—3+/5
Upper trapezius—3+/5
Middle trapezius—3/5
Lower trapezius—3/5
Serratus anterior—3/5
Rhomboids/levator scapula—5/5
Biceps—4−/5
Triceps—5/5

Resisted Tests

General abduction, outer-range lateral rotation, and supraspinatus are weak and painful.

Palpation

Tenderness was elicited over the tenoperiosteal and musculotendinous junction of the supraspinatus and AC joint.

Special Tests

Positive impingement sign

Assessment of Findings

Assessment

This patient appears to have stage II impingement pathology. His impairments include

- Altered mobility in periarticular soft tissues limiting posterior and inferior glide of the GH joint
- Reduced muscular extensibility in GH lateral rotators, further contributing limited GH posterior glide
- Decreased posterior and inferior glide of the head of the humerus, affecting joint arthrokinematics and thereby affecting joint osteokinematics
- Reduced muscular extensibility in scapular downward rotators, limiting scapular upward rotation
- Lengthened scapular elevator or upward rotator group, affecting length-tension properties of the muscle, which affect the muscle's participation in active force couples
- Decreased muscle force or torque capability of the elevator or upward rotator, affecting the muscle's participation in the active force couples
- Positive signs of injury to subacromial tissue, particularly supraspinatus (ie, positive impingement sign, weak and painful resisted tests, palpation).

Summary of Pathomechanics

This patient is vulnerable to developing impairments that contribute to impingement syndrome. The prolonged faulty posture he sustains during an 8- to 10-hour workday can lead to altered base, modulator, and biomechanical elements of the movement system. The faulty joint alignment (biomechanical), can contribute to GH impingement due to the altered relationship between the ST and GH joints. Prolonged faulty postures can lead to altered muscle length-tension properties (base), which can contribute to altered movement patterns (modulator). For example, if the scapula is chronically abducted, downwardly rotated, depressed, and anteriorly tilted at rest, the axioscapular upward rotators could adaptively lengthen and the axioscapular downward rotators and scapulohumeral muscles could adaptively shorten. When he raises the arm overhead, as is required for rock climbing and kayaking, the scapula may not sufficiently upwardly rotate, or the humeral head may translate excessively superior in the glenoid fossa. This movement pattern results in impingement of subacromial structures against the AC ligament and possibly the acromion process.

Therapeutic Exercise Intervention for Impairments

- Pain and inflammation: Short-term resolution as described under "First Aid" in Display 26-10; long-term resolution requires addressing the remaining impairments.

- ***Improve mobility***
  - Passive manual stretch to rhomboids (see Fig. 26-13)
  - Self-stretch to GH lateral rotators (see Management: Lateral Rotator and Posterior Capsule Stretch)
- ***Improve force or torque production and endurance; alter length-tension properties***

  Strengthen middle and lower trapezius in a short range (see Self-Management: Facelying Arm Lifts)
  Strengthen serratus anterior in the short range (see Self-Management: Serratus Anterior-Progression)
  Strengthen rotator cuff (see Self Management: Facelying Shoulder Rotation)
- ***Posture and movement***

  Ergonomic modifications at VDT workstation
  Transitional exercises to improve PICR of GH and ST joints in elevation (see Fig. 26-14)
  Functional retraining for ADLs
  Functional retraining for instrumental ADLs (sports and recreation)
  Alter sport-specific training

excessive anterior translation during lateral rotation and abduction. Specific joint mobilization of the posterior capsule combined with passive self-stretching is the best treatment for the hypomobility (see Self-Management: Lateral Rotator and Posterior Capsule Stretch).

As passive mobility is restored, the restoration of precise active mobility must closely follow. The glenohumeral joint needs to be trained to move in a precise PICR pattern without abnormal or excessive anterior translations. This often must occur in conjunction with restoring normal PICRs of the scapulothoracic joint (explained later in this section). The subluxating shoulder may require a period of immobilization to allow stiffening of lax structures. Abduction and lateral rotation positions must be avoided to prevent stretching of the anterior capsule. The immobilization period should last no longer than 3 weeks, and pain-free isometric exercises should begin as soon as tolerated to avoid the effects of prolonged immobilization. Active pen-

DISPLAY 26-10

Treatment for Primary Impingement Syndrome

First Aid: During the early stages, easy self-management measures can assist in decreasing inflammation and pain and promoting early healing.

- **Medications:** Antiinflammatory medications may be prescribed by the physician to assist in reducing inflammation to the acromial and subacromial tissues.
- **Rest:** The patient avoids postures or movements that trigger pain and inflammation. This may require absolute restriction of overhead activity, reduced activity, or modification of the technique used during overhead activity.
- **Resting position:** This position provides the greatest amount of volume in the shoulder joint, assisting in blood flow and decreasing pain. The patient should use pillows to support the arm in slight elevation, abduction, and neutral rotation while sitting, driving, or sleeping. The patient should avoid sleeping on the involved side. If sleeping on the uninvolved side, pillows should be used to support the shoulder as described.
- **Ice:** Ice can reduce inflammation and relieve pain. Choices include cold packs, bags of chipped ice, or ice massage. Ice should be applied directly to the affected tissues. This may require special positioning to expose the affected tissues.[43]

Supervised Treatment: After a thorough examination and evaluation, a plan of care is developed based on the presenting functional limitations and related impairments.

- **Pain and inflammation:** In addition to instructing the patient in first aid self-management, the physical therapist can use physical agents such as ultrasound, phonophoresis, or interferential stimulation.[113]
- **Mobility:** Exercise and joint mobilization can be prescribed to increase mobility in periarticular tissues and improve muscle extensibility. Education and exercise can be prescribed to normalize length-tension properties of adaptively shortened and lengthened muscles.
- **Force or torque production and endurance:** Exercise can be prescribed to improve force or torque capability, length-tension properties, and endurance of the rotator cuff and scapular upward rotators. Dosage parameters should be adjusted according to the goal of the exercise as outlined in Chapter 2.
- **Posture and movement:** For the tissue to heal and to prevent recurrence, the mechanical causes of the impingement must be eliminated. During the early phases of intervention, posture and movement must be addressed to the greatest possible extent given the presenting impairments in force or torque, endurance, and mobility. After the underlying foundation in physiologic capabilities has improved, long-term management requires specific retraining in posture and movement habits to eliminate the mechanical cause of impingement during function, including ergonomic modifications, alterations in training techniques, and specific movement retraining during ADLs and instrumental ADLs.

Surgery: If supervised treatment fails (in some stage II cases and most stage III cases), surgery to remove subacromial spurring and increase space for the subacromial tissues may be necessary. Surgery should be considered only when symptoms have persisted despite conservative treatment for more than 1 year. Anterior acromioplasty is the recommended choice for decompression of the rotator cuff from impingement.[58] The posterior half of the acromion is not involved in the impingement process and, therefore, lateral or complete acromionectomy is thought to weaken the deltoid unnecessarily.[113] In many cases, repair of the rotator cuff is necessary.

Prevention: Prevention of stage II and III disease is the best treatment. Prevention lies in early recognition (during stage I) and prompt and comprehensive treatment of the presenting functional limitations and related impairments.

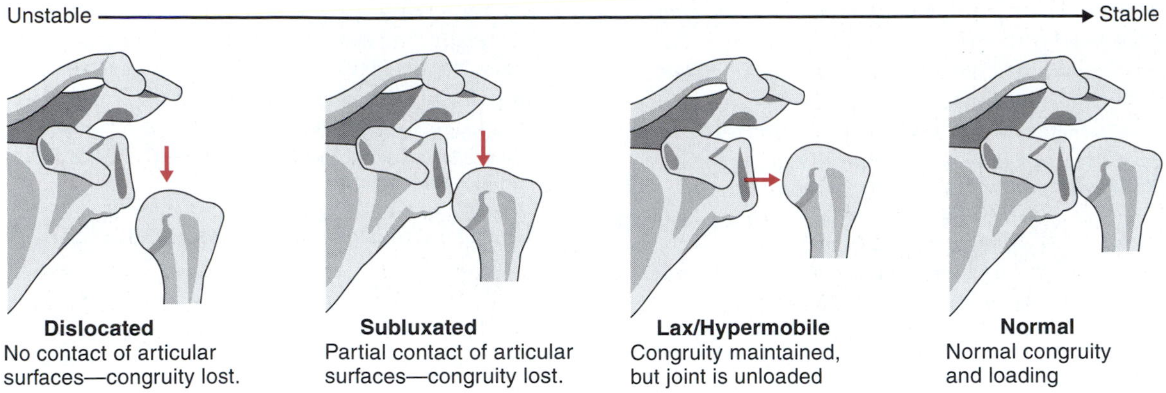

FIGURE 26-28 Continuum of shoulder stability. (From Strauss MB, Wrobel LJ, Neff RS, Cady GW. The shrugged-off shoulder: a comparison of patients with recurrent shoulder subluxations and dislocations. *Physician Sports Med.* 1983;11:96.)

dulum exercises (see Fig. 26-22) may be used immediately after immobilization to help increase ROM and stimulate contraction of the rotator cuff muscles. Active ROM exercises can be initiated against gravity as the patient regains strength and motor control. Abnormal movement patterns should be discouraged; therefore, ROM is progressed only within the ROMs with optimal PICRs.

Restore Impairments in Muscle Performance

Gradually, resistive exercises can be initiated targeting the pectoralis major, latissimus dorsi, teres major, and subscapularis to provide dynamic restraint to anterior translation into the anterior capsule. However, the main target muscle should be the subscapularis because of its insertion anterior to the glenohumeral joint and its proximity to the axis of rotation of the glenohumeral joint. Careful observation of the PICR during medial rotation is a good indicator of the participation of the subscapularis in the medial rotation force couple. Anterior translation of the humerus should not take place during medial rotation because it is a sign of insufficient subscapularis participation. Exercises should be prescribed to isolate subscapularis function as much as possible (see Self-Management: Subscapularis Isometric Exercise).

Infraspinatus and teres minor strengthening can be targeted to prevent excessive anterior translation of the head of the humerus.[89] For the infraspinatus and teres minor to provide a stabilizing force on the glenohumeral joint, stability of the scapulothoracic joint is required. If the scapula is not stabilized by the axioscapular muscles and the infraspinatus and teres minor contract, instead of providing a posterior restraint to the glenohumeral joint, contraction of the infraspinatus and teres minor can contribute to further anterior displacement. This occurs by reverse action on the scapula, and instead of compressing the glenohumeral joint into the glenoid fossa, the resultant force pulls the scapula toward the humerus and forces the head of the humerus anteriorly. During any lateral rotation exercise, care must be taken to ensure that motion is prevented at the scapulothoracic joint and that lateral rotation occurs at the glenohumeral joint without excessive anterior translation.

Isokinetic or plyometric upper extremity exercises (see Fig. 26-27) can be incorporated into the resistive training program of individuals returning to a high level of function.

Retrain the Precise Path of Instant Center of Rotation During the Activities of Daily Living

If the PICR is closely monitored, movements into full lateral rotation and abduction should not be contraindicated, because this motion does not excessively stretch the anterior capsule. If excessive anterior translation occurs because of lack of force-generating capability from the axioscapular or rotator cuff muscles and poor motor control, extremes of ROM should be avoided.

Sport-specific exercises can be gradually incorporated into the treatment program to prepare the patient for transition to functional activity (Fig. 26-29). Attention to the PICR of the glenohumeral joint is the guide to progression. Control over the translatory motions of the glenohumeral joint should be emphasized over general strength gains.

The literature supports the notion that motor control is more critical in restoring function to the unstable shoulder than general strength gains.[90] Research indicates that peak torque gains occur in persons trained with electromyographic biofeedback in purely functional patterns with no emphasis on "strength exercising." Functional gains and abolition of pain was greater and occurred earlier in the group trained functionally with electromyographic biofeedback than the group trained in more traditional strength regimens.

Rotator Cuff Tear

Rupture of the rotator cuff may be more frequent than suspected, and this diagnosis should be considered for individuals engaged in strenuous occupations or sports activities who sustain violent trauma, usually a fall. However, minor stress can easily cause a partial or complete tear of a tissue already weakened by degenerative changes caused by chronic impingement syndrome.

ETIOLOGY AND DIAGNOSIS

The four categories of rotator cuff pathology are summarized in Display 26-11.[91] Neer states that "impingement tears" comprise 90% of tears of the rotator cuff.[92] Because the diagnosis and treatment of primary and secondary impingement were addressed earlier, this discussion focuses on tensile disease or injury tears and macrotraumatic failure.

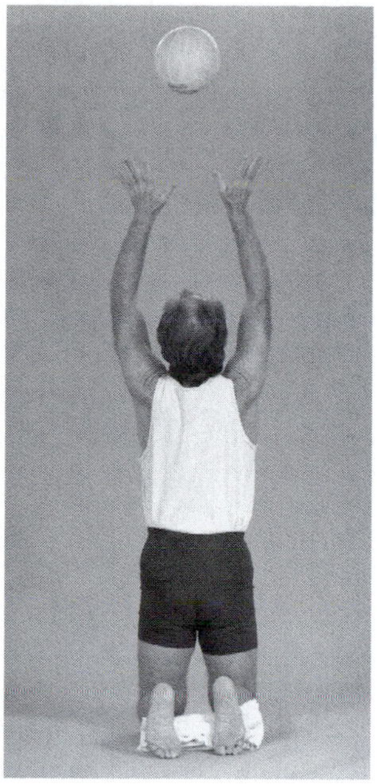

FIGURE 26-29 Sport-specific exercise for someone with glenohumeral hypermobility: ball tossing upward to simulate a set in volleyball.

Tensile disease or injury tears are a result of repetitive, intrinsic tension overload. The pathologic changes referred to as "angiofibroblastic hyperplasia" by Nirschl[93] occur in the early stages of tendon injury and can progress to rotator cuff tears from the continued tensile overload.[94] Throwing or racket sport athletes are at high risk for this type of rotator cuff injury because of the high, repetitive eccentric forces incurred by the posterior rotator cuff musculature during the deceleration and follow-through phases of overhead sport activities.

Macrotraumatic tendon failure is the result of a single traumatic event. Forces encountered in the traumatic event are greater than the normal tendon can tolerate. Full-thickness tears of the rotator cuff with bony avulsions of the greater tuberosity can occur from single traumatic episodes. Although a single traumatic event can result in tendon failure, normal tendons do not tear.[95] Repeated microtrauma and resulting tendon degeneration must create a substantially weakened tendon for it to fail.

Tears can be classified as partial or incomplete, complete, or massive.[92] Incomplete tears do not extend through the complete thickness of the tendon. Three types are recognized: superficial surface, deep surface, and intratendinous. Complete tears extend through the complete thickness of the tendon or muscle. A massive tear indicates more than one rotator cuff tendon or muscle is torn.

DISPLAY 26-11

Mechanisms of Rotator Cuff Pathology

- Primary impingement syndrome
- Secondary impingement syndrome
- Tensile disease or injury
- Macrotraumatic failure

A history of injury is not a prerequisite for the diagnosis of a rotator cuff tear. A mild incident such as pulling a cable to start a lawn mower or lifting a suitcase onto a shelf can complete a partial tear in a degenerated tendon or muscle. Symptoms can vary from mild and intermittent to constant and unbearable, depending on the use of the arm and the severity of the tear.

Incomplete tears may resemble the signs and symptoms of primary or secondary impingement syndrome. Resisted tests reveal weakness and pain, palpation elicits tenderness over the greater tuberosity, and active ROM demonstrates a painful arc. Mobility may not be disrupted, but the PICR is altered by an excessive superior translation of the humeral head.

It is typical for shoulders with complete cuff tears to remain mobile passively, but individuals who avoid glenohumeral movements for a long time, because of pain and decreased force or torque capability, may develop stiffness. Rupture of the long head of the biceps suggests the presence of a large cuff tear. Progressive grades of weakness caused by rotator cuff tears are summarized in Display 26-12.

Differentiation of an incomplete tear from a complete tear may require a radiologic test, such as arthrography, bursography, ultrasonography, or magnetic resonance imaging. None of these radiologic tests can be considered an infallible diagnostic method for incomplete tears, but they are reliable in diagnosing complete tears.[96] Arthroscopy can be used to inspect the rotator cuff and document the location and extent of pathologic changes that cannot be seen through diagnostic imaging techniques.[96]

TREATMENT

Incomplete Tears

Incomplete tears often are undiagnosed and are instead treated as impingement syndrome cases. An incomplete tear may be diagnosed by an arthrogram. Incomplete tears can be treated conservatively with physical therapy or with anterior acromioplasty and repair.

Two schools of thought are diametrically opposed with respect to conservative treatment of incomplete tears. One advocates immobilization of the arm in 90 degrees of scaption (ie, scapular plane) and lateral rotation to approximate the torn fibers. No motion is allowed for 8 weeks.[97] The other, more common school of thought advocates immediate active

DISPLAY 26-12

Progressive Weakness Caused by Rotator Cuff Tears

Initial subtle weakness → Spinatus atrophy * → Shrugging sign † → Dropping sign ‡

** Atrophy in the supraspinous and infraspinous fossa.*

† Positive when the infraspinatus is involved. Depicted by excessive scapular elevation during arm elevation.

‡ The "dropping sign" is elicited by the examiner passively rotating the arm into lateral rotation with the arm at the side and asking the patient to maintain that position after the examiner lets go. Inability to maintain the arm in lateral rotation indicates a large tear involving the infraspinatus or paralysis of the C5-C6 nerve root.

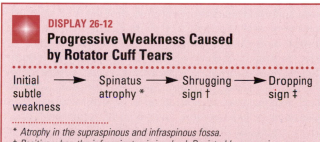

motion as soon as pain permits. If abduction from a dependent position is weak, an abduction splint is applied, and abduction exercises are started from that level of abduction. The splint is used for 3 weeks, and the goal is full active mobility within 8 weeks. This active concept is especially advocated for older patients, for whom even brief immobilization can lead to adhesive capsulitis (ie, frozen shoulder).[98]

Complete Tears

Traumatic tears in younger patients and tears after dislocations can be treated conservatively initially. Neer recommends reducing the activity level of the patient (ie, prohibiting throwing, lifting, and impact loads) for 9 to 12 months.[92] If healing has occurred at that time, progressive return to full activity is allowed.

Most tears are managed by surgical decompression and repair. Details of the surgical techniques are well documented in the literature.[92] The postoperative exercise regimen after anterior acromioplasty and repair of the rotator cuff is determined by the strength of the rotator cuff. Methodical planning and cooperation by the patient, surgeon, and physical therapist are necessary to plan a program with a successful outcome. The patient will have greater confidence if clear objectives are developed. Preoperatively, the surgeon and physical therapist should explain to the patient that it will take up to 12 months for mature healing of the tendons. However, during this time, activities will be progressively advanced, and strict adherence to the physical therapist's instructions will ensure the most successful outcome. The physical therapist must understand the specific anatomic considerations and limitations to plan a safe and effective postoperative rehabilitation program. Only the surgeon knows the strength and stability of the repair and therefore should closely supervise the aftercare program of each patient.

The algorithm shown in Display 26-13 provides guidance for rehabilitation after a standard rotator cuff repair.[92] Because of the unique anatomic arrangement and function of the rotator cuff, rehabilitation after surgery is considered to be more difficult than that of any other joint. In most patients, the muscles involved in the precisely integrated force couples used in upper extremity movements have suffered from months of atrophy and disuse. Early in the rehabilitation process, careful exercises may be prescribed to prevent severe atrophy of the scapular upward rotators (Fig. 26-30). Toward the latter stages of rehabilitation, precise integration and coordination of motor control must be restored to all the muscles involved in the functional movements used by the individual. Postoperative care after repair for a massive rotator cuff tear is far more conservative, requiring longer periods of immobilization and slower return to function. The overall postoperative prognosis for individuals with massive tears is considered to be satisfactory (ie, some weakness, good function, and no pain) compared with the often excellent (ie, essentially normal shoulder) prognosis for the individual with a complete tear.

Adhesive Capsulitis

Adhesive capsulitis is an unusual condition that occurs most often in the nondominant shoulder of individuals between the ages of 40 and 60. Seventy percent of these patients are women. The term adhesive capsulitis, also called frozen shoulder syndrome, describes a stiff shoulder in which active and passive movements are restricted primarily at the glenohumeral joint. Lateral rotation and elevation are the most marked limitations, followed by limitation of medial rotation. Any cause of pain in the shoulder may initiate a stiff shoulder, but frozen shoulder occurs most commonly when the following features of disuse exist:

- Tension
- Anxiety
- Passive apathy (ie, periarthritic personality)[99]
- Low pain threshold

Self-immobilization causes venous stasis and secondary congestion, and when combined with vasospastic anoxia, they lead to production of a protein-rich, edematous exudate and ultimately to a fibrous reaction. The progression of disability is illustrated in Figure 26-31.[98]

DIAGNOSIS

Adhesive capsulitis can occur in three phases, with each phase lasting approximately 4 months. The initial phase is called the freezing phase, which is characterized by painful limitation in motion. This is followed by a frozen phase, which is characterized by decreasing pain but increasingly greater limitation of motion. As the glenohumeral joint becomes less mobile, the scapulothoracic joint often compensates to allow the individual to elevate the arm. The most typical compensation is excessive scapulothoracic elevation and abduction. As the shoulder becomes more frozen, pain is typically minimal or absent when the arm is immobile, but stretching pain accompanies attempts to move the arm away from the dependent position. Various degrees of limitation exist during this phase, but the ultimate result of untreated adhesive capsulitis is significant glenohumeral hypomobility and limited scapulothoracic upward rotation mobility.

Because this condition is considered self-limited, the final phase is called the thawing phase, during which physical therapy can be most useful in restoring mobility and function to the affected shoulder. A frozen shoulder may last as long as 1 year; rarely, it may last as long as 3 years, causing stiffness, discomfort, and decreased function during the entire time. Fortunately, the disorder rarely recurs.

TREATMENT

The best approach to adhesive capsulitis is prevention. Although this syndrome is considered a self-limited process, complete recovery with no residual limitation and disability is neither ensured nor common. Fibrosis, secondary arthritis, myofascial contracture, disuse atrophy, and altered motor control patterns may be permanent. Only active use of the arm and full maintenance of glenohumeral and scapulothoracic active mobility with precise PICRs at all four shoulder girdle articulations can reverse these changes.

Local treatment of the shoulder requires a commitment of active participation and treatment carried out long enough to adequately restore active mobility. The patient must be able and willing to cooperate with the physical

DISPLAY 26-13
Rehabilitation After Rotator Cuff Repair

Protective Phase (1–6 weeks)

- Sling protection is used for 2 to 3 days and up to 6 weeks at night.
- Pendulum exercises (see Fig. 26-22) are initiated within the first 48 hours.
- Self-assisted ROM exercises are initiated at the end of the first week (A,B,C).

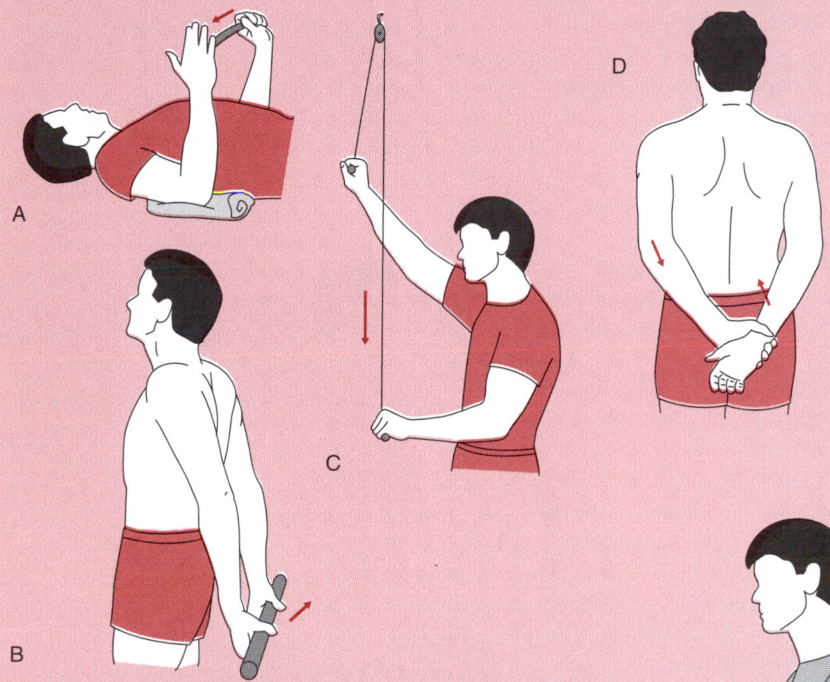

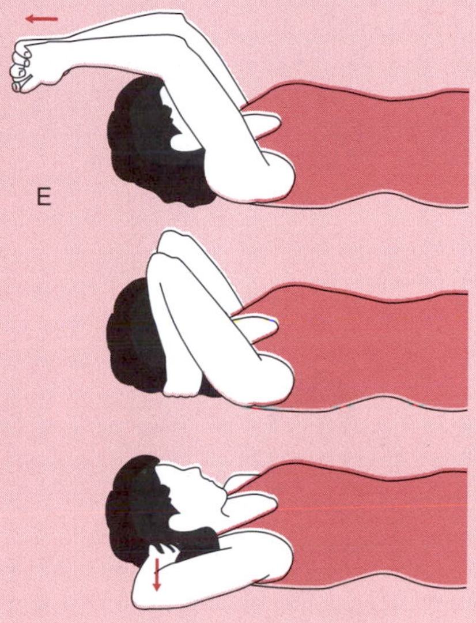

(A) Assisted lateral rotation in supine. A towel is placed under the elbow to keep the humerus in neutral and prevent excessive anterior displacement. The patient pushes the involved arm into lateral rotation, using the uninvolved arm to supply the power. ***(B)*** Assisted extension. The patient pushes backward into extension, using the uninvolved arm to supply the power. Caution should be used to prevent excessive glenohumeral (GH) extension and anterior displacement of the GH joint. ***(C)*** Pulley-assisted elevation. The uninvolved arm supplies the power to raise the involved arm. Caution should be used to prevent excessive scapular elevation as compensation for lack of GH mobility. The motion should be stopped as soon as a deviation in the path of instant center of rotation of the GH or sternothoracic joint is noted. This exercise can be progressed to active assisted elevation when directed by the physician.

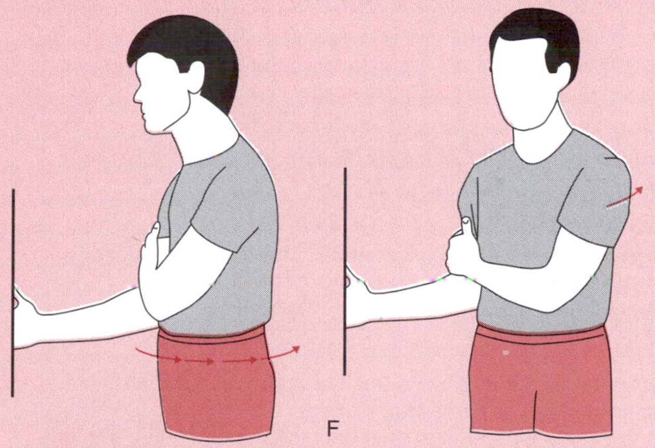

(D) Assisted medial rotation. The patient is instructed to medially rotate the arm by pushing the arm backward, followed by pulling the hand upward toward the scapula. Cautions should be used to prevent excessive scapular anterior tilt and GH anterior displacement. ***(E)*** Assisted abduction. The patient is instructed to (1) lie on the back, (2) lock the fingers together and stretch the arms overhead (the uninvolved arm powers the involved arm), (3) bring the hands behind the neck, (4) flatten the elbows (Reverse by sliding the hands overhead and down). Caution should be taken while abducting to ensure the scapulae are in a neutral position and adduct as the arm abducts. ***(F)*** Assisted lateral rotation in a doorway. The patient is instructed to stand in a doorway facing the door frame. The elbow is flexed to 90 degrees. The palm is on wall. The elbow is held in adduction. The body turns gradually until the patient faces into the room. Caution should be taken to ensure proper scapular alignment during the lateral rotation process.

Early Intermediate Phase (6 weeks–3 months)

- Additional self-assisted ROM exercises are prescribed 6 weeks after surgery (D,E,F).
- If motion is restricted at this time, *gentle* passive stretching by the physical therapist is indicated.

Late Intermediate Phase (3 months–5 months)

- Isometric exercise may be introduced 3 months after surgery.
- Isometric exercise is progressed to dynamic exercise based on the physician's recommendations (K,L).

(continued)

DISPLAY 26-13

Rehabilitation After Rotator Cuff Repair (Continued)

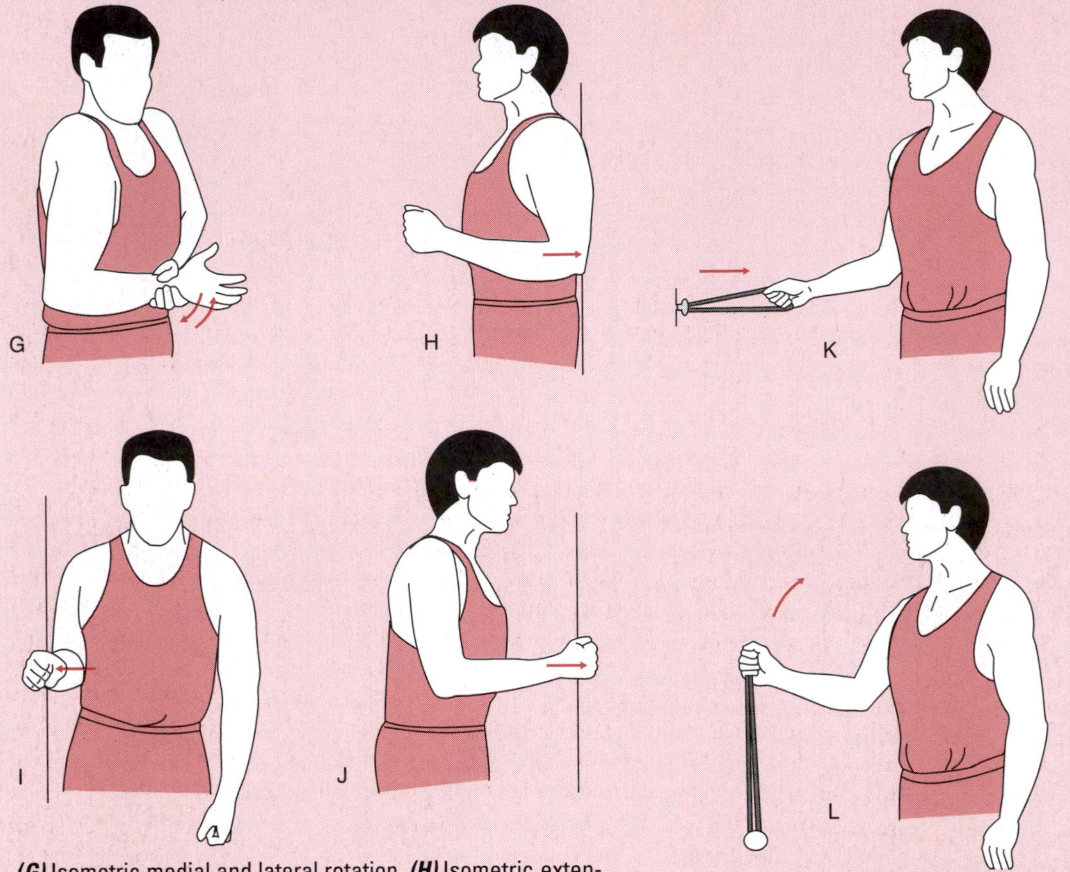

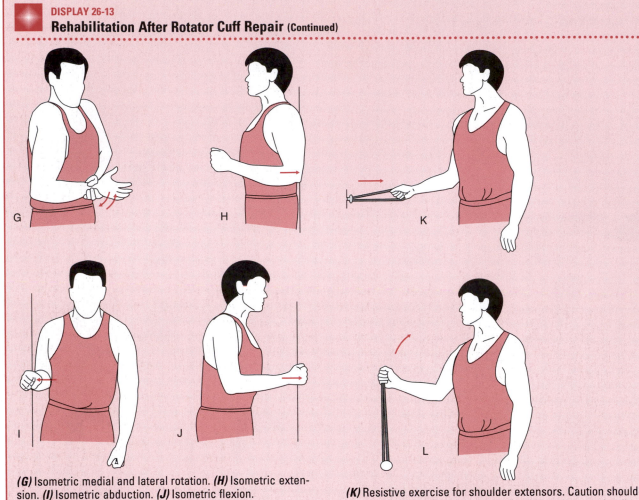

(G) Isometric medial and lateral rotation. ***(H)*** Isometric extension. ***(I)*** Isometric abduction. ***(J)*** Isometric flexion.

(K) Resistive exercise for shoulder extensors. Caution should be taken to prevent thoracic flexion or scapular anterior tilt. The range should be limited to extension to the midaxillary line to prevent contractions of the rhomboid in the short range. ***(L)*** Resistive exercise for shoulder flexion. The motion is upward into flexion as if throwing an "upper cut" punch. Caution should be taken to monitor the ST PICR.

- Active movement of the arm overhead is introduced based on the physician's recommendations.
- Swimming is allowed at 5 months after surgery.

Advanced Rehabilitation Phase (5 months–1 year)

- Submaximal sport-specific training is progressed to maximal training by the end of 1 after surgery.

General Precautions and Contraindications

- Flexion should precede abduction when restoring active motion.
- The patient should avoid leaning on the arm or carrying more than 5 pounds of weight in the early and intermediate phases of rehabilitation.
- Patients with complete tears of the supraspinatus should avoid lifting more than 15 pounds in the first year postoperatively.
- Skiing, skating, roller-blading, and other such activities are forbidden in the first year after surgery to avoid reinjury from a fall.

therapist and deal with psychological barriers. Treatment of anxiety, dependency, apathy, or a low pain threshold may be necessary for full resolution of the syndrome. Appropriate referral should be made to a practitioner educated to handle such impairments in the cognitive or affective element of the movement system.

Medications may be indicated to treat pain and muscle tension. A local injection of procaine and steroids may help relieve pain when it is severe. Nerve blocks may facilitate active exercise. A method of joint distention through a process of injecting contrast medium (used in arthrography) into the subscapular bursa can enlarge the bursa and relieve joint restrictions caused by adhesions within the bursa.[100] Other treatments such as manipulation under anesthesia and arthroscopy may be necessary. These treatments should be approached with substantial caution, because frozen shoulder is often a self-limited process. Overly aggressive surgical treatment may cause more problems than a nonoperative program of medication and physical therapy.[101]

Exercise is the recommended treatment, which may or may not be augmented by the aforementioned medical interventions. Exercises to promote mobility at all affected

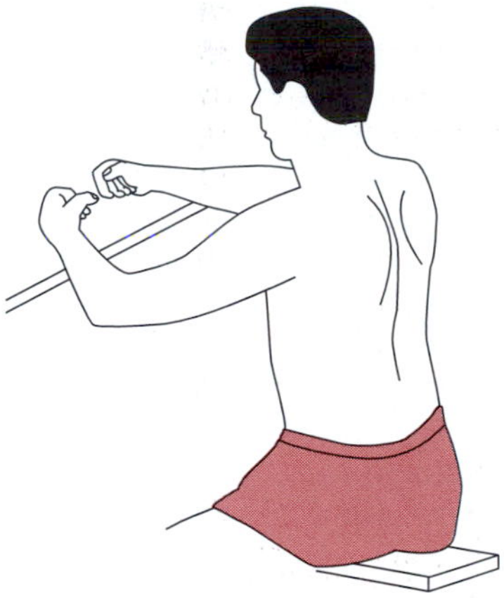

FIGURE 26-30 Alternative isometric scapular upward rotation. The arms can be positioned in as much elevation as is available. The cue should be to "*gently* squeeze your shoulder blades together." Caution should be taken to prevent excessive rhomboid or latissimus contribution.

joints are critical. Modalities such as ultrasound or moist hot packs placed around the entire glenohumeral joint may encourage maximal tissue elasticity by increasing tissue temperature. They are used most effectively before active or passive manual stretching or self-stretching. Manual or self-mobilization techniques directed at any or all four articulations in the shoulder girdle complex may be necessary to improve arthrokinematic mobility in the specific directions necessary to improve osteokinematic ROM. Figure 26-32 provides an example of a self-mobilization technique. Full active ROM is the goal, because any residual limitation may reinitiate the cycle. Active resistive exercises must closely follow ROM gains to restore strength and endurance lost during the immobilized period.

Despite decreased pain, improved mobility, and improved force-generating capacity, faulty movement patterns may persist. The individual may learn to use scapulothoracic, elbow, or trunk motions to substitute for lost glenohumeral motions.[102] Taping the scapulothoracic joint can significantly help to limit scapular substitution patterns and force greater mobility at the glenohumeral joint during functional activity (see the Adjunctive Interventions: Taping section).[103] Taping the scapulothoracic joint may transfer improvements made in mobility and force or torque production with specific exercise to ADLs and instrumental ADLs, including specific movement patterns necessary for sport.

Thoracic Outlet Syndrome

Mechanical, nontraumatic brachial plexus compression can be caused by bony, ligamentous, or muscular obstacles anywhere between the cervical spine and lower border of the axilla. Compression of the brachial plexus is commonly referred to as thoracic outlet syndrome (TOS). All the symptoms attributed to TOS imply compression of the brachial plexus, subclavian artery and vein, or both areas. Common sites of compression include the anterior scalene, between the clavicle and first rib, and under the pectoralis minor. Several types of anatomic impairments, such as a cervical rib, a J-curve structural variation of the first rib, and a long transverse process of C7, may predispose the neurovascular bundle to compression. Fibrous bands between the cervical vertebrae and first rib may also be a source of compression. Less commonly, a tumor in the thoracic outlet may compress the neurovascular bundle.

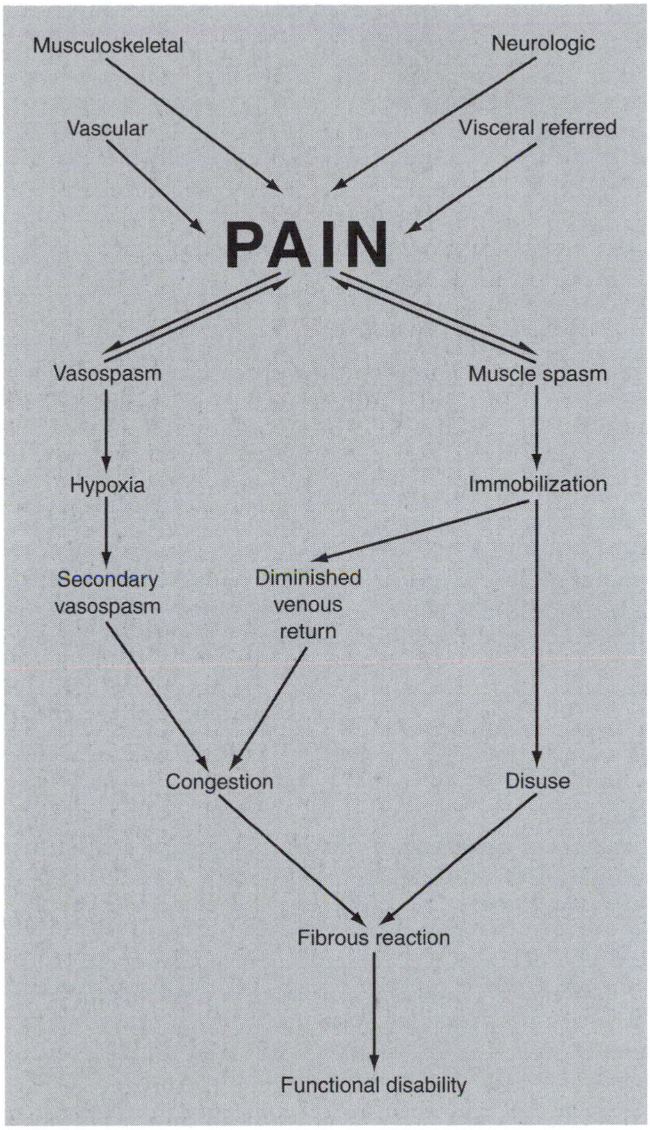

FIGURE 26-31 Schematic stages toward functional disability in adhesive capsulitis. (Redrawn with permission from Caillet R. *Shoulder Pain.* Philadelphia, FA Davis 1978.)

DIAGNOSIS

A careful evaluation is necessary to diagnose TOS and to differentiate it from a spinal tumor, multiple sclerosis, cervical disk pathology, carpal tunnel syndrome, angina, tendinitis, and other brachial plexus injuries. Typically, patients complain of pain and paresthesia (ie, numbness and tingling) involving the neck, shoulder, arm, forearm, or wrist and hand. Sensory and motor loss most commonly involves the C8-T1 segmental innervation regions. Because of the C8-T1 sensory and motor changes, fine coordination may be affected, and patients may complain of symptoms when holding a newspaper, combing hair, or buttoning clothes. The pain is often worse after the arm is used than

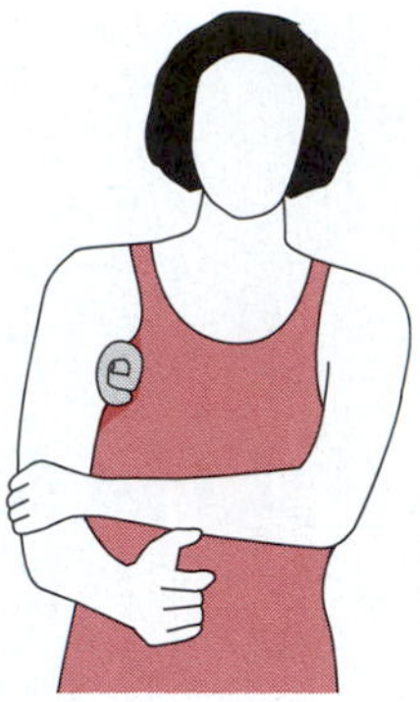

FIGURE 26-32 Self-mobilization of the glenohumeral joint into lateral distraction.

during use, and it is particularly disturbing at night. Some patients have complaints similar to intermittent claudication from the subclavian artery or vein compression, including diffuse pain, numbness, coolness, and fatigue of upper extremity musculature. Symptoms are eased by avoiding aggravating activity and through support of the involved extremity, such as supportive taping or keeping the hand in a pocket.

Diagnosis of vascular TOS is made by duplex scanning (ie, ultrasound combined with Doppler velocity waveforms), angiography, or venography. Electrodiagnostic tests can reveal chronic, severe lower trunk brachial plexopathy. Many TOS patients have normal electrodiagnostic study findings, possibly because of the position-specific onset of symptoms. Tests conducted with patients in the symptom-provoked positions may reveal positive findings.

Reproduction of a patient's symptoms by systematically positioning the head, neck, and upper extremity helps in diagnosing TOS and in determining at what sites compression is occurring. Although it is beyond the scope of this text to describe all the tests needed to diagnosis TOS, the following special tests should be included in differential diagnosis of TOS:

- Adson's maneuver: The Adson's maneuver result may be positive in many asymptomatic persons and therefore it should not be used exclusively as an indicator, but in conjunction with other objective testing,[104] this test is used to implicate the anterior scalene muscle's role in obliterating the pulse when the muscle is put on stretch.
- Costoclavicular maneuver: This test lowers the clavicle onto the first rib, causing compression.
- Hyperextension and hyperabduction: This test compresses the neurovascular bundle between the pectoralis minor and coracoid process.
- Hyperabduction and external rotation[105,106]: Tests produce an scissors-like compression of the neurovascular bundle between the clavicle and first rib. However, when pulse obliteration is used as the critical sign, the traditional tests produce too many false-positive results to be considered valid; most persons have pulse changes with these maneuvers.[107] Reproduction of symptoms with these tests is a more reliable sign of TOS.[106]
- Upper limb tension testing[108]

TREATMENT

The goal of treatment of TOS, regardless of the site of compression or the cause of compression, is to increase the space of the affected regions of the thoracic outlet and reduce pressure on the neurovascular bundle. Ultimately, the patient must be instructed in self-management techniques that treat the site and cause of compression and prevent recurrences.[109] Most authorities support the conservative approach using physical therapy interventions. Only after the individual has failed to respond to conservative measures and experiences persistent incapacitating symptoms should surgery be considered.

The treatment requires active patient participation and close attention to correcting factors contributing to neurovascular compression. Careful examination and evaluation and diagnosis by the involved practitioners are necessary to identify the contributing impairments. The conservative treatment approach is based on the following concepts:

- Correct posture and movement impairments relevant to neurovascular compression, such as correcting a depressed and anterior tilted scapula at rest, because this may cause costoclavicular or pectoralis minor compression on the neurovascular bundle.
- Taping the scapula into elevation (Fig. 26-33) often reduces compression and alleviates symptoms until the related impairments are remedied.
- Alter sleep habits such as sleeping on the stomach with the neck extended and rotated, because this may cause increased tension on the scalenes and pectoral region.
- Improve diaphragmatic breathing patterns. Accessory breathing patterns using scalenes and pectoralis minor may elevate the first rib and pull the scapula, and therefore the clavicle, closer to the first rib, causing compression of the fibers of the anterior scalene, within the costoclavicular space, or under the pectoralis minor.
- Correct faulty movement patterns, which can lead to muscle imbalances and predispose the neurovascular bundle to compression from excessive scapular tilting or depression.
- Correct physiologic impairments linked to posture and movement impairments, such as improving the length of the scalenes and pectoralis minor to increase the space of the thoracic outlet and mobility of the first rib; force-generating capacity or length–tension properties of underused synergists or antagonists such as the upper trapezius to alleviate a depressed scapula or lower trapezius and offset a short pectoralis minor; and recruitment of the diaphragm instead of accessory muscles for breathing.
- Alter movement patterns during instrumental ADLs. Examples include changing work station ergonomics, body mechanics, or sport-specific movements.
- Appropriately refer for treatment of any patients with cognitive-affective elements or exacerbating health habits that may be causing tension in the relevant musculature. For example, anxiety may cause cervical or brachial tension, or smoking may cause poor breathing habits.

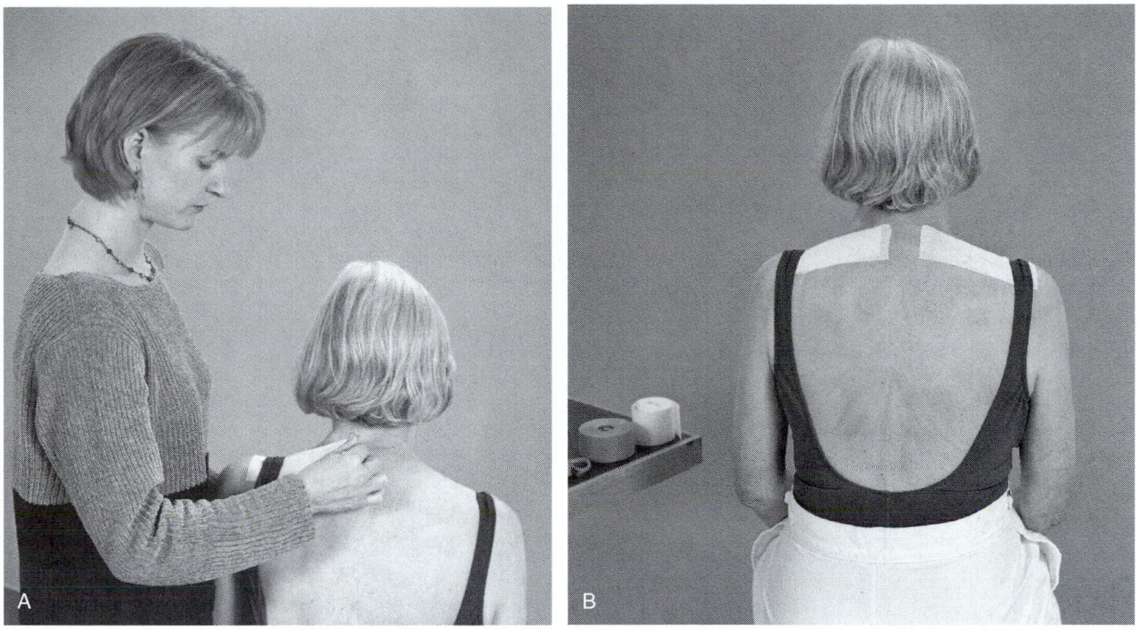

FIGURE 26-33 Taping the scapula into elevation. Use the following technique to correct scapular depression. ***(A)*** Anchor the tape to the lateral edge of the acromion process. ***(B)*** Tape bilateral scapula to prevent cervical shearing.

ADJUNCTIVE INTERVENTIONS: TAPING

Complex muscular relationships exist among the scapula, humerus, cervical, thoracic spine, lumbar spine, and pelvis. Faulty scapular alignment contributes to a variety of syndromes affecting the upper quadrant. Scapular taping can improve the resting alignment of the scapula on the thorax, thereby improving joint alignment of the related joints and length–tension properties of the shared musculature between the scapula and other regions of the upper quadrant. Scapular taping can be a useful adjunctive intervention when used with therapeutic exercise for the treatment of many upper quadrant diagnoses:

- Shoulder impingement syndrome[110]
- TOS
- Frozen shoulder
- Glenohumeral hypermobility
- Cervical sprain or strain
- Middle or lower trapezius strain
- Upper trapezius dominance[104]
- Neural entrapment syndromes in the region of the shoulder girdle contributing to distal upper extremity neuropathies (eg, carpal tunnel syndrome)

Patients can perform exercises and ADLs or instrumental ADLs while taped with the added benefit of improved joint alignment and length–tension properties of the scapular musculature. The benefit of scapular taping over an off-the-shelf brace is that taping allows the specific three-dimensional correction of each patient's unique alignment faults. Short-term taping (2 to 3 weeks) may assist in improved neuromuscular control of faulty movement patterns, whereas long-term taping (8 to 12 weeks) may affect muscle length–tension properties. Taping the scapulothoracic joint has several goals:

- To improve initial alignment, which promotes improved movement patterns
- To alter length–tension properties by stretching tissues that are too short and reducing tension placed on tissues that are too long
- To provide support and reduce stress to myofascial tissues under chronic tension
- To provide kinesthetic awareness of scapular position during rest and movement
- To guide the PICR during movement

Each piece of tape provides a specific corrective force on the scapula. Any one piece can be used in conjunction with other directional pieces to provide a multidimensional correction of the alignment of the scapula. The goal is to tape the scapula into improved alignment. If, however, the patient has significant kyphosis, forward-head, or forward-shoulder posture, 100% correction should not be attempted. It is instead recommended to moderately correct the faulty alignment, because too much change in such a short period may not be well tolerated by an individual with a chronic postural problem.

The tape product is specialized for taping the body for alignment and movement. It has the best combination of adhesive, extensible, yet stiff properties. The undertape is called Coverroll stretch, a hypoallergenic tape applied to protect the patient's skin from the overtape, called Leukotape (Beirsdorf Inc., Norwalk, CT). On the shoulder girdle, the Coverroll stretch often is adequate alone, particularly on a small-framed person with minimal to moderate postural faults.

The description of taping that follows details one method of taping, but other methods of taping can be used on the scapula and the humerus.[110] The goals of improved alignment and function are common to various techniques. Improved alignment and function during ADLs and instrumental ADLs and exercise can be achieved with proper taping techniques, and therefore taping can be a useful adjunctive intervention to therapeutic exercise and functional retraining.

Scapular Corrections

If the scapula is depressed at rest, apply the first set of instructions before any other.

Correcting Scapular Depression and Improving Scapular Elevation

- Apply the tape to the lateral edge of the acromion process, and passively elevate the scapula, ensuring that the acromial end rotates upward (see Fig. 26-33*A*). Pull the tape medially toward the cervical spine in the suprascapular space, following the fiber direction of the upper trapezius.
- Do not cross the cervical spine.
- Apply a piece in a similar direction without the forceful elevation and upward rotation on the opposite side to prevent lateral shearing across the cervical spine from a unilateral pull on the neck (Fig. 26-33*B*).
- Repeat the application until the correction is made. Often, if tape is applied to correct additional alignment faults, this piece needs to be repeated to ensure that other tape applications have not pulled the scapula into depression.

Correcting Scapular Downward Rotation and Improving Scapular Upward Rotation

- Anchor the tape slightly lateral to the root of the scapula (see Fig. 26-20*A*).
- Passively elevate the arm into full flexion. Pull the tape medially and caudally toward T10 (see Fig. 26-20*B*). Attach the tape to the lower thoracic spine as you maintain the scapula upwardly rotated (see Fig. 26-20*C*).

Correcting Scapular Abduction and Improving Scapular Adduction

- Anchor the tape to the root of the scapula.
- Passively elevate the arm into full flexion in the sagittal plane (see Fig. 26-20*B*).
- Pull the tape medially and slightly caudally, following the fiber direction of the middle trapezius. The emphasis should be on adducting the scapula while the scapula is fully upwardly rotated so as not to limit upward rotation excursion of the scapula. Attach the tape at about the level of T6 (Fig. 26-34).
- A second piece of tape can be used to prevent excessive abduction if the first technique alone is not sufficient.
- Apply the anchor piece just lateral to the axillary border of the scapula as proximal in the axilla as possible (Fig. 26-35*A*).
- Pull the tape posteriorly and slightly caudally while adducting and upwardly rotating the scapula. Attach the tape to the medial border of the inferior scapula (Fig. 26-35*B*). Be sure the tape is pulled caudally so as not to pull the scapula into downward rotation (Fig. 26-35*C*).

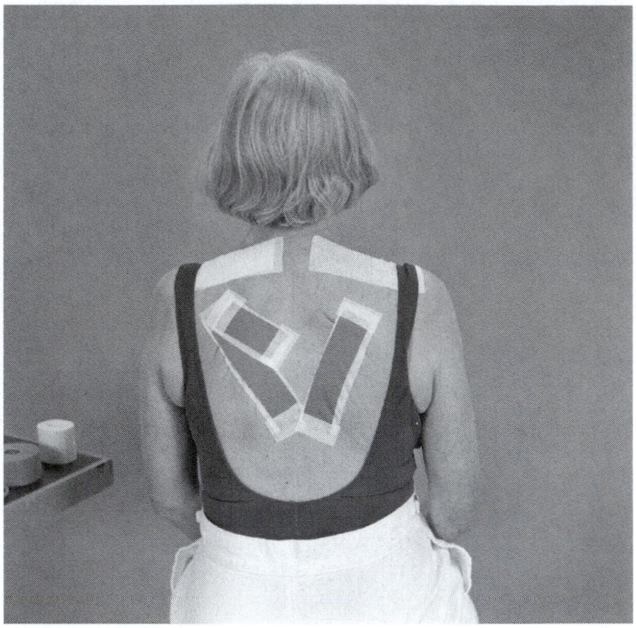

FIGURE 26-34 Taping the scapula into adduction. Use this technique to correct scapular abduction.

Correcting Scapular Winging

- Tape as for correction of scapular downward rotation (see Fig. 26-20) and abduction (see Fig. 26-34).
- Be sure to cover the medial border of the scapula.

Correction of Scapular Anterior Tilting

- Anchor the tape to the coracoid process (see Fig. 26-19*A*), and while tilting the scapula posteriorly, pull the tape over the upper trapezius in a medial and caudal direction (see Fig. 26-19*B*), and attach the tape to the root of the scapula.
- Tape as for correction of scapular abduction (see Fig. 26-34) and downward rotation (see Fig. 26-20), being sure to cover the inferior pole of the scapula to control tilt.

Correcting Scapular Elevation

- Anchor the tape to the anterior border of the upper trapezius and while depressing the scapula (see Fig. 26-21*A*), pull the tape over the upper trapezius and attach it to the spine of the scapula (see Fig. 26-21*B*).[104]
- Apply the tape as for correction of scapular downward rotation (see Fig. 26-20) while depressing and upwardly rotating the scapula.

Prevention of Allergic Reaction

A common side effect of taping is an allergic reaction to the tape adhesive or skin breakdown. The following are troubleshooting tips to help prevent adverse reactions to taping:

- Use only Coverroll stretch, which is hypoallergenic. The allergic reaction is usually to the adhesive in the Leukotape.
- Use a skin preparation solution before application of the tape. A recommended skin preparation solution is

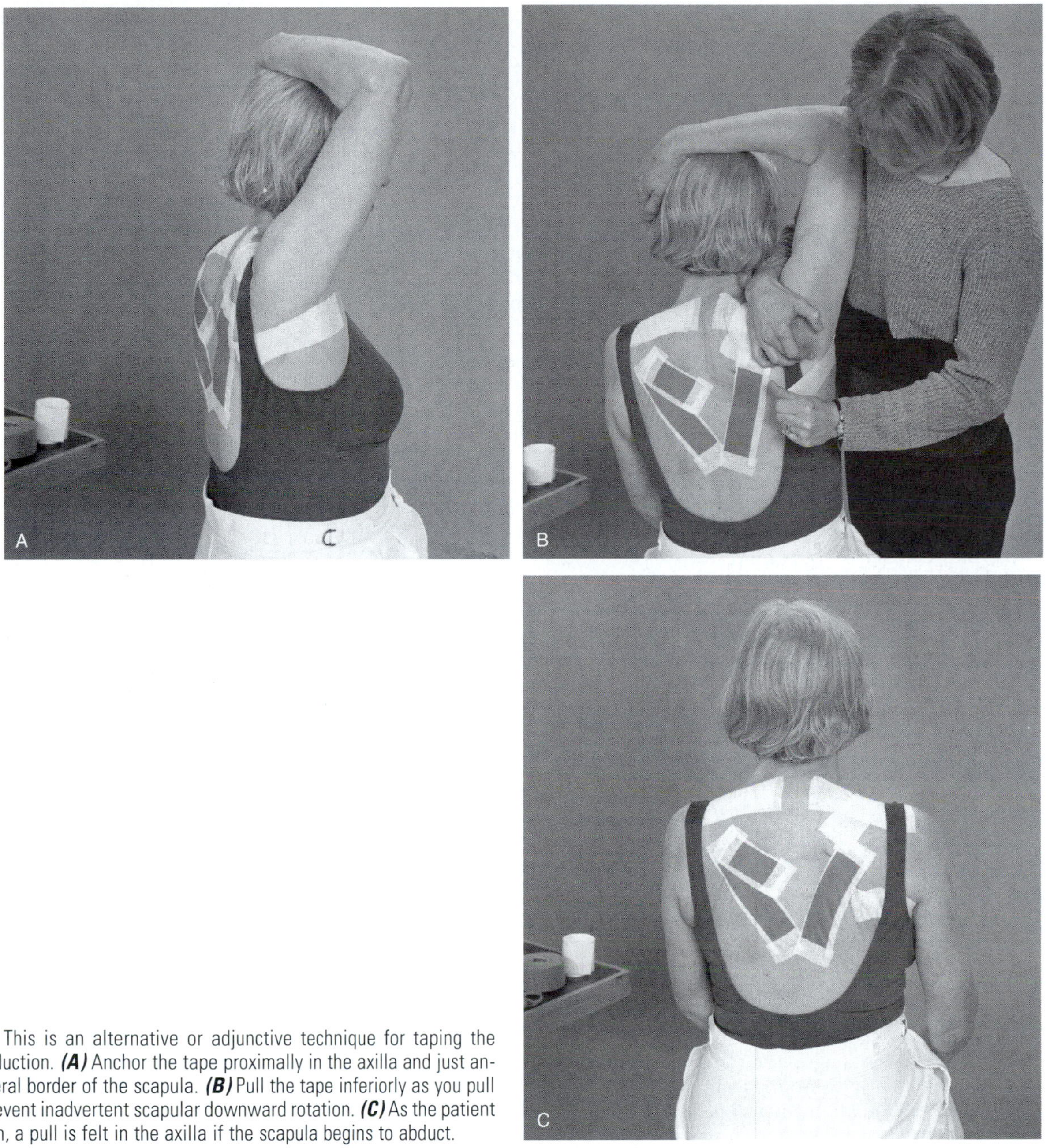

FIGURE 26-35 This is an alternative or adjunctive technique for taping the scapula into adduction. ***(A)*** Anchor the tape proximally in the axilla and just anterior to the lateral border of the scapula. ***(B)*** Pull the tape inferiorly as you pull it medially to prevent inadvertent scapular downward rotation. ***(C)*** As the patient elevates the arm, a pull is felt in the axilla if the scapula begins to abduct.

Milk of Magnesia. A thin coat applied to the skin should completely dry before the tape is applied to allows easier tape removal.

- Ensure that all tape residue is removed before the next tape application.
- Warn patients of potential skin irritation. Instruct patients to remove the tape immediately if any itching or burning sensations develop.

Prevention of Skin Breakdown

Skin breakdown often occurs because of excessive friction between the skin and the tape. Follow these guidelines to minimize skin breakdown:

- Do not cross the midline of the spine with the tape.
- Do not cross more than one joint at a time.
- Tape the scapulae bilaterally, particularly in elevation.
- Use a skin preparation solution before taping.
- Remove all tape residue before the next taping. Use Leukotape to dab off most of the residue, and follow up with adhesive tape remover.
- If skin breakdown occurs, allow the skin to heal fully before reapplying the tape. This may take 1 week or longer.

If taped properly, patients can often tolerate taping for 3 to 5 days. Showering with the tape is allowed, but soaking the tape is not recommended. For a person engaged in aggressive activities, the tape is more likely to loosen and

LAB ACTIVITIES

1. Medially rotate your arm, with your arm at your side and your elbow flexed 90 degrees. Raise your arm overhead in the sagittal plane. Now lower your arm in the frontal plane. What glenohumeral rotation are you in?
2. Depress your scapula, and rotate your head. Release the depression, and rotate your head. Which scapular position allowed you the greatest cervical rotation?
3. Sit in thoracic kyphosis, and raise your arm in the sagittal plane. Sit upright, and raise your arm. Which sitting posture allowed you the greatest upper extremity motion?
4. Assume a forward shoulder posture with the scapula abducted. With your arm at your side and elbow flexed 90 degrees, laterally rotate your shoulder. Assume a posture with scapular adduction, and laterally rotate your shoulder. Which scapular position allowed you the greatest lateral rotation?
5. Abduct your scapula, and horizontally abduct your shoulder. Adduct your scapula, and move your shoulder into horizontal abduction. What difference did your scapular position make on the arthrokinematic motion of your humerus?
6. Practice the manual stretch techniques for the pectoralis minor and rhomboid.
7. Analyze the PICR of the head of the humerus during prone glenohumeral medial rotation (see Self-Management: Subscapularis Isometric Exercise). Teach your partner how to prevent anterior translation of the head of the humerus during glenohumeral medial rotation.
8. During the prone lower trapezius progression (see Self-Management: Lower Trapezius Progression), why is it important to barely lift the elbows? What happens when your partner maximally lifts the elbows? Why is this not a desired response?
9. Attempt the hand-knee progression and the push-up progression (see Fig. 26-20) for serratus anterior strengthening. What signs indicate an individual is ready to progress to the next level? What signs indicate the individual is working at too high a level or has fatigued at any given level?
10. Teach your partner to move the scapula with the correct PICR during standing wall slides (see Fig. 26-14).

not be as effective for as many days as it is for a less active individual.

Key Points

- Critical to the management of the shoulder girdle complex is a thorough understanding of the anatomy and kinesiology of each of the four articulations comprising the complex.
- Precise PICRs at each of the four articulations and the integration of all four articulations with respect to joint function, force couples, and precise motor control to coordinate motion are required for optimal function of the shoulder complex.
- Because the shoulder girdle is one link in a kinetic chain, the function of the shoulder girdle affects and is affected by the function of other regions of the upper and lower quadrants.
- Treatment of impairments, although often necessary for improved function, should be complemented by functional retraining modified to the level of ability at a given time in the rehabilitation process.
- Ideal total body posture is a prerequisite for optimal movement in the shoulder girdle complex.
- Scapular taping can improve resting posture and thereby affect movement of the shoulder girdle complex.

Critical Thinking Questions

1. What glenohumeral motion is a prerequisite to restoring
   a. Full sagittal plane motion to the glenohumeral joint?
   b. Full frontal plane motion to the glenohumeral joint?
2. Why is the rotator cuff–deltoid function contingent on the scapular upward rotation force couple?
3. What structures can limit scapular upward rotation mobility?
4. Which muscles must have normal force or torque and length–tension relationships to achieve full upward scapular rotation ROM?
5. What is the timing of onset of the scapular muscles during scapular upward rotation to produce the ideal PICR for scapular rotation?
6. What musculature is shared by the shoulder girdle and cervical spine? What joints are linked by the shared musculature?
7. If the upper trapezius is overstretched, as in a depressed scapula, in what direction is cervical spine rotation limited? What treatment do you propose to correct this problem?
8. If the levator scapula is adaptively shortened, as in a downwardly rotated scapula, in what direction is cervical spine rotation limited? What treatment do you propose to correct this problem?

9. How can cervical nerve root involvement affect the function of the shoulder girdle?
10. Using the case described in Display 26-9, determine the dosage parameters for improving muscular force or torque of the rotator cuff (using the exercise described in Self-Management: Prone Rotator Cuff Strengthening).
11. Name one abnormal scapular movement pattern that should be considered a potential cause of glenohumeral anterior hypermobility.
12. What is the most critical intervention to promote healing of a strained muscle caused by adaptive lengthening from faulty postures?
13. How can poor technique during a biceps curl contribute to an anterior tilted scapula?
14. Adapt Self-Management: Prone Rotator Cuff Strengthening dosage parameters to focus on endurance.
15. In what alignment does the scapula rest to develop an elongated serratus anterior? How does this elongation contribute to a faulty PICR of the scapula during scapular upward rotation?
16. What intrinsic and extrinsic factors predispose an individual to impingement syndrome? Why is restoring the scapular PICR important in the long-term recovery of impingement syndrome?
17. With reference to Fig. 26-27, describe the beginning and ending positions, movement, and dosage parameters for an individual with anterior glenohumeral hypermobility (see Fig. 26-24). Write this as a self-management program for a patient.
18. When is active motion overhead introduced for a patient after rotator cuff repair? As a physical therapist, what physiologic capabilities do you consider to be minimal expectations for exercise progression to overhead positions?
19. How can taping the scapula help adhesive capsulitis to recover? What taping techniques would you use?
20. How can taping help treat TOS? What taping techniques would you use?
21. Using Case Study #4 in Unit 7, develop a comprehensive exercise program. Describe each exercise according to the therapeutic exercise intervention model described in Chapter 2. You can follow the format used in the Selective Intervention at the end of Chapter 27.

REFERENCES

1. Goss C, ed. *Gray's Anatomy of the Human Body.* 27th ed. Philadelphia: Lea & Febiger; 1959.
2. DePalma A. Surgical anatomy of the acromioclavicular and sternoclavicular joints. *Surg Clin North Am.* 1963;43: 1541–1550.
3. Sarrafian SK. Gross and functional anatomy of the shoulder. *Clin Orthop.* 1983;173:11–18.
4. Quiring D, Boroush EL. Functional anatomy of the shoulder girdle. *Arch Phys Med.* 1946;27:90–96.
5. Zuckerman JD, Matsen FA III. Biomechanics of the shoulder. In: Nordin M, Frankel VH, eds. *Basic Biomechanics of the Musculoskeletal System.* 2nd ed. Philadelphia: Lea & Febiger; 1989:225–247.
6. Inman V, Saunders M, Abbott LC. Observations on the function of the shoulder joint. *J Bone Joint Surg Am.* 1944;26:1–30.
7. Dawson DM, Hallett M, Millender LH. *Entrapment Neuropathies.* 2nd ed. Boston: Little, Brown; 1990.
8. Hadley MN, Sonntag VKH, Pittman HW. Suprascapular nerve entrapment. *J Neurosurg.* 1986;64:843–848.
9. Conway SR, Jones HR. Entrapment and compression neuropathies. In: Tollison CD, ed. *Handbook of Chronic Pain Management.* Baltimore: Williams & Wilkins; 1989.
10. Ludewig PM, Cook TM, Nawoczenski DA. Three-dimensional scapular orientation and muscle activity at selected positions of arm elevation. *J Orthop Sports Phys Ther.* 1996;24:57–65.
11. Bagg SD, Forrest WJ. A biomechanical analysis of scapular rotation during arm abduction in the scapular plane. *Am J Phys Med Rehabil.* 1988;67:238–245.
12. Basmajjian JV, Bazant FJ. Factors preventing downward dislocation of the adducted shoulder. *J Bone Joint Surg Am.* 1959;41:1182.
13. Saha AK. *Recurrent Anterior Dislocation of the Shoulder: A New Concept.* Calcutta: Academic Publications; 1969.
14. Saha AK. Dynamic stability of the glenohumeral joint. *Acta Orthop Scand.* 1971;42:491–505.
15. Freedman L, Munro RR. Abduction of the arm in the scapular plane: scapular and glenohumeral movements. *J Bone Joint Surg Am.* 1966;48:1503–1510.
16. Poppen NK, Walker PS. Normal and abnormal motion of the shoulder. *J Bone Joint Surg Am.* 1976;58:195–201.
17. Rothman RH, Marvel JP Jr, Heppenstall RB. Anatomic considerations in the glenohumeral joint. *Orthop Clin North Am.* 1975;6:341–352.
18. Kapandji IA. *Physiology of the Joints.* London: E&S Livingstone; 1970.
19. Kent BE. Functional anatomy of the shoulder complex: a review. *Phys Ther.* 1971;51:867–947.
20. Mosely HP, Overgaard B. The anterior capsular mechanism in recurrent anterior dislocations of the shoulder: morphological and clinical studies with special reference to the glenoid labrum and glenohumeral ligaments. *J Bone Joint Surg Br.* 1962;44:913.
21. Reeves B. Experiments in the tensile strength of the anterior capsular structures of the shoulder in man. *J Bone Joint Surg Br.* 1968;50:858–865.
22. Matsen FA, Lippitt SB, Slidles JA, et al, eds. *Practical Evaluation and Management of the Shoulder.* Philadelphia: WB Saunders; 1993.
23. Basmajian J. The surgical anatomy and function of the arm-trunk mechanism. *Surg Clin North Am.* 1963;43:1475.
24. Turkel SJ, Panio MW, Marshall JL, Girgis FG. Stabilizing mechanisms preventing anterior dislocation of the glenohumeral joint. *J Bone Joint Surg Am.* 1981;63:1208.
25. Johnston TB. The movements of the shoulder joint. A plea for the use of the "plane of the scapula" as the name of reference for movements occurring at the humeroscapular joint. *Br J Surg.* 1937;25:252–260.
26. Saha AK. Mechanism for shoulder movements and a plea for the recognition of "zero position" of glenohumeral joint. *Indian J Surg.* 1950;12:153–165.
27. Doody SG, Freedman L, Waterland JC. Shoulder movements during abduction in the scapular plane. *Arch Phys Med Rehabil.* 1970;51:595–604.
28. Sahrmann SA. *Diagnosis and Exercise Management of Musculoskeletal Pain Syndromes.* St. Louis: Mosby; 1999.
29. DePalma AF. *Surgery of the Shoulder.* 3rd ed. Philadelphia: JB Lippincott; 1983.
30. Palmer ML, Blakely RL. Documentation of medial rotation accompanying shoulder flexion. *Phys Ther.* 1986;66:55–58.
31. Codman EA. *The Shoulder.* Boston: Thomas Todd; 1934.

32. Cathcart CW. Movements of the shoulder girdle involved in those of the arm and trunk. *J Anat Physiol.* 1884;18:211–218.
33. Quain J. Bones of the superior extremity. In: Schafer EA, Thane GD, eds. *Elements of Anatomy.* 10th ed. London: Longmans, Green; 1892:169.
34. Morris H. Bones of the upper limb. In: Jackson CM, ed. *Human Anatomy.* 5th ed. Philadelphia: P. Blakiston's Son; 1914:257–258.
35. McKendrick A, Whittaker CR. *An X-ray Atlas of the Normal and Abnormal Structures of the Body.* Edinburgh: E&S Livingston; 1925:2–5.
36. Yamshon LJ, Bierman W. Kinesiological electromyography, 2: the trapezius. *Arch Phys Med.* 1948;29:647–651.
37. Saha AK. *Theory of Shoulder Mechanism: Descriptive and Applied.* Springfield, IL: Charles C Thomas; 1961:15–55.
38. Kronberg M, Nemeth G, Brostrom L. Muscle activity and coordination in the normal shoulder. *Clin Orthop.* 1990;8: 76–85.
39. Dvir Z, Berme N. The shoulder complex in elevation of the arm: a mechanism approach. *J Biomech.* 1978;11:219–225.
40. Engin AE. On the biomechanics of the shoulder complex. *J Biomech.* 1980;13:575–590.
41. Bagg SD, Forrest WJ. Electromyographic study of the scapular rotators during arm abduction in the scapular plane. *Am J Phys Med.* 1986;65:111–124.
42. Norlander S, Gustavsson BA, Lindell J, Noedgren B. Reduced mobility in the cervico-thoracic motion segment—a risk factor for musculoskeletal neck-shoulder pain: a two year prospective follow-up study. *Scand J Rehabil Med.* 1977;29: 167–174.
43. Cyriax J. *Textbook of Orthopedic Medicine.* 8th ed. London: Bailliere Tindall; 1982:127–158.
44. Sarhmann SA. *Diagnosis and Treatment of Movement Impairment Syndromes.* (Course outline). St. Louis, MO: Washington University; 1998.
45. Kendall FP, McCreary EK, Provance PG. *Muscle Testing and Function.* 4th ed. Baltimore, MD: Williams & Wilkins; 1993.
46. Daniels L, Worthingham C. *Muscle Testing: Techniques of Manual Examination.* 4th ed. Philadelphia: WB Saunders; 1980.
47. Kelly BT, Kirkendall DT, Levy AS, Speer KP. Current research on muscle activity about the shoulder. *Instr Course Lect.* 1977;46:53–66.
48. Maitland GD. *Vertebral Manipulation.* 5th ed. London: Butterworths; 1986.
49. Duncan GH, Bushnell MC, Lavigne GJ. Comparison of verbal and visual analogue scales for measuring the intensity and unpleasantness of experimental pain. *Pain.* 1989;37:295–303.
50. Hoppenfeld S. *Physical Examination of the Spine and Extremities.* New York: Appleton-Century-Crofts; 1976.
51. Ludington NA. Rupture of the long head of the biceps flexor cubite muscle. *Ann Surg.* 1923:77:358.
52. Jobe FW, Jobe C. Painful athletic injuries of the shoulder. *Clin Orthop Rel Res.* 1983;173:117–124.
53. Davies GJ, Gould JA, Larson RL. Functional examination of the shoulder girdle. *Phys Sports Med.* 1981;6:82.
54. Donatelli RA. *Physical Therapy of the Shoulder.* 3rd ed. New York: Churchill Livingstone; 1997.
55. Jackson P. Thoracic outlet syndrome: evaluation and treatment. *Clin Manag.* 1987;7:6–10.
56. Butler D. *Mobilization of the Nervous System.* Melbourne: Churchill Livingstone; 1991.
57. Maitland GD. *Peripheral Manipulation.* 2nd ed. London: Butterworths; 1977.
58. Neer CS. Impingement lesions. *Clin Orthop Rel Res.* 1963; 173:70–77.
59. Hawkins RJ, Kennedy JC. Impingement syndrome in athletes. *Am J Sports Med.* 1980;8:151.
60. Roach KE, Budiman-mak E, Songsiridej N, Lertratanakul Y. Development of a shoulder pain and disability index. *Arthritis Care Res.* 1991;4:143–149.
61. Williams JW, Holleman DR, Simel DL. Measuring shoulder function with the shoulder pain and disability index. *J Rheumatol.* 1995;22:727–732.
62. Travell JG, Simons DG. *Myofascial Pain and Dysfunction.* Baltimore: Williams & Wilkins; 1983.
63. DiGiovine NM, Jobe FW, Pink M, Perry J. An electromyographic analysis of the upper extremity in pitching. *J Shoulder Elbow Surg.* 1992;1:15–25.
64. Basmajian JV, DeLuca CJ. *Muscles Alive.* 5th ed. Baltimore: Williams & Wilkins; 1985.
65. Westgaard RH. Measurement and evaluation of postural load in occupational work situations. *Eur J Appl Physiol.* 1988;57:291–304.
66. Jensen C, Nilsen K, Hansen K, Westgaard RH. Trapezius muscle load as a risk indicator for occupational shoulder-neck complaints. *Int Arch Occup Environ Health.* 1993;64: 415–423.
67. Veiersted KB, Westgaard RH, Anderson P. Pattern of muscle activity during stereotyped work and its relationship to muscle pain. *Int Arch Occup Environ Health.* 1990;62:31–41.
68. Veiersted KB, Westgaard RH, Andersen P. Electromyographic evaluation of muscular work pattern as a predictor of trapezius myalgia. *Scand J Work Environ Health.* 1993;19: 284–290.
69. Veiersted KB, Westgaard RH. Development of trapezius myalgia among female workers performing light manual work. *Scand J Work Environ Health.* 1993;19:277–283.
70. Christensen H. Muscle activity and fatigue in the shoulder muscles of assembly plant employees. *Scand J Work Environ Health.* 1986;12:582–587.
71. Toivanen H, Helin P, Hanninen O. Impact of regular relaxation training and psychosocial working factors on neck-shoulder tension and absenteeism in hospital cleaners. *J Occup Med.* 1993;35:1123–1130.
72. Greico A, Occhipinti E, Colombini D, et al. Muscular effort and musculoskeletal disorders in piano students: electromyographic, clinical and preventive aspects. *Ergonomics.* 1989;32:697–716.
73. Sundelin G, Hagberg M. The effects of different pause types on neck and shoulder EMG activity during VDU work. *Ergonomics.* 1989;32:527–537.
74. Schuldt K, Ekholm J, Harms Ringdahl K, et al. Effects of arm support or suspension on neck and shoulder muscle activity during sedentary work. *Scand J Rehabil Med.* 1988;19:77–84.
75. McQuade KJ, Wei SH, Smidt GL. Effects of local muscle fatigue on three-dimensional scapulohumeral rhythm [abstract]. *Phys Ther.* 1993;73:S109.
76. Rathbun JB, Macnab I. The microvascular pattern of the rotator cuff. *J Bone Joint Surg Am.* 1972;54:41–50.
77. Lohr JF, Uhthoff HK. The microvascular pattern of the supraspinatus tendon. *Clin Orthop.* 1990;254:35–38.
78. Sarkar K, Taine W, Uhthoff HK. The ultrastructure of the coracoacromial ligament in patients with chronic impingement syndrome. *Clin Orthop.* 1990;254:49–54.
79. Ogata S, Uhthoff HK. Acromial enthesopathy and rotator cuff tear. *Clin Orthop.* 1990;254:39–48.
80. Ozaki J, Fujimoto S, Yoahiyuki N, et al. Tears of the rotator cuff of the shoulder associated with pathological changes in the acromion. *J Bone Joint Surg Am.* 1988;70:1224–1230.
81. Morrison DS, Bigliani LU. The clinical significance of variations in acromial morphology. *Orthop Trans.* 1987;11:234.

82. Neer CS. Anterior acromioplasty for the chronic impingement syndrome in the shoulder. *J Bone Joint Surg Am.* 1972;54:41–50.
83. Jobe FW, Pink M. Classification and treatment of shoulder dysfunction in the overhead athlete. *J Orthop Sports Phys Ther.* 1993;18:427–432.
84. Strauss MB, Wrobel LJ, Neff RS, Cady GW. The shrugged-off shoulder: a comparison of patients with recurrent shoulder subluxations and dislocations. *Physician Sports Med.* 1983;11:85–97.
85. Chandler TJ, Kibler B, Stracener EC, et al. Shoulder strength, power, and endurance in college tennis players. *Am J Sports Med.* 1992;20:455–458.
86. Smith RL, Brunolli J. Shoulder kinesthesia after anterior glenohumeral joint dislocation. *Phys Ther.* 1980;69:106–112.
87. Warren R. Subluxation of the shoulder in athletes. *Clin Sports Educ.* 1983;2:339–354.
88. Matthews LS, Oweida SJ. Glenohumeral instability in athletes: spectrum, diagnosis, and treatment. *Adv Orthop Surg.* 1985;8:236–248.
89. Perry J. Anatomy and biomechanics of the shoulder in throwing, swimming, gymnastics and tennis. *Clin Sports Med.* 1983;2:247–270.
90. Reid DC, Saboe LA, Chepeha JC. Anterior shoulder instability in athletes: comparison of isokinetic resistance exercises and an electromyographic biofeedback reeducation program a pilot program. *Physiother Can.* 1996;Fall:251–256.
91. Ellenbecker TS. Etiology and evaluation of rotator cuff pathology and rehabilitation. In: Donatelli RA, ed. *Physical Therapy of the Shoulder.* 3rd ed. New York: Churchill Livingstone; 1997.
92. Neer CS. *Shoulder Reconstruction.* Philadelphia: WB Saunders; 1990.
93. Nirschl RP. Shoulder tendinitis, In: Pettrone FP, ed. *Upper Extremity Injuries in Athletes: American Academy of Orthopedic Surgeons Symposium.* St. Louis: Mosby; 1988.
94. Andrews JR, Alexander EJ. Rotator cuff injury in throwing and racket sports. *Sports Med Arthrosc Rev.* 1995;3:30.
95. Cofield RH. Current concepts review of rotator cuff disease of the shoulder. *J Bone Joint Surg Am.* 1985;67:974.
96. Ellman H. Diagnosis and treatment of incomplete rotator cuff tears. *Clin Orthop.* 1990;254:64–74.
97. Watson-Jones R. *Fractures and Joint Injuries,* vol 11. 4th ed. Baltimore: Williams & Wilkins; 1955.
98. Caillet R. *Shoulder Pain.* Philadelphia: FA Davis; 1966.
99. Coventry MB. Problem of the painful shoulder. *JAMA.* 1953;151:177–185.
100. Andren L, Lundberg BJ. Treatment of rigid shoulders by joint distention during arthrography. *Acta Orthop Scand.* 1965;36:45.
101. The Center for Orthopedics and Sports Medicine. Frozen shoulder (adhesive capsulitis). http:/www.arthroscopy.com; July 31, 1997.
102. Baybar SR. Excessive scapular motion in individuals recovering from painful and stiff shoulders: causes and treatment strategies. *Phys Ther.* 1996;76:226–238.
103. Bush TA, Mork DO, Sarver KK, et al. The effectiveness of shoulder taping in the inhibition of the upper trapezius as determined by the electromyogram [abstract]. *Phys Ther.* 1996;76:S17.
104. Jackson P. Thoracic outlet syndrome: evaluation and treatment. *Clin Manag.* 1987;7:6–10.
105. Smith KF. The thoracic outlet syndrome: a protocol of treatment. *J Sports Med Phys Ther.* 1979;1:89–99.
106. Hirsh LF, Thanki A. The thoracic outlet syndrome: meeting the diagnostic challenge. *Postgrad Med.* 1985;77:197–207.
107. Sunderland S. Traumatized nerves, roots, and ganglia: musculoskeletal factors and neuropathological consequences. In: Korr IM, ed. *The Neurobiologic Mechanisms in Manipulative Therapy.* New York: Plenum; 1978:137.
108. Butler D. *Mobilization of the Nervous System.* Melbourne: Churchill Livingstone; 1991.
109. Edgelow PI. Neurovascular consequences of cumulative trauma disorders affecting the thoracic outlet: a patient-centered approach. In: Donatelli RA, ed. *Physical Therapy of the Shoulder.* 3rd ed. New York: Churchill Livingstone; 1997.
110. Host HH. Scapular taping in the treatment of anterior shoulder impingement. *Phys Ther* 1995;75:803–812.
111. Miklovitz SL. *Thermal Agents in Rehabilitation.* 2nd ed. Philadelphia: FA Davis; 1991.
112. Neer CS, Marberry TA. On the disadvantages of radical acromionectomy. *J Bone Joint Surg Am.* 1981;63:416.
113. Moseley HF. The clavicle: its anatomy and function. *Clin Orthop.* 1958;58:17–27.
114. Morris J. Joints of the shoulder girdle. *Aust J Physiol.* 1978;24.
115. Steindler A. *Kinesiology of the Human Body.* Springfield, IL: Charles C Thomas; 1955.

RECOMMENDED READINGS

DiGiovine NM, Jobe FW, Pink M, Perry J. An electromyographic analysis of the upper extremity in pitching. *J Shoulder Elbow Surg.* 1992;1:15–25.

Donatelli RA. *Physical Therapy of the Shoulder.* 3rd ed. New York: Churchill Livingstone; 1997.

Glousman R. Electromyographic analysis and its role in the athletic shoulder. *Clin Orthop Rel Res.* 1993;288:27–34.

Glousman R, Jobe FW, Tibone JE, et al. Dynamic electromyographic analysis of the throwing shoulder with glenohumeral instability. *J Bone Joint Surg Am.* 1988;70:220–226.

Perry J, Pink M, Jobe FW, et al. The painful shoulder during the backstroke: an electromyographic and cinematographic analysis of 12 muscles. *Clin J Sport Med.* 1992;2:13–20.

Pink M, Perry J, Browne A, et al. The normal shoulder during freestyle swimming. *Am J Sports Med.* 1991;19:569–575.

Pink M, Jobe FW, Perry J. The normal shoulder during the butterfly stroke: an electromyographic and cinematographic analysis of twelve muscles. *Clin Orthop Rel Res.* 1993;288:48–59.

Pink M, Jobe FW, Perry J. The painful shoulder during the butterfly stroke: an electromyographic and cinematographic analysis of twelve muscles. *Clin Orthop Rel Res.* 1993;288:60–72.

Scovazzo ML, Browne A, Pink M. The painful shoulder during freestyle swimming: an electromyographic and cinematographic analysis of 12 muscles. *Am J Sports Med.* 1991;19:577–582.

CHAPTER 27

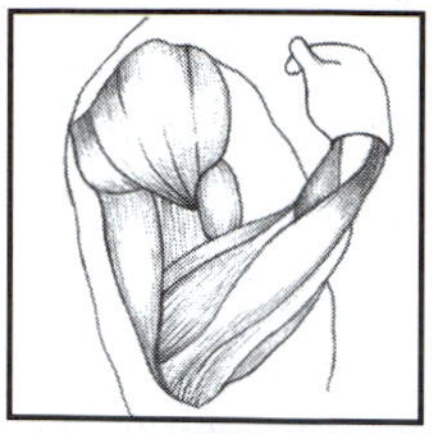

The Elbow, Forearm, Wrist, and Hand

Lori Thein Brody

Therapeutic exercise texts have often minimized or excluded the elbow, wrist, and hand, deferring evaluation of this region to other health care providers. This complex region has become a challenging and specialized area of rehabilitation. Although numerous texts describe the anatomy, kinesiology, pathology, and surgical repair of this area, few sources relate pathology, impairments, and functional limitations with physical therapy intervention at the distal upper extremity level.[1] This chapter discusses common impairments and functional limitations of the elbow, wrist, and hand and the related therapeutic interventions. A brief review of anatomy and kinesiology provides the basis for the interventions chosen.

ANATOMY*

Although the anatomy of a given joint is closely related to anatomy of adjacent joints, the elbow, wrist, and hand are discussed separately in the following sections.

Elbow and Forearm

OSTEOLOGY

The articulation of the humerus with the ulna and the radius forms the elbow joint, which is a hinge joint. The spool-shaped trochlea of the humerus articulates with the trochlear notch of the ulna, and the rounded humeral capitulum (capitellum) articulates with the radial head laterally (Fig. 27-1). During elbow extension, the trochlear notch contacts the inferoposterior aspect of the trochlea, and while in flexion, the trochlear notch slides over and articulates with the anterior trochlea. This movement uncovers the trochlea posteriorly, making it vulnerable to trauma from falls or blows. The nonarticulating portion of the humerus includes the medial and lateral epicondyles and the radial, coronoid, and olecranon fossae. The medial epicondyle is a subcutaneous, blunt projection that is easily palpable during flexion of the elbow.[2] The ulnar nerve passes along its posterior surface through a shallow groove. The medial supracondylar ridge forms the medial border of the humerus. The lateral epicondyle forms the distal end of the lateral humeral border, inferior to the lateral supracondylar ridge. The lateral epicondyle has an impression on the anterolateral surface for the origin of the forearm extensor muscles. When in full flexion, the radial fossa accommodates the margin of the radial head, and the coronoid fossa accommodates the margin of the ulnar coronoid process.[2]

The radius is the shorter and more lateral of the two forearm bones. It is narrower proximally than it is distally, and it contains the radial head, a cylindrical neck, and the oval radial tuberosity. The head's shape is discoid, and it articulates with the capitulum on the humerus and the radial notch on the ulna. The radial tuberosity is distal and medial relative to the neck, and it serves as the distal attachment of the biceps brachii. The radial shaft is convex laterally and triangular. The distal end is four sided with a lateral distally projecting styloid. A dorsal tubercle, called Lister's tubercle, is found on the distal dorsum of the radius.

The ulna is the longer of the two forearm bones and is the major distal component of the elbow joint proper. The trochlear notch comprises the proximal end of the ulna, and its articular surface is hook shaped with an anterior concavity. The trochlear notch forms the major articulation with the humeral trochlea. At the proximal end of the hook, the olecranon articulates with the olecranon fossa on the posterior aspect of the humerus when the elbow is extended. The more proximal and anterior aspect of the hook contains the coronoid process and radial notch. The coronoid process

*Portions of this section are from Brody LT. Athletic injuries about the elbow. In: Wadsworth C, ed. *The Elbow, Forearm, and Wrist* [home study course]. LaCross, WI: Orthopedic Section, APTA; 1997. Reproduced with permission.

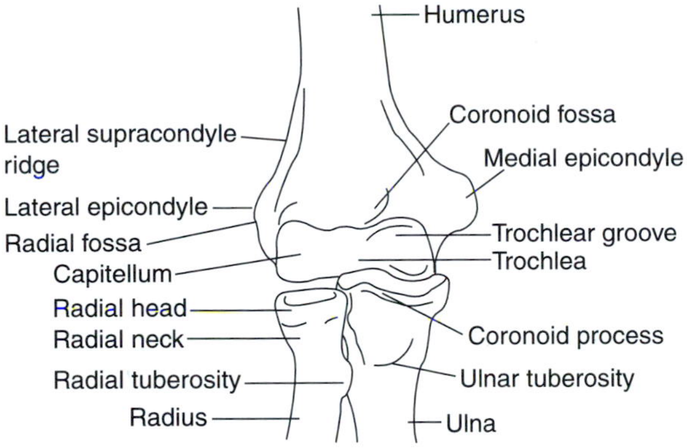

FIGURE 27-1 Elbow osteology with significant bony landmarks. (From Stroyan, Wilk KE. The functional anatomy of the elbow complex. *J of Orthop Sports Phys Ther.* 1993;17[6]:280.)

forms the inferior aspect of the trochlear notch and articulates with the coronoid fossa in full elbow flexion. On the lateral aspect of the coronoid process, the radial notch provides an articular surface for the radial head. Just distal to the coronoid process is a slight depression that accommodates the radial tuberosity during pronation. Posteriorly, the olecranon is smooth, and with the elbow in extension, it falls in a line between the medial and lateral epicondyles. During elbow flexion, the olecranon moves inferiorly, forming a triangle with the epicondyles.

The shaft of the ulna is triangular through most of its length, changing to a cylinder shape in its distal 25%. Distally, the ulna is slightly flared and contains a head and a styloid process. The head is prominent on the dorsal aspect of the wrist when the forearm is pronated. The lateral ulna articulates with the radius at the ulnar notch, but the ulna does not directly articulate with the carpal bones. The styloid process is a distal, rounded projection most easily palpated with the forearm in supination.[2]

ARTHROLOGY

The elbow joint contains at least two articulations, the humeroulnar and the humeroradial, and the ulna and radius have two articulations, the proximal and distal radioulnar articulations. The elbow is a compound synovial joint because of the multiple articulations. The primary articulating surfaces are the humeral trochlea and capitulum and the ulnar trochlear notch and radial head.

The humeroulnar joint is a hinge joint, although the arthrokinematics are more complex than simple gliding. The humeroradial joint functions as a hinge-type joint during elbow flexion and extension, but it functions as a pivot joint during forearm pronation and supination. The proximal radioulnar joint operates as a pivot joint, permitting rotation of the radius about the ulna.

The ulnar collateral ligament (UCL) is continuous with the articular capsule on the medial aspect of the humeroulnar joint (Fig. 27-2). Proximally, it attaches to the medial epicondyle of the humerus and descends inferiorly in a triangular, fan-shaped fashion. The anterior portion is a strong cordlike structure that attaches on the coronoid process of the ulna.[2] This portion serves as the primary stabilizer against valgus forces throughout most of the elbow's range of motion (ROM). The posterior portion is triangular and attaches to the medial margin of the olecranon. The thick anterior and posterior portions are united by a thin, oblique band spanning the olecranon and coronoid processes. The oblique band converts a depression on the medial trochlear notch into a foramen, where the intracapsular fat pad is continuous with the extracapsular fat found medial to the joint.[2] The ulnar nerve passes posterior to the medial epicondyle in proximity to the UCL.

The radial collateral ligament is also a triangular, fan-shaped band originating proximally at the lower portion of the lateral epicondyle, blending distally with the annular ligament. Its fibers blend with the origins of the extensor carpi radialis brevis (ECRB) and supinator muscles.[3]

The annular ligament is a strong band that nearly fully encircles the radial head to attach to the radial notch anteriorly and posteriorly. Anteriorly, the annular ligament blends with the articular capsule, but posteriorly, the capsule passes deep to the ligament. Several bands of the ligament extend to the lateral trochlear notch and structures posteriorly. The ligament's fibers blend with the radial collateral ligament and serve as a portion of the supinator muscle attachment.

The interosseous membrane is a broad, thin fascial sheath that attaches to the medial and lateral borders of the ulna and radius, respectively. The fibers of this membrane are oriented distomedially, functioning to connect the two forearm bones and to provide attachments for the deep forearm muscles. The distal surfaces of the radius and ulna at the distal radioulnar joint are enclosed by joint capsule and connected by the articular disk. This disk plays an important role at the wrist and is discussed in greater detail in the Wrist section.

MYOLOGY

Despite only a few muscles having a direct action at the humeroulnar joint, numerous muscles attach about the elbow and can be a source of pain and disability. Although many muscles perform multiple actions, they are classified by the articulation of their primary action.

Muscles Acting at the Humeroulnar Joint

The biceps brachii muscle originates from two heads, with the long head arising from the supraglenoid tubercle at

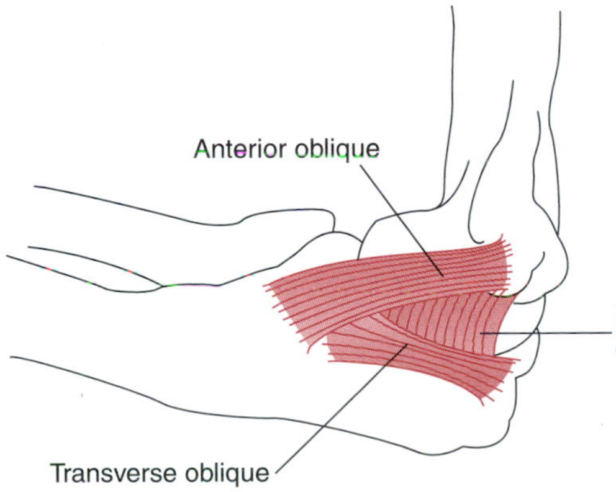

FIGURE 27-2 Ulnar collateral ligaments of the elbow (From Zarin B, Andrews J, Carson W. *Injuries to the Throwing Arm.* Philadelphia: WB Saunders;1985:196).

the shoulder and the short head arising from the coracoid process. Distally, the separate bellies form a common tendon that attaches after it twists to the posterior aspect of the radial tuberosity. This twisting rotates its anterior surface more laterally toward the distal attachment site. The tendon has a broad medial expansion known as the bicipital aponeurosis, which courses distally to blend with the deep fascia of the forearm flexors.[2] The biceps muscle is the primary flexor at the humeroulnar joint and a powerful supinator at the proximal radioulnar joint. The biceps is innervated by the musculocutaneous nerve originating from C5 and C6.

Secondary flexors at the humeroulnar joint include the brachialis and the brachioradialis muscles. The brachialis muscle originates from the distal one half of the anterior surface of the humerus and the lateral intermuscular septa, and it attaches distally to the ulnar tuberosity and the coronoid process. Its primary action is elbow flexion, and like the biceps brachii muscle, it receives innervation from the musculocutaneous nerve originating from C5-C6. The brachioradialis muscle receives its innervation through the radial nerve, which also originates from C5-C6. It is the more superficial than the biceps brachii muscle and forms the lateral border of the cubital fossa. The proximal origin of the brachioradialis muscle is the proximal two thirds of the lateral supracondylar ridge of the humerus and the lateral intermuscular septum. The distal attachment is to the lateral base of the radial styloid process.[4] It flexes the elbow and is most effective when the forearm is in neutral.

On the posterior surface, the triceps brachii muscle is composed of long, lateral, and medial heads. The long head originates from a flat tendon attached at the infraglenoid tubercle and the glenohumeral capsule. The lateral head arises from a flat tendon along a linear posterior humeral ridge and the lateral intermuscular septum. The medial head lies deep to the lateral and long heads, and it originates from the distal two thirds of the posterior and medial aspects of the humerus. The three heads converge distally to form a common tendon that descends posteriorly to attach to the posterior surface of the olecranon. The radial nerve supplies the triceps brachii muscle.

Blending with the triceps muscle is the small and triangular anconeus muscle. The anconeus originates from the lateral epicondyle of the humerus and inserts on the lateral aspect of the olecranon and the posterior surface of the ulna. It assists the triceps muscle with elbow extension.

Muscles Acting at the Radioulnar Joints

The primary muscles acting at the proximal radioulnar joint are the pronator and supinator muscles. The supinator muscle originates from the lateral epicondyle of the humerus, radial collateral ligament, annular ligament, and supinator crest of the ulna. Distally, the supinator muscle inserts into the lateral surface of the proximal third of the radius and extends onto the anterior and posterior surfaces. The posterior interosseous nerve supplies the supinator muscle. The biceps is also a major forearm supinator.

The pronator teres muscle proximally and the pronator quadratus muscle distally serve as the primary forearm pronator muscles. The pronator teres muscle originates from the humerus and the ulna. The larger, more superficial humeral head attaches proximally to the medial epicondyle, to the common flexor tendon, and to the deep antebrachial fascia. The ulnar head arises from the medial coronoid process. In approximately 83% of persons, the median nerve enters the forearm between these two heads.[2] Inserting along the lateral surface of the radial shaft, the pronator teres is innervated by the median nerve. The pronator quadratus is the primary forearm muscle acting at the distal radioulnar joint. The pronator quadratus is flat and quadrilateral, extending obliquely distolaterally from the ulna to the radius. It receives its nerve supply from the anterior interosseous brand of the median nerve.

Wrist

The bony structures of the carpal bones indicate their roles. The outer bones generally have half of their surfaces covered with articular cartilage (inner surfaces), and their outer surfaces are rough, providing attachment for connective tissues. The inner bones have two thirds of their surfaces covered by articular cartilage, and only the palmar and dorsal surfaces are irregular, providing for ligamentous attachments.

OSTEOLOGY

The wrist joint is a complex area that includes eight carpal bones, the distal radius and ulna, and the bases of the metacarpal bones (Fig. 27-3). Proximally, the distal radius and radioulnar disk articulate with the scaphoid, lunate, and triquetrum. Laterally, the scaphoid is the largest bone in the proximal carpal row. The scaphoid spans the intercarpal joint, linking the proximal and distal rows, and this position makes it susceptible to injury. This bone is divided into segments, including the proximal and distal poles and the middle, or waist, area. The proximal surface articulates with the radius, and the distal surface has two facets. Falls on an outstretched hand with the wrist extended place the scaphoid at risk for fracture. The scaphoid receives most of its blood supply from a single vessel, making the proximal pole susceptible to avascular necrosis after a fracture. Approximately 70% of fractures occur through the middle third, 20% through the proximal third, and 10% through the distal third.[5]

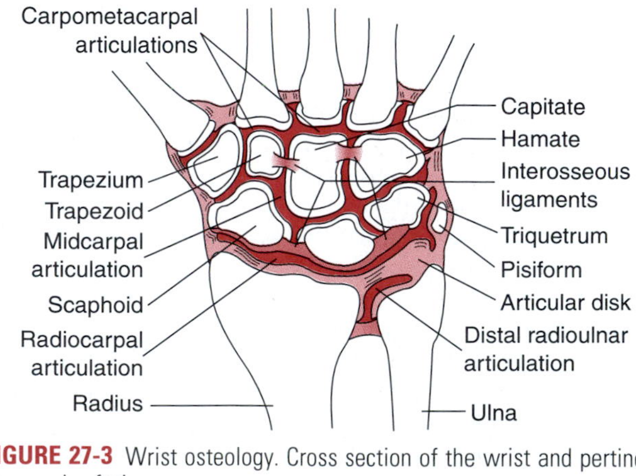

FIGURE 27-3 Wrist osteology. Cross section of the wrist and pertinent bony and soft tissues.

The lunate bone articulates between the scaphoid and the triquetrum laterally and medially, respectively. It is quadrangular, although semilunar in the sagittal plane. The proximal lunate articulates with the radius and articular disk and connects with the capitate distally. The lunate is the most frequently dislocated bone in the wrist. Perilunate instability is most common at the scaphoid-lunate joint (ie, scapholunate instability), followed in frequency by the triquetrum-lunate joint (ie, triquetrolunate instability).[6,7]

The triquetrum articulates laterally with the lunate, proximally with the articular disk, and distally and laterally with the hamate. It has a somewhat pyramidal shape and bears an oval, isolated facet for articulation with the pisiform on its palmar surface.[2] The pisiform is a pea-shaped bone that has sesamoid bone attributes and several soft tissue attachments. Among the attachments are the tendons of the flexor carpi ulnaris and abductor digiti minimi, the flexor and extensor retinacula, and stabilizing ligaments.

In the distal carpal row, the trapezium articulates distolaterally with the first metacarpal and distomedially with the second metacarpal. This surface is saddle shaped to allow a large arc of motion at the first carpometacarpal (CMC) joint. The trapezium bears a large, concave medial surface that articulates with the trapezoid. The palmar surface contains a groove through which the tendon of the flexor carpi radialis tendon passes.

The trapezoid is a small, irregularly shaped bone nesting between the trapezium laterally and the capitate medially. It articulates with the scaphoid proximally and the second metacarpal distally. Its palmar and dorsal surfaces are rough, allowing for attachment of connective tissues.

The capitate is the central and largest of all carpal bones. Its central position allows articulation with seven other bones, and it serves as a central site for ligamentous attachment. It is generally divided into head, neck, and body regions. Its large triangular distal body bears a concavoconvex surface to articulate with the third metacarpal.[2] The waist divides the distal body from the proximal head. The proximal head articulates with the lunate and scaphoid. Because of its central location, the capitate is the keystone is the proximal transverse arch.[8]

The hamate is cuneiform, with the exception of its prominent hook (ie, hamulus) from which it derives its name.[2] The lateral surface articulates with the capitate, and medially, the hamate articulates with the triquetrum. Distally, the hamate bears facets that articulate with the fourth and fifth metacarpals. The hook protrudes from its palmar surface and serves as the origin and attachment for several soft tissue structures. The ulnar nerve also passes beneath the hook as it courses distally to the hand.

ARTHROLOGY

The wrist is generally divided into radiocarpal, midcarpal, and intercarpal joints. The radiocarpal joint is biaxial and ellipsoid, and it is formed by the articulations of the distal radius and the triangular articular disk with the scaphoid, lunate, and triquetrum bones.[2] The articular disk accounts for approximately 11% of the articular surface, and the radial facets account for 89% (Fig. 27-4).[9]

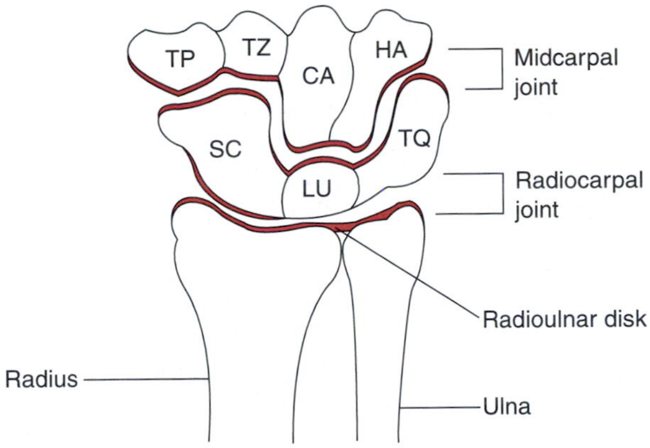

FIGURE 27-4 Wrist complex. The radiocarpal joint is composed of the radius and the articular disk, with the scaphoid (SC), lunate (LU), and triquetrum (TQ) bones. The midcarpal joint is composed of the scaphoid, lunate, and triquetrum with the trapezium (TP), trapezoid (TZ), the capitate (CA) and hamate (HA) bones.

The medial portion of the radiocarpal joint includes a network of structures called the triangular fibrocartilage complex (Fig. 27-5).[9] Structures included in the triangular fibrocartilage complex are the articular disk, dorsal and volar radioulnar ligaments, meniscus homolog, ulnar collateral and radioulnar ligaments, and the sheath of the extensor carpi ulnaris (ECU) tendon.[9] The articular disk and meniscus homolog continue their attachments distally with these ligaments and tendon to attach to the triquetrum, hamate, and base of the fifth metacarpal.

The radiocarpal joint is surrounded by an articular capsule that is lined with a synovial membrane and reinforced by several ligaments. These ligaments are true intracapsular ligaments, and the radiocarpal and ulnocarpal joints are considered to be extrinsic because of attachments outside the wrist. Ligaments at this joint include the palmar radiocarpal, palmar ulnocarpal, dorsal radiocarpal, and ulnar and radial collateral carpal ligaments (Fig. 27-6).[2]

The intercarpal joints consist of articulations between individual bones within the proximal carpal row and the distal carpal row. The midcarpal joint is the articulation between the proximal and distal rows. The ligaments in this area are

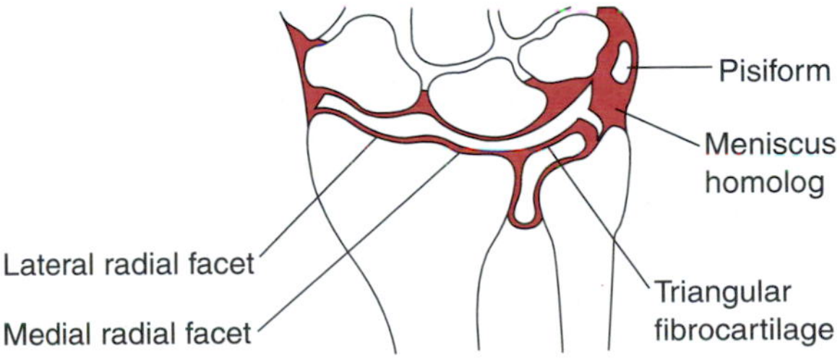

FIGURE 27-5 The proximal surface of the radiocarpal joint is formed by the medial and lateral facets of the distal radius and by the triangular fibrocartilage or articular disk. The articular disk and meniscus homolog are together part of the triangular fibrocartilage complex.

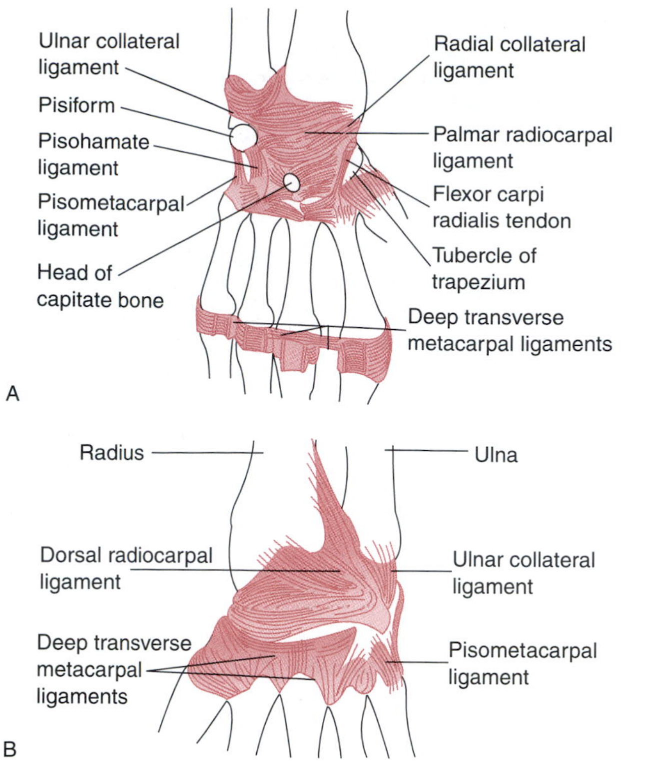

FIGURE 27-6 ***(A)*** Palmar aspect of the ligaments of the left wrist and metacarpal area. ***(B)*** Dorsal aspect of the ligaments of the left wrist.

considered to be intrinsic and are divided into interosseous and midcarpal ligaments. Interosseous ligaments occur within the proximal or distal row, and midcarpal ligaments span the proximal and distal rows on the palmar and dorsal surfaces.[10] The specific ligaments are listed in Table 27-1.

Table 27-1. INTRINSIC LIGAMENTS OF THE WRIST

CLASSIFICATION OF INTRINSIC LIGAMENTS	LIGAMENT NAMES
Interosseous	
Distal row	Trapezium-trapezoid Trapezoid-capitate Capitohamate
Proximal row	Scapholunate Lunotriquetral
Midcarpal	
Dorsal*	Scaphotriquetral Dorsal intercarpal
Palmar*	Scaphotrapeziotrapezoid Scaphocapitate Triquetrocapitate Triquetrohamate

* Midcarpal ligaments span the proximal and distal rows on the palmar or dorsal surfaces.

From Berger RA. The anatomy and basic biomechanics of the wrist joint. *J Hand Ther.* 1996;9:84–93.

The CMC joints are also enclosed in an articular capsule that is somewhat loose. The first metacarpal and trapezium are connected by this capsule and by the lateral, palmar, and dorsal ligaments. The second through fifth CMC joints also contain dorsal and palmar ligaments and the interosseous ligaments. The interosseous ligaments are short, thick fibrous bands connecting the distal margins of the capitate and hamate with the articulating surfaces of the third and fourth metacarpal bones.[2] The second to fifth metacarpal bases are connected by dorsal, palmar, and interosseous ligaments.

MYOLOGY: MUSCLES ACTING AT THE WRIST JOINT

Several important muscles that function at the wrist have their origin at the elbow. These are the major wrist flexors and extensors. Originating at the lateral aspect of the humerus are the common wrist extensors and the ECU and ECRB muscles. The extensor carpi radialis longus (ECRL) muscle originates in proximity to the common extensor origin. The extensor digitorum functions primarily at the hand and is discussed in the Hand section.

Also arising from the common extensor tendon is the ECU muscle. It attaches to the antebrachial fascia and to the posterior ulnar border by the common flexor aponeurosis. It courses distally to attach at the ulnar side of the base of the fifth metacarpal. The ECU muscle is innervated by the radial nerve and functions to extend and adduct the wrist.

The ECRB muscle originates from the common extensor tendon, the radial collateral ligament, and the adjacent intermuscular septa. The distal insertion is on the dorsum of the base of the third metacarpal bone. The ECRB muscle extends and abducts the wrist and is innervated by the radial nerve. Although the ECRL muscle arises from the distal third of the lateral supracondylar ridge and lateral intermuscular septa rather than the common extensor tendon, its proximity to this tendon and its similar function make it a significant structure. This muscle inserts distally at the dorsal surface of the base of the second metacarpal bone. Like the ECRB muscle, the innervation is from the radial nerve, and it functions to extend and abduct the wrist.

On the medial humerus, the flexor digitorum superficialis (FDS), flexor carpi ulnaris, flexor carpi radialis, and palmaris longus muscles originate from the common flexor tendon on the medial epicondyle. In addition to this common origin, the humeroulnar head of the FDS originates from the anterior band of the UCL, the adjacent intermuscular septa, and the medial coronoid process. The radial head arises from the anterior radial border. The median nerve and the ulnar artery descend between these two heads.[2] The muscle courses distally to insert by means of four tendons on the middle phalanges of digits two through five. The function of the FDS is to flex the proximal interphalangeal joints of the second through fifth digits and to assist in flexion of the metacarpophalangeal (MCP) and wrist joints. The median nerve innervates the muscle.

The flexor carpi radialis muscle originates from the deep antebrachial fascia and the common flexor tendon. Distally, the muscle inserts on the base of the second metacarpal and a slip of the base of the third metacarpal. It is innervated by the median nerve. In combination with the flexor carpi ulnaris muscle, it flexes the wrist. In combination with the ECR muscle, it abducts the wrist.

The humeral head of the flexor carpi ulnaris muscle originates from the common flexor tendon. The ulnar head originates from an aponeurosis from the medial margin of the olecranon and proximal two thirds of the posterior ulnar border. Distally, it inserts on the pisiform bone, and it attaches through ligaments to the hamate and fifth metacarpal bones. The flexor carpi ulnaris muscle flexes the wrist, and in combination with the ECU muscle, it adducts the wrist. The ulnar nerve innervates the muscle.

The variably found palmaris longus muscle originates from the common flexor tendon, the adjacent intermuscular septa, and the antebrachial fascia. The tendon extends distally to insert in the flexor retinaculum and palmar aponeurosis. The palmaris longus muscle tenses the palmar fascia and flexes the wrist, and it is innervated by the median nerve.

Hand

OSTEOLOGY

Five metacarpals and 14 phalanges comprise the bony structure of the hand. Each metacarpal has a distal head, shaft, and base.[2] The medial four metacarpals have rounded heads articulating with their respective proximal phalanges. The metacarpal's articular surface is convex, forming the rounded "knuckles" on the hand's dorsum. The medial four metacarpals articulate proximally with each other and with the distal row of carpal bones. The first and second metacarpals do not articulate with each other. Of the metacarpal bones, the third has the longest shaft and the largest base.[2] The first metacarpal is saddle shaped proximally to articulate with the trapezium, and the distal end is pulley shaped, with two small condyles.

There are three phalanges in each finger and two in the thumb. Each phalanx has a distal head, shaft, and proximal base. The base of the proximal metacarpals contains concave facets to articulate with the pulley-shaped, convex metacarpal heads. Likewise, the bases of the middle phalanges have two concave facets separated by a smooth ridge to articulate with the heads of the proximal phalanges. The phalanges provide numerous attachments for ligaments and muscles. The thumb contains two sesamoid bones at the MCP joint.

ARTHROLOGY

The MCP and interphalangeal (IP) joints have similar arthrologic structures. Each is composed of an articular capsule and synovial lining. The MCP joints contain volar ligaments, which are thick and fibrocartilaginous, loosely attached to the metacarpal, and firmly attached at the phalangeal bases.[2] Because of the incongruence of the MCP joints, the volar ligament (ie, volar plate) does more than reinforce joint capsule. Its fibrocartilaginous structure adds surface area to the base of the proximal phalanx to more closely approximate the size of the larger metacarpal head. This plate also checks hyperextension. Its flexible attachments permits motion into flexion without restricting motion or impinging the long flexor tendons.[9] The transverse metacarpal ligament connects the volar ligaments of the second through fifth MCP joints. Collateral ligaments are found on either side of the joint and are strong, rounded cords.[2] The capsular, volar, and collateral ligament arrangement at the MCP joints is the same structure found in the IP joints (Fig. 27-7).

MYOLOGY: MUSCLES ACTING AT THE HAND

The muscular anatomy of the hand can be classified as thumb and finger musculature. Finger flexion is produced by extrinsic and intrinsic flexor musculature. The FDS and the flexor digitorum profundus (FDP) originate outside the hand. The FDS originates from the common flexor tendon from the medial epicondyle of the humerus, the medial side of the coronoid process, and the oblique line of the radius. Its distal attachment is through four tendons into the sides of the middle phalanges of the second through fifth digits.[4] The FDS flexes the proximal IP joints and assists in flexion of the MCP and wrist joints. The FDP arises from the anterior and medial surfaces of the proximal ulna, interosseous membrane, and deep antebrachial fascia and, like the FDS, inserts through four tendons. The FDP tendons insert into the bases of the distal phalanges of the second through fifth digits. The FDP flexes the distal IP joints and assists in flexion of the proximal interphalangeal (PIP) and MCP joints.

The FDP and the FDS lie under the flexor retinaculum, a thick, fibrous band that converts the volar concavity of the wrist into a carpal tunnel. Within the tunnel lie the tendons of the flexor pollicis longus (FPL), FDS, and FDP and the median nerve. A portion of this retinaculum passes medially to attach to the pisiform and the hook of the hamate. This expansion forms the roof of Guyon's canal, through which the ulnar nerve and artery pass. The first and second FDP muscles are innervated by the median nerve, and the third and fourth are innervated by the ulnar nerve.

On the dorsum, the extrinsic finger flexors are the extensor digitorum (ED), extensor indicis, and the extensor digiti minimi. The ED originates from the humeral lateral epicondyle from the common extensor tendon and from the adjacent intermuscular septa and antebrachial fascia. Insertion is accomplished by means of four tendons, which divide into a medial and two lateral bands. The medial band

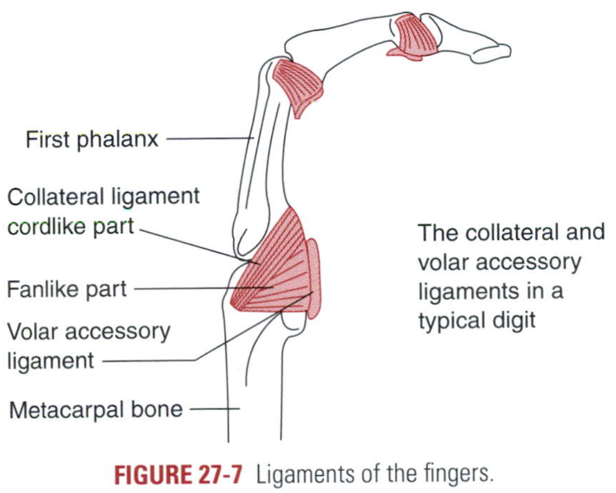

FIGURE 27-7 Ligaments of the fingers.

inserts into the base of the middle phalanx, and the lateral bands rejoin over the middle phalanx and eventually insert into the base of the distal phalanx (Fig. 27-8). The ED is innervated by the radial nerve and has several functions; the primary one is extension of the MCP joint. In conjunction with the lumbricals and interossei, the ED assists interphalangeal joint extension.[2,4] The ED is assisted at the index finger by the extensor indicis. The extensor indicis originates from the posterior surface of the ulna and interosseous membrane and inserts distally into the extensor expansion of the index finger along with the ED. Its function is the same as the ED at the index finger, although it allows independent extension of the index MCP joint while the other fingers are flexed. The ED is also assisted in its function at the fifth digit by the extensor digiti minimi. The extensor digiti minimi originates from the same common extensor tendon as the ED and inserts into the extensor expansion of the fifth digit, along with the ED.[4] It also allows independent extension of the fifth digit.

Like the extrinsic flexor muscles, the extrinsic extensor muscles are stabilized by a retinaculum called the extensor retinaculum. The extensor retinaculum is a strong, fibrous band that courses obliquely from the anterior border of the radius medially to the triquetrum and pisiform bones.[2] This retinaculum contains vertical septa that divide the dorsal musculature into six compartments.

The primary intrinsic muscles of the hand include the dorsal and palmar interossei and the lumbricales (Fig. 27-9). The dorsal interossei originate at the radial and ulnar border of the metacarpals and insert on the respective radial and ulnar borders of the extensor expansion and base of the proximal phalanges. The dorsal interossei abduct and assist in MCP flexion and IP extension of the second, third, and fourth fingers. The first dorsal interossei assists in adduction of the thumb.[4] The palmar interossei originate from the ulnar and radial metacarpal shafts (base in the case of the first) and insert into the extensor expansion of the respective digit. The palmar interossei adduct the thumb and the second, fourth and fifth digits, and they assist in flexion of the MCP and extension of the IP joints of fingers two through four. The lumbricales originate from the FDP tendons of adjacent fingers and insert into the radial border of the extensor expansion on the dorsum of the respective finger.[4] The lumbricales function to extend the IP and flex the MCP joints of the second through fifth digits. They also extend the IP joints when the MCP joints are extended through their attachment to the dorsal hood mechanism of the ED.

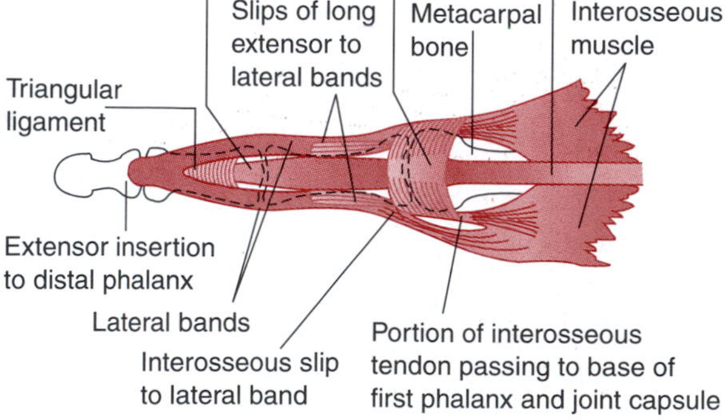

FIGURE 27-8 Dorsal view of extensor mechanism of the fingers.

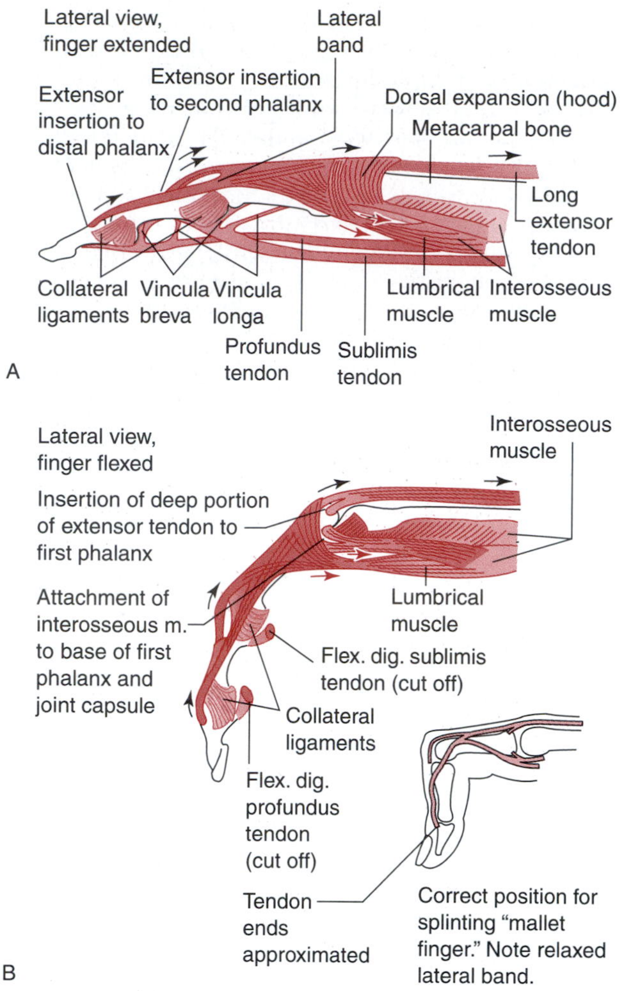

FIGURE 27-9 Intrinsic muscle anatomy. ***(A)*** Extended position. ***(B)*** Flexed position.

The thumb is supplied by extrinsic and intrinsic muscles. Extrinsic muscles include the abductor pollicis longus (APL), the extensor pollicis longus, extensor pollicis brevis (EPB), and the FPL. The APL originates from the posterior aspect of the ulna, the interosseous membrane, and posterior aspect of the middle third of the radius, and it inserts at the radial side of the first metacarpal base. It abducts and extends the CMC joint and assists in radial deviation and flexion of the wrist.[4] The APL and EPB make up the first dorsal compartment. The extensor pollicis longus originates from the middle one third of the posterior surface of the ulna and the interosseous membrane, passes around Lister's tubercle, and inserts on the dorsal surface of the base of the distal phalanx. Found in the third dorsal compartment, the extensor pollicis longus extends the IP joint and assists in extending the MCP and CMC joints of the thumb. The EPB originates on the posterior surface of the radius and interosseous membrane and inserts distally on the dorsal aspect of the base of the proximal phalanx. It extends the MCP joint and extends and abducts the CMC joint. The FPL arises from the anterior aspect of the radius and interosseous membrane, inserts on the palmar aspect of the base of the thumb's distal phalanx, and flexes the IP joint. It also assists in flexion of the MCP and CMC joints.[4]

The intrinsic muscles of the thumb consist of the flexor pollicis brevis, the adductor and abductor pollicis and opponens pollicis. The flexor pollicis brevis originates from the flexor retinaculum and the trapezium and trapezoid and capitate bones, and it inserts on the radial side of the base of the proximal phalanx. It flexes the MCP and CMC joints and assists in opposition. The adductor pollicis arises from the capitate bone and the bases of the second and third metacarpals, and it inserts on the ulnar side of the base of the proximal phalanx. It adducts the CMC and MCP joints and assists in flexion of the MCP joint. The abductor pollicis originates laterally on the flexor retinaculum and the trapezium and scaphoid bones and inserts on the radial side of the base of the proximal phalanx. It abducts the CMC and MCP joints of the thumb. The opponens pollicis originates from the flexor retinaculum and the trapezium bone and inserts along the entire length of the radial side of the first metacarpal. It flexes, abducts, and medially rotates (opposes) the CMC joint, bringing the pads of the thumb in contact with the pads of the four fingers.[4]

Regional Neurology

Several important nerves serve the elbow, wrist, and hand. These nerves may be injured locally by trauma, stretched during activities, or compressed within a confined space. Understanding the area anatomy aids the clinician in determining the source of symptoms.

The median nerve originates from two roots from the lateral (C5, C6, C7) and medial (C8, T1) cords. It descends along the brachial artery to enter the distal arm of the cubital fossa. It passes between the brachialis posteriorly and the bicipital aponeurosis anteriorly. At the elbow, the median nerve passes under the ligament of Struthers and the lacertus fibrosus and then enters the forearm between the heads of the pronator teres. This nerve can be injured or entrapped in any of these areas. It continues distally behind and adhered to the FDS and anterior to the FDP. As the median nerve passes the distal margin of the pronator teres muscle, it divides into the median nerve and the anterior interosseous nerve.[2] The anterior interosseous nerve supplies the first and second FDP, FPL, and pronator quadratus. Just proximal to the flexor retinaculum, the median nerve becomes superficial and then passes deep to the flexor retinaculum into the palm. It then passes through the carpal tunnel, where it may become compressed. After passing through the tunnel, the median nerve divides into five or six branches, providing motor and sensory innervation to the hand.

The ulnar nerve arises from the medial cord (C8, T1) of the brachial plexus, but it may receive fibers from the ventral ramus of C7. Because of its location and anatomic relationships, the ulnar nerve is susceptible to compression, traction, and friction. The ulnar nerve courses distally through the axilla along with the axillary artery and vein and the brachial artery. At the middle of the humerus, it moves medially, descending anterior to the medial head of the triceps. The ulnar nerve can become entrapped here by the arcade of Struthers, approximately 8 cm proximal to the medial epicondyle.[2] At the elbow, the ulnar nerve passes superficially through a groove on the dorsum of the medial epicondyle, entering the forearm in the cubital tunnel between the two heads of the flexor carpi ulnaris. The ulnar nerve can become entrapped here as well, because the cubital tunnel narrows 55% during elbow flexion.[11] Traction across an unstable medial elbow joint can also injure the ulnar nerve. Through the forearm, the ulnar nerve descends along the medial side of the FDP. Just proximal to the wrist, it sends off a dorsal branch that continues distally across the flexor retinaculum. The ulnar nerve continues distally with the ulnar artery, beneath the most superficial aspect of the flexor retinaculum, and divides into superficial and deep terminal branches. The ulnar nerve can be compressed as it crosses the distal edge of the pisohamate portion of the retinaculum. The superficial and deep branches provide motor and sensory innervation to the hand.

The radial nerve arises from the posterior cord (C5, C6, C7, C8) and is the largest branch of the brachial plexus. It courses distally between the medial and long heads of the triceps and then passes obliquely posterior to the humerus and deep to the lateral head of the triceps to the lateral aspect of the humerus to penetrate the anterior compartment.[2] Its proximity to the humerus makes it susceptible to injury in mid-humeral fractures. As the radial nerve continues distally, it bifurcates to become the posterior interosseous and superficial radial nerves. The superficial radial nerve has only sensory fibers. The posterior interosseous nerve is analogous to its anterior correlate (ie, anterior interosseous nerve) in that is has only motor fibers. The posterior interosseous nerve passes through the supinator muscle, around the proximal radius, and beneath the extensor muscle mass, and the superficial radial nerve passes beneath the brachioradialis muscle and continues distally to the hand. The superficial radial nerve continues distally along the anterolateral aspect of the forearm. Proximal to the wrist, it passes deep to curve around the radius and divides into four or five dorsal digital nerves. This nerve innervates the skin of the dorsolateral hand. It is susceptible to injury in the distal forearm and hand, where it lies superficially. Compression can by caused by casts, watchbands, and similar items.[12]

KINESIOLOGY

Elbow and Forearm

Normal ROM at the elbow joint is 0 to 135 degrees actively and 0 to 150 degrees passively. Much of this mobility is necessary for the normal activities of daily living (ADLs). For example, putting on a shirt requires a range of 15 to 140 degrees, and drinking from a cup requires range of 72 to 130 degrees.[13] ROM in flexion is limited by anterior muscle bulk, and ROM in extension is limited by the bony articulation of the olecranon in the olecranon fossa. The extended position of the humeroulnar joint is the close-packed position; additional inherent stability occurs in extreme flexion. Motion occurs primarily by gliding of the ulna on the trochlea.

Pronation and supination technically occur through the forearm at the proximal and distal radioulnar joints. The normal range of pronation and supination is 0 to 80 degrees in each direction. Pronation occurs as the radius crosses over the ulna at the proximal radioulnar joint. Although most ADLs occur with the forearm in a middle position, some activities, such as receiving change in the palm of the hand, require full supination.

Resistance to valgus stress in full extension is limited equally by the UCL, bony congruity, and the anterior capsule.[9] As the elbow moves into flexion, most of the resistance to valgus stress is provided by the anterior band of the UCL. Morrey and An[14] found the UCL to contribute approximately 54% of the resistance to valgus stress in flexion. The joint articulation contributed 33% of the resistance to valgus.

Resistance to varus in full extension is provided by the bony congruity and by the radial collateral ligament and capsule.[9] Resistance to distraction is provided by soft tissue components, and the anterior portion of the joint capsule provides the primarily resistance to anterior displacement.

A cadaveric study of the flexor pronator group relative to the UCL throughout the ROM has significant implications for rehabilitation of individuals with medial elbow injuries. At 30 degrees of elbow flexion, the pronator teres and flexor carpi radialis muscles were entirely anterior to the UCL, and the flexor carpi ulnaris muscle was found over or posterior to the UCL.[15] The FDS muscle was over the UCL in most cases. The findings were similar at 90 degrees, except the flexor carpi ulnaris muscle was completely over the UCL, and the FDS muscle was anterior to the UCL in most cases. At 120 degrees, the pronator teres, flexor carpi radialis, and FDS muscles were all anterior to the UCL, and only the flexor carpi ulnaris muscle was over the UCL. This pattern suggests that the flexor carpi ulnaris muscle is the primary dynamic medial elbow stabilizer throughout the ROM and particularly at 120 degrees of flexion.[15]

Wrist

The normal wrist ROM is from 80 degrees of flexion to 70 degrees of extension. The resting position of the wrist is between 20 and 35 degrees of extension and 10 to 15 degrees of ulnar deviation while in the close-packed position.[16] The wrist functions primarily through a range of 10 degrees of flexion to 35 degrees of extension when performing most ADLs.[17] However, some activities, such as rising from a chair, require significantly more extension.[17] Movement at the radiocarpal joint is predominantly a gliding movement of the concave distal radius and articular disk on the convex proximal carpal row. The proximal carpal row is considered to be an intercalated segment, a relatively unattached middle segment of a three-segment link, because of its position between the radius and distal carpus.[9]

Mechanically, the scaphoid plays a critical role in stabilizing this segment by means of its position bridging the proximal and distal carpal rows (ie, the midcarpal joint). The radiocarpal and midcarpal joints provide variable proportions of the motion during wrist extension and flexion. When the proportion contributed by radiocarpal joint exceeds that of the midcarpal joints in one direction, this pattern reverses in the other direction.[9] Wrist extension is initiated at the distal carpal row, with this row gliding on the relatively stable proximal row. As the wrist passes into extension, these rows begin to move together, with the scaphoid intervening as the bridge to this process.[9] Full extension is the close-packed position of the wrist.

In general, the distal carpal row functions as a unit because of the interlocking of articular surfaces and the ligamentous connections between the distal row and the metacarpals distally.[10] The distal row tends to move in unison with the second and third metacarpals, palmar flexing when these metacarpals palmar flex and dorsal flexing when they dorsally flex.

The proximal carpal row differs in its movement pattern from the distal row. In general, the bones in the proximal row move together, although greater motion occurs between the bones in the proximal row than in the distal row. This is true of the direction and magnitude of motion between the bones in the proximal row. The proximal row tends to move in the same direction as the distal row and therefore in the same direction as the second and third metacarpals.[10] Between-bone motion also occurs, and during wrist extension, the scaphoid supinates while the lunate pronates, functionally separating these bones. This motion underlies perilunate instabilities occurring as a result of forceful extension.

Frontal plane motion is normally from 15 degrees of radial deviation to 30 degrees of ulnar deviation. The ulnar styloid is shorter than the radial styloid, accounting for the greater range in ulnar deviation than radial. Greater ulnar and radial deviation is possible when the wrist is in a neutral flexion-extension position. Arthrokinematic motion in radial and ulnar deviation is more complex than in flexion and extension. During radial deviation, the proximal carpal row glides ulnarly and flexes while the distal row pivots radially. During ulnar deviation, the proximal row glides radially and moves into extension while the distal row moves ulnarly.[10]

The mobility of the wrist depends on the position of the fingers because of the length of extrinsic tendons crossing the wrist and hand joints. For example, wrist flexion is decreased when the fingers are simultaneously flexed because of the length of the extrinsic finger extensor muscles. Likewise, the mobility of the fingers depends on the position of the wrist, as evidenced by the inability to fully flex the fingers when the wrist is flexed.

Load transmission across the wrist is significant and varies with wrist position. With the wrist and forearm in neutral, approximately 80% of the force is transmitted across the radiocarpal joint and 20% across the ulnocarpal joint.[18] Further breakdown of the radiocarpal loads shows that approximately 45% of these forces are transmitted across the radioscaphoid joint and 35% across the radiolunate joint.[18] Forearm pronation increases the load transmitted across the ulnocarpal joint to approximately 37%, with a proportional reduction of load at the radiocarpal joint. Radiocarpal forces increase to 87% when the wrist is in radial deviation.[10]

Hand

CARPOMETACARPAL JOINTS

CMC joints two through five are similar in structure and function, but the first CMC is different. The second through fourth CMC joints permit one degree of freedom in flexion and extension, and the fifth CMC allows some abduction and adduction as well. Motion at the CMC joints is limited primarily by the ligamentous structure. Motion increases at the CMC joints from the radial to the ulnar side of the hand.[9] Almost no motion occurs at the second and third CMC joints, the fourth is slightly more mobile, and the fifth moves through a range of nearly 10 to 20 degrees.[9]

The first CMC joint is saddle shaped and has two degrees of freedom and some axial rotation. This mobility allows for opposition, a key function of the thumb. The thumb is involved in nearly all forms of prehension, or handling activities, and loss of the thumb accounts for the greatest portion of disability in the hand.[19] ROM is approximately from 20 degrees of flexion to 45 degrees of extension and from 0 degrees of adduction to 40 degrees of abduction. Mobility at the CMC is limited by the ligamentous and interposed soft tissues.

A primary role of the CMC joints is to contribute to cupping of the hand, forming palmar arches. This hollowing allows the hand to conform to the shape of the object being held. Two arches are visible: the longitudinal arch that spans the length of the hand and the metacarpal arch that transverses the palm.

METACARPOPHALANGEAL JOINT

The four medial MCP joints possess two degrees of freedom, flexion and extension, and abduction and adduction. The mobility at these joints increases from the radial to ulnar sides of the hand, with an active ROM from 90 degrees of flexion to 10 degrees of extension. Passively, variable amounts of extension are available. Functional flexion at the MCP joint is approximately 60 degrees.[16] The range in abduction and adduction is approximately 20 degrees in each direction. The range in the frontal plane is limited by articular surface geometry, and the range in flexion is limited by joint geometry and capsule, and the range in extension is limited by the volar plates.

The MCP joint of the thumb also possesses two degrees of freedom. The ROM is more limited here than in fingers two through five. Almost no hyperextension is available in normal hands, and only approximately 50 degrees of flexion can be obtained. Extension at this joint is further limited by the presence of two sesamoid bones, stabilized by collateral and intersesamoid ligaments. The primary function of MCP mobility of the thumb is providing additional range for opposition and prehension activities.

INTERPHALANGEAL JOINTS

The IP joints of the fingers and thumb are similar in function. Each is a hinge joint with one degree of freedom. ROM at the IP joints, like the other joints in the hand, increases from the radial to the ulnar side of the hand. This is easily observed when making a fist. The ROM at the PIP is from 0 degrees of extension to 100 degrees of flexion at the radial side of the hand and nearly 135 degrees of flexion at the ulnar side. Little hyperextension is available because of the volar plates. The distal interphalangeal (DIP) joint demonstrates less ROM, from 10 degrees of extension to 80 degrees of flexion. Functional flexion at the PIP joints is approximately 60 degrees, and functional flexion at the DIP joints is 40 degrees.[16]

EXTENSOR MECHANISM

The extensor mechanism of the fingers is composed of the extensor hood (ie, extensor expansion or dorsal aponeurosis) and the ED, palmar interossei, dorsal interossei, and lumbrical muscles. Each finger contains a similar mechanism that is necessary for successful extension of the finger. As the ED courses distally, it flattens into an aponeurotic hood over the metacarpal, and just distal to the MCP joint, the ED is joined by tendon fibers from the interossei muscles. The interossei arise from the lateral borders of the metacarpals (see Fig. 27-9). This aponeurosis formed by the ED and interossei continues distally, where, proximal to the PIP, the hood splits into three branches. All three branches receive fibers from the interossei, and the medial branch also receives fibers from the lumbricals. A central tendon continues distally and crosses the PIP to insert at the base of the middle phalanx. Two lateral bands on either side continue distally, cross the PIP joint, and reunite into a single tendon that terminates at the distal phalanx. Several local ligaments attach to the extensor hood and prevent bowstringing during movement. The oblique retinacular ligaments are important in simultaneous PIP and DIP extension.

A complete description of the mechanics of the extensor hood is beyond the scope of this text, but a few generalizations can be made. At the MCP joint, contraction of the of the ED produces extension while activation of the lumbricals and interossei produce flexion. The torque produced by the ED exceeds the that of others, and extension results. At the PIP joint, the ED, interossei, and lumbricals together produce extension. Isolated contraction of the ED causes the finger to claw or to produce MCP hyperextension with IP flexion[9] because of the passive pull of the long finger flexors at the IP joints. Extension of the PIP joint also produces DIP extension (and vice versa), and when the PIP is held in flexion, the DIP is incapable of isolated extension. This mechanism is finely tuned to produce fine movements and strong grip. Any imbalance in the lateral slips disrupts this mechanism and significantly alters hand function.

GRIP

The hand is well suited for the major task of gripping. Grip can be divided into power grip and prehension grip, or pinching. The power grip is used for developing firm control, and the prehension grip is used when accuracy and precision are needed. Examples of power grip include hook, spherical, cylinder, and fist grasps, and examples of prehension grip include the three-fingered, key, and tip pinches.

Grip activity has been broken down into four stages. In the first step, the hand opens by simultaneous action of the long extensor and hand intrinsic muscles. The fingers then close about the object, requiring activity of the intrinsic and extrinsic flexor and opposition muscles. The third step is an increase in force in these same muscles to a level appropriate for the task. The hand again opens to release the object.[16] While the flexors are grasping the object, the wrist extensor muscles must fire simultaneously to prevent the long flexors from producing wrist flexion.

The innervation of the hand is related to the two types of grip. The ulnar nerve controls the motor and sensory distribution of the medial digits, and these digits are used more for the power grip. The median nerve controls the lateral digits, which are used more for the prehensile grip. The thumb musculature, used in both types of grip, is innervated by both nerves.[16]

The power grip is used when force generation is the primary objective (Fig. 27-10*A*). Carrying a suitcase, climbing on a jungle gym, making a fist, and grasping a baseball to throw are all examples of power grip. In this situation, the ulnar digits stabilize the object, holding it against the palm, with or without the assistance of the thumb. The fingers are fully flexed while the wrist is extended and ulnarly deviated.

The prehension grip is used when fine control is necessary. This grip is used when holding a writing implement, putting a key in the door, or holding a piece of paper between two fingers (Fig. 27-10*B*). The prehension grip includes primarily the MCP joints and the radial side of the hand. The index and middle fingers work with the thumb to create a tripod. In contrast with the power grip, the object in a prehension grip may never come in contact with the palm.

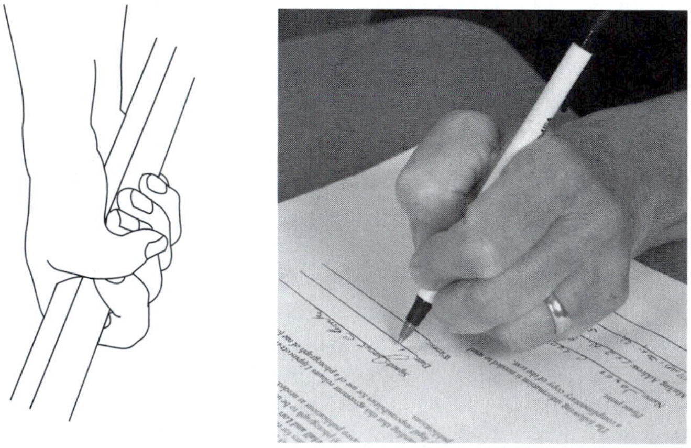

FIGURE 27-10 ***(A)*** Power grip. ***(B)*** Prehension grip used while writing.

EXAMINATION AND EVALUATION

Examination and evaluation of the elbow, wrist, and hand must include a comprehensive assessment of the upper quarter. The upper extremity relationships between the cervical spine and distal joints requires a full examination to ensure identification of the problem source. Many of the examination techniques depend on the situation. The presence of comorbidities such as diabetes or rheumatoid arthritis necessitates different examination techniques from those used for the patient without such additional issues. The following sections address the key aspects of elbow, wrist, and hand examinations.

History

The history and subjective information focuses the remainder of the examination. In addition to the medical history and evaluation of the current problem, subjective information about the signs and symptoms after the injury is valuable. Information is gathered about the functional limitations (eg, inability to manipulate buttons, zippers and other small objects, inability to carry out hygiene activities, difficulty writing or typing, problems opening jars) and disability (eg, unable to work because of inability to type, unable to care for child because of pain and weakness in elbow) associated with the current complaint. This information, along with data gathered during the objective examination, forms the basis for the interventions chosen. Information to differentiate primary elbow, wrist, and hand problems from those referred from the cervical spine must be ascertained.

Observation and Clearing Tests

Observation of posture and position of the limb and clearing tests for the cervical spine and shoulder are essential parts of the examination and evaluation. The following are components of general observation:

- Posture of the head and neck
- Muscle tone throughout upper extremity, including thenar and hypothenar eminences
- Quality, color, and temperature of the skin
- Quality of the nails
- Carrying angle of the elbow
- Swelling, ecchymosis
- Resting position of the elbow, forearm, and wrist
- Ability to use limb during examination

The resting position of the hand also should be evaluated, including these deformities:

- Swan-neck deformity
- Boutonniére deformity
- Ulnar drift
- Clubbing of DIPs
- Heberden's or Bouchard's nodes
- Claw fingers
- Dupuytren's contracture
- Mallet or trigger finger

Mobility Examination

Mobility examination of the elbow, wrist, and hand includes osteokinematic and arthrokinematic testing and tests of muscle extensibility. It is particularly important to find the sources of mobility loss in the hand, because this impairment is associated with significant functional limitations and disability. Examination procedures should distinguish between contractile and noncontractile tissues and between intrinsic and extrinsic muscle limitations. In most cases, the following tests of mobility should be performed:

Elbow and Forearm

- Active range of motion (AROM), passive range of motion (PROM), and overpressure for flexion, extension, pronation, and supination
- Distraction and anterior, medial, and lateral glides

Wrist

- AROM, PROM, and overpressure for flexion, extension, and radial and ulnar deviation
- Distraction and anterior, posterior, radial, and ulnar glides
- Radiocarpal, midcarpal, intercarpal, and carpometacarpal assessment

Hand

- AROM, PROM, and overpressure for flexion, extension, abduction, and adduction (at appropriate joints)
- Distraction and anterior, posterior, radial, and ulnar glides (at appropriate joints)

Muscle Extensibility

- All muscles crossing the elbow, wrist, and hand
- Intrinsic muscles of the hand

Muscle length testing is performed for the extrinsic forearm flexors and extensors. Forearm extensor muscle length is assessed during passive wrist flexion ROM bilaterally with the elbows extended, forearms pronated, wrists flexed, and fingers fisted. Forearm flexor muscle length is assessed during passive wrist extension bilaterally with the elbows extended, forearms supinated, and wrists and fingers extended.

Muscle Performance Examination

Muscles functioning at the elbow, wrist, and hand should be tested in a logical order on the basis of the subjective information provided, history, and the results of the examination. Many of the hand muscles are quite small, and therapists must consider their relative strength when applying traditional manual muscle testing criteria. Stabilization, particularly when trying to isolate small intrinsic muscles of the hand, ensures that the muscle of interest is being tested. The number of muscles in this area is too extensive to list, but Kendall[4] has described the testing procedures for the relevant muscles in the region.

Pain and Inflammation Examination

The initial pain examination is performed as part of the subjective history. The patient is asked about the level of pain and the pattern of that pain over 24 hours. During the objective examination, a visual analog scale or similar tool can provide objective information about pain. Inflammation can be detected by palpation for warmth and specific tenderness. Swelling can be detected by volumetric measurement.

Special Tests

Many special tests assess the integrity of tissues throughout the upper quarter. These tests examine ligament stability, soft tissue mobility, neurologic status, and functional tasks. Magee[16] has provided a complete listing and description of special tests. Some of the more common tests used are listed in Display 27-1.

DISPLAY 27-1

Special Tests at the Elbow, Wrist, and Hand

Elbow

- Valgus stress test (0 and 30 degrees)
- Varus stress test (0 and 30 degrees)
- Tinel's sign
- Pinch grip
- Tennis elbow tests
  - Resisted wrist extension
  - Passive wrist flexion
  - Resisted 3rd finger extension
- Golfer's elbow
  - Resisted wrist flexion
  - Passive wrist extension

Wrist and Hand

- Carpal tunnel tests
  - Phalen's test
  - Tinel sign
  - Three jaw chuck test
- Allen's test
- Finkelstein's test
- Brunnel-Littler test
- Retinacular test
- Froment's sign
- Ligamentous instability testing for the fingers
- Thumb ulnar collateral ligament testing
- Lunatotriquetral ballottement test
- Scaphoid stress test
- Hand function tests
- Grip strength test
- Reflexes and sensation
- Upper limb tension tests

THERAPEUTIC EXERCISE INTERVENTIONS FOR COMMON PHYSIOLOGIC IMPAIRMENTS

Mobility Impairment

Impaired mobility in the distal upper extremity can be very disabling. Fine motor skills are necessary for the simplest of daily activities. Mobility activities must restore full ROM throughout the distal segments to maintain independence in many household tasks. Impaired mobility in this region is treated with a combination of therapeutic modalities, exercise, and splinting.

HYPOMOBILITY

Hypomobility in this region can occur for a number of reasons. Injuries that necessitate a period of immobilization can produce profound mobility loss. Surgery, neurologic injuries, burns, and falls can significantly impair mobility. Because of the mobility required for functional use of the upper limb, loss of motion in this region can be quite disabling.

Intervention for mobility loss requires a thorough evaluation to determine the structures responsible for or contributing to the motion loss. The joint capsule, short musculotendinous structures, immobile fascial tissues, or restricted nervous tissues are a few examples of tissues that may be at fault. Evaluation techniques aimed at differentiating contractile from noncontractile tissues, followed by specific tension testing, can pinpoint the source of limitation. Only then can appropriate intervention be initiated.

Mobility impairment at the elbow includes loss of flexion and extension. Loss of elbow extension occurs frequently after fractures or dislocations at the elbow. Loss of motion occurs rapidly at the elbow, and therefore immobilization is kept to the minimum acceptable time. Degenerative joint disease has a lower impact on the upper extremity joints than the lower, and loss of motion because of arthritic changes at the elbow therefore is less common than at the knee. Loss of motion at the elbow is often compensated by trunk, shoulder, and wrist motion, all of which may place additional loads on these structures.

Mobility loss at the forearm includes loss of pronation and supination. The capsular pattern shows equal loss of pronation and supination. Loss of motion at the forearm is common after immobilization for wrist and hand fractures. The distal radioulnar joint is affected in individuals with rheumatoid arthritis. Disease may cause the ulna to dorsally subluxate on the radius at the distal radioulnar joint. Loss of pronation and supination results in difficulties with turning knobs, opening jars, receiving change, and turning a key. These motions are frequently transferred to the shoulder, with the person performing external and internal rotation to compensate. Restoration of motion is important to prevent secondary injury to the shoulder.

Loss of motion at the wrist is common after falls or fractures injuring the wrist. Rheumatoid arthritis also affects the wrist joint. The patient with rheumatoid arthritis often has a wrist deformity of flexion, radial deviation, and volar subluxation of the carpal bones.[19] Ankylosis may eventually ensue, severely restricting mobility at the wrist. This motion loss is particularly disabling for the individual with rheumatoid arthritis, because adjacent joints are also affected and unable to compensate for wrist immobility.

Loss of motion in the hand is frequently caused by rheumatoid arthritic changes. This disease produces MCP joint ulnar deviation and volar subluxation of the proximal phalanges. Swan-neck deformity, or hyperextension of the PIP and flexion of the DIP, results from flexor and extensor imbalance and PIP joint laxity.[19] Loss of motion in the hand may result from osteoarthritis, and this process tends to affect the PIP and DIP joints but not the MCP joints (see Self-Management: Proximal and Distal Interphalangeal Joint Flexion). The thumb CMC is significantly affected by osteoarthritis and rheumatoid arthritis. Injuries such as fractures, dislocations, and burns produce limitations in mobility after treatment. Dupuytren's contraction, or contraction of the palmar fascia, usually affects the fourth or fifth fingers, where the skin is adherent to the underlying fascia. This progressive fibrosis of the palmar fascia has no known cause and affects men older than 40 years of age more than women.[16] These impairments can lead to functional limitations (eg, inability to grasp a pen) and therefore disability (eg, unable to work because of inability to grasp objects).

Activities to increase mobility begin with an adjunctive agent such as heat, followed by joint mobilization if capsular restriction is the cause of immobility. For example, limited motion because of capsular restriction at the elbow may be treated with humeroulnar distraction techniques and some anterior and posterior glides. After mobilization techniques, passive prolonged stretching in the direction of limitation may be performed along with concurrent application of heat or cold. Active mobility in the new range should follow (Fig. 27-11). For example, active pronation and supination may be followed by active hand to mouth exercises or

SELF-MANAGEMENT: *Proximal and Distal Interphalangeal Joint Flexion*

Purpose: To increase the mobility in the joints and tendons of your fingers

Starting position: Start with all the joints of your fingers as straight as possible.

Movement technique: Keeping your knuckle joints (MCP) straight, bend the middle and fingertip joints (PIP and DIP) as far as possible. Return to the starting position.

Repeat ____ times

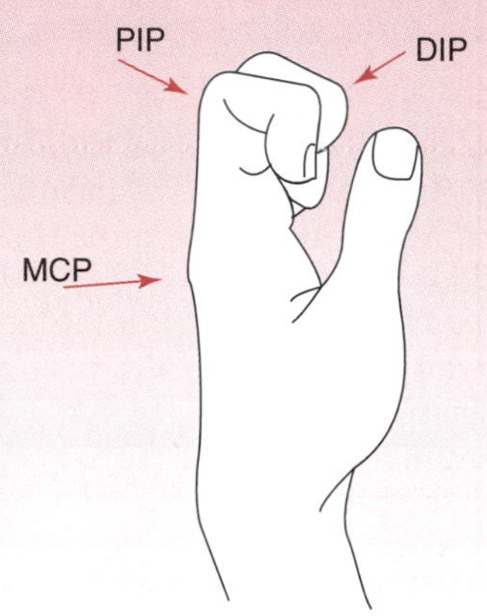

active forward reaching. When immobility is caused by a short or stiff extrinsic muscle or intrinsic muscles, traditional stretching techniques may be employed. At the same time, postural correction and strengthening of the antagonist (which is often weak because of its lengthened position) must occur. Immobile fascial connective tissues are mobilized by manual techniques such as massage and manual deep pressure application. As with stretching, this intervention should be followed with active use of the limb (Fig. 27-12) (see Self-Management: Metacarpophalangeal and Proximal Interphalangeal Joint Flexion With Distal Interphalangeal Joint Extension).

Treatment for immobility of the hand of a patient with rheumatoid arthritis depends on the acuteness of the situation and the degree of deformity. Immobilization may be the treatment of choice in some phases of this disease process (see the Stiff Hand and Restricted Motion section). Neural gliding techniques are employed when neural tension test reveals immobility of neural tissue to be the source of the patient's symptoms.

HYPERMOBILITY

Hypermobility is an uncommon problem at the elbow and forearm; hypomobility is a much more common complaint. Elbow hyperextension ROM is one criteria for a diagnosis of systemic hypermobility. However, hypermobility at this

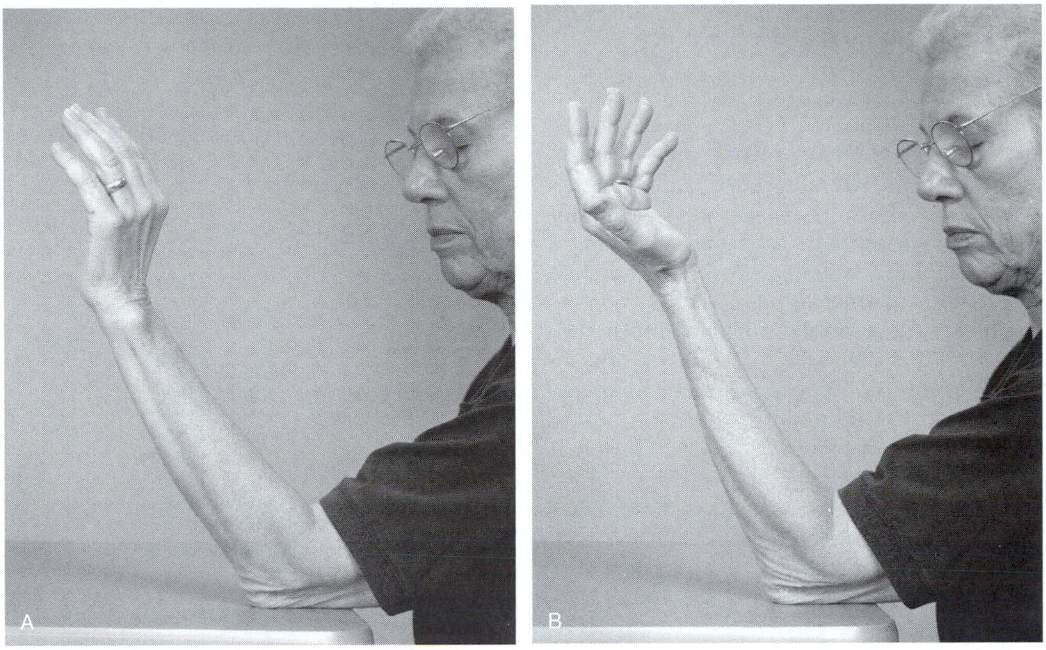

FIGURE 27-11 Active motion of the forearm. ***(A)*** Pronation. ***(B)*** Supination.

joint is rarely symptomatic because of the limited weight bearing occurring in the upper extremities. Individuals participating in upper extremity weight-bearing sports such as gymnastics or wrestling may have difficulty associated with elbow hyperextension during sports.

Similarly, hypermobility is uncommon at the wrist and hand. Hypermobility should not be confused with instability. Instabilities occur in the wrist and the hand. Lunate dislocation with perilunate instability and scapholunate dissociation are common, and instability in the fingers is evident in the hand of the patient with rheumatoid arthritis. However, physiologic hypermobility rarely exists without pathol-

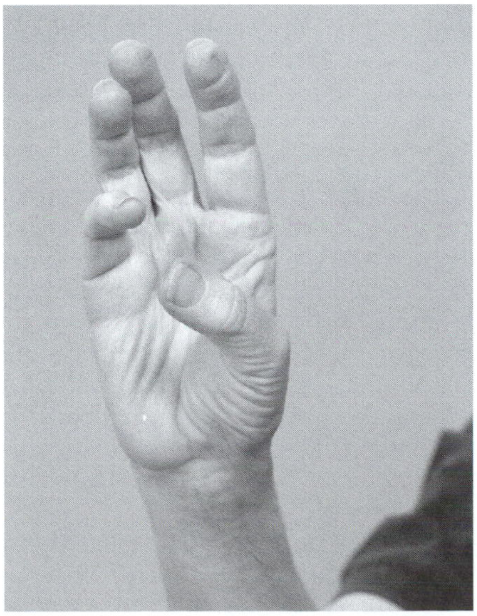

FIGURE 27-12 Active pinch exercise.

SELF-MANAGEMENT: *Metacarpophalangeal and Proximal Interphalangeal Joint Flexion With Distal Interphalangeal Joint Extension*

Purpose: To increase the mobility of your finger joints and tendons

Starting position: Start with all joints of your fingers as straight as possible.

Movement technique: Bend your knuckle (MCP) and middle (PIP) joints while keeping the fingertip joints (DIP) straight. Return to the starting position.

Repeat ____ times

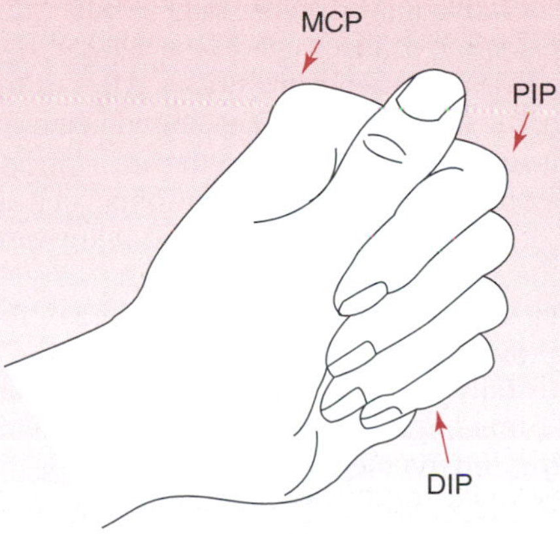

ogy or injury, and if hypermobility is present, it rarely produces symptoms.

Impaired Muscle Performance

Several injuries or pathologies can impair a patient's ability to produce torque in the distal upper extremity. Fractures, dislocations, contusions, sprains, tendon lacerations, burns, nerve entrapments, and crush injuries are some of the conditions that can limit a person's torque-producing ability. An evaluation to determine the source of impairment and an understanding of the healing process can guide intervention to improve torque production. The relationship between the force or torque impairment and functional limitations or disability must be established to justify and guide treatment. Although specific muscular strengthening exercises are employed, these activities must be progressed to activities that reproduce the function of the upper extremity. This approach may include self-care activities such as dressing, grooming, and bathing and work activities such as grasping, pinching, typing, and other dexterous movements.

Any strengthening exercises for the elbow, wrist, and hand must consider the kinetic chain relationship across these joints. The joints are interconnected and related, and the muscular anatomy often crosses several joints. Strengthening exercises for the elbow often load the wrist and finger muscles as the individual holds a weight or other resistive equipment in the hand. The difference between strengthening exercises requiring a grip and those using resistance around the wrist (eg, a cuff weight) must be considered. For example, strengthening exercises for lateral epicondylitis focus on strengthening the wrist extensor muscles in their roles as active wrist extensors (concentrically and eccentrically) and as stabilizers against finger flexor activity such as gripping or shaking hands. Any wrist extension exercise that concurrently requires gripping may overload these muscles (Fig. 27-13). This relationship is one reason why prescribing shoulder exercises while holding a 16-ounce can in the hand often produces lateral epicondylitis in previously asymptomatic individuals.

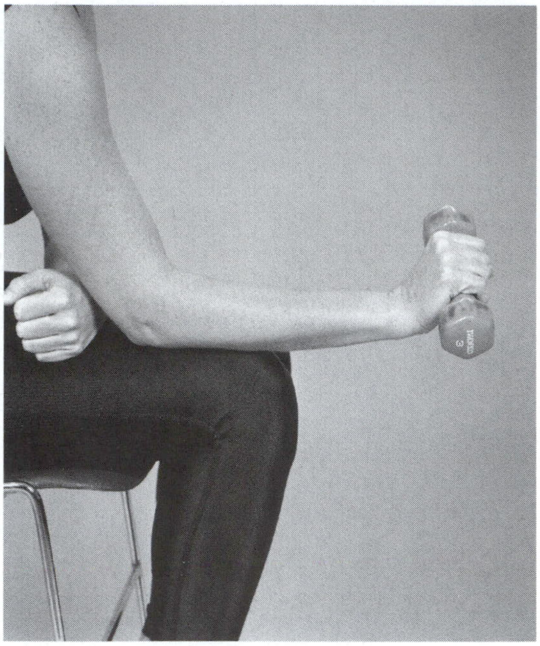

FIGURE 27-13 Resisted wrist extension with free weights.

NEUROLOGIC CAUSES

Neurologic pathology or injury is a common source of impaired muscle function in the distal upper extremity. Cervical degenerative joint disease, degenerative disk disease, and cervical spine injuries can cause symptoms distally in the respective nerve root distributions. After exiting the cervical spine, the nerves may be entrapped in a number of locations throughout the neck and thorax. Entrapment may produce distal neurovascular symptoms such as thoracic outlet syndrome. In this situation, the neurovascular bundle is compressed at one or more sites (eg, cervical rib, scalene muscles) producing a variety of intermittent to constant symptoms.

More distally, the radial nerve may be compressed in the radial tunnel, the ulnar nerve at the medial elbow or at the pisiform, and the median nerve in the carpal tunnel. The ulnar nerve is also subject to traction injuries at the medial elbow in the thrower. Similarly, the mobility of any nerve within its nerve sheath may become restricted.

Injury, compression, traction, or ischemia of these nerves, proximally or distally, results in various symptoms, including loss of the ability to produce torque in the muscles served by the damaged nerve. Treatment for a limited ability to produce torque depends on the specific situation. For example, the individual with distal weakness caused by cervical spine disk herniation may benefit from traction, postural retraining, and cervical spine exercises, followed by progressive resistive exercises for distal musculature only after the proximal symptoms have resolved. Nerve entrapments at the elbow, wrist, or hand must be treated first by release techniques to mobilize the nerve. In contrast, traction injuries to the ulnar nerve at the elbow should be initially treated with stabilization techniques. Only then can strengthening exercises be initiated. These exercises may be performed in positions or postures that minimize the traction or compressive forces on the nerve. Progression to more provocative and functional patterns should follow.

MUSCULAR CAUSES

Muscle injuries in this region range from tendinopathies at the elbow (ie, medial and lateral epicondylitis) and wrist (ie, de Quervain's tenosynovitis) to tendon lacerations in the hand. Intervention to increase the ability to produce torque after injury to the muscle depends on the location and severity of injury, the role of that muscle in functional activities, and the stages of healing. The ability of the muscle to tolerate loads, whether stretching loads or isometric during shortening or lengthening muscle contractions, is the first step in determining an individual's readiness for strengthening exercises.

After the appropriate level of load is determined, progressive isometric to dynamic exercises may be initiated for elbow musculature (eg, extensors, flexors), forearm musculature (eg, pronators, supinators), and wrist and hand (eg, flexors, extensors, ulnar and radial deviators). Exercises may be performed in an open chain, using light weights, bands, or other functional objects (Fig. 27-14). Closed chain activity is also appropriate, such as leaning against a wall or on a countertop to provide resistance. In the hand, manual resistance is often used. After surgery for tendon repairs, PROM in the direction of pull of the lacerated tendon is allowed first, followed by AROM and assisted AROM when sufficient healing allows. Mobilization occurs early to prevent adhesions of the tendon within the sheath. However, resistance is applied only after satisfactory healing at the surgical site (about 8 weeks). At that point, simple gripping exercises using sponges, putty, or other small resistive objects may be initiated (Fig. 27-15). Resistance to extension can be provided manually or by using small resistive bands. In addition to restoring torque producing abilities, the fine motor function of the muscles must be retrained. A variety of dexterity tasks are available for training these skills (see Self-Management: Finger Pinch With Putty).

DISUSE AND DECONDITIONING

Proximal muscle deconditioning can lead to distal muscle overuse injuries. This occurs with repetitive work or activity and reinforces the importance of a thorough upper quarter examination. Effective repetitive distal activity requires proximal stabilization, maintaining posture within a neutral range. When the proximal muscles fatigue, posture is compromised, and a greater load is placed on the distal muscles. For example, as the rotator cuff fatigues during a repetitive lifting task, more of the lifting may be performed by the elbow flexors and wrist extensors, predisposing the individual to lateral epicondylitis. As one group of distal muscles fatigues, the load is shifted to alternate muscle groups, overworking these muscles. Appropriate muscle endurance for the required task is necessary throughout the kinetic chain.

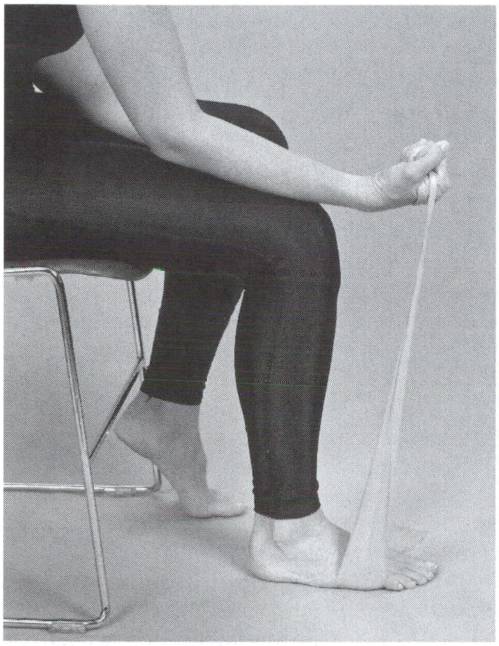

FIGURE 27-14 Resisted wrist flexion with a resistive band.

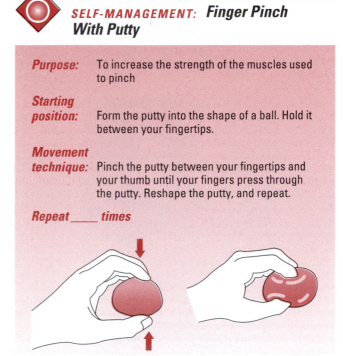

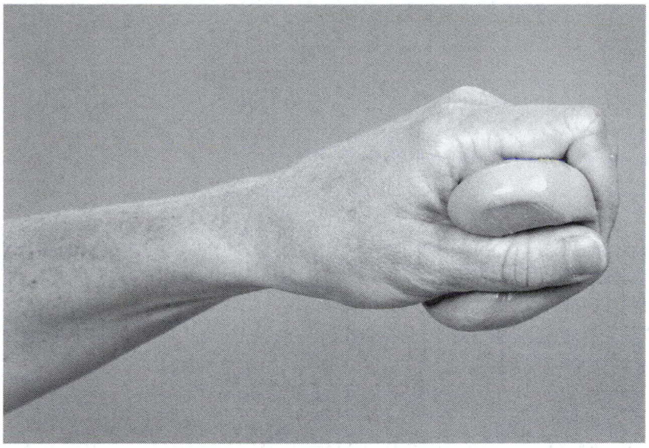

FIGURE 27-15 Grip strengthening using putty.

Endurance Impairment

Muscular endurance impairment is often seen at the wrist and hand in individuals who perform repetitive work with their hands. Imbalance between the endurance of wrist flexors and extensors, along with a number of other factors, contribute to forearm, wrist, and hand pain. Forms of epicondylitis at the elbow may be considered forms of endurance impairment as well. Epicondylitis may develop as an acute injury because of a muscular strain, or it may result from fatigue of the relative musculature. In this situation, impaired muscle endurance is contributing to the situation.

SELF-MANAGEMENT: *Finger Pinch With Putty*

Purpose: To increase the strength of the muscles used to pinch

Starting position: Form the putty into the shape of a ball. Hold it between your fingertips.

Movement technique: Pinch the putty between your fingertips and your thumb until your fingers press through the putty. Reshape the putty, and repeat.

Repeat ____ times

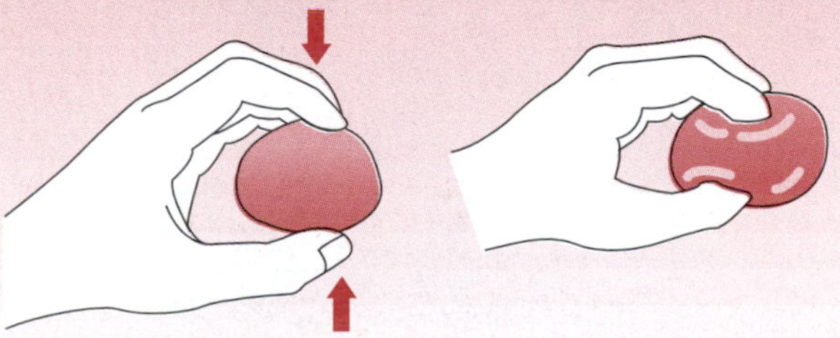

Intervention for muscle endurance impairment focuses on high-repetition, low-resistance exercises for the involved muscles, with appropriate rest periods between sets and repetitions. Particular attention should be given to the posture assumed during performance of these exercises. Wrist extensor strengthening exercises should focus on the position of interest; if the individual functions at work with the wrist in a specific posture, that posture should be assessed and corrected if necessary. Subsequent exercises should focus on strengthening the muscle at the length it will be during functional activity. In contrast, training the wrist extensor muscles in the case of lateral epicondylitis probably must focus on a dynamic range of strengthening, given the wide ROM for most activities producing lateral epicondylitis (eg, tennis, painting, hammering) (see Self-Management: Wrist Extension Exercise With Grocery Bag).

SELF-MANAGEMENT: *Wrist Extension Exercise With Grocery Bag*

Purpose: To increase the strength of your forearm, wrist and hand muscles

Starting position: Find a bag or purse with a narrow handle. A large-handled object can increase your pain. Place objects such as cans or bags of beans in the bag according to the weight recommendations of your clinician. Hold the handle of the bag over the edge of a table with your palm down.

Movement technique:
Level 1: Hold the bag for a count of 10. Rest by setting the bag down or by holding it with your other hand.
Level 2: Raise and lower the bag through a comfortable range.

Repeat ____ times

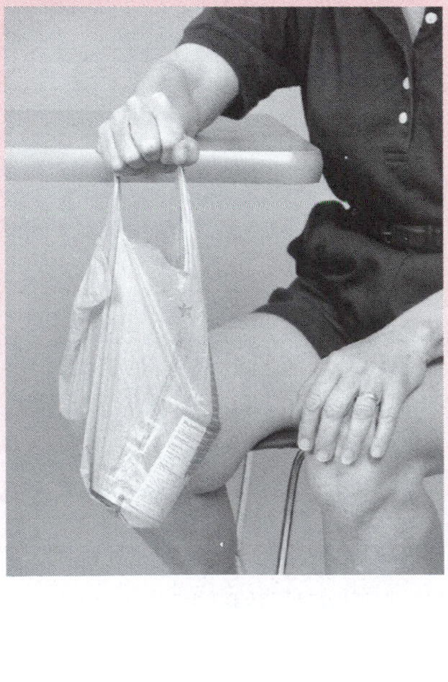

Pain and Inflammation Impairment

Pain and inflammation occur throughout the distal upper extremity for a variety of reasons. Injury or surgery can result in pain and inflammation. Central or local nerve compression usually produces pain locally and pain radiating from the site of compression. Inflammatory conditions such as rheumatoid arthritis or osteoarthritis produce pain and inflammation in the affected joints, and tendinopathies also are painful.

Inflammation is easily detected in this region because of the superficial nature of the structures. The MCP, PIP, and DIP joints in the hand are easily observed for swelling and redness and palpated for warmth and tenderness. Crepitus in tendons such as the APL and EPB tendons in a person with de Quervain's syndrome is readily palpable, as is the local tenderness associated with medial and lateral epicondylitis.

Intervention for inflammation is based on the acuteness of the inflammation (see Chapter 10). Gentle active, active assisted, or passive motion to maintain mobility during the acute phase may be indicated. In some situations, immobilization with splints may be necessary, with occasional removal for gentle mobility activities. After the acute phase has passed, more aggressive activities may be initiated.

Gentle grade I oscillations may be used to decrease pain in some situations. This approach along with ice and other adjunctive agents can decrease pain enough to allow resumption of a therapeutic exercise program.

Posture and Movement Impairment

The most common posture and movement impairments in this region are work- and hobby-related cumulative injuries. Lateral and medial epicondylitis at the elbow and carpal tunnel syndrome (CTS) and de Quervain's tendinitis at the wrist result from impairments in posture and movement. The posture of the wrist and hand influences symptoms at the elbow. Grasping and pinching always cause a flexion moment at the wrist that must be offset by extensor muscle activity. This places loads on the common extensor tendon at the elbow. Hand grip strength is a function of the object's size and the posture of the wrist. For a given size of object, an optimal wrist position for maximum grip strength exists.[20] In the examination of the individual with a disorder related to work or hobbies, the size of the tool and its impact on elbow, wrist, and posture must be considered. These tools can be hobby related (eg, golf club, racquet, gardening tools, knitting needles) or work related (eg, hammers, screwdrivers, shovels, welding tools, sewing tools). When grip is involved, the posture of the upper quarter relative to that tool must be examined. Posture during nongrip activities such as keyboard operating also is important. The guidelines for posture while sitting at a computer work terminal can be found in the Patient-Related Instruction: Computer Workstation Posture.

Movement factors may contribute to injuries in this region. Fatigue during repetitive activity produces changes in movement patterns and subsequent overuse injuries. As

Patient-Related Instruction

Computer Workstation Posture

The following information can help you to evaluate your computer workstation. If you have specific medical problems, consult your clinician for any special needs you may have.

Computer

Correct keyboard position

- Elbows bent at 90 degrees
- Wrists straight or slightly bent up
- Try placing the keyboard on a commercially available keyboard tray with a wrist rest.

Correct monitor position

- About 16 to 22 inches away (about an arm's length)
- Top of the screen even with top of forehead
- Use a stand or adjustable monitor arm to regulate height.

Mouse

Correct mouse position

- Elbows bent at 90 degrees
- Wrist straight or slightly bent up
- Shoulders relaxed and arm at your side
- Elbow supported on armrest if available

Your Work

- Your document and screen should be at similar heights.
- Use a document holder.
- Sit directly in front of the keyboard, monitor, and document holder.

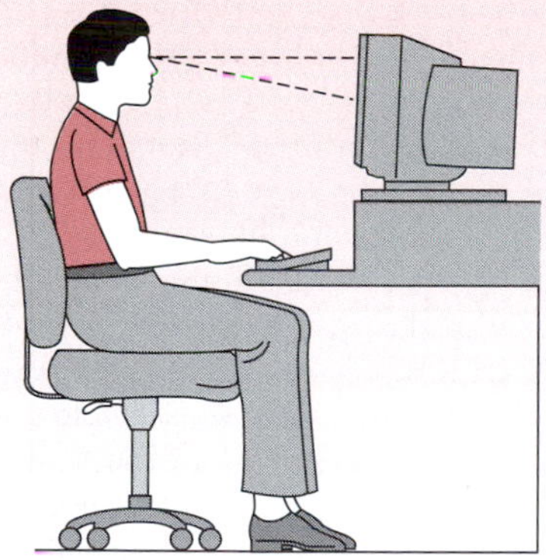

muscles begin to fatigue, the individual has more difficulty controlling force production, and substitution occurs. Substitution may occur with a synergistic muscle or a muscle group more proximal or distal in the kinetic chain. In either case, the primary muscle and the substituting group are vulnerable to overuse injuries. Allowing adequate rest time, using proper tool size, reinforcing good posture, and controlling cycle time, recovery time, and exertion frequency can decrease repetitive loads.

THERAPEUTIC EXERCISE INTERVENTIONS FOR COMMON DIAGNOSES

Cumulative Trauma Disorders

Most musculoskeletal injuries that occur in the workplace are not caused by accidents or acute injuries that sprain ligaments; they result from wear and tear stresses on the musculoskeletal system. Wear and tear injuries are frequently referred to as cumulative trauma disorders (CTDs). There has been a significant increase in the number of reported cases of CTDs in the workplace (Display 27-2). According to the Bureau of Labor Statistics, 23,800 cases were reported in 1972, a number that steadily increased to 332,000 in 1994. In 1995, the number of cases decreased by 7% to 308,000.[21] The clinician working in an outpatient setting may see many patients with this type of disorder.

CTDs are by definition work-related phenomena, although these disorders may also occur with certain hobbies and other nonwork-related activities. The World Health Organization has defined CTDs as being multifactorial in nature, indicating that a number of risk factors contribute to these disorders, including physical risk factors, environment, work organization, and psychosocial, sociocultural, and individual risk factors. Because of the multifactorial nature of CTDs, there is some controversy about the role these risk factors play in the development of CTDs.

Physical risk factors include repetition, awkward postures, prolonged activities, forceful exertions, and fatigue (Display 27-3).[22] The magnitude, duration, and repetition need to be considered for each of these risk factors. Environmental risk factors, such as vibration and cold, may also be present, further complicating the picture. The worker exposed to these factors and not given adequate recovery time may develop a CTD. The worker is unable to recover from the microinjuries or microtrauma that occurs at the tissue level over time. CTDs typically have a slow onset, with only minimal symptoms noticed initially. Many people ignore the early symptoms and do not seek medical attention until the symptoms prevent them from participating in work or in recreational or home activities.

Work may also aggravate or exacerbate an existing health or musculoskeletal problem. For example, forceful gripping

DISPLAY 27-2

Factors Contributing to the Increase in Cumulative Trauma Disorders

- Work pace
- Same task, little variability
- Concentrated forces on smaller physiologic elements
- Decreased time for rest
- Increase in service and high-tech jobs
- Aging workforce
- Reduction in staff turnover
- Increased awareness of the problem

DISPLAY 27-3
Common Characteristics Associated With Cumulative Trauma Disorders

- Work-related: intensity, duration, repetition or cycle time, posture, vibration, force, contact stress, tool geometry
- Mechanical and physiologic processes
- Exacerbation of an existing health problem (eg, rheumatoid arthritis, osteoarthritis)
- Recovery requiring weeks, months, or years
- Multifactorial: work + recreational activity + hobbies
- Fatigue
- Symptoms often poorly localized, nonspecific, and episodic

at work may aggravate a previous sport injury at the elbow, such as lateral epicondylitis. The diagnosis of lateral epicondylitis is frequently used to describe a CTD injury at the elbow involving the lateral extensor mechanism.

Acting alone or in combination, awkward postures, excessive forces, and frequent repetitions may cause mechanical and physiologic stress on the soft tissues. When a person is positioned in an awkward posture, the body is unable to function at an optimal level. For example, wrist deviations may stretch the soft tissue, irritating the tendons and tendon sheaths. When in a lengthened position, the wrist muscles may be unable to exert the required force for the task. When the wrist is in a 45-degree flexed position, the grip strength may be reduced by 40%.[23] The individual may be functioning at a greater percentage of their maximum capabilities. Fatigue is more likely to occur when functioning at a higher percentage of the maximum voluntary contraction. Fatigue, coupled with excessive repetitive motions, may exceed the tendon sheath's capacity to lubricate the tendon, causing increased friction and eventual wear and tear of the tendon.

Workplace design and ergonomics must be carefully evaluated when a patient is diagnosed with a CTD. Ergonomics is the study of fitting the job to the individual. Certain occupational risk factors such as repetitive gripping or forceful pushing with the wrist in an ulnar-deviated position may prevent the person from successfully returning to that job without symptoms recurring. A job analysis or ergonomic analysis should be completed to assess the risk factors present in the individual's work environment. An example is an individual grasping a straight-handled tool such as a knife. This tool and activity places the wrist in an ulnar-deviated position. By angling the tool handle instead of the wrist, the wrist's position is improved. By ensuring appropriate preventive maintenance (eg, sharpening the knife on a timely basis), the stress on the tool operator is decreased.

Nerve Injuries

A variety of nerve injuries occur throughout the elbow, wrist, and hand because of the anatomic structures in the upper extremity and the functional demands in the region. A thorough knowledge of the local anatomy provides a foundation for understanding the impairments found with these nerve injuries.

CARPAL TUNNEL SYNDROME

CTS at the wrist is the most common peripheral compression neuropathy.[19] The carpal tunnel is a small tunnel on the volar aspect of the wrist that is occupied by the median nerve and by nine tendons. The base of the carpal tunnel is formed by the carpal arch, one of three concave arches on the volar aspect of the wrist and hand. The carpal arch is concave on its palmar surface and is spanned by the flexor retinaculum. At this level, the median nerve contains motor fibers innervating the abductor pollicis brevis, the superficial head of the flexor pollicis brevis, the opponens pollicis, and the first and second lumbrical muscles. Sensory fibers provide innervation to the volar thumb and to the index, middle, and one half of the ring fingers.

The average cross-sectional area of the carpal tunnel is 1.7 cm^2 with the wrist in neutral. Pressure in the carpal tunnel varies with wrist position. Normal tissue fluid pressure with the wrist in neutral is 2.5 mm Hg. Passive flexion and extension of the wrist has been shown to increase carpal tunnel pressure significantly.[24] With the wrist in 40 degrees of flexion, the carpal tunnel pressure increases to 47 mm Hg.[24] The mean wrist position associated with the lowest carpal tunnel pressure is approximately 2 degrees of flexion and 3 degrees of ulnar deviation. Wrist extension increases carpal tunnel pressure more than wrist flexion.[24,25] Digital fingertip pressure also increases carpal tunnel pressure.

CTS is caused by a decrease in the size of the carpal tunnel or an increase in the size of its contents, which compresses the median nerve. A single insult (eg, Colles fracture), systemic conditions or disease (eg, pregnancy, diabetes, rheumatoid arthritis), anomalous anatomy, and cumulative trauma within the carpal tunnel (eg, flexor tenosynovitis) can compress the median nerve. Physical factors associated with CTS include repetitive motion, force, mechanical stresses, posture, vibration and temperature. CTS most commonly occurs in women between 40 and 60 years of age.

CTS can manifest with sensory or motor impairments of the median nerve. Diagnosis is based on the presence of one or more common symptoms and on the results of provocative tests. Electrodiagnostic studies can be valuable in confirming the diagnosis and detecting other neuropathies. Associated impairments can include nocturnal pain and numbness, clumsiness when holding small objects, paresthesias in the median nerve distribution, and occasionally pain that radiates proximally. Symptoms of shoulder pain or upper arm pain are not uncommon.[25] Diagnosis is based on the history, a positive Tinel test result, direct compression tests, Phalen's sign, manual muscle testing, sensation testing, upper limb tension tests, and extrinsic muscle length tests.

Intervention for CTS is multifaceted and may include a trial of nonsteroidal antiinflammatory medication, night (and occasionally day) wrist splints positioned at 0 to 15 degrees of extension, patient education regarding body mechanics and ergonomics, and therapeutic exercise (Fig. 27-16). Exercise intervention for CTS focuses on mobility and strengthening without producing an exacerbation. Stretches for the extrinsic and intrinsic muscles are prescribed for several times each day (Fig. 27-17). If working, a patient should perform them before work, on breaks, or after work. They

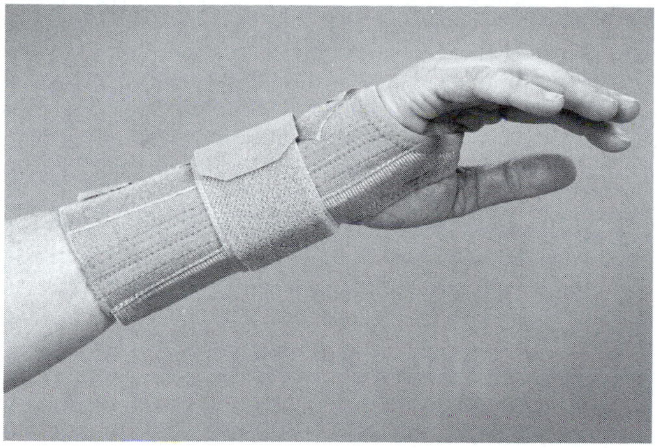

FIGURE 27-16 A wrist splint is used to rest the forearm and wrist musculature.

should be performed slowly and gently; the patient should feel only a gentle stretching sensation. Differential tendon gliding exercises are performed to lubricate and increase gliding of the FPL, FDS, and FDP tendons. These are best performed with the hand elevated to concurrently control local edema. Median nerve gliding exercises and the upper limb tension test with median nerve bias can be used as treatment techniques. The upper limb tension test with median nerve bias requires a position of shoulder girdle depression, shoulder abduction to approximately 110 degrees, forearm supination, wrist and finger extension, and shoulder lateral rotation.[1] After assuming this stretch position while standing, the patient should perform repetitions of elbow flexion and extension or wrist flexion and extension. Strengthening is generally not prescribed for patients with CTS who also have flexor tenosynovitis. If the precipitating factors have been eliminated and weakness creates a functional limitation, resistive exercises are closely monitored. The focus should be on balancing mobility and strength about the wrist.

Patient education is a key intervention in the treatment and prevention of CTS. Patients are instructed to maintain a neutral upper extremity joint position during seated or standing work. This position is accomplished with the wrist in neutral, elbow flexed in the middle range, shoulders relaxed in adduction, scapula slightly depressed and adducted, and the cervical spine positioned with the earlobe in line with the glenohumeral joint. The patient is also instructed to avoid a sustained pinch and grip, especially with the wrist in flexion, and to avoid repetitive overuse of the wrist and fingers. Patients should avoid direct pressure over the carpal tunnel by using a wrist rest or padded table edge (see Patient-Related Instruction: Computer Workstation Posture).

Ergonomic intervention includes use of ergonomic tools that are padded with appropriately sized grips and handles. Data processing station revision should allow an adjustable chair height and keyboard height and tilt. Antivibration gloves are helpful for preoperative and postoperative carpal tunnel release to pad and protect the carpal tunnel and flexor tendons (Fig. 27-18).[25,26]

Modality treatment can also control symptoms and enhance the therapeutic exercise program. Patients may find a decrease in symptoms with use of contrast baths once daily at home. Patients with acute flexor tenosynovitis are seen for several clinic visits that may include phonophoresis of the finger flexor muscles before stretching exercises.

Patients treated acutely for CTS related to flexor tenosynovitis often respond well to conservative treatment without recurrence of symptoms if finger and wrist position and activities are monitored.[25] Conservative treatment is rec-

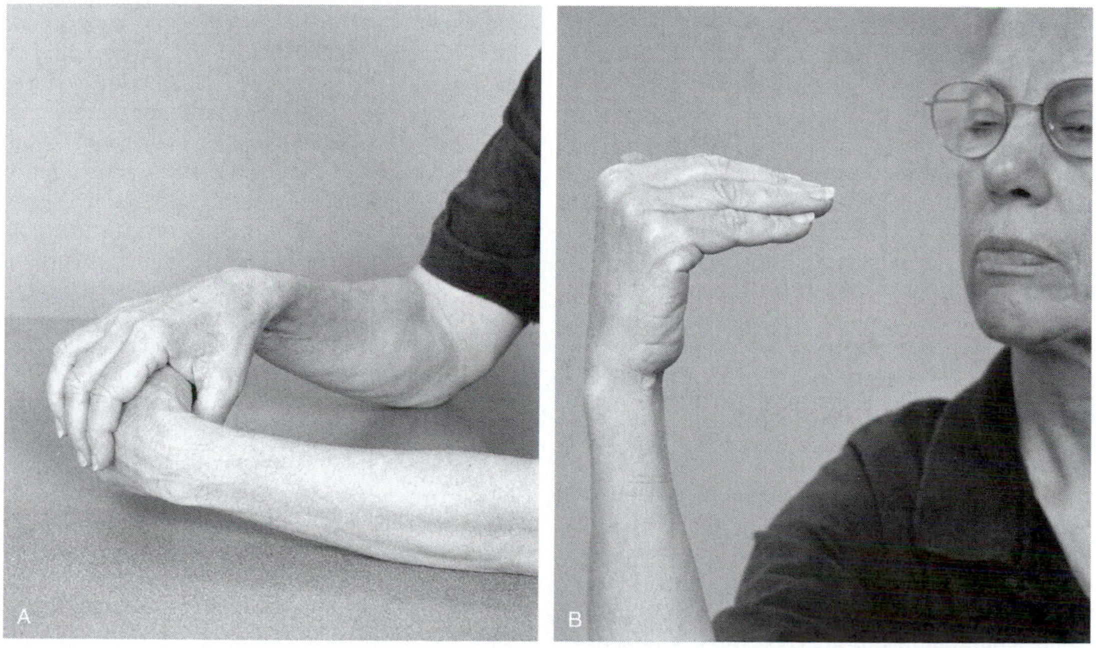

FIGURE 27-17 ***(A)*** Stretching exercise for wrist extensor muscles. ***(B)*** Flexion at the metacarpal joints with extension at the interphalangeal joints can maintain mobility in the extensor digitorum tendon and the collateral ligaments.

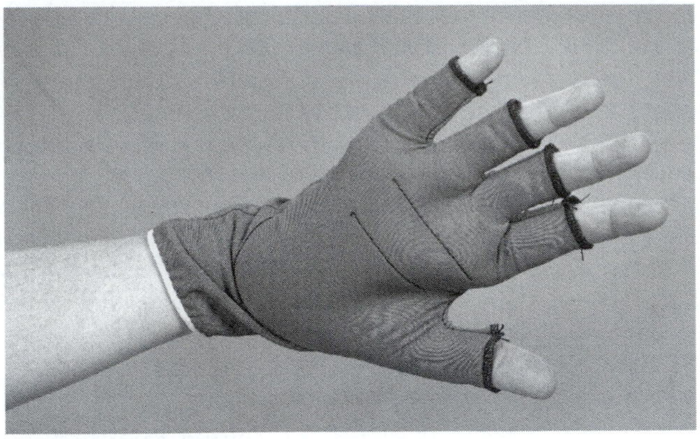

FIGURE 27-18 Antivibration gloves.

ommended for patients with transient symptoms and negative nerve study results. Patients who fail conservative treatment (usually a 3-month trial) often require carpal tunnel release surgery. Studies have shown that the carpal tunnel increases in size with the release of the volar carpal ligament. Symptoms often improve immediately after surgery in mild to moderate cases.

CUBITAL TUNNEL SYNDROME

Cubital tunnel syndrome is the second most common entrapment neuropathy in the upper extremity.[26] This syndrome is characterized by ulnar nerve pathology at the elbow in the absence of trauma. The cubital tunnel is formed by the medial epicondyle, olecranon, medial collateral ligament of the elbow, and a fibrous band called the arcade of Struthers.[27] Several muscles in the wrist and hand are innervated by the ulnar nerve, and the ulnar nerve provides sensation to the dorsal and volar ulnar side of the hand, the fifth finger, and the ulnar half of the ring finger.

Ulnar nerve entrapment may produce nerve injury through ischemia or mechanical deformation of the nerve. These forces can occur from trauma to the elbow, external compression, repetitive elbow motion, or prolonged elbow flexion. The more superficial positions of the sensory fibers within the ulnar nerve at the elbow make them susceptible to compression. With elbow motion, normal nerve excursion has been reported to be as great as 10 mm. Traction on the nerve may occur with repetitive activities such as throwing. The nerve may also undergo increases in traction forces when its excursion is limited by posttraumatic adhesions.[26] Intraneural pressure increases in the cubital tunnel from 7 to 24 mm Hg when moving from elbow extension to flexion. Pressure as high as 209 mm Hg has been recorded in a cubital tunnel patient with elbow flexion and flexor carpi ulnaris contraction.[27]

Symptoms of cubital tunnel syndrome can include aching in the medial forearm and ulnar side of the hand. The aching can radiate proximally or distally. Paresthesias or anesthesias in the ulnar nerve distribution often accompany the pain.[27] Prolonged or repeated end-range elbow flexion tends to exacerbate symptoms. Functional activities eliciting symptoms include sleeping with the elbow flexed at night, combing the hair, driving, or holding the telephone. Leaning on the medial elbow can directly compress the ulnar nerve. Early in the syndrome, patients typically find the paresthesias can be controlled by repositioning the elbow in a more extended position. As the syndrome progresses, functional limitations caused by motor changes cause functional limitations such as difficulty in turning keys, a weak grip and pinch, and dropping objects held in the ulnar side of the hand.

Physical examination focuses on Tinel testing over the ulnar nerve, provocative elbow flexion testing (including direct compression over the cubital tunnel), upper limb tension testing with ulnar nerve bias, observation of muscle bulk and clawing in the fourth and fifth digits, muscle testing, Froment's sign, and sensory testing. The differential diagnoses include C8-T1 nerve root pathology, thoracic outlet syndrome, and compression of the ulnar nerve at Guyon's canal.

Conservative management of cubital tunnel syndrome consists of eliminating all sources of external and dynamic ulnar nerve compression at the elbow, antiinflammatory medication, elbow splinting in 40 to 60 degrees at night, elbow pads, and stretching exercises. Stretching exercises focus on extrinsic flexor and extensor muscles along with ulnar nerve–innervated intrinsic muscle stretches. Nerve gliding techniques may be appropriate for patients with intermittent symptoms. The ulnar nerve's normal longitudinal excursion can be limited by adherence to adjacent structures. Nerve gliding can be achieved by assuming a modified ulnar nerve bias tension test position while standing. This position requires shoulder depression and abduction, wrist extension, and forearm supination, followed by elbow extension.[1] Several repetitions of elbow or wrist flexion and extension can be performed. This intermittent stretch is usually better tolerated than a prolonged stretch (Fig. 27-19).

Key adjunctive interventions are focused on patient education. Posture correction and any necessary proximal stretching or strengthening to maintain posture is indicated when the patient has faulty posture. Short pectoralis minor and weak scapular stabilizers are often observed in individuals working at computers or on assembly lines. The ADLs can be modified to allow rest of the involved arm. Use of the uninvolved arm is encouraged to wash and comb hair, eat, or perform any activity requiring prolonged or repeated elbow flexion. Use of a telephone headset is helpful in cases of frequent or prolonged telephone use. A transcutaneous electrical nerve stimulation unit may provide some relief. Four electrodes can be placed along the ulnar nerve, with two proximal to the cubital tunnel and two distal.

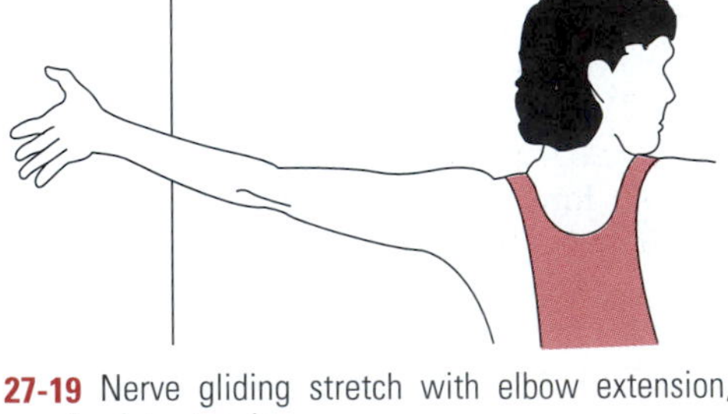

FIGURE 27-19 Nerve gliding stretch with elbow extension, forearm supination, and wrist extension.

If conservative treatment of cubital tunnel syndrome does not reduce or resolve symptoms in 3 months, surgical treatment may be considered. In the absence of clinically identifiable sensory loss or muscle weakness, conservative treatment may be continued indefinitely in the form of a home exercise program. Ulnar nerve transposition surgery involves mobilizing the ulnar nerve at the ulnar groove and anteriorly transposing it subcutaneously, intramuscularly, or submuscularly to the flexor pronator muscle group.

RADIAL TUNNEL SYNDROME

Radial nerve entrapment at the elbow, also called radial tunnel syndrome, is entrapment of the posterior interosseous nerve in one of five locations within the radial tunnel:

- The entrance to the tunnel where fibrous bands encircle the nerve
- The leash of Henry, where the radial recurrent vessels supply the brachioradialis and the ECRL muscles
- The fascia and medial portion of the ECRB tendon
- The arcade of Frohse
- Distally between the tendinous origins of the supinator muscle[11,27]

Radial nerve entrapment occurs much less frequently than median and ulnar nerve compressions. Radial nerve compression may be caused by direct trauma or anatomic structures compressing the nerve. Nerve compression commonly results from repetitive pronation and supination or wrist flexion and extension activities. Occasionally, a single strenuous effort initiates the problem, and subsequent repetitive motion perpetuates it.

The patient with radial tunnel syndrome often has symptoms similar to those produced by lateral epicondylitis. Frequently, these persons have undergone unsuccessful treatment for lateral epicondylitis. Tennis elbow straps may increase symptoms because of additional compression. The most common symptom is that of aching in the extensor-supinator muscle mass that is distal to the lateral epicondyle. Tenderness is approximately 3 inches distal to the lateral epicondyle, with occasional pain radiating distally. No overt sensory deficits are found, because the posterior interosseous nerve contains only motor fibers. A brachial plexus or C7 nerve root injury should be excluded in the differential diagnosis. The upper limb tension test with radial nerve bias may provide additional information.

Intervention for radial tunnel syndrome is conservative, including rest, antiinflammatory medication, therapeutic exercise, and wrist cock-up splinting for 3 to 6 months. The goal of stretching is to restore full extrinsic wrist extensor and flexor muscle length and tendon excursion. If extensor stretches are painful, initial stretches can be performed with the elbow flexed and forearm supinated, followed by fisted wrist flexion. The exercise is progressed until full elbow extension and forearm pronation are achieved with fisted wrist flexion without forcing through pain. Radial nerve gliding techniques may be helpful to encourage adequate nerve gliding from the cervical spine to the wrist and hand level.

Adjunctive treatments include iontophoresis or phonophoresis applied over the supinator or moist heat before stretching. Soft tissue massage to the forearm flexors and extensors may help to relax involved muscles and improve the extensibility and circulation in the area. Activity modifications necessary to prevent recurrence of radial tunnel syndrome include upper extremity use with the forearm in neutral to prevent prolonged stretching or overuse of the supinator muscle. This revision is particularly important in lifting tasks. Job rotation or diversification can prevent prolonged use of the extensor-supinator muscle group.

Functional outcomes after conservative management of radial tunnel syndrome are difficult to determine because of the challenge in identifying the correct diagnosis, the relative rarity of the syndrome, and the frequent surgical intervention in clearly diagnosed cases. The clinician should be alert to radial tunnel syndrome as a differential diagnosis in cases of recalcitrant lateral epicondylitis. When radial tunnel is properly diagnosed, surgery is often the treatment of choice. Patients commonly are seen postoperatively for scar and pain management, stretching, and strengthening programs.

Musculoskeletal Disorders

LATERAL EPICONDYLITIS

Lateral epicondylitis is the most common problem seen in the lateral elbow. The incidence of lateral epicondylitis in recreational and professional tennis players is 39% to 50%.[28] Although "tennis elbow" is the common name for this problem, lateral epicondylitis is seen as frequently in persons who are not tennis players. Any individual using hand tools for work or an avocation are susceptible to developing symptoms. The combination of continuous grip along with repeated wrist and elbow activity precipitates symptoms.

Wrist extension is accomplished by the combined actions of the ECRL, ECRB, and ECU. These muscles all originate on the lateral epicondyle of the humerus, including the supracondylar ridge. These wrist extensors insert distal to the carpus onto the second, third, and fifth metacarpal bones, respectively. The lateral epicondyle is also the origin of the extensor digitorum and extensor digiti minimi, which insert into the extensor mechanism.

Of the extensor muscles involved in lateral epicondylitis, the ECRB is generally the greatest contributor to symptoms.[29] The ECRB may be involved in 100% of cases, and the EDC is involved in 30% of cases.[29] The wrist is stabilized by the extensors working in synergy with the flexors. Biomechanical models have shown that grasping and pinching tasks always produce a flexion moment at the wrist that must be countered by the wrist extensors. Many tasks requiring use of hand tools or writing instruments require wrist extensor activity. Because optimal hand function occurs when the hand is in a complete fist and the wrist is extended 15 to 20 degrees, the grip size of the implement and the resting posture of the wrist can have a great impact on producing and alleviating symptoms.

Individuals with lateral epicondylitis describe pain with any activity that requires gripping and lifting, such as shaking hands, lifting a carton of milk, or turning doorknobs. Use of hand tools, writing, and lifting bags also produce common symptoms. Tenderness to palpation over the lateral epicondyle is common, and pain with resisted wrist extension is painful.

The treatment of choice for lateral epicondylitis is conservative, consisting of relative rest, occasional bracing, inflammation control, and therapeutic exercise. Exercise includes stretching to restore the normal length of the musculotendinous unit. Stretching the wrist into flexion and pronation should reproduce a sensation of tightness in the forearm. Reproduction of pain at the elbow indicates that stretching is too vigorous. Strengthening should be initiated at a level that keeps loading within the optimal loading zone (see Chapter 10). Because the wrist extensors work during wrist extension and gripping, the clinician must approach use of hand-held weights cautiously. The initial strengthening program may include gripping and wrist extension as separate exercises, gradually progressing to concurrent wrist extension and gripping (Fig. 27-20). Depending on the symptoms, the program may begin with isometric muscle contractions and progress to dynamic concentric and eccentric exercises.

Adjunctive interventions include therapeutic modalities such as ice, phonophoresis, or iontophoresis and as cross-friction massage and bracing. Bracing may include a counterforce brace such as a tennis elbow strap or a wrist splint (Fig. 27-21). A counterforce brace decreases loads on the extensor origin by creating a new origin of the muscle that bypasses the inflamed portion of the tendon. Counterforce bracing also limits the maximum contraction of the muscles, thereby decreasing forces. A wrist splint can limit wrist extensor activity necessary by providing an external stabilization to the wrist. Patient education regarding home and work ergonomics should be provided. Lifting with the forearm supinated decreases wrist extensor muscle activity. Tasks should be modified to limit repetitive elbow and wrist motion when possible. Judicious use of cortisone injections by the physician can decrease inflammation.

When conservative management of lateral epicondylitis fails, surgical management may be considered. Nirschl[28] observed that most patients have inadequate and fragmented conservative treatment plans. Good documentation and appropriate follow-up care are necessary to ensure that all conservative measures have been appropriately exhausted before surgery is considered.

MEDIAL EPICONDYLITIS

Medial epicondylitis is encountered less frequently than lateral epicondylitis and accounts for 10% to 20% of all epicondylitis cases.[27] The muscles involved are the flexor-pronator group, including the flexor carpi radialis, palmaris longus, pronator teres, and flexor carpi ulnaris. Repetitive wrist flexion in recreational activities such as golf or fly fishing or at work subject the common wrist extensors to overuse. Affected persons usually describe pain at the medial epicondyle with resisted wrist flexion and forearm pronation. Passive stretch into extension and supination also may reproduce symptoms.

Management of medial epicondylitis is conservative, with a focus on controlled activity matched with appropriate rest, stretching and strengthening exercises, and interventions to reduce pain and inflammation. Therapeutic exercises include stretching for the flexor and pronator muscles, as long as stretching does not reproduce elbow symptoms (Fig. 27-22). As symptoms resolve, a progressive strengthening program with an emphasis on the demands specific to the individual patient is implemented. Therapeutic modalities such as ice, iontophoresis, and phonophoresis and physician-prescribed medications (when indicated) can provide relief from the pain and inflammation. This intervention creates a better environment in which the therapeutic exercise program can be more effective. When conservative management fails, surgical resection of the diseased portion of the tendon may be undertaken.

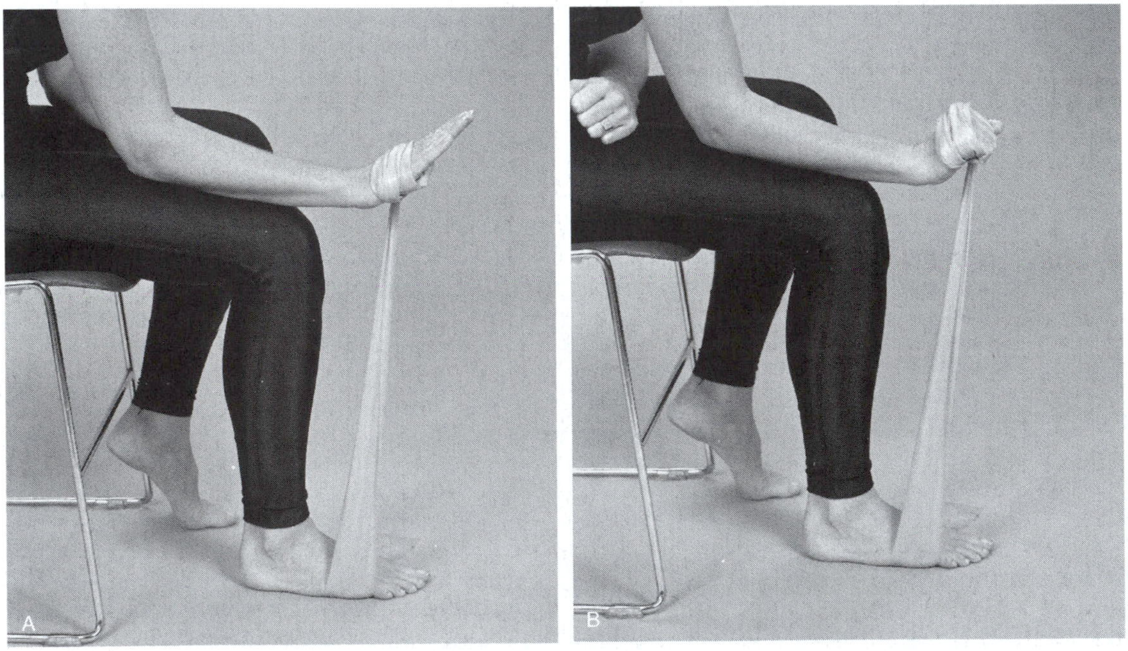

FIGURE 27-20 Wrist extension exercises. ***(A)*** Without grip. ***(B)*** With grip.

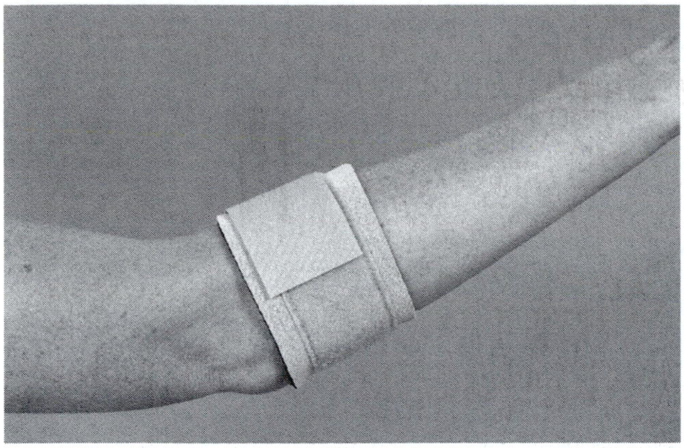

FIGURE 27-21 Tennis elbow strap.

DE QUERVAIN'S SYNDROME

De Quervain's syndrome, also called stenosing tenosynovitis, is an inflammation of the tendons of the first dorsal wrist compartment. The muscles in this compartment are the EPB and APL. The most common cause is overuse of the hand and wrist, particularly in movements requiring radial deviation while the thumb is stabilized in a grip.[30] Women are affected about 3 to 10 times more often than men.

Persons with de Quervain's syndrome notice pain on the radial aspect of the wrist in the region of the radial styloid. Flexing the thumb across the palm is quite painful, and resisted extension and abduction may be painful as well. Palpable tenderness and bogginess may be noticed over the tendons of the first compartment. Radial and ulnar deviation may produce clicking or pain. The Finkelstein test is the most commonly used test to diagnose de Quervain's syndrome. Measurements may reveal that pinch and grip are weak and painful.

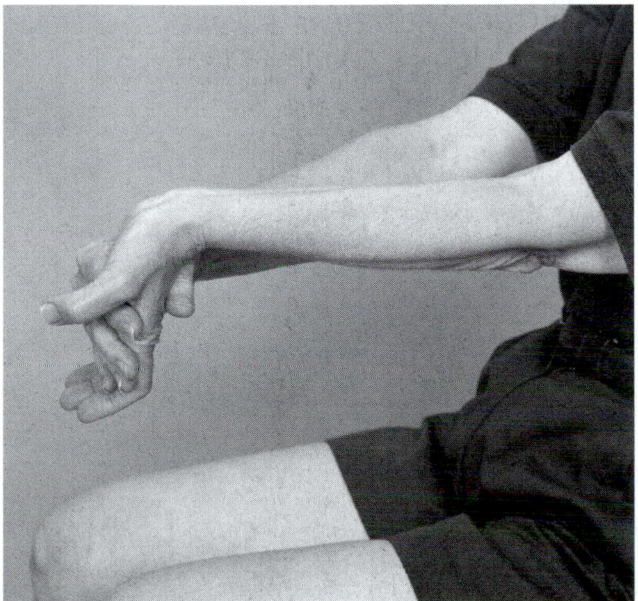

FIGURE 27-22 Wrist flexor stretch.

Therapeutic exercise intervention for de Quervain's syndrome includes stretching for the EPB and APL and the extrinsic wrist flexor and extensor muscles. Strengthening should be initiated after full pain-free ROM has been achieved. Strengthening includes the thumb and wrist musculature and full gripping exercises. To prevent further overuse to these tendons during the initiation of a rehabilitation program, immobilization using a forearm base thumb spica splint may be necessary. The splint should be worn during symptomatic times or periods of high activity. The splint is removed to perform exercises throughout the day.

Other adjunctive measures include cross-friction massage over the first dorsal compartment. Work, hobby, or sport modifications to decrease the frequency and forces involved with wrist and thumb motion may be necessary. Therapeutic modalities to reduce inflammation such as ice and iontophoresis may be helpful. The physician may place the patient on an antiinflammatory medication, inject the area with steroid or analgesic medication, or surgically release of the first dorsal compartment. Patient education to avoid or limit situations contributing to the symptoms is essential to prevention of recurrence.

TRIGGER FINGER

Trigger finger, also known as digital tenovaginitis stenosans, is a result of thickening of the flexor tendon sheath. Thickening causes catching of the tendon as the finger actively flexes.[16] The flexor tendons of the fingers have an intricate anatomy that includes a synovial sheath extending from the mid-metacarpal area to the DIP joints. Overlying the sheath are a series of annular and cruciform fibrous bands or pulleys. These pulleys hold the flexor tendons close to the metacarpals and phalangeal bones, thereby improving the efficiency of motion. Thickening of the sheath at the A-1 pulley (ie, fibrous band that overlays the synovial sheath at the MCP joint level) and enlargement of the flexor tendons are the basis for the symptoms found. This thickening may be cause by repetitive trauma or by direct pressure over the MCP joint in the palm, as when grasping.

Impairments associated with trigger finger include pain and tenderness in the finger from the volar MCP to the PIP level and intermittent triggering or "snapping" of the finger. The triggering usually occurs with flexion, and it may require passive assist to fully extend the finger.

Intervention for trigger finger is usually conservative and involves active IP flexion and tendon gliding exercises on an hourly basis. Ultrasound, massage, and icing can be used to relieve symptoms of pain and swelling. Splinting is common, and the hand-based splint or digital splint holds the MCP joint at full extension while leaving all other joints free. The splint is worn at all times for 1 to 3 weeks. Thereafter, it is worn for periods of high activity. The splint prevents triggering at the A-1 pulley and rest to minimize inflammation. The physician may inject into the synovial sheath at the level of the A-1 pulley to decrease local inflammation.

If conservative management is unsuccessful, surgery may be performed to release the A-1 pulley. Postoperative therapeutic intervention includes the same active exercise program and potential splinting as conservative management. Progressive grip strengthening may be required to return the patient to full functional use of the hand for work and ADLs. Education and work modification to avoid or limit repetitive grasping and releasing activities of the hand also are necessary.

TENDON LACERATION

Tendon lacerations and repair require a complex series of treatments that must account for wound healing, tendon healing, and surgical techniques. Tendon repair treatment is complicated by the need for tendon excursion to prevent adhesions while allowing stability and protection to the healing tendon. Controlled motion helps prevent tendon adhesion, which limits motion and therefore limits function. Too much motion may compromise the repair. The clinician must provide a system of controlled motion, based on physician preference, surgical technique, mechanism of injury, and patient adherence.

The extensor tendons are divided into 8 zones, which determine treatment protocol used. Because of the extensiveness of each protocol, we review only the highlights for each zone (Fig. 27-23).[31] In zones I and II, laceration causes a mallet finger. A mallet finger splint is fitted to the patient's DIP joint in 0 to 15 degrees of hyperextension from postoperative day 1 through 6 weeks. The PIP joint is left free to allow movement at the PIP level and proximally. The DIP joint should not be allowed to flex during this time. AROM exercises are initiated at 6 weeks, with PROM started at 7 to 8 weeks. Strengthening is started after 8 weeks with monitoring for an extensor lag. If a lag is present, the patient returns to wearing the splint and AROM.

For zones III and IV, a digital gutter splint is fabricated to include the DIP and PIP joints (MCP is left free) at 2 weeks after surgery. At 4 weeks, AROM is begun, and a 6 weeks, PROM is begun. Treatment must be modified if an extensor lag develops. Gentle strengthening is begun after 8 weeks.

For zone V (distal to tendonae junctionae), a hand-based splint is custom fabricated at 3 days to 1 week. This hand-based splint holds the MCP in 70 to 80 degrees of flexion and the digit in full extension. This position prevents contracture of the lateral bands at the MCP. AROM, PROM, and strengthening are continued as for zones III and IV.

For zones V (proximal to tendonae junctionae), VI, VII, and VIII, a volar forearm splint is fabricated at 3 to 5 days postoperatively. This splint extends from just proximal to the PIP joint, crosses the MCP joint, and continues two thirds of the way up the forearm, with the wrist positioned in 30 degrees of extension. This allows controlled movement of the extensor tendons through PIP and DIP joint movement, which prevents tendon adhesions. AROM, PROM, and strengthening exercises are continued as for the more distal zones.

Flexor tendon repairs also rely on zones to determine the appropriate protocol. There are five flexor tendon zones (see Fig. 27-23*B*). Current treatment protocols focus on controlled motion to prevent scar adhesions that limit functional movement. They also rely on the use of a dorsal blocking splint to prevent disruption of the surgical repair. This dorsal blocking splint is custom fabricated with the wrist in 20 degrees of flexion, the MCPs in 50 degrees of flexion, and the PIP and DIPs in full extension.[31]

The program for zones I, II, and III consists of passive flexion and extension motion at the PIP and DIP joints and composite passive flexion and extension at the MCP, PIP,

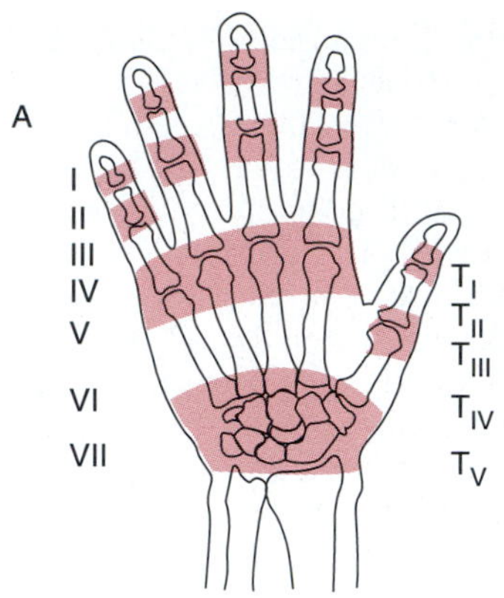

Zones of extensor tendon injury:

I — DIP joint and distal phalanx
II — Middle phalanx
III — PIP joint
IV — Proximal phalanx
V — MP joint
VI — Metacarpal bone
VII — Wrist
T_I — IP joint and distal phalanx of the thumb
T_{II} — Proximal phalanx of the thumb
T_{III} — Thumb MP joint
T_{IV} — Metacarpal bone of the thumb
T_V — Wrist

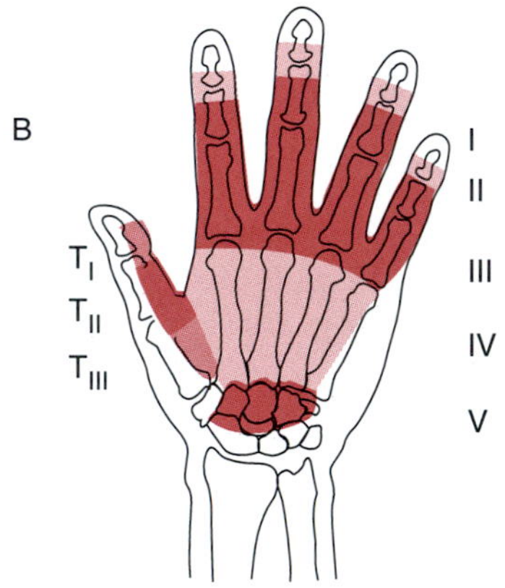

Zones of flexor tendon injury:

I — Distal to the FDS insertion
II — Between the A_1 pulley and the FDS insertion
III — Area between the distal carpal tunnel border and the A_1 pulley
IV — Within the carpal tunnel
V — Proximal to the carpal tunnel
T_I — From the thumb IP joint distally
T_{II} — Between the thumb A_1 pulley and the IP joint
T_{III} — Area of the first metacarpal bone

FIGURE 27-23 ***(A)*** Extensor tendon zones of the hand. ***(B)*** Flexor tendon zones of the hand.

and DIP joints within the confines of the splint. This program is started on postoperative day 1 or 2 and continued through week 5.[31] AROM is started at 3.5 weeks, PROM into extension is begun at 6 weeks, and strengthening is started at 8 weeks. Full functional use is allowed at 10 to 12 weeks postoperatively. The program for zones I, II, and III uses the dorsal blocking splint with rubber-band traction. The addition of a palmar pulley allows for greater FDP tendon excursion. The rubber band traction holds the digit into near full composite flexion, and the patient is instructed to extend the finger against the force of the rubber band to the dorsal blocking splint. The patient is instructed to do this 20 to 30 times per hour. This protocol is initiated 2 to 6 days postoperatively. AROM is started 5 weeks postoperatively, with PROM into extension started 7 to 8 weeks postoperatively. Strengthening is performed after 8 weeks.[31]

For zones IV and V, both protocols are overall as previously delineated, but they progress faster. AROM is initiated at 3 weeks within the dorsal blocking splint. AROM out of the splint occurs at 4 weeks. PROM into extension and strengthening is initiated at 6 weeks. A four-strand suture technique allows controlled active movement beginning on postoperative day 2. A wrist-hinged dorsal blocking splint is used to allow a tenodesis movement where the digits are held at the end range by active digit contraction. PROM may be used to achieve full composite flexion. This splint and active motion is continued until week 8, with full active and passive exercise and strengthening started at that time.[31]

Bone and Joint Injuries

MEDIAL ELBOW INSTABILITY

Medial elbow instability is seen in children and adults and is found most often in individuals involved in throwing. High forces on the medial elbow structures during the cocking and acceleration phases can result in attenuation and rupture of the static ligamentous structures. In the adult, acute rupture of the UCL can occur. More often, continued valgus loading and loss of dynamic muscular support places loads on the UCL, leading to gradual instability. Progressive instability can lead to rupture or tension of the ulnar nerve.

In the child or adolescent, medial elbow instability is commonly known as "little league elbow." The growth plate and associated ligamentous and tendinous structures are at risk until the fusion at the growth plate is complete. In the child, the valgus stress on the medial side of the elbow is countered with a compressive force on the lateral side at the radiocapitellar joint. This can lead to compression and shearing of the radial head on the capitellum. Osteochondrosis of the capitellum can occur with loose body formation.

Treatment of the child or adult with valgus instability depends on the pathologic stage. Controlled rest is essential, along with strengthening exercises for the involved musculature. Dynamic support of the medial elbow to minimize loads on the static structures is a critical component of the treatment program. This approach includes strengthening the trunk, shoulder, elbow, forearm, and wrist muscles (Fig. 27-24). Proximal weakness can transfer loads distally, and a rotator cuff problem can produce instability problems at the elbow. In addition to strengthening, consideration of throwing form and the throwing schedule (eg, number of throws, games, inning) is important to prevent a recurrence of the problem.

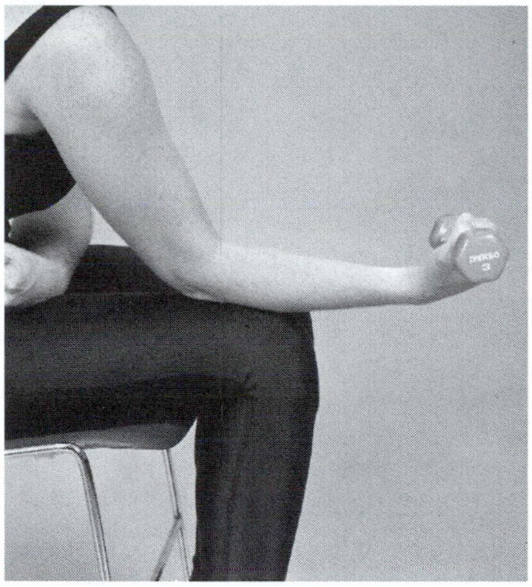

FIGURE 27-24 Wrist flexor muscle strengthening.

ELBOW DISLOCATIONS

Elbow dislocations are second in incidence only to dislocations of the shoulder in the adult population. The elbow is the most frequently dislocated joint in children younger than 10 years of age.[32] Elbow dislocations are classified by the direction of movement of the radius and ulna on the humerus, and most are posterior. A fall on an outstretched hand or hyperextension are the most common mechanisms of injury. Dislocation also can injure the UCL, the lateral collateral ligament, the anterior capsule, and common flexor and extensor muscle origins or fracture the medial epicondyle. The ulnar, median, or radial nerves may be injured. After dislocation, the elbow is reduced (and stabilized if necessary) and immobilized for 1 to 2 weeks.

Impairments after dislocation include loss of motion, pain, inability to produce torque, and occasionally neurovascular problems. Restoration of full motion may be difficult and should be a priority in the treatment program. Many patients retain a residual loss of extension of 10 to 15 degrees, and full recovery of motion and strength took 3 to 6 months for most patients.[33]

Intervention after dislocation include AROM and assisted AROM initiated 2 to 7 days after the dislocation and PROM 2 weeks after the dislocation. Motion should be performed in a variety of shoulder positions. Dynamic splinting may be necessary to restore motion. Prefabricated splints are available to restore flexion or extension. A static night splint can maintain current range if a dynamic splint cannot be tolerated all night. Caution is necessary to avoid overly aggressive PROM, because it may contribute to heterotopic bone formation. Individuals with head injuries or those with a combined fracture-dislocation with prolonged immobilization face the greatest risk of heterotopic bone formation.

Isometric muscle contractions are initiated early and progressed to dynamic contractions as tolerated (Fig. 27-25). Open and closed chain exercises and proprioceptive neuro-

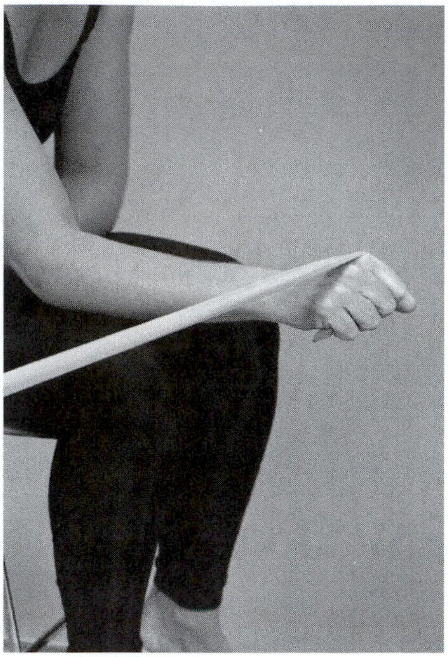

FIGURE 27-25 Resisted pronation using a band.

muscular facilitation techniques are useful for restoration of function. If instability is present, a hinged elbow support with extension blocks may allow functional use of the elbow within a limited range. Exercises are performed throughout the day, in or out of the brace. If the patient has hypomobility, joint mobilization techniques can help restore full elbow and forearm mobility.

CARPAL INSTABILITY

The body and ligamentous anatomy of the wrist is intricately balanced to allow flexibility and stability. Williams[2] observed that the carpal bones are spring loaded like a jack-in-the-box and kept under control by ligament restraints. The palmar ligaments are very substantial compared with the dorsal wrist ligaments. An area between the capitate and lunate where no ligamentous support is maintained is an area of potential weakness.

Many types and descriptions of static and dynamic carpal patterns exist. Static instability patterns demonstrate radiographic changes such as abnormal gapping between carpal bones. A static instability generally indicates a significant injury such as a complete ligament tear. Dynamic instability patterns are detected during the physical examination or with special imaging techniques. Dynamic instability patterns generally indicate increased laxity or partial ligament tears. Scapholunate dissociation is the most common form of carpal instability and occurs when ligaments from the proximal pole of the scaphoid are torn. This injury can occur from a fall on an extended, ulnarly deviated wrist; degeneration due to rheumatoid arthritis; a direct blow to the wrist; or in association with a distal radius fracture, carpal fracture, or carpal dislocation.

Impairments associated with a scapholunate dissociation include point tenderness over the involved ligament, swelling of the dorsal wrist, pain or limited AROM and PROM of the wrist, a painful click or clunk with radial deviation, grip weakness, and decreased wrist and hand function because of pain. In addition to routine examination procedures such as documentation of pain with rest and functional activities, ROM, and strength of the forearm, wrist, and hand musculature, the clinician should assess grip and pinch strength. Grip strength is performed with a dynamometer at the standard setting, with five settings used to demonstrate a bell-shaped curve and rapid alternating grip strength. Lateral and three-point pinch strength is also assessed.

Severe instabilities are treated with surgical reduction and ligament reconstruction. Fusions may also be performed for a number of carpal instability patterns. After surgery or for mild cases of instability, the patient is referred for rehabilitative management.

Therapeutic exercises for carpal instability include grip and pinch strengthening exercises. Putty exercises and isolated muscle strengthening exercises are incorporated to restore strength and dynamic function throughout the region. With a lunate dislocation and ligament injury, a painful grip may indicate instability leading to lunate destruction. In this situation, grip strengthening should be avoided. Any mobility deficits are treated with active, passive, and active assisted ROM.

Intervention for carpal instability also includes protective splinting of the wrist. The thumb MCP is included in cases of scaphoid involvement, such as scapholunate dissociation. If the ligament disruption is on the ulnar side of the wrist, a wrist cock-up or ulnar gutter splint suffices. Therapeutic modalities may be used for pain and inflammation, and patient education is a critical component of successful management.

GAMEKEEPER'S THUMB

The MCP joint of the thumb functions primarily in flexion and extension because of the condyloid shape of the joint surface. Small degrees of abduction, adduction, and rotation also occur. Tautness in the UCL limits abduction and extension and adds stability to the joint in a functional position. However, this functional position also places the UCL at risk for injury. The most common injuries to the thumb MCP involve the UCL.

Gamekeeper's thumb, or a sprain to the UCL of the MCP joint, is the result of abduction or hyperextension forces. This injury occurs frequently in skiing when a fall catches the thumb in the strap of the ski pole, pulling the thumb into abduction. Complete ruptures lead to instability and significant disability. A thorough examination, with valgus stress performed in extension (collateral ligament and volar plate) and flexion (collateral ligament only), should be done to differentiate partial from complete tears. Impairments associated with gamekeeper's thumb include tenderness along the ulnar aspect of the MCP joint, localized edema, and instability of the joint.

Treatment of partial tears requires immobilization in a thumb spica cast for 3 weeks, followed by a thumb spica splint (Fig. 27-26). The splint is removed throughout the day to allow exercise of the wrist and hand. Acute injuries with gross instability require surgical stabilization. Therapeutic exercise after immobilization after surgical and nonsurgical treatment include pain-free thumb MCP flexion

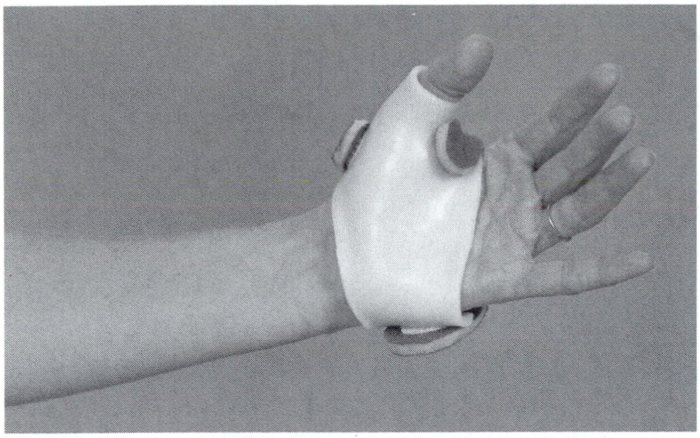

FIGURE 27-26 Thumb spica splint.

and extension and gradually adding pain-free rotation and opposition. After 4 to 6 weeks, grip and pinch strengthening exercises are initiated with putty or gripper equipment (see Self-Management: Thumb Press). Lateral (key) pinch is initiated, but the patient should be instructed to limit or avoid tip pinch stress until 6 to 8 weeks. Exercises should be progressed to activities pertinent to the patient's lifestyle as quickly as possible within the constraints of healing.

OLECRANON FRACTURES

Olecranon fractures are generally the result of a direct blow or a fall. A fall on an outstretched hand with the elbow in flexion, followed by a strong contraction of the triceps, can cause an olecranon fracture. A nondisplaced fracture is immobilized in 45 to 90 degrees of flexion for a short time. A displaced fracture may be treated with open reduction and internal fixation (ORIF) using tension band wiring or plate and screw fixation. A small comminuted fracture may be excised with reattachment of the triceps tendon. Excision of loose bodies is required during surgery to prevent a loss of mobility from these fragments. The impairments seen after fracture or surgery are pain, limited ROM, and loss of the ability to produce torque. The proximity of the ulnar nerve makes it vulnerable to injury in a olecranon fracture. Close examination is necessary to assess the status of the nerve.

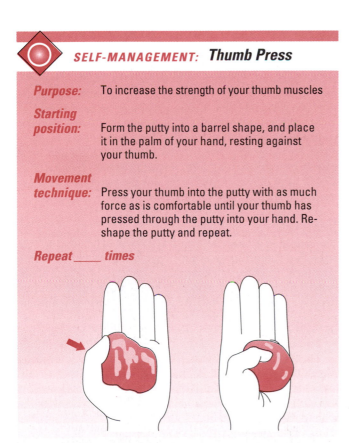

Intervention after fracture begins with AROM in a forearm neutral position. AROM and assisted AROM may be initiated as early as 2 days after fracture. These individuals usually are immobilized, and the immobilization is removed for ROM activities. The length of immobilization is decreased for the elderly, and ROM exercise is initiated sooner.[25,34] Active ROM is progressed to assisted AROM and PROM.

The biceps muscle often shortens because of the flexed elbow position during immobilization or protection periods. Suggested forms of exercise to restore muscle length include elbow and shoulder extension, walking with a normal arm swing, and contract-relax stretching.

The adaptive shortening may result in weakness, and strength should be addressed concurrently. Suggested strengthening exercises include isometric contractions throughout the available range for all major muscle groups, resistive band exercises for shoulder musculature, resisted elbow flexion in a variety of forearm positions, resisted elbow extension, and resisted wrist and forearm exercises. A stationary bicycle with combined arm movements or a cross-country ski machine allowing repetitive elbow flexion and extension is helpful to restore motion and strength. If forearm rotation strength is limited, a light hammer can be used to train pronation and supination (Fig. 27-27).

Adjunctive interventions include elevation, ice, and active shoulder, wrist, and finger exercises to control edema. Scar massage should be initiated early after surgical stabilization. Generally, the scar is mature enough to tolerate massage 10 to 14 days postoperatively. The triceps may become adherent to the scar and should be treated with cross-friction massage and triceps resistive exercises. Joint mobilization with distraction may be initiated in later stages if loss of motion is a problem. The prognosis after an olecranon fracture is good, but loss of terminal extension is a common residual impairment.

RADIAL HEAD FRACTURE

Radial head fractures occur most often as a result of falls on an outstretched hand with the forearm in supination. These fractures also occur in combination with dislocation. The individual with a radial head fracture has pain over the radial head in the lateral elbow, and forearm rotation is painful. A nondisplaced fracture can be treated with sling immobilization for 1 to 2 days, while a displaced fracture may be treated with ORIF. For severe fractures, the radial head may be excised. Any pathology at the distal radioulnar joint can complicate this form of treatment. The patient

SELF-MANAGEMENT: **Thumb Press**

Purpose: To increase the strength of your thumb muscles

Starting position: Form the putty into a barrel shape, and place it in the palm of your hand, resting against your thumb.

Movement technique: Press your thumb into the putty with as much force as is comfortable until your thumb has pressed through the putty into your hand. Reshape the putty and repeat.

Repeat ____ times

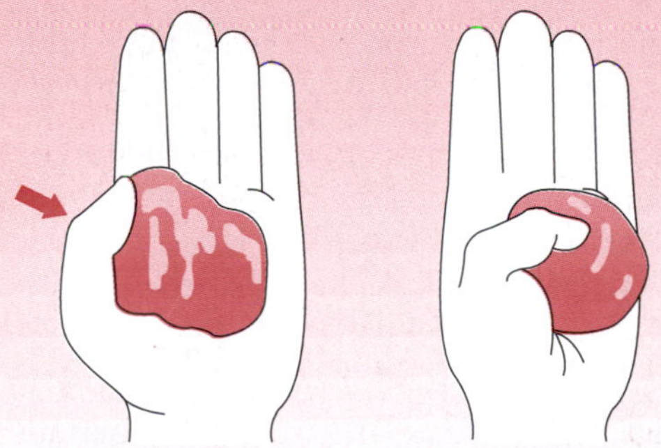

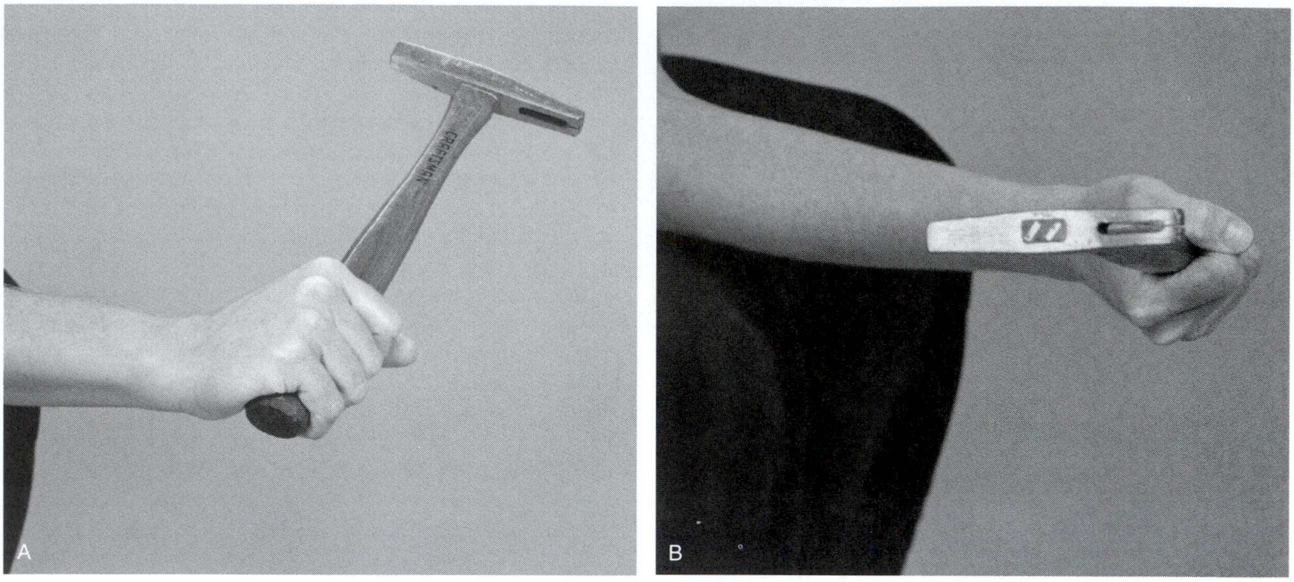

FIGURE 27-27 Range of motion of the forearm using a hammer. ***(A)*** Pronation. ***(B)*** Supination.

may be immobilized with the forearm in neutral but allowing elbow ROM (ie, sugar tong or Muenster splint) for 2 to 3 weeks.

The most common impairment after a radial head fracture is a loss of 10 to 20 degrees of elbow extension. Crepitus or clicking at the radial head may occur with supination and pronation.

Treatment of a nondisplaced radial head fracture includes initiation of elbow and forearm AROM 1 week after injury. Successful treatment demands early ROM. The progression is similar to that for olecranon fractures. After ORIF of displaced fractures, motion may begin immediately postoperatively, barring any secondary injuries. Strengthening and functional use of the limb should be progressed as for other upper extremity injuries.

COLLES FRACTURE

The distal radius is fractured more frequently than any other bone in the body.[19] The Colles fracture is a dorsally angulated fracture of the distal radius with or without concurrent ulnar fracture. This fracture occurs most often from falling on an outstretched hand. The volarly angulated distal radius fracture is known as a Smith's fracture. The Colles fracture is initially treated with closed reduction and cast immobilization in an above-elbow cast to prevent pronation and supination or with ORIF. If healing is progressing well, a short forearm cast may be applied after 2 weeks.

The major impairments after cast removal are pain, decreased mobility and strength, and swelling. Control of edema is critical to prevent a stiff hand. Elevation, ice, edema massage, and compression garments can be used to reduce edema. Education about controlling edema must be emphasized to prevent further complications.

Restoration of mobility is essential for full functioning of the hand. The priority in the early phase of mobility exercises should be to regain wrist flexion, extension, and supination, because these are usually the most limited motions and important for a functional outcome (see Self-Management: Finger and Wrist Flexor Stretching). Exercises should include AROM and self-PROM techniques using the opposite extremity. If mobility remains limited, joint mobilization may facilitate gains in ROM. When dealing with complicated Colles fractures, splinting may be necessary to maintain gains in ROM achieved while at rest or at night or to assist in increasing mobility. Static splinting provides support and maintains range between exercise sessions. This may be supplied by prefabricated wrist supports or custom-made splints. Dynamic splinting may also be of value in cases of limited mobility. These splints include a constant or variable tension across the wrist, forearm, or both areas to facilitate increasing motion in the direction desired. Many commercial devices are available, or a custom splint may be fabricated.

Strengthening exercises may be initiated with isometric contractions, grip strengthening, and resisted elbow exercises. As range improves, dynamic exercises for the wrist may be employed using free weights or resistive bands (Fig. 27-28). The clinician must consider the patient's preinjury status to establish relevant goals.

SCAPHOID FRACTURE

The scaphoid is often fractured as a result of a fall on an outstretched hand but goes unrecognized. Individuals often pass these fractures off as sprains because of the lack of obvious deformity. The scaphoid is highly susceptible to injury because of its shape and its position. Its narrow midline makes it more vulnerable to stress, and its position crosses the two rows of carpal bones, predisposing it to more frequent injury.

The individual with a scaphoid fracture relates a history of a fall on or other trauma to an extended wrist, with subsequent pain and loss of motion. Pain is particularly apparent with any overpressure in extension, such as in pushing a heavy door open. Athletes are unable to bench press because of the pressure into wrist extension. Palpable tenderness over the anatomic snuffbox and painful extension warrant medical evaluation.

SELF-MANAGEMENT: *Finger and Wrist Flexor Stretching*

Purpose: To increase the mobility of the soft tissues in your wrist and hand

Starting position: With your palm facing up and wrist at the edge of a table

Movement technique: Using your other hand, gently press your wrist and fingers down toward the floor. Hold 15 to 30 seconds, relax, and repeat.

Repeat ____ times

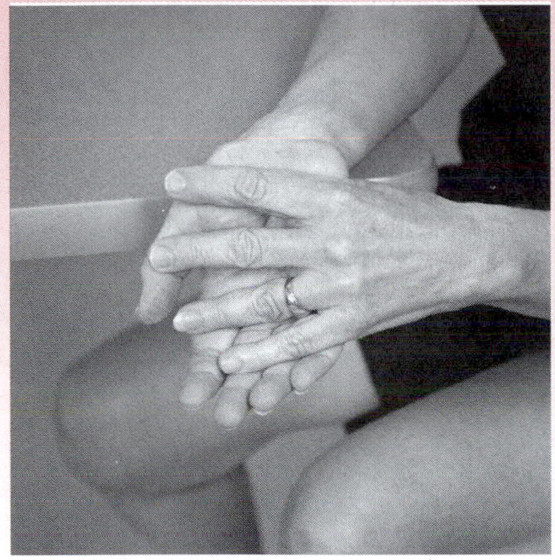

Medical intervention for scaphoid fractures is immobilization for 8 to 12 weeks. Because the poor vascular supply predisposes the scaphoid to nonunion, these fractures are treated conservatively. If the fracture is severe or displaced, ORIF with a Herbert screw may be used. Because of the importance of the scaphoid in providing stability to the wrist, healing of this fracture is important. A bone stimulator may be used to facilitate bone healing. The thumb is immobilized along with the wrist because of its involvement in thumb mobility.

The rehabilitation after immobilization is similar to that for a Colles fracture. Edema control and restoration of mobility, strength, and function relative to the individual's needs are the primary goals. Self-stretching exercises, mobilization, and strengthening exercises are indicated (Fig. 27-29). Specific thumb AROM and PROM exercises should also be included. Specific grip, pinch, and thumb opposition strengthening exercises also are important after a scaphoid fractures. Putty or other household products (eg, racquetball, nerf ball, clothespin, rubber bands) may be used. Include the patient in discovering objects at home or work that may be used to accomplish the established goals (Fig. 27-30).

METACARPAL FRACTURE

The MCP joints of fingers two through five are essentially ball and socket joints with a slack joint capsule in extension and taut collateral ligaments in flexion. The dorsal and palmar interossei muscles arise from the metacarpal bones and insert into the extensor mechanism. These muscle groups need special attention during evaluation, because their length and strength may be affected after injury or immobilization for metacarpal fractures.

Metacarpal fractures can occur from a fall onto an outstretched hand with initial ground contact along the metacarpals, from industrial accidents (eg, punch press machines), or from fist fights. When the fifth metacarpal is the only involved bone, it is commonly referred to as a boxer's

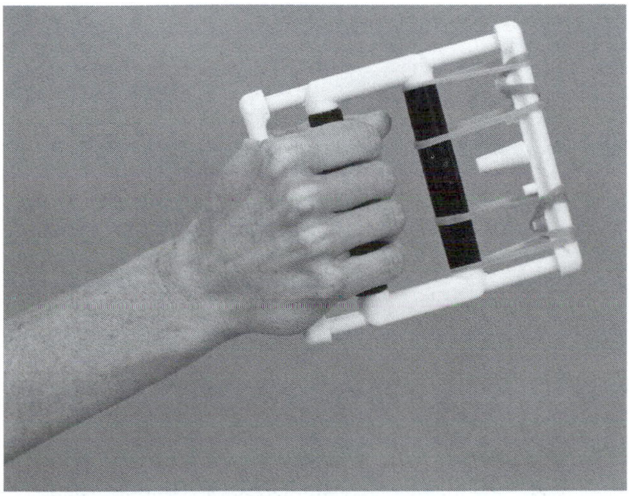

FIGURE 27-28 Grip strengthening exercises. Resistance is easily altered by increasing or decreasing the number of bands.

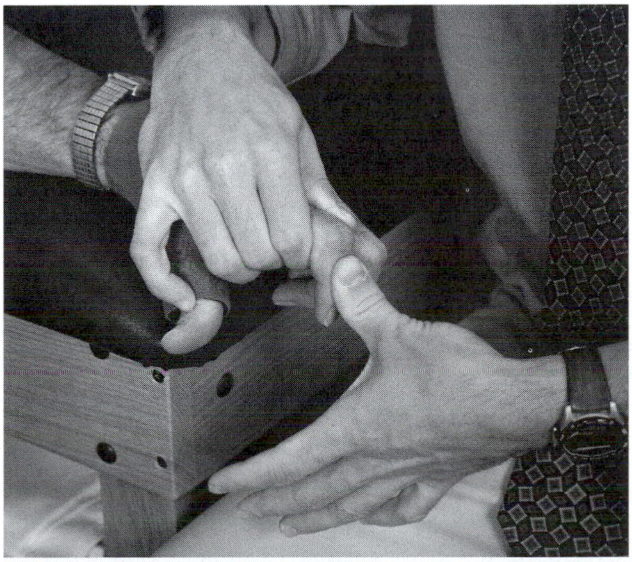

FIGURE 27-29 Resisted finger extension at the proximal interphalangeal joint.

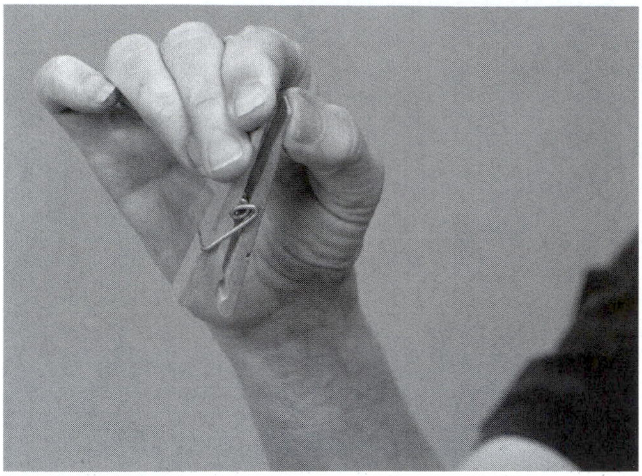

FIGURE 27-30 Resisted pinching using a clothespin.

fracture. Metacarpal fractures account for approximately 30% to 35% of all hand fractures.[35] Impairments associated with fracture in the acute stage include pain, swelling, loss of motion and strength, and deformity.

Medical intervention depends on the severity of the fracture. If the fracture is nondisplaced, it is usually casted for 2 to 3 weeks. A custom static splint that crosses the wrist and includes only the affected MCP joints up the PIP level may be worn for 2 to 3 weeks. If the MCP joint is flexed during immobilization, the position can prevent collateral ligament contracture. If the fracture is displaced, surgical fixation with pins, Kirschner wires, or a plate is indicated.

The start of rehabilitation depends on the medical intervention. If the fracture is surgically stabilized, treatment begins as early as 1 to 3 days after surgery. Early intervention avoids associated impairments of dorsal hand edema, extensor tendon adhesions, MCP collateral ligament adhesions, and intrinsic muscle contractures. Exercises in the first phase emphasize gentle AROM of the wrist and all fingers and blocked MCP flexion and extension exercise (see Self-Management: Metacarpophalangeal Joint Extension With Distal Interphalangeal Joint Flexion). This specific exercise prevents collateral ligament adhesions and encourages extensor tendon gliding with minimal stress placed on the fracture site. Aggressive interosseous and lumbrical stretching along with thumb-index web space stretching also should be initiated in this phase. Intrinsic muscle stretching can only be accomplished by maintaining the MCP in neutral or hyperextension while flexing at both IP joints (Fig. 27-31).

At 2 weeks, scar mobilization may begin, and at 4 to 6 weeks after surgery, passive MCP flexion may be initiated. At 6 to 8 weeks after surgery, intervention may focus on aggressive MCP flexion (ie, joint mobilizations), wrist strengthening, and grip and pinch strengthening, including the intrinsic muscles (eg, putty exercises for finger abduction and adduction).

The patient treated with immobilization may begin after cast removal at 2 to 3 weeks after the injury. Gentle AROM of the wrist and MCP joints is initiated at this time. PROM is initiated after 4 to 6 weeks. All other noninvolved joints and

SELF-MANAGEMENT: Metacarpophalangeal Joint Extension With Proximal and Distal Interphalangeal Joint Flexion

Purpose: To increase the mobility in your finger extensor tendon

Starting position: Keep the middle (PIP) and end (DIP) joints flexed.

Movement technique: Keeping those joints flexed, actively extend at your knuckle joints.

Repeat ____ times

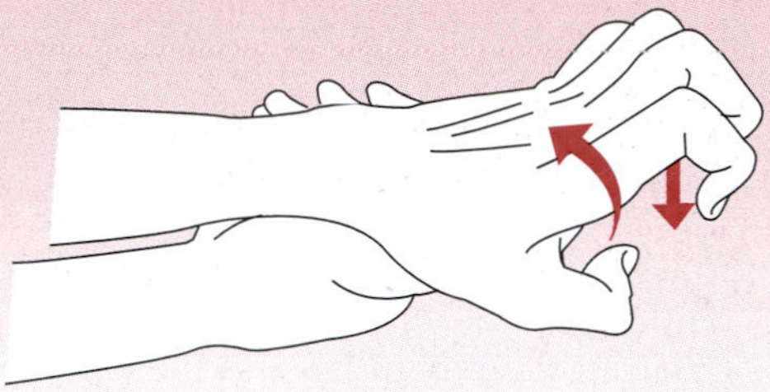

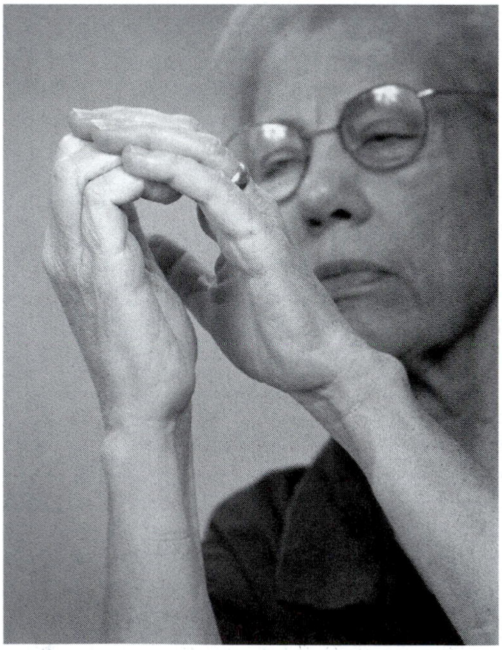

FIGURE 27-31 Stretching exercises at the proximal and distal interphalangeal joints.

fingers should be completing AROM exercises from the beginning of immobilization to prevent functional loss. The program is progressed similar to that for surgical management.

Adjunctive agents include education, elevation, ice, and compression garments to control edema. Dynamic splinting may be used to promote passive stretching of the MCP joints for 20-minute sessions performed 6 to 8 times per day. Massage is used to manage scar formation in the operative cases.

PHALANGEAL FRACTURE

Phalangeal fractures usually occur as a result of trauma. Approximately 45% to 50% of all hand fractures involve the distal phalanx, 15% to 20% the proximal phalanx, and 8% to 12% the middle phalanx.[35] Impairments observed in the acute stage include localized swelling, pain, and tenderness over the fractures; hypomobility at IP joints and possibly MCP joint; and abnormal alignment of the IP joint. Associated impairments after immobilization usually include restricted PIP joint extension (from volar plate contracture) and flexor tendon adhesions.

Like metacarpal fractures, the intervention depends on the severity of the fracture. If nondisplaced, the immobilization is accomplished by a custom splint or foam-covered metal splint. The period of immobilization varies according to the location of the fracture. If located at proximal or distal ends, only 3 to 4 weeks are required because of the good vascularity in cancellous bone. Mid-shaft middle phalangeal fractures require 10 to 14 weeks or longer because of the poor blood supply in the bony cortex. Displaced fractures require internal fixation with Kirschner wires or pinning. Extreme care is taken to avoid rotation, and often a buddy splint or buddy taping technique is used to help minimize this complication.

Intervention after nonsurgical postimmobilization care of phalangeal fractures is usually initiated at 3 to 6 weeks after injury or when immobilization is no longer necessary. Exercises of active and passive motion for all MCP, PIP, and DIP joints should be initiated along with tendon gliding exercises. For PIP joint restrictions of 20 degrees or more, dynamic PIP extension splinting may be required. Several commercial prefabricated splints are available, or custom splints can be fabricated. Static progressive splinting can be used at night. The finger splint is fabricated in full extension, and tension-adjustable straps are used to allow gradual fingers extension toward the splint.

After surgical internal fixation, intervention may begin as early as 2 days after surgery. Gentle AROM of the MCP, PIP, and DIP joints, with emphasis on full PIP joint motion, is initiated. Tendon gliding, scar management, and edema control also should be encouraged. At 4 to 8 weeks after surgery, dynamic PIP extension splinting may be initiated, along with buddy taping during exercises or ADLs.

Complex Regional Pain Syndrome

Reflex sympathetic dystrophy (RSD) is a term used to describe a cluster of signs and symptoms, including pain disproportionate to the injury, vasomotor and trophic changes, stiffness, swelling, and decreased function. Other terms for RSD have included sympathetically maintained pain, causalgia, sympathetic dystrophy without pain, shoulder-hand syndrome, and Sudeck's atrophy. The uncertain role of the sympathetic nervous system in RSD led the International Association for the Study of Pain and the American Pain Association to recommend use of the term complex regional pain syndrome (CRPS) to replace the term RSD.[36]

Several common features and two classifications of CRPS have been identified. The common features are local tissue damage or nerve damage that initiates a reflex response in the peripheral and central nervous systems. A variety of disorders with the same abnormal clinical findings share these criteria with CRPS. The two types have been classified by the absence or presence of nerve involvement, the first resembling RSD (without nerve involvement) and the second equivalent to causalgia (with nerve involvement).[36] A number of impairments are associated with CRPS and may include pain and inflammation, swelling, stiffness, vasomotor disturbances, trophic changes, bone demineralization, and dystonia.[36] Initial functional limitations are numerous and are based on pain-limited use of the extremity. An ADL checklist is helpful to monitor even small improvements in functional tasks.

Pain disproportionate to the injury severity is the primary clinical feature of CRPS. In the upper extremity, the pain is found throughout a large part of the arm, from the upper arm distally to and fully including the hand. The pain is often described as burning initially and eventually changing to pressure, aching, and binding sensations. Pain is often constant, staring locally at the original injury site and spreading throughout the extremity. The pain often leads to disuse and self-immobilization of the extremity, along with the known consequences of this response. In addition to constant pain, hypersensitivity to touch occurs, with extreme sensitivity to any kind of tactile stimulation. Occasionally, sympathetic and trophic changes occur with minimal complaints of pain or pain related only to motion of stiff joints.

Excessive swelling at the injury site is often the first objective sign noticed in the early phase. Swelling can subsequently spread throughout the distal upper extremity. Initially, it has a fusiform and pitting appearance, but it later takes on a hard and brawny character that contributes to joint stiffness. Periarticular thickening is observed at the IP joints. Edema is difficult to control even with otherwise successful intervention techniques.

Joint restriction with CRPS is often more profound than expected for the associated diagnosis. Unlike the traditional joint stiffness experienced after injury that decreases with ROM and functional use, individuals with CRPS tend to lose motion over time and seem to be refractory to improvement with traditional active and passive exercises and dynamic splinting. Fibrosis of ligaments limits motion about joints, and adhesions in tendon sheaths limit the gliding properties of the tendon, producing inflammation and pain. These changes contribute to the vicious circle of pain and inflammation. Palmar fascitis can be seen, and nodules and thickening of the palmar fascia can be palpated. This stiffness contributes to limited MCP and IP extension.

Discoloration of various degrees occurs with vasomotor instability. Pallor results from with vasoconstriction of the arterial and venous systems. Redness is evident when there is dilation of both sides of the vascular tree. Blueness (cyanosis) is usually present with vasoconstriction of the venous system.[37] Sudomotor changes occurring include hyperhidrosis (excessive sweating) early and dryness in later stages.

Bone demineralization is a reliable sign of CRPS and assists in making the diagnosis. Although some demineralization takes place with immobilization, the bulk of calcium loss results from increased blood flow in the periarticular bone.[37] Sudeck[38] described the condition as "inflammatory bone atrophy." Untreated cases progress from "spotty" osteoporosis to diffuse osteoporosis.

Trophic changes in the skin are initially caused by swelling and later by nutritional changes in the hand. The skin appears glossy or shiny, and evidence of subcutaneous tissue atrophy is present. Excessive and dark hair growth may be present. The nails become coarse, rigid, and curved.[37]

Intervention for CRPS must be approached practically and cautiously. Traditional exercises for restricted joints are often painful and exacerbate the pain cycle and vasomotor instability. Pain must be controlled before progressing to other treatment techniques. Modalities such as heat and cold may be helpful in reducing pain but must not aggravate the vasomotor tone. Elevation and moist heat before edema massage and exercise can improve tissue extensibility and tolerance to exercise.

Therapeutic exercise interventions include AROM, joint mobilization techniques, and continuous passive motion (CPM) devices. Exercise is best tolerated if initiated at proximal and less painful joints. Supine shoulder flexion or simple posture correction with the patient's back against a wall promotes upper extremity blood flow and improved proximal joint alignment. Active exercise of the wrist and hand should be performed elevated and directed to individual joints and motions. Blocked finger flexion exercises encourage more complete joint motion and specific tendon gliding (see Self-Management: Blocked Finger Extension). Holding a towel or soft ball while gripping can improve motor function by the assistance of palmar sensory stimulation (Fig. 27-32). Patients are encouraged to keep the wrist in slight extension during gripping exercises to ensure maximal efficiency of the flexor tendons.

A three-component stress-loading program has been a successful technique for treatment of CRPS. The components include compressive loading of the upper extremity, distraction, and use of other modalities, including splinting.[39] The object is to provide stress to the tissues while minimizing painful joint motion. Loading activities can include rocking on hands and knees or standing with weight applied through the upper extremity by leaning on a table (Fig. 27-33). Therapy putty or a foam ball under the palm can be used to allow feedback on the pressure being applied with the weight-bearing activities. Fingers can be flexed over the edge of the table if composite finger extension is painful. Resistive band exercises can also be used to provide stress to upper extremity joints without introducing painful joint motion.

Other interventions may be used to decrease pain and edema and to improve mobility. Joint mobilization techniques specific to pain control, such as joint distraction and volar-dorsal glides, are often tolerated well and promote normal joint proprioceptive sensory input (Fig. 27-34). End-range techniques may produce pain early with increased local inflammation and a resulting loss of joint motion. These techniques should be introduced gradually and instructed

SELF-MANAGEMENT: Blocked Finger Extension

Purpose: To increase the mobility of your finger joints and tendons

Starting position:
Level 1: Hold the knuckle joint of your finger straight.
Level 2: Hold the knuckle and middle joints of your finger straight.

Movement technique:
Level 1: Bend your middle joint, keeping your fingertip joint straight.
Level 2: Bend only your fingertip joint.

Repeat ____ times

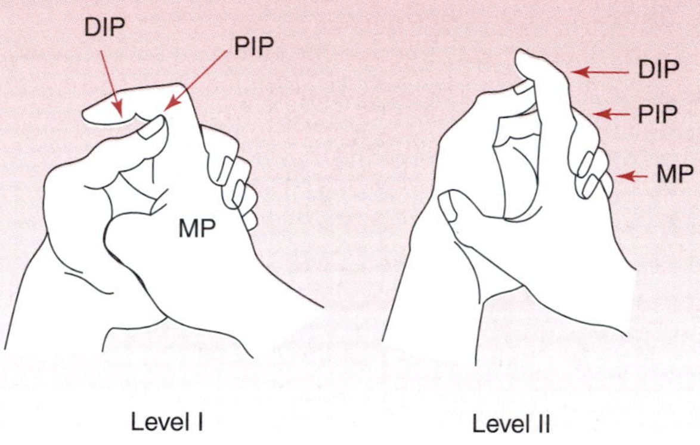

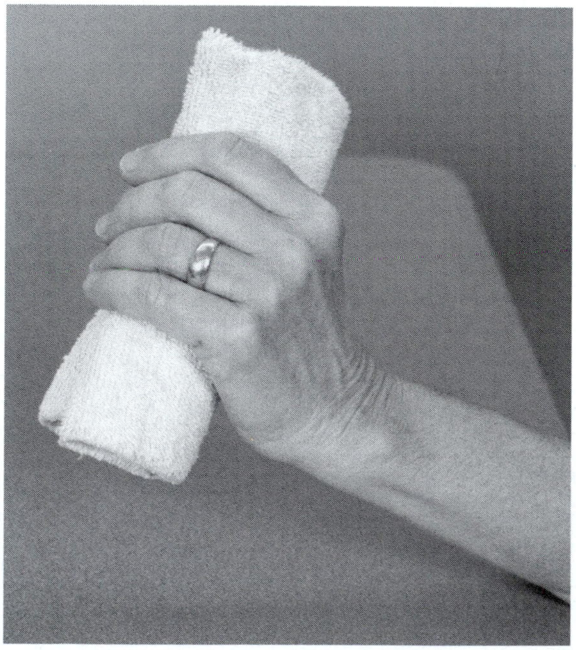

FIGURE 27-32 Grasping exercise using a towel.

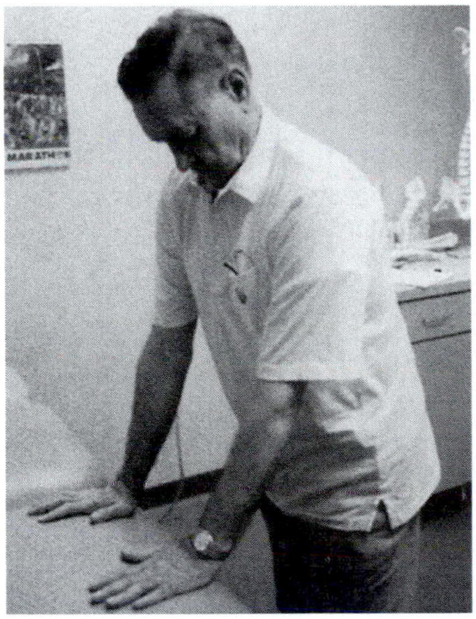

FIGURE 27-33 Leaning on a table can facilitate weight bearing through the wrist.

for home use when tolerated. CPM devices can be used periodically, alternating with active use and exercises. The device can be adjusted and controlled by the patient to allow slow and repetitive joint motion in pain-free ranges. The CPM may also contribute to pain relief (ie, gate control theory) and improve periarticular and cartilage nutrition.

Splinting can be an effective technique to maintain or regain joint motion. Tissue responds positively to the appropriate amount of force and negatively to excessive force. Static splinting can be effective in early stages to maintain the joints of the hand in their functional positions at rest. The functional position is described as the wrist in mid-extension, the thumb abducted, the MCP joints flexed 60 to 70 degrees, and the IP joints near full extension. A resting-hand splint for an entire hand or a joint-specific PIP extension splint can prevent anticipated development of joint motion restrictions. Dynamic splinting may be tolerated when edema is stabilized to allow a slow and gradual stretch of contracted joint tissues. Dynamic splinting should be done intermittently with gentle tension provided for 20 to 30 minutes. Vascularity should be monitored closely. Increases in edema or pain indicate the need to decrease tension or wearing time.

Hypersensitivity leads to disuse and tactile overprotection, and desensitization programs can be designed on the initial visit. These programs allow the patient a graded and controlled series of activities to improve tactile tolerance and raise the sensory pain threshold. The program can include textures (eg, denim, terrycloth, corduroy), massage or percussion (eg, light progressing to firm) with the opposite hand, and tapping a sensitive finger tip on a table (Fig. 27-35). Effort should be made to avoid cyclic stimulation to avoid increased pain. Protective padding or splinting may be helpful for temporary and intermittent use to protect a hypersensitive area from repeated painful environmental stimuli.

Transcutaneous electrical nerve stimulation has been effective for pain modulation, vasodilation, and vasoconstriction. Reports describe improvement in RSD pain as high as 90%.[40] Electrode placement and stimulating parameters may vary in effectiveness. Effective sites may include direct placement over the anatomic pain site, over peripheral or superficial cutaneous nerves, or proximal to the area of discomfort. The initial home program should promote pain relief to ensure adherence.

Elevation to decrease arterial hydrostatic pressure and assist in lymphatic and venous damage, elevated massage, and compression are techniques used to decrease edema. Elevated massage from distal to proximal aspects can mobilize edema, assist in pain relief, and improve ROM and desensitization. Maintaining continuous contact with the skin can decrease the chance for pain exacerbation during massage. Compression can be performed by intermittent sequential compression pumps and continuous compression devices. Acute edema may require only 2 hours of sequential compression pump use daily to be effective in edema reduction. Chronic fibrotic edema may require

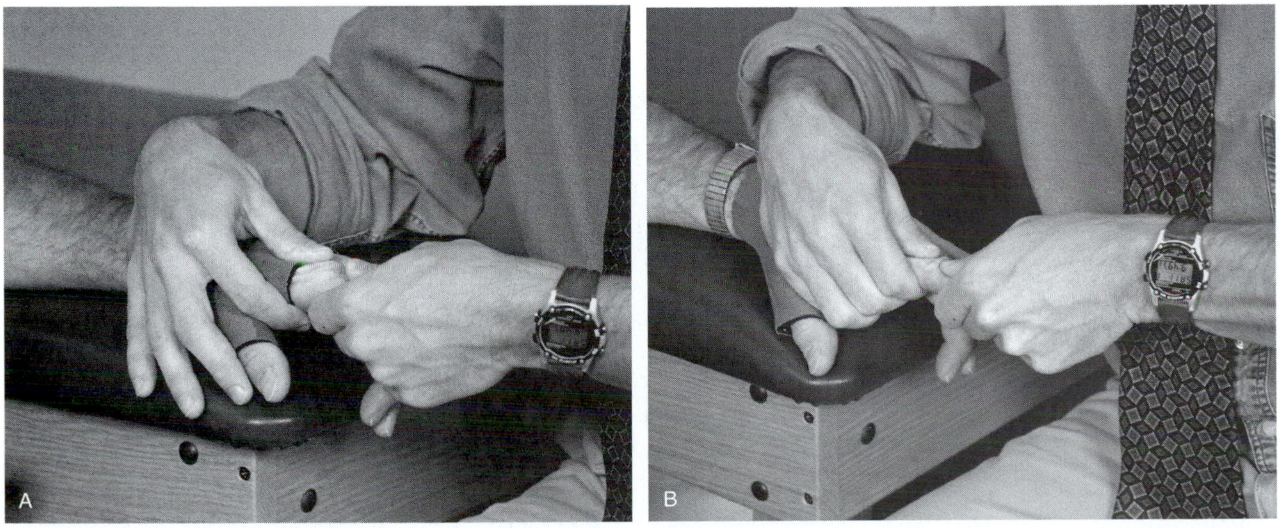

FIGURE 27-34 Mobilization at the metacarpaphalangeal joint. ***(A)*** Dorsal glides. ***(B)*** Volar glides.

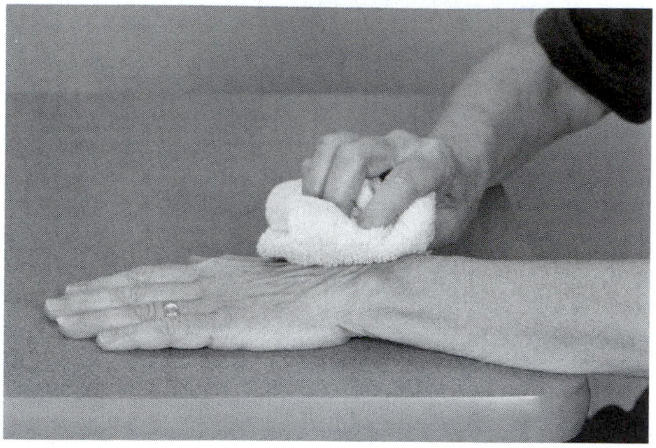

FIGURE 27-35 A variety of textures can be used to desensitize the hand.

more prolonged use. Acute edema may require near continuous use of external compression. Compression gloves with exposed fingertips allow use of the hand while controlling edema. A light, self-adhering wrap can be used for individual finger edema reduction.

Stellate ganglion blocks are often performed by physicians in the treatment of CRPS. These procedures block all efferent sympathetic impulses. After a successful block, the patient may find significant relief and be more successful in exercise attempts. The sympathetic block is therapeutic and helps to confirm the diagnosis.

Treatment of a patient with CRPS must be approached with patience, sympathy, and flexible planning. Improvement is often slow, and the stiffness and pain may worsen before improving. Psychological help is often necessary to assist with pain management. Individuals with acute symptoms often respond quickly with a decrease in pain and swelling after one treatment. Those in latter stages respond slowly and often unpredictably. Their impairments and functional limitations can be overwhelming. Keeping their program focused on one or two priority activities at a time increases adherence and the ability to assess the effectiveness of each treatment.

Stiff Hand and Restricted Motion

The diagnosis of the "stiff hand" is often used to describe joint limitation from a variety of causes. The primary diagnosis can include lacerations, burns, fractures, soft tissue crush injuries, and nerve and vascular trauma. The common cause is tissue trauma resulting in an inflammatory response. The resulting edema, fibrosis, and collagen alteration limits tissue gliding (ie, tendons) and extensibility (ie, skin, ligament, and joint capsule). Restricted motion is categorized by the tissue causing the limitation as articular or extraarticular. Joint stiffness that follows simple immobilization is attributable to fixation of the joint ligaments to bone in areas normally meant to be free from such fixation and shortening of the ligament by new collagen synthesis.

Knowledge of the normal anatomy and kinesiology of the wrist and hand help to understand, predict, and effectively treat limited mobility. At the MCP joints, the capsule is very elastic dorsally to allow for full MCP joint flexion. The extensor expansion glides over the dorsal capsule. With dorsal hand swelling, the MCP joints often lose joint flexion. This is initially caused by limited extensibility of the dorsal skin and progressively by adhesions of the collateral ligaments in their position of joint extension. The PIP and DIP joints are similar to the MCP joints with two exceptions. First, the collateral ligaments at the IP joints do not become slack in flexion; they remain taut throughout joint range, preventing lateral motion of the IP joints. Second, unlike the MCP joint, the loose-packed position for the IP joints is flexion. The volar plate becomes slack with IP joint flexion and taut in extension, preventing hyperextension, as seen at the MCP joint. After prolonged local swelling, the IP joints tend to lose joint extension, and the volar plate can become adhered in its slack position, preventing the necessary lengthening for full IP joint extension.

Structures outside the joint such as muscle, tendon, or skin adhesions can also limit joint motion. After prolonged immobilization in wrist and finger flexion, the flexor muscles become shortened. After tendon repair or fractures adjacent to tendons, tendon gliding is often limited by scar tissue or fracture calluses. For complete finger flexion, 7.0 cm of excursion is needed in the FDP tendons.[3] After a dorsal hand burn, metacarpal fracture, or prolonged dorsal hand edema resulting in decreased skin mobility, adjacent joint motions may be lost. Approximately 4 cm of dorsal skin laxity is needed for full MCP joint flexion and complete fisting.

Patients with articular and extraarticular tissue restriction describe functional limitations such as an inability to hold a fork or grip a steering wheel and difficulty getting into their pockets. Examination must distinguish between articular and extraarticular sources of limited motion. A thorough evaluation, performed with an understanding of the local anatomy and kinesiology, can result in effective intervention.

Interventions for articular limitations include heat before joint mobilization, strengthening, and splinting. Splinting can include dynamic splints (worn for 20 to 30 minutes six to eight times each day or 2 to 3 hours for one or two times each day) or static splints (worn at night). A flexion glove can apply nonspecific tension to the dorsal tissue of the fingers, with an elastic strap used to increase forces at the IP joints (Fig. 27-36).

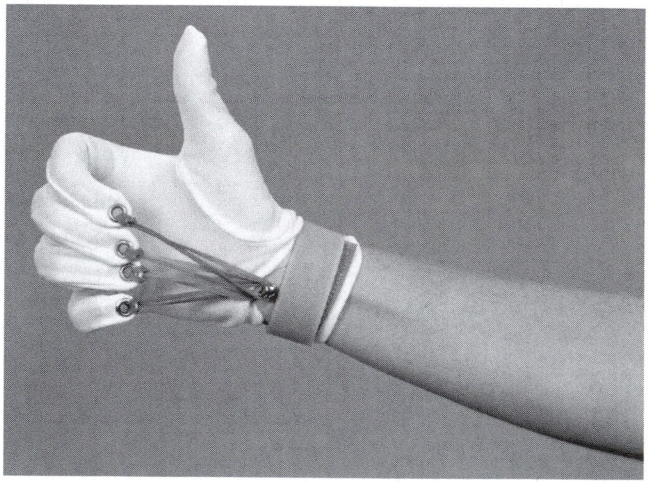

FIGURE 27-36 A flexion glove can improve the range of motion into flexion.

LAB ACTIVITIES

For each of the following case scenarios, evaluate your patient, design and execute and exercise program. Teach your patient a home exercise program.

1. A 56-year-old woman sustained an ulnar shaft fracture when she slipped and fell on the ice 6 weeks ago. She was casted for 3 weeks above the elbow and then recasted with a below-elbow cast. Her cast was removed 3 days ago. Evaluation reveals loss of AROM and PROM for elbow extension, pronation, and supination, wrist flexion and extension, and radial and ulnar deviation. Strength testing was not performed. She had no edema. Joint play assessment was not performed, but atrophy was visible.
2. A 12-year-old boy complains of medial elbow pain. He is active in Little League and pitched 14 innings over the weekend. He complains of pain along the medial collateral ligament, pain with passive elbow extension, flexion, pronation, and supination (with a guarded end feel). A mild effusion is observed, and there is increased laxity with valgus stressing. Radiographic findings are negative.
3. A 44-year-old patient presents with lateral elbow pain after shoveling wet, heavy snow. He complains of pain with activities such as picking up his briefcase, turning the doorknob, and grasping objects. He also has difficulty using the mouse on his computer. Examination reveals a loss of AROM and PROM of wrist flexion (and finger flexion increases symptoms), decreased strength with wrist extension and supination, and pain with palpation at the lateral epicondyle. There is no effusion, but slight warmth is noticed.
4. Three weeks ago, a 22-year-old collegiate gymnast dislocated her elbow (the olecranon displaced posteriorly) from a fall on an outstretched hand when she missed grasping the high bar and fell to the floor. She was in a sling for 2 weeks and out of the sling for 1 week, but she is carrying her arm in a guarded position. Examination reveals a loss of elbow extension (actively and passively with a springy end feel), full anteroposterior flexion, and a loss of pronation and supination anteroposteriorly. Joint play assessment reveals decreased humeroulnar joint distraction.
5. A 70-year-old woman fell on the ice and sustained a Colles fracture 8 weeks ago. She underwent a closed reduction and was immobilized in a series of casts. She also has insulin-dependent diabetes mellitus and has decreased sensation over for distal forearm, wrist, and hand. Examination reveals a loss of all active and passive wrist motion, decreased joint play in the inferior radioulnar joint, visible atrophy, and a loss of strength with resisted movements in neutral.
6. A 32-year-old man sustained a scaphoid fracture 10 weeks ago when he fell on an outstretched hand while skiing downhill. He was casted for 8 weeks, and periodic radiographs revealed nonunion of his scaphoid. He underwent surgical stabilization of the fracture using a bone graft from his iliac spine. He has been immobilized for 12 weeks since surgery. He is referred to physical therapy to begin ROM out of the splint four times each day. Examination reveals a loss of all wrist motions, decreased thumb flexion and extension, and decreased opposition.
7. A 40-year-old meat cutter sustained a laceration of his finger extensors (proximal to his MCP joints) while working. He underwent surgical fixation and was allowed to actively contract only the finger flexors. He has been removed from his splint and is allowed to begin active finger extension. Examination reveals decreased active finger extension (at the MCP joints) from weakness but full passive finger extension. Mobility of the MCP joints is decreased.
8. A 50-year-old man sustained a crush injury to his hand when his shirt sleeve got caught in a printing press and pulled his hand in. He sustained multiple metacarpal and carpel fractures, some of which were surgically stabilized through pinning. He has been casted for 8 weeks and presents to physical therapy today. Examination reveals a massive loss of motion of all wrist and fingers joints, atrophy in the thenar and hypothenar eminence, and decreased joint mobility in the carpal and MCP joints and all finger joints.

Extra-articular restriction rely heavily on tendon gliding activities such as differential tendon gliding and blocked IP flexion. As with articular restrictions, static or dynamic splinting plays a role in improving mobility. When intrinsic muscles are shortened or the tendons adhere to surrounding tissues, stretching, gliding, and splinting are the treatments of choice. Along with exercise and splinting, edema can be controlled with compression gloves, compression pumps, elevation, and wraps. Scar massage is important in treating surgical or burn cases.

Key Points

- The ulnar nerve may become entrapped in the cubital tunnel, the median nerve compressed in the carpal tunnel, and the radial nerve entrapped in any of several locations at the lateral elbow.
- The UCL is the primary static stabilizer and the flexor carpi ulnaris muscle the primary dynamic stabilizer of the medial elbow.

- The carpal tunnel is located on the volar aspect of the wrist and contains nine tendons and the median nerve.
- Grip is generally divided in power grip, used when force generation is the primary objective, and prehension grip, used when precision is the main goal.
- Activities to increase mobility include traditional stretching exercises, joint mobilization, and tendon and nerve gliding exercises.
- CTDs are usually the result of a combination of factors such as work pace, decreased rest intervals, and little variability in the task.
- Conservative management of CTS is often successful if hand and wrist postures and hand activities are monitored.
- Radial tunnel syndrome is often misdiagnosed as lateral epicondylitis.
- Cases of lateral and medial epicondylitis often result from repetitive wrist and hand activities at work, at home, or during recreation.
- Medial elbow instability occurs in children and adults who participate in throwing sports. Progressive instability in the child can lead to osteochondrosis of the capitellum and loose body formation.
- Sprain of the thumb's UCL (or gamekeeper's thumb) can result in degenerative joint disease of the CMC joint if instability continues.
- The anatomy of the scaphoid predisposes it to nonunion after a fracture. Any individual with wrist pain and wrist extension loss after a fall on an outstretched hand should be evaluated for fracture of the scaphoid.
- Individuals with complex regional pain syndrome have various degrees of pain, trophic changes, loss of mobility, and a variety of functional limitations and disability.
- Interventions for individuals with a stiff hand include mobility activities, splinting, and strengthening exercises.

Critical Thinking Questions

1. Consider Case Study #8 in Unit 7. Design a workstation for this individual given his physical examination and subjective history. How would your treatment differ if the patient's occupation was
   a. A carpenter
   b. A house painter
   c. A portrait painter
   d. A violinist
   e. A pianist
2. Consider potential reasons why this patient's symptoms did not resolve after his work station update several months ago.
3. Discuss the relationship between this patient's head and neck examination and his distal complaints.

REFERENCES

1. Butler DS. *Mobilisation of the Nervous System.* New York: Churchill Livingstone; 1991.
2. Williams PL, Warwick R, Dyson M, Bannister LH, eds. *Gray's Anatomy*. 37th ed. New York, NY: Churchill Livingstone; 1989.
3. Tubiana R. Architecture and functions of the hand. In: Thomine JM, Mackin EJ, eds. *Examination of the Hand and Upper Limb*. Philadelphia: WB Saunders; 1984.
4. Kendall FP, McCreary EK, Provance PG. *Muscles Testing and Function*. 4th ed. Baltimore: Williams & Wilkins; 1993.
5. Russe O. Fracture of the carpal navicular. *J Bone Joint Surg Am.* 1960;42:759–768.
6. Ambrose L, Posner MA. Lunate-triquetral and midcarpal joint instability. *Hand Clin*. 1992;8:653–668.
7. Culver JE. Instabilities of the wrist. *Clin Sports Med*. 1986;5:725–740.
8. Chase RA. Anatomy and kinesiology of the hand in rehabilitation of the hand. In: Hunter JM, Mackin EJ, Callahan AD, eds. *Rehabilitation of the Hand: Surgery and Therapy*. 4th ed. St. Louis: CV Mosby; 1995.
9. Norkin CC, Levangie PK. *Joint Structure and Function: A Comprehensive Analysis*. 2nd ed. Philadelphia: FA Davis; 1992.
10. Berger RA. The anatomy and basic biomechanics of the wrist joint. *J Hand Ther.* 1996;9:84–93.
11. Safran MR. Elbow injuries in athletes: A review. *Clin Orthop*. 1995;310:257–277.
12. Pratt NE. *Clinical Musculoskeletal Anatomy*. Philadelphia: JB Lippincott; 1991.
13. Morrey BF, Askew KN, Chao EYS. A biomechanical study of normal functional elbow motion. *J Bone Joint Surg Am.* 1981:63:872–887.
14. Morrey BF, An KN. Articular and ligamentous contributions to the stability of the elbow joint. *Am J Sports Med.* 1983; 11:315–319.
15. Davidson PA, Pink M, Perry J, Jobe FW. Functional anatomy of the flexor pronator muscle group in relation to the medial collateral ligament of the elbow. *Am J Sports Med*. 1995;23: 245–250.
16. Magee D. *Orthopedic Physical Assessment.* 3rd ed. Philadelphia: WB Saunders; 1997.
17. Brumfield RH, Champoux JA. A biomechanical study of normal functional wrist motion. *Clin Orthop*. 1984;187:23–25.
18. Viegas SF, Tencer AF, Cantrell J, et al. Load transfer characteristics of the wrist: Part I. The normal joint. *J Hand Surg*. 1987;12:971–978.
19. Wadsworth C. The wrist and hand. In: Malone TR, McPoil T. Nitz AJ, eds. *Orthopedic and Sports Physical Therapy*. 3rd ed. St. Louis: CV Mosby; 1997.
20. O'Driscoll SW, Horii E, Ness R, et al. The relationship between wrist position, grasp size and grip strength. *J Hand Surg Am.* 1992;17:169–177.
21. National Institute for Occupational Safety and Health. *Musculoskeletal Disorders and Workplace Factors: A Critical Review of Epidemiologic Evidence for Work-Related Musculoskeletal Disorders of the Neck, Upper Extremity, and Low Back*. NIOSH Publication No. 97-141. Cincinnati, OH: NIOSH; 1997.
22. Putz-Anderson V. *Cumulative Trauma Disorders: A Manual for Musculoskeletal Diseases of the Upper Limbs.* Bristol, PA: Taylor & Francis; 1992.
23. Eastman Kodak Company. *Ergonomic Design for People at Work*, vol 2. New York: Van Nostrand Reinhold; 1986.
24. Rempel D. Musculoskeletal loading and carpal tunnel pressure. In: Gordon SL, Blair SJ, Fine LJ, eds. *Repetitive Motion Disorders of the Upper Extremity*. Rosemont, IL: American Academy of Orthopaedic Surgeons; 1995.
25. Ditmars DM, Hovin HP. Carpal tunnel syndrome. *Hand Clin*. 1986;2(3)525–532.
26. Idler RS. Anatomy and biomechanics of the digital flexor tendons. *Hand Clin*. 1985;1(1)3–11.

27. Plancher KD, Peterson RK, Steichen JB. Compressive neuropathies and tendinopathies in the athletic elbow. *Clin Sports Med.* 1996;15:331–372.
28. Nirschl RP. Soft tissue injuries about the elbow. *Clin Sports Med.* 1986;5:637–652.
29. Kibler WB. Pathophysiology of overload injuries around the elbow. Clin Sports Med. 1995;15:447–457.
30. Kirkpatrick WH. De Quervain's disease. In: Hunter JM, Schneider LH, Mackin EF, Callahan AD, eds. *Rehabilitation of the Hand.* 3rd ed. St. Louis: CV Mosby; 1990.
31. Cannon NM, ed. *Diagnosis and Treatment Manual for Physicians and Therapists.* 3rd. ed. Indianapolis: Hand Rehabilitation Center of Indiana; 1991.
32. Sobel J, Nirschl RP. Elbow injuries. In: Zachazewski JE, Magee DJ, Quillen WS, eds. *Athletic Injuries and Rehabilitation.* Philadelphia: WB Saunders; 1996.
33. Josefsson PO, Johnell O, Gentz CF. Long term sequelae of simple dislocation of the elbow. *J Bone Joint Surg Am.* 1984; 66:927–930.
34. Rowe C. The management of fractures in elderly patients is different. *J Bone Joint Surg Am.* 1965;47:1043–1059.
35. Meyer FN, Wilson RL. Management of nonarticular fractures of the hand. In: Hunter JM, Schneider LH, Mackin EF, Callahan AD, eds. *Rehabilitation of the Hand.* 4th ed. St. Louis: CV Mosby; 1995.
36. Stralka SW, Akin K. Reflex sympathetic dystrophy syndrome. In: *Orthopaedic Section Home Study Course.* LaCrosse, WI: Orthopaedic Section, APTA; December 1997.
37. Lankford LL. Reflex sympathetic dystrophy. In: Hunter JM, Schneider LH, Mackin EF, Callahan AD, eds. *Rehabilitation of the Hand.* 3rd ed. St. Louis: CV Mosby; 1990.
38. Sudeck PMH. Ueber die acute entzundliche Knockenatrophie. *Arch Klin Chir.* 1900:62:147–156.
39. Watson HK, Ryu J. Degenerative disorders of the carpus. *Orthop Clin North Am.* 1984;15:337–354.
40. Lee VH, Reynolds CC. Clinical application of transcutaneous electrical nerve stimulator in patients with upper extremity pain. In: Hunter JM, Schneider LH, Mackin EF, Callahan AD, eds. *Rehabilitation of the Hand.* 3rd ed. St. Louis: CV Mosby; 1990.
41. Cram JR, Kasmann GS, Holtz J. *Introduction to Surface Electromyography.* Rockville, MD: Aspen Publishers; 1998.
42. Kasman GS, Cram JR, Wolf SL. *Clinical Applications in Surface Electromyography.* Rockville, MD: Aspen Publishers; 1998.

SELECTED INTERVENTION

Upper Quadrant

See Case Study #8

Although this patient requires comprehensive intervention, one specific exercise addressing motor control is described.

ACTIVITY: Simulated typing with surface electromyography (SEMG)

PURPOSE: Develop motor control strategy to use appropriate levels of wrist extensor activation, wrist flexor relaxation, production of microrests, and complete baseline recovery between timed bouts of data entry

RISK FACTORS: Watch for cervical posture as part of repetitive strain; injury to extensor group may be secondary to cervical dysfunction.

ELEMENT OF MOVEMENT SYSTEM EMPHASIZED: Modulator

STAGE OF MOTOR CONTROL: Skill

MODE: Isometric wrist extensor and flexors, concentric and eccentric finger flexors and extensors

POSTURE: Sitting at a simulated workstation in optimal ergonomic posture, with SEMG appropriately placed on right and left forearm flexor and extensor groups[41]

MOVEMENT: While simulated typing is performed on a keyboard using a palm and wrist rest and optimal ergonomic posture, SEMG monitors forearm flexor and extensor activity bilaterally. The right forearm attempts to follow the template developed by the left forearm. Random stopping is called out to determine the spontaneous speed and level of recovery to baseline. Timed rest breaks are scheduled to determine planned speed and level of recovery to baseline.

SPECIAL CONSIDERATIONS: Closely monitor cervical position and paracervical muscle tension.

DOSAGE

Special Considerations

Anatomic: Lateral epicondyle, musculotendinous and tenoperiosteal junction of wrist and finger extensor group

Physiologic: Subacute strain

Learning capability: May be difficult as patient works up to 60 hours a week at visual display terminal. Probably has strong patterns of overuse of wrist and finger extensors.

Repetitions/sets: Five minutes of typing form one repetition. Perform up to five sets.

Rest period: Random 5-second rest breaks are called out during each repetition; 15-second breaks are taken after each 5-minute bout of exercise.

Frequency: If SEMG is rented, practice should be twice daily for 2–4 weeks. If only used in clinic, recommend three times a week for 3 to 6 weeks. For cost effectiveness, unit rental is preferred.

Sequence: Perform after stretching exercises are performed, but not after muscle performance exercises so as not to overly fatigue muscles.

Speed: Functional speed

Environment: Initially in quiet home environment; then progress to work environment

Feedback: Initially, continuous audio feedback from the SEMG unit. Threshold is set so as not to exceed left side wrist and finger extensor activity. Visual feedback is used to see the speed and level of recovery to baseline during microrests and rest breaks. The patient is reassessed once each week, and the decision to progressively fade feedback is based on performance. Progressive fading of feedback occurs during exercise sessions to eliminating either audio or visual feedback every third set, to every other set, and so forth. A second party relaying the results between sets provides verbal knowledge of the results.

Functional movement pattern to reinforce goal of exercise: In addition to using an improved motor strategy during data entry, the patient is encouraged to use elbow flexors instead of forearm extensors during lifting tasks (eg, lift in forearm supination versus pronation) to reduce the strain to the wrist/finger extensors.

Rationale for exercise choice: This exercise was chosen as a skill-level activity to reduce the overuse of the wrist and finger extensors during a highly repetitive functional activity. Through the use of SEMG feedback with a proper faded feedback schedule,[42] the patient can develop an intrinsic reference for muscle activation and error detection to improve motor control strategies to reduce recruitment effort and improve the speed and level of relaxation to baseline.

SELECTED INTERVENTION
Total Body

See Case Study #10

Although this patient requires comprehensive intervention, one specific exercise prescribed in the intermediate stage of recovery is described.

ACTIVITY: Step-ups; swing phase, with counterrotation (see Fig. 25–29 in Chapter 25)

PURPOSE: Incorporate proper total-body movements in a functional context

RISK FACTORS: None

ELEMENT OF THE MOVEMENT SYSTEM EMPHASIZED: Modulator

STAGE OF MOTOR CONTROL: Controlled mobility

POSTURE: Standing in front of a 6-inch step in front of a mirror

MOVEMENT: Lift the right leg onto the step with simultaneous right thoracic rotation and left forward arm swing

SPECIAL CONSIDERATIONS: Be sure the patient does not hike his right hip during the hip flexion phase and does not drop his right shoulder (right thoracic lateral flexion) or adduct his right scapula instead of right thoracic rotation during the upper body counterswing maneuver.

DOSAGE

Special considerations

Anatomic: Right hamstring and adductor, right subscapularis, right glenohumeral joint

Physiologic: chronic moderate strain and tendinitis, questionable instability of right glenohumeral joint

Learning capability: Very engrained movement pattern from a long history of high-mileage running; may require high repetitions and significant feedback in early stages of learning

Repetitions/sets: Initially to form fatigue as evidenced by hip hike, shoulder drop, and scapula adduction; work up to 3 sets of 20–30 repetitions

Frequency: 6–7 days each week

Duration: Expect at least 2 weeks before evidence of motor control changes and 6–8 weeks before skill level is achieved.

Sequence: Perform after specific exercises for psoas muscle performance, thoracic rotation mobility, and abdominal muscle performance exercises have been performed. Follow with step-up: stance phase.

Speed: Slow progressed to functional speed

Environment: home in front of a mirror

Feedback: Initially in clinic with mirror providing visual feedback and clinician providing verbal feedback. Taper to continued use of mirror, but with knowledge of results of verbal feedback after every 3–4 repetitions. Withdraw mirror and verbally provide KR every 3–4 repetitions. Progress toward skill.

FUNCTIONAL MOVEMENT PATTERN TO REINFORCE GOAL OF EXERCISE: Ascending stairs, gait.

RATIONALE FOR EXERCISE CHOICE: The total-body movement pattern of right hip hike and right shoulder drop during swing phase of gait may be perpetuating the upper and lower extremity conditions. Without adequate hip flexion, the gluteus maximus is less efficient at assisting the stance phase of gait or step up; the persistent right shoulder drop and scapula adduction and downward rotation can perpetuate posture and movement impairments consistent with glenohumeral impingement and hypermobility. As a result, this pattern of movement must be altered to fully recover from the upper and lower body conditions.

UNIT 7

Case Studies

Dorothy Berg, Carrie Hall, and Lori Thein Brody

CASE STUDY #1

Lisa is a 17-year-old high school student who complains of right (R) ankle pain and swelling. She describes injuring herself yesterday during basketball practice. Coming down after a rebound attempt, she landed on the foot of another player, twisting her ankle and falling to the ground. Immediately after the injury, she was able to move her ankle and walk off the court. Now Lisa reports difficulty bearing full weight on her R foot and is unable to walk or run without a significant limp. Her team is contending for the state championship in 6 weeks, and Lisa hopes to play.

EXAMINATION

Pain: 4/10 at rest, constant in nature in non–weight-bearing: 6/10 with weight bearing

Gait: R foot flat, "step to" pattern with use of axillary crutches.

Active Range of Motion: Plantar flexion/dorsiflexion 20–5 degrees; foot inversion/eversion 3–5 degrees with pain end range

Passive Range of Motion: Plantar flexion/dorsiflexion 40–15 degrees; foot inversion/eversion 3–8 degrees with muscle guarding

Accessory Motion: Subtalar and talocrural distraction hypomobile; subtalar medial/lateral glide hypomobile with muscle guarding; talonavicular, cuboid/navicular and cuneiform/navicular all hypomobile

Palpation: Moderate localized swelling in region distal to R lateral malleolus; marked tenderness and early signs of ecchymosis in same region

Strength Testing: Anterior tibialis 4/5 (pain elicited); posterior tibialis 5/5; gastrocnemius/soleus 5/5; peroneus longus 4–/5 (pain elicited)

Resisted Testing: Dorsiflexors and evertors weak and painful

Balance: Unable to assess because of patient discomfort in weight bearing

EVALUATION: Acute, traumatic ligamentous injury to the R ankle.

Impairment

- Localized pain, and swelling of lateral R ankle
- Decreased active and passive range of motion for R ankle
- Midfoot hypomobility
- Faulty R foot alignment in stance into calcaneal eversion
- Decreased static and dynamic standing balance
- Weakness in ankle evertors and dorsiflexors

Functional Limitation

- Limited weight bearing and movement tolerance in standing and walking, necessitating the use of crutches
- Unable to run or jump on R foot

Disability

- Unable to play basketball

DIAGNOSIS: Second degree sprain of the R calcaneofibular ligament

PROGNOSIS

Short Term Goals (7–10 days)

1. Ambulate without an assistive device, step-through pattern, 15 minutes, no ankle pain
2. Tolerate low-intensity running and jumping

Long Term Goals (3–4 weeks)

1. Ambulate unlimited, no ankle pain
2. Return to full-intensity basketball practice

CASE STUDY #2

Sarah is a 69-year-old, retired college professor with a medical diagnosis of osteoarthritis in both knees. She is widowed and living alone in a third-floor apartment with elevator access. Yesterday, Sarah underwent elective surgery for bilateral (B) total-knee arthroplasties. Her medical history includes emphysema, myocardial infarct 2 years ago, moderate obesity, and hypertension. She lives independently but has a maximum walking tolerance of one-half block when using a cane for support.

EXAMINATION

Arousal/Cognition: Alert and oriented; follows complex commands; motivated to get out of bed

Cardiovascular: Pale with complaints of nausea; short of breath with exertion; diaphoretic in sitting; vital signs: pulse 96 supine, 108 sitting; blood pressure 144/66 mm Hg supine, 126/64 mm Hg sitting

Wounds: Dressed with gauze and clear tape, moderately soaked with bloody drainage; periwound regions warm to touch, hypererythemic, and swollen

Pain: 3/10 at rest, 8/10 with movement

Active Range of Motion: R knee extension/flexion 20–47 degrees (pain elicited); L knee extension/flexion 15–52 degrees (pain elicited)

Endurance: Maximum sitting tolerance 15 minutes; maximum standing tolerance 20 seconds

Strength Testing: Iliopsoas (B) 2+/5; gluteus maximus(B) 4/5; gluteus medius (B) 2+/5; quadriceps (R) 2/5, (L) 3–/5; hamstrings (R) 2+/5, (L) 3–/5

Resisted Testing: Shoulder girdle extension and depression, elbow extension all strong and pain free

Posture: Semiflexed both knees, with L > R valgus knee deformity

Gait: Wide base of support, stiff knees, flexed trunk, maximum upper extremity support on walker

EVALUATION: Acute, postoperative pain, inflammation, muscle weakness, and decreased active motion of both knees

Impairment

- Bilateral decreased knee active range of motion
- Bilateral weak quadriceps and hamstrings
- Postoperative pain and inflammatory response
- Markedly limited activity tolerance

Functional Limitation

- Required moderate assist for bed mobility and basic sit to stand transfer
- Unable to sit >15 minutes
- Unable to stand >20 seconds
- Unable to walk

Disability

- Unable to resume independent basic and instrumental activities of daily living
- Unable to walk household distances
- Unable to resume teaching and writing interests
- Unable to access family, church, and clubs for social interaction

DIAGNOSIS: Postoperative day 1 after bilateral total knee arthroplasties

PROGNOSIS

Short Term Goals (7–10 days)

1. Independent bed mobility and basic transfer with walker
2. Independent ambulation 30 meters with walker
3. Active knee range of motion >10–70 degrees to enable up/down stairs
4. Out of bed and up in chair >5 hours per day

Long Term Goals (12 weeks)

1. Ambulation >100 meters, rest breaks as needed, allowing for baseline compromised cardiopulmonary status
2. Return to independent driving for community access
3. Return to preoperative vocational routine

CASE STUDY #3

Cathy is a 61-year-old journalist with a number of complaints, including trunk weakness, leg weakness, and generalized fatigue. She has a history of osteoporosis, osteoarthritis, and a recent 2-week bout with diarrhea caused by her medication. Recently, Cathy has had difficulty managing a 40–50-hour work week. She has no history of regular exercise nor any home exercise equipment. Her maximum walking tolerance is reportedly one block, limited by shortness of breath, general fatigue, and hip discomfort.

EXAMINATION

Posture/Alignment: Long kyphosis with posterior displacement of the upper trunk and a forward head. Lumbar spine is flattened. Posterior pelvic tilt. B hips extended and internally rotated. B knees in recurvatum; tibial external rotation; scapulae abducted and elevated.

Muscle Length: Hamstrings: passive straight-leg raise to 50 degrees (B)

Strength Testing: Trunk curl 3–/5; leg lowering 2–/5; iliopsoas (R) 3/5 degrees, (L) 3–/5; gluteus medius (R) 3/5, (L) 2+/5; gluteus maximus (B) 3+/5; quadriceps (R) 4/5, (L) 4–/5; hamstrings (R) 4–/5, (L) 3+/5

Active and Passive Range of Motion:

Thoracolumbar spine: forward bend thoracic > lumbar flexion with lumbar spine remaining in neutral; back bend with excessive extension at thoracolumbar junction;

Hip: internal rotation (R) 0–20 degrees, (L) 0–15 degrees, external rotation (R) 0–35 degrees, (L) 0–33 degrees, flexion (bent knee) 0–85 degrees, extension 0–25 degrees

Shoulder: flexion in scapular plane 0–140 degrees, with early upward rotation of scapulae and lacking thoracic extension component at end range

Endurance: Standardized 12-minute walk test completed with subjective complaints of shortness of breath and lower extremity muscle fatigue; distance, 900 meters; standing rest required at 10 minutes, peak heart rate of 132, blood pressure of 153/88 mm Hg

EVALUATION: Generalized deconditioning with gradual onset of faulty alignment because of changes in joint mobility and muscle strength and length, compounded by recent illness

Impairment

- Muscle weakness pelvic girdle
- Faulty spinal, pelvic and lower extremity alignment
- Muscle shortening of hamstrings and rectus abdominis
- Decreased cardiovascular endurance
- Decreased lower extremity muscle endurance
- Restrictions at thoracolumbar spine intervertebral and thoracic spine costovertebral joints
- Faulty shoulder girdle movement patterns
- Hip joint restrictions

Functional Limitation

- Unable to walk >10 minutes without shortness of breath and fatigue
- Stairs require rail support
- Difficulty getting up from low chairs
- Rest breaks required during AM and PM self-care routine

Disability

- Unable to tolerate exertion of a full work week
- Unable to complete basic and instrumental activities of daily living in a timely manner
- Avoidance to social activities because of fatigue

DIAGNOSIS: Generalized deconditioning superimposed on baseline medical diagnoses of osteoporosis and osteoarthritis

PROGNOSIS

Short Term Goals (2 weeks)

1. Demonstration of energy conservation and pacing techniques to maximize activity tolerance at work and home

Long Term Goals (4–6 months)

1. Increase in musculoskeletal and cardiovascular endurance to allow resumption of full duties at work and home

CASE STUDY #4

Jack is a 58-year-old, retired banker who presented with complaints of right (R) shoulder pain that was most noticeable when reaching overhead or behind. His pain occasionally wakes him at night. Jack's medical history is significant for a nonspecific R shoulder injury sustained playing tennis 2 years ago. This went untreated, and the symptoms resolved. Jack has been refurbishing his 35-foot wooden sailboat and noticed the onset of shoulder pain after sanding the deck. He is R-hand dominant.

EXAMINATION

Posture/Alignment: Forward head with upper cervical extension, cervical-thoracic junction flexion, and flattened thoracolumbar spine; scapulae elevated, abducted, and downwardly rotated R > L; R humerus anteriorly displaced in the glenohumeral joint

Active Range of Motion: R shoulder flexion 0–90 degrees, extension 0–30 degrees, abduction 0–100 degrees, external rotation 0–25 degrees, internal rotation 0–50 degrees; pain elicited end range all directions

Passive Range of Motion: R shoulder flexion 0–110 degrees, extension 0–33 degrees, abduction 0–110 degrees, external rotation 0–25 degrees, internal rotation 0–55 degrees; end-range pain elicited in all directions

Accessory Motion Testing:
Glenohumeral: diffusely hypomobile, especially posterior and inferior glides
Scapulothoracic: hypomobile medial glide and upward rotation; hypermobile lateral/cephalic glides
Upper thoracic: hypomobile segmental anterior/posterior glides T2-T8

Strength Testing: Upper trapezius/levator scapula (R) 5/5, (L) 5/5; middle trapezius (R) 2/5, (L) 3/5; lower trapezius (R) 1/5, (L) 3/5; rhomboids (R) 3/5, (L) 4/5; serratus anterior (R) 4/5, (L) 5/5

Resisted Testing (neutral position): Strong and painless R shoulder flexion, extension, internal rotation, abduction and adduction; weak and painless external rotation

Quality of Movement: Glenohumeral flexion/abduction achieved through 30 degrees of glenohumeral motion, followed by 1:1 scapulohumeral rhythm to roughly 90 degrees; remaining motion achieved through shoulder girdle elevation

EVALUATION: Decreased osteokinematic and arthrokinematic motion of R shoulder girdle and cervical-thoracic spine, resulting in faulty movement patterns and pain with end-range shoulder function

Impairment
- Decreased physiologic and accessory motion
- Faulty scapulothoracic, glenohumeral and cervical-thoracic spine alignment
- Faulty shoulder girdle movement patterns
- Pain with end-range shoulder girdle motion, especially forward flexion

Functional Limitation
- Unable to reach, lift, or pull overhead
- Disturbed sleep

Disability
- Difficulty retrieving wallet from back pocket
- Difficulty unlocking car passenger door from driver's seat
- Unable to complete moderate- or heavy-duty boat refurbishing tasks

DIAGNOSIS: Subacute R shoulder adhesive capsulitis

PROGNOSIS

Short Term Goals (3 weeks)
1. Decrease night pain by 50%
2. Light weight lifting and reaching activities up to shoulder height without pain

Long Term Goals (3–4 months)
1. No night pain
2. Ability to tolerate resisted motion at end range of shoulder motion; thus able to complete heavy-duty jobs on boat

CASE STUDY #5

Irene is an 85-year-old woman who fell at home, resulting in acute low back pain and right more than left (R > L) lower extremity radiculopathy and necessitating bed rest for more than 2 weeks. She is weak, deconditioned, unsteady on her feet, and fearful of falling. She now uses a walker for ambulation. Her back still gives her pain, although she no longer suffers lower extremity symptoms. Irene lives in her own apartment in an assisted-living environment. Before the fall, she independently handled her basic activities of daily living and was socially active with fellow residents.

EXAMINATION

Posture: Kyphotic/ lordodic thoracolumbar alignment; anterior pelvic tilt; hips slightly flexed

Strength Testing: Leg lowering 2/5; gluteus maximus (R) 2+/5, (L) 3+/5; gluteus medius (R) 2/5, (L) 3/5; iliopsoas (R) 3/5, (L) 4–/5; quadriceps (R) 4/5, (L) 4+/5; hamstrings (R) 3–/5, (L) 3+/5

Muscle Length: Moderate shortening of quads > iliopsoas, R > L; (B) hamstrings unremarkable

Functional Movement Testing: Pain with standing or walking (4/10). Pain relief with sitting or sidelying. Standing forward bend at 20 degrees; standing backward bend trace with reproduction of symptoms

Gait: Positive Trendelenburg with stance R > L; wide base of support; flexed at hips with forward displaced trunk over pelvis; markedly diminished lumbopelvic rhythm

Balance: Standardized stand reach test of 6 inches; provoked balance response demonstrates delayed step response with hip > ankle strategies

Reflexes: Knee jerk (B) 2+; ankle jerk (R) 1+, (L) 2+

Sensory: Light touch intact, mildly decreased proprioception R > L

EVALUATION:

Fixed kyphosis and lordosis malalignment, with corresponding muscle length and tension changes; painful with active or passive extension, affecting static and dynamic standing balance, and standing tolerance

Impairment
- Fixed kyphotic-lordotic alignment of thoracolumbar spine
- Muscle weakness, especially trunk and proximal lower extremity
- Shortened iliopsoas and quadriceps, R > L
- Decreased static and dynamic standing balance
- Fear of falling
- Pain with lumbar extension

Functional Limitation
- Assist required to get out of bed or up from a chair
- Inability to stand >2 minutes
- Inability to walk >10 meters
- Mobility avoidance

Disability
- Loss of independence performing basic activities of daily living
- Loss of independence with ambulation
- Unable to walk to dining room
- Reluctant to participate in usual social activities (bridge, films, out for dinner with family)

DIAGNOSIS:

Lumbar spinal stenosis exacerbated by fall. Now with subacute pain, deconditioning, balance deficits and increased fear of falling.

PROGNOSIS

Short Term Goals (2 weeks)
1. Independent ambulation with walker, 25 meters
2. Independent transfer out of bed
3. Independent stand for 10 minutes for morning self-care routine

Long Term Goals (8 weeks)
1. Independent ambulation within building complex; no assistive device
2. Resume all previous social activities with friends and family

CASE STUDY #6

Scott, a 32-year-old man, presented 1 week after right (R) anterior cruciate ligament autograft reconstruction. He is on medical leave of absence from his position as a full-time driver and delivery man for a shipping company. Scott is an outdoor enthusiast and has hopes of returning to rock climbing, kayaking, and skiing after his rehabilitation.

EXAMINATION

Gait: Toe-touch pattern with use of axillary crutches; knee held semiflexed

Active Range of Motion: Knee extension/flexion 15–60 degrees with subjective sensation of "tightness" at both extremes

Passive Range of Motion: Knee extension/flexion 12–70 degrees with spasm end feel

Palpation: Moderate suprapatellar swelling; posterior capsule distention; girth (3 cm proximal to superior patellar pole) R = 44 cm, L = 38 cm; moderate joint line tenderness

Strength Testing: Resisted testing contraindicated; surface electromyographic testing confirms 35% decreased vastus medialis oblique recruitment relative to nonsurgical leg

Accessory Motion: Hypomobile patellar glides, all directions

EVALUATION: Postoperative R knee joint effusion, pain, decreased range of motion, and altered muscle recruitment patterns

Impairment

- Localized swelling in suprapatellar and posterior capsule regions
- Acute surgical pain with end-range knee motion
- Impaired vastus medialus recruitment
- Decreased patello-femoral accessory joint mobility
- Loss of R lower extremity coordination

Functional Limitation

- Unable to tolerate foot flat stance on R with a step through pattern
- Crutches required secondary to above gait problems
- Unable to tolerate prolonged static extension

Disability

- Unable to lift from floor height or drive, therefore unable to work
- Unable to participate in usual outdoor sports

DIAGNOSIS: R knee dysfunction from primary structural injury and corrective surgery

PROGNOSIS

Short Term Goals (2–4 weeks)

1. Ambulate without assistive device
2. Return to modified work routine

Long Term Goals (6–12 months)

1. Return to preoperative work routine
2. Resume low-to-moderate-intensity sports

CASE STUDY #7

Mary is a 36-year-old wife and mother of two young children. She has a 6-month history of chronic back, hip, neck, and shoulder pain, recently diagnosed as fibromyalgia. She is not working, although she is trained as a research lab technician. Mary reports she's having a hard time keeping up with her husband and children and increasing difficulty managing her home. Even minor activities such as lifting or carrying her children can result in profound pain, fatigue, or weakness just a few hours later. She once was very active and now is skeptical but hopeful that she can return to a regular exercise program. Ultimately, she would like to return to part-time work.

EXAMINATION

Posture and Observation: Tall, slim build; stands in ankle plantar flexion, knee recurvatum, anterior pelvic sway relative to thorax, posterior pelvic tilt with lumbar flexion and thoracic kyphosis. Cervical spine in R sidebend. Resting muscle tension apparent in facial, neck, and shoulder muscles. Upper chest breathing pattern; respiratory rate 24 at rest.

Active Range of Motion:

Cervical: flexion 0–30 degrees; extension 0–25 degrees; rotation (R) 0–40 degrees, (L) 0–28 degrees; sidebending (R) 0–30 degrees, (L) 0–22 degrees

Thoracolumbar: flexion to floor with lumbar > hip motion, pain elicited at initial and end range; extension, rotation, and sidebending all mildly decreased with guarding

Muscle Length: Shortened hamstrings; shortened gastroc/soleus; shortened two joint hip flexors; shortened pectoralis major and minor; lengthened middle and lower trapezius; shortened latissimus dorsi

Strength Testing: Upper trapezius (B) 5/5; middle trapezius (R) 3–/5, (L) 2/5; lower trapezius (B) 2/5; sternocleidomastoid (R) 2–/5, (L) 2+/5; trunk curl 3–/5; leg lowering 2/5; gluteus maximus (B) 3+/5; gluteus medius (R) 3–/5, (L) 3/5; iliopsoas (B) 3+/5; quads (R) 4/5, (L) 4–/5; hamstrings (R) 4+/5, (L) 4–/5

Surface Electromyography: Elevated resting muscle tension prevalent (temporalis, upper trapezius, sternocleidomastoid, lumbar paraspinals); same groups demonstrate erratic and asymmetric recruitment with static and active range of motion testing

Palpation: Tender to light pressure in suboccipital region, medial upper trapezius, sternocleidomastoid origin and insertion R > L, interscapular region, anterior thigh and posterior iliac crest

EVALUATION: Diffuse soft tissue and muscle pain, weakness, and fatigue

Impairment

- Multifocal soft tissue pain, aggravated with activity
- Profound muscle fatigue
- Abnormal static and dynamic muscle tension and recruitment patterns, generally elevated
- Mild diffuse loss of active physiologic range of motion, especially spine and hips

Functional Limitation

- Unable to sit >10 minutes
- Unable to stand >15 minutes
- Unable to walk >½ mile
- Unable to lift >10 pounds from floor height

Disability

- Unable to play on the floor with children
- Unable to tolerate sexual intercourse
- Unable to return to work as lab technician

DIAGNOSIS: Chronic pain of fibromyalgia with secondary weakness, fatigue, loss of motion, and abnormal motor recruitment

PROGNOSIS

Short Term Goals (6–8 weeks)

1. Ambulate 15 minutes twice per day without residual symptoms
2. Lift 20 pounds from floor height
3. Static lift 20 pounds for 3 minutes

Long Term Goals (1 year)

1. Return to work part time
2. Continuous ambulation for 30–40 minutes without residual pain or fatigue

CASE STUDY #8

George is a 35-year-old computer data entry specialist with a 9-month history of multiple complaints, including interscapular pain, head and neck pain with associated headaches, and right (R) lateral forearm pain. No specific traumatic event preceded these symptoms, although they have progressively worsened over the last couple months such that they now interfere with his ability to work. His employer completed a workstation assessment several months ago and provided state-of-the-art office equipment, but this has provided no significant relief of George's symptoms. Typically, he can spend several uninterrupted hours on the computer without awareness of time passed. A typical work week is 60 hours. George is moderately obese and admits to a sedentary lifestyle.

EXAMINATION

Posture/Alignment: Forward head, elevated shoulders L > R, excessive lumbar lordosis with anterior pelvic tilt. Scapulae excessively abducted and downwardly rotated L > R. Cubital fossa oriented medially bilaterally. Laterally rotated femurs with hyperextended knees in postural knock-knees

Active Range of Motion:

Cervical: flexion 0–25 degrees; extension 0–60 degrees, pain elicited; rotation (R) 0–55 degrees, (L) 0–60 degrees; sidebend (R) 0–35 degrees, (L) 0–45 degrees

Shoulder: forward flexion (R) 0–120 degrees, (L) 0–140 degrees; extension (R) 0–30 degrees, (L) 0–45 degrees; external rotation (R) 0–35 degrees, (L) 0–50 degrees

Hip: hip external rotation (B) 0–45 degrees, internal rotation (B) 0–10 degrees

Muscle Length: Shortened latissimus dorsi; lengthened rhomboids and mid-lower trapezius; shortened pectoralis major

Strength Testing: Serratus anterior 3/5; rhomboid major 4/5; upper trapezius 5/5; middle and lower trapezius 1–2/5; infraspinatus/teres minor 4/5; anterior/middle deltoid 5/5; biceps (R) 4–/5, (L) 5/5; triceps (B) 5/5; flexor carpi radialis/ulnaris (R) 4/5, (L) 5/5; extensor carpi radialis longus brevis (R) 3+/5, pain elicited, (L) 5/5; pronator teres/supinator (R) 4–/5, (L) 5/5; trunk curl 3/5; leg lowering 2/5; iliopsoas (R) 3+/5, (L) 4/5

Accessory Motion Testing: Cervical: L > R hypomobile posterior/anterior and rotation segmental testing at C1/2 and C2/3; shoulder girdle: decreased anterior/inferior glenohumeral glides; decreased scapulothoracic inferior glide and downward rotation; excessive scapulothoracic lateral glide and upward rotation

Palpation: Suboccipital region moderately tender; diffusely tender interscapular L > R; tender R lateral epicondyle

Deep Tendon Reflexes: Biceps (R) 1+, (L) 2+; triceps 2+ and symmetric

Sensation: Diminished light touch R lateral forearm and thumb

EVALUATION: Chronic postural malalignment resulting in multifocal postural and movement dysfunction most evident in overstretched and weakened scapular stabilizers and upper cervical segmental hypomobility; subsequent musculoskeletal pain and headaches; subacute overuse injury to R wrist extensor group

Impairment
- Upper cervical, asymmetric facet joint motion dysfunction
- Painful and shortened deep suboccipital extensors
- Faulty shoulder girdle alignment
- Overstretched and weakened shoulder girdle adductors, upward rotators, and depressors
- Postural muscle weakness and fatigue
- Pain and inflammation R extensor carpi radialis longus

Functional Limitation
- Unable to sit >30 minutes
- Daily headaches limiting concentration
- Difficulty keying with right hand because of forearm pain

Disability
- Unable to complete job requirements
- Loss of job satisfaction

DIAGNOSIS: Chronic grade 1 muscle strain of middle and lower trapezius; upper cervical facet joint movement dysfunction and possible fixed deformity; R extensor carpi radialis longus tendonitis

PROGNOSIS

Short Term Goals (2–4 weeks)
1. Reduce headache frequency and intensity by 50%
2. Increase sitting tolerance to 60 minutes, incorporating postural adjustments and short breaks

Long Term Goals (6 months)
1. Reduce headache frequency and intensity by 75–100%
2. Return to baseline work level

CASE STUDY #9

Janet is a 47-year-old nurse with primary complaints of posterolateral right (R) thigh pain. The pain is worse with weight bearing first thing in the morning, gets better with limited activity, but worsens by the end of the day—especially if she has been on her feet quite a bit during the day. Secondary complaints include intermittent, dull low back pain and occasional bouts of sharp pain in the arch of her R foot.

EXAMINATION

Posture and Alignment: Thoracic kyphosis, lumbar lordosis, posterior pelvic tilt with anterior displacement of pelvis over base of support; elevated iliac crest R > L; medially rotated femurs R > L; laterally rotated tibias R > L; foot pronation R > L

Active Range of Motion: Hip internal rotation 0–55 degrees, external rotation 0–30 degrees; thoracolumbar flexion full and pain free with reversal of lumbar lordosis

Muscle Length: Shortened tensor fascia lata/iliotibial band (TFL/ITB) with end-range stretch pain; shortened hamstrings (medial > lateral); shortened gastroc/soleus

Strength Testing: Leg lowering 2/5; trunk curl 4/5; gluteus medius (R) 2+/5, (L) 3/5; gluteus maximus (R) 3/5, (L) 3+/5; TFL (R) 3+/5 (pain elicited), (L) 4/5; iliopsoas (R) 2+/5, (L) 3+/5; quadriceps (R) 4–/5, (L) 4+/5; hamstrings (R) 4+/5, (L) 4+/5; posterior tibialis (B) 5/5 (R > L muscle fatigue)

Accessory Motion Testing: Hypermobile posterior/anterior glides T10-L2 with relative hypomobility of lower lumbar segments; hypomobile dorsal glide great toe R > L

Movement Testing: Single-leg stance (R) with pain and excessive medial rotation of femur; decreased pain when femur held in lateral rotation

Gait: Positive Trendelenburg (R), medial rotation of femur midstance (R), excessive foot pronation early and late stance R > L

Palpation: Tender along R ITB; slight tenderness to deep palpation of plantar fascia at calcaneus origin

EVALUATION:

Acute, easily irritable pain arising from R ITB due to compensatory TFL patterns associated with weakness and length/tension imbalance of TFL synergists; intermittent bouts of foot pain arising from plantar fascia, excessive pronation, and great toe hypomobility, currently nonsymptomatic

Impairment

- Postural alignment fault of posterior pelvic tilt, medially rotated femur, and foot pronation
- Muscle weakness of tensor fascia lata synergists, including gluteus medius, iliopsoas, and quadriceps
- Shortened iliotibial band
- Lengthened gluteus medius
- Faulty movement patterns during gait

Functional Limitation

- Unable to walk 20 minutes without onset of R leg pain

Disability

- Unable to perform all job requirements for full 8-hour shift
- Unable to walk for fitness
- Difficulty performing household tasks because of leg pain

DIAGNOSIS:

ITB fascitis and intermittent plantar fascitis

PROGNOSIS

Short Term Goals (4–6 weeks)

1. Perform light duty work 40 hours per week
2. Walk 1.5 miles per day, paced at 20 minutes per mile, without leg or foot pain
3. Perform housework without leg pain if paced at 30–40-minute work intervals

Long Term Goals (12–16 weeks)

1. Resume full duty work at 40 hours per week
2. Walk 3 miles per day, paced at 20 minutes per mile, without leg or foot pain
3. Perform all housework without limitations

CASE STUDY #10

Pete is a 38-year-old man with complaints of right (R) shoulder and hip pain. He fell onto his R shoulder 6 months ago. He complains of clicking and instability, particularly during movements of hand behind back. He also has impingement pain at the middle to end range of arm elevation. He is an avid runner (30–40 miles per week) and has posterior, superior, and medial hip pain after about 2 miles of running. The hip pain resolves about 45–60 minutes after the run. His occupation requires prolonged sitting at a computer, and he has increased hip pain after 45–60 minutes of sitting. His shoulder also begins to ache after approximately the same time period.

EXAMINATION

Alignment: Slight forward head and head tilt to left (L); R head of humerus slightly anterior displaced; R scapula in moderate depression, tilt, downward rotation, adduction; R iliac crest elevated relative to left; R femur adducted and in slight medial rotation relative to L; R tibia slightly laterally rotated; R foot in slight abduction and pronation. Total body posture is a classic swayback. Sitting alignment is with pelvis in posterior tilt and R trunk sidebending with R scapula depressed, downwardly rotated, and tilted.

Gait: At loading response, R trunk is in R sidebending with R scapula depressed, downwardly rotated, and adducted; throughout R stance phase, the pelvis demonstrates a compensated Trendelenburg on the right; throughout swing phase on the L, the pelvis moves in excessive R forward rotation (clockwise approximately 12 degrees); foot mechanics appear unremarkable with exception of slight excessive supination at terminal stance.

Lumbar and Cervical Scan Examinations: Negative for reproduction of symptoms or neurologic signs

Range of Motion:
Right shoulder: flexion 0–150 degrees, scaption 0–150 degrees, lateral rotation/medial rotation (with arm abducted 90 degrees) 90–40 degrees
Right hip: flexion/extension 95–10 degrees, abduction/adduction 30–5 degrees, lateral/medial rotation (prone) 50–20 degrees;
Thoracic rotation: 25% limitation right rotation

Scapulohumeral Rhythm: During arm elevation, scapula is slow to upwardly rotate; most of rotation occurs in last phase of arm elevation; reduced overall scapulothoracic (ST) upward rotation on R relative to L; scapular winging on return from elevation

Muscle Length: Moderate shortness in right medial hamstrings, R tensor facia lata/iliotibial band (TFL/ITB), excessive length of R iliopsoas, moderate shortness in R rhomboid, significant shortness in (R) infraspinatous/teres minor, excessive length in R trapezius and serratus anterior.

Strength Testing (short range positional strength): Gluteus medius (R) 3+/5, (L) 4+/5; gluteus maximus (R) 4–/5, (L) 4+5; iliopsoas (R) 3/5, (L) 4/5; medial hamstrings (R) 4–/5 (pain elicited), (L) 5/5; adductors (R) 4–/5 (pain elicited), (L) 5/5; hip lateral rotators (R) 3+/5, (L) 4+/5; subscapularis (R) 3+/5, (L) 4+/5; infraspinatus/teres minor (R)/(L) 5/5; upper trapezius (R) 4–/5, (L) 5/5; middle trapezius (R) 3+/5, (L) 4/5; lower trapezius (R) 3+/5, (L) 4/5; serratus anterior (R) 3–/5, (L) 4/5; trunk curl 5/5; leg lowering 3/5

Joint Mobility: Moderate restriction in glenohumeral (GH) posterior and inferior glide (capsular end feel, pain after resistance), moderate excessive mobility in GH anterior glide (capsular end feel); moderate restriction in ST upward rotation (muscular end feel), and acromioclavicular joint anterior glide (capsular end feel); moderate restriction in hip posterior and inferior glide (capsular end feel, pain after resistance).

Resisted Tests: Weak and painful R medial hamstrings, adductors, and subscapularis

Special Tests: Positive apprehension and relocation signs R shoulder, positive impingement sign for R shoulder, positive slump test R lower extremity (pain reproduced in posterior, superior, and medial hip)

Palpation: Tenderness over subscapularis and supraspinatus insertions; tenderness in region of medial ischial tuberosity and inferior pubic ramus

Functional Tests: Pain and apprehension with reaching R hand behind back; painful arc with touching R hand to head; during hand behind back maneuver, R scapula fails to adduct, and humeral head translates excessively anteriorly when compared with L. Step-ups illustrate hip hike with hip flexion phase on R and compensated R Trendelenburg with R stance limb; squats reveal asymmetrical hip flexion with R hip hike at end range.

EVALUATION: Chronic strain to R hamstring and adductor muscles; chronic strain to R subscapularis; impingement R shoulder; questionable R shoulder instability

(continued)

CASE STUDY #10 (Continued)

Impairment

- Localized pain R anterior and superior shoulder and right hip
- Hypermobility/instability(?) of R shoulder
- Capsular restriction R hip
- Short ST downward rotators, GH lateral rotators, medial hamstrings, TFL/ITB, R adductors
- Long ST upward rotators, subscapularis, iliopsoas
- Thoracic spine, GH, ST, hip joint restrictions
- Weakness in R shoulder upward rotators, subscapularis, gluteus medius, gluteus maximus, iliopsoas, hip lateral rotators

Functional Limitation

- Unable to reach R hand behind back or overhead without discomfort or unstable feeling
- Unable to sit, climb more than 5 flights of stairs, or run 2 miles without right hip discomfort

Disability

- Unable to sit at computer for more than 45–60 minutes at a time at work
- Unable to participate in recreational activity of running at desired level

DIAGNOSIS: R shoulder impingement with hypermobility or instability; R subscapularis strain; R medial hamstrings and adductor magnus strain with secondary sciatic nerve injury or entrapment. Need to rule out R glenoid lebrum tear and long thoracic nerve injury, which may have occurred during the fall.

PROGNOSIS

Short Term Goals (2–3 months)

1. Elevate R arm through full range of motion and reach behind back without pain or instability
2. Sit 45 minutes without R hip pain
3. Climb 5 flights of stairs without R hip pain
4. Run 15 miles per week without increased right hip pain

Long Term Goals (6–8 months)

1. Unlimited use of right arm without pain or instability
2. Sit unlimited periods (in good alignment) without R hip pain
3. Climb up to 10 flights of stairs without R hip pain
4. Run 30 miles per week without R hip pain

CASE STUDY #11

Mr. Lawn, a 67-year-old man, had a right (R) total hip replacement (THR) 4 years ago. He also has left (L) hip degenerative joint disease (DJD). For the last 4 months he has been noticing increasing L hip pain and is beginning to have pain in the R hip as well if he attempts to play more than 9 holes of golf. He states that 18 holes is usual, and he pulls his own cart. Recent muddy conditions seem to have made symptoms worse. His main concern is that R low back pain will be triggered by R hip pain, as it has been in the past. During the last episode of low back pain, he had to sleep sitting up in his chair, because it was the only place he could get comfortable. Mr. Lawn lives with his wife, who is in the early stages of Alzheimer's disease, and his golf games are his main social contact with friends. He is otherwise healthy and does all the driving, shopping, and housework.

EXAMINATION

Pain: L hip at rest 2/10, after 18 holes of golf 7/10; R hip at rest 1/10, after golf 3/10; R low back at rest 0/10, after golf 1/10

Posture: In standing: bilateral (B) supinated feet; marked B tibial bowing; B femoral internal rotation; high L iliac crest; anterior tilted pelvis; mild hip flexion; supine apparent short R leg; R iliac crest and ischial tuberosity high compared with L

Gait: Marked B trunk sidebend to side of stance leg, decreased hip and knee flexion; slight circumduction B; decreased pronation B feet; R stance time decreased compared with L

Active Range of Motion (open chain):

	R hip	*L hip*
Extension/flexion	5–110 degrees	5–115 degrees (pain)
Internal/external rotation	20–25 degrees	20–15 degrees (pain)
Abduction	30 degrees	20 degrees
Knee flexion/extension	2–125 B degrees	
Lumbar flexion	Hands 4 inches below knees	
Lumbar extension	25% normal range (pain)	

Accessory Motion: L Hip: hypomobile in distal glide, capsular tightness in internal and external passive rotation. Lumbar spine: extension and right sidebend with overpressure restricted and painful compared with L

Palpation: B rectus femoris, iliopsoas, hip adductors, and R quadratus lumborum dense/tender

Strength Testing: Rectus femoris (B) 5/5; iliopsoas (R) 4–/5, (L) 5/5; gluteus maximus (R) 4–/5, (L) 4/5; gluteus medius (R) 4–/5, L 3+/5; quadriceps (B) 5/5; gastroc/soleus (B) 5/5; abdominals 4–/5 by leg lowering test

Balance: R single-leg stance time; 5 seconds; L single-leg stance time: 12 seconds

Neurologic Signs: Normal for L3-S1 light touch, deep tendon reflexes, and key muscle strength.

Active Movement Testing (open chain): Pain is elicited with L hip flexion. Internal rotation and abduction at end of available range in each motion. Standing lumbar sidebend and R rotation is painful. Single-leg stance (R) causes R hip pain, and closed chain testing was deferred because of initial apprehension and balance deficits.

EVALUATION: DJD-related hip muscle strength and range deficits leading to gait and pelvic asymmetry and hip joint pain and to R L5/S1 compression and irritation.

Impairment
- B hip range of motion restriction
- B hip joint muscle weakness
- Abdominal muscle overstretch
- Frontal plane pelvic asymmetry
- Sagittal plane lumboplevic asymmetry
- Decreased standing balance
- Gait abnormality
- Unable to maintain neutral pelvis

Functional Limitation
- Pain limits walk endurance

Disability
- Unable to play golf
- Unable to socialize and restore self mentally and emotionally for wife's care

DIAGNOSIS: Condition after R hip THR; L hip DJD with muscle imbalance leading to probable R L5-S1 facet compression irritation

(continued)

CASE STUDY #11 (Continued)

PROGNOSIS

Short Term Goals (14–21 days)

1. Regain sagittal and frontal plane alignment in standing and walking
2. Regain at least 4/5 strength in all hip and abdominal muscle groups
3. Equalize L hip range of motion to that of R hip
4. Able to balance 30 seconds in single-leg stance (B)

Long Term Goals (4–6 weeks)

1. Ambulate with normal gait pattern
2. Walk 18 holes of golf, pulling cart, without pain in hips or low back

APPENDIX 1

Red Flags: Recognizing Signs and Symptoms

David Musnick* and Carrie Hall

Because therapists often have consistent daily or weekly contact with patients, they may be the health professionals to recognize serious neuromusculoskeletal pathology or systemic disease requiring medical referral. A thorough history, carefully conducted interview, systems review, and screening examinations must be completed during the initial evaluation. Any red flags—signs or symptoms that signal pathologic conditions—may indicate serious somatic or visceral disease or disorders that are beyond the scope of physical therapy intervention. The information outlined in this appendix delineates signs and symptoms of somatic and visceral origin.

Physical therapists often perform interventions, such as therapeutic exercise, to alleviate pain. The physical therapist must be sure that the pain is of neuromusculoskeletal origin and is within the scope of physical therapy practice. A patient with pain that may be caused by serious pathology or referred from a visceral source should be immediately referred to a medical physician for further testing.

Visceral structures can be a source of referred pain to musculoskeletal regions, particularly to the shoulder, back, chest, hip, or groin. The mechanism by which visceral structures refer pain to musculoskeletal regions are twofold:

1. Visceral afferents that supply internal organs transmit impulses to the dorsal horn in which somatic and visceral pain fibers share second-order neurons. Impulses from visceral nerve endings arrive at similar interneuron pools as impulses from somatic origin. Visceral pain may then be felt in somatic segments and skin areas with which it shares neurons in the dorsal horn. This pattern is called referred visceral sensation. Broader pain referral from visceral structures can occur with multiple-segment overlap. Referred visceral sensation may coexist with reflex muscle spasm and vasomotor changes.
2. Visceral structures in the thoracic and abdominal cavities have free nerve endings in loose connective tissue in epithelial and serous linings and in blood vessels. Neural afferent information is transmitted along small, unmyelinated, type C nerve fibers within sympathetic and parasympathetic nerves of the autonomic nervous system. The pain is usually not well localized by the patient and is usually described as vague, deep, and aching.

Signs and symptoms associated with referred visceral pain are the most common red flags signaling the need for further evaluation. The cause of this pain is related to the pathologic function of the primary visceral structure involved. Viscera may refer pain caused by tissue ischemia, obstruction, mechanical distention, or inflammation. Tables 1 and 2 describe the sources and characteristics of somatic and visceral pain. Tables 3 and 4 review the signs and symptoms associated with referred visceral pain. Whenever a patient reports symptoms described in Tables 3 and 4, screening for systemic disease is appropriate. The decision to screen for systemic disease may be even more critical if the patient is older than 45 years of age and the symptoms have an insidious onset.

Table 5 describes systemic, visceral, or nonmechanical causes of regional musculoskeletal pain. The physical therapist should be aware of constant, severe pain with increases in intensity, nonmechanical patterns, or the symptoms or signs described in Table 4 in association with regional musculoskeletal pain. Referral of the patient to a physician is indicated when pain in a musculoskeletal region is accompanied by symptoms and signs indicating systemic or nonmechanical disease. Some types of referred visceral pain are made worse with mechanical stress. Mechanical exacerbation on examination is not 100% specific and cannot alone be used for diagnosing mechanical problems.

Female patients, persons older than 50 years of age, and children may present with symptoms about which the practitioner should be aware:

- Female patients with new-onset thoracolumbar, lumbosacral, or sacroiliac pain should be screened through a renal and reproductive history and lumbar scanning examination. Prompt medical screening is indicated if the person has fever, costovertebral angle tenderness, urinary symptoms, pelvic or suprapubic pain or tenderness, tachycardia, orthostatic changes, or an unclear diagnosis. Renal and reproductive organ disease can cause significant morbidity if not treated quickly.
- Malignant disease should be suspected in patients older than 50 years of age who have constant back pain that is increased with recumbency, history of primary tumor, pathologic fractures, night pain, or mul-

* *David Musnick, MD, is an Internal Medicine/Sports Medicine physician in Seattle and Bellevue, Washington. He teaches seminars in Differential Diagnosis to physical therapists. He has taken numerous courses in exercise and manual therapy topics taught by physical therapists. He has written a book on functional exercise, Conditioning for Outdoor Fitness, published by Mountaineers Books in Seattle.*

Table 1. SOURCES AND CHARACTERISTICS OF SOMATIC AND VISCERAL PAIN

Somatic Sources

Superficial Somatic Cutaneous Pain

- Localized but may refer within 6–12 inches
- Aching
- Burning
- Throbbing (eg, abscesses)
- Neck, hip, or elbow pain with reactive lymph nodes
- Reactive lymph glands are aggravated by pressure or stretching

Deep Somatic Pain*

Muscles

- Localized or may be in referred patterns
- Increases with direct pressure on a tender area or site of lesion, locally or in a referral pattern

Joints

- Deep aching that is vague within the area (more common with peripheral joints) and a referred pattern that is felt more distally from the area (especially spinal joints)
- May decrease with rest or when stressful action has stopped
- May increase with activity
- Increases with stress testing or palpation

Ligaments

- Deep aching in the region of the ligament but may also be perceived distally
- Increases with stress testing or palpation

Neurologic Pain

- Characteristic pain referral patterns based on the site of the lesion
- May be associated with bone pain if the origin of neurologic compression is bone

Bone Pain

- Perceived close to the bone (see Table 2)
- Constant and not relieved by rest
- May be worse with walking, jumping, or other impact
- If a tumor is growing in a bone the pain will be gradually increasing and may be worse at night when the patient is trying to sleep

Visceral Sources

- Vague pain
- Deep pain
- Aching pain
- Boring pain
- Tearing pain
- If a hollow organ is involved, pain may be more colicky (ie, crescendo and decrescendo)
- May involve visceral symptoms (see Table 4)
- May be felt deep or referred superficially to a somatic site (see Table 5)

* Pain may originate in muscles, ligaments, joints, periosteum, vessels, dura, and fascia.

Table 2. CAUSES OF BONE PAIN AND ASSOCIATED SIGNS AND SYMPTOMS

CAUSES	ASSOCIATED CONDITIONS AND SYMPTOMS
• Stress and compression fractures	• Overuse • Osteoporosis • Evaluate for menstrual and eating disorders in young females
• Avascular necrosis (wrist, femoral head, shoulders, feet)	• Corticosteroid use • Trauma
• Osteomyelitis	• Fever or other source of infection
• Hematologic disorders of the bone marrow	• Fatigue • Multiple areas of bone pain, especially in the spine and pelvis
• Paget's disease	• Cranial neuropathies • Leg deformities • Warm bones on examination
• Benign tumor	• Scoliosis if in the spine, especially in a child
• Cancer (primary or metastatic)	• Symptoms of the primary cancer • Fatigue • Pain of bone origin in more than one spine site; a spine site combined with a rib or long bone site may be metastatic cancer and should be referred for evaluation

Table 3. CHARACTERISTICS OF SYSTEMIC SYMPTOMS

Data Obtained From the History

- Insidious onset or no known cause (or both)
- Pattern of presentation: gradual, progressive, cyclical
- Constant
- Intense
- Bilateral
- Unrelieved by rest or change of position
- Night pain
- History of infection
- Migratory arthralgias

Constitutional Symptoms

- Fever
- Chills
- Malaise
- Fatigue
- Night sweats
- Gastrointestinal symptoms
- Skin rash
- Weight loss
- Dyspnea (ie, shortness of breath)
- Diaphoresis at rest or with minimal exertion

tiple painful areas in the spine. The axial skeleton is involved more commonly than the appendicular skeleton, with the lumbar and thoracic spine affected similarly (incidence of approximately 45% to 50%). Cord compression signs require immediate referral to a physician.

- Back pain is rare in patients younger than 16 years of age, especially in nongymnasts and in patients without trauma. Pediatric patients with low back pain and without history of trauma or overuse should be screened by a medical practitioner.
- Pediatric patients with hip pathology may complain of knee or hip pain or a vague pain with walking. Any pediatric patient seen for recent-onset, undiagnosed limping should be evaluated with a medical history and scan of the lumbar spine, hip, knee, and lower extremity (including temperature). Patients with these complaints should be seen promptly by a medical practitioner and have an x-ray examination to evaluate the hip, if indicated.

Table 4. VISCERAL SYMPTOMS AND SIGNS CATEGORIZED BY ORIGIN

Infection

- Fever
- Chills
- Malaise
- Fatigue
- Night sweats
- Red rash
- Swelling
- Purulence
- Constant pain
- Painful, enlarged lymph nodes
- Superficial palpation or percussion tenderness
- Root or cord compression by space-occupying lesion in spine

Pulmonary

- Cough
- Sputum
- Wheezing
- Shortness of breath
- Chest pain
- Pain worsened by deep inspiration
- Hemoptysis (ie, coughing up blood)
- Decreased aerobic exercise capacity

Cardiac

- Arrhythmia (fast >120, slow <40)
- Pauses
- Irregular pulse
- Chest, jaw, scapular, or left arm pain
- High or low blood pressure (>180 or <85)
- Dizziness
- Syncope (ie, fainting)
- Bilateral leg and foot swelling
- Shortness of breath

Vascular

- Low-amplitude pulse
- Coldness
- Paleness
- Swelling
- Constant pain
- Tearing or boring pain
- Color change

Gastrointestinal

- Nausea
- Vomiting
- Bloating
- Weight loss
- Loss of appetite
- Change in stools
- Bloody stools
- Diarrhea
- Absence of bowel movement
- Abdominal pain
- Yellow eyes or skin
- Food may help or aggravate

Renal

- Costovertebral angle tenderness
- Hematuria (ie, red urine)
- Painful or frequent urination

Endocrine

- Energy or temperature changes
- Urinary volume change
- Possible bone pain

Neoplastic

- Constant or night pain
- Age >45 years
- Myelopathy signs (eg, spinal cord compression)
- Previous primary tumor
- Pathologic fracture
- Generalized weakness
- Pain in multiple bony locations

Gynecologic

- Pelvic or low back pain
- Menstrual abnormalities
- Pelvic mass

Rheumatologic

- Peripheral joint swelling
- Deformity
- Redness or pain
- Rash
- Proximal weakness

Table 5. SYSTEMIC DISEASE OR VISCERAL PAIN REFERRED FROM THE MUSCULOSKELETAL REGION

Headache

- Intracranial tumor (U)
- Meningitis (U)
- Subarachnoid hemorrhage (U)
- Sinus infection
- Temporal arteritis; refer patients with visual problems immediately to prevent blindness (U)

Cervical Spine Region Pain

Visceral Referred Pain

Thoracic Origin

- Cardiac ischemia or infarction (U)
- Pneumomediastinum (U)
- Pericarditis (U)
- Aortic arch dissection (U)

(continued)

Table 5. SYSTEMIC DISEASE OR VISCERAL PAIN REFERRED FROM THE MUSCULOSKELETAL REGION (Continued)

- Pancoast tumor
- Pleuritis

Infectious Origin
- Meningitis (U)
- Epidural abscess (U)
- Osteomyelitis (U)
- Disk space infection (U)
- Transverse myelitis (U)
- Lyme disease

Neoplastic Causes
- Metastatic tumor
- Intramedullary or extramedullary tumor
- Epidural hematoma (U)

Vascular Origin
- Subarachnoid hemorrhage (U)
- Vertebral artery dissection (U)
- Carotid artery thrombosis (U)

Other Visceral Referred Pain
- Sphenoid sinusitis
- Thyroiditis
- Parotitis
- Cervical lymphadenitis (from a throat or skin source)
- Pharyngeal space infection (P) (U)
- Cysts (P)

Nonviscerogenic Referred Pain

Rheumatologic Disease
- Fibromyalgia
- Polymyalgia rheumatica
- Rheumatoid arthritis
- Ankylosing spondylitis
- Gout or other crystal-induced inflammation

Shoulder Pain

Visceral Referred Pain

Neoplastic Causes
- Metastatic lesions
- Breast
- Prostate
- Kidney
- Lung
- Thyroid
- Cervical cord or root compression
- Pancoast's tumor
- Lung cancer

Cardiac Origin (left shoulder)
- Angina or myocardial infarction (U)
- Pericarditis (U)
- Aortic aneurysm (U)

Pulmonary Origin
- Empyema and lung abscess
- Pulmonary tuberculosis
- Spontaneous pneumothorax (U)
- Lung cancer

Breast Origin
- Mastodynia
- Primary or secondary cancer

Abdominal Origin
- Liver disease
- Ruptured spleen (U)
- Gallbladder disease
- Subphrenic abscess

Systemic Disease
- Collagen vascular disease
- Gout
- Syphilis, gonorrhea
- Sickle cell anemia
- Hemophilia
- Rheumatic disease

Thoracic-Scapular Region Pain

Visceral Referred Pain

Cardiac Origin
- Myocardial ischemia or infarction (U)
- Dissecting aortic aneurysm (U)

Pulmonary Origin
- Pneumonia (U)
- Pleuritis
- Pulmonary embolism (U)
- Pneumothorax (U)
- Empyema (U)

Neoplastic Causes
- Mediastinal tumors
- Pancreatic carcinoma

Neck Origin
- Esophagitis

Abdominal Origin
- Liver disease (eg, hepatitis, cirrhosis, metastatic tumors)
- Gallbladder disease

Anterior or Lateral Chest Pain

Serious Causes (U)

Pulmonary Origin
- Pulmonary embolism
- Pneumothorax
- Pneumomediastinum
- Pneumopericardium
- Mediastinal tumor
- Asthma
- Pneumonia (if respiratory rate >20 and short of breath)

Cardiac Origin
- Pericarditis
- Dissecting coronary artery or aorta (eg, Marfan's syndrome)
- Cardiac hypertrophy
- Primary pulmonary hypertension
- Myocarditis
- Tachycardia (heart rate >140–160 at rest)
- Suspected myocardial infarction (may occur in younger patient using cocaine)

Less Serious Causes

Infectious Origin
- Herpes zoster infection
- Pneumonia (if no respiratory compromise)
- Pleurisy
- Bronchitis

Gastrointestinal Origin
- Esophageal tear
- Spasm
- Reflux

(continued)

Table 5. SYSTEMIC DISEASE OR VISCERAL PAIN REFERRED FROM THE MUSCULOSKELETAL REGION (Continued)

Thoracolumbar Spine and Sacroiliac Region Pain

Visceral Referred Pain

Neoplastic Causes

- Malignant tumors of the spinal cord or meninges (neurologic deficit)
- Lymphoma (night sweats, weight loss, lymphadenopathy)
- Multiple myeloma (>40 years of age, moderately severe bone pain, multiple osteopenic spine lesions, kidney disease, fatigue from excessive calcium)
- Metastatic tumors (eg, prostate, breast, lung, kidney, thyroid, colon)
- Pediatric malignancies (eg, Ewing's sarcoma, osteosarcoma, lymphoma, leukemia, skeletal metastasis from Wilms' tumor, neuroblastoma, rhabdomyosarcoma) (P)

Abdominal Origin

- Abdominal aortic aneurysm (U)
- Peptic ulcer
- Pancreatic disorders
- Pyelonephritis (U)
- Nephrolithiasis (renal stone) (U)
- Hydronephrosis
- Renal tumor
- Renal infarction (U)

Pelvic Origin

- Urinary bladder retention
- Crohn's disease of the rectum
- Chronic prostatitis
- Uterine masses
- Retroverted or prolapsed uterus
- Endometriosis
- Pelvic inflammatory disease (fever, nausea, pelvic pain) (U)
- Ectopic pregnancy (missed menstrual cycle, pelvic pain) (U)
- Benign ovarian tumor
- Colon diverticulitis
- Retroperitoneal fibrosis

Rheumatologic Causes

- Ankylosing spondylitis
- Reiter's syndrome
- Psoriatic arthritis

Infectious Origin (U)

- Osteomyelitis
- Disk space infection
- Epidural abscess
- Pyogenic sacroiliitis

Endocrine and Metabolic Causes

- Osteoporosis with compression fracture

Hip, Groin, and Thigh Pain

Visceral Referred Pain

Neoplastic Causes

- Bone tumors
- Spinal metastasis

Abdominal Origin

- Inguinal or femoral hernia
- Appendicitis (U)
- Crohn's disease
- Ureteral colic

Pelvic Origin

- Pelvic inflammatory disease (P)

Thrombosis Syndromes (U)

- Deep venous thrombosis with proximal extension to femoral vein and/or pelvic veins (calf pain and swelling)
- Greater saphenous vein phlebitis (superficial, may progress to deep vein thrombosis)

Arthritis

- Osteoarthritis
- Gout, pseudogout
- Rheumatoid arthritis
- Ankylosing spondylitis (degenerative joint disease of hip in a younger male)
- Reiter's syndrome

Pediatric Hip Disease (P)

- Legg-Calve-Perthes (proximal femoral epiphyseal blood flow interruption and necrosis; collapse of femoral head; hip pain, limp, adductor and iliopsoas spasm, possible Trendelenburg sign; child 4–8 years old)
- Slipped capital femoral epiphysis (hip, thigh, or knee pain; hip hypomobility especially in medial rotation; older child or adolescent)
- Transient synovitis (hip, thigh, or knee pain; difficulty walking and possible fever, 2–12 years of age with peak incidence at 6–7 years)

Infectious Origin

- Lymphadenitis caused by cellulitis distally or abdominal wall, perineum, or genital areas or other infections, including sexually transmitted diseases (U)
- Iliopsoas abscess (retroperitoneal infection or inflammation) (U)

Systemic disease

- Sickle cell anemia, avascular necrosis
- Hemophilia (hemarthrosis, bleeding in iliopsoas)
- Tuberculosis

Lower Leg, Knee, and Ankle Region Pain

Visceral Referred Pain

Arterial Compromise

- Occlusion of the popliteal artery from trauma, thrombosis, or knee dislocation (U)
- Claudication syndromes (age >55, coronary disease, diabetes, calf pain with walking)
- Arterial occlusion (acute leg pain, pulseless, cold extremity) (U)

Venous Syndromes

- Venous thrombosis (deep venous thrombosis of the veins in the calf, calf pain, enlarged calf, midline tenderness) (U)
- Thrombophlebitis of the greater saphenous vein (medial leg pain) (U)

Infectious Syndromes (U)

- Cellulitis
- Erysipelas
- Necrotizing fascitis
- Gas gangrene
- Other myositis syndromes, including streptococcal

Rheumatologic Causes

- Reiter's syndrome
- Ankylosing spondylitis (chronic ankle or foot tendinitis, bursitis)

Other Causes

- Sarcoidosis (ankle or knee swelling, chest symptoms)

P, pediatric; U, urgent.

APPENDIX 2

Red Flags: Potentially Serious Symptoms and Signs in Exercising Patients

David Musnick and Carrie Hall

Certain symptoms occurring during exercise may indicate significant medical problems and may be the reason for referral. Display 1 lists the symptoms associated with comorbidities and the tests that should be performed to exclude a medical emergency. Display 2 lists signs indicating medical problems that necessitate medical referral.

During supervised exercise, a patient may develop serious signs and symptoms. Display 3 describes the signs and symptoms related to exercise and the appropriate course of action with respect to various comorbidities:

- Asthma or other pulmonary disease
- Cough
- Cardiovascular disorders
- Syncope
- Hypoglycemia
- Allergic reactions
- Deep vein thrombosis
- Pulmonary embolus
- Spinal cord compression from metastatic disease

DISPLAY 1

Symptoms Associated With Medical Conditions

CONDITION	SYMPTOMS	TESTS
Bronchial or lung tissue	• Wheezing • Pleuritic pain (chest pain increased by a deep breath) • Cough • Significant shortness of breath	• Pulse • Respiratory rate • Blood pressure • Peak flow
Coronary artery, heart valve, cardiac tissue	• Tightness or pain in the left chest, jaw, scapula, or left arm • Lightheadedness • Nausea	• Pulse • Blood pressure in both arms to determine differential
Cardiac rhythm disturbance	• Lightheadedness • Fainting • Bradycardia (heart rate less than 50) • Pauses between beats, especially if associated with lightheadedness	• Postural pulse • Blood pressure • Neurologic screen
Cardiac or pulmonary condition	• Severe intolerance to aerobic or strength training	• Pulse • Respiratory rate • Blood pressure
Chronic fatigue or fibromyalgia	• Flare-up of fatigue after exercise • Intolerance to aerobic or strength training	• Screen for tender points
Cervical or intracerebral pathologies	• Exercise-induced headaches	• Complete neurologic and cervical screen
Neurogenic, vascular claudication, or deep venous thrombosis	• Calf pain with exercise	• Peripheral pulses • Straight-leg raise • Neurologic screen • Homans' test • Calf circumference

DISPLAY 2
Signs Associated With Medical Conditions

SIGNS	CONDITION
Heart Rate	
Less than 50 beats per minute (unless very aerobically fit individual)	• Bradycardia
Pauses greater than 3 seconds between beats (especially if associated with lightheadedness)	• Diseased sinus node • Serious bradycardia
Moderately elevated heart rates during and after cessation of exercise	• Chronic pulmonary or cardiac disease • Arrhythmia
Elevated heart rate before exercise	• Fever • Pulmonary compromise • Hyperthyroidism • Volume depletion (from bleeding or other fluid loss)
Heart rate elevation greater than 120 beats per minute 5 minutes after exercise; if heart rate is greater than 140 beats per minute and accompanied by chest pain, considered a medical emergency	• Possible myocardial infarction • Fever • Hyperthyroidism • Arrhythmia (tachycardia) • Volume depletion
Blood Pressure	
Systolic blood pressure less than 85 mm Hg (exercise is contraindicated)	• Hypotension
Systolic blood pressure greater than 140 (exercise not contraindicated until systolic reaches 170; isometric exercise contraindicated)	• Hypertension
Respiratory Rate	
Greater than 20 (exercise contraindicated unless there is a known chronic lung condition)	• Asthma • Pulmonary infections • Chronic lung conditions • Acute pain • Fever

DISPLAY 3
Common Medical Conditions That May Produce Serious Signs and Symptoms During Exercise

Asthma, Pulmonary Diseases, and Shortness of Breath

If a patient has a history of asthma, chronic pulmonary disease, or recent upper respiratory tract infection with any of the symptoms listed below during or after exercise, he may have an asthma flare, temporary bronchospasm, or another pulmonary problem (eg, bronchitis, pneumonia). Any patient with active asthma should be managed by a physician and encouraged to bring his asthma inhaler and peak flow meter to the therapy department.

SYMPTOMS AND SIGNS

- Coughing
- Wheezing
- Substernal chest tightness
- Mild shortness of breath at rest or precipitated by exercise or cold weather
- Use of accessory muscles of respiration (eg, scalenes, pectoralis minor, intercostals)
- Elevated respiratory rate (>18 breaths per minute) 5 minutes after cessation of exercise
- Low peak flow level for age, sex, and height

CLINICAL ACTIONS

- Administer the patient's bronchospasm inhaler. A second inhalation should be administered after 1 to 2 minutes. Recheck signs and symptoms within 5 to 10 minutes.
- Peak flow of less than 80% of predicted indicates asthma or chronic obstructive pulmonary disease (COPD), indicating referral for a medical evaluation.
- Peak flow of less than 250 indicates severe airway obstruction and is reason for referral to the emergency room.
- Respiratory rate greater than 24, resting heart rate greater than 100, and a peak flow of less than 200 to 250 are signs of pulmonary compromise or a severe exacerbation and poor clinical response to the medication. If the patient is not improved significantly after the inhalation of medication, his physician should be called immediately. If the patient appears to be in respiratory distress, he should be transferred to an emergency room.
- Exercise can be continued if the patient responds well to the medication. The physician should be called regarding management of the medications to prevent future exacerbations.

(continued)

DISPLAY 3 (Continued)

Common Medical Conditions That May Produce Serious Signs and Symptoms During Exercise

Cough

ASSOCIATED CONDITIONS

- Pulmonary infection (accompanied by colored sputum, fever, chills)
- Medication side effect
- Serious lung disorder
- Asthma
- Reactive airway disease
- Congestive heart failure
- Mild respiratory tract infection

Increased intraabdominal and intrathoracic pressure induced by coughing can greatly exacerbate spine pain conditions of a mechanical nature. Patients with spinal disorders should be advised to suppress cough with over-the-counter medications and consult their physician to determine the cause and receive definitive treatment. Patients with a persistent cough should be referred to a physician.

Cardiovascular Disorders

SYMPTOMS

- Chest, substernal, left arm, anterior neck, jaw, and periscapular pain
- Headache, blurred vision, exacerbation of neck pain (symptoms of severe hypertension)
- Uncontrolled hypertension that exacerbates headache and neck pain
- Chest pain, lightheadedness, fainting, and perceptions of strong beats or irregularity (symptoms of heart rhythm abnormalities)

CLINICAL ACTIONS

- If heart rate is less than 45 or greater than 150 beats per minute after cessation of exercise for more than 5 minutes, refer the patient immediately or call 911.
- If the patient has a heart rate greater than 150 and is younger than 50 years old, an attempt to decrease the heart rate by putting slight pressure on the carotid body can be made by massaging the carotid pulse just inferior to the angle of the jaw. The radial pulse can be monitored with another hand, and if it begins to slow, pressure can be taken off the carotid body. If there is no effect within 10 to 15 seconds, this procedure should be stopped.
- If the patient has angina symptoms (ie, severe, constricting chest pain) with known coronary disease, administer his own nitroglycerin while he is sitting or lying down. You may repeat this after 5 minutes. If no relief occurs after a total of three doses in 15 minutes, call 911.
- If systolic blood pressure is greater than 180 or diastolic pressure is greater than 110, the therapy appointment should be terminated and the patient referred to his physician.
- If the systolic blood pressure is greater than 220 and the diastolic pressure is greater than 130, the patient should go to the emergency room, and the referring physician should be called.
- High blood pressure, midline thoracic pain, and between-arm blood pressure differences of 10 mm Hg should be referred immediately.
- A patient with a history of coronary disease should be referred immediately if he is experiencing arrhythmia and has chest pain.
- If the patient is unconscious, call 911 and begin cardiopulmonary resuscitation.

Syncope

Syncope is defined as a sudden and reversible loss of consciousness and decrease or loss of postural muscle tone. It can be caused by transient cerebral ischemia (a total loss of cerebral flow for 10 seconds leads to a blood pressure <70) or altered chemical composition of blood flow to the brain (brain cells depend on a constant level of glucose for energy).

SYMPTOMS

- Changes in vision
- Nausea
- Sweating
- Feeling of dizziness
- Feeling of leg or trunk postural weakness
- Palpitations or chest pain if tachycardia
- Calf or chest pain if pulmonary embolism

To determine if the syncope is caused by postural changes, the blood pressure and heart rate are taken in three positions: supine, sitting, and standing. The blood pressure is assessed in each position. If the systolic pressure lowers by more than 20 points or the heart rate elevates by more than 20 points with each positional change, the patient can be determined to have posturally related syncope.

CLINICAL ACTIONS

- The patient should be positioned in supine with legs elevated for at least 3 minutes to increase venous return of blood.
- A patient with posturally related syncope and a history of vomiting or diarrhea is usually dehydrated and requires significant rehydration with more than 2 L of fluid. The patient should have arrangements made for transportation to a physician's office or a medical facility. It may be possible for the patient to take in enough fluid orally. Rehydration may be started in the therapy department, but it should not be completed in the therapy department.

(continued)

DISPLAY 3 (Continued)

Common Medical Conditions That May Produce Serious Signs and Symptoms During Exercise

- Syncope that occurs more than one time requires termination of the therapy appointment and transportation to the emergency room (unless it is clearly a vasovagal faint). A vasovagal faint is one in which there is no ongoing pathology and the blood pressure and pulse become normal after 3–5 minutes in all positions. A patient who faints more than one time should not be allowed to transport himself to a medical facility.

Hypoglycemic Episodes

Hypoglycemic episodes most commonly occur in patients with diabetes. The causes vary, including improper timing of meals or snacks, excessive insulin or improper dosing or timing of insulin, and excessive or unplanned exercise coupled with inadequate food intake.

SYMPTOMS AND SIGNS

- Shakiness
- Weakness
- Sweaty
- Blurred vision
- Excessive anxiety
- Irritability
- Lightheadedness
- Confusion
- Decreased cognitive abilities
- Unconsciousness
- Blood sugar levels less than 50 to 60

All diabetes patients should be asked to bring their meters with strips to every therapy visit in case of a hypoglycemic episode. Any of the above symptoms should prompt blood sugar assessment.

CLINICAL ACTIONS

- If the glucose level is less than 60, and the patient is awake, give a carbohydrate snack of three glucose tablets, a tube of Instaglucose gel, *or* a ½ to 1 cup of juice. Ask the patient to take a snack including carbohydrate and protein or fat.
- Do not begin any aerobic exercise.
- Recheck the serum glucose level in 30 minutes. If the patient feels significantly better, he can resume exercise.
- If the patient is unconscious, administer glucagon immediately. Mix the liquid in the syringe with the powder in the bottle, and then inject the whole clear solution that is in the syringe into the deltoid muscle or the quadriceps muscle. Place the patient in a sidelying position to protect the airway. When the patient awakens and is fully conscious, give a glucose snack and protein, refer the patient to the emergency room, and call the primary physician.

INSTRUCTIONS FOR DIABETIC PATIENTS BEFORE EXERCISE

- If the glucose level is 100 to 180, administer 15 g of carbohydrate.
- If the glucose level is 180 to 250, it is not necessary to increase food intake.
- If the glucose level is more than 250, do not start aerobic exercise.

Allergic Reactions

Patients may develop allergic reactions to exercise that can occur for the first time in the therapy department:

- Exercise-related hives (ie, itchy, raised skin areas filled with fluid)
- Angioedema (ie, swelling in the subcutaneous tissues around the eyes, lips, hands, and feet, and possibly in the tongue and posterior pharynx and airway)
- Anaphylactic shock (ie, associated with decreased blood pressure, increased pulse, sweatiness, pallor, angioedema, and asthma symptoms)

Anaphylactic shock may occur as a reaction to a medication such as antibiotics, angiotensin-converting enzyme inhibitors, aspirin, or nonsteroidal anti-inflammatory drugs. Exercise-induced anaphylaxis may occur with vigorous aerobic exercise as the only precipitating factor. Any patient with a history of exercise-induced shock should always exercise with another person and should always carry an epinephrine kit.

A patient may also develop any of these reactions in response to Latex gloves or another allergen that he is severely allergic to that may be used in the therapy department. A patient may also react to his medications.

CLINICAL ACTIONS

- Hives usually do not cause emergent problems unless this condition progresses to other, more serious problems. Stop exercise, and consider having the patient take an antihistamine such as Benadryl. Call his primary physician.
- Angioedema is an emergency if it involves swelling of the tongue and airway. If the patient displays difficulty controlling saliva or breathing, the treatment of choice is to administer one dose of epinephrine (0.3 mL of 1 : 1000 solution) in the deltoid area. If a qualified person is not on the premises to administer this treatment, call 911.

(continued)

DISPLAY 3 (Continued)

Common Medical Conditions That May Produce Serious Signs and Symptoms During Exercise

- Anaphylactic shock is a **severe, life-threatening emergency.** Blood pressure and pulse should be taken, although blood pressure may be difficult to detect. The patient should lie down with legs elevated. A dose of epinephrine should be administered immediately and 911 called.

Deep Venous Thrombosis

Individuals at risk for DVT include those who have sustained local trauma to a vessel, have a hypercoagulable disorder, or have been immobilized by bed rest or casts. The most common locations of DVT include the calf, thigh, arms, and pelvis.

SYMPTOMS AND SIGNS

- Pain in the calf or thigh
- Swelling of the calf (circumferential tape measurements are indicated to verify swelling)
- Pain in the calf with walking
- Tenderness with palpation of the deep calf along the midline
- Positive Homans' sign (ie, pain on dorsiflexion of the ankle)

Any patient complaining of calf pain or swelling should be evaluated for DVT.

CLINICAL ACTIONS

- Suspicion of DVT warrants referral to a physician or emergency room within the next few hours.
- The patient should walk minimally, because there is a danger of the clot breaking off from the vessel.

Pulmonary Embolus (PE)

Pulmonary embolus is an **urgent condition** in which an area of lung is infarcted as a result of a thrombus occluding a pulmonary artery. The thrombus usually originates in a deep vein of the leg and travels through the venous return circulation into the right side of the heart and out through the pulmonary circulation to occlude a pulmonary artery. Small thrombi may progress to the periphery of the lung and infarct the peripheral lung tissue, with resultant inflammation and pleuritic pain. Large thrombi may occlude the pulmonary circulation and lead to severe cardiac compromise.

SYMPTOMS AND SIGNS

- Pleuritic pain with referred areas of pain
- Shortness of breath
- Fast respiratory rate
- Coughing up blood
- Rapid pulse rate

Suspicion of PE requires immediate referral to the emergency room. If not on the hospital premises, call 911.

Spinal Cord Compression and Metastatic Disease

Patients with metastatic spine lesions can develop cord compression that is manifested by sensory, motor, or bladder symptoms. For a patient with multisite bone pain and new-onset neurologic symptoms, a complete neurologic examination is indicated. If you suspect a cord compression syndrome, check for upper motor neuron (UMN) signs on examination (eg, clonus, Babinski, hypertonicity). If UMN signs and motor, sensory, or bladder symptoms are present, refer the patient immediately.

Index

Page numbers followed by *f* indicate figures; those followed by *t* indicate tables; those followed by *b* indicate boxed material.

B

C

D

E

F

G

H

I

J

K

L

M

Q

R